Professional Guide to
PATHOPHYSIOLOGY

THIRD EDITION

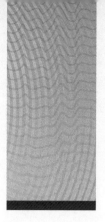

Professional Guide to
Pathophysiology

THIRD EDITION

. Wolters Kluwer | Lippincott Williams & Wilkins
Health

Philadelphia • Baltimore • New York • London
Buenos Aires • Hong Kong • Sydney • Tokyo

STAFF

Executive Publisher
Judith A. Schilling McCann, RN, MSN

Clinical Director
Joan M. Robinson, RN, MSN

Art Director
Elaine Kasmer

Product Manager
Diane Labus

Editor
Margaret Eckman

Clinical Editor
Joanne M. Bartelmo, RN, MSN

Copy Editor
Heather Ditch

Design Assistant
Kate Zulak

Associate Manufacturing Manager
Beth J. Welsh

Editorial Assistants
Karen J. Kirk, Jeri O'Shea, Linda K. Ruhf

PGPATHO3E010210-060915

**Library of Congress
Cataloging-in-Publication Data**

Professional guide to pathophysiology. — 3rd ed.
   p. ; cm.
   Includes bibliographical references and index.
   ISBN 978-1-60547-766-4 (alk. paper)
   1.   Physiology, Pathological.   I. Lippincott
Williams & Wilkins.
   [DNLM: 1.   Pathology.   2.   Physiological
Phenomena.   QZ 140 P9647 2011]
   RB113.P76 2011
   616.07—dc22
                                          2009031489

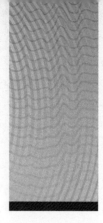

TABLE OF CONTENTS

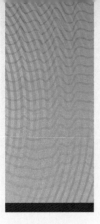

CONTRIBUTORS AND CONSULTANTS

Diane D. Abercrombie, PA-C, MA, MMSc
Academic Coordinator and Assistant Professor
University of South Alabama
Dept. of Physician Assistant Studies
Mobile, Ala.

Sally W. Aboelela, PhD
Assistant Professor
Columbia University School of Nursing
New York

Cheryl L. Brady, RN, MSN
Assistant Professor
Kent State University
Salem, Ohio

Natalie Burkhalter, RN, MSN, FNP,
ACNP, CCRN
Interim Dean of the College of Nursing and
Health Sciences
Associate Professor
Texas A&M International University
Laredo, Tex.

Ruth A. Chaplen, RN, MSN, APRN-BC, AOCN
Nurse Practitioner
Karmanos Cancer Institute
Clinical Instructor
Wayne State University College of Nursing
Detroit

Lillian Craig, RN, MSN, FNP-C
Family Nurse Practitioner
Adjunct Faculty
Oklahoma Panhandle State University
Goodwell, Okla.

J. Kenneth Ehlers, MPAS, PA-C
Physician Assistant
Naval School of Health Sciences
San Diego

Nancy H. Haynes, RN, PhD, CCRN
Associate Professor
Saint Luke's College
Kansas City, Mo.

Lieutenant Commander Manuel Leal,
PA-C, MPAS
Department Head
Naval School of Health Sciences
San Diego

Judith A. Lewis, RN, PhD, WHNP-BC, FAAN
Professor Emerita
Virginia Commonwealth University
Richmond, Va.

Karen L. Madsen, RN, MSN, FNP-BC
Assistant Professor
Cox College
Springfield, Mo.

E. Ann Myers, MD, FACP, FACE
Physician Administrative Consultant in
Endocrinology
St. Mary's Medical Center
San Francisco

Donna L. Van Houten, RN, BSN, MS
Nursing Faculty
GateWay Community College (Maricopa
Community College District)
Phoenix, Ariz.

Colleen R. Walsh, RN, MSN, ONC, CS, ACNP-BC
Instructor, Graduate Nursing
University of Southern Indiana
College of Nursing and Health Professions
Evansville, Ind.

Sarah Yuan, MD, PhD
Professor of Surgery
University of California at Davis Medical Center
Sacramento, Calif.

vi

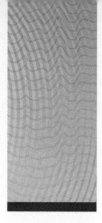

FOREWORD

Although pathology changes very little, our understanding of pathophysiology is constantly changing as it's enriched by new scientific research. Indeed, research has contributed greatly to our knowledge base regarding normal physiology as well as disease states. This third edition of *Professional Guide to Pathophysiology* reflects such recent advances in medical knowledge. Discoveries of new disease processes, which cause unique patterns of pathology, are clearly described in this updated text.

The first chapter lays a foundation for normal cellular physiology and pathologic deviations of disease. Following that, cancer, infection, and fluid and electrolytes each deserve a specific chapter because of their ubiquitous effects. Since the Human Genome project, our understanding of genetic links has exploded with new insight and data. This new edition expands on such recent genetic discoveries, not only in the chapter on genetics, but also in subsequent chapters pertaining to specific systems. The remainder of the book is organized by body system, with an initial discussion of normal anatomy and physiology as a background for pathology specific to that area. Subsequent disease entries cover causes, pathophysiology, signs and symptoms, complications, diagnosis, treatment, and special considerations.

Parallel to the text, "banners" draw the attention to potentially life-threatening disorders, "Clinical alert" highlights important complications and critical interventions that may be required, "Closer look" illustrations provide rich visual detail of physiologic and pathophysiologic processes, and "Disease block" flowcharts show points where treatment halts disease progression. "Genetic link" highlights information about gene-related discoveries in specific disorders; "Age alert" presents age-related differences in pathophysiologic processes, incidences, onset, and clinical findings in various disorders; and "Multisystem disorder" discusses a collaborative approach to disorders affecting multiple body systems.

The new full-color design serves to enhance a greater understanding of pathology and also provides a visual for teaching patients as well as students. Additionally, a new "Prevention" icon provides valuable health promotion and diseases prevention tips for selected disorders.

Professional Guide to Pathophysiology, Third Edition, readily provides the vital information needed, helping the clinician keep current and helping the student emerge more knowledgeable.

Richard R. Roach, MD
Assistant Professor of Medicine
Kalamazoo (Mich.) Center for Medical
  Studies

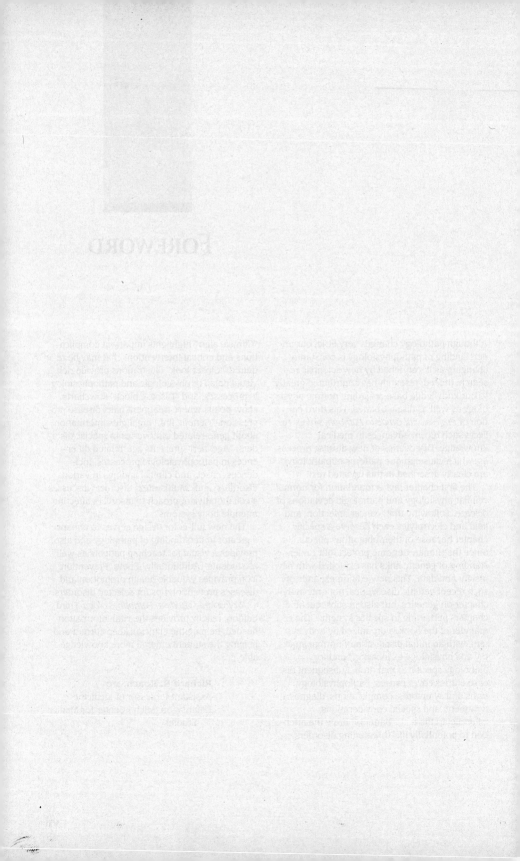

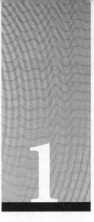

FUNDAMENTALS OF PATHOPHYSIOLOGY

An understanding of pathophysiology requires a review of normal physiology—how the body functions day to day, minute to minute—at the levels of cells, tissues, and organs, and as a whole organism.

Homeostasis

Every cell in the body is involved in maintaining a dynamic, steady state of internal balance called *homeostasis*. Any change or damage at the cellular level can affect the entire body. When homeostasis is disrupted by an external stressor—such as injury, lack of nutrients, or invasion by parasites or other organisms—illness may occur. Many external stressors affect the body's internal equilibrium throughout a person's life. Pathophysiology can be considered as what happens when normal defenses fail.

MAINTAINING BALANCE
Three structures in the brain are responsible for maintaining the body's homeostasis:
◆ *medulla oblongata,* the part of the brain stem associated with vital functions, such as respiration and circulation
◆ *pituitary gland,* which regulates the function of other glands and thereby a person's growth, maturation, and reproduction
◆ *reticular formation,* a network of nerve cells (nuclei) and fibers in the brain stem and spinal cord that help control vital reflexes, such as cardiovascular function and respiration.

Homeostasis is maintained by self-regulating feedback mechanisms. These mechanisms have three components:
◆ a sensor that detects disruptions in homeostasis (caused by nerve impulses or changes in hormone levels)
◆ a central nervous system control center that receives signals from the sensor and regulates the body's response to those disruptions (by initiating the effector mechanism)
◆ an effector that acts to restore homeostasis.
Feedback mechanisms exist in two varieties:
◆ A *positive* feedback mechanism moves the system away from homeostasis. It takes the original response to the sensed change and exaggerates it. This amplified response proceeds in the same direction as the initial disturbance, causing a further deviation from homeostasis. For example, a positive feedback mechanism is responsible for intensifying labor contractions during childbirth.
◆ A *negative* feedback mechanism works to restore homeostasis by correcting a deficit in the system.
An effective negative feedback mechanism must sense a change in the body, such as a high blood glucose level, and attempt to return body functions to normal. In the case of a high blood glucose level, the effector mechanism triggers increased insulin production by the pancreas, returning the blood glucose level to normal and restoring homeostasis.

Disease and illness

Although *disease* and *illness* are commonly used interchangeably, they aren't synonyms. Disease occurs when homeostasis isn't maintained. Illness occurs when a person is no longer in a state of perceived "normal" health. For example, a person may have coronary artery disease, diabetes, or asthma but not be ill all the time because his body has adapted to the disease. In such a situation, a person can perform necessary activities of daily living. Illness usually refers to subjective symptoms that may indicate the presence of disease.

The course and outcome of a disease are influenced by genetic factors (such as a tendency toward obesity), unhealthy behaviors (such as smoking), attitudes (such as being a type A personality), and even the person's perception of the disease (such as acceptance or denial). Diseases are dynamic and may be manifested in various ways, depending on the patient and his environment.

CAUSE

The cause of disease may be intrinsic or extrinsic. Genetic factors, age, sex, infectious agents, or behaviors (such as being inactive, smoking, or abusing illegal drugs) can cause disease. Diseases that have no known cause are called *idiopathic*.

DEVELOPMENT

A disease's development is called its *pathogenesis*. Unless identified and successfully treated, most diseases progress according to a typical pattern of symptoms. Some diseases are self-limiting or resolve quickly with limited or no intervention; others are chronic and are never resolved. Patients with chronic diseases may undergo periodic remissions and exacerbations.

A disease is usually detected when it causes a change in metabolism or cell division that causes signs and symptoms. Manifestations of disease may include hypofunction (such as constipation), hyperfunction (such as increased mucus production), or increased mechanical function (such as a seizure).

How the cells respond to disease depends on the causative agent and the affected cells, tissues, and organs. The resolution of disease depends on many factors functioning over time, such as extent of disease and the presence of other diseases.

STAGES

Typically, diseases progress through these stages:
◆ *Exposure or injury*—Target tissue is exposed to a causative agent or is injured.

◆ *Latent phase or incubation*—No signs or symptoms are evident.
◆ *Prodromal period*—Signs and symptoms are usually mild and nonspecific.
◆ *Acute phase*—The disease reaches its full intensity, possibly resulting in complications. This phase is called the *subclinical acute phase* if the patient can still function as though the disease weren't present.
◆ *Remission*—This second latent phase occurs in some diseases and is usually followed by another acute phase.
◆ *Convalescence*—The patient progresses toward recovery after the disease is terminated.
◆ *Recovery*—The patient regains health or normal functioning. No signs or symptoms of disease remain.

STRESS

When a stressor, such as a life change, occurs, a person can respond in one of two ways: by adapting successfully or by failing to adapt. A maladaptive response to stress may result in disease.

Stressors may be physical or psychological. Physical stressors, such as exposure to a toxin, may elicit a harmful response leading to an identifiable illness or set of signs and symptoms. Psychological stressors, such as the death of a loved one, may also cause a maladaptive response.

Hans Selye, a pioneer in the study of stress and disease, describes the following stages of adaptation to a stressful event: alarm, resistance, and recovery or exhaustion. (See *Physical response to stress*.) In the alarm stage, the body senses stress and arouses the central nervous system. The body releases chemicals to mobilize the fight-or-flight response. In this dual effort, the sympathoadrenal medullary response causes the release of epinephrine and the hypothalamic-pituitary adrenal axis causes the release of glucocorticoids. These systems work together to enable the body to respond to stressors. This release is the adrenaline rush associated with panic or aggression. In the resistance stage, the body either adapts and achieves homeostasis or it fails to adapt and enters the exhaustion stage, resulting in disease.

The stress response is controlled by actions that take place in the cells of the nervous and endocrine systems. These actions try to redirect energy to the organ that's most affected by stress, such as the heart, lungs, or brain.

Stressful events can exacerbate some chronic diseases, such as diabetes or multiple sclerosis. Effective coping strategies can prevent or reduce the harmful effects of stress.

Cell physiology

The cell is the smallest living component of a living organism. Organisms may be made up of a single cell, such as bacteria, or billions of cells, such as human beings. In large organisms, highly specialized cells that perform an identical function are organized into tissue, such as epithelial tissue, connective tissue, nerve tissue, and muscle tissue. Tissues, in turn, form organs (such as the skin, skeleton, brain, and heart), which are integrated into body systems, such as the central nervous system (CNS), cardiovascular system, and musculoskeletal system.

CELL COMPONENTS
Like organisms, cells are complex units of specialized components, each component having its own function. A normal cell's largest components are the cytoplasm, the nucleus, and the cell membrane, which surrounds the internal components and holds the cell together. (See *Cell components and structures,* page 4.)

Cytoplasm
The gel-like cytoplasm consists primarily of cytosol, a viscous, semitransparent fluid that's 70% to 90% water plus various proteins, salts, and sugars. Suspended in the cytosol are many tiny structures called *organelles.*

Organelles are the cell's metabolic machinery. Each performs a function to maintain the cell's life. Organelles include mitochondria, ribosomes, endoplasmic reticulum, Golgi apparatus, lysosomes, peroxisomes, cytoskeletal elements, centrosomes, microfilaments, and microtubules.

◆ *Mitochondria* are spherical or rod-shaped structures that produce most of the body's adenosine triphosphate (ATP). ATP contains high-energy phosphate chemical bonds that fuel many cellular activities. Mitochondria are the sites of cellular respiration—the metabolic use of oxygen to produce energy, carbon dioxide, and water.
◆ *Ribosomes* are the sites of protein synthesis.
◆ The *endoplasmic reticulum* is an extensive network of two varieties of membrane-enclosed tubules. The rough endoplasmic reticulum is covered with ribosomes. The smooth endoplasmic reticulum contains enzymes that synthesize lipids.
◆ The *Golgi apparatus* synthesizes carbohydrate molecules that combine with protein produced by the rough endoplasmic reticulum and lipids produced by the smooth endoplasmic reticulum to form such products as lipoproteins, glycoproteins, and enzymes.

 CLOSER LOOK

Physical response to stress

According to Hans Selye's General Adaptation Model, the body goes through the following stages when reacting to stress.

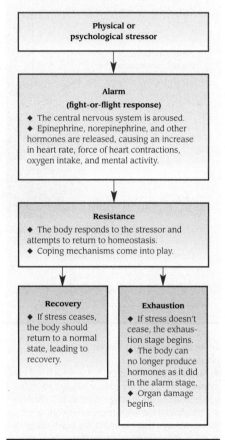

◆ *Lysosomes* are digestive bodies that break down nutrient material as well as foreign or damaged material in cells. A membrane surrounding each lysosome separates its digestive enzymes from the rest of the cytoplasm. The enzymes digest nutrient matter brought into the cell by means of endocytosis, in which a portion of the cell membrane surrounds and engulfs matter to form a membrane-bound intracellular vesicle. The membrane of the lysosome fuses with the membrane of the vesicle surrounding the endocytosed material. The lysosomal enzymes then digest the engulfed material. Lysosomes digest the foreign matter ingested by

CLOSER LOOK

Cell components and structures

Cells differ in size and shape, but all consist of the same components and structures. The illustration below shows the composition of a cell. Each part has a function in maintaining the cell's life and homeostasis.

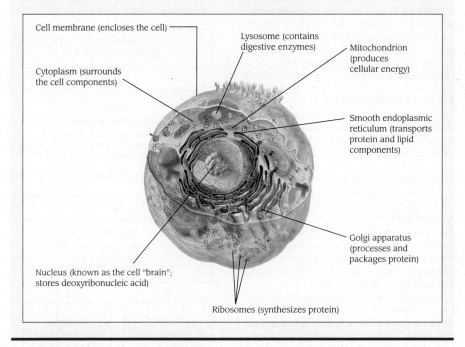

Cell membrane (encloses the cell)

Cytoplasm (surrounds the cell components)

Lysosome (contains digestive enzymes)

Mitochondrion (produces cellular energy)

Smooth endoplasmic reticulum (transports protein and lipid components)

Golgi apparatus (processes and packages protein)

Nucleus (known as the cell "brain"; stores deoxyribonucleic acid)

Ribosomes (synthesizes protein)

white blood cells by a similar process called *phagocytosis*.

◆ *Peroxisomes* contain oxidases, which are enzymes that chemically reduce oxygen to hydrogen peroxide and hydrogen peroxide to water.

◆ *Cytoskeletal elements* form a network of protein structures that maintain the cell's shape.

◆ *Centrosomes* contain centrioles, which are short cylinders adjacent to the nucleus that take part in cell division.

◆ *Microfilaments* and *microtubules* enable the movement of intracellular vesicles (allowing axons to transport neurotransmitters) and the formation of the mitotic spindle, the framework for cell division.

Nucleus

The cell's control center is the nucleus, which plays a role in cell growth, metabolism, and reproduction. Within the nucleus, one or more nucleoli (dark-staining intranuclear structures) synthesize ribonucleic acid, a complex polynucleotide that controls protein synthesis. The

nucleus also stores deoxyribonucleic acid (DNA), the double helix that carries genetic material and is responsible for cell reproduction, or division.

Cell membrane

The semipermeable cell membrane forms the cell's external boundary, separating it from other cells and from the external environment. Roughly 75Å (³⁄₁₀ millionths of an inch) thick, the cell membrane consists of a double layer of phospholipids with protein molecules embedded in it. These protein molecules act as receptors, ion channels, or carriers for specific substances.

CELL DIVISION

Each cell must replicate itself for life to continue. Cells replicate by division in one of two ways: mitosis (division that results in two daughter cells with the same DNA and chromosome content as the mother cell) or meiosis (division that creates four gametocytes, each containing one-half the number of chromosomes of the original cell). Most cells undergo mitosis; meiosis occurs only in reproductive cells.

Mitosis

Mitosis, the type of cell division that leads to tissue growth, creates an equal division of material in the nucleus (karyokinesis) followed by division of the cell body (cytokinesis). This process yields two duplicates of the original cell. (See chapter 5, Genetics, for a detailed discussion of mitosis and meiosis.)

CELL FUNCTIONS

A cell's basic functions are movement, conduction, absorption, secretion, excretion, respiration, and reproduction. In the human body, different cells are specialized to perform only one function; muscle cells, for example, are responsible for movement. However, respiration and reproduction occur in all cells.

Movement

Some cells, such as muscle cells, work together to produce movement of a specific body part, the contents within an organ, or the entire organism. Muscle cells attached to bone move the extremities. When muscle cells that envelop hollow organs or cavities contract, they produce movement of contents, such as the peristaltic movement of the intestines or the ejection of blood from the heart.

Conduction

Conduction is the transmission of a stimulus, such as a nerve impulse, heat, or sound wave, from one body part to another.

Absorption

The absorption process occurs as substances move through a cell membrane. For example, food is broken down into amino acids, fatty acids, and glucose in the digestive tract. Specialized cells in the intestine then absorb the nutrients and transport them to blood vessels, which carry them to other cells of the body. These target cells, in turn, absorb the substances, using them as energy sources or as building blocks to form or repair structural and functional cellular components.

Secretion

Some cells, such as those in the glands, release substances that are used in another part of the body. The beta cells of the islets of Langerhans of the pancreas, for example, secrete insulin, which is transported by the blood to its target cells, where the insulin facilitates the movement of glucose across cell membranes.

Excretion

Cells excrete the waste generated by normal metabolic processes. This waste includes such substances as carbon dioxide and certain acids and nitrogen-containing molecules.

Respiration

Cellular respiration occurs in the mitochondria, where ATP is produced. The cell absorbs oxygen; it then uses the oxygen and releases carbon dioxide during cellular metabolism. The energy stored in ATP is used in other reactions that require energy.

Reproduction

New cells are needed to replace older cells for tissue and body growth. Most cells divide and reproduce through mitosis. However, some cells, such as nerve and muscle cells, typically lose their ability to reproduce after birth.

CELL TYPES

Each of the four types of tissue (epithelial, connective, nerve, and muscle) consists of several specialized cell types, which perform specific functions.

Epithelial cell

Epithelial cells line most of the body's internal and external surfaces, such as the skin's epidermis, internal organs, blood vessels, body cavities, glands, and sensory organs. Epithelial cells have various functions, including support, protection, absorption, excretion, and secretion.

Connective tissue cell

Connective tissue cells are found in the skin, the bones and joints, the artery walls, the fascia around organs, the nerves, and body fat. The types of connective tissue cells include fibroblasts (such as collagen, elastin, and reticular fibers), adipose (fat) cells, mast cells (which release histamines and other substances during inflammation), and bone. The major functions of connective tissues are protection, metabolism, support, temperature maintenance, and elasticity.

Nerve cell

Two types of cells—neurons and neuroglial cells—comprise the nervous system. Neurons have a cell body, dendrites, and an axon. The dendrites carry nerve impulses to the cell body from the axons of other neurons. Axons carry impulses away from the cell body to other neurons or organs. A myelin sheath around the axon facilitates rapid conduction of impulses by

keeping them within the nerve cell. Neurons perform the following functions:
♦ generate electrical impulses
♦ conduct electrical impulses
♦ influence other neurons, muscle cells, and cells of glands by transmitting those impulses.

Neuroglial cells support, nourish, and protect the neurons. There are four types:
♦ *Oligodendroglia* produce myelin within the CNS.
♦ *Astrocytes* provide essential nutrients to neurons and assist neurons in maintaining the proper bioelectrical potentials for impulse conduction and synaptic transmission.
♦ *Ependymal cells* are involved in the production of cerebrospinal fluid.
♦ *Microglia* ingest and digest tissue debris when nerve tissue is damaged.

Muscle cell

Muscle cells contract to produce movement or tension. The intracellular proteins actin and myosin interact to form cross-bridges that result in muscle contraction. An increase in intracellular calcium is necessary for muscle to contract.

There are three basic types of muscle cells:
♦ *Skeletal (striated) muscle cells* are long, cylindrical cells that extend along the entire length of the skeletal muscles. These muscles, which attach directly to the bone or are connected to the bone by tendons, are responsible for voluntary movement. By contracting and relaxing, striated muscle cells alter the muscle's length. Contraction shortens the muscle; relaxation permits the muscle to return to its resting length.
♦ *Smooth (nonstriated) muscle cells* are present in the walls of hollow internal organs, such as the GI and genitourinary tracts, and of blood vessels and bronchioles. Unlike striated muscle, these spindle-shaped cells contract involuntarily. By contracting and relaxing, they change the hollow structure's luminal diameter and thereby move substances through the organ.
♦ *Cardiac muscle cells* branch out across the smooth muscle of the heart's chambers and contract involuntarily. They produce and transmit cardiac action potentials, which cause cardiac muscle cells to contract. Impulses travel from cell to cell as though no cell membrane existed.

AGE ALERT *In older adults, skeletal muscle cells become smaller and many are replaced by fibrous connective tissue. The result is loss of muscle strength and mass.*

Pathophysiologic changes

The cell faces several challenges through its life. Stressors, changes in the body's health, disease, and other extrinsic and intrinsic factors can change the cell's normal functioning (homeostasis).

CELL ADAPTATION

Cells can generally continue functioning despite changing conditions or stressors. However, severe or prolonged stress or changes may injure or even destroy cells. When cell integrity is threatened—for example, by hypoxia, anoxia, chemical injury, infection, or temperature extremes—it reacts in one of two ways:
♦ by drawing on its reserves to keep functioning
♦ by adaptive changes or cellular dysfunction.

If enough cellular reserve is available and the body doesn't detect abnormalities, the cell adapts by atrophy, hypertrophy, hyperplasia, metaplasia, or dysplasia. (See *Adaptive cell changes,* page 7.) If cellular reserve is insufficient, cell death (necrosis) occurs. Necrosis is usually localized and easily identifiable.

Atrophy

Atrophy is a reduction in the size of a cell or organ that may occur when cells face reduced workload or disuse, insufficient blood flow, malnutrition, or reduced hormonal and nerve stimulation. Examples of atrophy include loss of muscle mass and tone after prolonged bed rest.

Hypertrophy

In contrast, hypertrophy is an increase in the size of a cell or organ caused by an increase in workload. The three basic types of hypertrophy are *physiologic, compensatory,* and *pathologic.*
♦ *Physiologic hypertrophy* reflects an increase in workload that isn't caused by disease—for example, the increase in muscle size caused by hard physical labor or weight training.
♦ *Compensatory hypertrophy* takes place when cell size increases to take over for nonfunctioning cells. For instance, one kidney will enlarge when the other isn't functioning or is removed.
♦ *Pathologic hypertrophy* is a response to disease. An example is thickening of the heart muscle as the muscle pumps against increasing resistance in patients with hypertension.

Hyperplasia

Hyperplasia is an increase in the number of cells caused by increased workload, hormonal stimulation, or decreased tissue density. Like hypertrophy, hyperplasia may be *physiologic, compensatory,* or *pathologic.*
♦ *Physiologic hyperplasia* is an adaptive response to normal changes. An example is the monthly increase in the number of uterine cells that occurs

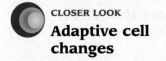

CLOSER LOOK
Adaptive cell changes

Cells adapt to changing conditions and stressors within the body in the ways illustrated below.

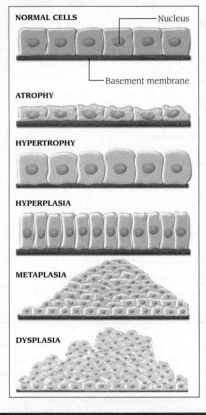

Metaplasia

Metaplasia is the replacement of one cell type with another cell type (one that can better endure the change or stressor). A common cause of metaplasia is constant irritation or injury that initiates an inflammatory response. The new cell type can better endure the stress of chronic inflammation. Metaplasia may be either *physiologic* or *pathologic.*

◆ *Physiologic metaplasia* is a normal response to changing conditions and is generally transient. For example, in the body's normal response to inflammation, monocytes that migrate to inflamed tissues transform into macrophages.

◆ *Pathologic metaplasia* is a response to an extrinsic toxin or stressor and is generally irreversible. For example, after years of exposure to cigarette smoke, stratified squamous epithelial cells replace the normal ciliated columnar epithelial cells of the bronchi. Although the new cells can better withstand smoke, they don't secrete mucus nor do they have cilia to protect the airway. If exposure to cigarette smoke continues, the squamous cells can become cancerous.

Dysplasia

In dysplasia, abnormal differentiation of dividing cells results in cells that are abnormal in size, shape, and appearance. Although dysplastic cell changes aren't cancerous, they can precede cancerous changes. Common examples include dysplasia of epithelial cells of the cervix or the respiratory tract.

CELL INJURY

Injury to any cellular component can lead to illness as the cells lose their ability to adapt. One early indication of cell injury is a biochemical lesion that forms on the cell at the point of injury. For example, in a patient with chronic alcoholism, biochemical lesions on the cells of the immune system may increase the patient's susceptibility to infection, and cells of the pancreas and liver are affected in a way that prevents their reproduction. These cells can't return to normal functioning.

Intrinsic and extrinsic causes

Cell injury may result from any of several intrinsic or extrinsic causes:

◆ *Toxins.* Substances that originate in the body (endogenous factors) or outside the body (exogenous factors) may cause toxic injuries. Common endogenous toxins include products of genetically determined metabolic errors, gross malformations, and hypersensitivity reactions.

in response to estrogen stimulation of the endometrium after ovulation.

◆ *Compensatory hyperplasia* occurs in some organs to replace tissue that has been removed or destroyed. For example, liver cells regenerate when part of the liver has been surgically removed.

◆ *Pathologic hyperplasia* is a response to either excessive hormonal stimulation or abnormal production of hormonal growth factors. Examples include acromegaly, in which excessive growth hormone production causes bones to enlarge, and endometrial hyperplasia, in which excessive secretion of estrogen causes heavy menstrual bleeding and possibly malignant changes.

Exogenous toxins include alcohol, lead, carbon monoxide, and drugs that alter cellular function. Examples of such drugs are chemotherapeutic agents used for cancer and immunosuppressants used to prevent rejection in organ transplant recipients.

♦ *Infection.* Viruses, fungi, protozoa, and bacteria can cause cell injury or death. These organisms affect cell integrity, usually by interfering with cell division, producing nonviable, mutant cells. For example, human immunodeficiency virus alters the cell when the virus is replicated in the cell's ribonucleic acid.

♦ *Physical injury.* Physical injury results from a disruption in the cell or in the relationships of the intracellular organelles. Two major types of physical injury are thermal and mechanical. Causes of thermal injury include burns, radiation therapy for cancer, X-rays, and ultraviolet radiation. Causes of mechanical injury include surgery, trauma from motor vehicle accidents, and frostbite.

♦ *Deficit injury.* When a deficit of water, oxygen, or nutrients occurs, or if constant temperature and adequate waste disposal aren't maintained, normal cellular metabolism can't take place. A lack of just one of these basic requirements can cause cell disruption or death. Causes of deficit include hypoxia (inadequate oxygen), ischemia (inadequate blood supply), and malnutrition.

Irreversible cell injury occurs when the cell membrane or the organelles can no longer function.

CELL DEGENERATION

Degeneration is a type of nonlethal cell damage that generally occurs in the cytoplasm and that doesn't affect the nucleus. It usually affects organs with metabolically active cells, such as the liver, heart, and kidneys, and is caused by these problems:

♦ increased water in the cell or cellular swelling
♦ fatty infiltrates
♦ atrophy
♦ autophagocytosis (that is, the cell absorbs some of its own parts)
♦ pigmentation changes
♦ calcification
♦ hyaline infiltration
♦ hypertrophy
♦ dysplasia (related to chronic irritation)
♦ hyperplasia.

When changes in cells are identified, prompt health care can slow degeneration and prevent cell death. An electron microscope can reveal cellular changes, and thus aid in the diagnosis

---

Factors that affect cell aging

Cell aging can be affected by the intrinsic and extrinsic factors listed below.

Intrinsic factors
♦ Congenital
♦ Degenerative
♦ Immunologic
♦ Inherited
♦ Metabolic
♦ Neoplastic
♦ Nutritional
♦ Psychogenic

Extrinsic factors
Physical agents
♦ Chemicals
♦ Electricity
♦ Force
♦ Humidity
♦ Radiation
♦ Temperature

Infectious agents
♦ Bacteria
♦ Fungi
♦ Insects
♦ Protozoa
♦ Viruses
♦ Worms

---

of disease, before the patient complains of symptoms. Unfortunately, many cell changes remain unidentifiable even under a microscope, making early detection of disease impossible. An example of reversible degenerative change is cervical dysplasia. Examples of irreversible degenerative diseases include Huntington's disease and amyotrophic lateral sclerosis.

CELL AGING

During the normal process of aging, cells lose structure and function. Atrophy, a decrease in size or wasting away, may indicate loss of cell structure. Hypertrophy or hyperplasia is characteristic of lost cell function. (See *Factors that affect cell aging.*)

Signs of aging occur in all body systems. Examples include diminished elasticity of blood vessels, bowel motility, muscle mass, and subcutaneous fat. Cell aging can slow down or speed up, depending on the number and extent of injuries and the amount of wear and tear on the cell.

CLOSER LOOK
Biological theories of aging

Various theories have been proposed to explain the process of normal aging. Biological theories attempt to explain physical aging as an involuntary process that eventually leads to cumulative changes in cells, tissues, and fluids.

Theory	Sources	Retardants
Cross-link theory		
Strong chemical bonding between organic molecules in the body causes increased stiffness, chemical instability, and insolubility of connective tissue and deoxyribonucleic acid.	Lipids, proteins, carbohydrates, and nucleic acids	Restricting calories and sources of lathyrogens (antilink agents) such as chickpeas
Free-radical theory		
An increased number of unstable free radicals produces effects harmful to biological systems, such as chromosomal changes, pigment accumulation, and collagen alteration.	Environmental pollutants; oxidation of dietary fats, proteins, carbohydrates, and elements	Improving environmental monitoring; decreasing intake of foods that stimulate free radicals; increasing intake of vitamins A and C (mercaptans) and vitamin E
Immunologic theory		
An aging immune system is less able to distinguish body cells from foreign cells; as a result, it begins to attack and destroy body cells as if they were foreign. This autoagression may explain the adult onset of such conditions as diabetes mellitus, rheumatic heart disease, and arthritis. Theorists have speculated about the existence of several erratic cellular mechanisms that can precipitate attacks on various tissues through autoaggression or immunodeficiencies.	Alteration of B and T cells of the humoral and cellular systems	Immunoengineering— selective alteration and replenishment or rejuvenation of the immune system
Wear-and-tear theory		
Body cells, structures, and functions wear out or are overused through exposure to internal and external stressors. Effects of the residual damage accumulate, the body can no longer resist stress, and death occurs.	Repeated injury or overuse; internal and external stressors (physical, psychological, social, and environmental), including trauma, chemicals, and buildup of naturally occurring wastes	Reevaluating and possibly adjusting lifestyle

The cell aging process limits the human life span (of course, many people die of disease before they reach the maximum life span of about 110 years). Several theories attempt to explain the reasons behind cell aging. (See *Biological theories of aging.*)

CELL DEATH

Like disease, cell death may be caused by internal (intrinsic) factors that limit the cell's life span or external (extrinsic) factors that contribute to cell damage and aging. When a stressor is severe or prolonged, the cell can no longer adapt and it dies.

Cell death, or *necrosis,* may manifest in different ways, depending on the tissues or organs involved.

◆ *Apoptosis* is genetically programmed cell death. This process accounts for the constant cell turnover in the skin's outer keratin layer and the eye's lens.

◆ *Liquefaction necrosis* occurs when a lytic (dissolving) enzyme liquefies necrotic cells. This type of necrosis is common in the brain, which has a rich supply of lytic enzymes.

◆ In *caseous necrosis,* the necrotic cells disintegrate but the cellular pieces remain undigested for months or years. This type of necrotic tissue gets its name from its crumbly, cheeselike (caseous) appearance. It commonly occurs in pulmonary tuberculosis.

◆ In *fat necrosis,* enzymes called *lipases* break down intracellular triglycerides into free fatty acids. These free fatty acids combine with sodium, magnesium, or calcium ions to form soaps. The tissue becomes opaque and chalky white.

◆ *Coagulative necrosis* commonly occurs when the blood supply to any organ (except the brain) is interrupted. It typically affects the kidneys, heart, and adrenal glands. Lytic (lysosomal) enzyme activity in the cells is inhibited, so the necrotic cells maintain their shape, at least temporarily.

◆ *Gangrenous necrosis,* a form of coagulative necrosis, results from a lack of blood flow and is complicated by an overgrowth and invasion of bacteria. It commonly occurs in the lower legs as a result of arteriosclerosis or in the GI tract. Gangrene can occur in one of three forms: *dry, moist (or wet),* or *gas.*

– *Dry gangrene* occurs when bacterial invasion is minimal. It's marked by dry, wrinkled, dark brown or blackened tissue on an extremity.

– *Moist (or wet) gangrene* develops with liquefaction necrosis that includes extensive lytic activity from bacteria and white blood cells to produce a liquid center in an affected area. It can occur in the internal organs as well as the extremities.

– *Gas gangrene* develops when anaerobic bacteria of the genus *Clostridium* infect tissue. It's more likely to occur with severe trauma and may be fatal. The bacteria release toxins that kill nearby cells and the gas gangrene rapidly spreads. Release of gas bubbles from affected muscle cells indicates that gas gangrene is present.

Necrotic changes

When a cell dies, enzymes inside it are released and start to dissolve cellular components. This dissolution triggers an acute inflammatory reaction in which white blood cells migrate to the necrotic area and begin to digest the dead cells. At this point, the dead cells begin to change morphologically in one of three ways:

◆ *pyknosis,* in which the nucleus shrinks, becoming a dense mass of genetic material with an irregular outline

◆ *karyorrhexis,* in which the nucleus breaks up, strewing pieces of genetic material throughout the cell

◆ *karyolysis,* in which hydrolytic enzymes released from intracellular structures called *lysosomes* dissolve the nucleus.

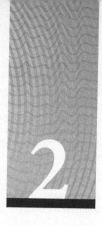

CANCER

Cancer, also called *malignant neoplasia,* refers to a group of more than 100 different diseases that are characterized by deoxyribonucleic acid (DNA) damage that causes abnormal cell growth and development. Malignant cells have two defining characteristics: They can no longer divide and differentiate normally, and they have acquired the ability to invade surrounding tissues and travel to distant sites.

Cancer ranks second to cardiovascular disease as the leading cause of death in the United States. One in four deaths is due to cancer. Some epidemiologists predict that it will outrank cardiovascular disease in the near future. Every year, more than 1 million cancer cases are diagnosed in the United States, and 550,000 people die of cancer-related causes. One-third of these deaths are related to nutrition problems, physical inactivity, obesity, and other lifestyle factors that are preventable in most cases.

Cancer development

The most widely held theory about carcinogenesis involves a three-stage process: initiation, promotion, and progression.

INITIATION
Initiation refers to the damage to or mutation of DNA that occurs when the cell is exposed to an initiating substance or event (such as chemicals, a virus, or radiation) during DNA replication (transcription). Usually, enzymes detect errors in transcription and remove or repair them. Sometimes, however, an error is missed. If regulatory proteins recognize the error and block further division, then the error may be repaired or the cell may self-destruct, a process known as *apoptosis.* If these proteins miss the error, it becomes a permanent mutation that's passed on to future generations of cells.

PROMOTION
Promotion involves the mutated cell's exposure to factors (*promoters*) that enhance its growth. This exposure may occur shortly after initiation or years later.

Promoters may be hormones such as estrogen, food additives such as nitrates, or drugs such as nicotine. They can affect the mutated cell by altering:
♦ the function of genes that control cell growth and replication
♦ cell response to growth stimulators or inhibitors
♦ intercellular communication.

PROGRESSION
Progression occurs as tumor cells acquire additional mutations, enabling the tumor to invade adjacent tissue, metastasize to distant sites, and become resistant to therapy. This step is irreversible.

Causes

The healthy body is well equipped to defend itself against cancer. Only when the immune system and other defenses fail does cancer prevail.

Evidence suggests that cancer develops from a complex interaction of exposure to carcinogens and accumulated mutations in genes that control cell growth. Researchers have identified approximately 100 control genes, which fall into four types: *proto-oncogenes, tumor-suppressor genes, DNA repair genes,* and *apoptosis genes.*

Each of the four types of genes plays a role. When proto-oncogenes mutate, they become oncogenes, leading to uncontrolled cell death growth. Mutated tumor-suppressor genes lose the ability to stop abnormal cell growth. Mutations in DNA repair genes allow damage to go unrepaired, and mutations in apoptosis genes result in damaged cells losing the ability to self-destruct.

Common causes of acquired genetic damage are viruses, radiation, environmental and dietary carcinogens, and hormones. Other factors that interact to increase a person's likelihood of developing cancer are age, nutritional status, hormonal balance, and response to stress.

GENETICS

Although cancers may be considered genetic in nature because they result from mutations in genes, only about 10% are inherited. When mutations occur in reproductive cells (germline), damage can be passed on to future generations. This results in a predisposition to develop the cancer.

GENETIC LINK *The discovery of cancer-related genes has enhanced the identification, guidance, and management of persons at high risk for common cancers associated with inheritance of cancer-predisposing, genetic mutations. Recent discoveries include:*

◆ *Breast and ovarian cancers — Women with a BRCA 1 or BRCA 2 gene alteration have a 36% to 85% lifetime risk of developing breast cancer and a 16% to 60% lifetime risk of developing ovarian cancer.*

◆ *Colon cancer — In a gene alteration, the helicase-like transcription factor gene (one of the genes that helps stabilize DNA and regulates protein production in the cell) is inactivated, which contributes to the transformation of normal colon cells into cancer cells.*

◆ *Melanoma — The p16 gene causes some melanomas that run in certain families.*

Common characteristics of genetically predisposed cancer include:

◆ early onset of malignant disease

◆ increased incidence of bilateral cancer in paired organs (breasts, adrenal glands, kidneys, and eighth cranial nerve [acoustic neuroma])

◆ increased incidence of multiple primary cancers in nonpaired organs

◆ increased risk of development of a less differentiated tumor

◆ abnormal chromosome complement in tumor cells.

VIRUSES

Viral proto-oncogenes typically contain DNA that's identical to that of human oncogenes. In animal studies of viral ability to transform cells, some viruses that infect people have demonstrated the potential to cause cancer. For example, the Epstein-Barr virus, which causes infectious mononucleosis, has been linked to Burkitt's lymphoma and nasopharyngeal carcinoma.

IMMUNOSURVEILLANCE FAILURE

Research suggests that cancer cells develop continually, but the immune system recognizes these cells as foreign and destroys them. This defense mechanism, termed *immunosurveillance,* has two major components: *cell-mediated* immune response and *humoral* immune response. Together these two components interact to promote antibody production, cellular immunity, and immunologic memory. Researchers believe that an intact immune system is responsible for spontaneous regression of tumors. Thus, cancer development is a concern for patients who are immunodeficient or who must take an immunosuppressant.

Cell-mediated immune response

Cancer cells carry cell-surface antigens (specialized protein molecules that trigger an immune response) called *tumor-associated antigens* (TAAs) and *tumor-specific antigens* (TSAs). The cell-mediated immune response begins when T lymphocytes encounter a TAA or a TSA and become sensitized to it. After repeated contacts, the sensitized T cells release chemical factors called *lymphokines,* some of which begin to destroy the antigen. This reaction triggers the transformation of a different population of T lymphocytes into "killer T lymphocytes" targeted to cells carrying the specific antigen — in this case, cancer cells.

Humoral immune response

The humoral immune response reacts to a TAA by triggering the release of antibodies from plasma cells and activating the serum-complement system to destroy the antigen-bearing cells. However, an opposing immune factor, a "blocking antibody," may enhance tumor growth by protecting malignant cells from immune destruction.

Disruption of the immune response

Immunosurveillance isn't a fail-safe system. If the immune system fails to recognize tumor cells as foreign, the immune response won't activate. The tumor will continue to grow until it's beyond the immune system's ability to destroy it. In addition to this failure of surveillance, other mechanisms may come into play.

The tumor cells may suppress the immune defenses. The tumor antigens may combine with humoral antibodies to form complexes that essentially hide the antigens from the normal immune defenses. These complexes could also depress further antibody production. Tumors also may change their antigenic "appearance" or produce substances that impair usual immune defenses. The tumor growth factors not only promote the growth of the tumor but also increase the person's risk of infection. Finally, prolonged exposure to a tumor antigen may deplete the patient's lymphocytes and further impair the ability to mount an appropriate response.

The patient's population of suppressor T lymphocytes may be inadequate to defend against malignant tumors. Suppressor T lymphocytes usually assist in regulating antibody production; they also signal the immune system when an immune response is no longer needed. Certain carcinogens, such as viruses or chemicals, may weaken the immune system by destroying or damaging suppressor T cells or their precursors, and subsequently allow for tumor growth.

Theoretically, cancer develops when any of several factors disrupts the immune response:

◆ *Aging cells.* As cells age, errors in copying genetic material during cell division may give rise to mutations. If the aging immune system doesn't recognize these mutations as foreign, the mutated cells may proliferate and form a tumor.

◆ *Cytotoxic drugs or steroids.* These agents decrease antibody production and destroy circulating lymphocytes.

◆ *Extreme stress or certain viral infections.* These conditions may depress the immune response, thus allowing cancer cells to proliferate.

◆ *Suppression of immune system.* Radiation, cytotoxic drug therapy, and lymphoproliferative and myeloproliferative diseases (such as lymphatic and myelocytic leukemia) depress bone marrow production and impair leukocyte function.

◆ *Acquired immunodeficiency syndrome.* This condition weakens the cell-mediated immune response.

◆ *Cancer.* The disease itself is immunosuppressive. Advanced disease exhausts the immune system, leading to anergy (the absence of immune reactivity).

Risk factors

Many cancers are related to specific environmental or lifestyle factors that predispose a person to develop cancer. Accumulating data suggest that some of these risk factors initiate carcinogenesis, other risk factors act as promoters, and some risk factors initiate and promote the disease process.

AIR POLLUTION

Air pollution has been linked to the development of cancer, particularly lung cancer. Persons living near industries that release toxic chemicals have an increased risk of cancer. Many outdoor air pollutants—such as arsenic, benzene, hydrocarbons, polyvinyl chlorides, and other industrial emissions as well as vehicle exhaust—have been studied for their carcinogenic properties.

Indoor air pollution, such as from cigarette smoke and radon, also poses an increased risk of cancer. In fact, indoor air pollution is considered to be more carcinogenic than outdoor air pollution.

TOBACCO

Cigarette smoking increases the risk of lung cancer more than tenfold over that of nonsmokers by late middle age. Tobacco smoke contains nitrosamines and polycyclic hydrocarbons, two carcinogens that are known to cause mutations. The risk of lung cancer from cigarette smoking correlates directly with the duration of smoking and the number of cigarettes smoked per day. Tobacco smoke is also associated with laryngeal cancer and is considered a contributing factor in cancer of the bladder, pancreas, kidney, and cervix. Research also shows that smoking cessation may decrease a person's risk of lung cancer.

Although the risk associated with pipe and cigar smoking is similar to that of cigarette smoking, some evidence suggests that the effects are less severe. Smoke from cigars and pipes is more alkaline. This alkalinity decreases nicotine absorption in the lungs and is more irritating to the lungs, so the smoker doesn't inhale as readily.

Inhalation of secondhand smoke, or *passive smoking,* by nonsmokers also increases the risk of lung and other cancers. Use of smokeless tobacco, in which the oral tissue directly absorbs nicotine and other carcinogens, is linked to an increase in oral cancers that seldom occur in persons who don't use the product.

Preventing cervical cancer

The human papillomavirus (HPV), types 16 and 18, causes 70% of cervical cancer cases. To prevent this disorder, encourage the patient to do the following:

Get vaccinated
Since 2006, the quadrivalent HPV recombinant vaccine (Gardasil) has been available to reduce cervical cancer. This vaccine is recommended for girls and women ages 9 to 26. The vaccine is most effective if given before the patient is sexually active. Remind the patient that Pap tests are still recommended.

Have Pap test screenings
The most effective way to screen for cervical cancer is the Pap test. Screenings should be conducted as follows:
◆ every year or every 2 years using liquid-based Pap tests, beginning approximately 3 years after onset of vaginal intercourse, but no later than age 21
◆ every 2 to 3 years at or older than age 30 for women who have had three consecutive normal Pap test results (more frequent

screening may be indicated with certain risk factors)
◆ every 3 years after age 30 (but not more frequently) with either conventional or liquid-based Pap tests, plus the human papillomavirus deoxyribonucleic acid test. Screening may stop for women age 70 and older who have had three consecutive normal Pap tests in 10 years.

Be careful with sexual activity
Having sexual intercourse at a young age increases the risk for contracting HPV. Advise your patient that delaying first intercourse may help reduce this risk. Also, having fewer sexual partners may decrease the risk.

Don't smoke
Chances of developing cervical cancer can be reduced by not smoking.

ALCOHOL
Alcohol consumption, especially in conjunction with cigarette smoking, is commonly associated with cirrhosis of the liver, a precursor to hepatocellular cancer. The risk of breast and colorectal cancers also increases with alcohol consumption. Possible mechanisms for breast cancer development include impaired removal of carcinogens by the liver, impaired immune response, and interference with cell membrane permeability of the breast tissue. Alcohol stimulates rectal cell proliferation in rats, an observation that may help explain the increased incidence of colorectal cancer in humans who regularly consume alcohol.

Heavy use of alcohol and cigarette smoking synergistically increase the incidence of cancers of the mouth, larynx, pharynx, and esophagus. Alcohol probably acts as a solvent for the carcinogenic substances found in smoke, enhancing their absorption.

SEXUAL BEHAVIOR
Sexual practices have been linked to specific types of cancer. The age of first sexual intercourse and the number of sexual partners are positively correlated with a woman's risk of cervical cancer. Furthermore, a woman who has had only one sexual partner is at higher risk if that partner has had

multiple partners. The suspected underlying mechanism here involves virus transmission, most likely human papillomavirus (HPV). HPV types 6 and 11 are associated with genital warts. HPV is the most common cause of abnormal Papanicolaou smears, and cervical dysplasia is a direct precursor to squamous cell carcinoma of the cervix, both of which have been linked to HPV (especially types 16 and 18). (See *Preventing cervical cancer.*)

OCCUPATION
Because of exposure to specific substances, certain occupations increase the risk of cancer. People exposed to asbestos, such as insulation installers and miners, are at risk for a type of lung cancer called *mesothelioma*. Asbestos also may act as a promoter for other carcinogens. Workers involved in the production of dyes, rubber, paint, and beta-naphthylamine are at increased risk for bladder cancer.

ULTRAVIOLET RADIATION
Exposure to ultraviolet B (UVB) radiation can damage the skin and increase the risk of skin cancer development. UVB is known to cause damage to the DNA of skin cells. Specifically, it causes a genetic mutation in the P53 tumor-suppressor gene. Recent evidence shows that

PREVENTION

Preventing basal cell carcinoma

Most basal cell carcinomas can be prevented through lifestyle changes. Teach your patient to do the following:

Avoid the midday sun

Sunlight is strongest between 10 a.m. and 4 p.m. Outdoor activities should be scheduled for other times of the day, even in winter or when it's cloudy. Advise your patient that sunlight is more intense when it reflects off water, sand, and snow.

Use sunscreen year-round

Sunscreens don't filter out all harmful UV radiation, but they're helpful for sun protection. Advise your patient to wear a broad-spectrum sunscreen with a sun protection factor (SPF) of at least 15 when he goes outside, year-round. He should use about 1 ounce—the amount that fits in his palm—to cover his entire body, including lips, ears, and the backs of hands and neck. Sunscreen should be applied 20 to 30 minutes before sun exposure and reapplied every 2 hours throughout the day, as well as after swimming or exercising.

Wear protective clothing

Sunscreens shouldn't be relied on as the sole means of sun protection. It's important to also wear tightly woven clothing that covers the arms and legs and a broad-brimmed hat rather than a baseball cap or visor. Sunglasses that provide full protection from both UVA and UVB rays should also be worn.

Be careful with medications

Some common prescription and over-the-counter drugs make skin more sensitive to sunlight. These include antibiotics; certain cholesterol, high blood pressure, and diabetes medications; ibuprofen (Advil, Motrin); and the acne medication isotretinoin (Accutane).

Perform regular skin checks

Encourage your patient to examine his skin often for new growths or changes in existing moles, freckles, bumps, and birthmarks, including on the scalp, ears, and buttocks, and to be vigilant about checking for recurring tumors.

Get enough vitamin D

This vitamin may help lower the risk of certain cancers. Although it's normally produced by sunlight on the skin, many experts recommend getting the daily requirement of vitamin D through food or supplements.

---

exposure to ultraviolet A (UVA) radiation from sunlamps and tanning booths also contributes to skin cancer development. The damaging effects of UVA are thought to be indirect, occurring as a result of energy transferred through reactive oxygen intermediates (free radicals).

The amount of exposure to ultraviolet radiation also correlates with the type of cancer that develops. For example, cumulative exposure to ultraviolet radiation is associated with basal and squamous cell skin cancer, and severe episodes of burning and blistering at a young age are associated with melanoma. (See *Preventing basal cell carcinoma*.)

IONIZING RADIATION

Ionizing radiation (such as X-rays) is associated with acute leukemia, thyroid, breast, lung, stomach, colon, and urinary tract cancers as well as multiple myeloma. Low doses can cause DNA mutations and chromosomal abnormalities, and large doses can inhibit cell division. This damage can directly affect carbohydrate, protein, lipid, and nucleic acids (macromolecules), or it can act on intracellular water to produce free radicals that damage the macromolecules.

Ionizing radiation can also enhance the effects of genetic abnormalities. For example, it increases the risk of cancer in people with a genetic abnormality that affects DNA repair mechanisms. Other compounding variables include the area and percentage of the body exposed, the person's age, hormonal balance, prescribed drugs, and preexisting or concurrent conditions.

HORMONES

Hormones—specifically the sex steroid hormones estrogen, progesterone, and testosterone—have been implicated as promoters of breast, endometrial, ovarian, and prostate cancers.

Estrogen, which stimulates the proliferation of breast and endometrial cells, is considered a promoter for breast and endometrial cancers. Prolonged exposure to estrogen, as in women with early menarche and late menopause, increases the risk of breast cancer. Likewise,

American Cancer Society recommendations for cancer prevention

The recommendations listed below from the American Cancer Society focus on nutrition and physical activity prevention measures.

♦ Eat a variety of healthful foods, with an emphasis on plant sources.

♦ Eat five or more servings of a variety of vegetables and fruits each day. Choose whole grains in preference to processed (refined) grains and sugars.

♦ Limit consumption of red meats, especially processed ones and those high in fat.

♦ Choose foods that can help you maintain a healthful weight.

♦ Adopt a physically active lifestyle.

♦ Adults: Engage in at least moderate activity for 30 minutes or more on 5 or more days of the week; 45 minutes or more of moderate to vigorous activity on 5 or more days per week may further reduce the risk of breast and colon cancer.

♦ Children and adolescents: Engage in at least 60 minutes/day of moderate-to-vigorous physical activity at least 5 days/ week.

♦ Maintain a healthful weight throughout life.

♦ Balance caloric intake with physical activity.

♦ Lose weight if currently overweight or obese.

♦ Don't smoke, and limit or abstain from consumption of alcoholic beverages.

---

long-term use of estrogen replacement therapy without progesterone supplementation for menopausal symptoms increases a woman's risk of endometrial cancer. Progesterone may play a protective role, counteracting estrogen's stimulatory effects.

The male sex hormones stimulate the growth of prostatic tissue. However, research fails to show an increased risk of prostate cancer in men who take exogenous androgens.

DIET

Numerous aspects of diet are linked to an increase in cancer, including:

♦ obesity (in women only, possibly related to production of estrogen by fatty tissue), which is linked to a suspected increased risk of endometrial cancer

♦ high consumption of dietary fat, which is linked to endometrial, breast, prostate, ovarian, and rectal cancers

♦ high consumption of smoked foods, salted fish or meats, and foods containing nitrites, which may be linked to gastric cancer

♦ naturally occurring carcinogens (such as hydrazines and aflatoxin) in foods, which are linked to liver cancer

♦ carcinogens produced by microorganisms stored in foods, which are linked to stomach cancer

♦ diet low in fiber (which slows transport through the gut), which is linked to colorectal cancer.

The American Cancer Society has developed specific nutritional guidelines for cancer prevention. (See *American Cancer Society recommendations for cancer prevention*.)

Pathophysiologic changes

Cancer's characteristic features are uncontrollable proliferation of cells and independent spread from a primary site (site of origin) to other tissues where it establishes secondary foci (metastasis). This spread occurs through circulation in the blood or lymphatic fluid, by unintentional transplantation from one site to another during surgery, and by local extension. Thus, cancer cells differ from normal cells in terms of cell size, shape, number, differentiation, and purpose or function. In addition, cancer cells can travel to distant tissues and organ systems. (See *Cancer cell characteristics*.)

CELL GROWTH

Typically, each of the billions of cells in the human body has an internal clock that tells the cell when it's time to reproduce. Mitotic reproduction occurs in a sequence called the *cell cycle*. Normal cell division occurs in direct proportion to cells lost, thus providing a mechanism for controlling growth and differentiation. These controls are absent in cancer cells, and cell production exceeds cell loss. Consequently, cancer cells enter the cell cycle more frequently and at different rates. They're most commonly found in the synthesis and mitosis phases of the cell cycle, and they spend very little time in the resting phase.

Normal cells reproduce at a rate controlled through the activity of specific control or regulator genes (called *proto-oncogenes* when they function normally). These genes produce proteins that act as on-and-off switches. There's no generalized control gene; different cells respond to specific control genes. The P53 and c-myc genes are two examples of control genes: P53 is a tumor-suppressor gene that can stop DNA replication if the cell's DNA has been damaged; c-myc helps initiate DNA replication and if it senses an error in DNA replication, it can cause the cell to self-destruct.

Hormones, growth factors, and chemicals released by neighboring cells or by immune or inflammatory cells can affect control gene activity. These substances bind to specific receptors on the cell membranes and send out signals causing the control genes to stimulate or suppress cell reproduction. Examples of hormones and growth factors that affect control genes include:
◆ erythropoietin, which stimulates red blood cell (RBC) proliferation
◆ epidermal growth factor, which stimulates epidermal cell proliferation
◆ insulin-like growth factor, which stimulates fat and connective tissue proliferation
◆ platelet-derived growth factor, which stimulates connective tissue cell proliferation.

Substances released by injured or infected nearby cells or by cells of the immune system also affect cellular reproduction. For example, interleukin, released by immune cells, stimulates cell proliferation and differentiation. Interferon, released from virus-infected and immune cells, may affect the cell's rate of reproduction.

Additionally, cells that are close to one another appear to communicate with each other through gap junctions (channels through which ions and other small molecules pass). This communication provides information to the cell about the neighboring cell types and the amount of space available. The nearby cells send out physical and chemical signals that control the reproduction rate. For example, if the area is crowded, the nearby cells will signal the same type of cells to slow or cease reproduction, thus allowing the formation of only a single layer of cells. This feature is called *density-dependent growth inhibition*.

In cancer cells, the control genes fail to function normally. The control may be lost or the gene may become damaged. An imbalance of growth factors may occur, or the cells may fail to respond to the suppressive action of the growth factors. Any of these mechanisms may lead to uncontrolled cellular reproduction.

One striking characteristic of cancer cells is that they fail to recognize the signals emitted by nearby cells about available tissue space. Instead of forming only a single layer, cancer cells continue to accumulate in a disorderly array.

The loss of control over normal growth is termed *autonomy*. This independence is further evidenced by the ability of cancer cells to break off and travel to other sites.

Cancer cell characteristics

Cancer cells, which undergo uncontrolled cellular growth and development, typically exhibit these characteristics:
◆ Vary in size and shape
◆ Undergo abnormal mitosis
◆ Function abnormally
◆ Don't resemble the cell of origin
◆ Produce substances not usually associated with the original cell or tissue
◆ Aren't encapsulated
◆ Can spread to other sites

CELL DIFFERENTIATION

Usually, cells become specialized during development. That is, the cells develop highly individualized characteristics that reflect their specific structure and functions in their corresponding tissue. For example, all blood cells are derived from a single stem cell that differentiates into RBCs, white blood cells (WBCs), platelets, monocytes, and lymphocytes. As the cells become more specialized, their reproduction and development slow down. Eventually, highly differentiated cells become unable to reproduce and some — skin cells, for example — are programmed to die and be replaced.

Cancer cells lose the ability to differentiate — that is, they enter a state, called *anaplasia*, in which they no longer appear or function like the original cell. (See *Understanding anaplasia,* page 18.)

Anaplasia occurs in varying degrees. The less the cells resemble the cell of origin, the more anaplastic they're said to be. As the anaplastic cells continue to reproduce, they lose the typical characteristics of the original cell.

Some anaplastic cells begin functioning as another type of cell, possibly becoming a site for hormone production. For example, small-cell lung cancer cells often produce antidiuretic hormone, which is produced by the hypothalamus but stored in and secreted by the posterior pituitary gland.

When anaplasia occurs, cells of the same type in the same site exhibit many different shapes and sizes. Mitosis is abnormal and chromosome defects are common.

INTRACELLULAR CHANGES

The abnormal and uncontrolled cell proliferation of cancer cells is associated with numerous changes within the cancer cell itself. These changes affect the cell membrane, cytoskeleton, and nucleus.

Understanding anaplasia

Anaplasia refers to the loss of differentiation, a common characteristic of cancer cells. As differentiation is lost, the cancer cells no longer demonstrate the appearance and function of the original cell.

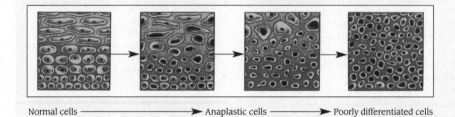

Normal cells ⟶ Anaplastic cells ⟶ Poorly differentiated cells

Cell membrane

The cell membrane is a thin, dynamic, semipermeable structure that separates the cell's internal environment from its external environment. It consists of two layers of lipid molecules (called the *lipid bilayer*) with protein molecules attached to or embedded in each layer. The bilayer is composed of phospholipids, glycolipids, and other lipids, such as cholesterol.

The protein molecules help stabilize the structure of the membrane and participate in the transport and exchange of material between the cell and its environment. Large glycoproteins, called *fibronectin,* are responsible for holding the cells in place and maintaining the specific arrangement of the receptors to allow for the exchange of material.

In the cancer cell, fibronectin is defective or is broken down as it's produced, thus affecting the organization, structure, adhesion, and migration of the cells. Some of the other proteins and glycolipids are also absent or altered. These changes affect the density of the receptors on the cell membrane and the cell's shape. Communication between the cells becomes impaired, response to growth factors is enhanced, and recognition of other cells is diminished. The result is uncontrolled growth.

Permeability of the cancer cell membrane is also altered. During its uncontrolled, rapid proliferation, the cancer cell has a much greater metabolic demand for nutrients to sustain its growth.

During normal development, cell division can occur only when the cells are anchored to nearby cells or to extracellular molecules via anchoring junctions. In cancer cells, anchoring junctions need not be present. Thus, they continue to divide and can metastasize.

Disruption or blockage of gap junctions interferes with intercellular communication. This may be the underlying mechanism by which cancer cells continue to grow and migrate, forming layers of undifferentiated cells, even in a crowded environment.

Cytoskeleton

The *cytoskeleton* is composed of protein filament networks including actin and microtubules. Usually, actin filaments exert a pull on the extracellular organic molecules that bind cells together. Microtubules control cell shape, movement, and division. In cancer cells, the functions of these components are altered. Additionally, cytoplasmic components are fewer and abnormally shaped. Less cellular work occurs because of a decrease in endoplasmic reticulum and mitochondria.

Nucleus

In cancer cells, nuclei are pleomorphic, meaning enlarged and of various shapes and sizes. They're also highly pigmented and have larger and more numerous nucleoli than normal. The nuclear membrane is typically irregular and commonly has projections, pouches, or blebs, and fewer pores. Chromatin (uncoiled chromosomes) may clump along the outer areas of the nucleus. Breaks, deletions, translocations, and abnormal karyotypes (chromosome shape and number) are common changes in the chromosomes. The chromosome defects seem to stem from the increased mitotic rate in cancer cells. The appearance of the mitotic cancer cell under light microscopy is commonly described as atypical and bizarre.

TUMOR DEVELOPMENT AND GROWTH

Typically, a long time passes between the initiating event and the appearance of cancer. During this time, the cancer cells continue to grow, develop, and replicate, each time undergoing successive changes and further mutations.

How fast a tumor grows depends on specific characteristics of the tumor and its host.

Tumor growth needs

For a tumor to grow, an initiating event or events must cause a mutation that will transform the normal cell into a cancer cell. After the initial event, the tumor continues to grow only if available nutrients, oxygen, and blood supply are adequate and the immune system fails to recognize or respond to the tumor.

Location and blood supply

Two important tumor characteristics affecting growth are tumor location and available blood supply. The location determines the originating cell type, which in turn determines the cell cycle time. For example, epithelial cells have a shorter cell cycle than that of connective tissue cells. Thus, tumors arising from epithelial cells (such as squamous cell carcinomas and adenocarcinomas) grow more rapidly than tumors arising from connective tissue cells (such as fibrosarcomas).

Tumors need an available blood supply to provide nutrients and oxygen for continued growth and to remove wastes; however, a tumor larger than 1 to 2 mm in size has typically outgrown its available blood supply. Some tumors secrete tumor angiogenesis factors, which stimulate the formation of new blood vessels, to meet the demand.

The degree of anaplasia also affects tumor growth. Remember that the more anaplastic the tumor's cells, the less differentiated the cells and the more rapidly they divide.

Many cancer cells also produce their own growth factors. Numerous growth factor receptors are present on the cell membranes of rapidly growing cancer cells. This increase in receptors, in conjunction with the changes in the cell membranes, further enhances cancer cell proliferation.

Host characteristics

Several important characteristics of the host affect tumor growth. These characteristics include age, sex, overall health status, and immune system function.

🔳 **AGE ALERT** *Age is an important factor affecting tumor growth. Relatively few cancers are found in children. Yet the incidence of cancer* correlates directly with increasing age. This correlation suggests that numerous or cumulative events are necessary for the initial mutation to continue, eventually forming a tumor.

Certain cancers are more prevalent in one sex than in the other. For example, sex hormones influence tumor growth in breast, endometrial, cervical, and prostate cancers. Researchers believe that the hormone sensitizes the cell to the initial precipitating factor, thus promoting carcinogenesis.

Overall health status also is an important host characteristic. As tumors obtain nutrients for growth from the host, they can alter normal body processes and cause cachexia. Conversely, if the person is nutritionally depleted, tumor growth may slow. Chronic tissue trauma also has been linked with tumor growth because healing involves increased cell division. The more rapidly cells divide, the greater the likelihood of mutations.

SPREAD OF CANCER

Between the initiating event and the emergence of a detectable tumor, some or all of the mutated cells may die. The survivors, if any, reproduce until the tumor reaches a diameter of 1 to 2 mm. New blood vessels form to support continued growth and proliferation. As the cells further mutate and divide more rapidly, they become more undifferentiated. The number of cancerous cells soon begins to exceed the number of normal cells. Eventually, the tumor mass extends, spreading into local tissues and invading the surrounding tissues. When the local tissue is blood or lymph, the tumor can gain access to the circulation. Once access is gained, tumor cells that detach or break off travel to distant sites in the body, where they can survive and form a new tumor in that secondary site. This process is called *metastasis*.

Dysplasia

Not all cells that proliferate rapidly go on to become cancerous. Throughout a person's life span, various body tissues experience periods of benign rapid growth such as during wound healing. Sometimes changes in the size, shape, and organization of the cells lead to a condition called *dysplasia*.

Exposure to chemicals, viruses, radiation, or chronic inflammation causes dysplastic changes that may be reversed by removing the initiating stimulus or treating its effects. However, if the stimulus isn't removed, precancerous or dysplastic lesions can progress and give rise to cancer. For example, actinic keratoses, thickened patches on the skin of the face and hands

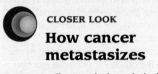

CLOSER LOOK
How cancer metastasizes

Cancer usually spreads through the bloodstream to other organs and tissues, as shown below.

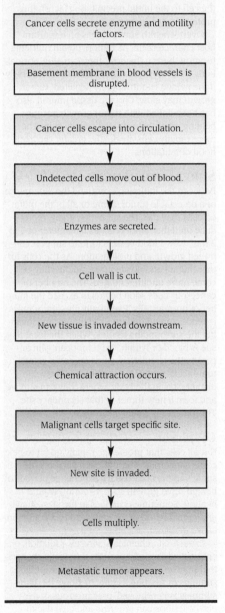

Cancer cells secrete enzyme and motility factors.

↓

Basement membrane in blood vessels is disrupted.

↓

Cancer cells escape into circulation.

↓

Undetected cells move out of blood.

↓

Enzymes are secreted.

↓

Cell wall is cut.

↓

New tissue is invaded downstream.

↓

Chemical attraction occurs.

↓

Malignant cells target specific site.

↓

New site is invaded.

↓

Cells multiply.

↓

Metastatic tumor appears.

of people exposed to sunlight, are associated with the development of skin cancer. Removal of the lesions and use of sunblock help minimize the risk that the lesions will progress to skin cancer. Knowledge about precancerous lesions and promoter events provide the rationale for early detection and screening as important preventive measures.

Localized tumor

Initially, a tumor remains localized. Recall that cancer cells communicate poorly with nearby cells. As a result, the cells continue to grow and enlarge, forming a mass or clumps of cells. The mass exerts pressure on the neighboring cells, blocking their blood supply, and subsequently causing their death.

Invasive tumor

Invasion is growth of the tumor into surrounding tissues. It's the first step in metastasis. Five mechanisms are linked to invasion: cellular multiplication, mechanical pressure, lysis of nearby cells, reduced cell adhesion, and increased motility. Experimental data indicate that the interaction of all five mechanisms is necessary for invasion.

By their very nature, cancer cells multiply rapidly (cellular replication). As they grow, they exert pressure on surrounding cells and tissues, which eventually die because their blood supply has been cut off or blocked (mechanical pressure). Loss of mechanical resistance leads the way for the cancer cells to spread along the lines of least resistance and occupy the space once filled by the dead cells.

Vesicles on the cancer cell surface contain a rich supply of receptors for laminin, a complex glycoprotein that's a major component of the basement membrane, a thin sheet of noncellular connective tissue upon which cells rest. These receptors permit the cancer cells to attach to the basement membrane, forming a bridgelike connection (lysis of nearby cells). Some cancer cells produce and excrete powerful proteolytic enzymes; other cancer cells induce normal host cells to produce them. These enzymes, such as collagenases and proteases, destroy the normal cells and break through their basement membrane, enabling the cancer cells to enter.

Reduced cell adhesion also is seen with cancer cells. As discussed in the section on intracellular changes, reduced cell adhesion likely results when the cell-stabilizing glycoprotein fibronectin is deficient or defective.

Cancer cells also secrete a chemotactic factor that stimulates and increases motility. Thus, the cancer cells can move independently into adjacent tissues and into the circulation, and then on to a secondary site. Finally, cancer cells develop fingerlike projections called *pseudopodia* that facilitate cell movement. These projections injure and kill neighboring cells and attach to vessel walls, enabling the cancer cells to enter.

Metastatic tumor
Metastatic tumors are those in which the cancer cells have traveled from the original or primary site to a second or more distant site. Most commonly, metastasis occurs through the blood vessels and lymphatic system. Tumor cells also can be transported from one body location to another by external means, such as carriage on instruments or gloves during surgery.

Hematogenous metastasis
Invasive tumor cells break down the basement membrane and walls of blood vessels, and the tumor sheds malignant cells into the circulation. Most of the cells die, but a few escape the host defenses and the turbulent environment of the bloodstream. From here, the surviving mass of tumor cells, called a *tumor cell embolus,* travels downstream and commonly lodges in the first capillary bed it encounters. For example, blood from most organs next enters the capillaries of the lungs, which are the most common sites of metastasis.

Once lodged, the tumor cells develop a protective coat of fibrin, platelets, and clotting factors to evade detection by the immune system. Then they become attached to the epithelium, ultimately invading the vessel wall, interstitium, and parenchyma of the target organ. (See *How cancer metastasizes.*) To survive, the new tumor develops its own vascular network and may ultimately spread again.

Lymphatic metastasis
The lymphatic system is the most common route for distant metastasis. Tumor cells enter the lymphatic vessels through damaged basement membranes and are transported to regional lymph nodes. In this case, the tumor becomes trapped in the first lymph node it encounters. The consequent enlargement, possibly the first evidence of metastasis, may be caused by increased tumor growth within the node or a localized immune reaction to the tumor. The lymph node may filter out or contain some of the tumor cells, limiting further spread. The cells that escape can enter the blood from the lymphatic circulation through plentiful connections between the venous and lymphatic systems.

Metastatic sites
Typically, the first capillary bed, whether lymphatic or vascular, encountered by the circulating tumor mass determines the location of the metastasis. For example, because the lungs receive all of the systemic venous return, they're a common site for metastasis. In breast cancer, the axillary lymph nodes, which are close to the breast, are a common site of metastasis. Other types of cancer seem most likely to spread to specific organs. This organ tropism may be a result of growth factor or hormones secreted by the target organ or chemotactic factors that attract the tumor. (See *Common sites of metastasis,* page 22.)

Signs and symptoms

In most patients, the earlier the cancer is found, the more effective treatment is likely to be and the better the prognosis. Some cancers may be diagnosed on a routine physical examination, even before the person develops signs or symptoms. Others may display early warning signals. The American Cancer Society developed a mnemonic device to help identify cancer warning signs. (See *Cancer's seven warning signs,* page 23.)

Unfortunately, a person may not notice or heed the warning signs. These patients may present with some of the more common signs and symptoms of advancing disease, such as anemia, cachexia, fatigue, infection, leukopenia and thrombocytopenia, and pain. These signs and symptoms are nonspecific and can be attributed to other disorders.

ANEMIA
Cancer of the blood-forming cells, WBCs or RBCs may directly cause anemia. Anemia in patients with metastatic cancer is commonly the result of chronic bleeding, severe malnutrition, chemotherapy, or radiation.

CACHEXIA
Unexplained weight loss is generally a sign of advanced disease. When weight loss is severe, cachexia—a generalized wasting of fat and protein—occurs. Cachexia is common in individuals with cancer. A person with cachexia typically appears emaciated and experiences an overall deterioration in physical status. Cachexia is characterized by anorexia (loss of appetite), alterations in taste perception, early satiety, weight loss, anemia, marked weakness, and altered metabolism of proteins, carbohydrates, and lipids.

Common sites of metastasis

The chart below lists some of the more common sites of metastasis for selected cancers.

Cancer type	Sites for metastasis
Breast	Axillary lymph nodes, lung, liver, bone, brain
Colorectal	Liver, lung, peritoneum
Lung	Liver, brain, bone, adrenal glands
Ovarian	Peritoneum, diaphragm, liver, lungs
Prostate	Bone
Testicular	Lungs, liver

Anorexia may accompany pain or adverse reactions to chemotherapy or radiation therapy. Diminished perception of sweet, sour, or salty sensations also contribute to anorexia. Food that once seemed seasoned and palatable now tastes bland.

Protein-calorie malnutrition may cause hypoalbuminemia, edema (the lack of serum proteins, which usually keep fluid in the blood vessels, enables fluid to escape into the tissues), muscle wasting, and immunodeficiency.

The high metabolic activity of malignant tumor cells carries with it the need for nutrients above those required for normal metabolism. As cancer cells appropriate nutrients to fuel their growth, normal tissue becomes starved and depleted, and wasting begins. Under normal circumstances, when starvation occurs, the body spares protein, relying on carbohydrates and fats for energy production. However, cancer cells metabolize both protein and fatty acids to produce energy.

The patient with cancer commonly feels sated after eating only a few bites of food. This feeling is believed to be the result of metabolites released from the tumor. Also, tumor necrosis factor, which the body produces in response to cancer, contributes to cachexia.

FATIGUE

Patients commonly describe fatigue as feelings of weakness, being tired, and lacking energy or the ability to concentrate. The underlying mechanism for fatigue isn't known, but it's believed to be the combined result of several pathophysiologic mechanisms.

The very existence of the cancerous tumor may contribute to fatigue. A malignant tumor needs oxygen and nutrients to grow. Thus, it depletes the surrounding tissues of blood and oxygen. For example, a vascular tumor can cause lethargy secondary to inadequate oxygen supply to the brain. Lung cancer can interfere with gas exchange and oxygen supply to the heart and peripheral tissues. Accumulating waste products and muscle loss from the release of toxic products of metabolism or other substances from the tumor further add to the fatigue.

Other factors also play a role in fatigue. Pain can be physically and emotionally draining. Stress, anxiety, and other emotional factors further compound the problem. If the person lacks the energy required for self-care, malnutrition, consequent lack of energy reserves, and anemia can contribute to complaints of fatigue.

INFECTION

Infection is common in the patient with advanced cancer, particularly if he has myelosuppression from treatment, direct invasion of the bone marrow, development of fistulas, or immunosuppression from hormonal release in response to chronic stress. Malnutrition and anemia further increase the patient's risk of infection. Also, obstructions, effusions, and ulcerations may develop, creating a favorable environment for microbial growth.

LEUKOPENIA AND THROMBOCYTOPENIA

Typically, leukopenia and thrombocytopenia occur when cancer invades the bone marrow. Chemotherapy and radiation therapy to the bones result in decreased numbers of WBCs and platelets.

Leukopenia greatly increases the patient's risk of infection. The patient with thrombocytopenia is at risk for hemorrhage. Even when the platelet count is normal, platelet function may be impaired in certain hematologic cancers.

PAIN

The presence of pain depends on the location of the growing tumor. In cancer's early stages, pain is often absent or mild; as cancer progresses, however, the pain's severity usually increases. Generally, pain is the result of one or more of the following:
♦ pressure
♦ obstruction

Cancer's seven warning signs

The American Cancer Society has developed a simple way to remember the seven warning signs of cancer. Each letter in the word *caution* represents a possible warning sign that should prompt an individual to seek medical attention.

C hange in bowel or bladder habits

A sore that doesn't heal

U nusual bleeding or discharge

T hickening or lump in the breast or elsewhere

I ndigestion or difficulty swallowing

O bvious change in a wart or mole

N agging cough or hoarseness

◆ invasion of sensitive tissue
◆ visceral surface stretching
◆ tissue destruction
◆ inflammation.

Pressure on or obstruction of nerves, blood vessels, or other tissues and organs leads to tissue hypoxia, accumulation of lactic acid, and possibly cell death. In areas where space for tumor growth is limited, such as in the brain or bone, compression is a common cause of pain. Additionally, pain occurs when the viscera, which is usually hollow, is stretched by a tumor, as in GI cancer.

Cancer cells also release proteolytic enzymes that directly injure or destroy neighboring cells. This injury sets up a painful inflammatory response.

Diagnosis

A thorough history and physical examination should precede sophisticated diagnostic tests. The choice of diagnostic tests is determined by the patient's presenting signs and symptoms and the suspected body system involved. Diagnostic tests serve several purposes, including:
◆ establishing tumor presence and extent of disease
◆ determining possible sites of metastasis

◆ evaluating affected and unaffected body systems
◆ identifying the stage and grade of tumor.

SCREENING TESTS

Useful tests for early detection and staging of tumors include screening tests, X-rays, radioactive isotope scanning (nuclear medicine imaging), computed tomography (CT) scanning, endoscopy, ultrasonography, magnetic resonance imaging (MRI), and positron emission tomography (PET) scanning. The single most important diagnostic tool is the biopsy for direct histologic study of the tumor tissue.

Screening tests are perhaps the most important diagnostic tools in the prevention and early detection of cancer. They may provide valuable information about the possibility of cancer even before the patient develops signs and symptoms. The American Cancer Society has recommended specific screening tests to aid in the early detection of cancer. (See *American Cancer Society guidelines: Early cancer detection,* pages 24 and 25.)

X-rays

Most commonly, X-rays are ordered to identify and evaluate changes in tissue densities. The type and location of the X-ray is determined by the patient's signs and symptoms and the suspected location of the tumor or metastasis. For example, a chest X-ray may be indicated to identify lung cancer if the patient is an older smoker or to rule out lung metastasis if the patient has colorectal cancer.

Some X-rays, such as those of the GI tract (barium enema) and the urinary tract (excretory urography), involve the use of contrast agents. Radiopaque substances can also be injected into the lymphatic system, and their flow can be monitored by lymphangiography. This specialized X-ray technique is helpful in evaluating tumors of the lymph nodes and metastasis. Because lymphangiography is invasive and may be difficult to interpret, CT scanning and MRI have largely replaced it.

Radioactive isotope scanning

A specialized camera detects radioactive isotopes that are injected into the bloodstream or ingested. The radiologist evaluates their distribution (uptake) throughout tissues, organs, and organ systems. This type of scanning provides a view of organs and regions within the organ that can't be seen with a simple X-ray. The area of uptake is termed a *hot spot* or a *cold spot* (an area of decreased uptake). Typically, tumors are revealed as cold spots; the exception is the bone

American Cancer Society guidelines: Early cancer detection

For people having periodic health examinations, a cancer-related checkup should include health counseling and specific examinations for malignant and nonmalignant disorders. The recommendations listed below from the American Cancer Society focus on five common cancers whose survival rates can be improved if the cancer is detected early. People who are at increased risk for certain cancers may require a different screening schedule, such as beginning at an earlier age or being screened more often.

Screening area	Recommendations
Breast	
♦ Mammogram	♦ Every year age 40 and older
♦ Clinical breast examination	♦ Every year age 40 and older (part of every health examination); every 3 years for ages 20 to 39
♦ Breast self-examination (BSE)	♦ Optional; suggested monthly for age 20 and older*
♦ Magnetic resonance imaging	♦ Every year for women at high risk (greater than 20% lifetime risk)
Cervix	
♦ Papanicolaou (Pap) test	♦ Every year or every 2 years using liquid-based Pap tests, beginning approximately 3 years after onset of vaginal intercouse, but no later than age 21
	♦ Every 2 to 3 years at or older than age 30 for women who have had three consecutive normal Pap test results (more frequent screening may be indicated with certain risk factors)
	♦ Every 3 years after age 30 (but not more frequently) with either conventional or liquid-based Pap test, plus the human papillomavirus deoxyribonucleic acid test
	♦ Screening may stop for women age 70 and older who have had three consecutive normal Pap tests in 10 years
	♦ Not necessary after a total hysterectomy (with removal of the cervix), unless surgery was done as a treatment for cervical cancer

scan, in which hot spots indicate the presence of disease. Examples of areas commonly evaluated with radioactive isotope scanning include thyroid, liver, spleen, brain, and bone.

CT scanning

CT scanning evaluates successive layers of tissue by using narrow-beam X-ray to provide a cross-sectional view of the structure. It can also reveal different characteristics of tissues within a solid organ. CT scans are commonly obtained of the brain and head, body, and abdomen to evaluate for neurologic, pelvic, abdominal, and thoracic cancers and metastases.

Endoscopy

Endoscopy provides a direct view of a body cavity or passageway to detect abnormalities. Common endoscopic sites include the upper and lower GI tract and the bronchial tree. During endoscopy, the physician can excise small tumors, aspirate fluid, or obtain tissue samples for histologic examination.

Ultrasonography

Ultrasonography uses high-frequency sound waves to detect tissue density changes that are difficult or impossible to observe by radiology or endoscopy. Ultrasound helps differentiate cysts from solid tumors and is commonly used to provide information about breast, abdominal, and pelvic cancer.

MRI

MRI uses magnetic fields and radio frequencies to show a cross-sectional view of the body organs and structures. Like CT scanning, it's commonly used to evaluate neurologic, pelvic, abdominal, and thoracic cancers. MRI is now undergoing clinical trials as a diagnostic tool for breast cancer. Preliminary findings have concluded that, in women with a high genetic risk

American Cancer Society guidelines: Early cancer detection *(continued)*

Screening area	Recommendations
Endometrium	
Women at risk for hereditary nonpolyposis colon cancer	
◆ Endometrial biopsy	◆ Annually, beginning at age 35
Prostate	
Men age 50 and older (with life expectancy of at least 10 years), men age 45 and older (at high risk), or men age 40 and older (at even higher risk)	
◆ Prostate-specific antigen	◆ Annually
◆ Digital rectal examination	◆ Annually
Colon and rectum (one of the tests below)	
Men and women age 50 and older	
◆ Fecal occult blood test (FOBT) or fecal immunochemical test (FIT)**,***	◆ Every year
◆ Stool DNA test***	◆ Interval uncertain
◆ Flexible sigmoidoscopy***	◆ Every 5 years
◆ Double-contrast barium enema***	◆ Every 5 years
◆ Colonoscopy	◆ Every 10 years
◆ Computed tomography colonography (virtual colonoscopy)***	◆ Every 5 years

* Women in their 20s should be instructed about the benefits and limitations of BSE; women have the option of not performing BSE or performing it only occasionally.

** For FOBT or FIT, the take-home multiple sample method should be used.

*** Colonoscopy should be performed if test results are positive.

for breast cancer, MRI is a more sensitive screening tool than mammography, ultrasound, or clinical breast examinations. However, its high cost and high false-positive rate (which can lead to unnecessary biopsies) prohibit it from being recommended for routine use, although it may be used in combination with other techniques.

PET scanning

PET scans use radioisotope technology to create a picture of the body in action. They use computers to construct images from the emission of positive electrons (positrons) by radioactive substances administered to the patient. Unlike other diagnostic methods that simply create images of how the body looks, PET scans provide real-time imaging of the body while it functions. Using PET scans to study the spread of cancer involves injecting the cancer patient with a small amount of radioactive glucose. Cancer cells metabolize sugar more quickly than healthy cells do, and this increase can be seen in the image. The three-dimensional PET scan pictures show malignancies as having a greater concentration of sugar.

Biopsy

A biopsy, the removal of a portion of suspicious tissue, is the only definitive method to diagnose cancer. Biopsy tissue samples can be taken by curettage; fluid aspiration (pleural effusion); fine-needle aspiration, core needle biopsy, stereotactic needle biopsy, vacuum-assisted biopsy, or large core biopsy (breast); dermal punch (skin or mouth); endoscopy (rectal polyps and esophageal lesions); and surgical excision (visceral tissue and nodes). The specimen is examined by a pathologist to determine cell type, grade, and other characteristics necessary for accurate staging of the tumor.

Common tumor cell markers

Tumor cell markers may be used to detect, diagnose, or treat cancer. Alone, however, they aren't sufficient for a diagnosis. Tumor cell markers may also be associated with other benign (nonmalignant) conditions. The chart below highlights some of the more commonly used tumor cell markers and their associated malignant and nonmalignant conditions.

Marker	Malignant conditions	Nonmalignant conditions
Alpha-fetoprotein (AFP)	♦ Endodermal sinus tumor ♦ Liver cancer ♦ Ovarian germ cell cancer ♦ Testicular germ cell cancer (specifically embryonal cell carcinoma)	♦ Ataxia-telangiectasia ♦ Cirrhosis ♦ Hepatitis ♦ Pregnancy ♦ Wiskott-Aldrich syndrome
Carcinoembryonic antigen (CEA)	♦ Bladder cancer ♦ Breast cancer ♦ Cervical cancer ♦ Colorectal cancer ♦ Kidney cancer ♦ Liver cancer ♦ Lung cancer ♦ Lymphoma ♦ Melanoma ♦ Ovarian cancer ♦ Pancreatic cancer ♦ Stomach cancer ♦ Thyroid cancer	♦ Inflammatory bowel disease ♦ Liver disease ♦ Pancreatitis ♦ Tobacco use
CA 15-3	♦ Breast cancer (usually advanced) ♦ Lung cancer ♦ Ovarian cancer ♦ Prostate cancer	♦ Breast disease (benign) ♦ Endometriosis ♦ Hepatitis ♦ Lactation ♦ Ovarian disease (benign) ♦ Pelvic inflammatory disease ♦ Pregnancy
CA 19-9	♦ Bile duct cancer ♦ Colorectal cancer ♦ Pancreatic cancer ♦ Stomach cancer	♦ Cholecystitis ♦ Cirrhosis ♦ Gallstones ♦ Pancreatitis
CA 27-29	♦ Breast cancer ♦ Colon cancer ♦ Kidney cancer ♦ Liver cancer ♦ Lung cancer ♦ Ovarian cancer ♦ Pancreatic cancer ♦ Stomach cancer ♦ Uterine cancer	♦ Breast disease (benign) ♦ Endometriosis ♦ Kidney disease ♦ Liver disease ♦ Ovarian cysts ♦ Pregnancy (first trimester)
CA 125	♦ Breast cancer ♦ Colorectal cancer ♦ Endometrial cancer ♦ Lung cancer ♦ Ovarian cancer ♦ Pancreatic cancer	♦ Endometriosis ♦ Liver disease ♦ Menstruation ♦ Pancreatitis ♦ Pelvic inflammatory disease ♦ Peritonitis ♦ Pregnancy

Common tumor cell markers *(continued)*

Marker	Malignant conditions	Nonmalignant conditions
Human chorionic gonadotropin (HCG)	◆ Breast cancer ◆ Choriocarcinoma ◆ Embryonal cell carcinoma ◆ Gestational trophoblastic disease ◆ Liver cancer ◆ Lung cancer ◆ Pancreatic cancer ◆ Specific dysgerminomas of the ovary ◆ Stomach cancer ◆ Testicular cancer	◆ Marijuana use ◆ Pregnancy
Lactate dehydrogenase (LDH)	◆ Almost all cancers ◆ Ewing's sarcoma ◆ Leukemia ◆ Non-Hodgkin's lymphoma ◆ Testicular cancer	◆ Anemia ◆ Heart failure ◆ Hypothyriodism ◆ Liver disease ◆ Lung disease
Neuron-specific enolase	◆ Kidney cancer ◆ Melanoma ◆ Neuroblastoma ◆ Pancreatic cancer ◆ Small-cell lung cancer ◆ Testicular cancer ◆ Thyroid cancer ◆ Wilm's tumor	◆ Unknown
Prostatic acid phosphatase	◆ Prostate cancer	◆ Prostatic conditions (benign)
Prostate-specific antigen (PSA)	◆ Prostate cancer	◆ Prostatic hyperplasia (benign) ◆ Prostatitis

TUMOR CELL MARKERS

Some cancer cells release substances that usually aren't present in the body or are present only in small quantities. These substances, called *tumor markers* or *biologic markers,* are produced by the cancer cell's genetic material during growth and development or by other cells in response to the presence of cancer. (See *Common tumor cell markers,* pages 26 and 27.)

Markers may be found on the tumor's cell membrane or in the blood, cerebrospinal fluid, or urine. Tumor cell markers include hormones, enzymes, genes, antigens, and antibodies. They have many clinical uses, for example:
◆ screening people who are at high risk for cancer
◆ diagnosing a specific type of cancer in conjunction with clinical manifestations
◆ monitoring therapy's effectiveness
◆ detecting recurrence.

Tumor cell markers provide a method for detecting and monitoring the progression of certain types of cancer. Unfortunately, several disadvantages of tumor markers may preclude their use alone. For example:
◆ By the time the tumor cell marker level is elevated, the disease may be too far advanced to cure.
◆ Most tumor cell markers aren't specific enough that a certain type of cancer can be identified.
◆ Some nonmalignant diseases, such as pancreatitis or ulcerative colitis, also are associated with tumor cell markers.

Perhaps the worst drawback is that the absence of a tumor cell marker doesn't mean that a person is free from cancer. For example, mucinous ovarian cancer tumors typically don't express the ovarian cancer marker CA 125, so a negative test result doesn't eliminate the possibility of ovarian malignancy.

Understanding TNM staging

The TNM (tumor, node, and metastasis) system developed by the American Joint Committee on Cancer provides a consistent method for classifying malignant tumors based on the extent of the disease. It also offers a convenient structure to standardize diagnostic and treatment protocols. Differences in classification may occur, depending on the primary cancer site.

T for primary tumor
The anatomic extent of the primary tumor depends on its size, depth of invasion, and surface spread. Tumor stages progress from TX to T4 as follows:
TX — Primary tumor can't be assessed
T0 — No evidence of primary tumor
Tis — Carcinoma in situ
T1, T2, T3, T4 — Increasing size or local extent (or both) of primary tumor

N for nodal involvement
Nodal involvement reflects the tumor's spread to the lymph nodes as follows:
NX — Regional lymph nodes can't be assessed
N0 — No evidence of regional lymph node metastasis
N1, N2, N3 — Increasing involvement of regional lymph nodes

M for distant metastasis
Metastasis denotes the extent (or spread) of disease. Levels range from MX to M4 as follows:
MX — Distant metastasis can't be assessed
M0 — No evidence of distant metastasis
M1 — Single, solitary, distant metastasis
M2, M3, M4 — Multiple foci or multiple organ metastasis

Tumor classification

Tumors are initially classified as benign or malignant depending on the specific features they exhibit. Typically, benign tumors are well differentiated — that is, their cells closely resemble those of the tissue of origin. Commonly encapsulated with well-defined borders, benign tumors grow slowly, usually displacing but not infiltrating surrounding tissues and, therefore, causing only slight damage. Benign tumors don't metastasize.

Conversely, most malignant tumors are undifferentiated to varying degrees, having cells that may differ considerably from those of the tissue of origin. They're seldom encapsulated and are commonly poorly delineated. They rapidly expand in all directions, causing extensive damage as they infiltrate surrounding tissues. Most malignant tumors metastasize through the blood or lymph to secondary sites.

Malignant tumors are further classified by tissue type, degree of differentiation (grading), and extent of the disease (staging). High-grade tumors are poorly differentiated and are more aggressive than low-grade tumors. Early-stage cancers carry a more favorable prognosis than later-stage cancers that have spread to nearby or distant sites.

TISSUE TYPE
Histologically, malignant tumors are classified by the type of tissue in which the growth origi-

nates. Three cell layers form during the early stages of embryonic development:
◆ *Ectoderm* primarily forms the external embryonic covering and the structures that will come into contact with the environment.
◆ *Mesoderm* forms the circulatory system, muscles, supporting tissue, and most of the urinary and reproductive systems.
◆ *Endoderm* gives rise to the internal linings of the embryo, such as the epithelial lining of the pharynx and respiratory and GI tracts.

Carcinomas are tumors of epithelial tissue. They may originate in endodermal tissues, which develop into internal structures, such as the stomach and intestine, or in ectodermal tissues, which develop into external structures such as the skin. Tumors arising from glandular epithelial tissue are commonly called *adenocarcinomas*.

Sarcomas originate in the mesodermal tissues, which develop into supporting structures, such as the bone, muscle, or fat. Sarcomas may be further classified based on the specific cells involved. For example, malignant tumors arising from fat cells are called *liposarcomas*, and those arising from bone cells, *osteosarcomas*. *Leukemias* originate in the blood and bone marrow, whereas *lymphomas* arise from the lymphatic system.

GRADING
Histologically, malignant tumors are classified by their degree of differentiation. The greater

their differentiation, the greater the tumor cells' similarity to the tissue of origin. Typically, a malignant tumor is graded on a scale of 1 to 4, in order of increasing clinical severity.

◆ Grade 1 — Well differentiated; cells closely resemble the tissue of origin and maintain some specialized function.

◆ Grade 2 — Moderately well differentiated; cells vary somewhat in size and shape with increased mitosis.

◆ Grade 3 — Poorly differentiated; cells vary widely in size and shape with little resemblance to the tissue of origin; mitosis is greatly increased.

◆ Grade 4 — Undifferentiated; cells exhibit no similarity to tissue of origin.

STAGING

Malignant tumors are staged (classified anatomically) by the extent of the disease. The most commonly used method for staging is the TNM staging system, which evaluates **T**umor size, **N**odal involvement, and **M**etastatic progress. This classification system provides an accurate tumor description that's adjustable as the disease progresses. TNM staging enables reliable comparison of treatments and survival rates among large population groups; it also identifies nodal involvement and metastasis to other areas. (See *Understanding TNM staging*.)

Treatment

Cancer treatments include surgery, radiation therapy, chemotherapy, hormonal therapy, and immunotherapy (also called *biotherapy*). Each may be used alone or in combination (called *multimodal therapy*), depending on the tumor's type, stage, localization, and responsiveness and on limitations imposed by the patient's clinical status. Cancer treatment has four goals:

◆ cure, to eradicate the cancer and promote long-term patient survival

◆ control, to arrest tumor growth

◆ palliation, to alleviate symptoms when the disease is beyond control

◆ prophylaxis, to provide treatment when no tumor is detectable, but the patient is known to be at high risk for tumor development or recurrence.

Cancer treatment is further categorized by type according to when it's used, as follows:

◆ primary, to eradicate the disease

◆ adjuvant, in addition to primary, to eliminate microscopic disease and promote cure or improve the patient's response

◆ salvage or palliative, to manage recurrent disease.

As with any treatment regimen, complications may arise. Indeed, many complications of cancer are related to the adverse effects of treatment, such as fluid and electrolyte imbalances secondary to anorexia, vomiting, or diarrhea; bone marrow suppression, including anemia, leukopenia, thrombocytopenia, and neutropenia; and infection. Hypercalcemia is the most common metabolic abnormality experienced by cancer patients. Pain, which accompanies many progressing cancers, can reach intolerable levels.

Certain complications are life-threatening and require prompt intervention. These oncologic emergencies may result from the tumor's effects or its by-products, secondary involvement of other organs due to disease spread, or adverse effects of treatment. (See *Common cancer emergencies,* pages 30 and 31.)

SURGERY

Surgery, once the mainstay of cancer treatment, is now typically combined with other therapies. It may be performed to aid diagnosis of the disease, initiate primary treatment, or achieve palliation, and is occasionally done for prophylaxis. The surgical biopsy procedure is diagnostic surgery, and continuing surgery then removes the bulk of the tumor. When used as a primary treatment method, surgery is an attempt to remove the entire tumor (or as much as possible, by a procedure called *debulking*), along with surrounding tissues, including lymph nodes.

A common method of surgical removal of a small tumor mass is called *wide and local excision.* The tumor mass is removed along with a small or moderate amount of easily accessible surrounding tissue that's normal. A radical or modified radical excision removes the primary tumor along with lymph nodes, nearby involved structures, and surrounding structures that may be at high risk for disease spread. Typically a radical excision results in some degree of disfigurement and altered functioning. Today's less radical surgical procedures, such as a lumpectomy instead of mastectomy, are more acceptable to the patient. The health care professional and the patient should discuss the types of surgery available. Ultimately the choice belongs to the patient.

Palliative surgery is used to relieve complications, such as pain, ulceration, obstruction, hemorrhage, or pressure. Examples include a cordotomy to relieve intractable pain and bowel resection or ostomy to remove a bowel obstruction. Additionally, surgery may be performed to remove hormone-producing glands, thereby limiting the growth of a hormone-sensitive tumor.

Common cancer emergencies

This chart lists certain oncologic emergencies that may arise and the associated malignancy.

Emergency and cause	Associated malignancy
Cardiac tamponade	
Fluid accumulation around pericardial space or pericardial thickening secondary to radiation therapy	♦ Breast cancer ♦ Leukemia ♦ Lung cancer ♦ Lymphoma ♦ Melanoma
Disseminated intravascular coagulation	
Widespread clotting in arterioles and capillaries and simultaneous hemorrhage	♦ Hematologic malignancies ♦ Mucin-producing adenocarcinomas
Hypercalcemia	
Increased bone resorption due to bone destruction or tumor-related elevation of parathyroid hormone, osteoclast-activating factor, or prostaglandin levels	♦ Breast cancer ♦ Lung cancer ♦ Multiple myeloma ♦ Renal cancer
Malignant peritoneal infusion	
Seeding of tumor into the peritoneum, excess intraperitoneal fluid production or release of humoral factors by the tumor	♦ Colon cancer ♦ Mesothelioma ♦ Ovarian cancer
Malignant pleural effusion	
Implantation of cancer cells on pleural surface, tumor obstruction of lymphatic channels or pulmonary veins, shedding of necrotic tumor cells into the pleural space or thoracic duct perforation	♦ Breast cancer ♦ GI tract cancer ♦ Leukemia ♦ Lung cancer (most common) ♦ Lymphoma ♦ Mesothelioma ♦ Testicular cancer
Spinal cord compression	
Encroachment on spinal cord or cauda equina due to metastasis or vertebral collapse and displacement of bony elements	♦ Breast, cervical, GI tract, kidney, lung, or prostate cancer ♦ Lymphoma ♦ Melanoma
Superior vena cava syndrome	
Impaired venous return secondary to occlusion of vena cava	♦ Breast cancer ♦ Lung cancer ♦ Lymphoma

Common cancer emergencies *(continued)*

Emergency and cause	Associated malignancy
Syndrome of inappropriate antidiuretic hormone	
Ectopic production by tumor; abnormal stimulation of hypothalamus-pituitary axis; mimicking or enhanced effects on kidney; may be induced by chemotherapy	◆ Bladder cancer ◆ GI tract cancer ◆ Hodgkin's disease ◆ Prostate cancer ◆ Sarcomas ◆ Small-cell lung cancer
Tumor lysis syndrome	
Rapid cell destruction and turnover caused by chemotherapy or rapid tumor growth	◆ Leukemias ◆ Lymphomas

Prophylactic surgery may be done if a patient has personal or familial risk factors for a particular type of cancer. Here, nonvital tissues or organs with a high potential for developing cancer are removed. One example is prophylactic mastectomy. Much controversy exists over this type of surgery because of the possible long-term physiologic and psychological effects, although potential benefits may significantly outweigh the downside.

RADIATION THERAPY

Radiation therapy involves the use of high-energy radiation to treat cancer. Used alone or in conjunction with other therapies, it aims to destroy dividing cancer cells while damaging normal cells as little as possible. Two types of radiation are used to treat cancer: ionizing radiation and particle beam radiation. Both target the cellular DNA. Ionizing radiation deposits energy that damages the genetic material inside the cancer cells. Normal cells are also affected but can recover. Particle beam radiation uses a special machine and fast-moving particles to treat the cancer. The particles can cause more cell damage than ionizing radiation does.

The guiding principle for radiation therapy is that the dose administered be large enough to eradicate the tumor, but small enough to minimize the adverse effects to the surrounding normal tissue. How well the treatment meets this goal is known as the *therapeutic ratio*.

Radiation interacts with oxygen in the nucleus to break strands of DNA and interacts with water in body fluids (including intracellular fluid) to form free radicals, which also damage the DNA. If this damage isn't repaired, the cells die, either immediately or when they attempt to di-

vide. Radiation may also render tumor cells unable to enter the cell cycle. Thus, cells most vulnerable to radiation therapy are those that undergo frequent cell division — for example, cells of the bone marrow, lymph, GI epithelium, and gonads.

Therapeutic radiation may be delivered by external beam radiation or by intracavitary or interstitial implants. Use of implants requires that the therapy be done on an inpatient basis and that anyone who comes in contact with the patient while the internal radiation implants are in place must wear radiation protection. High-dose-rate remote brachytherapy, a temporary form of radiation implantation (it's in place for only a few minutes), delivers powerful radiation directly to the tumor through several hollow catheters, while minimizing damage to the surrounding tissues. This therapy is typically done on an outpatient basis. It has been used to treat breast, cervical, esophageal, lung, pancreatic, and prostate cancers.

Normal and malignant cells respond to radiation differently, depending on blood supply, oxygen saturation, previous irradiation, and immune status. Generally, normal cells recover from radiation faster than malignant cells do. Success of treatment and damage to normal tissue also vary with the radiation's intensity. Although a large, single dose of radiation has greater cellular effects than do fractions of the same amount delivered sequentially, a protracted schedule allows time for normal tissue to recover between doses.

Adverse effects

Radiation may be used palliatively to relieve pain, obstruction, malignant effusions, cough, dyspnea, ulcerations, and hemorrhage. It can also promote healing of pathologic fractures after surgical stabilization and delay metastasis.

Combining radiation and surgery can minimize the need for radical surgery, prolong survival, and preserve anatomic function. For example, preoperative doses of radiation shrink a large tumor to operable size while preventing further spread of the disease during surgery. After the wound heals, postoperative doses prevent residual cancer cells from multiplying or metastasizing.

Radiation therapy has local and systemic adverse effects, affecting both normal and malignant cells. Systemic adverse effects, such as weakness, fatigue, anorexia, nausea, vomiting, and anemia may respond to antiemetics, steroids, frequent small meals, fluid maintenance, and rest. They're seldom severe enough to require discontinuing radiation but they may mandate a dosage adjustment. (For localized adverse effects, see *Radiation's adverse effects*.)

Patients receiving radiation therapy must have frequent blood counts, particularly of WBCs and platelets if the target site involves areas of bone marrow production. Radiation also requires special skin care measures, such as covering the irradiated area with loose cotton clothing to protect it from light and avoiding deodorants, colognes, and other topical agents during treatment.

CHEMOTHERAPY

Chemotherapy includes a wide range of antineoplastic drugs, which may induce regression of a tumor and its metastasis. It's particularly useful in controlling residual disease and as an adjunct to surgery or radiation therapy. It can be curative in highly responsive cancers, such as childhood leukemia, Hodgkin's disease, choriocarcinoma, and testicular cancer. As a palliative treatment, chemotherapy aims to improve the patient's quality of life by temporarily relieving pain and other symptoms.

Every dose of a chemotherapeutic agent destroys only a percentage of tumor cells. Therefore, regression of the tumor requires repeated doses of drugs. The goal is to eradicate enough of the tumor so that the immune system can destroy the remaining malignant cells.

The *growth fraction* is the proportion of cells within a tumor that are actively dividing. Tumors with large growth fractions are more responsive to chemotherapy than those with smaller growth fractions. Nondividing cells are the least sensitive and thus are the most potentially dangerous. They must be destroyed to eradicate a malignancy. Therefore, repeated cycles of chemotherapy are used to destroy nondividing cells as they enter the cell cycle to begin active proliferation.

Depending on the type of cancer, one or more different categories of chemotherapeutic agents may be used. The most commonly used types of chemotherapeutic agents are:
◆ Alkylating agents and nitrosoureas inhibit cell growth and division by reacting with DNA at any phase of the cell cycle. They prevent cell replication by breaking and cross-linking DNA.
◆ Antimetabolites prevent cell growth by competing with metabolites in the production of nucleic acid, substituting themselves for purines and pyrimidines, which are essential for DNA and ribonucleic acid (RNA) synthesis. They exert their effect during the S phase of the cell cycle.
◆ Antitumor antibiotics block cell growth by binding with DNA and interfering with DNA-dependent RNA synthesis. Acting in any phase of the cell cycle, they bind to DNA and generate toxic oxygen free radicals that break one or both strands of DNA.
◆ Plant (Vinca) alkaloids prevent cellular reproduction by disrupting mitosis. Acting primarily in the M phase of the cell cycle, they interfere with the formation of the mitotic spindle by binding to microtubular proteins.

Other chemotherapeutic agents include epipodophyllotoxins and taxanes which, like plant alkaloids, interfere with formation of the mitotic spindle, and miscellaneous agents, such as hydroxyurea and L-asparaginase, which seem to be cell cycle–specific agents but whose mode of action is unclear. (See *Chemotherapy's action in the cell cycle,* page 34.)

A combination of drugs from different categories may be used to maximize the number of tumor cells destroyed. Combination therapy typically includes drugs with different toxicities and synergistic actions. Use of combination therapy also helps prevent the development of drug-resistant mechanisms by the tumor cells.

Adverse effects

Chemotherapy causes numerous adverse effects that reflect the drugs' mechanism of action. Although antineoplastics are toxic to cancer cells, they can also cause transient changes in normal tissues, especially those with proliferating cells. For example, antineoplastics typically cause anemia, leukopenia, and thrombocytopenia because they suppress bone marrow function; vomiting because they irritate the GI epithelial cells and stimulate the vomiting center in the brain; and alopecia and dermatitis because they destroy hair follicles and skin cells. Many antineoplastics are given I.V., and they can cause

Radiation's adverse effects

Radiation therapy can cause local adverse effects, depending on the area irradiated. The chart below highlights some of the more commonly seen local effects and the measures to manage them.

Area irradiated	Adverse effect	Management
Head and neck	♦ Alopecia	♦ Gentle combing and grooming of scalp ♦ Soft head cover
	♦ Mucositis	♦ Cool carbonated drinks ♦ Ice; ice pops ♦ Soft, nonirritating diet ♦ Non-alcohol-based mouthwash with viscous lidocaine ♦ Soft toothbrushes or swabs
	♦ Xerostomia (dry mouth)	♦ Good oral hygiene ♦ Oral saliva replacement ♦ Hard candy to stimulate secretions
	♦ Dental caries	♦ Gingival care ♦ Prophylactic fluoride to teeth
Chest	♦ Lung tissue irritation	♦ Avoidance of persons with upper respiratory tract infections ♦ Humidifier if necessary ♦ Steroid therapy
	♦ Pericarditis ♦ Myocarditis	♦ Antiarrhythmics
	♦ Esophagitis	♦ Analgesia ♦ Fluid maintenance ♦ Total parenteral nutrition or enteral feedings
Kidneys	♦ Anemia ♦ Azotemia ♦ Edema ♦ Headache ♦ Hypertensive nephropathy ♦ Lassitude ♦ Nephritis	♦ Fluid and electrolyte maintenance ♦ Monitoring for signs of renal failure
Abdomen and pelvis	♦ Cramps ♦ Diarrhea	♦ Fluid and electrolyte maintenance ♦ Loperamide and diphenoxylate with atropine ♦ Low-residue diet

venous sclerosis and pain when administered. If extravasated, they may cause deep cutaneous necrosis, requiring debridement and skin grafting. To minimize the risk of extravasation, most drugs with the potential for direct tissue injury are now given through a central venous catheter.

The pharmacologic action of a given drug determines whether it's administered orally, subcutaneously, I.M., I.V., intracavitarily, intrathe-cally, or by arterial infusion. Dosages are calculated according to the patient's body surface area, with adjustments made for general condition and degree of myelosuppression.

Many patients approach chemotherapy apprehensively. They need to be allowed to express their concerns and be provided with simple and truthful information. Explanations about what to expect, including possible adverse effects, can help minimize fear and anxiety.

Chemotherapy's action in the cell cycle

Some chemotherapeutic agents are cell cycle–specific, impairing cellular growth by causing changes in the cell during specific phases of the cell cycle. Other agents are cell cycle–nonspecific, affecting the cell at any phase during the cell cycle. The illustration below shows where the cell cycle–specific agents work to disrupt cancer cell growth.

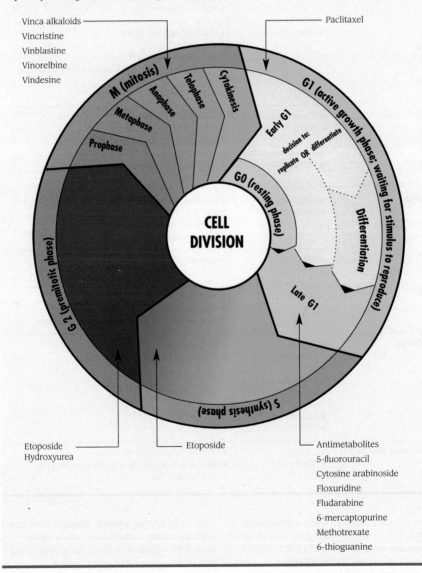

Vinca alkaloids
Vincristine
Vinblastine
Vinorelbine
Vindesine

Paclitaxel

M (mitosis)
Anaphase
Metaphase
Prophase
Telophase
Cytokinesis

G1 (active growth phase; waiting for stimulus to reproduce)
Early G1
decision to:
replicate OR differentiate
Differentiation

G0 (resting phase)

CELL DIVISION

Late G1

G 2 (premitotic phase)

S (synthesis phase)

Etoposide
Hydroxyurea

Etoposide

Antimetabolites
5-fluorouracil
Cytosine arabinoside
Floxuridine
Fludarabine
6-mercaptopurine
Methotrexate
6-thioguanine

HORMONAL THERAPY

Hormonal therapy is based on studies showing that certain hormones can inhibit the growth of certain cancers. For example, the luteinizing hormone–releasing hormone analogue, leuprolide, is used to treat prostate cancer. With long-term use, this hormone inhibits testosterone release and tumor growth. Tamoxifen, an antiestrogen hormonal agent, blocks estrogen receptors in breast tumor cells that require estrogen to thrive. Additionally, tamoxifen can be given prophylactically to women at high risk for breast cancer. Adrenocortical steroids are effective in treating leukemias and lymphomas because they suppress lymphocytes.

Adverse effects

Hormonal agents have certain adverse effects, including hot flashes, sweating, impotence, decreased libido, nausea and vomiting, and blood dyscrasias (with tamoxifen).

IMMUNOTHERAPY

Immunotherapy (also known as *biotherapy*) relies on treatment agents known as *biological response modifiers*. Biological agents are usually combined with chemotherapeutic drugs or radiation therapy. Drugs in this category are used both for treatment of the cancer and supportive therapy during treatment.

The main biotherapy agent classifications include interferons, interleukins, tyrosine kinase inhibitors, antiangiogenic agents, and monoclonal antibodies. Interferons have antiviral, antiproliferative, and immunomodulary effects. The interleukins exert their effects on the T lymphocytes. Tyrosine kinase inhibitors block the signal that tells the cell nucleus to start dividing. Antiangiogenic agents inhibit formation of blood vessels necessary to nourish and oxygenate the tumor. Monoclonal antibodies, such as rituximab, provide targeted therapy for cancer by selectively binding to tumor cell surfaces. (See *Understanding monoclonal antibodies.*)

Although not used to treat cancer directly, hematopoietic growth factors such as erythropoietin are used to increase the patient's blood counts when chemotherapy or radiation has caused a decrease.

Adverse effects

Adverse effects of biotherapeutic agents mimic the body's normal immune response, with flu-like symptoms being the most common.

Understanding monoclonal antibodies

Monoclonal antibodies are a major advance in overall cancer therapy. They're used in combination with chemotherapy to achieve partial or complete response.

In the human body, B cells (a class of white blood cells) produce endogenous antibodies in response to foreign stimuli, such as bacteria. The antibodies bind to markers (antigens) on the surfaces of foreign cells and mark the cell for destruction by other parts of the immune system.

Monoclonal antibodies are exogenous antibodies genetically engineered in the laboratory to function as endogenous antibodies. An antibody against a specific antigen is made by combining an antibody-producing B cell with a cancer cell. This combination creates a new cell, a hybridoma, which will produce multiple copies or clones of a single antibody, thus the name *monoclonal antibody*.

Researchers are currently investigating monoclonal antibodies for almost every type of cancer. Many have been approved for use by the U.S. Food and Drug Administration. Information is available on their website (www.fda.gov).

Common cancers

Worldwide, the most common malignancies include skin cancer, leukemias, lymphomas, and cancers of the breast, bone, GI tract and associated structures, thyroid, lung, urinary tract, and reproductive tract. (See *Reviewing common cancers*, pages 36 to 45.) In the United States, the most common forms of cancer are skin, prostate, breast, lung, and colorectal. Some cancers, such as ovarian germ-cell tumors and retinoblastoma, occur predominantly in younger patients; yet, more than two-thirds of the patients who develop cancer are older than age 65.

Reviewing common cancers

This chart highlights the important signs and symptoms and diagnostic test results for some of the most common cancers.

Type and findings	Diagnostic test results
Acute leukemia	
♦ Sudden onset of high fever resulting from bone marrow invasion and cellular proliferation within bone marrow ♦ Thrombocytopenia and abnormal bleeding secondary to bone marrow suppression ♦ Weakness and lassitude related to anemia from bone marrow invasion ♦ Pallor and weakness related to anemia ♦ Chills and recurrent infections related to proliferation of immature nonfunctioning white blood cells (WBCs) ♦ Bone pain from leukemic infiltration of bone ♦ Neurologic manifestations, including headache, papilledema, facial palsy, blurred vision and meningeal irritation secondary to leukemic infiltration or cerebral bleeding ♦ Liver, spleen, and lymph node enlargement related to leukemic cell infiltration	♦ Bone marrow aspiration reveals proliferation of immature WBCs. ♦ Complete blood count (CBC) shows thrombocytopenia and neutropenia. ♦ Differential WBC count reveals cell type. ♦ Lumbar puncture reveals leukemic infiltration to cerebrospinal fluid (CSF). ♦ Computed tomography (CT) scan shows affected organs.
Basal cell carcinoma	
♦ Noduloulcerative lesions usually on face (forehead, eyelid regions, and nasolabial folds) appearing as small, smooth, pinkish and translucent papules with telangiectactic vessels crossing surface; occasionally pigmented; depressed centers with firm elevated borders with enlargement resulting from basal cell proliferation in the deepest layer of epidermis with local invasion ♦ Superficial basal cell epitheliomas, commonly on chest and back, appearing as oval or irregularly shaped, lightly pigmented scaly plaques with sharply defined, threadlike elevated borders resembling psoriasis or eczema resulting from basal cell proliferation ♦ Sclerosing basal cell epitheliomas occurring on the head and neck and appearing as waxy, sclerotic yellow to white plaques without distinct borders resulting from basal cell proliferation	♦ All types diagnosed by clinical appearance, incisional or excisional biopsy, and histologic study.
Bladder cancer	
Early stage ♦ Commonly asymptomatic ***Later stage*** ♦ Gross, painless, intermittent hematuria secondary to tumor invasion ♦ Suprapubic pain after voiding from pressure exerted by the tumor or obstruction ♦ Bladder irritability and frequency related to tumor compression and invasion	♦ Cystoscopy and biopsy confirm cell type. ♦ Urinalysis reveals hematuria and malignant cytology. ♦ Excretory urography identifies large, early-stage tumor or infiltrating tumor. ♦ Retrograde cystography reveals changes in bladder structure and bladder wall integrity. ♦ Pelvic arteriography confirms tumor invasion into bladder wall.

Reviewing common cancers *(continued)*

Type and findings	Diagnostic test results

Bladder cancer *(continued)*

	♦ CT scan reveals thickened bladder wall and enlarged retroperitoneal lymph nodes.
	♦ Ultrasonography detects metastasis beyond bladder; differentiates presence of tumor from cyst.

Bone cancer *(osteosarcoma or Ewing's sarcoma)*

♦ Possibly asymptomatic	♦ Incisional or aspiration biopsy confirms cell type.
♦ Bone pain, especially at night, from tumor disruption of normal structural integrity and pressure on surrounding tissues	♦ Bone X-rays, radioisotope bone scan, and CT scan reveal tumor size.
♦ Tender, swollen, possibly palpable mass resulting from tumor growth	♦ Blood studies reveal elevated serum alkaline phosphatase level.
♦ Pathologic fractures secondary to tumor invasion and destruction of bone causing weakening	
♦ Hypercalcemia from ectopic parathyroid hormone production by the tumor or increased bone resorption	
♦ Limited mobility (late in the disease) from continued tumor growth and disruption of bone strength	

Breast cancer

♦ Hard stony mass in the breast related to cellular growth	♦ Breast examination reveals lump or mass in breast.
♦ Change in symmetry of breast secondary to growth of tumor on one side	♦ Mammography reveals presence of mass and location.
♦ Skin thickening or dimpling, scaly skin around nipple or changes in nipple, edema or ulceration related to tumor cell infiltration to surrounding tissues	♦ Needle or surgical biopsy confirms the cell type.
	♦ Ultrasonography reveals solid tumor, differentiating it from a fluid-filled cyst.
♦ Warm, hot, pink area from inflammation and infiltration of surrounding tissues	♦ Bone scan and CT scan reveal metastasis.
♦ Unusual discharge or drainage indicating tumor invasion and infiltration into the ductal system	♦ Elevated alkaline phosphatase level, liver biopsy, and liver function studies reveal liver metastasis.
♦ Pain related to enlarging tumor and subsequent pressure	♦ Hormonal receptor assay identifies tumor as hormonal dependent.
♦ Hypercalcemia or pathologic fractures secondary to metastasis to bone	♦ Ductoscopy reveals small intraductal lesions that aren't palpable or visible on mammography.
	♦ Ductal lavage identifies cancerous cells in the milk ducts of the breast.
	♦ Axillary lymph node dissection or sentinal lymph node biopsy reveals metastasis to local or regional lymph nodes.

Cervical cancer

♦ No symptoms or other clinically apparent changes in preinvasive cervical cancer	♦ Papanicolaou (Pap) test reveals malignant cellular changes.
♦ Abnormal vaginal bleeding with persistent vaginal discharge and postcoital pain and bleeding related to cellular invasion and erosion of the cervical epithelium	♦ Colposcopy identifies the presence and extent of early lesions.
	♦ Biopsy confirms cell type.

(continued)

Reviewing common cancers (continued)

Type and findings	Diagnostic test results

Cervical cancer (continued)

♦ Pelvic pain secondary to pressure on surrounding tissues and nerves from cellular proliferation
♦ Vaginal leakage of urine and stool from fistulas due to erosion and necrosis of cervix
♦ Anorexia, weight loss, and anemia related to the hypermetabolic activity of cellular proliferation and increased tumor growth needs

♦ CT scan, nuclear imaging scan, and lymphangiography identify metastasis.

Chronic lymphocytic leukemia

♦ Gradual onset of fatigue related to anemia
♦ Splenomegaly secondary to increased numbers of lysed red blood cells being filtered
♦ Hepatomegaly and lymph node enlargement from infiltration by leukemic cells
♦ Bleeding tendencies secondary to thrombocytopenia
♦ Infections related to deficient humoral immunity

♦ Lymph node biopsy distinguishes between benign and malignant tumors.
♦ CBC reveals:
– numerous abnormal lymphocytes with mild but persistently elevated WBC count
– granulocytopenia common but WBC count increasing as disease progresses
– hemoglobin level below 11 g/dl
– neutropenia (under 1,500/µl)
– lymphocytosis (over 10,000/µl)
– thrombocytopenia (under 150,000/µl).
♦ Blood studies reveal decreased serum globulin levels.
♦ Bone marrow aspiration and biopsy show lymphocytic invasion.

Colorectal cancer

Tumor in right colon (ascending)
♦ Black, tarry stools secondary to tumor erosion and necrosis of the intestinal lining
♦ Anemia secondary to increased tumor growth needs and bleeding resulting from necrosis and ulceration of mucosa
♦ Abdominal aching, pressure, or cramps secondary to pressure from tumor
♦ Weakness, fatigue, anorexia, weight loss secondary to increased tumor growth needs
♦ Vomiting and constipation as disease progresses related to possible obstruction

Tumor in left colon (descending)
♦ Intestinal obstruction including abdominal distention, pain, vomiting, cramps, and rectal pressure related to increasing tumor size and ulceration of mucosa
♦ Constipation, diarrhea, or "ribbon" or pencil-shaped stools as disease progresses
♦ Dark red or bright red blood in stools secondary to erosion and ulceration of mucosa

♦ Digital rectal examination reveals mass.
♦ Fecal occult blood test detects blood in stools.
♦ Proctoscopy or sigmoidoscopy reveals tumor mass.
♦ Colonoscopy visualizes tumor location up to the ileocecal valve.
♦ CT scan reveals areas of possible metastasis.
♦ Barium X-ray shows location and size of lesions not manually or visually detectable.
♦ Blood studies reveal elevated carcinoembryonic antigen (tumor marker).

Reviewing common cancers *(continued)*

Type and findings	Diagnostic test results

Esophageal cancer

♦ No early symptoms
♦ Dysphagia secondary to tumor interfering with passageway
♦ Weight loss resulting from dysphasia, tumor growth and increasing obstruction, and anorexia related to tumor growth needs
♦ Ulceration and subsequent hemorrhage from erosive effects (fungating and infiltrative) of the tumor
♦ Fistula formation and possible aspiration secondary to continued erosive tumor effects

♦ Esophageal X-ray with barium swallow and motility studies reveals structural and filling defects and reduced peristalsis.
♦ Endoscopic examination with punch and brush biopsies confirms cancer cell type.

Hodgkin's disease

♦ Painless swelling in one lymph node (usually the cervical region) with a history of upper respiratory infection
♦ Persistent fever, night sweats, fatigue, weight loss, and malaise related to hypermetabolic state of cellular proliferation and defective immune function
♦ Pruritus that becomes acute as the disease progresses
♦ Extremity pain, nerve irritation, or absence of pulse due to rapid enlargement of lymph nodes
♦ Pericardial friction rub, pericardial effusion, and neck vein engorgement secondary to direct invasion from mediastinal lymph nodes
♦ Enlargement of retroperitoneal nodes, spleen, and liver related to progression of disease and cellular infiltration

♦ Lymph node biopsy confirms presence of Reed-Sternberg cells, nodular fibrosis, and necrosis.
♦ Bone marrow, liver, mediastinal, lymph node, and spleen biopsies reveal histologic presence of cells.
♦ Chest X-ray, abdominal CT scan, lung scan, bone scan, and lymphangiography detect lymph and organ involvement.
♦ Hematologic tests show:
– mild to severe normocytic anemia
– normochromic anemia
– elevated, normal, or reduced WBC count
– differential with any combination of neutrophilia, lymphocytopenia, monocytosis, and eosinophilia.
♦ Blood studies reveal elevated serum alkaline phosphatase, indicating bone or liver involvement.

Laryngeal cancer

♦ Hoarseness persisting longer than 3 weeks related to encroachment on the true vocal cord
♦ Lump in the throat or pain or burning when drinking citrus juice or hot liquids related to tumor growth
♦ Dysphagia secondary to increasing pressure and obstruction with tumor growth
♦ Dyspnea and cough related to progressive tumor growth and metastasis
♦ Enlargement of cervical lymph nodes and pain radiating to ear related to invasion of lymphatic tissue and subsequent pressure

♦ Laryngoscopy shows presence of tumor.
♦ Xeroradiography, biopsy, laryngeal tomography, CT scan, or laryngography identifies borders of the lesion.
♦ Chest X-ray reveals metastasis.

(continued)

Reviewing common cancers *(continued)*

Type and findings	Diagnostic test results

Liver cancer

♦ Mass in right upper quadrant with a tender nodular liver on palpation secondary to tumor cell growth
♦ Severe pain in epigastrium or right upper quadrant related to tumor size and increased pressure on surrounding tissue
♦ Bruit, hum, or rubbing sound if tumor involves a large part of the liver
♦ Weight loss, weakness, anorexia related to increased tumor growth needs
♦ Dependent edema secondary to tumor invasion and obstruction of portal veins

♦ Needle or open biopsy of the liver confirms cell type.
♦ Serum liver funtion studies reveal elevated levels of alanine transaminase and aspartate transaminase, alkaline phosphatase, lactic dehydrogenase, and bilirubin, indicating abnormal liver function.
♦ Blood studies reveal elevated alpha-fetoprotein levels.
♦ Chest X-ray reveals possible metastasis.
♦ Liver scan may show filling defects.
♦ Serum electrolyte studies reveal hypernatremia and hypercalcemia; serum laboratory studies reveal hypoglycemia, leukocytosis, or hypocholesterolemia.

Lung cancer

♦ Cough, hoarseness, wheezing, dyspnea, hemoptysis, and chest pain related to local infiltration of pulmonary membranes and vasculature
♦ Fever, weight loss, weakness, anorexia related to increased tumor growth needs from hypermetabolic state of cellular proliferation
♦ Bone and joint pain from cartilage erosion due to abnormal production of growth hormone
♦ Cushing's syndrome related to abnormal production of corticotropin
♦ Hypercalcemia related to abnormal production of parathyroid hormone or bone metastasis
♦ Hemoptysis, atelectasis, pneumonitis, and dyspnea from bronchial obstruction related to increasing growth
♦ Shoulder pain and unilateral paralysis of diaphragm due to phrenic nerve involvement
♦ Dysphagia related to esophageal compression
♦ Vein distention and facial, neck, and chest edema secondary to obstruction of vena cava
♦ Piercing chest pain, increasing dyspnea, severe arm pain secondary to invasion of the chest wall

♦ Chest X-ray shows an advanced lesion, including size and location.
♦ Sputum cytology reveals possible cell type.
♦ CT scan of the chest delineates tumor size and relationship to surrounding structures.
♦ Bronchoscopy locates tumor; washings reveal malignant cell type.
♦ Needle lung biopsy confirms cell type.
♦ Mediastinal and supraclavicular lymph node biopsies reveal possible metastasis.
♦ Thoracentesis shows malignant cells in pleural fluid.
♦ Bone scan, bone marrow biopsy, and magnetic resonance imaging (MRI) of the brain reveal metastasis.
♦ Position emission tomography scanning shows increased uptake of glucose in malignant tissue.

Malignant brain tumor

♦ Headache, dizziness, vertigo, nausea and vomiting, and papilledema secondary to increased intracranial pressure from tumor invasion and compression of surrounding tissues
♦ Cranial nerve dysfunction secondary to tumor invasion or compression of cranial nerves
♦ Focal deficits including motor deficits (weakness, paralysis, or gait disorders), sensory disturbances (anesthesia, paresthesia, or disturbances of vision or hearing) secondary to tumor invasion or compression of motor or sensory control areas of the brain

♦ Stereotactic tissue biopsy confirms cell type.
♦ Neurologic assessment reveals manifestations of lesion affecting specific lobe.
♦ Skull X-ray, CT scan, MRI, and cerebral angiography identify location of mass.
♦ Brain scan reveals area of increased uptake in location of tumor.
♦ Lumbar puncture shows increased pressure and protein level, decreased glucose level, and, occasionally, tumor cells in CSF.

Reviewing common cancers *(continued)*

Type and findings	Diagnostic test results

Malignant brain tumor (continued)

♦ Disturbances of higher function including defects in cognition, learning, and memory

Local
♦ Dementia, personality or behavioral changes, gait disturbances, seizures, language disorders
♦ Sensory loss, hemianopia, cranial nerve dysfunction, ataxia, pupillary abnormalities, nystagmus, hemiparesis, and autonomic dysfunction depending on location of tumor

Malignant melanoma

♦ Enlargement of skin lesion or nevus accompanied by changes in color, inflammation or soreness, itching, ulceration, bleeding, or textural changes secondary to malignant transformation of melanocytes in the basal layer of the epidermis or within the aggregated melanocytes of an existing nevus

Superficial spreading melanoma
♦ Red, white, and blue color over a brown or black background with an irregular, notched margin typically on areas of chronic irritation

Nodular melanoma
♦ Polypoidal nodule with uniformly dark discoloration appearing as a blackberry, but possibly flesh-colored with flecks of pigment around base

Lentigo maligna melanoma
♦ Large flat freckle of tan, brown, black, whitish, or slate color with irregularly scattered black nodules on surface

♦ Skin biopsy with histologic examination confirms cell type and tumor thickness.
♦ Chest X-ray, gallium scan, MRI, and CT scans of the chest, abdomen, or brain reveal metastasis.
♦ Bone scan reveals bone metastasis.

Multiple myeloma

♦ Severe, constant back and rib pain that increases with exercise secondary to invasion of bone
♦ Arthritic symptoms including achiness, joint swelling, and tenderness possibly from vertebral compression
♦ Pathologic fractures resulting from invasion of bone causing loss of structural integrity and strength
♦ Azotemia secondary to tumor proliferation to the kidney and pyelonephritis due to subsequent tubular damage from large amounts of Bence Jones protein, hypercalcemia, and hyperuricemia
♦ Anemia, bleeding, and infections secondary to tumor effects on bone marrow cell production

♦ CBC shows moderate to severe anemia; differential may show 40% to 50% lymphocytes but seldom more than 3% plasma cells.
♦ Differential smear reveals rouleaux formation from elevated erythrocyte sedimentation rate.
♦ Urine studies reveal Bence Jones protein, proteinuria, and hypercalciuria.
♦ Bone marrow aspiration detects myelomatous cells (abnormal number of immature plasma cells).
♦ Serum electrophoresis shows elevated globulin spike that is electrophoretically and immunologically abnormal.

(continued)

Reviewing common cancers *(continued)*

Type and findings	Diagnostic test results

Multiple myeloma *(continued)*

♦ Thoracic deformities and increasing vertebral complaints secondary to extension of tumor and continued vertebral compression
♦ Loss of 5″ (12.7 cm) or more of body height due to vertebral collapse

♦ Bone X-rays (in early stages) reveal diffuse osteoporosis; in later stages, they show multiple sharply circumscribed osteolytic lesions, particularly in the skull, pelvis, and spine.

Non-Hodgkin's lymphoma

♦ Swelling of the lymph glands, enlarged tonsils and adenoids, and painless, rubbery nodes in the cervical supraclavicular areas from cellular proliferation
♦ Dyspnea and coughing related to lymphocytic infiltration of oropharynx
♦ Abdominal pain and constipation secondary to mechanical obstruction of surrounding tissues

♦ Lymph node biopsy reveals cell type.
♦ Biopsy of tonsils, bone marrow, liver, bowel, or skin reveals malignant cells.
♦ CBC may show anemia.
♦ Blood studies reveal elevated or normal uric acid level and elevated serum lactic dehydrogenase level.
♦ Electrolyte studies reveal elevated serum calcium level if bone lesions are present.
♦ Blood studies reveal normal serum protein level.
♦ Bone and chest X-rays, lymphangiography, liver and spleen scans, abdominal CT scan, and excretory urography show evidence of metastasis.

Ovarian cancer

♦ Vague abdominal discomfort, dyspepsia and other mild GI complaints from increasing size of tumor exerting pressure on nearby tissues
♦ Urinary frequency, constipation from obstruction resulting from increased tumor size
♦ Pain from tumor rupture, torsion, or infection
♦ Feminizing or masculinizing effects secondary to cellular type
♦ Ascites related to invasion and infiltration of the peritoneum
♦ Pleural effusions related to pulmonary metastasis

♦ Pap test may be normal.
♦ Abdominal ultrasound, CT, or X-ray delineates tumor presence and size.
♦ CBC may show anemia.
♦ Excretory urography reveals abnormal renal function and urinary tract abnormalities or obstruction.
♦ Chest X-ray reveals pleural effusion with distant metastasis.
♦ Barium enema shows obstruction and size of tumor.
♦ Lymphangiography reveals lymph node involvement.
♦ Mammography reveals no abnormalities, eliminating breast cancer as the primary site.
♦ Liver function studies reveal abnormal results with ascites.
♦ Paracentesis fluid aspiration reveals malignant cells.
♦ Tumor markers such as carcinoembryonic antigen (CA)125 are elevated.

Pancreatic cancer

♦ Jaundice with clay-colored stools and dark urine secondary to obstruction of bile flow from tumor in head of pancreas
♦ Recurrent thrombophlebitis from tumor cytokines acting as platelet aggregating factors
♦ Nausea and vomiting secondary to duodenal obstruction

♦ Laparotomy with biopsy confirms cell type.
♦ Ultrasound identifies location of mass.
♦ Angiography reveals vascular supply of the tumor.
♦ Endoscopic retrograde cholangiopancreatography identifies tumor area.

Reviewing common cancers *(continued)*

Type and findings	Diagnostic test results
Pancreatic cancer *(continued)*	
♦ Weight loss, anorexia, and malaise, secondary to effects of increased tumor growth needs ♦ Abdominal or back pain secondary to tumor pressure ♦ Blood in the stools from ulceration of GI tract or ampulla of Vater	♦ CT scan and MRI identify tumor location and size. ♦ Serum laboratory test results reveal increased levels of serum bilirubin, serum amylase, and serum lipase. ♦ Clotting study reveals prolonged prothrombin time (PT). ♦ Blood studies reveal elevated levels of aspartate aminotransferase and alanine aminotransferase, indicating necrosis of liver cells. ♦ Blood studies reveal markedly elevated levels of alkaline phosphatase, indicating biliary obstruction. ♦ Tumor markers such as CA 19-9 are elevated. ♦ Plasma insulin immunoassay shows a measurable serum insulin level in the presence of islet cell tumors. ♦ CBC reveals decreased hemoglobin and hematocrit levels, showing mild anemia. ♦ Fasting blood glucose level may reveal hypoglycemia or hyperglycemia.
Prostate cancer	
♦ Symptoms appearing only in late stages ♦ Difficulty initiating a urine stream, dribbling, urine retention secondary to obstruction of urinary tract from tumor growth ♦ Hematuria (rare) from infiltration of bladder	♦ Biopsy confirms cell type. ♦ DRE reveals a small hard nodule. ♦ Blood studies reveal elevated prostatic surface antigen level. ♦ Blood studies reveal elevated serum acid phosphatase level. ♦ MRI, CT scan, transrectal prostatic ultrasonography, and excretory urography identify tumor mass. ♦ Blood studies reveal elevated alkaline phosphatase level and positive bone scan, indicating bone metastasis
Renal cancer	
♦ Pain resulting from tumor pressure and invasion ♦ Hematuria secondary to tumor spreading to renal pelvis ♦ Smooth, firm, nontender mass palpable over affected kidney due to tumor growth ♦ Possible fever from hemorrhage or necrosis ♦ Hypertension from compression of renal artery with renal parenchymal ischemia and renin excess ♦ Polycythemia secondary to erythropoietin excess ♦ Hypercalcemia from ectopic parathyroid hormone production by the tumor or bone metastasis ♦ Urine retention secondary to obstruction of urinary flow ♦ Pulmonary embolism secondary to renal venous obstruction	♦ CT scan, I.V. and retrograde pyelography, ultrasound, cystoscopy (to rule out associated bladder cancer), nephrotomography, and renal angiography identify presence of tumor and help differentiate it from a cyst. ♦ Liver function studies show increased levels of alkaline phosphatase, bilirubin, alanine aminotransferase, and aspartate aminotransferase; clotting studies reveal prolonged PT. ♦ Urinalysis reveals gross or microscopic hematuria. ♦ CBC shows anemia, polycythemia, and increased erythrocyte sedimentation rate. ♦ Electrolyte studies reveal elevated serum calcium level.

(continued)

Reviewing common cancers *(continued)*

Type and findings	Diagnostic test results
Squamous cell carcinoma	
♦ Lesions on skin of the face, ears, dorsa of hands and forearms from cell proliferation in sun-damaged areas ♦ Induration and inflammation as cell changes from nonmalignant to malignant cell ♦ Ulceration and invasion of underlying tissues from continued cell proliferation	♦ Excisional biopsy confirms cell type.
Stomach cancer	
♦ Chronic dyspepsia and epigastric discomfort related to tumor growth in gastric cells and destruction of mucosal barrier ♦ Weight loss, anorexia, feelings of fullness after eating, anemia, and fatigue secondary to increased tumor growth needs ♦ Blood in stools from erosion of gastric mucosa by tumor	♦ Barium X-ray with fluoroscopy shows tumor or filling defects in outline of stomach, loss of flexibility and distensibility, and abnormal mucosa with or without ulceration. ♦ Gastroscopy with fiberoptic endoscopy visualizes gastric mucosa, including presence of gastric lesions for biopsy. ♦ CT scans, X-rays, liver and bone scans, and liver biopsy reveal metastasis.
Testicular cancer	
♦ Firm, painless, smooth testicular mass and occasional complaints of heaviness secondary to tumor growth ♦ Gynecomastia and nipple tenderness related to tumor production of chorionic gonadotropin or estrogen ♦ Urinary complaints related to ureteral obstruction ♦ Cough, hemoptysis, and shortness of breath from invasion of the pulmonary system	♦ Testicular palpation reveals detectable mass. ♦ Transillumination of testicles reveals tumor that doesn't transilluminate. ♦ Surgical excision and biopsy reveal cell type; inguinal exploration determines the extent of nodal involvement. ♦ Excretory urography detects ureteral deviation from para-aortic node involvement. ♦ Blood studies reveal elevated serum alphafetoprotein and beta human chorionic gonadotropin levels as tumor markers. ♦ Lymphangiography, ultrasound, and abdominal CT scan reveal mass and possible metastasis.
Thyroid cancer	
♦ Painless nodule or hard nodule in an enlarged thyroid gland or palpable lymph nodes with thyroid enlargement reflecting tumor growth ♦ Hoarseness, dysphagia, and dyspnea from increased tumor growth and pressure on surrounding structures ♦ Hyperthyroidism from excess thyroid hormone production from tumor ♦ Hypothyroidism secondary to tumor destruction of the gland	♦ Thyroid scan reveals hypofunctional nodes or cold spots. ♦ Needle biopsy confirms cell type. ♦ CT scan, ultrasound, and chest X-ray reveal medullary cancer.

Reviewing common cancers *(continued)*

Type and findings	Diagnostic test results

Uterine (endometrial) cancer

♦ Uterine enlargement secondary to tumor growth
♦ Postmenopausal bleeding or persistent and unusual premenopausal bleeding from erosive effects of tumor growth
♦ Pain and weight loss related to progressive infiltration and invasion of tumor cells and continued cellular proliferation

♦ Endometrial, cervical, and endocervical biopsies are positive for malignant cells, revealing cell type.
♦ Dilatation and curettage identifies malignancy in patients whose biopsies were negative.
♦ Multiple cervical biopsies and endocervical curettage pinpoint cervical involvement.
♦ Schiller's test reveals cervix resistant to staining (indicating cancerous tissues).
♦ Chest X-ray and CT scan reveal metastasis.
♦ Barium enema identifies possible bladder or rectal involvement.

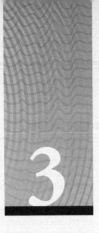

3

INFECTION

The 20th century encompassed astonishing advances in treating and preventing infection, such as potent antibiotics, complex immunizations, and modern sanitation, yet infection remains the most common cause of human disease. Even in countries with advanced medical care, infectious disease remains a major cause of serious illness. In developing countries, infection is one of the most critical health problems.

Understanding infection

Infection is the invasion and multiplication of microorganisms in or on body tissue that produce signs and symptoms as well as an immune response. Such reproduction injures the host by causing cell damage from microorganism-produced toxins or from intracellular multiplication, or by competing with host metabolism. Infectious diseases range from relatively mild illnesses to debilitating and lethal conditions: from the common cold through chronic hepatitis to acquired immunodeficiency syndrome. The severity of the infection varies with the pathogenicity and number of the invading microorganisms and the strength of host defenses. The very young and the very old are especially susceptible.

For infection to be transmitted, these factors must be present: causative agent, infectious reservoir with a portal of exit, mode of transmission, a portal of entry into the host, and a susceptible host.

RISK FACTORS

A healthy person can usually ward off infections with the body's own built-in defense mechanisms that include:
◆ intact skin
◆ normal flora that inhabit the skin and various organs (see *How microbes interact with the body*)
◆ lysozymes (enzymes that can kill microorganisms or microbes) secreted by eyes, nasal passages, glands, stomach, and genitourinary organs
◆ defensive structures, such as the cilia, that sweep foreign matter from the airways
◆ a healthy immune system.

However, if an imbalance develops, the potential for infection increases. Risk factors for the development of infection include weakened defense mechanisms, environmental and developmental factors, and pathogen characteristics.

WEAKENED DEFENSE MECHANISMS

The body has many defense mechanisms for resisting entry and multiplication of microbes. However, a weakened immune system makes it easier for these pathogens to invade the body and launch an infectious disease. This weakened state is referred to as *immunodeficiency* or *immunocompromise*.

Impaired function of white blood cells (WBCs) and low levels of T and B cells characterize immunodeficiencies. An immunodeficiency may be congenital (caused by a genetic defect and present at birth) or acquired (developed after birth). Acquired immunodeficiency may result from infection, malnutrition, chronic stress, or pregnancy. Diabetes, renal failure, and cirrhosis can suppress the immune response, as can corticosteroids and chemotherapeutic drugs.

Regardless of cause, the result of immunodeficiency is the same. The body's ability to recognize and fight pathogens is impaired. People who are immunodeficient are more susceptible to all infections, are more acutely ill when they become infected, and require a much longer time to heal.

ENVIRONMENTAL FACTORS

Other conditions that may weaken a person's immune defenses include poor hygiene, malnutrition, inadequate physical barriers, emotional and physical stressors, chronic diseases, medical and surgical treatments, and inadequate immunization.

Good hygiene promotes normal host defenses; poor hygiene increases the risk of infection. Unclean skin harbors microbes and offers an environment for them to colonize, and untended skin is more likely to allow invasion. Frequent washing removes surface microbes and maintains an intact barrier to infection, but it may damage the skin. To maintain skin integrity, lubricants and emollients may be used to prevent cracks and breaks.

The body needs a balanced diet to provide the nutrients, vitamins, and minerals that an effective immune system needs. Protein malnutrition inhibits the production of antibodies, without which the body can't mount an effective attack against microbe invasion. Malnutrition is directly related to incidence of nosocomial infections. Along with a balanced diet, the body needs adequate vitamins and minerals to use ingested nutrients.

Dust can facilitate transportation of pathogens. For example, dust-borne spores of the fungus *Aspergillus* transmit the infection. If the inhaled spores become established in the lungs, they're notoriously difficult to expel. Fortunately, persons with intact immune systems can usually resist infection with *Aspergillus,* which is usually dangerous only in the presence of severe immunosuppression.

DEVELOPMENTAL FACTORS

The very young and very old are at higher risk for infection. The immune system doesn't fully develop until about age 6 months. An infant exposed to an infectious agent usually develops an infection. The most common type of infection in toddlers affects the respiratory tract. When young children put toys and other objects in their mouths, they increase their exposure to various pathogens.

Exposure to communicable diseases continues throughout childhood, as children progress from day-care facilities to schools. Skin diseases, such

How microbes interact with the body

Microbes interact with their host in various ways.

Double benefit

Some of the microorganisms of the normal human flora interact with the body in ways that mutually benefit both parties. *Escherichia coli* organisms, part of the normal intestinal flora, obtain nutrients from the human host; in return, they secrete vitamin K, which the human body needs for blood clotting.

Single benefit

Other microbes of the normal flora have a commensal interaction with the human body—an interaction that benefits one party (in this case, the microbes) without affecting the other.

Parasitic interaction

Some pathogenic microbes, such as helminths (worms), are parasites, meaning that they harm the host while they benefit from their interaction with it.

as impetigo and lice infestation, commonly pass from one child to the next at this age. Accidents are common in childhood as well, and broken or abraded skin opens the way for bacterial invasion. Lack of immunization also contributes to incidence of childhood diseases.

Advancing age, on the other hand, is associated with a declining immune system, partly as a result of decreasing thymus function. Chronic diseases, such as diabetes and atherosclerosis, can weaken defenses by impairing blood flow and nutrient delivery to body systems.

PATHOGEN CHARACTERISTICS

A microbe must be present in sufficient quantities to cause a disease in a healthy human. The number needed to cause a disease varies from one microbe to the next and from host to host, and may be affected by the mode of transmission. The severity of an infection depends on several factors, including the microbe's pathogenicity—that is, the likelihood that it will cause pathogenic changes or disease. Factors that affect pathogenicity include the microbe's specificity, invasiveness, quantity, virulence, toxigenicity, adhesiveness, antigenicity, and viability. (See *Chain of infection,* pages 48 and 49.)

Chain of infection

An infection can occur only if the six components depicted below are present. Removing one link in the chain prevents infection.

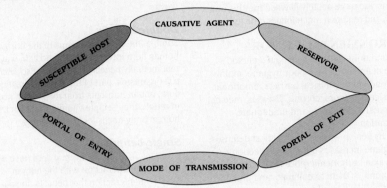

Causative agent

A *causative agent* for infection is any microbe that can produce disease.

Reservoir

The *reservoir* is the environment or object in or on which a microbe can survive and, in some cases, multiply. Inanimate objects, human beings, and other animals can all serve as reservoirs, providing the essential requirements for a microbe to survive at specific stages in its life cycle.

Portal of exit

The *portal of exit* is the path by which an infectious agent leaves its reservoir. Usually, this portal is the site where the organism grows. Common portals of exit associated with human reservoirs include the respiratory, genitourinary, and GI tracts; the skin and mucous membranes; and the placenta (in transplacental disease transmission from mother to fetus). Blood, sputum, vomitus, stool, urine, wound drainage, and genital secretions also serve as portals of exit. The portal of exit varies from one infectious agent to the next.

Mode of transmission

The *mode of transmission* is the means by which the infectious agent passes from the portal of exit in the reservoir to the susceptible host. Infections can be transmitted through one of four modes: contact, airborne, enteric, and vector-borne. Some organisms use more than one mode of transmission to get from the reservoir to a new host. As with portals of exit, the mode of transmission varies with the specific microbe.

Contact transmission is subdivided into direct contact, indirect contact, and droplet spread (contact with droplets that enter the environment).

◆ *Specificity* is the range of hosts to which a microbe is attracted. Some microbes may be attracted to a wide range of humans and animals, whereas others select only human or only animal hosts.

◆ *Invasiveness* (sometimes called *infectivity*) is a microbe's ability to invade and multiply in the host tissues. Some microbes can enter through intact skin; others can enter only if the skin or mucous membrane is broken. Some microbes produce enzymes that enhance their invasiveness.

◆ *Quantity* refers to the number of microbes that succeed in invading and reproducing in the body.

◆ *Virulence* is the severity of the disease a pathogen can produce. Virulence can vary depending on the host defenses; any infection can be life-threatening in an immunodeficient patient. Infection with a pathogen known to be particularly virulent requires early diagnosis and treatment.

◆ *Toxigenicity* is related to virulence. It describes a pathogen's potential to damage host tissues by producing and releasing toxins.

◆ *Adhesiveness* is the ability of the pathogen to attach to host tissue. Some pathogens secrete a sticky substance that helps them adhere to tissue

Direct contact refers to person-to-person spread of organisms through physical contact.

Indirect contact occurs when a susceptible person comes in contact with a contaminated object.

Droplet transmission results from contact with contaminated respiratory secretions. It differs from airborne transmission in that the droplets don't remain suspended in the air but settle on surfaces.

Airborne transmission occurs when fine microbial particles containing pathogens remain suspended in the air for a prolonged period, and then are spread widely by air currents and inhaled.

Enteric (oral-fecal) transmission occurs when infecting organisms found in stool are ingested by susceptible victims, in many cases, through fecally contaminated food or water.

Vector-borne transmission occurs when an intermediate carrier, or vector, such as a flea or a mosquito, transfers a microbe to another living organism. This type of transmission is of most concern in tropical areas, where insects commonly transmit disease.

Portal of entry

Portal of entry refers to the path by which an infectious agent invades a susceptible host. Usually, this path is the same as the portal of exit.

Susceptible host

A *susceptible host* is also required for the transmission of infection to occur. The human body has many defense mechanisms for resisting the entry and multiplication of pathogens. When these mechanisms function normally, infection doesn't occur. However, in a weakened host, an infectious agent is more likely to invade the body and launch an infectious disease.

while protecting them from the host's defense mechanisms.

♦ *Antigenicity* is the degree to which a pathogen can induce a specific immune response. Microbes that invade and localize in tissue initially stimulate a cellular response; those that disseminate quickly throughout the host's body generate an antibody response.

♦ *Viability* is the ability of a pathogen to survive outside its host. Most microbes can't live and multiply outside a reservoir.

Stages of infection

Development of an infection usually proceeds through four stages. The first stage, *incubation*, may be almost instantaneous or last for years. During this time, the pathogen is replicating, and the infected person is contagious and can transmit the disease. The *prodromal stage* (stage two) follows incubation, and the still-contagious host makes vague complaints of feeling unwell. In stage three, *acute illness*, microbes are actively destroying host cells and affecting specific host systems. The patient recognizes which area of the body is affected and voices complaints that are more specific. Finally, the *convalescent stage* (stage four) begins when the body's defense mechanisms have confined the microbes and healing of damaged tissue is progressing.

Infection-causing microbes

Microorganisms that are responsible for infectious diseases include bacteria, viruses, fungi, parasites, mycoplasmas, rickettsia, and chlamydiae.

BACTERIA

Bacteria are simple one-celled microorganisms with a cell wall that protects them from many of the human body's defense mechanisms. Although they lack a nucleus, bacteria possess all the other mechanisms they need to survive and rapidly reproduce.

Bacteria can be classified according to shape—rod shaped bacilli, spherical cocci, and spiral-shaped spirilla. (See *Comparing bacterial shapes,* page 50.) Bacteria can also be classified according to their need for oxygen (aerobic or anaerobic), their mobility (motile or nonmotile), and their tendency to form protective capsules (encapsulated or nonencapsulated) or spores (sporulating or nonsporulating).

Bacteria damage body tissues by interfering with essential cell function or by releasing exotoxins or endotoxins, which cause cell damage. (See *How bacteria damage tissue,* page 51.) During bacterial growth, the cells release exotoxins, enzymes that damage the host cell, altering its function or killing it. Enterotoxins are a specific type of exotoxin secreted by bacteria that infect the GI tract; they affect the vomiting center of the brain and cause gastroenteritis. Exotoxins also can cause diffuse reactions in the host, such as inflammation, bleeding, clotting, and fever. Endotoxins are contained in the cell walls of gram-negative bacteria, and they're released during lysis of the bacteria.

Comparing bacterial shapes

Bacteria exist in three basic shapes: rods (bacilli), spheres (cocci), and spirals (spirilla)

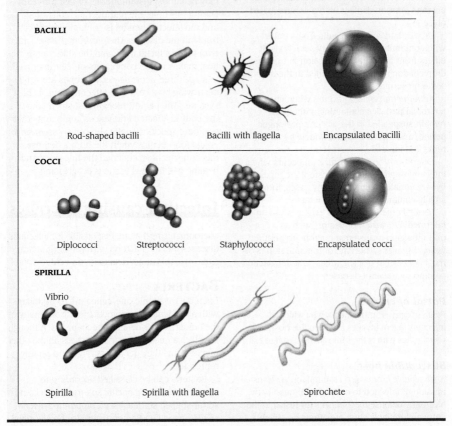

BACILLI

| Rod-shaped bacilli | Bacilli with flagella | Encapsulated bacilli |

COCCI

| Diplococci | Streptococci | Staphylococci | Encapsulated cocci |

SPIRILLA

Vibrio

| Spirilla | Spirilla with flagella | Spirochete |

Examples of bacterial infection include staphylococcal wound infection, cholera, and streptococcal pneumonia. (See *Gram-positive and gram-negative bacteria,* page 52.)

VIRUSES

Viruses are subcellular organisms made up of only a ribonucleic acid (RNA) nucleus or a deoxyribonucleic acid (DNA) nucleus covered with proteins. They're the smallest known organisms, so tiny that only an electron microscope can make them visible. (See *How viruses size up,* page 53.) Independent of the host cells, viruses can't replicate. Rather, they invade a host cell and stimulate it to participate in forming additional virus particles. Some viruses destroy surrounding tissue and release toxins. (See *Viral infection of a host cell,* page 53.) Viruses lack the genes necessary for energy production. They depend on the ribosomes and nutrients of infected host cells for protein production. The estimated 400 viruses that infect humans are classified according to their size, shape, and means of transmission (respiratory, fecal, oral, sexual).

Most viruses enter the body through the respiratory, GI, and genital tracts. A few, such as human immunodeficiency virus (HIV), are transmitted through blood, broken skin, and mucous membranes. Viruses can produce a wide variety of illnesses, including the common cold, herpes simplex, herpes zoster, chickenpox, infectious mononucleosis, hepatitis B and C, and rubella. Signs and symptoms depend on the host cell's status, the specific virus, and whether the intracellular environment provides good living conditions for the virus.

Retroviruses are a unique type of virus that carry their genetic code in RNA rather than in the more common carrier, DNA. These RNA viruses contain the enzyme reverse transcriptase,

CLOSER LOOK

How bacteria damage tissue

Bacteria and other infectious organisms constantly infect the human body. Some, such as the intestinal bacteria that produce vitamins, are beneficial. Others are harmful, causing illnesses ranging from the common cold to life-threatening septic shock.

To infect a host, bacteria must first enter it. They do this by adhering to the mucosal surface and directly invading the host cell or by attaching to epithelial cells and producing toxins, which invade host cells. To survive and multiply within a host, bacteria or their toxins adversely affect biochemical reactions in cells. The result is a disruption of normal cell function or cell death (see illustration below). For example, the diphtheria toxin damages heart muscle by inhibiting protein synthesis. In addition, as some organisms multiply, they extend into deeper tissue and eventually gain access to the bloodstream.

Some toxins cause blood to clot in small blood vessels. The tissues supplied by these vessels may be deprived of blood and damaged (see illustration below).

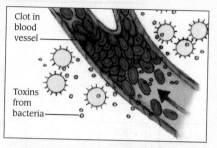

Other toxins can damage the cell walls of small blood vessels, causing leakage. This fluid loss results in decreased blood pressure, which in turn impairs the heart's ability to pump enough blood to vital organs (see illustration below).

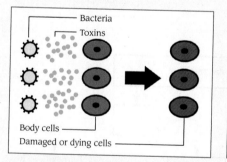

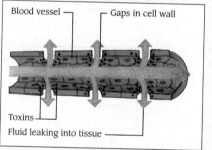

---

which changes viral RNA into DNA. The host cell then incorporates the alien DNA into its own genetic material. The most notorious retrovirus today is HIV.

FUNGI

Fungi have rigid walls and nuclei that are enveloped by nuclear membranes. They occur as yeast (single-cell, oval-shaped organisms) or molds (organisms with hyphae, or branching filaments). Depending on the environment, some fungi may occur in both forms. Found almost everywhere on earth, fungi live on organic matter, in water and soil, on animals and plants, and on a wide variety of unlikely materials. They can live inside and outside their host. Superficial fungal infections cause athlete's foot and vaginal infec-

tions. *Candida albicans* is part of the body's normal flora but under certain circumstances it can cause yeast infections of virtually any part of the body but especially the mouth, skin, vagina, and GI tract. For example, antibiotic treatment or a change in the pH of the susceptible tissues (because of a disease such as diabetes, or use of certain drugs, such as hormonal contraceptives) can wipe out the normal bacteria that keep the yeast population in check.

PARASITES

Parasites are unicellular or multicellular organisms that live on or within another organism and obtain nourishment from the host. They take only the nutrients they need and usually don't kill their hosts. Examples of parasites that

Gram-positive and gram-negative bacteria

This flowchart highlights the different types of gram-positive and gram-negative bacteria.

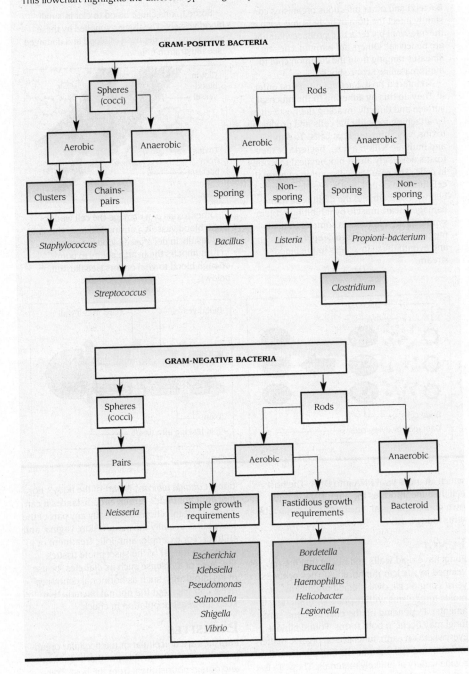

How viruses size up

Viruses vary in size, appearance, and behavior. This illustration compares the sizes of selected viruses with the size of a typical bacterium, *Escherichia coli.*

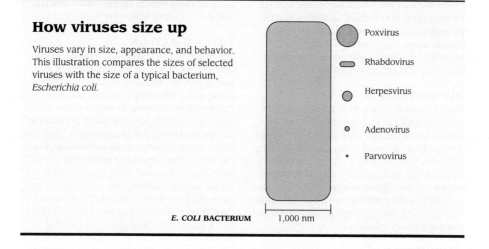

Poxvirus

Rhabdovirus

Herpesvirus

Adenovirus

Parvovirus

E. COLI BACTERIUM   1,000 nm

CLOSER LOOK

Viral infection of a host cell

The virion (A) attaches to receptors on the host-cell membrane and releases enzymes (called *absorption*) (B) that weaken the membrane and enable the virion to penetrate the cell. The virion removes the protein coat that protects its genetic material (C), replicates (D), and matures, and then escapes from the cell by budding from the plasma membrane (E). The infection can then spread to other host cells.

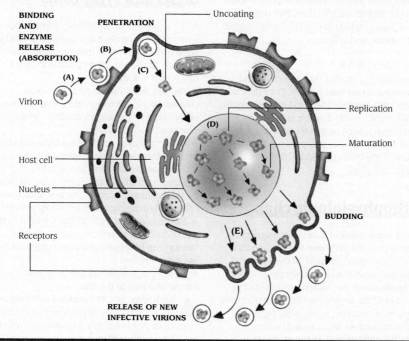

BINDING AND ENZYME RELEASE (ABSORPTION)

PENETRATION

Uncoating

(B)

(A)

(C)

Virion

Replication

(D)

Maturation

Host cell

Nucleus

BUDDING

Receptors

(E)

RELEASE OF NEW INFECTIVE VIRIONS

can produce an infection if they cause cellular damage to the host include helminths, such as pinworms and tapeworms, and arthropods, such as mites, fleas, and ticks. Helminths can infect the human gut; arthropods commonly cause skin and systemic disease.

MYCOPLASMAS

Mycoplasmas are bacteria-like organisms, the smallest of the cellular microbes that can live outside a host cell, although some may be parasitic. Lacking cell walls, they can assume many different shapes ranging from coccoid to filamentous. The lack of a cell wall makes them resistant to penicillin and other antibiotics that work by inhibiting cell wall synthesis. Mycoplasmas can cause primary atypical pneumonia and many secondary infections.

RICKETTSIA

Rickettsia are small, gram-negative, bacteria-like organisms that can cause life-threatening illness. They may be coccoid, rod-shaped, or irregularly shaped. Because they're live viruses, rickettsia require a host cell for replication. They have no cell wall, and their cell membranes are leaky; thus, they must live inside another, better protected cell. Rickettsia are transmitted by the bites of arthropod carriers, such as lice, fleas, and ticks, and through exposure to their waste products. Rickettsial infections that occur in the United States include Rocky Mountain spotted fever, typhus, and Q fever.

CHLAMYDIAE

Chlamydiae are smaller than rickettsia and bacteria but larger than viruses. They depend on host cells for replication and are susceptible to antibiotics. Chlamydiae are transmitted by direct contact, such as that which occurs during sexual activity. They're a common cause of infections of the urethra, bladder, fallopian tubes, and prostate gland.

Pathophysiologic changes

Clinical expressions of infectious disease vary, depending on the pathogen involved and the organ system affected. Most of the signs and symptoms result from host responses, which may be similar or very different from host to host. During the prodromal stage, a person will complain of common, nonspecific signs and symptoms, such as fever, muscle aches, headache, and lethargy. In the acute stage, signs and symptoms that are more specific provide evidence of the microbe's target. However, some illnesses remain asymptomatic and are discovered only by laboratory tests.

INFLAMMATION

The inflammatory response is a major reactive defense mechanism in the battle against infective agents. Inflammation may be the result of tissue injury, infection, or allergic reaction. Acute inflammation has two stages: vascular and cellular. In the vascular stage, arterioles at or near the injury's site briefly constrict and then dilate, causing fluid pressure to increase in the capillaries. The consequent movement of plasma into the interstitial space causes edema. At the same time, inflammatory cells release histamine and bradykinin, which further increase capillary permeability. Red blood cells and fluid flow into the interstitial space, contributing to edema. The extra fluid arriving in the inflamed area dilutes microbial toxins.

During the cellular stage of inflammation, WBCs and platelets move toward the damaged cells. Phagocytosis of the dead cells and microorganisms begins. Platelets control any excess bleeding in the area, and mast cells arriving at the site release heparin to maintain blood flow to the area. (See *Blocking inflammation*.)

Signs and symptoms

Acute inflammation is the body's immediate response to cell injury or cell death. The cardinal signs and symptoms of inflammation include redness, heat, pain, edema, and decreased function of a body part.

◆ *Redness* results when arterioles dilate and circulation to the site increases. Filling of previously empty or partially distended capillaries causes a localized blush.

◆ *Heat* in the area results from local vasodilation, fluid leakage into the interstitial spaces, and increased blood flow to the area.

◆ *Pain* occurs when pain receptors are stimulated by swollen tissue, local pH changes, and chemicals excreted during the inflammatory process.

◆ *Edema* is caused by local vasodilation, leakage of fluid into interstitial spaces, and the blockage of lymphatic drainage to help wall off the inflammation.

◆ *Loss of function* occurs primarily as a result of edema and pain at the site.

⚠ **CLINICAL ALERT** *Localized infections produce a rapid inflammatory response with obvious signs and symptoms. Disseminated infections have a slow inflammatory response and take longer to identify and treat, thereby increasing morbidity and mortality.*

DISEASE BLOCK
Blocking inflammation

Several substances act to control inflammation. The flowchart below shows the progression of inflammation and the points ✳ at which drugs can reduce inflammation and pain.

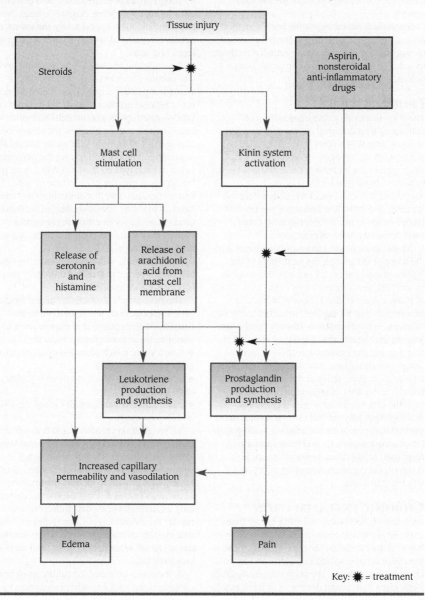

Key: ✳ = treatment

FEVER

Fever occurs with the introduction of an infectious agent. An elevated temperature helps fight an infection because many microorganisms can't survive in a hot environment. When body temperature rises too high, body cells can be damaged, particularly those of the nervous system.

Diaphoresis (sweating) is the body's method of cooling itself and returning the temperature to "normal" for that individual. Artificial methods to reduce a slight fever can impair the body's defenses against infection.

LEUKOCYTOSIS

The body responds to the introduction of pathogens by increasing the number and types of circulating WBCs. This process is called *leukocytosis*. In the acute or early stage, the neutrophil count increases. Bone marrow begins to release immature leukocytes, because existing neutrophils can't meet the body's demand for defensive cells. The immature neutrophils (called *bands* in the differential WBC count) can't serve any defensive purpose.

As the acute phase comes under control and the damage is isolated, the next stage of the inflammatory process takes place. Neutrophils, monocytes, and macrophages begin the process of phagocytosis of dead tissue and bacteria. Neutrophils and monocytes, attracted to the site of infection by chemotaxis, identify the foreign antigen and attach to it. Then they engulf, kill, and degrade the microorganism that carries antigen on its surface. Macrophages, a mature type of monocyte, arrive at the site later and remain in the area of inflammation longer than the other cells. Besides phagocytosis, macrophages play several other key roles at the site, such as preparing the area for healing and processing antigens for a cellular immune response. An elevated monocyte count is common during resolution of an injury and in chronic infections.

CHRONIC INFLAMMATION

An inflammation reaction lasting longer than 2 weeks is referred to as *chronic inflammation.* It may follow an acute process. A poorly healed wound or an unresolved infection can lead to chronic inflammation. The body may encapsulate a pathogen that it can't destroy in order to isolate it. An example of such a pathogen is *Mycobacterium tuberculosis*, the cause of tuberculosis; encapsulated mycobacteria appear in X-rays as identifiable spots in the lungs. With chronic inflammation, permanent scarring and loss of tissue function can occur.

Diagnosis

Accurate assessment helps identify infectious diseases, appropriate treatment, and avoidable complications. It begins with obtaining the patient's complete medical history, performing a thorough physical examination, and performing or ordering appropriate diagnostic tests. Tests that can help identify and gauge the extent of infection include laboratory studies, radiographic tests, and scans.

Typically, the first test is a WBC count and a differential. Elevation in overall number of WBCs is a positive result. The differential count is the relative number of each of five types of WBCs—neutrophils, eosinophils, basophils, lymphocytes, and monocytes. It's obtained by classifying 100 or more WBCs in a stained film of peripheral blood. Multiplying the percentage value of each type by the total WBC count gives the absolute number of each type of WBC. This test recognizes only that something has stimulated an immune response. Bacterial infection usually causes an elevation in the counts; viruses may cause no change or a decrease in normal WBC level.

An erythrocyte sedimentation rate test may be done to reveal that an inflammatory process is occurring within the body.

The next step is to obtain a stained smear from a specific body site to determine the causative agent. Stains that may be used to visualize the microorganism include:
♦ Gram stain, which identifies gram-negative or gram-positive bacteria
♦ acid-fast stain, which identifies mycobacteria and *Nocardia*
♦ silver stain, which identifies fungi, *Legionella*, and *Pneumocystis.*

Although stains provide rapid and valuable diagnostic information, they only tentatively identify a pathogen. Confirmation requires culturing. Any body substance can be cultured, but enough growth to identify the microbe may occur in as few as 8 hours (streptococcal) or as long as several weeks, depending on how rapidly the microbe replicates. Types of cultures that may be ordered are blood, urine, sputum, throat, nasal, wound, skin, stool, and cerebrospinal fluid.

A specimen obtained for culture must not be contaminated with any other substance. For example, a urine specimen must not contain debris from the perineum or vaginal area. If obtaining a clean urine specimen isn't possible, the patient must be catheterized to make sure that only the urine is being examined.

Contaminated specimens may mislead and prolong treatment.

Additional tests that may be requested include magnetic resonance imaging to locate infection sites, chest X-rays to search the lungs for respiratory changes, and gallium scans to detect abscesses.

Treatment

Treatment of infections can vary widely. Vaccines may be administered to induce a primary immune response under conditions that won't cause disease. If infection occurs, treatment is tailored to the specific causative organism. Drug therapy should be used only when it's appropriate. Supportive therapy can play an important role in fighting infections.

◆ Antibiotics work in various ways, depending on the antibiotic class. Their action is bactericidal (killing the bacteria) or bacteriostatic (preventing the bacteria from multiplying). Antibiotics may inhibit cell wall synthesis, protein synthesis, bacterial metabolism, or nucleic acid synthesis or activity, or they may increase cell membrane permeability. (See *Antimicrobial drugs and chemicals*.)

◆ Antifungals destroy the invading microbe by increasing cell membrane permeability. The antifungal binds sterols in the cell membrane, resulting in leakage of intracellular contents, such as potassium, sodium, and nutrients.

◆ Antivirals stop viral replication by interfering with deoxyribonucleic acid synthesis.

The overuse of antimicrobials has created widespread resistance to some drugs. Some pathogens that were once well controlled by medicines are again surfacing with increased virulence. One such pathogen known to cause tuberculosis is *Mycobacterium tuberculosis*.

Some diseases, including most viral infections, don't respond to available drugs. Supportive care is the only recourse while the host defenses repel the invader. To help the body fight an infection, the patient should:

◆ use standard precautions to avoid spreading the infection

◆ drink plenty of fluids

◆ get plenty of rest

◆ avoid people who may have other illnesses

◆ take over-the-counter medications appropriate for his symptoms only with full knowledge about dosage, actions, and possible adverse effects or reactions

◆ follow the physician's orders for taking prescription drugs and be sure to finish all medication

◆ not share the prescription with others.

Antimicrobial drugs and chemicals

The following drugs or chemicals prevent growth of microorganisms or destroy them by a specific action.

Mechanisms of action	Agent
Inhibition of cell-wall synthesis	Bacitracin Carbapenems Cephalosporins Cycloserine Fosfomycin Monobactams Penicillins Vancomycin
Damage to cytoplasmic membrane	Imidazoles Polyene antifungals Polymyxins
Metabolism of nucleic acid	Nitrofurans Nitroimidazoles Quinolones Rifampin
Protein synthesis	Aminoglycosides Chloramphenicol Clindamycin Macrolides Mupirocin Spectinomycin Tetracyclines
Modification of energy metabolism	Dapsone Isoniazid Sulfonamides Trimethoprim

Differentiating infections

Infection can strike any part of the body. The accompanying chart describes various infections along with their signs and symptoms and appropriate diagnostic tests. (See *Reviewing infections*, pages 58 to 73.)

Reviewing infections

Infection and findings	Diagnosis

Bacterial infections

Anthrax

Cutaneous anthrax
♦ Small, elevated, itchy lesion that resembles an insect bite, develops into a vesicle, and finally becomes a small, painless ulcer with a necrotic (black) center
♦ Enlarged lymph glands

♦ Isolation of *Bacilllus anthracis* from cultures of the blood, skin lesions, or sputum confirms the diagnosis.
♦ Specific antibodies may be detected in the blood; the Anthrax Quick enzyme-linked immunosorbent assay (ELISA) test detects antibodies to anthrax in 1 hour (four times faster than previous tests).

Inhalational anthrax
♦ Initial flulike symptoms, such as malaise, fever, headache, myalgia, and chills
♦ Progression to severe respiratory difficulties, such as dyspnea, stridor, chest pain, and cyanosis
♦ Onset of shock

Gastrointestinal anthrax
♦ Nausea and vomiting
♦ Decreased appetite
♦ Fever
♦ Progression to abdominal pain, bloody emesis, and severe diarrhea

Botulism

♦ Initial signs and symptoms include dry mouth, sore throat, weakness, dizziness, vomiting, and diarrhea
♦ Cardinal sign: acute symmetrical cranial nerve impairment (ptosis, diplopia, and dysarthria)
♦ Descending weakness or paralysis of muscles in the extremities or trunk
♦ Dyspnea from respiratory muscle paralysis

♦ Identification of the offending toxin in the patient's serum, stool, gastric contents, or the suspected food confirms the diagnosis.
♦ Electromyogram showing diminished muscle action potential after a single supramaximal nerve stimulus is also diagnostic.

Infant botulism
♦ Generalized muscle weakness, hypotonia, and feeble cry
♦ Constipation
♦ Depressed gag reflex and inability to suck
♦ Flaccid facial expression, ptosis, and ophthalmoplegia due to cranial nerve deficits
♦ Areflexia and loss of head control

Chlamydial infections

Cervicitis
♦ Cervical erosion
♦ Dyspareunia
♦ Micropurulent discharge
♦ Pelvic pain

♦ Swab from site of infection establishes a diagnosis of urethritis, cervicitis, salpingitis, endometritis, or proctitis.
♦ Culture of aspirated material establishes a diagnosis of epididymitis.
♦ Antigen-detection methods are the diagnostic tests of choice for identifying chlamydial infection.
♦ Polymerase chain reaction (PCR) test is highly sensitive and specific.

Endometritis or salpingitis
♦ Pain and tenderness of the lower abdomen, cervix, uterus, and lymph nodes
♦ Chills, fever

Reviewing infections *(continued)*

Infection and findings

Diagnosis

Bacterial infections (continued)

Chlamydial infections *(continued)*
♦ Breakthrough bleeding, bleeding after intercourse, and vaginal discharge
♦ Dysuria

Epididymitis
♦ Painful scrotal swelling
♦ Urethral discharge

Proctitis
♦ Diarrhea
♦ Tenesmus
♦ Pruritus
♦ Bloody or mucopurulent discharge
♦ Diffuse or discrete ulceration in the rectosigmoid colon

Prostatitis
♦ Low back pain
♦ Urinary frequency, nocturia, and dysuria
♦ Painful ejaculation

Urethral syndrome
♦ Dysuria, pyuria, and urinary frequency

Urethritis
♦ Dysuria, erythema, tenderness of the urethral meatus
♦ Urinary frequency
♦ Pruritus and urethral discharge (copious and purulent or scant and clear or mucoid)

Conjunctivitis*
♦ Hyperemia of the conjunctiva
♦ Discharge
♦ Tearing
♦ Pain
♦ Photophobia (with corneal involvement)
♦ Itching and burning

♦ Culture from the conjunctiva identifies the causative organism.
♦ In stained smears, predominance of lymphocytes indicates viral infection; of neutrophils, bacterial infection; of eosinophils, an allergy-related infection.

Gonorrhea
In males
♦ May be asymptomatic
♦ Urethritis, including dysuria and purulent urethral discharge, with redness and swelling at the site of infection

♦ Culture from the site of infection, grown on a Thayer-Martin or Transgrow medium, establishes the diagnosis by isolating *Neisseria gonorrhoeae*.
♦ Gram stain shows gram-negative diplococci.
♦ Complement fixation and immunofluorescent assays of serum reveal antibody titers four times the normal rate.

In females
♦ May be asymptomatic
♦ Inflammation and a greenish yellow discharge from the cervix

(continued)

Note: May also result from viral infection.

Reviewing infections *(continued)*

Infection and findings	Diagnosis

Bacterial infections (continued)

Gonorrhea *(continued)*
In males or females
♦ Pharyngitis or tonsillitis
♦ Rectal burning, itching, and bloody muco-purulent discharge

Clinical features (vary according to the site involved)
♦ Urethra: dysuria, urinary frequency and incontinence, purulent discharge, itching, red and edematous meatus
♦ Vulva: occasional itching, burning, and pain due to exudate from an adjacent infected area
♦ Vagina: engorgement, redness, swelling, and profuse purulent discharge
♦ Liver: right-upper-quadrant pain
♦ Pelvis: severe pelvic and lower abdominal pain, muscle rigidity, tenderness, and abdominal distention; nausea, vomiting, fever, and tachycardia (may develop in patients with salpingitis or pelvic inflammatory disease)

Listeriosis
♦ Commonly causes asymptomatic carrier state
♦ Malaise
♦ Chills
♦ Fever
♦ Back pain

In fetuses
♦ Abortion
♦ Premature delivery or stillbirth
♦ Organ abscesses

In neonates
♦ Meningitis, resulting in tense fontanels
♦ Irritability
♦ Lethargy
♦ Seizures
♦ Coma

♦ *Listeria monocytogenes* is identified by its diagnostic tumbling motility on a wet mount of the culture.
♦ Positive culture of blood, spinal fluid, drainage from cervical or vaginal lesions, or lochia from a mother with an infected infant.

Lyme disease
Stage 1
♦ Erythema chronicum migrans (ECM): red macule or papule, commonly on the site of a tick bite, which grows to over 2" (5 cm), feels hot and itchy, and resembles a bull's eye or target; after a few days, more lesions erupt and a migratory, ringlike rash appears
 ♦ Conjunctivitis
 ♦ Diffuse urticaria occurs
 ♦ Lesions are replaced by small red blotches in 3 to 4 weeks

♦ Because *Borrelia burgdorferi* is unusual in humans and indirect immunofluorescent antibody tests are marginally sensitive, diagnosis is usually based on the characteristic ECM lesion and related clinical findings.
♦ Serology reveals mild anemia and elevated erythrocyte sedimentation rate, white blood cell (WBC) count, serum immunoglobulin (Ig) M level, and aspartate aminotransferase.
♦ Cerebrospinal fluid (CSF) analysis reveals presence of antibodies to *B. burgdorferi* if the disease has affected the central nervous system (CNS).

Reviewing infections *(continued)*

Infection and findings   **Diagnosis**

Bacterial infections (continued)

Lyme disease *(continued)*
♦ Malaise and fatigue
♦ Intermittent headache
♦ Neck stiffness
♦ Fever, chills, and achiness
♦ Regional lymphadenopathy

Stage 2
♦ Neurologic abnormalities—fluctuating menin-
goencephalitis with peripheral and cranial neuropathy; begins weeks to months later
♦ Facial palsy
♦ Cardiac abnormalities: brief, fluctuating atrioventricular heart block, left ventricular dysfunction, cardiomegaly

Stage 3
♦ Arthritis with marked swelling begins weeks
or years later
♦ Neuropsychiatric symptoms, such as psychotic
behavior, memory loss, dementia, and depression
♦ Encephalopathic symptoms, such as headache,
confusion, and difficulty concentrating
♦ Ophthalmic manifestations, such as iritis, ker-
atitis, renal vasculitis, optic neuritis

Meningitis**
♦ Fever
♦ Chills
♦ Headache
♦ Nuchal rigidity
♦ Vomiting
♦ Photophobia
♦ Lethargy
♦ Coma
♦ Positive Brudzinski's and Kernig's signs
♦ Exaggerated and symmetrical deep tendon
reflexes and opisthotonos
♦ Wide pulse pressure
♦ Bradycardia
♦ Occasional rash

♦ Lumbar puncture isolates the infecting organism (usually *Neisseria meningitidis, Haemophilus
influenzae* [in children and young adults], or
Streptococcus pneumoniae [in adults]) from CSF
and shows increased CSF cell count and protein
level and decreased CSF glucose level.
♦ Blood culture isolates the infecting organism.

Otitis media
♦ Ear pain
♦ Ear drainage
♦ Hearing loss
♦ Fever
♦ Lethargy
♦ Irritability
♦ Vertigo
♦ Signs of upper respiratory tract infection
(such as sneezing and coughing)
♦ Tinnitus

♦ Otoscopy reveals obscured or distorted bony
landmarks of the tympanic membrane.
♦ Pneumatoscopy can show decreased tympanic
membrane mobility.
♦ Culture of the ear drainage identifies the
causative organism.

(continued)

***Note:* May also result from viral, protozoal, or fungal infection.

Reviewing infections *(continued)*

Infection and findings	Diagnosis

Bacterial infections *(continued)*

Peritonitis
♦ Sudden, severe, and diffuse abdominal pain that tends to intensify and localize in the area of the underlying disorder with associated rebound tenderness
♦ Weakness and pallor
♦ Excessive sweating
♦ Cold skin
♦ Decreased intestinal motility and paralytic ileus
♦ Intestinal obstruction causes nausea, vomiting, and abdominal rigidity
♦ Hypotension
♦ Tachycardia
♦ Fever
♦ Abdominal distention

♦ Abdominal X-ray shows edematous and gaseous distention of the small and large bowel or in the case of visceral organ perforation, air lying under the diaphragm.
♦ Chest X-ray may show elevation of the diaphragm.
♦ Blood studies show leukocytosis.
♦ Paracentesis reveals bacteria, exudate, blood, pus, or urine.
♦ Laparotomy may be necessary to identify the underlying cause.

Plague
Bubonic plague
♦ Malaise and fever
♦ Pain or tenderness in regional lymph nodes, possibly associated with swelling
♦ Painful, inflamed, and possibly suppurative buboes; classic sign is an excruciatingly painful bubo
♦ Hemorrhagic areas that become necrotic; such areas appear dark, hence the name "black death"
♦ Restlessness, disorientation, delirium, toxemia, and staggering gait

Primary pneumonic plague
♦ Acute onset of high fever, chills, severe headache, tachycardia, tachypnea, and dyspnea
♦ Productive cough (first mucoid sputum, later frothy pink or red)
♦ Severe prostration, respiratory distress and, usually, death

Secondary pneumonic plague
♦ Pulmonary extension of the bubonic form
♦ Cough producing bloody sputum
♦ Severe prostration, respiratory distress and, usually, death

Septicemic plague
♦ Toxicity, hyperpyrexia, seizures, prostration, shock, and disseminated intravascular coagulation
♦ Widespread, nonspecific tissue damage

♦ Characteristic buboes and a history of exposure to rodents are strongly suggestive of diagnosis.
♦ Stained smears and cultures of *Yersinia pestis* obtained from a needle aspirate of a small amount of fluid from skin lesions confirms the diagnosis.
♦ Other laboratory findings include elevated WBC count with increased polymorphonuclear leukocytes and hemoagglutination reaction (antibody titer) studies.
♦ In pneumonic plague, chest X-ray shows fulminating pneumonia and stained smear and culture of sputum identify *Y. pestis.*
♦ In septicemic plague, stained smear and blood culture containing *Y. pestis* are diagnostic.
♦ For a presumptive diagnosis of plague, a fluorescent antibody test may be ordered.

Reviewing infections *(continued)*

Infection and findings   **Diagnosis**

Bacterial infections (continued)

Pneumonia***
♦ High temperature
♦ Cough with purulent, yellow or bloody sputum
♦ Dyspnea
♦ Crackles and decreased breath sounds
♦ Pleuritic pain
♦ Chills
♦ Malaise
♦ Tachypnea

♦ Chest X-rays confirm the diagnosis by disclosing infiltrates.
♦ Sputum specimen, Gram stain and culture, and sensitivity tests help differentiate the type of infection and the drugs that are effective.
♦ WBC count indicates leukocytosis in bacterial pneumonia, and a normal or low count in viral or mycoplasmal pneumonia.
♦ Blood cultures reflect bacteremia and are used to determine the causative organism.
♦ Arterial blood gas levels vary, depending on severity of pneumonia and underlying lung state.
♦ Bronchoscopy or transtracheal aspiration allows the collection of material for culture.
♦ Pulse oximetry may show a reduced oxygen saturation level.

Salmonellosis
♦ Fever
♦ Abdominal pain, severe diarrhea with entero-colitis

Typhoidal infection
♦ Headache
♦ Increasing fever
♦ Constipation

♦ Blood cultures isolate the organism in typhoid fever, paratyphoid fever, and bacteremia.
♦ Stool cultures isolate the organism in typhoid fever, paratyphoid fever, and enterocolitis.
♦ Cultures of urine, bone marrow, pus, and vomitus may show the presence of *Salmonella.*

Shigellosis
In children
♦ High fever
♦ Diarrhea with tenesmus
♦ Nausea, vomiting, and abdominal pain and distention
♦ Irritability
♦ Drowsiness
♦ Stool may contain pus, mucus, or blood
♦ Dehydration and weight loss

♦ Microscopic examination of a fresh stool may reveal mucus, red blood cells (RBCs), and poly-morphonuclear leukocytes; direct immunofluo-rescence with specific antisera may reveal *Shigella.*
♦ Severe infection increases hemagglutinating antibodies.
♦ Sigmoidoscopy or proctoscopy may reveal typical superficial ulcerations.

In adults
♦ Sporadic, intense abdominal pain
♦ Rectal irritability
♦ Tenesmus
♦ Headache and prostration
♦ Stool may contain pus, mucus, and blood

(continued)

***Note: May also result from fungal or protozoal infection.

Reviewing infections *(continued)*

Infection and findings	Diagnosis

Bacterial infections (continued)

Syphilis

Primary syphilis
♦ Chancres (small, fluid-filled lesions) on the anus, fingers, lips, tongue, nipples, tonsils, or eyelids
♦ Regional lymphadenopathy

Secondary syphilis
♦ Symmetrical mucocutaneous lesions
♦ General lymphadenopathy
♦ Rash may be macular, papular, pustular, or nodular
♦ Headache
♦ Malaise
♦ Anorexia, weight loss, nausea, and vomiting
♦ Sore throat and slight fever
♦ Alopecia
♦ Brittle and pitted nails

Late syphilis
♦ Gumma lesion (benign) found on any bone or organ
♦ Gastric pain, tenderness, enlarged spleen
♦ Anemia
♦ Involvement of the upper respiratory tract, perforation of the nasal septum or palate, and destruction of bones and organs
♦ Fibrosis of elastic tissue of the aorta
♦ Aortic insufficiency
♦ Aortic aneurysm
♦ Meningitis
♦ Paresis
♦ Personality changes
♦ Arm and leg weakness

♦ Dark field examination of a lesion identifies *Treponema pallidum.*
♦ Fluorescent treponemal antibody absorption tests identifies antigens of *T. pallidum* in tissue, ocular fluid, CSF, tracheobronchial secretions, and exudates from lesions.
♦ Venereal Disease Research Laboratory slide test and rapid plasma reagin test detect nonspecific antibodies.

Tetanus

Localized
♦ Spasm and increased muscle tone near the wound

Systemic
♦ Marked muscle hypertonicity
♦ Hyperactive deep tendon reflexes
♦ Tachycardia
♦ Profuse sweating
♦ Low-grade fever
♦ Painful, involuntary muscle contractions

♦ Diagnosis may rest on clinical features, a history of trauma, and no previous tetanus immunization.
♦ Blood cultures and tetanus antibody tests are often negative; only one-third of patients have a positive wound culture.
♦ CSF pressure may rise above normal.

Toxic shock syndrome
♦ Intense myalgias
♦ Fever over 104° F (40° C)
♦ Vomiting and diarrhea
♦ Headache
♦ Decreased level of consciousness (LOC)
♦ Rigor

♦ Diagnosis is based on clinical findings and body system involvement.
♦ Isolation of *Staphylococcus aureus* from vaginal discharge or lesions.

Reviewing infections *(continued)*

Infection and findings   **Diagnosis**

Bacterial infections (continued)

Toxic shock syndrome *(continued)*
♦ Conjunctival hyperemia
♦ Vaginal hyperemia and discharge
♦ Deep red rash (especially on the palms and
soles) that later desquamates
♦ Severe hypotension

♦ Negative results on blood tests for Rocky
Mountain spotted fever, leptospirosis, and
measles help rule out these disorders.

Tuberculosis
♦ Fever and night sweats
♦ Productive cough lasting longer than 3 weeks
♦ Hemoptysis
♦ Malaise
♦ Adenopathy
♦ Weight loss
♦ Pleuritic chest pain
♦ Symptoms of airway obstruction from lymph
node involvement

♦ Chest X-ray shows nodular lesions, patchy
infiltrates (mainly in upper lobes), cavity formation,
scar tissue, and calcium deposits.
♦ Tuberculin skin test reveals infection at some
point, but doesn't indicate active disease.
♦ Stains and cultures of sputum, CSF, urine,
drainage from abscesses, or pleural fluid show
heat-sensitive, nonmotile, aerobic, acid-fast
bacilli; deoxyribonucleic acid (DNA) probe testing
of young growth from the cultured specimen is
used to detect the bacteria. If no bacteria is
detected, the specimen is sent to the appropriate
laboratory for identification.
♦ Computed tomography (CT) scan or magnetic
resonance imaging (MRI) allow the evaluation of
lung damage and may confirm a difficult diagnosis.
♦ Bronchoscopy shows inflammation and altered
lung tissue. It also may be performed to obtain
sputum if the patient can't produce an adequate
sputum specimen.

Tularemia
♦ Signs and symptoms appearing 3 to 14 days
after exposure
♦ Reddened skin area progressing to an ulcer
♦ Inguinal or axillary lymphadenopathy
♦ Headache
♦ Muscle pains
♦ Shortness of breath
♦ Dry cough
♦ Hemoptysis
♦ Fever
♦ Chills
♦ Sweating
♦ Weight loss
♦ Joint stiffness
♦ Progressive weakness
♦ Pneumonia

♦ Serology is positive for tularemia.
♦ Blood culture is positive for tularemia.
♦ Chest X-ray reveals infiltrate pneumonia.

Urinary tract infections
Acute pyelonephritis
♦ Fever and shaking chills
♦ Nausea, vomiting, and diarrhea
♦ Symptoms of cystitis may be present
♦ Tachycardia
♦ Generalized muscle tenderness

♦ Urine culture reveals microorganism.
♦ Urinary microscopy is positive for pyuria,
hematuria, or bacteriuria.

(continued)

Reviewing infections *(continued)*

Infection and findings

Diagnosis

Bacterial infections (continued)

Urinary tract infections *(continued)*
Cystitis
♦ Dysuria, urinary frequency, urgency, and suprapubic pain
♦ Cloudy, malodorous and, possibly, bloody urine
♦ Fever
♦ Nausea and vomiting
♦ Costovertebral angle tenderness

Urethritis
♦ Dysuria, urinary frequency, and pyuria

Whooping cough (Pertussis)
♦ Irritating, hacking cough characteristically ending in a loud, crowing, inspiratory whoop that may expel tenacious mucus
♦ Anorexia
♦ Sneezing
♦ Listlessness
♦ Infected conjunctiva
♦ Low-grade fever

♦ Classic clinical findings suggest the disease.
♦ Nasopharyngeal swabs and sputum cultures show *Bordetella pertussis*.
♦ Fluorescent antibody screening of nasopharyngeal smears is less reliable than cultures.
♦ Serology shows an elevated WBC count.

Viral infections

Chickenpox (Varicella)
♦ Pruritic rash of small, erythematous macules that progresses to papules and then to clear vesicles on an erythematous base
♦ Slight fever
♦ Malaise and anorexia

♦ Characteristic clinical signs suggest the virus.
♦ Isolation of virus from vesicular fluid helps confirm the virus; Giemsa stain distinguishes varicella-zoster from vaccinia and variola viruses.

Congenital varicella
♦ Hypoplastic deformity and scarring of a limb, retarded growth, and CNS and eye manifestations

In an immunocompromised patient with progressive varicella
♦ Lesions and a high fever for over 7 days

Cytomegalovirus (CMV) infection
♦ Mild, nonspecific complaints
♦ Immunodeficient population: pneumonia, chorioretinitis, colitis, encephalitis, abdominal pain, diarrhea, or weight loss
♦ Infants ages 3 to 6 months appear asymptomatic but may develop hepatic dysfunction, hepatosplenomegaly, spider angiomas, pneumonitis, and lymphadenopathy

♦ Virus isolated in urine, saliva, throat, cervix, WBC and biopsy specimens. Complement fixation studies, hemagglutination inhibition antibody tests, and indirect immunofluorescent test for CMV IgM antibody (congenital infections) aid diagnosis.
♦ CMV DNA detection by PCR demonstrates viral presence in organs, blood, urine, or respiratory secretions.

Congenital infection
♦ Jaundice, petechial rash, hepatosplenomegaly, thrombocytopenia, hemolytic anemia

Reviewing infections *(continued)*

Infection and findings	Diagnosis

Viral infections (continued)

H1N1 flu (swine flu)
♦ Fever and chills
♦ Cough
♦ Sore throat
♦ Headache and body aches
♦ Fatigue and malasie

♦ Real-time polymerase chain reaction test positive for H1N1 virus
♦ Viral culture positive for H1N1 virus

Herpes simplex
Type 1
♦ Fever
♦ Sore, red, swollen throat
♦ Submaxillary lymphadenopathy
♦ Increased salivation, halitosis, and anorexia
♦ Severe mouth pain
♦ Edema of the mouth
♦ Vesicles (on the tongue, gingiva, and cheeks, or anywhere in or around the mouth) on a red base that eventually rupture, leaving a painful ulcer and then yellow crusting

♦ Tzanck smear shows multinucleated giant cells.
♦ Herpes simplex virus culture is positive.
♦ Virus is isolated from local lesions.
♦ Tissue biopsy aids in diagnosis.
♦ Elevated antibodies and increased WBC count indicate primary infection.

Type 2
♦ Tingling in the area involved
♦ Malaise
♦ Dysuria
♦ Dyspareunia (painful intercourse)
♦ Leukorrhea (white vaginal discharge containing mucus and pus cells)
♦ Localized, fluid-filled vesicles that are found on the cervix, labia, perianal skin, vulva, vagina, glans penis, foreskin, and penile shaft, mouth or anus; inguinal swelling may be present

Herpes zoster
♦ Pain within the dermatome affected
♦ Fever
♦ Malaise
♦ Pruritus
♦ Paresthesia or hyperesthesia in the trunk, arms, or legs may also occur
♦ Small, red, nodular skin lesions on painful areas (nerve specific) that change to pus or fluid-filled vesicles

♦ Staining antibodies from vesicular fluid and identification under fluorescent light differentiates herpes zoster from localized herpes simplex.
♦ Examination of vesicular fluid and infected tissue shows eosinophilic intranuclear inclusions and varicella virus.
♦ Lumbar puncture shows increased pressure; CSF shows increased protein levels and possibly pleocytosis.

Human immunodeficiency virus infection
♦ Rapid weight loss
♦ Dry cough
♦ Recurring fever or profuse night sweats
♦ Profound and unexplained fatigue
♦ Swollen lymph glands in the armpits, groin, or neck
♦ Diarrhea that lasts for more than a week
♦ White spots or unusual blemishes on the tongue, in the mouth, or in the throat

♦ Two ELISA tests are positive.
♦ Western blot test is positive.

(continued)

Reviewing infections *(continued)*

Infection and findings	Diagnosis

Viral infections *(continued)*

Human immunodeficiency virus infection *(continued)*
♦ Pneumonia
♦ Red, brown, pink, or purplish blotches on or under the skin or inside the mouth, nose, or eyelids
♦ Memory loss, depression, and other neurologic disorders

Infectious mononucleosis
♦ Headache
♦ Malaise and fatigue
♦ Sore throat
♦ Cervical lymphadenopathy
♦ Temperature fluctuations with an evening peak
♦ Splenomegaly
♦ Hepatomegaly
♦ Stomatitis
♦ Exudative tonsillitis, or pharyngitis
♦ Maculopapular rash

♦ Monospot test is positive.
♦ WBC count is abnormally high (10,000 to 20,000/mm³) during the second and third weeks of illness. From 50% to 70% of the total count consists of lymphocytes and monocytes, and 10% of the lymphocytes are atypical.
♦ Heterophil antibodies in serum drawn during the acute phase and at 3- to 4-week intervals increase to four times normal.
♦ Indirect immunofluorescence shows antibodies to Epstein-Barr virus and cellular antigens.

Monkeypox
♦ Signs and symptoms appearing after an incubation period of about 12 days
♦ Fever
♦ Headache, muscle aches, backache
♦ Lymphadenopathy
♦ General feeling of discomfort and exhaustion
♦ Papular rash beginning on the face or other area of the body within 1 to 3 days after onset of fever; lesions eventually crust and fall off

♦ Diagnosis is based on history and presenting signs and symptoms.
♦ Monkeypox virus may be isolated from vesicular fluid to aid in diagnosis.

Mumps
♦ Myalgia
♦ Malaise and fever
♦ Headache
♦ Earache aggravated by chewing
♦ Parotid gland tenderness and swelling, and pain when chewing or when drinking sour or acidic liquids
♦ Swelling of the other salivary glands

♦ Virus is isolated from throat washings, urine, blood, or spinal fluid.
♦ Serologic antibody testing shows a rise in paired antibodies.
♦ Clinical signs and symptoms, especially parotid gland enlargement are characteristic.

Rabies
Prodromal symptoms
♦ Local or radiating pain or burning and a sensation of cold, pruritus, and tingling at the bite site
♦ Malaise and fever
♦ Headache
♦ Nausea
♦ Sore throat and persistent loose cough
♦ Nervousness, anxiety, irritability, hyperesthesia, sensitivity to light and loud noises
♦ Excessive salivation, tearing and perspiration

♦ Virus is isolated from saliva or throat.
♦ Fluorescent rabies antibody test is positive.
♦ WBC count is elevated.
♦ Histologic examination of brain tissue from human rabies victims shows perivascular inflammation of the gray matter, degeneration of neuron, and characteristic minute bodies, called *Negri bodies,* in the nerve cells.

Reviewing infections *(continued)*

Infection and findings

Diagnosis

Viral infections (continued)

Rabies *(continued)*
Excitation phase
♦ Intermittent hyperactivity, anxiety, apprehension
♦ Shallow respirations
♦ Altered LOC
♦ Ocular palsies
♦ Strabismus
♦ Asymmetrical pupillary dilation or constriction
♦ Absence of corneal reflexes
♦ Facial muscle weakness
♦ Forceful, painful pharyngeal muscle spasms
that expel fluids from the mouth, resulting in
dehydration
♦ Swallowing problems cause frothy drooling
and soon the sight, sound, or thought of water
triggers uncontrollable pharyngeal muscle
spasms and excessive salivation
♦ Nuchal rigidity
♦ Seizures
♦ Cardiac arrhythmias

Terminal phase
♦ Gradual, generalized, flaccid paralysis
♦ Peripheral vascular collapse
♦ Coma and death

Respiratory syncytial virus infection
Mild disease
♦ Nasal congestion
♦ Coughing and wheezing
♦ Malaise
♦ Sore throat
♦ Earache
♦ Dyspnea
♦ Fever

♦ Cultures of nasal and pharyngeal secretions
may reveal the virus; however, this infection is
so labile that cultures aren't always reliable.
♦ Serum antibody titers may be elevated.
♦ Recently developed serologic techniques are
the indirect immunofluorescent and ELISA
methods.
♦ Chest X-rays help detect pneumonia.

Bronchitis, bronchiolitis, pneumonia
♦ Nasal flaring, retraction, cyanosis, and
tachypnea
♦ Wheezes, rhonchi, and crackles
♦ Signs, such as weakness, irritability, and
nuchal rigidity, of CNS infection may be
observed

Rubella
♦ Maculopapular, mildly itchy rash usually
beginning on the face and then spreading
rapidly, often covering the trunk and extremities
♦ Small, red macules on the soft palate
(Forschheimer spots)
♦ Low-grade fever
♦ Headache
♦ Malaise

♦ Clinical signs and symptoms are usually sufficient to make a diagnosis.
♦ Cell cultures of the throat, blood, urine, and
CSF, along with convalescent serum that shows
a fourfold rise in antibody titers, confirms the
diagnosis.

(continued)

Reviewing infections *(continued)*

Infection and findings　　　　　　**Diagnosis**

Viral infections *(continued)*

Rubella *(continued)*
♦ Anorexia
♦ Sore throat
♦ Cough
♦ Postauricular, suboccipital, and posterior
cervical lymph node enlargement

Rubeola
♦ Fever
♦ Photophobia
♦ Malaise
♦ Anorexia
♦ Conjunctivitis, puffy red eyes, and rhinorrhea
♦ Coryza
♦ Hoarseness, hacking cough
♦ Koplik's spots (tiny, bluish white specks surrounded by a red halo), pruritic macular rash becoming papular and erythematous

♦ Diagnosis rests on distinctive clinical features.
♦ Measles virus may be isolated from the blood, nasopharyngeal secretions, and urine during the febrile stage.
♦ Serum antibodies appear within 3 days.

Smallpox
♦ Abrupt onset of chills (and possible seizures in children)
♦ High fever (above 104° F [40° C])
♦ Headache, backache, severe malaise, vomiting (especially in children), and marked prostration
♦ Occasionally, violent delirium, stupor, or coma
♦ Sore throat and cough as well as lesions on the mucous membranes of the mouth, throat, and respiratory tract
♦ Skin lesions progressing from macular to papular, vesicular, and pustular, with eventual desquamation causing intense pruritus and permanently disfiguring scars
♦ In fatal cases, death typically resulting from encephalitic manifestations, extensive bleeding from orifices, or secondary bacterial infections

♦ Most conclusive laboratory test is culture of variola virus isolated from an aspirate of vesicles and pustules.
♦ Microscopic examination of smears from lesion scrapings and complement fixation detect virus or antibodies to the virus in the patient's blood.

West Nile virus infection
Mild infection (more common than severe infection)
♦ Fever
♦ Headache and body aches
♦ Swollen lymph glands
♦ Skin rash

Severe infection (producing neurologic illnesses including meningitis and encephalitis)
♦ Headache
♦ High fever
♦ Neck stiffness
♦ Disorientation, stupor, or coma
♦ Tremors and occasional convulsions
♦ Paralysis
♦ Rarely, death

♦ IgM antibody capture-ELISA performed on serum or CSF specimens detects antibodies specific to West Nile virus and confirms the diagnosis.

Reviewing infections *(continued)*

Infection and findings

Diagnosis

Fungal infections

Histoplasmosis
African histoplasmosis
♦ Cutaneous nodules, papules, and ulcers
♦ Lesions of the skull and long bones
♦ Lymphadenopathy and visceral involvement without pulmonary lesions

Chronic pulmonary histoplasmosis
♦ Productive cough, dyspnea, and occasional hemoptysis
♦ Weight loss
♦ Extreme weakness
♦ Breathlessness and cyanosis

Primary acute histoplasmosis
♦ May be asymptomatic or may cause symptoms of a mild respiratory illness similar to a severe cold or influenza
♦ Fever
♦ Malaise
♦ Headache
♦ Myalgia
♦ Anorexia
♦ Cough
♦ Chest pain
♦ Anemia, leukopenia, or thrombocytopenia
♦ Oropharyngeal ulcers

Progressive disseminated histoplasmosis
♦ Hepatosplenomegaly
♦ General lymphadenopathy
♦ Anorexia and weight loss
♦ Fever and, possibly, ulceration of the tongue, palate, epiglottis, and larynx, with resulting pain, hoarseness, and dysphagia

♦ Culture or histology reveals the organism.
♦ Stained biopsies using Gomori's stains or periodic acid-Schiff reaction give a fast diagnosis of the disease.
♦ Positive histoplasmin skin test or urine antigen test indicates exposure to histoplasmosis.
♦ Rising complement fixation and agglutination titers (more than 1:32) strongly suggest histoplasmosis.

Protozoal infections

Malaria
Benign form
♦ Chills
♦ Fever
♦ Headache and myalgia

Acute attacks (occur when erythrocytes rupture)
♦ Chills and shaking
♦ High fever (up to 107° F [41.7° C])
♦ Profuse sweating
♦ Hepatosplenomegaly
♦ Hemolytic anemia

Life-threatening form
♦ Persistent high fever
♦ Orthostatic hypotension

♦ Peripheral blood smears of RBCs identify the parasite.
♦ Indirect fluorescent serum antibody tests are unreliable in the acute phase.
♦ Hemoglobin level is decreased.
♦ Leukocyte count is normal to decreased.
♦ Protein and leukocytes are present in urine sediment.

(continued)

Reviewing infections *(continued)*

Infection and findings	**Diagnosis**

Protozoal infections *(continued)*

Malaria *(continued)*
♦ RBC sludging that leads to capillary obstruction at various sites
♦ Hemiplegia
♦ Seizures
♦ Delirium and coma
♦ Hemoptysis
♦ Vomiting
♦ Abdominal pain, diarrhea, and melena
♦ Oliguria, anuria, uremia

Schistosomiasis
♦ Transient pruritic rash at the site of cercariae penetration
♦ Fever
♦ Myalgia
♦ Cough

♦ Typical symptoms and a history of travel to endemic areas suggest the diagnosis.
♦ Ova in the urine or stool or a mucosal lesion biopsy confirm diagnosis.
♦ WBC count shows eosinophilia.

Later signs and symptoms
♦ Hepatomegaly, splenomegaly, and lymphadenopathy

Schistosoma mansoni *and* S. japonicum
♦ Irregular fever
♦ Malaise, weakness
♦ Weight loss
♦ Diarrhea
♦ Ascites, hepatosplenomegaly
♦ Portal hypertension
♦ Fistulas, intestinal stricture

S. haematobium
♦ Terminal hematuria dysuria
♦ Ureteral colic

Toxoplasmosis
Acquired toxoplasmosis
♦ Malaise, myalgia, headache
♦ Fatigue
♦ Sore throat
♦ Fever
♦ Cervical lymphadenopathy
♦ Maculopapular rash

♦ Identification of *Toxoplasma gondii* in an appropriate tissue specimen confirms diagnosis.
♦ CT scans and MRI disclose lesions in patients with toxoplasmosis encephalitis.

Congenital toxoplasmosis
♦ Hydrocephalus or microcephalus
♦ Seizures
♦ Jaundice
♦ Purpura and rash

Ocular toxoplasmosis
♦ Chorioretinitis
♦ Yellow-white elevated cotton patches
♦ Blurred vision
♦ Scotoma
♦ Pain
♦ Photophobia

Reviewing infections *(continued)*

Infection and findings   **Diagnosis**

Protozoal infections (continued)

Trichinosis

Stage 1 (enteric phase)
♦ Anorexia
♦ Nausea, vomiting, diarrhea
♦ Abdominal pain and cramps

Stage 2 (systemic phase) and stage 3 (muscular encystment phase)
♦ Edema (especially of the eyelids or face)
♦ Muscle pain
♦ Itching and burning skin
♦ Sweating
♦ Skin lesions
♦ Fever
♦ Delirium and lethargy in severe respiratory, cardiovascular, or CNS infection

♦ Stools may contain mature worms and larvae during the invasion stage.
♦ Skeletal muscle biopsies can show encysted larvae 10 days after ingestion.
♦ Skin testing may show a positive histaminelike reactivity.
♦ Elevated acute and convalescent antibody titers confirm the diagnosis.
♦ Serology results indicate elevated aspartate aminotransferase, alanine aminotransferase, creatine kinase, and lactate dehydrogenase levels during the acute stages and an elevated eosinophil count.
♦ Lumbar puncture demonstrates CNS involvement with normal or elevated CSF lymphocytes and increased protein levels.

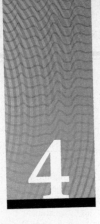

FLUIDS AND ELECTROLYTES

The body is mostly liquid — various electrolytes dissolved in water. Electrolytes are ions (electrically charged versions) of essential elements — predominantly sodium (Na^+), chloride (Cl^-), hydrogen (H^+), bicarbonate (HCO_3^-), calcium (Ca^{2+}), potassium (K^+), sulfate (SO_4^{2-}), magnesium (Mg^+), and phosphate (PO_4^{3-}). Only ionic forms of elements can dissolve or combine with other elements. Electrolyte balance must remain in a narrow range for the body to function. The kidneys maintain chemical balance throughout the body by producing and eliminating urine. They regulate the volume, electrolyte concentration, and acid-base balance of body fluids; detoxify and eliminate wastes; and regulate blood pressure by regulating fluid volume. The skin and lungs also play a role in fluid and electrolyte balance. Sweating results in loss of sodium and water; every breath contains water vapor.

Fluid balance

The kidneys maintain fluid balance in the body by regulating the amount and components of fluid inside and around the cells.

INTRACELLULAR FLUID

The fluid inside each cell is called *intracellular fluid* (ICF). Each cell has its own mixture of components in ICF, but the amounts of these substances are similar in every cell. ICF contains large amounts of potassium, magnesium, and phosphate ions.

EXTRACELLULAR FLUID

The fluid in the spaces outside the cells, called *extracellular fluid* (ECF), is constantly moving. Normally, ECF includes blood plasma and interstitial fluid (the fluid between cells in tissues); in some pathologic states it accumulates around organs in the chest or abdomen (sometimes referred to as third spacing). However, this fluid isn't available to expand ICF.

ECF is rapidly transported through the body by circulating blood and between blood and tissue fluids by fluid and electrolyte exchange across the capillary walls. It contains large amounts of sodium, chloride, and bicarbonate ions, plus such cell nutrients as oxygen, glucose, fatty acids, and amino acids. ECF also contains carbon dioxide, transported from the cells to the lungs for excretion, and other cellular products, transported from the cells to the kidneys for excretion.

The kidneys maintain the volume and composition of ECF and, to a lesser extent, ICF by continually exchanging water and ionic solutes, such as hydrogen, sodium, potassium, chloride, bicarbonate, sulfate, and phosphate ions, across the cell membranes of the renal tubules.

FLUID EXCHANGE

Two sets of forces determine the exchange of fluid between blood plasma and interstitial fluid. All four forces act to equalize concentrations of fluids, electrolytes, and proteins on both sides of the capillary wall.

Forces that tend to move fluid from the vessels to the interstitial fluid include:

◆ hydrostatic pressure of blood (the outward pressure of plasma against the walls of capillaries)
◆ osmotic pressure of tissue fluid (the tendency of ions to move across a semipermeable membrane—the capillary wall—from an area of greater concentration to one of lower concentration).

Forces that tend to move fluid into vessels include:
◆ oncotic pressure of plasma proteins (similar to osmosis, but because proteins can't cross the vessel wall, they attract fluid into the area of greater concentration)
◆ hydrostatic pressure of interstitial fluid (inward pressure against the capillary walls).

Hydrostatic pressure at the arteriolar end of the capillary bed is greater than it is at the venular end. Oncotic pressure of plasma increases slightly at the venular end as fluid escapes. When the endothelial barrier (capillary wall) is normal and intact, fluid escapes at the arteriolar end of the capillary bed and is returned at the venular end. The small amount of fluid lost from the capillaries into the interstitial tissue spaces is drained off through the lymphatic system and returned to the bloodstream.

Acid-base balance

Regulation of the extracellular fluid environment involves the ratio of acid to base, measured clinically as pH. In physiology, all positively charged ions are acids and all negatively charged ions are bases. To regulate acid-base balance, the kidneys secrete hydrogen ions (acid), reabsorb sodium (acid) and bicarbonate ions (base), acidify phosphate salts, and produce ammonium ions (acid). This keeps blood at its normal pH of 7.35 to 7.45. The following are important pH boundaries:
◆ less than 6.8 = incompatible with life
◆ less than 7.2 = cell function seriously impaired
◆ less than 7.35 = acidosis
◆ 7.35 to 7.45 = normal
◆ greater than 7.45 = alkalosis
◆ greater than 7.55 = cell function seriously impaired
◆ greater than 7.8 = incompatible with life.

Pathophysiologic changes in electrolyte imbalance

The regulation of intracellular and extracellular electrolyte concentrations depends on:

◆ balance between the intake of substances containing electrolytes and the output of electrolytes in urine, stool, and sweat
◆ transport of fluid and electrolytes between ECF and ICF.

Fluid imbalance occurs when regulatory mechanisms can't compensate for abnormal intake and output at any level from the cell to the organism. Fluid and electrolyte imbalances include edema, isotonic alterations, hypertonic alterations, hypotonic alterations, and electrolyte imbalances. Disorders of fluid volume or osmolarity (concentration of electrolytes in the fluid) result. Many conditions also affect capillary exchange, resulting in fluid shifts.

EDEMA

Despite almost constant interchange through the endothelial barrier, the body maintains a steady state of extracellular water balance between the plasma and interstitial fluid. Increased fluid volume in the interstitial spaces is called *edema,* and is classified as localized or systemic. Obstruction of the veins or lymphatic system or increased vascular permeability usually causes localized edema in the affected area such as the swelling around an injury. Systemic, or generalized, edema may be due to heart failure or renal disease. Massive systemic edema is called *anasarca.*

Edema results from abnormal expansion of the interstitial fluid or the accumulation of fluid in a third space, such as the peritoneum (ascites), pleural cavity (hydrothorax), or pericardial sac (pericardial effusion). (See *Causes of edema,* page 76.)

TONICITY

Many fluid and electrolyte disorders are classified according to how they affect osmotic pressure, or tonicity. Tonicity describes the relative concentrations of electrolytes (osmotic pressure) on both sides of a semipermeable membrane (the cell wall or the capillary wall). The word *normal* in this context refers to the usual electrolyte concentration of physiologic fluids. Normal saline has a sodium chloride concentration of 0.9%.
◆ Isotonic solutions have the same electrolyte concentration and therefore the same osmotic pressure as ECF.
◆ Hypertonic solutions have a greater-than-normal concentration of some essential electrolyte, usually sodium.
◆ Hypotonic solutions have a lower-than-normal concentration of some essential electrolyte, also usually sodium.

Causes of edema

Edema results when excess fluid accumulates in the interstitial spaces. This chart shows the causes and effects of this fluid accumulation.

Cause	Underlying condition
Hypoproteinemia	Cirrhosis Gastroenteropathy Malnutrition Nephrotic syndrome
Increased endothelial permeability	Allergic or immunologic reactions Burns Inflammation Trauma
Increased hydrostatic pressure	Cirrhosis Constrictive pericarditis Heart failure Venous thrombosis
Lymphatic obstruction	Cancer Inflammatory scarring Radiation
Sodium retention	Excessive salt intake Increased tubular reabsorption of sodium Reduced renal perfusion

Isotonic alterations

Isotonic alterations or disorders don't make the cells swell or shrink because osmosis doesn't occur. They occur when ICF and ECF have equal osmotic pressure, but there's a dramatic change in total-body fluid volume. Examples include blood loss from penetrating trauma or expansion of fluid volume if a patient receives too much normal saline solution.

Hypertonic alterations

Hypertonic alterations occur when ECF is more concentrated than ICF. Water flows out of the cell through the semipermeable cell membrane, causing cell shrinkage. This shrinkage can occur when a patient is given hypertonic (greater than 0.9%) saline, when severe dehydration causes hypernatremia (high sodium concentration in blood), or when renal disease causes sodium retention.

Hypotonic alterations

When ECF becomes hypotonic, osmotic pressure forces some ECF into the cells, causing them to swell. Overhydration is the most common cause; as water dilutes ECF, it becomes hypotonic with respect to ICF. Water moves into the cells until balance is restored. In extreme hypotonicity, cells may swell until they burst and die.

ALTERATIONS IN ELECTROLYTE BALANCE

Major electrolytes include the cations (positively charged ions) sodium, potassium, calcium, and magnesium and the anions (negatively charged ions) chloride, phosphate, and bicarbonate. The body continuously attempts to maintain intracellular and extracellular equilibrium of electrolytes. Too much or too little of any electrolyte will affect most body systems.

Sodium and potassium

Sodium is the major cation in ECF, and potassium is the major cation in ICF. Especially in nerves and muscles, communication within and between cells involves changes (repolarization and depolarization) in surface charge on the cell membrane. During repolarization, an active transport mechanism in the cell membrane, called the *sodium-potassium pump*, continually shifts sodium into and potassium out of cells; during depolarization, the process is reversed.

Fluid and electrolyte implications of blood pressure findings

Blood pressure reflects changes in fluid and electrolyte status.

Blood pressure	Fluid and electrolyte status
Normal	◆ Hemodynamic stability ◆ Initial hemodynamic instability
Hypotension	◆ Fluid volume deficit ◆ Potassium imbalance ◆ Calcium imbalance ◆ Magnesium imbalance ◆ Acidosis
Hypertension	◆ Fluid volume excess ◆ Hypernatremia

Physiologic roles of sodium cations include:
◆ maintaining tonicity of ECF
◆ regulating acid-base balance by renal reabsorption of sodium ion (base) and excretion of hydrogen ion (acid)
◆ facilitating nerve conduction and neuromuscular function
◆ facilitating glandular secretion
◆ maintaining water balance.

Physiologic roles of potassium include:
◆ maintaining cell electrical neutrality
◆ facilitating cardiac muscle contraction and electrical conductivity
◆ facilitating neuromuscular transmission of nerve impulses
◆ maintaining acid-base balance.

Calcium

Calcium is indispensable in cell permeability, bone and teeth formation, blood coagulation, nerve impulse transmission, and normal muscle contraction. Hypocalcemia can cause tetany and seizures; hypercalcemia can cause cardiac arrhythmias and coma.

Magnesium

Magnesium is present in a smaller quantity, but physiologically it's as significant as the other major electrolytes. Its major function is to enhance neuromuscular communication. Other functions include: ·
◆ stimulating parathyroid hormone secretion, which regulates intracellular calcium
◆ activating many enzymes in carbohydrate and protein metabolism
◆ facilitating cell metabolism

◆ facilitating sodium, potassium, and calcium transport across cell membranes
◆ facilitating protein transport.

Chloride

Chloride is mainly an extracellular anion; it accounts for two-thirds of all serum anions. Secreted by the stomach mucosa as hydrochloric acid, it provides an acid medium for digestion and enzyme activation. Chloride also:
◆ helps maintain acid-base and water balances
◆ influences the tonicity of ECF
◆ facilitates exchange of oxygen and carbon dioxide in red blood cells
◆ helps activate salivary amylase, which triggers the digestive process.

Phosphate

The anion phosphate is involved in cellular metabolism as well as neuromuscular regulation and hematologic function. Phosphate reabsorption in the renal tubules is inversely related to the calcium level, which means that an increase in urinary phosphorus triggers calcium reabsorption and vice versa.

EFFECTS OF ELECTROLYTE IMBALANCE

Electrolyte imbalances can affect all body systems. Too much or too little potassium or too little calcium or magnesium can increase the excitability of the cardiac muscle, causing arrhythmias. Multiple neurologic symptoms may result from electrolyte imbalance, ranging from disorientation or confusion to a completely depressed central nervous system. Too much or too little sodium or too much potassium can cause

oliguria. Blood pressure may be increased or decreased. (See *Fluid and electrolyte implications of blood pressure findings*.) The GI tract is particularly susceptible to electrolyte imbalance:
♦ too much potassium — abdominal cramps, nausea, and diarrhea
♦ too little potassium — paralytic ileus
♦ too much magnesium — nausea, vomiting, and diarrhea
♦ too much calcium — nausea, vomiting, and constipation.

Disorders of fluid and electrolyte balance

Fluid and electrolyte balance is essential for health. Many factors, such as illness, injury, (from trauma or burns), medications, nutritional imbalance, surgery, and treatments, can disrupt a patient's fluid and electrolyte balance. Even a patient with a minor illness is at risk for fluid and electrolyte imbalance. (See *Electrolyte imbalances*, pages 79 to 81.)

HYPOVOLEMIA
Water content of the human body progressively decreases from birth to old age, as follows:
♦ in neonates, as much as 75% of body weight
♦ in adults, about 60% of body weight
♦ in elderly patients, about 55%.
Most of the decrease occurs in the first 10 years of life. Hypovolemia, or extracellular fluid (ECF) volume deficit, is the isotonic loss of body fluids — that is, relatively equal losses of sodium and water.

AGE ALERT *Infants are at risk for hypovolemia because their bodies need to have a higher proportion of water to total body weight.*

Causes
Excessive fluid loss, reduced fluid intake, third-space fluid shift, or a combination of these factors can cause ECF volume loss.
Causes of fluid loss include:
♦ abdominal surgery
♦ diabetes mellitus with polyuria or diabetes insipidus
♦ excessive diuretic therapy
♦ excessive perspiration
♦ excessive use of laxatives
♦ fever
♦ fistulas
♦ hemorrhage
♦ nasogastric drainage
♦ renal failure with polyuria
♦ vomiting or diarrhea.
Possible causes of reduced fluid intake include:
♦ coma

♦ dysphagia
♦ environmental conditions preventing fluid intake
♦ psychiatric illness.
Fluid shift may be related to:
♦ acute intestinal obstruction
♦ acute peritonitis
♦ burns (during the initial phase)
♦ crushing injury
♦ hip or pelvic fracture (1.5 to 2 L of blood may accumulate in tissues around the fracture)
♦ pancreatitis
♦ pleural effusion.

Pathophysiology
Hypovolemia is an isotonic disorder. Fluid volume deficit decreases capillary hydrostatic pressure and fluid transport. Cells are deprived of normal nutrients that serve as substrates for energy production, metabolism, and other cellular functions. Decreased renal blood flow triggers the renin-angiotensin system to increase sodium and water reabsorption. The cardiovascular system compensates by increasing heart rate, cardiac contractility, venous constriction, and systemic vascular resistance, thus increasing cardiac output and mean arterial pressure. Hypovolemia also triggers the thirst response, releasing more antidiuretic hormone and producing more aldosterone.
When compensation fails, hypovolemic shock occurs in this sequence:
♦ decreased intravascular fluid volume
♦ diminished venous return, which reduces preload and decreases stroke volume
♦ reduced cardiac output
♦ decreased mean arterial pressure
♦ impaired tissue perfusion
♦ decreased oxygen and nutrient delivery to cells
♦ multisystem organ failure.

Signs and symptoms
Signs and symptoms depend on the amount of fluid loss. (See *Estimating fluid loss*, page 82.) These may include:
♦ orthostatic hypotension due to increased systemic vascular resistance and decreased cardiac output
♦ tachycardia induced by the sympathetic nervous system to increase cardiac output and mean arterial pressure
♦ thirst to prompt ingestion of fluid (increased ECF osmolality stimulates the thirst center in the hypothalamus)

AGE ALERT *Elderly patients have a diminished thirst sensitivity due to aging. As a result, they may not realize their need for fluid, predisposing them to further hypervolemia. Check for signs of deficient fluid volume in these patients by looking for dry mouth and longitudinal furrows over the tongue.*

Electrolyte imbalances

Signs and symptoms of electrolyte imbalance are often subtle. Blood chemistry tests help diagnose and evaluate electrolyte imbalances.

Electrolyte imbalance	Signs and symptoms	Diagnostic test results
Hyponatremia	♦ Muscle twitching and weakness due to osmotic swelling of cells ♦ Lethargy, confusion, seizures, and coma due to altered neurotransmission ♦ Hypotension and tachycardia due to decreased extracellular circulating volume ♦ Nausea, vomiting, and abdominal cramps due to edema affecting receptors in the brain or vomiting center of the brain stem ♦ Oliguria or anuria due to renal dysfunction	♦ Serum sodium < 135 mEq/L ♦ Decreased urine specific gravity ♦ Decreased serum osmolality ♦ Urine sodium > 100 mEq/24 hours ♦ Increased red blood cell count
Hypernatremia	♦ Agitation, restlessness, fever, and decreased level of consciousness due to altered cellular metabolism ♦ Hypertension, tachycardia, pitting edema, and excessive weight gain due to water shift from intracellular to extracellular fluid ♦ Thirst, increased viscosity of saliva, rough tongue due to fluid shift ♦ Dyspnea, respiratory arrest, and death from dramatic increase in osmotic pressure	♦ Serum sodium > 145 mEq/L ♦ Urine sodium < 40 mEq/24 hours ♦ High serum osmolality
Hypokalemia	♦ Dizziness, hypotension, arrhythmias, electrocardiogram (ECG) changes, and cardiac arrest due to changes in membrane excitability ♦ Nausea, vomiting, anorexia, diarrhea, decreased peristalsis, and abdominal distention due to decreased bowel motility ♦ Muscle weakness, fatigue, and leg cramps due to decreased neuromuscular excitability	♦ Serum potassium < 3.5 mEq/L ♦ Coexisting low serum calcium and magnesium levels not responsive to treatment for hypokalemia usually suggest hypomagnesemia ♦ Metabolic alkalosis ♦ ECG changes include flattened T waves, elevated U waves, depressed ST segment
Hyperkalemia	♦ Tachycardia changing to bradycardia, ECG changes, and cardiac arrest due to hypopolarization and alterations in repolarization ♦ Nausea, diarrhea, and abdominal cramps due to smooth-muscle hyperactivity in the GI tract ♦ Muscle weakness and flaccid paralysis due to inactivation of membrane sodium channels	♦ Serum potassium > 5 mEq/L ♦ Metabolic acidosis ♦ ECG changes include tented and elevated T waves, widened QRS complex, prolonged PR interval, flattened or absent P waves, depressed ST segment
Hypochloremia	♦ Muscle hypertonicity and tetany due to increased neuromuscular irritability ♦ Shallow, depressed breathing as the body attempts to compensate for alkalosis ♦ Usually associated with hyponatremia and its characteristic symptoms, such as muscle weakness and twitching	♦ Serum chloride < 98 mEq/L ♦ Serum pH > 7.45 (supportive value) ♦ Serum carbon dioxide (CO_2) > 32 mEq/L (supportive value)

(continued)

Electrolyte imbalances *(continued)*

Electrolyte imbalance	Signs and symptoms	Diagnostic test results
Hyperchloremia	♦ Major signs and symptoms are due to metabolic acidosis ♦ Deep, rapid breathing ♦ Weakness ♦ Diminished cognitive ability, possibly leading to coma	♦ Serum chloride > 108 mEq/L ♦ Serum pH < 7.35, serum CO_2 < 22 mEq/L (supportive values)
Hypocalcemia	♦ Anxiety, irritability, twitching around the mouth, laryngospasm, seizures, positive Chvostek's and Trousseau's signs due to enhanced neuromuscular irritability ♦ Hypotension and arrhythmias due to decreased calcium influx	♦ Serum calcium < 8.5 mg/dl ♦ Low platelet count ♦ ECG shows lengthened QT interval, prolonged ST segment, arrhythmias ♦ Possible changes in serum protein because half of serum calcium is bound to albumin
Hypercalcemia	♦ Drowsiness, lethargy, headaches, irritability, confusion, depression, or apathy due to decreased neuromuscular irritability (increased threshold) ♦ Weakness and muscle flaccidity due to depressed neuromuscular irritability and release of acetylcholine at the myoneural junction ♦ Bone pain and pathological fractures due to calcium loss from bones ♦ Heart block due to decreased neuromuscular irritability ♦ Anorexia, nausea, vomiting, constipation, and dehydration due to hyperosmolarity ♦ Flank pain due to kidney stone formation	♦ Serum calcium > 10.5 mg/dl ♦ ECG shows signs of heart block and shortened QT interval ♦ Azotemia ♦ Decreased parathyroid hormone level ♦ Sulkowitch urine test shows increased calcium precipitation
Hypomagnesemia	♦ Nearly always coexists with hypokalemia and hypocalcemia ♦ Hyperirritability, tetany, leg and foot cramps, positive Chvostek's and Trousseau's signs, confusion, delusions, and seizures due to alteration in neuromuscular transmission ♦ Arrhythmias, vasodilation, and hypotension due to enhanced inward sodium current or concurrent effects of calcium and potassium imbalance	♦ Serum magnesium < 1.5 mEq/L ♦ Coexisting low serum potassium and calcium levels
Hypermagnesemia	♦ Hypermagnesemia is uncommon, caused by decreased renal excretion (renal failure) or increased intake of magnesium ♦ Diminished reflexes, muscle weakness to flaccid paralysis due to suppression of acetylcholine release at the myoneural junction, blocking neuromuscular transmission and reducing cell excitablity ♦ Respiratory distress secondary to respiratory muscle paralysis	♦ Serum magnesium > 2.5 mEq/L ♦ Coexisting elevated potassium and calcium levels

Electrolyte imbalances *(continued)*

Electrolyte imbalance	Signs and symptoms	Diagnostic test results
	♦ Heart block, bradycardia due to decreased inward sodium current ♦ Hypotension due to relaxation of vascular smooth muscle and reduction of vascular resistance by displacing calcium from the vascular wall surface	
Hypophosphatemia	♦ Muscle weakness, tremor, and paresthesia due to deficiency of adenosine triphosphate ♦ Peripheral hypoxia due to 2,3-diphosphoglycerate deficiency	♦ Serum phosphate < 2.5 mg/dl ♦ Urine phosphate > 1.3 g/ 24 hours
Hyperphosphatemia	♦ Usually asymptomatic unless leading to hypocalcemia, with tetany and seizures	♦ Serum phosphate > 4.5 mg/dl ♦ Serum calcium < 9 mg/dl ♦ Urine phosphorus < 0.9 g/ 24 hours

♦ flattened neck veins due to decreased circulating blood volume
♦ sunken eyeballs due to decreased volume of total-body fluid and consequent dehydration of connective tissue and aqueous humor
♦ dry mucous membranes due to decreased body fluid volume (glands that produce fluids to moisten and protect the vascular mucous membranes fail, so they dry rapidly)
♦ diminished skin turgor due to decreased fluid in the dermal layer (making skin less pliant)
♦ rapid weight loss due to acute loss of body fluid

AGE ALERT *In infants younger than age 4 months with hypovolemia, the posterior and anterior fontanels are sunken when palpated. Between ages 4 and 18 months, the posterior fontanel is normally closed; however, in infants with hypovolemia, the anterior fontanel is sunken.*

♦ decreased urine output due to decreased renal perfusion from renal vasoconstriction
♦ prolonged capillary refill time due to increased systemic vascular resistance.

Complications
♦ Shock
♦ Acute renal failure
♦ Death

Diagnosis
No single diagnostic finding confirms hypovolemia, but these diagnostic test results are suggestive:
♦ Increased blood urea nitrogen level (early sign)
♦ Elevated serum creatinine level (late sign)

♦ Increased serum protein, hemoglobin, and hematocrit (unless caused by hemorrhage, when loss of blood elements causes subnormal values)
♦ Rising blood glucose level
♦ Elevated serum osmolality; except in hyponatremia, where serum osmolality is low
♦ Serum electrolyte and arterial blood gas analysis may reflect associated clinical problems due to underlying cause of hypovolemia or treatment regimen

If the patient has no underlying renal disorder, typical urinalysis findings include:
♦ Urine specific gravity greater than 1.030
♦ Increased urine osmolality
♦ Urine sodium level less than 50 mEq/L

Treatment
♦ Oral fluids (may be adequate in mild hypovolemia if the patient is alert enough to swallow and can tolerate it)
♦ Parenteral fluids to supplement or replace oral therapy (moderate to severe hypovolemia; choice of parenteral fluid depends on type of fluids lost, severity of hypovolemia, and patient's cardiovascular, electrolyte, and acid-base status)
♦ Fluid resuscitation by rapid I.V. administration (severe volume depletion; depending on patient's condition, 100 to 500 ml of fluid over 15 minutes to 1 hour; fluid bolus may be given more quickly if needed)
♦ Blood or blood products (with hemorrhage)
♦ An antidiarrheal as needed
♦ An antiemetic as needed

Estimating fluid loss

The following assessment parameters indicate the severity of fluid loss.

Minimal fluid loss
Intravascular volume loss of 10% to 15% is considered minimal. Signs and symptoms include:
◆ slight tachycardia
◆ normal supine blood pressure
◆ positive postural vital signs, including a decrease in systolic blood pressure more than 10 mm Hg or an increase in pulse rate more than 20 beats/minute
◆ increased capillary refill time (> 3 seconds)
◆ urine output greater than 30 ml/hour
◆ cool, pale skin on arms and legs
◆ anxiety.

Moderate fluid loss
Intravascular volume loss of about 25% is considered moderate. Signs and symptoms include:
◆ rapid, thready pulse
◆ supine hypotension
◆ cool truncal skin
◆ urine output of 10 to 30 ml/hour
◆ severe thirst
◆ restlessness, confusion, or irritability.

Severe fluid loss
Intravascular volume loss of 40% or more is considered severe. Signs and symptoms include:
◆ marked tachycardia
◆ marked hypotension
◆ weak or absent peripheral pulses
◆ cold, mottled, or cyanotic skin
◆ urine output less than 10 ml/hour
◆ unconsciousness.

◆ I.V. dopamine (Intropin) or norepinephrine (Levophed) to increase cardiac contractility and renal perfusion (if patient remains symptomatic after fluid replacement)
◆ Oxygen therapy to ensure sufficient tissue perfusion
◆ Autotransfusion (for some patients with hypovolemia caused by trauma)

Special considerations
◆ I.V. infusions should be started with the shortest, largest-bore catheters possible be-cause they offer less resistance to fluid flow than that of long, thin catheters.
◆ The patient's mental status and vital signs should be monitored closely, including orthostatic blood pressure measurements when appropriate.
◆ If the blood pressure doesn't respond to interventions as expected, the patient should be reassessed for a bleeding site that may have been missed. (Remember, a patient can lose a large amount of blood internally from a fractured hip or pelvis.)

HYPERVOLEMIA
The expansion of extracellular fluid (ECF) volume, called *hypervolemia*, may involve the interstitial or intravascular space. Hypervolemia develops when excess sodium and water are retained in about the same proportions. It's always secondary to an increase in total-body sodium content, which causes water retention. Usually, the body can compensate and restore fluid balance.

Causes
Conditions that increase the risk of sodium and water retention include:
◆ cirrhosis of the liver
◆ corticosteroid therapy
◆ heart failure
◆ low dietary protein intake
◆ nephrotic syndrome
◆ renal failure.
  Sources of excessive sodium and water intake include:
◆ blood or plasma replacement
◆ dietary intake of water, sodium chloride, or other salts
◆ parenteral fluid replacement with normal saline or lactated Ringer's solution.
  Fluid shift to the ECF compartment may follow:
◆ colloid oncotic fluids such as albumin
◆ hypertonic fluids, such as mannitol (Osmitrol) or hypertonic saline solution
◆ remobilization of fluid after burn treatment.

Pathophysiology
Increased ECF volume causes this sequence of events:
◆ circulatory overload
◆ increased cardiac contractility and mean arterial pressure
◆ increased capillary hydrostatic pressure
◆ shift of fluid to the interstitial space
◆ edema.
  Elevated mean arterial pressure inhibits secretion of antidiuretic hormone and aldosterone and consequent increased urinary elimination of water and sodium. These compensatory

mechanisms usually restore normal intravascular volume. If hypervolemia is severe or prolonged or the patient has a history of cardiovascular dysfunction, compensatory mechanisms may fail, and heart failure and pulmonary edema may ensue.

Signs and symptoms
◆ Rapid breathing due to fewer red blood cells per milliliter of blood (dilution causes a compensatory increase in respiratory rate to increase oxygenation)
◆ Dyspnea (labored breathing) due to increased fluid volume in pleural spaces
◆ Crackles (gurgling or bubbling sounds on auscultation) due to elevated hydrostatic pressure in pulmonary capillaries
◆ Rapid, bounding pulse due to increased cardiac contractility (from circulatory overload)
◆ Hypertension (unless heart is failing) due to circulatory overload (causes increased mean arterial pressure)
◆ Distended neck veins due to increased blood volume and increased preload
◆ Moist skin (compensatory to increase water excretion through perspiration)
◆ Acute weight gain due to increased volume of total-body fluid from circulatory overload (best indicator of ECF volume excess)
◆ Edema (increased mean arterial pressure leads to increased capillary hydrostatic pressure, causing fluid shift from plasma to interstitial spaces)
◆ S_3 gallop (abnormal heart sound due to rapid filling and volume overload of the ventricles during diastole)

Complications
◆ Skin breakdown
◆ Acute pulmonary edema with hypoxemia

Diagnosis
No single diagnostic test confirms the disorder, but these findings indicate hypervolemia:
◆ Decreased serum potassium and blood urea nitrogen (BUN) levels due to hemodilution (increased serum potassium and BUN levels usually indicate renal failure or impaired renal perfusion)
◆ Decreased hematocrit due to hemodilution
◆ Normal serum sodium (unless associated sodium imbalance is present)
◆ Low urine sodium excretion (usually less than 10 mEq/day because the edematous patient is retaining sodium or because cardiovascular dysfunction is triggering sodium resorption in the kidneys)

◆ Increased hemodynamic values (including pulmonary artery, pulmonary artery wedge, and central venous pressures)

Treatment
◆ Restricted sodium and water intake
◆ Preload reduction agents, such as morphine, furosemide (Lasix), and nitroglycerin (Nitro-Bid), and afterload reduction agents, such as hydralazine (Apresoline) and captopril (Capoten) for pulmonary edema

⚠ **CLINICAL ALERT** *Carefully monitor I.V. fluid administration rate and patient response, especially in elderly patients or those with impaired cardiac or renal function, who are particularly vulnerable to acute pulmonary edema.*

For severe hypervolemia or renal failure, the patient may undergo renal replacement therapy, including:
◆ hemodialysis or peritoneal dialysis
◆ continuous arteriovenous hemofiltration (allows removal of excess fluid from critically ill patients who may not need dialysis; the patient's arterial pressure serves as a natural pump, driving blood through the arterial line)
◆ continuous venovenous hemofiltration (similar to arteriovenous hemofiltration, but a mechanical pump is used when mean arterial pressure is less than 60 mm Hg).

Supportive measures include:
◆ oxygen administration
◆ use of thromboembolic disease support hose to help mobilize edematous fluid
◆ bed rest with head of bed elevated
◆ treatment of underlying condition that caused or contributed to hypervolemia.

Special considerations
◆ If the patient is prone to hypervolemia, an infusion pump should be used with any infusions to prevent the administration of too much fluid.
◆ The patient's vital signs and hemodynamic status should be assessed to note his response to therapy. Signs of hypovolemia indicate overcorrection. Elderly, pediatric, and otherwise compromised patients are at higher risk for complications with therapy.
◆ If the patient with hypervolemia isn't responding to diuretic therapy, his kidney function may be impaired. Dialysis is typically the next step. If the patient can't tolerate dialysis, continuous arteriovenous hemofiltration may be used.

Pathophysiologic changes in acid-base imbalance

Acid-base balance is essential to life. Concepts related to imbalance include acidemia, acidosis, alkalemia, alkalosis, and compensation.

ACIDEMIA

Acidemia is an arterial pH of less than 7.35, which reflects a relative excess of acid in the blood. The hydrogen ion content in extracellular fluid (ECF) increases, and the hydrogen ions move to the intracellular fluid (ICF). To keep ICF electrically neutral, an equal amount of potassium leaves the cell, creating relative hyperkalemia.

ACIDOSIS

Acidosis is a systemic increase in hydrogen ion concentration. If the lungs fail to eliminate carbon dioxide (CO_2) or if volatile (carbonic) or nonvolatile (lactic) acid products of metabolism accumulate, hydrogen ion concentration rises. Acidosis can also occur if persistent diarrhea causes loss of basic bicarbonate anions or the kidneys fail to reabsorb bicarbonate or secrete hydrogen ions.

ALKALEMIA

Alkalemia is arterial blood pH greater than 7.45, which reflects a relative excess of base in the blood. In alkalemia, an excess of hydrogen ions in the ICF forces them into the ECF. To keep ICF electrically neutral, potassium moves from ECF to ICF, creating a relative hypokalemia.

ALKALOSIS

Alkalosis is a bodywide decrease in hydrogen ion concentration. An excessive loss of CO_2 during hyperventilation, loss of nonvolatile acids during vomiting, or excessive ingestion of base may decrease hydrogen ion concentration.

COMPENSATION

The lungs and kidneys, along with a number of chemical buffer systems in the intracellular and extracellular compartments, work together to maintain plasma pH in the range of 7.35 to 7.45 (through mechanisms of compensation). For a description of acid-base values and compensatory mechanisms, see *Interpreting arterial blood gas values*.

Buffer systems

A buffer system consists of a weak acid (that doesn't readily release free hydrogen ions) and a corresponding base such as sodium bicarbonate. These buffers resist or minimize a change in pH when an acid or base is added to the buffered solution. Buffers work in seconds.

The four major buffers or buffer systems include:
◆ carbonic acid–bicarbonate system (the most important, works in lungs)
◆ hemoglobin–oxyhemoglobin system (works in red blood cells) hemoglobin binds free hydrogen, blood flows through lungs, hydrogen combines with CO_2
◆ other protein buffers (in ECF and ICF)
◆ phosphate system (primarily in ICF).

When primary disease processes alter either the acid or base component of the ratio, the lungs or kidneys (whichever isn't affected by the disease process) act to restore the ratio and normalize pH. Because the body's mechanisms that regulate pH occur in stepwise fashion over time, the body tolerates gradual changes in pH better than abrupt ones.

Kidney compensation

If a respiratory disorder causes acidosis or alkalosis, the kidneys respond by altering their handling of hydrogen and bicarbonate ions to return the pH to normal. Renal compensation begins hours to days after a respiratory alteration in pH. Despite this delay, renal compensation is powerful.
◆ Acidemia — the kidneys excrete excess hydrogen ions, which may combine with phosphate or ammonia to form titratable acids in the urine. The net effect is to *raise* the concentration of bicarbonate ions in the ECF and so restore acid-base balance.
◆ Alkalemia — the kidneys excrete excess bicarbonate ions, usually with sodium ions. The net effect is to *reduce* the concentration of bicarbonate ions in the ECF and restore acid-base balance.

Lung compensation

If acidosis or alkalosis results from a metabolic or renal disorder, the respiratory system regulates the respiratory rate to return the pH to normal. The partial pressure of arterial CO_2 ($Paco_2$) reflects CO_2 levels proportionate to blood pH. As the concentration of the gas increases, so does its partial pressure. Within minutes after the slightest change in $Paco_2$, central chemoreceptors in the medulla that regulate the rate and depth of ventilation detect the change.
◆ Acidemia increases respiratory rate and depth to eliminate CO_2.
◆ Alkalemia decreases respiratory rate and depth to retain CO_2.

Interpreting arterial blood gas values

This chart compares abnormal arterial blood gas values and their significance for patient care.

	pH	Paco$_2$ (mm Hg)	HCO$_3^-$ (mEq/L)	Compensation
Normal	7.35 to 7.45	35 to 45	22 to 26	
Respiratory acidosis	< 7.35	> 45	◆ Acute: may be normal ◆ Chronic: > 26	◆ Renal: increased secretion and excretion of acid; compensation takes 24 hours to begin ◆ Respiratory: rate increases to expel CO$_2$
Respiratory alkalosis	> 7.45	< 35	◆ Acute: may be normal ◆ Chronic: < 22	◆ Renal: decreased H$^+$ secretion and active secretion of HCO$_3^-$ into urine
Metabolic acidosis	< 7.35	< 35	< 22	◆ Respiratory: lungs expel more CO$_2$ by increasing rate and depth of respirations ◆ Renal: increased H$^+$ (acid) secretion and resoprtion of HCO$_3^-$ (base) from the renal tubules
Metabolic alkalosis	> 7.45	> 45	> 26	◆ Respiratory: hypoventilation is immediate but limited because of ensuing hypoxemia ◆ Renal: more effective but slow to excrete less acid and more base

Disorders of acid-base balance

Acid-base disturbances can cause respiratory acidosis or alkalosis or metabolic acidosis or alkalosis.

RESPIRATORY ACIDOSIS

Respiratory acidosis is an acid-base disturbance characterized by reduced alveolar ventilation. The patient's pulmonary system can't clear enough carbon dioxide (CO$_2$) from the body. This leads to hypercapnia (partial pressure of arterial carbon dioxide [Paco$_2$] greater than 45 mm Hg) and acidosis (pH less than 7.35). Respiratory acidosis can be acute (due to a sudden failure in ventilation) or chronic (in long-term pulmonary disease). Any compromise in the essential components of breathing — ventilation, perfusion, and diffusion — may cause respiratory acidosis.

Prognosis depends on the severity of the underlying disturbance as well as the patient's general clinical condition. The prognosis is least optimistic for a patient with a debilitating disorder.

Causes

◆ Airway obstruction or parenchymal lung disease (interferes with alveolar ventilation)
◆ Cardiac arrest (acute)
◆ Central nervous system (CNS) trauma (injury to the medulla may impair ventilatory drive)
◆ Chronic bronchitis
◆ Chronic metabolic alkalosis as respiratory compensatory mechanisms try to normalize pH by decreasing alveolar ventilation
◆ Chronic obstructive pulmonary disease (COPD) or asthma
◆ Drugs (opioids, general anesthetics, hypnotics, alcohol, and sedatives, including some of the newer "designer" drugs, such as MCMA or "ecstasy," decrease the sensitivity of the respiratory center)
◆ Extensive pneumonia
◆ Large pneumothorax
◆ Neuromuscular diseases, such as myasthenia gravis, Guillain-Barré syndrome, and

poliomyelitis (respiratory muscles can't respond properly to respiratory drive)
♦ Pulmonary edema
♦ Severe adult respiratory distress syndrome (reduced pulmonary blood flow and poor exchange of CO_2 and oxygen between the lungs and blood)
♦ Sleep apnea
♦ Ventilation therapy (use of high-flow oxygen in patients with chronic respiratory disorders suppresses the patient's hypoxic drive to breathe; high positive end-expiratory pressure in the presence of reduced cardiac output may cause hypercapnia due to large increases in alveolar dead space)

Pathophysiology

When pulmonary ventilation decreases, $Paco_2$ is increased, and the CO_2 level rises in all tissues and fluids, including the medulla and cerebrospinal fluid. Retained CO_2 combines with water to form carbonic acid. The carbonic acid dissociates to release free hydrogen and bicarbonate (HCO_3^-) ions. Increased $Paco_2$ and free hydrogen ions stimulate the medulla to increase respiratory drive and expel CO_2.

As pH falls, 2,3-diphosphoglycerate accumulates in red blood cells, where it alters hemoglobin so it releases oxygen. This reduced hemoglobin, which is strongly alkaline, picks up hydrogen ions and CO_2 and removes them from the serum.

As respiratory mechanisms fail, rising $Paco_2$ stimulates the kidneys to retain bicarbonate and sodium ions and excrete hydrogen ions. As a result, more sodium bicarbonate ($NaHCO_3$) is available to buffer free hydrogen ions. Some hydrogen is excreted in the form of ammonium ion, neutralizing ammonia, which is an important CNS toxin.

As the hydrogen ion concentration overwhelms compensatory mechanisms, hydrogen ions move into the cells and potassium ions move out. Without enough oxygen, anaerobic metabolism produces lactic acid. Electrolyte imbalances and acidosis critically depress neurologic and cardiac functions.

Signs and symptoms

Clinical features vary according to the severity and duration of respiratory acidosis, the underlying disease, and the presence of hypoxemia. CO_2 and hydrogen ions dilate cerebral blood vessels and increase blood flow to the brain, causing cerebral edema and depressing CNS activity.

Possible signs and symptoms include:
♦ restlessness or apprehension caused by hypoxemia

♦ changes in level of consciousness, such as confusion, somnolence, or coma, caused by hypoxemia
♦ headaches resulting from cerebral vasodilation
♦ fine or flapping tremor (asterixis) caused by continued elevation of CO_2 levels
♦ papilledema caused by increased intracranial pressure as a result of cerebral vasodilation
♦ depressed reflexes related to elevated CO_2 levels and CNS depression.

Respiratory acidosis may also cause cardiovascular abnormalities, including:
♦ tachycardia and hypertension, caused by sudden onset of hypercapnia and effects of hypoxemia
♦ atrial and ventricular arrhythmias secondary to development of hyperkalemia
♦ hypotension with vasodilation (bounding pulses and warm periphery, in severe acidosis).

Complications

♦ Profound CNS and cardiovascular deterioration due to dangerously low blood pH (less than 7.15)
♦ Myocardial depression (leading to shock and cardiac arrest)
♦ Elevated $Paco_2$ despite optimal treatment (in chronic lung disease)

Diagnosis

♦ Arterial blood gas (ABG) analysis, showing $Paco_2$ greater than 45 mm Hg; pH less than 7.35; and normal HCO_3^- in the acute stage and elevated HCO_3^- in the chronic stage (confirms the diagnosis)
♦ Chest X-ray (often shows such causes as heart failure, pneumonia, COPD, and pneumothorax)
♦ Potassium level greater than 5 mEq/L
♦ Low serum chloride level
♦ Acidic urine pH (as the kidneys excrete hydrogen ions to return blood pH to normal)
♦ Drug screening (may confirm suspected drug overdose)

Treatment

Effective treatment of respiratory acidosis requires correction of the underlying source of alveolar hypoventilation. Treatment of pulmonary causes of respiratory acidosis includes:
♦ removal of a foreign body from the airway
♦ artificial airway through endotracheal intubation or tracheotomy and mechanical ventilation (if the patient can't breathe spontaneously)
♦ increasing the partial pressure of arterial oxygen to at least 60 mm Hg and pH greater than 7.2 to avoid cardiac arrhythmias

◆ aerosolized or I.V. bronchodilators to open constricted airways
◆ an antibiotic to treat pneumonia
◆ chest tubes to correct pneumothorax
◆ positive end-expiratory pressure to prevent alveolar collapse
◆ thrombolytic or anticoagulant therapy for massive pulmonary emboli
◆ positioning patient to maximize air exchange
◆ bronchoscopy to remove excessive retained secretions.

Treatment for patients with COPD includes:
◆ a bronchodilator
◆ oxygen at low flow rates (more oxygen than the person's normal flow rate removes the hypoxic drive, further reducing alveolar ventilation)
◆ a corticosteroid
◆ gradual reduction in $Paco_2$ to baseline to provide sufficient chloride and potassium ions to enhance renal excretion of bicarbonate (in chronic respiratory acidosis).

Other treatments include:
◆ drug therapy for such conditions as myasthenia gravis
◆ dialysis or charcoal to remove toxic drugs
◆ correction of metabolic alkalosis
◆ careful administration of I.V. sodium bicarbonate.

Special considerations
◆ Be alert for critical changes in the patient's respiratory, CNS, and cardiovascular functions. Report such changes as well as any variations in ABG levels or electrolyte status immediately. Also, maintain adequate hydration.
◆ Maintain a patent airway and provide adequate humidification if acidosis requires mechanical ventilation. Perform tracheal suctioning regularly and vigorous chest physiotherapy if ordered. Continuously monitor ventilator settings and respiratory status.
◆ To prevent respiratory acidosis, closely monitor patients with COPD and chronic CO_2 retention for signs of acidosis. Also, administer oxygen at low flow rates.
◆ Closely monitor all patients who receive narcotics and sedatives. Instruct the patient who has received a general anesthetic to turn, cough, and perform deep-breathing exercises frequently to prevent the onset of respiratory acidosis.

RESPIRATORY ALKALOSIS
Respiratory alkalosis is an acid-base disturbance characterized by a partial pressure of arterial carbon dioxide ($Paco_2$) less than 35 mm Hg and blood pH greater than 7.45; alveolar hyperventilation is the cause. Hypocapnia (below

normal $Paco_2$) occurs when the lungs eliminate more carbon dioxide (CO_2) than the cells produce.

Respiratory alkalosis is the most common acid-base disturbance in critically ill patients and, when severe, has a poor prognosis.

Causes
◆ Pulmonary—severe hypoxemia, pneumonia, interstitial lung disease, pulmonary vascular disease, and acute asthma
◆ Nonpulmonary—anxiety, fever, aspirin toxicity, metabolic acidosis, central nervous system (CNS) disease (inflammation or tumor), sepsis, hepatic failure, and advanced pregnancy

Pathophysiology
When pulmonary ventilation increases more than needed to maintain normal CO_2 levels, excessive amounts of CO_2 are exhaled. The consequent hypocapnia leads to a chemical reduction of carbonic acid, excretion of hydrogen and bicarbonate ions, and a rising pH.

In defense against the increasing serum pH, the hydrogen-potassium buffer system pulls hydrogen ions out of the cells and into the blood in exchange for potassium ions. The hydrogen ions entering the blood combine with available bicarbonate ions to form carbonic acid, and the pH falls.

Hypocapnia stimulates the carotid and aortic bodies as well as the medulla, increasing the heart rate (which hypokalemia can further aggravate) but not the blood pressure. At the same time, hypocapnia causes cerebral vasoconstriction and decreased cerebral blood flow. It also overexcites the medulla, pons, and other parts of the autonomic nervous system. When hypocapnia lasts more than 6 hours, the kidneys secrete more bicarbonate and less hydrogen. Full renal adaptation to respiratory alkalosis requires normal volume status and renal function, and it may take several days.

Continued low $Paco_2$ and the vasoconstriction it causes increases cerebral and peripheral hypoxia. Severe alkalosis inhibits calcium ionization; as calcium ions become unavailable, nerves and muscles become progressively more excitable. Eventually, alkalosis overwhelms the CNS and heart.

Signs and symptoms
◆ Deep, rapid breathing (possibly more than 40 breaths/minute and much like the Kussmaul's respirations that characterize diabetic acidosis) usually causing CNS and neuromuscular disturbances (cardinal sign of respiratory alkalosis)

◆ Light-headedness or dizziness due to decreased cerebral blood flow
◆ Circumoral and peripheral paresthesias caused by hypokalemia
◆ Carpopedal spasms, twitching (possibly progressing to tetany), and muscle weakness caused by overstimulation of autonomic nervous system from hypocapnia

Complications
Possible complications of severe respiratory alkalosis include:
◆ cardiac arrhythmias that may not respond to conventional treatment as the hemoglobin-oxygen buffer system becomes overwhelmed
◆ hypocalcemic tetany, seizures
◆ periods of apnea if pH remains high and $Paco_2$ remains low.

Diagnosis
◆ Arterial blood gas (ABG) analysis showing $Paco_2$ less than 35 mm Hg; elevated pH in proportion to decrease in $Paco_2$ in the acute stage but decreasing toward normal in the chronic stage; normal bicarbonate (HCO_3^-) in the acute stage but less than normal in the chronic stage (confirms respiratory alkalosis, rules out respiratory compensation for metabolic acidosis)
◆ Serum electrolyte studies (detect metabolic disorders causing compensatory respiratory alkalosis)
◆ Electrocardiogram findings (may indicate cardiac arrhythmias)
◆ Low chloride (in severe respiratory alkalosis)
◆ Toxicology screening (for salicylate poisoning)
◆ Basic urine pH as kidneys excrete HCO_3^- to raise blood pH

Treatment
Possible treatments to correct the underlying condition include:
◆ removal of ingested toxins, such as salicylates, using gastric lavage
◆ treatment of fever or sepsis
◆ oxygen for acute hypoxemia
◆ treatment of CNS disease
◆ having patient breathe into a paper bag to increase CO_2 and help relieve anxiety (for hyperventilation caused by severe anxiety)
◆ adjustment of tidal volume and minute ventilation in patients on mechanical ventilation to prevent hyperventilation (by monitoring ABG analysis results).

Special considerations
◆ Watch for and report changes in neurologic, neuromuscular, or cardiovascular functions.

◆ Remember that twitching and cardiac arrhythmias may be associated with alkalemia and electrolyte imbalances. Monitor ABG and serum electrolyte levels closely, reporting any variations immediately.
◆ Explain all diagnostic tests and procedures to reduce anxiety.

METABOLIC ACIDOSIS
Metabolic acidosis is an acid-base disorder characterized by excess acid and deficient bicarbonate (HCO_3^-) caused by an underlying non-respiratory disorder. A primary decrease in plasma HCO_3^- causes pH to fall. It can occur with increased production of a nonvolatile acid (such as lactic acid), decreased renal clearance of a nonvolatile acid (as in renal failure), or loss of HCO_3^- (as in chronic diarrhea). Symptoms result from action of compensatory mechanisms in the lungs, kidneys, and cells.

AGE ALERT *In children, metabolic acidosis is more prevalent among those who are vulnerable to acid-base imbalance because their metabolic rates are rapid and ratios of water to total-body weight are low.*

Severe or untreated metabolic acidosis can be fatal. The prognosis improves with prompt treatment of the underlying cause and rapid reversal of the acidotic state.

Causes
Metabolic acidosis usually results from excessive fat metabolism in the absence of usable carbohydrates. This can be caused by diabetic ketoacidosis, chronic alcoholism, malnutrition, or a low-carbohydrate, high-fat diet—all of which produce more ketoacids than the metabolic process can handle. Other causes include:
◆ anaerobic carbohydrate metabolism (decreased tissue oxygenation or perfusion—as in cardiac pump failure after myocardial infarction, pulmonary or hepatic disease, shock, or anemia—forces a shift from aerobic to anaerobic metabolism, causing a corresponding increase in lactic acid level)
◆ diarrhea, intestinal malabsorption, or loss of sodium bicarbonate from the intestines, causing bicarbonate buffer system to shift to the acidic side (for example, ureteroenterostomy and Crohn's disease can also induce metabolic acidosis)
◆ inhibited secretion of acid due to hypoaldosteronism or the use of potassium-sparing diuretics
◆ salicylate intoxication (overuse of aspirin), exogenous poisoning or, less frequently, Addison's disease (increased excretion of sodium and chloride and retention of potassium)

◆ underexcretion of metabolized acids or inability to conserve base due to renal insufficiency and failure (renal acidosis).

Pathophysiology

As acid (hydrogen) starts to accumulate in the body, chemical buffers (plasma HCO_3^- and proteins) in the cells and extracellular fluid (ECF) bind the excess hydrogen ions.

Excess hydrogen ions that the buffers can't bind decrease blood pH and stimulate chemoreceptors in the medulla to increase respiration. The consequent fall of $Paco_2$ frees hydrogen ions to bind with HCO_3^-. Respiratory compensation occurs in minutes but isn't sufficient to correct the acidosis.

Healthy kidneys try to compensate by secreting excess hydrogen ions into the renal tubules. These ions are buffered by either phosphate or ammonia and excreted into the urine in the form of weak acid. For each hydrogen ion secreted into the renal tubules, the tubules reabsorb and return to the blood one sodium and one HCO_3^-.

The excess hydrogen ions in ECF passively diffuse into cells. To maintain the balance of charge across the membranes, the cells release potassium ions. Excess hydrogen ions change the normal balance of potassium, sodium, and calcium ions and thereby impair neural excitability.

Signs and symptoms

In mild acidosis, symptoms of the underlying disease may hide the direct clinical evidence and include:
◆ headache and lethargy progressing to drowsiness, stupor, and (if condition is severe and untreated) coma and death caused by central nervous system (CNS) depression
◆ Kussmaul's respirations (as the lungs attempt to compensate by blowing off carbon dioxide)
◆ associated GI distress leading to anorexia, nausea, vomiting, diarrhea, and possibly dehydration
◆ warm, flushed skin due to a pH-sensitive decrease in vascular response to sympathetic stimuli
◆ fruity-smelling breath from fat catabolism and excretion of accumulated acetone through the lungs due to underlying diabetes mellitus.

Complications

Metabolic acidosis depresses the CNS and, if untreated, may lead to:
◆ weakness, flaccid paralysis
◆ coma

◆ ventricular arrhythmias, possibly cardiac arrest.

In the metabolic acidosis of chronic renal failure, HCO_3^- is drawn from bone to buffer hydrogen ions; the results include:
◆ growth retardation in children
◆ bone disorders such as renal osteodystrophy.

Diagnosis

The following test results confirm the diagnosis of metabolic acidosis:
◆ arterial pH less than 7.35 (as low as 7.10 in severe acidosis); $Paco_2$ normal or less than 34 mm Hg as respiratory compensatory mechanisms take hold; HCO_3^- may be 22 mEq/L).

The following test results support the diagnosis of metabolic acidosis:
◆ urine pH less than 4.5 in the absence of renal disease (as the kidneys excrete acid to raise blood pH)
◆ serum potassium greater than 5.5 mEq/L from chemical buffering
◆ glucose greater than 150 mg/dl
◆ serum ketone bodies in diabetes
◆ elevated plasma lactic acid in lactic acidosis
◆ anion gap greater than 14 mEq/L in high-anion gap metabolic acidosis, lactic acidosis, ketoacidosis, aspirin overdose, alcohol poisoning, renal failure, or other conditions characterized by accumulation of organic acids, sulfates, or phosphates
◆ anion gap 12 mEq/L or less in normal anion gap metabolic acidosis from HCO_3^- loss, GI or renal loss, increased acid load (hyperalimentation fluids), rapid I.V. saline administration, or other conditions characterized by loss of bicarbonate.

Treatment

Treatment aims to correct the acidosis as quickly as possible by addressing both the symptoms and underlying cause. Measures may include:
◆ sodium bicarbonate I.V. for severe high anion gap to neutralize blood acidity in patients with pH less than 7.20 and HCO_3^- loss; monitor plasma electrolytes, especially potassium, during sodium bicarbonate therapy (potassium level may fall as pH rises)
◆ I.V. lactated Ringer's solution to correct normal anion gap metabolic acidosis and ECF volume deficit
◆ evaluation and correction of electrolyte imbalances
◆ correction of the underlying cause (for example, in diabetic ketoacidosis, continuous low-dose I.V. insulin infusion)
◆ mechanical ventilation to maintain respiratory compensation if needed

🚫 **PREVENTION**

Preventing metabolic acidosis

To prevent metabolic acidosis, carefully observe patients receiving I.V. therapy or who have intestinal tubes in place as well as those suffering from shock, hyperthyroidism, hepatic disease, circulatory failure, or dehydration. Teach the patient with diabetes how to routinely test blood for glucose, and encourage strict adherence to diet, exercise, and medications (insulin or oral hypoglycemic therapy).

♦ antibiotic therapy to treat infection
♦ dialysis for patients with renal failure or certain drug toxicities
♦ antidiarrheal agents for diarrhea-induced HCO_3^- loss
♦ monitoring for secondary changes due to hypovolemia such as falling blood pressure (in diabetic acidosis).

Special considerations

♦ Frequently monitor vital signs, laboratory results, and level of consciousness because changes can occur rapidly.
♦ In diabetic acidosis, watch for secondary changes due to hypovolemia, such as decreasing blood pressure.
♦ Record intake and output accurately to monitor renal function. Watch for signs of excessive serum potassium—weakness, flaccid paralysis, and arrhythmias, possibly leading to cardiac arrest. After treatment, check for overcorrection to hypokalemia.
♦ Because metabolic acidosis commonly causes vomiting, position the patient to prevent aspiration. Prepare for possible seizures with seizure precautions.
♦ Provide good oral hygiene. Use sodium bicarbonate washes to neutralize mouth acids, and lubricate the patient's lips with lemon-glycerin swabs.
♦ Keep sodium bicarbonate available for administration as indicated based on ABG results. (See *Preventing metabolic acidosis*.)

METABOLIC ALKALOSIS

Metabolic alkalosis occurs when low levels of acid or high bicarbonate (HCO_3^-) cause metabolic, respiratory, and renal responses, producing characteristic symptoms (most notably, hypoventilation). This condition is always secondary to an underlying cause. With early diagnosis and prompt treatment, prognosis is good, but untreated metabolic alkalosis may lead to coma and death.

Causes

Metabolic alkalosis results from loss of acid, retention of base, or renal mechanisms associated with low serum levels of potassium and chloride.

Causes of critical acid loss include:
♦ chronic vomiting
♦ Cushing's disease, primary hyperaldosteronism, and Bartter's syndrome (lead to sodium and chloride retention and urinary loss of potassium and hydrogen)
♦ fistulas
♦ massive blood transfusions
♦ nasogastric tube drainage or lavage without adequate electrolyte replacement
♦ use of steroids and certain diuretics (furosemide [Lasix], thiazides, and ethacrynic acid [Edecrin]).

Excessive HCO_3^- retention causing chronic hypercapnia can result from:
♦ excessive intake of absorbable alkali (as in milk alkali syndrome, often seen in patients with peptic ulcers)
♦ excessive intake of bicarbonate of soda or other antacids (usually for treatment of gastritis or peptic ulcer)
♦ excessive amounts of I.V. fluids with high concentrations of bicarbonate or lactate
♦ respiratory insufficiency.

Alterations in extracellular electrolyte levels that can cause metabolic alkalosis include:
♦ low chloride (as chloride diffuses out of the cell, hydrogen diffuses into the cell)
♦ low plasma potassium causing increased hydrogen ion excretion by the kidneys.

Pathophysiology

Chemical buffers in the extracellular fluid (ECF) and intracellular fluid bind HCO_3^- that accumulates in the body. Excess unbound HCO_3^- raises blood pH, which depresses chemoreceptors in the medulla, inhibiting respiration and raising partial pressure of arterial carbon dioxide ($Paco_2$). Carbon dioxide combines with water to form carbonic acid. Low oxygen levels limit respiratory compensation.

When the blood HCO_3^- rises to 28 mEq/L or more, the amount filtered by the renal glomeruli exceeds the reabsorptive capacity of the renal tubules. Excess HCO_3^- is excreted in the urine, and hydrogen ions are retained. To maintain electrochemical balance, sodium ions and water are excreted with the bicarbonate ions.

When hydrogen ion levels in ECF are low, they diffuse passively out of the cells and, to maintain the balance of charge across the cell membrane, extracellular potassium ions move into the cells. As intracellular hydrogen ion levels fall, calcium ionization decreases, and nerve cells become more permeable to sodium ions. As sodium ions move into the cells, they trigger neural impulses, first in the peripheral nervous system and then in the central nervous system.

Signs and symptoms

Clinical features of metabolic alkalosis result from the body's attempt to correct the acid-base imbalance, primarily through hypoventilation. Signs and symptoms include:
◆ irritability, picking at bedclothes (carphology), twitching, and confusion due to decreased cerebral perfusion
◆ nausea, vomiting, and anorexia due to hypokalemia
◆ cardiovascular abnormalities due to hypokalemia and hypocalcemia
◆ respiratory disturbances (such as cyanosis and apnea) and slow, shallow respirations resulting from hypoventilation as a compensatory mechanism
◆ diminished peripheral blood flow during repeated blood pressure checks may provoke carpopedal spasm in the hand (Trousseau's sign, a possible sign of impending tetany) caused by hypocalcemia.

Complications
◆ Seizures
◆ Coma

Diagnosis
◆ Blood pH greater than 7.45 and HCO_3^- greater than 26 mEq/L (confirm diagnosis)
◆ $Paco_2$ greater than 45 mm Hg (indicates attempts at respiratory compensation)
◆ Low potassium (less than 3.5 mEq/L), calcium (less than 8.9 mg/dl), and chloride (less than 98 mEq/L)
◆ Urine pH about 7.0
◆ Alkaline urine after the renal compensatory mechanism begins to excrete bicarbonate
◆ Electrocardiogram may show low T wave, merging with a P wave, and atrial or sinus tachycardia

Treatment

The goal of treatment is to correct the underlying cause of metabolic alkalosis and includes:
◆ *cautious* use of ammonium chloride I.V. (rarely) or hydrochloric acid to restore ECF hydrogen and chloride levels

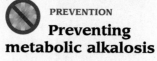

PREVENTION
Preventing metabolic alkalosis

To prevent metabolic alkalosis, warn patients against overusing alkaline agents. Irrigate nasogastric tubes with isotonic saline solution instead of plain water to prevent loss of gastric electrolytes. Monitor I.V. fluid concentrations of bicarbonate or lactate. Teach patients with ulcers to recognize symptoms of milk-alkali syndrome: a distaste for milk, anorexia, weakness, and lethargy.

◆ potassium chloride (KCl) and normal saline solution (except in heart failure); usually sufficient to replace losses from gastric drainage
◆ discontinuation of diuretics and supplementary KCl (metabolic alkalosis from potent diuretic therapy)
◆ oral or I.V. acetazolamide (Diamox; enhances renal bicarbonate excretion) to correct metabolic alkalosis without rapid volume expansion (acetazolamide also enhances potassium excretion, so potassium may be given before drug).

Special considerations
◆ Structure the patient's care plan around cautious I.V. therapy, keen observation, and strict monitoring of the patient's status.
◆ Dilute potassium when giving I.V. fluids containing potassium salts. Monitor the infusion rate to prevent damage to blood vessels; watch for signs of phlebitis.

⚠ **CLINICAL ALERT** *Carefully monitor patients receiving potassium infusions in concentrations greater than 60 mEq/L for cardiac arrhythmias.*
◆ When administering ammonium chloride 0.9%, limit the infusion rate to 1 L in 4 hours; faster administration may cause hemolysis of red blood cells. Avoid overdosage because it may cause overcorrection to metabolic acidosis. Don't give ammonium chloride with signs of hepatic or renal disease; instead, use hydrochloric acid.
◆ Watch closely for signs of muscle weakness, tetany, or decreased activity. Monitor vital signs frequently, and record intake and output to evaluate respiratory, fluid, and electrolyte status. Remember, respiratory rate usually decreases in an effort to compensate for alkalosis. Hypotension and tachycardia may indicate electrolyte imbalance, especially hypokalemia.
◆ Observe seizure precautions. (See *Preventing metabolic alkalosis*.)

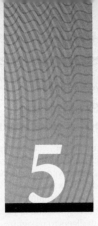

5

GENETICS

Genetics is the study of heredity—the passing of physical, biochemical, and physiologic traits from biological parents to their children. In this transmission, disorders can be transmitted and mistakes or mutations can result in disability or death.

The instructions for traits are carried within our genes. A gene is a segment of deoxyribonucleic acid (DNA) and serves as the template for eventual production of a protein. DNA is a double helix polymer (macromolecule) made up of individual units called nucleotides. Each nucleotide is composed of one sugar (deoxyribose), one phosphate, and one nitrogen-containing base. It's estimated that there are over 3 billion nucleotides within our human genome. Each gene can contain hundreds to thousands of nucleotides; yet, genes make up less than 5% of our DNA. Each DNA double helix is tightly wound around histone proteins to form a chromosome. Every normal human cell (except reproductive cells) has 46 chromosomes, 22 paired chromosomes called *autosomes*, and 2 sex chromosomes (a pair of Xs in females and an X and a Y in males). A representation of a person's individual set of chromosomes is called his *karyotype*. (See *Normal human karyotype*.)

Since 1990, the human genome has been studied to determine the exact order (sequence) of nucleotides in gene rich areas of the DNA. Human genome research continues to be of high importance in all areas of biomedical research as genes within the DNA sequence are identified, their function determined, and the consequences of genetic alterations and relationship to disease are studied. These areas of research continue to result in improved diagnostics and health outcomes for persons with or at risk for developing genetic diseases. (See *The genome at a glance*, page 94.)

A word of warning at the outset: For a wide variety of reasons, not every gene that might be expressed actually is expressed. Thus, the following chapter may seem to contain a great many "hedge" words, such as "may," "perhaps," and "some." Genetic principles are based on studies of thousands of individuals. Those studies have led to generalities that are usually true, but exceptions occur. Genetics is a young science.

Genetic components

The DNA within our human genome consists of over 3 billion nucleotides. Each nucleotide contains one of four possible nitrogenous bases: adenine (A), thymine (T), guanine (G) or cytosine (C). The two strands of a DNA helix in a chromosome are joined at the bases by weak hydrogen bonds. Adenine joins with thymine and guanine joins with cytosine. The looseness of the bonds allows the strands to separate easily during cell division. (See *DNA duplication: Two double helices from one,* page 95.) The genes carry a code for each trait a person inherits, from blood type to eye color to body shape and myriad of other traits.

DNA ultimately controls the formation of essential substances throughout the life of every cell in the body, and it does this through the genes. A gene ultimately determines the linear sequence of an amino acid chain. The amino acid chain is modified to produce a specific

Normal human karyotype

The illustration shows the arrangement of chromosomes (karyotype) in a normal male.

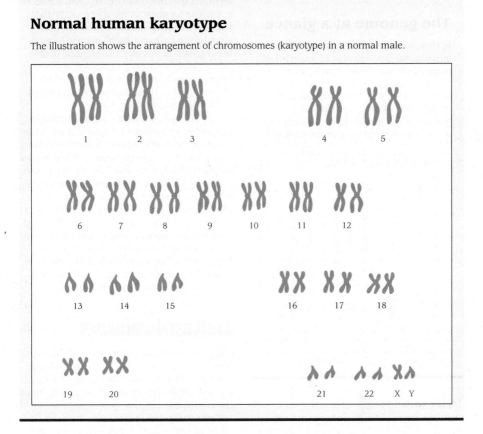

protein, which is necessary for cellular structure or function and contributes to a particular inherited trait, such as eye color or blood type. In the cell, a gene is transcribed within the nucleus into messenger ribonucleic acid (mRNA). This message leaves the nucleus and many different chemicals and cellular components within the cell cytoplasm are used to translate mRNA into an amino acid chain. A specific cellular component, called a ribosome, reads the message of three mRNA bases at a time. A sequence of three mRNA bases is called a codon, and there are 64 different codons within our genetic code. The ribosome reads the mRNA codons to determine and assemble the sequence of amino acids that will undergo further modification within the cell to become a functional protein. (See *How genes control cell function*, page 96.)

Trait transmission

Germ cells, or *gametes* (ovum and sperm), are one of two classes of cells in the body; each germ cell contains 23 chromosomes (called the *haploid* number) in its nucleus. All the other cells in the body are somatic cells, which are *diploid*, meaning they contain 23 *pairs* of chromosomes.

When ovum and sperm unite, the corresponding chromosomes pair up so that the fertilized cell and every somatic cell of the new person has 23 pairs of chromosomes in its nucleus.

GERM CELLS

The body produces germ cells through a type of cell division called *meiosis*. Meiosis occurs only when the body is creating haploid germ cells from their diploid precursors. Each of the 23 pairs of chromosomes in the germ cell separates so that, when the cell then divides, each new cell (ovum or sperm) contains one set of 23 chromosomes.

Most of the genes on one chromosome are identical or almost identical to the gene on its mate. (As we discuss later, each chromosome may carry a different version of the same gene.) The location (or locus) of a gene on a chromosome is specific and doesn't vary from person to person.

The genome at a glance

In 1998, a gene map was released by an international consortium of radiation hybrid mapping laboratories containing more than 30,000 distinct cyclic deoxyribonucleic acid–based markers. The particular makeup of an individual organism is called its *genome,* which is made up of the alleles (or different versions of the genes) it possesses.

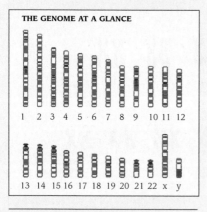

THE GENOME AT A GLANCE

1 2 3 4 5 6 7 8 9 10 11 12

13 14 15 16 17 18 19 20 21 22 x y

Source: *www.ncbi.nlm.nih.gov/genome/guide.*

Determining sex

Only one pair of chromosomes in each cell — pair 23 — is involved in determining a person's sex. These are the sex chromosomes; the other 22 numbered chromosome pairs are called *autosomes.* Females have two X chromosomes and males have one X and one Y chromosome.

Each gamete produced by a male contains either an X or a Y chromosome. When a sperm with an X chromosome fertilizes an ovum, the offspring is female (two X chromosomes); when a sperm with a Y chromosome fertilizes an ovum, the offspring is male (one X and one Y chromosome). Very rare errors in cell division can result in a germ cell that has no sex chromosome or two sex chromosomes. After fertilization with a gamete that contains a missing or extra sex chromosome, the zygote may have an XO, XXY, XXX, or XYY karyotype and still survive. Most other errors in sex chromosome division are incompatible with life.

MITOSIS

The fertilized ovum — now called a *zygote* — undergoes a type of cell division called *mitosis.* Before a cell divides, its chromosomes duplicate. During this process, the double helix of DNA

separates into two chains; each chain serves as a template for constructing a new chain. Individual DNA nucleotides are linked into new strands with bases complementary to those in the originals. In this way, two identical double helices are formed, each containing one of the original strands and a newly formed complementary strand. These double helices are duplicates of the original DNA chain.

The cell cycle within somatic cells consists of alternations between interphase and mitosis — protein synthesis and DNA replication occur during interphase. Mitosis consists of four phases: prophase, metaphase, anaphase and telophase. Following telophase, cytokinesis occurs resulting in two new daughter cells, each genetically identical to the original and to each other. (See *Five phases of mitosis,* page 97.) Each of the two resulting cells likewise divides, and so on, eventually forming a many-celled human embryo. Thus, each cell in a person's body (except ovum or sperm) contains an identical set of 46 chromosomes that are unique to that person.

Trait predominance

Each parent contributes one set of chromosomes (and therefore one set of genes) so that every offspring has two genes for every locus (location on the chromosome) on the autosomal chromosomes.

Some characteristics, or traits, are determined by one gene that may have many variants (alleles), such as the ability to roll the tongue. A person who has identical alleles on each chromosome is homozygous for that gene; if the alleles are different, they're said to be heterozygous.

Others, called *polygenic traits,* require the interaction of one or more genes. Recent research has revealed that eye color is a polygenic trait. Three different genes at three different chromosome locations influence eye color. In addition, environmental factors may affect how a gene or genes are expressed.

AUTOSOMAL INHERITANCE

For unknown reasons, on autosomal chromosomes, one allele may be more influential than the other in determining a specific trait. The more powerful, or *dominant,* allele is more likely to be expressed in the offspring than the less influential, or *recessive,* allele. Offspring will express a dominant allele when one or both chromosomes in a pair carry it. A recessive allele won't be expressed unless both chromosomes carry recessive alleles. For example, the

CLOSER LOOK
DNA duplication: Two double helices from one

The nucleotide, the basic structural unit of deoxyribonucleic acid (DNA), contains a phosphate group, deoxyribose, and a nitrogen base made of adenine (A), thymine (T), cystosine (C), and guanine (G). A DNA molecule's double helix forms from the twisting of nucleotide strands (shown below).

During duplication, a DNA chain separates and new complementary chains form and link to the separated originals (parents). The result is two identical double helices—each containing a parent and daughter strand.

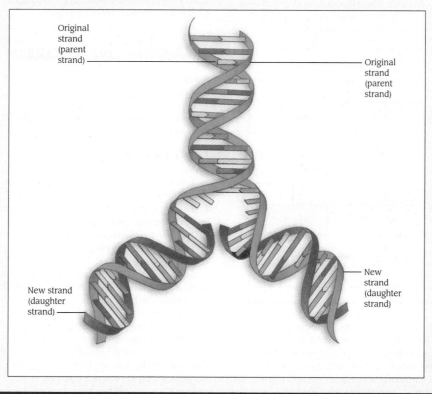

Original strand (parent strand)

Original strand (parent strand)

New strand (daughter strand)

New strand (daughter strand)

condition in which a person reflexively sneezes when quickly transitioning from a dark environment to intense bright light is thought to be dominant. A person who doesn't experience this has two recessive alleles, whereas a person who does reflexively sneeze has either one or both dominant alleles for the trait.

SEX-LINKED INHERITANCE
The X and Y chromosomes aren't literally a pair because the X chromosome is much larger than the Y. The male literally has less genetic material than the female, which means he has only one copy of most genes on the X chromosome. Inheritance of those genes is called *X-linked*.

A man will transmit one copy of each X-linked gene to his daughters and none to his sons. A woman will transmit one copy to each child, male or female.

Inheritance of genes on the X chromosomes is different in another way. Some recessive genes on the X chromosomes act like dominants in males. Remember, males have an X and a Y chromosome in each somatic cell and few genes are shared between these two very different sex chromosomes. Therefore, genes on the X chromosome that don't have partner genes on the Y chromosome will be expressed in males. In females, one of the two X chromosomes is randomly and permanently inactivated

CLOSER LOOK
How genes control cell function

This simplified diagram outlines how the genetic code directs formation of specific proteins. Some proteins are the building blocks of cell structure. Others, called enzymes, direct intracellular chemical reactions. Together, structural proteins and enzymes direct cell function.

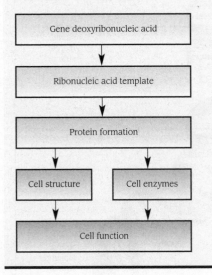

in somatic cells during early embryogenesis. This phenomenon is called X-inactivation or Lyonization. X-inactivation ensures that females, like males, have one functional copy of the X chromosome in each body cell. The process of inactivating either the paternally contributed X or the maternally contributed X is random in each cell. Due to X-inactivation, one recessive allele will be expressed in some somatic cells and the partner allele (whether dominant or recessive) in other somatic cells. The most common example occurs not in people but in cats. Only female cats have calico (tricolor) coat patterns. Dark and orange hair color in the cat is carried on the X chromosome. Some hair cells in females express the brown allele and others, the orange color. The white color results from an autosomal gene.

MULTIFACTORIAL INHERITANCE

Some traits require a combination of two or more genes and environmental factors to be expressed. This is called *multifactorial inheritance*. Height is a classic example of a multifactorial trait. In general, the height of offspring will be in a range between the height of the two parents. But the combination of multiple genes contributed by each parent, nutritional patterns, health care, and other environmental factors also influence development. The better-nourished, healthier children of two short parents may be taller than either. Common health problems, such as obesity, diabetes, and hypertension, are associated with effects from multiple genes that are modified from environmental and lifestyle factors.

Pathophysiologic changes

Autosomal, sex-linked, and multifactorial disorders originate from damage to genes or chromosomes. Some defects arise spontaneously, whereas others may be caused by environmental teratogens.

GENE ERRORS

A rare change in genetic material is a *mutation*, which occurs in less than 1% of the population. A change that occurs with greater frequency is known as *polymorphism*. A mutation may occur spontaneously or after exposure of a cell to radiation, certain chemicals, or viruses. Mutations can occur anywhere in the genome—the person's entire inventory of genes.

Every cell has built-in defenses against genetic damage. However, if a mutation isn't identified or repaired, the mutation may produce a trait different from the original trait and is transmitted to offspring during reproduction. The mutation initially causes the cell to produce some abnormal protein that makes the cell different from its ancestors. Mutations may have no effect, they may change expression of a trait, and others change the way a cell functions. Some mutations cause serious or deadly defects, such as cancer or congenital anomalies.

Autosomal disorders

In single-gene disorders, an error occurs at a single gene site on the DNA strand. A mistake may occur in the copying and transcribing of a single codon (nucleotide triplet) through additions, deletions, excessive repetitions, or base changes.

Single-gene disorders are inherited in clearly identifiable patterns that are the same as those seen in inheritance of normal traits. Because every person has 22 pairs of autosomes and only 1 pair of sex chromosomes, most hereditary disorders are caused by autosomal mutations.

CLOSER LOOK

Five phases of mitosis

In mitosis (used by all cells except gametes), the nuclear contents of a cell reproduce and divide, resulting in the formation of two daughter cells. The five steps, or phases, of this process are illustrated below.

Interphase

During interphase, protein synthesis and preparation for cell division take place. The nucleus and nuclear membrane are well defined and the nucleolus is prominent. Chromosomes replicate, each forming a double strand that remains attached at the center of each chromosome by a structure called the *centromere;* they appear as an indistinguishable matrix within the nucleus. Centrioles (in animal cells only, not plant cells) appear outside the nucleus.

Centrioles
Nucleus
Nucleolus

Prophase

In prophase, the nucleolus disappears and chromosomes become distinct. Halves of each duplicated chromosome (chromatids) remain attached by a centromere. Centrioles move to opposite sides of the cell and radiate spindle fibers.

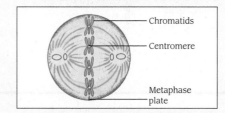

Centrioles
Spindle fibers

Metaphase

Chromosomes line up randomly in the center of the cell between spindles, along the metaphase plate. The centromere of each chromosome replicates.

Chromatids
Centromere
Metaphase plate

Anaphase

Centromeres move apart, pulling the separate chromatids (now called *chromosomes*) to opposite ends of the cell. In human cells, each end of the cell now contains 46 chromosomes. The number of chromosomes at each end of the cell equals the original number.

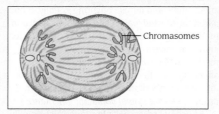

Chromasomes

Telophase

A nuclear membrane forms around each end of the cell, and spindle fibers disappear. The cytoplasm compresses and divides the cell in half. Each new cell contains the diploid number (46 in humans) of chromosomes.

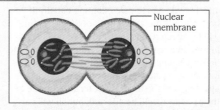

Nuclear membrane

Autosomal dominant inheritance

The diagram shows the inheritance pattern of a disorder when one parent has recessive normal genes (aa) and the other has a dominant gene associated with the disorder (Aa). Each child has a 50% chance of inheriting A.

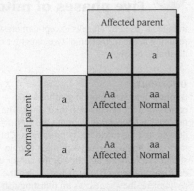

		Affected parent	
		A	a
Normal parent	a	Aa Affected	aa Normal
	a	Aa Affected	aa Normal

Autosomal recessive inheritance

The diagram shows the inheritance pattern of a disorder when both unaffected parents are heterozygous (Aa) for a recessive autosomal gene (a). As shown, each child has a one-in-four chance of being affected (aa), a one-in-four chance of having two normal genes (AA) and no chance of transmittal, and a 50% chance of being a carrier (Aa) who can transmit the altered gene.

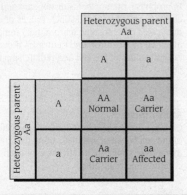

		Heterozygous parent Aa	
		A	a
Heterozygous parent Aa	A	AA Normal	Aa Carrier
	a	Aa Carrier	aa Affected

Autosomal dominant transmission usually affects male and female offspring equally. If one parent is affected, each child has one chance in two of being affected. If both parents are affected and each carries one dominant allele and one recessive allele for the disorder, they have affected or unaffected children. An example of this type of inheritance occurs in Marfan syndrome. (See *Autosomal dominant inheritance*.)

Autosomal recessive inheritance also usually affects male and female offspring equally. If both parents are affected, all of their offspring will be affected. If both parents are unaffected but are heterozygous for the trait (carriers of the defective gene), each child has one chance in four of being affected. If only one parent is affected, and the other is not a carrier, none of their offspring will be affected, but all will carry the defective gene. If one parent is affected and the other is a carrier, their offspring will have a 50% chance of being affected. (See *Autosomal recessive inheritance*.) Autosomal recessive disorders may occur when there is no family history of the disease.

Sex-linked disorders

Genetic disorders caused by genes located on the sex chromosomes are termed *sex-linked disorders*. Most sex-linked disorders are passed on the X chromosome, usually as recessive traits. Because males have only one X chromosome, a single X-linked recessive gene can cause disease to be exhibited in a male. Females receive two X chromosomes, so they can be homozygous for a disease allele, homozygous for a normal allele, or heterozygous (a carrier).

Most people who express X-linked recessive traits are males with unaffected parents. In rare

X-linked recessive inheritance

The diagram shows the children of a normal parent and a parent with a recessive gene on the X chromosome (shown by an open dot). All daughters of an affected male will be carriers. The son of a female carrier may inherit a recessive gene on the X chromosome and be affected by the disease. Unaffected sons can't transmit the disorder.

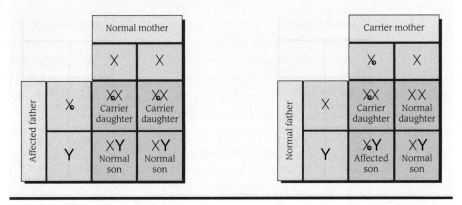

cases, the father is affected and the mother is a carrier. All daughters of an affected male will be carriers. Sons of an affected male will be unaffected, and the unaffected sons aren't carriers. Unaffected male children of a female carrier don't transmit the disorder. Hemophilia is an example of an X-linked inheritance disorder. (See *X-linked recessive inheritance*.)

Characteristics of X-linked dominant inheritance include evidence of the inherited trait in the family history. A person with the abnormal trait usually has one affected parent (except in the case of a new mutation occurring in a germ cell that conceived the individual). If the father has an X-linked dominant disorder, all his daughters and none of his sons will be affected. If a mother has an X-linked dominant disorder, each of her children has a 50% chance of being affected. (See *X-linked dominant inheritance*, page 100.)

Multifactorial disorders

Most multifactorial disorders result from the effects of several different genes and an environmental component. In polygenic inheritance, each gene has a small additive effect, and the effect of a combination of genetic errors in a person is unpredictable. Multifactorial disorders can result from a less-than-optimum expression of many different genes, not from a specific error.

Some multifactorial disorders are apparent at birth, such as cleft lip, cleft palate, congenital heart disease, anencephaly, clubfoot, and myelomeningocele. Others don't become apparent until later, such as type 2 diabetes mellitus, hypertension, hyperlipidemia, most autoimmune diseases, and many cancers. Multifactorial disorders that develop during adulthood are often believed to be strongly related to environmental factors, not only in incidence but also in the degree of expression.

Environmental teratogens

Teratogens are environmental agents that can harm the developing fetus by causing congenital structural or functional defects. Teratogens may also cause spontaneous miscarriage, complications during labor and delivery, hidden defects in later development (such as cognitive or behavioral problems), or neoplastic transformations. (See *Teratogens and associated disorders*, page 101.)

Environmental factors of maternal or paternal origin include the use of chemicals (such as drugs, alcohol, or hormones), exposure to radiation, general health, and age. Maternal factors include infections during pregnancy, existing diseases, nutritional factors, exposure to high altitude, maternal-fetal blood incompatibility, and poor prenatal care.

The embryonic period—the first 8 weeks after fertilization—is a vulnerable time when specific organ systems are actively differentiating. Exposure to teratogens usually kills the embryo. During the fetal period, organ systems are formed and continue to mature. Exposure during this time can cause intrauterine growth retardation, cognitive abnormalities, or structural defects.

X-linked dominant inheritance

The diagram shows the children of a normal parent and a parent with an abnormal, X-linked dominant gene on the X chromosome (shown by the dot on the X). When the father is affected, only his daughters have the abnormal gene. When the mother is affected, both sons and daughters may be affected.

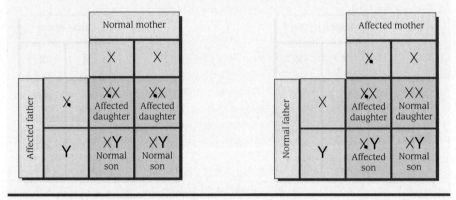

CHROMOSOME DEFECTS

Aberrations in chromosome structure or number cause a class of disorders called *congenital anomalies,* or *birth defects.* The aberration may be loss, addition, or rearrangement of genetic material. If the remaining genetic material is sufficient to maintain life, an endless variety of clinical manifestations may occur. Most clinically significant chromosome aberrations arise during meiosis. Meiosis is an incredibly complex process that can go wrong in many ways. Potential contributing factors include maternal age, radiation, and use of some therapeutic or recreational drugs.

Translocation, the shifting or moving of chromosomal material, occurs when chromosomes split apart and rejoin in an abnormal arrangement. The cells still have a normal amount of genetic material, so often there are no visible abnormalities. However, the children of parents with translocated chromosomes may have serious genetic defects, such as monosomies or trisomies. Parental age doesn't seem to be a factor in translocation.

Errors in chromosome number

During both meiosis and mitosis, chromosomes normally separate in a process called *disjunction.* Failure to separate, called *nondisjunction,* causes an unequal distribution of chromosomes between the two resulting cells. If nondisjunction occurs during mitosis soon after fertilization, it may affect all the resulting cells. Gain or loss of chromosomes is usually caused by nondisjunction of autosomes or sex chromosomes during meiosis. The incidence of nondisjunction increases with maternal age. (See *Chromosomal disjunction and nondisjunction,* page 103.)

The presence of one chromosome less than the normal number is called *monosomy;* an autosomal monosomy is nonviable. The presence of an extra chromosome is called a *trisomy,* the most common of which are trisomies 21, 18, and 13. Children with trisomy 18 or 13 usually don't survive beyond the first months of life. A mixture of both trisomic and normal cells results in mosaicism, which is the presence of two or more cell lines in the same person. The effect of mosaicism depends on the proportion and anatomic location of abnormal cells.

Disorders

This section discusses disorders in the context of their pattern of inheritance as well as environmental factors. The alphabetically listed disorders have these patterns of inheritance:
◆ Autosomal recessive—cystic fibrosis, sickle cell anemia, Tay-Sachs disease
◆ Autosomal dominant—Marfan syndrome
◆ X-linked recessive—hemophilia, fragile X syndrome
◆ Polygenic multifactorial—cleft lip and cleft palate, neural tube defects
◆ Chromosome number—Down syndrome, Klinefelter syndrome.

Teratogens and associated disorders

This chart lists common teratogens and their associated disorders.

Teratogens	Associated disorders
Infections	
Toxoplasmosis Rubella Cytomegalovirus Herpes simplex Other infections (syphilis, hepatitis B, mumps, gonorrhea, parvovirus, varicella)	◆ Growth deficiency ◆ Mental retardation ◆ Hepatosplenomegaly ◆ Hearing loss ◆ Cardiac and ocular defects ◆ Active infection ◆ Carrier state
Maternal disorders	
Diabetes mellitus	◆ Abnormalities of the spine, lower extremities, heart, kidney, or external genitalia
Phenylketonuria	◆ Mental retardation ◆ Microcephaly ◆ Congenital heart defects ◆ Intrauterine growth retardation
Hyperthermia	◆ Intrauterine growth retardation ◆ Central nervous system (CNS) and neural tube defects ◆ Facial defects
Drugs, chemicals, and physical agents	
Alcohol	◆ Fetal alcohol syndrome ◆ Learning disabilities
Anticonvulsants	◆ Intrauterine growth retardation ◆ Mental deficiency ◆ Facial abnormalities ◆ Cardiac defects ◆ Cleft lip and palate ◆ Malformed ears ◆ Genital defects
Cocaine	◆ Premature delivery ◆ Abruptio placentae ◆ Intracranial hemorrhage ◆ GI and genitourinary (GU) abnormalities
Diethylstilbestrol	◆ Clear-cell adenocarcinoma of vagina ◆ Structural and functional defects of female GU tract
Folate deficiency	◆ Neural tube defects
Lithium	◆ Congenital heart disease

(continued)

Teratogens and associated disorders *(continued)*

Teratogens	Associated disorders
Drugs, chemicals, and physical agents *(continued)*	
Methotrexate	♦ Intrauterine growth retardation ♦ Decreased ossification of skull ♦ Prominent eyes ♦ Limb abnormalities ♦ Mild developmental delay
Radiation	♦ Microcephaly ♦ Mental retardation
Tetracycline	♦ Brown staining of decidual teeth ♦ Dental caries ♦ Enamel hypoplasia
Vitamin A derivatives	♦ Facial defects ♦ Cardiac defects ♦ CNS defects ♦ Incomplete development of thymus
Warfarin (Coumadin)	♦ Intrauterine growth retardation ♦ Mental retardation ♦ Seizures ♦ Nasal hypoplasia ♦ Abnormal calcification of axial skeleton

Adapted from Hansen, M. *Pathophysiology: Foundations of Disease and Clinical Intervention.* Philadelphia: W.B. Saunders, 1998, with permission of the publisher.

CLEFT LIP AND CLEFT PALATE

Cleft lip and cleft palate may occur separately or in combination. They originate in the second month of pregnancy if the front and sides of the face and the palatine shelves fuse imperfectly. Cleft lip with or without cleft palate occurs twice as often in males than in females. Cleft palate without cleft lip is more common in females.

Cleft lip deformities can occur unilaterally, bilaterally or, rarely, in the midline. Only the lip may be involved, or the defect may extend into the upper jaw or nasal cavity. (See *Types of cleft deformities,* page 104.)

Incidence is highest in children with a family history of cleft defects.

Cleft lip with or without cleft palate occurs in about 1 in 1,000 births among Whites; the incidence is higher in Asians (1.7 in 1,000) and Native Americans (more than 3.6 in 1,000) but lower in Blacks (1 in 2,500).

Causes

♦ Chromosomal or Mendelian syndrome (cleft defects are associated with more than 300 syndromes)

♦ Exposure to teratogens during fetal development

♦ Combined genetic and environmental factors (accounts for 75% of isolated cleft cases)

Pathophysiology

During the second month of pregnancy, the front and sides of the face and the palatine shelves develop. Because of a chromosomal abnormality, exposure to teratogens, genetic abnormality, or environmental factors, the lip or palate fuses imperfectly.

The deformity may range from a simple notch to a complete cleft. A cleft palate may be partial or complete. A complete cleft includes the soft palate, the bones of the maxilla, and the alveolus on one or both sides of the premaxilla.

A double cleft is the most severe of the deformities. The cleft runs from the soft palate forward to either side of the nose. A double cleft separates the maxilla and premaxilla into freely moving segments. The tongue and other muscles can displace the segments, enlarging the cleft.

CLOSER LOOK

Chromosomal disjunction and nondisjunction

The illustration shows normal disjunction and nondisjunction of an ovum. When disjunction proceeds normally, fertilization with a normal sperm results in a zygote with the correct number of chromosomes. In nondisjunction, the sister chromatids fail to separate; the result is one trisomic cell and one monosomic cell.

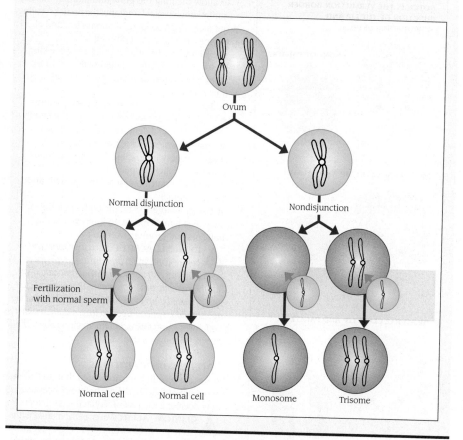

CLINICAL ALERT *Isolated cleft palate is more commonly associated with other congenital defects than isolated cleft lip with or without cleft palate. The constellation of U-shaped cleft palate, mandibular hypoplasia, and glossoptosis is known as Pierre Robin syndrome, or Robin syndrome. It can occur as an isolated defect or one feature of many different syndromes; therefore, a comprehensive genetic evaluation is suggested for infants with Robin sequence. Because of the mandibular hypoplasia and glossoptosis, careful evaluation and management of the airway are mandatory for infants with Robin sequence.*

Signs and symptoms
◆ Obvious cleft lip or cleft palate due to incomplete fusion of the lip or palate
◆ Feeding difficulties due to incomplete fusion of the palate

Complications
◆ Malnutrition, because the abnormal palate affects nutritional intake
◆ Hearing impairment, often due to middle-ear damage or recurrent infections
◆ Permanent speech impediment, even after surgical repair

Types of cleft deformities

The following illustrations show variations of cleft lip and cleft palate.

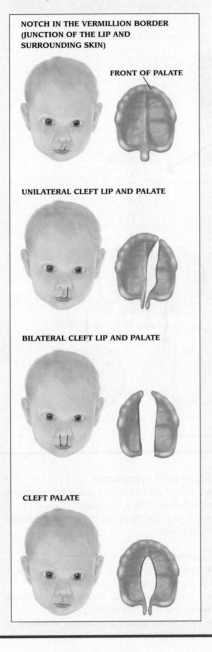

NOTCH IN THE VERMILLION BORDER (JUNCTION OF THE LIP AND SURROUNDING SKIN)

FRONT OF PALATE

UNILATERAL CLEFT LIP AND PALATE

BILATERAL CLEFT LIP AND PALATE

CLEFT PALATE

Diagnosis
◆ Clinical presentation, obvious at birth
◆ Prenatal targeted ultrasound

Treatment
◆ Surgical correction of cleft lip in the first few days of life to permit sucking, or delayed for 8 to 10 weeks (sometimes as long as 6 to 8 months) to allow the infant to grow and mature, thereby minimizing surgical and anesthesia risks, ruling out associated congenital anomalies, and allowing time for parental bonding
◆ Orthodontic prosthesis to improve sucking
◆ Surgical correction of cleft palate at 12 to 18 months, after the infant gains weight and is infection-free
◆ Speech therapy to correct speech patterns
◆ Use of a contoured speech bulb attached to the posterior of a denture to occlude the nasopharynx when a wide horseshoe defect makes surgery impossible (to help the child develop intelligible speech)
◆ Adequate nutrition for normal growth and development
◆ Use of a large soft nipple with large holes, such as a lamb's nipple, to improve feeding patterns and promote nutrition

⚠ **CLINICAL ALERT** *Daily use of folic acid before conception and during pregnancy decreases the risk for isolated (not associated with another genetic or congenital malformation) cleft lip or palate by up to 25%. Women of childbearing age should be encouraged to take a daily multivitamin containing folic acid until menopause or until they're no longer fertile.*

Special considerations
◆ Recent research has indicated that ingestion of 0.4 mg of folic acid daily before conception may decrease the risk of isolated cleft defects.

⚠ **CLINICAL ALERT** *Never place a child with Pierre Robin syndrome on his back because his tongue could fall back and obstruct his airway. Place the infant on his side for sleeping. Most other infants with a cleft palate can sleep on their backs without difficulty.*
◆ Maintain adequate nutrition to ensure normal growth and development. Experiment with feeding devices. An infant with a cleft palate typically has an excellent appetite but commonly has difficulty feeding because of air leaks around the cleft and nasal regurgitation. He usually feeds better from a bottle and nipple designed specifically for feeding infants with cleft defects. These bottles come with special nipples or regular nipples with enlarged holes and may be used with cleft palate bottles.

◆ Teach the parents how best to feed the infant. Advise them to hold the infant in a near-sitting position, with the flow directed to the side or back of the infant's tongue. Tell them to burp the infant frequently because he tends to swallow a lot of air. If the underside of the nasal septum becomes ulcerated and the child refuses to suck because of the pain, instruct the parents to direct the nipple to the side of the mouth to give the mucosa time to heal. Tell them to gently clean the palatal cleft with a cotton-tipped applicator dipped in half-strength hydrogen peroxide or water after each feeding.

◆ Encourage the mother of an infant with cleft lip to breast-feed if the cleft doesn't prevent effective sucking. Breast-feeding an infant with a cleft palate or one who has just had corrective surgery isn't usually possible. (Postoperatively, the infant can't suck for 6 to 10 weeks.) However, if the mother desires, suggest that she use a breast pump to express breast milk and then feed it to her infant from a bottle.

◆ After surgery, record intake and output and maintain good nutrition. To prevent atelectasis and pneumonia, the physician may gently suction the nasopharynx (this may be necessary before surgery, too). Restrain the infant to prevent him from hurting himself. Elbow restraints allow the infant to move his hands while keeping them away from his mouth. When necessary, use an infant seat to keep the child in a comfortable sitting position. Hang toys within reach of restrained hands.

◆ Surgeons sometimes place a curved metal bow over a repaired cleft lip to minimize tension on the suture line. Remove the gauze before feedings, and replace it often. Moisten it with normal saline solution until the sutures are removed. Check your facility's policy to confirm this procedure.

◆ Help the parents deal with their feelings about the child's deformity. Start by telling them about it and showing them their infant as soon as possible. Because some place undue importance on physical appearance, many parents feel shock, disappointment, and guilt when they see the child. Help them by being calm and providing positive information.

◆ Direct the parents' attention to their child's assets. Stress the fact that surgical repairs can be made. Include the parents in the care and feeding of the child right from the start to encourage normal bonding. Provide the instructions, emotional support, and reassurance that the parents will need to take proper care of the child at home.

◆ Refer them to a social worker who can guide them to community resources, if needed, and to a genetic counselor to determine the recurrence risk.

CYSTIC FIBROSIS

In cystic fibrosis, dysfunction of the exocrine glands affects multiple organ systems. The disease affects males as well as females and is the most common fatal genetic disease in white children.

Cystic fibrosis is accompanied by many complications and now carries an average life expectancy of 32 years. The disorder is characterized by chronic airway infection leading to bronchiectasis, bronchiolectasis, exocrine pancreatic insufficiency, intestinal dysfunction, abnormal sweat gland function, and reproductive dysfunction.

The incidence of cystic fibrosis varies with ethnic origin. It occurs in 1 of 2,000 births in Whites of North America and northern European descent, and 1 in 17,000 births in Blacks.

Causes

The responsible gene is on chromosome 7q; it encodes a membrane-associated protein called the cystic fibrosis transmembrane regulator (CFTR). The exact function of CFTR remains unknown, but it appears to help regulate chloride and sodium transport across epithelial membranes.

Causes of cystic fibrosis include:
◆ abnormal coding found on as many as 900 CFTR alleles
◆ autosomal recessive inheritance.

Pathophysiology

Most cases arise from the mutation that affects the genetic coding for a single amino acid, resulting in a protein (the CFTR) that doesn't function properly. The CFTR (resulting from this mutation) resembles other transmembrane transport proteins, but it lacks the phenylalanine in the protein produced by normal genes. This regulator interferes with cyclic adenosine monophosphate–regulated chloride channels and transport of other ions by preventing adenosine triphosphate from binding to the protein or by interfering with activation by protein kinase.

The mutation affects volume-absorbing epithelia (in the airways and intestines), salt-absorbing epithelia (in sweat ducts), and volume-secretory epithelia (in the pancreas). Lack of phenylalanine leads to dehydration, increasing the viscosity of mucus-gland secretions, leading to obstruction of glandular ducts. Cystic fibrosis has a varying effect on electrolyte and water transport. (See *How cystic fibrosis affects the body*, page 106)

MULTISYSTEM DISORDER

How cystic fibrosis affects the body

Because cystic fibrosis involves dysfunction of the exocrine glands, it affects multiple organ systems. The far-reaching effects prompt a multidisciplinary approach to the patient's care to allow for the best possible outcome.

Below is a summary of what cystic fibrosis does to the body, including collaborative management.

Effects on body systems
Respiratory system
♦ Thick secretions and dehydration occur as a result of ionic imbalance.
♦ Chronic airway infections by *Staphylococcus aureus*, *Pseudomonas aeruginosa*, and *Pseudomonas cepacia* may develop, possibly due to abnormal airway surface fluids and failure of lung defenses.
♦ Accumulation of thick secretions in the bronchioles and alveoli results in dyspnea.
♦ Stimulation of the secretion-removal reflex produces a paroxysmal cough.
♦ Barrel chest, cyanosis, and clubbing of fingers and toes result from chronic hypoxia.
♦ Obstructed glandular ducts occur leading to peribronchial thickening; this obstruction is due to increased viscosity of bronchial, pancreatic, and other mucous gland secretions.

Cardiovascular system
♦ Fatal shock and arrhythmias may result from hyponatremia and hypochloremia from sodium lost in sweat.
♦ Pulmonary hypertension can result in cardiac dysfunction in adult cystic fibrosis patients with severe lung disease.
♦ Pulmonary hypertension and cor pulmonale in cystic fibrosis are thought to be related to progressive destruction of the lung parenchyma and pulmonary vasculature and to pulmonary vasoconstriction secondary to hypoxemia.

Endocrine system
♦ Retention of bicarbonate and water due to the absence of cystic fibrosis transmembrane regulator chloride channel in the pancreatic ductile epithelia limits membrane function and leads to retention of pancreatic enzymes, chronic cholecystitis and cholelithiaisis, and the ultimate destruction of the pancreas.
♦ Diabetes, pancreatitis, and hepatic failure can develop because of the disease's effects on the intestines, pancreas, and liver.

GI system
♦ Obstruction of the small and large intestines results from inhibited secretion of chloride and water and excessive absorption of liquid.
♦ Biliary cirrhosis occurs because of retention of biliary secretions.
♦ Malnutrition and malabsorption of fat-soluble vitamins (A, D, E, and K) are caused by deficiencies of trypsin, amylase, and lipase from obstructed pancreatic ducts, preventing the conversion and absorption of fat and protein in the intestinal tract.

Genitourinary system
♦ In males, a bilateral congenital absence of the vas deferens is accompanied by a lack of sperm in the semen.
♦ In females, secondary amenorrhea and increased mucus in the reproductive tracts block the passage of ova.

Collaborative management
♦ Pulmonary specialists and respiratory therapists assist with clearing airway secretions and maintaining a patent airway.
♦ An endocrinologist may assist with managing diabetes as well as other pancreatic and reproductive disorders.
♦ Nutritional specialists may be consulted to help with dietary measures (such as providing high-calorie meals that include the appropriate level of salt needed) and fluid therapy.
♦ Physical and occupational therapists may be needed to help with activity management and energy conservation.

Signs and symptoms
♦ Thick secretions and dehydration due to ionic imbalance
♦ Chronic airway infections by *Staphylococcus aureus*, *Pseudomonas aeruginosa*, and *Pseudomonas cepacia*, possibly due to abnormal airway surface fluids and failure of lung defenses
♦ Dyspnea due to accumulation of thick secretions in bronchioles and alveoli
♦ Paroxysmal cough due to stimulation of the secretion-removal reflex
♦ Barrel chest, cyanosis, and clubbing of fingers and toes from chronic hypoxia
♦ Crackles on auscultation due to thick, airway-occluding secretions

◆ Wheezes heard on auscultation due to constricted airways
◆ Retention of bicarbonate and water due to the absence of the CFTR chloride channel in the pancreatic ductile epithelia; limits membrane function and leads to retention of pancreatic enzymes, chronic cholecystitis and cholelithiasis, and ultimate destruction of the pancreas
◆ Obstruction of the small and large intestine due to inhibited secretion of chloride and water and excessive absorption of liquid
◆ Biliary cirrhosis due to retention of biliary secretions
◆ Fatal shock and arrhythmias due to hyponatremia and hypochloremia from sodium lost in sweat
◆ Failure to thrive: poor weight gain, poor growth, distended abdomen, thin extremities, and sallow skin with poor turgor due to malabsorption
◆ Clotting problems, retarded bone growth, and delayed sexual development due to deficiency of fat-soluble vitamins
◆ Rectal prolapse in infants and children due to malnutrition and wasting of perirectal supporting tissues
◆ Esophageal varices due to cirrhosis and portal hypertension

Complications
◆ Obstructed glandular ducts (leading to peribronchial thickening) due to increased viscosity of bronchial, pancreatic, and other mucus gland secretions
◆ Atelectasis or emphysema due to respiratory effects
◆ Diabetes, pancreatitis, and hepatic failure due to effects on the intestines, pancreas, and liver
◆ Malnutrition and malabsorption of fat-soluble vitamins (A, D, E, and K) due to deficiencies of trypsin, amylase, and lipase (from obstructed pancreatic ducts, preventing the conversion and absorption of fat and protein in the intestinal tract)
◆ Lack of sperm in the semen (azoospermia) due to congenital bilateral absence of the vas deferens
◆ Secondary amenorrhea and increased mucus in the reproductive tracts, blocking the passage of ova

Diagnosis
The Cystic Fibrosis Foundation has developed criteria for a definitive diagnosis:
◆ The presence of one or more of the clinical findings typically associated with cystic fibrosis
◆ A history of cystic fibrosis in a sibling
◆ Identification of mutations in each CFTR gene
◆ Two elevated sweat chloride tests obtained on separate days

AGE ALERT *In very young infants, the sweat test may be inaccurate because they may not produce enough sweat for a valid test. The test may need to be repeated.*

These test results may support the diagnosis:
◆ Chest X-rays indicating early signs of obstructive lung disease.
◆ Stool specimen analysis indicating the absence of trypsin, suggesting pancreatic insufficiency.
◆ Deoxyribonucleic acid (DNA) testing can now locate the presence of the Delta F 508 deletion (found in about 70% of patients with cystic fibrosis, although the disease can stem from more than 100 other mutations). It allows prenatal diagnosis in families with a previously affected child. It's recommended that all pregnant couples receive screening for the disorder.
◆ Pulmonary function tests reveal decreased vital capacity, elevated residual volume due to air entrapments, and decreased forced expiratory volume in 1 second. This test is used if pulmonary exacerbation already exists.
◆ Liver enzyme tests may reveal hepatic insufficiency.
◆ Sputum culture reveals organisms that cystic fibrosis patients typically and chronically colonize, such as *Staphylococcus* and *Pseudomonas*.
◆ Serum albumin measurement helps assess nutritional status.
◆ Electrolyte analysis assesses hydration status.

Treatment
The aim of treatment is to help the child lead as normal a life as possible. The type of treatment depends on the organ system involved and may include:
◆ hypertonic radiocontrast materials delivered by enema to treat acute obstructions due to meconium ileus
◆ breathing exercises, postural drainage, and chest percussion to clear pulmonary secretions
◆ an antibiotic to treat lung infection, guided by sputum culture results
◆ drugs to increase mucus clearance
◆ an inhaled beta-adrenergic agonist to control airway constriction
◆ pancreatic enzyme replacement to maintain adequate nutrition
◆ a sodium-channel blocker to decrease sodium reabsorption from secretions and improve viscosity
◆ uridine triphosphate to stimulate chloride secretion by a non-CFTR channel
◆ a salt supplement to replace electrolytes lost through sweat
◆ Dornase alfa, a genetically engineered pulmonary enzyme, to help liquefy mucus

◆ recombinant alpha-antitrypsin to counteract excessive proteolytic activity produced during airway inflammation
◆ gene therapy to introduce normal CFTR into affected epithelial cells (researchers are currently working on developing efficient delivery methods)
◆ transplantation of heart or lungs in severe organ failure.

Special considerations
◆ Throughout this illness, teach the patient and his family about the disease and its treatment. The Cystic Fibrosis Foundation can provide educational and support services.
◆ Although many males with cystic fibrosis are infertile, females with the illness may become pregnant (due to increased life expectancies). As a result, more cystic fibrosis patients are now facing difficult reproductive decisions. Refer such patients (or the parents of an affected child) for genetic counseling so they can discuss family planning issues or prenatal diagnosis options if they're considering having more children.
◆ Be aware that some patients have recently undergone lung transplants to reduce the effects of the disease.
◆ Recent research indicates that the genetic defect responsible for cystic fibrosis has also been identified in individuals experiencing some forms of unexplained pancreatitis.

DOWN SYNDROME
Down syndrome, or *trisomy 21*, is a spontaneous chromosome abnormality that causes characteristic facial features, other distinctive physical abnormalities, and mental retardation; 60% of affected persons have cardiac defects. Down syndrome occurs in1 in 660 live births, but incidence increases with advanced maternal age. Improved treatment for heart defects, respiratory and other infections, and acute leukemia has significantly increased life expectancy. Fetal and neonatal mortality remain high, usually resulting from complications of associated heart defects.

Causes
◆ Advanced parental age (when the mother is age 35 or older at delivery or the father is age 42 or older)
◆ Cumulative effects of environmental factors, such as radiation and viruses

Pathophysiology
Nearly all cases of Down syndrome result from trisomy 21 (3 copies of chromosome 21). The result is a karyotype of 47 chromosomes instead of the usual 46. (See *Karyotype of Down syndrome*.)

In 4% of patients, Down syndrome results from an unbalanced translocation or chromosomal rearrangement in which the long arm of chromosome 21 breaks and attaches to another chromosome.

Some affected persons and some asymptomatic parents may have chromosomal mosaicism, a mixture of two cell types, some with the normal 46 and some with 47 (an extra chromosome 21).

Signs and symptoms
◼ **AGE ALERT** *At birth, the physical signs of Down syndrome are evident. The infant is hypotonic and has distinctive craniofacial features.*

Other signs and symptoms include:
◆ distinctive facial features (low nasal bridge, epicanthic folds, protruding tongue, and low-set ears); small open mouth and disproportionately large tongue
◆ single transverse crease on the palm (Simian crease)
◆ small white spots on the iris (Brushfield's spots)
◆ mental retardation (estimated IQ of 30 to 70)
◆ developmental delay due to hypotonia and decreased cognitive processing
◆ congenital heart disease, mainly septal defects and especially of the endocardial cushion
◆ impaired reflexes due to decreased muscle tone in limbs.

Complications
◆ Early death due to cardiac complications
◆ Increased susceptibility to leukemia
◆ Premature senile dementia, usually in the 4th decade if the patient survives
◆ Increased susceptibility to acute and chronic infections
◆ Strabismus and cataracts as the child grows
◆ Poorly developed genitalia and delayed puberty (females may menstruate and be fertile; males may be infertile with low serum testosterone levels and often with undescended testes)

Diagnosis
◆ Definitive karyotype
◆ Amniocentesis, chorionic villi sampling, or percutaneous umbilical blood sampling for prenatal diagnosis, recommended for pregnant women age 35 and older, even with a negative family history
◆ Prenatal targeted ultrasonography for duodenal obstruction or an atrioventricular canal defect (suggestive of Down syndrome)

Karyotype of Down syndrome

Each autosome is normally one of a pair. A patient with Down syndrome, *or trisomy 21*, has an extra chromosome 21.

MALE WITH DOWN SYNDROME

◆ Maternal blood tests during pregnancy that show low alpha-fetoprotein levels, low unconjugated estriol levels, and high human chorionic gonadotropin levels (all suggestive of Down syndrome)

Treatment

◆ Surgery to correct heart defects and other related congenital abnormalities
◆ An antibiotic for recurrent infections
◆ Plastic surgery to correct characteristic facial traits (especially protruding tongue; possibly improving speech, reducing susceptibility to dental caries, and resulting in fewer orthodontic problems)
◆ Early intervention programs and supportive therapies to maximize cognitive and physical capabilities
◆ Thyroid hormone replacement for hypothyroidism

Special considerations

Support for the parents of a child with Down syndrome is vital. Follow the guidelines listed here to help them meet their child's physical and emotional needs.

◆ Establish a trusting relationship with the parents and encourage communication during the difficult period soon after diagnosis. Recognize signs of grieving.
◆ Teach parents the importance of a balanced diet for the child. Stress the need for patience while feeding the infant, who may have difficulty sucking and may be less demanding and seem less eager to eat than other infants.
◆ Encourage the parents to hold and nurture their child.
◆ Emphasize the importance of adequate exercise and maximal environmental stimulation; refer the parents for infant stimulation classes, which may begin in the early months of life.
◆ Help the parents set realistic goals for their child. Explain that, although the child's mental

development may seem normal at first, they shouldn't view this early development as a sign of future progress. By the time he's age 1 the child's development may begin to lag behind that of other children.

◆ Refer the parents and older siblings for genetic and psychological counseling, as appropriate, to help them evaluate future reproductive risks. Discuss options for prenatal testing.

◆ Encourage the parents to remember the emotional needs of other children in the family.

◆ Refer the parents to national or local Down syndrome organizations and support groups.

FRAGILE X SYNDROME

Fragile X is the most common inherited cause of mental retardation. About 85% of males and 50% of females who inherit the fragile X mental retardation 1 (FMR1) mutation will demonstrate clinical features of the syndrome. Postpubescent males with fragile X syndrome often have distinct physical features, behavioral difficulties, and cognitive impairment. Females with fragile X syndrome tend to have more subtle symptoms.

Fragile X syndrome is estimated to occur in about 1 in 1,500 males and 1 in 2,500 females. It has been reported in almost all races and ethnic populations.

Causes
◆ Genetic defect on the X-chromosome
◆ Well-defined mutation at a specific location on the FMR1 gene

Pathophysiology
Fragile X syndrome is an X-linked condition that does not follow a simple X-linked inheritance pattern. The normal sequence of the FMR1 gene was identified at Xq27.3 in 1991. The unique mutation that results in fragile X syndrome consists of an expanding region of a specific triplet of nitrogenous bases: cytosine, guanine, guanine (CGG) within the gene's deoxyribonucleic acid (DNA) sequence. Normally, FMR1 contains 6 to 49 sequential copies of the CGG triplet. When the number of CGG triplets expands to the range of 50 to 200 repeats, the region of DNA becomes unstable and is referred to as a premutation. A full mutation consists of more than 200 CGG triplet repeats.

The full mutation typically causes abnormal methylation (methyl groups attach to components of the gene) of FMR1. Methylation inhibits gene transcription and, thus, protein production. The reduced or absent protein product is responsible for the clinical features of fragile X syndrome. Between 15% and 20% of males with a full mutation don't have the cognitive impair-

ment associated with fragile X. This lack may be explained by either the presence of unmethylated portions of their mutated FMR1 that can be transcribed for eventual protein production or the males are mosaic for the FMR1 premutation. In asymptomatic mosaic males it's believed that the cells with a premutation are able to produce enough protein to compensate for the cells that contain a full mutation and consequently produce no protein.

About 50% of females who inherit a full mutation from their mother have clinical features of fragile X syndrome. This incidence is primarily due to the normal process of random X inactivation. At the time of meiosis, both X chromosomes must be activated. However, shortly after the zygote stage, an X chromosome is inactivated in every cell. Clinically measurable effects of the full FMR1 mutation will be more likely in relevant tissues or organs that have a disproportionate number of cells in which the normal X chromosome has been inactivated.

Males with a premutation don't have fragile X. They're considered unaffected or normal-transmitting males. Because males have only one X chromosome, all daughters of a transmitting male will inherit their father's X chromosome with the premutation. None of the male's sons will inherit the premutation because they inherit their father's Y chromosome rather than the X chromosome.

Females with the premutation don't have fragile X syndrome. However, the premutation can expand into the full mutation range (greater than 200 CGG triplets) when it's transmitted from a premutation carrier mother to her offspring. This expansion can occur during or after maternal meiosis. Therefore, the following possibilities exist for every pregnancy of a mother with a premutation:

◆ A female receives the mother's X chromosome with the nonmutated FMR1 gene. She will not be affected with fragile X. None of her future offspring will be at risk for inheriting the syndrome from her.

◆ A male receives the mother's X with the nonmutated FMR1 gene. He won't be affected with fragile X. None of his future offspring will be at risk for inheriting the syndrome from him.

◆ A female receives the mother's X chromosome with the FMR1 premutation. She will be a carrier like her mother but won't have fragile X syndrome. Her future offspring will be at risk for inheriting a full mutation from her.

◆ A male receives the mother's X with the FMR1 premutation. He won't be affected with fragile X. All of his future daughters but none of his future sons will inherit the premutation from him.

♦ A female receives the mother's X chromosome with the FMR1 gene whose premutation expanded into a full mutation during or after maternal meiosis. Depending on the outcome of random X inactivation, the daughter may have clinically definable fragile X syndrome. Her future offspring will be at risk for inheriting the full mutation and, thus, the syndrome from her.

♦ A male receives the mother's X chromosome with the FMR1 gene whose premutation has expanded into a full mutation during or after maternal meiosis. In 85% of cases, the son in this situation will have fragile X syndrome. Evidence indicates, however, that the FMR1 gene in the son's gametes may have the CGG triplet repeat within the premutation range, not the full mutation range as in his somatic cells. Therefore, his future daughters wouldn't be expected to have fragile X syndrome.

It should be noted that most often the FMR1 status of a mother is determined after her son is clinically and later molecularly diagnosed with fragile X syndrome. Health care professionals need to be sensitive to the fact that the mother could find out she is a carrier of a premutation or she has a full mutation. Consequently, not only will she learn her son's diagnosis but she, too, could be diagnosed with fragile X if she has a full mutation and clinical symptoms.

Signs and symptoms

Small children may have relatively few identifiable physical characteristics; behavioral or learning difficulties may be the initial presenting features. Signs and symptoms in affected males include:

♦ a prominent jaw and forehead and a head circumference exceeding the 90th percentile

♦ a long, narrow face with long or large ears that may be posteriorly rotated

♦ connective tissue abnormalities, including hyperextension of the fingers, a floppy mitral valve (in 80% of adults), and mild to severe pectus excavatum

♦ unusually large testes, found in most affected males after puberty

♦ average IQ of 30 to 70

♦ hyperactivity, speech difficulties, language delay, and autistic-like behaviors, which may be attributed to other disorders, such as attention deficit hyperactivity disorder, and thus delay the diagnosis.

About 50% of females with the FMR1 full mutation will have clinical symptoms, although the degree of severity and number of symptoms vary widely among females with fragile X syndrome. Those who are symptomatic typically have a much milder clinical presentation than males due to having an unaffected X chromosome in addition to the one with a FMR1 full mutation. Signs and symptoms in females include:

♦ some degree of cognitive impairment, most commonly, learning disabilities (math difficulties, language deficits, and attentional problems)

♦ IQ scores in the mental retardation range

♦ autistic-like features (rare)

♦ excessive shyness or social anxiety

♦ prominent ears and connective tissue manifestations (possibly as significant as in males).

Although males with the FMR1 premutation are asymptomatic, some female carriers of a FMR1 premutation can have associated symptoms. These symptoms include significantly earlier menopause and a low-normal performance IQ.

Complications
♦ Behavioral or learning difficulties
♦ Cognitive impairment
♦ Connective tissue abnormalities

Diagnosis
♦ Identification of clinical symptoms
♦ Positive genetic test, preferably DNA analysis of blood or buccal samples to detect the size of the CGG repeat and the methylation status of FMR1

Before identification of the FMR1 mutation, a special cytogenetic (chromosome) blood test was used to microscopically detect the fragile site on the long arm of the affected X chromosome. It's now common knowledge that a full FMR1 mutation doesn't always result in a cytogenetically detectable fragile site. Therefore, chromosome analysis alone can provide false-negative results. Chromosome analysis still has utility together with FMR1 mutation analysis when performing a genetic evaluation on a male with mental retardation of unknown etiology.

In addition to diagnosing fragile X syndrome, genetic testing can determine whether the mother of a diagnosed individual is a carrier of the FMR1 premutation or has a full mutation. This information can be used for preconceptional genetic counseling by a trained professional and prenatal testing if the woman so chooses. FMR1 mutation analysis also can be subsequently performed on at-risk family members. It should be noted, however, that communication of genetic test results to at-risk family members constitutes a breach of patient confidentiality and privacy unless prior written permission to communicate results has been obtained from the previously tested patients.

Treatment

Fragile X syndrome has no known cure. Treatment is aimed at controlling individual symptoms. Most patients are on individualized pharmacotherapy for seizures, mood disorders, aggression, or sleep disorders. Surgery may be needed to repair a defective mitral valve.

Special considerations

◆ Individuals who have been identified as carriers may experience guilt and grief; provide support to help both the carrier and family members accept the diagnosis.

◆ Parents of an affected child may need help to deal with their grief over unmet expectations for the child; refer them for appropriate counseling if necessary.

◆ Refer the family (and possibly the extended family) to a professional trained in genetics to discuss the diagnosis, testing, and the risk of recurrence in future offspring.

◆ Recurrent otitis media is common. To maximize the affected child's potential for language development, early diagnosis and aggressive treatment of otitis media are essential.

◆ Throughout childhood, assess for seizure activity, hyperactivity, and attention deficit disorder, referring for appropriate therapy as necessary.

◆ Enroll infants and toddlers in early intervention programs.

◆ Advocate for special education services and individualized speech, language, and occupational therapy services during school years.

HEMOPHILIA

Hemophilia is an X-linked recessive bleeding disorder; the severity and prognosis of bleeding vary with the degree of deficiency, or nonfunction, and the site of bleeding. Hemophilia results from a deficiency of specific clotting factors.

Hemophilia A, or *classic hemophilia,* is a deficiency of clotting factor VIII; it's five times more common than type B, affecting 1 in 10,000 males worldwide. Hemophilia B, or *Christmas disease,* results from a deficiency of factor IX. There's no relationship between factor VIII and factor IX inherited defects.

Causes

◆ Defect in a specific gene on the X chromosome that codes for factor VIII synthesis (hemophilia A)

◆ More than 300 different base-pair substitutions involving the factor IX gene on the X chromosome (hemophilia B)

Pathophysiology

Hemophilia is an X-linked recessive genetic disease causing abnormal bleeding because of specific clotting factor malfunction. Factors VIII and IX are components of the intrinsic clotting pathway; factor IX is an essential factor and factor VIII is a critical cofactor. Factor VIII accelerates the activation of factor X by several thousand-fold. Excessive bleeding occurs when these clotting factors are reduced by more than 75%. A deficiency or nonfunction of factor VIII causes hemophilia A, while a deficiency or nonfunction of factor IX causes hemophilia B.

Hemophilia may be severe, moderate, or mild, depending on the degree of activation of clotting factors. Patients with severe disease have no detectable factor VIII or factor IX activity or less than 1% of normal. Moderately afflicted patients have 1% to 4% of normal clotting activity, and mildly afflicted patients have 5% to 25% of normal clotting activity.

A person with hemophilia forms a platelet plug at a bleeding site, but clotting factor deficiency impairs the ability to form a stable fibrin clot. Delayed bleeding is more common than immediate hemorrhage.

Signs and symptoms

◆ Spontaneous bleeding in severe hemophilia (prolonged or excessive bleeding after circumcision is often the first sign) because of absence of clotting factors

◆ Excessive or continued bleeding or bruising after minor trauma or surgery caused by inability to form a stable fibrin clot because of clotting factor deficiency

◆ Large subcutaneous and deep intramuscular hematomas due to bleeding into the tissue or muscle from mild trauma

◆ Prolonged bleeding in mild hemophilia after major trauma or surgery, but no spontaneous bleeding after minor trauma

◆ Pain, swelling, and tenderness due to bleeding into joints (especially weight-bearing joints)

◆ Internal bleeding, often manifested as abdominal, chest, or flank pain

◆ Hematuria from bleeding into kidney

◆ Hematemesis or tarry stools from bleeding into the GI tract

Complications

◆ Peripheral neuropathy, pain, paresthesia, and muscle atrophy due to bleeding near peripheral nerves

◆ Ischemia and gangrene due to impaired blood flow through a major vessel distal to bleed

◆ Decreased tissue perfusion and hypovolemic shock (shown as restlessness, anxiety, confusion, pallor, cool and clammy skin, chest pain, decreased urine output, hypotension, and tachycardia)

Diagnosis

◆ Specific coagulation factor assays to diagnose the type and severity of hemophilia
◆ Factor VIII assay of 0% to 30% of normal and prolonged activated partial thromboplastin time (hemophilia A)
◆ Deficient factor IX and normal factor VIII levels (hemophilia B)
◆ Normal platelet count and function, bleeding time, and prothrombin time (hemophilia A and B)
◆ Positive family history, prenatal diagnosis, and carrier testing (although nearly one-third of all patients have no family history)

Treatment

Hemophilia isn't curable, but treatment can prevent crippling deformities and prolong life expectancy. It includes:
◆ cryoprecipitate antihemophilic factor (AHF) (for hemophilia A) or lyophilized AHF VIII or IX to increase clotting factor levels and to permit normal hemostasis levels
◆ recombinant factor VIII and purified factor IX during bleeding episodes (hemophilia B)
◆ aminocaproic acid (Amicar) for oral bleeding (inhibits plasminogen activator substances)
◆ prophylactic desmopressin before dental procedures or minor surgery to release stored von Willebrand's factor and factor VIII (to reduce bleeding)
◆ an analgesic to control joint pain.
 AGE ALERT *Young children should wear clothing with padded patches on the knees and elbows to help prevent injury. Older children should avoid contact sports.*

Special considerations

During bleeding episodes:
◆ Give a clotting agent, as ordered. The body uses up antihemophilic factor in 48 to 72 hours, so repeat infusions as ordered until bleeding stops.
◆ Apply cold compresses or ice bags and raise the injured part.
◆ To prevent recurrence of bleeding, restrict activity for 48 hours after bleeding is under control.
◆ Control pain with an analgesic, such as acetaminophen, propoxyphene, codeine, or meperidine, as ordered. Avoid I.M. injections because of possible hematoma formation at the injection site. Aspirin and aspirin-containing medications are contraindicated because they decrease platelet adherence and may increase

the bleeding. Caution should be used when trying other nonsteroidal anti-inflammatory drugs — for example, ibuprofen or ketoprofen.
If the patient has bled into a joint:
◆ Immediately elevate the joint.
◆ To restore joint mobility, begin range-of-motion exercises, if ordered, at least 48 hours after the bleeding is controlled. Tell the patient to avoid weight bearing until bleeding stops and swelling subsides.
After bleeding episodes and surgery:
◆ Watch closely for signs of further bleeding, such as increased pain and swelling, fever, or symptoms of shock.
◆ Closely monitor partial thromboplastin time.
◆ Teach parents special precautions to prevent bleeding episodes.
◆ Refer a new patient to a hemophilia treatment center for evaluation. The center will devise a treatment plan for the patient's primary physician and is a resource for other medical and school personnel, dentist, and others involved in care.
◆ Persons who have been exposed to human immunodeficiency virus through contaminated blood products need special support.
◆ Refer patients and carriers for genetic counseling.

KLINEFELTER SYNDROME

Klinefelter syndrome, a relatively common genetic abnormality, results from an extra X chromosome — creating an XXY sex chromosome constitution — and affects only males. It usually becomes apparent at puberty, when the secondary sex characteristics develop. The testicles fail to mature and degenerative testicular changes begin that eventually result in irreversible infertility. Klinefelter syndrome commonly causes gynecomastia and is also associated with a tendency toward learning disabilities. Because not all patients with the extra X chromosome will display the same characteristics, the term *XXY male* has come into favor, as opposed to labeling all males with an extra X chromosome as having Klinefelter syndrome. Some of these XXY males may develop Klinefelter syndrome, and some may not.

The XXY chromosome arrangement, probably the most common cause of hypogonadism, appears in about 1 in every 500 males, and may be one of the most common genetic abnormalities.

Causes

◆ Cells with one extra X chromosome create a 47,XXY complement instead of the normal 46,XY (See *Spermatogenic mistake,* page 114.)

Spermatogenic mistake

Fertilization by a sperm with X and Y chromosomes produces an XXY zygote.

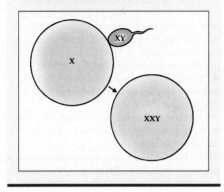

♦ In the rare mosaic form, only some cells contain the extra X chromosomes and others contain the normal XY complement
♦ Lack of one X chromosome, 45X (See *Turner's syndrome.*)

Pathophysiology

The extra chromosome responsible for Klinefelter syndrome probably results from either meiotic nondisjunction during parental gametogenesis or from mitotic nondisjunction in the zygote. The incidence of meiotic nondisjunction increases with maternal age.

Signs and symptoms

Klinefelter syndrome may not be apparent until puberty or later in mild cases. Because many of these patients are not mentally retarded, behavioral problems in adolescence or infertility may be the only presenting features initially.

The signs and symptoms exhibited are the result of the genetic defect involving the extra X chromosome. The syndrome's characteristic features include:
♦ a small penis and prostate gland
♦ small testicles
♦ sparse facial and abdominal hair
♦ feminine distribution of pubic hair (triangular shape)
♦ sexual dysfunction (impotence, lack of libido)
♦ in fewer than 50% of patients, gynecomastia
♦ in the mosaic form, delay of pathologic changes and resulting infertility
♦ abnormal body build (long legs with short, obese trunk)
♦ tall stature

♦ in some individuals, behavioral problems beginning in adolescence
♦ increased incidence of pulmonary disease and varicose veins.

Complications

♦ Aspermatogenesis and infertility, due to progressive sclerosis and hyalinization of the seminiferous tubules in the testicles and testicular fibrosis during and after puberty
♦ Learning disabilities and behavioral problems
♦ Osteoporosis
♦ Breast cancer because of the extra X chromosome

Diagnosis

♦ A karyotype (chromosome analysis) determined by culturing lymphocytes from the patient's peripheral blood
♦ A decreased urinary 17-ketosteroid level
♦ Increased excretion of follicle-stimulating hormone
♦ A decreased level of plasma testosterone after puberty

Treatment

Depending on the severity of symptoms, treatment may include:
♦ mastectomy in patients with persistent gynecomastia
♦ supplemental testosterone to induce secondary sexual characteristics of puberty
♦ psychological counseling for body image problems or emotional maladjustment due to sexual dysfunction.

Special considerations

♦ Genetic counseling is essential for patients with the mosaic form of the syndrome who are fertile; they may transmit this chromosomal abnormality as well as others.
♦ Encourage patients to discuss feelings of confusion and rejection that may arise, and try to reinforce their male identity.
♦ Improve the patient's compliance with hormone replacement therapy by making sure he understands the potential benefits and adverse effects of testosterone administration.

MARFAN SYNDROME

Marfan syndrome is a rare degenerative, generalized disease of the connective tissue. It results from elastin and collagen defects and causes ocular, skeletal, and cardiovascular anomalies. Death occurs from cardiovascular complications from early infancy to adulthood. The syndrome affects males and females equally.

Turner's syndrome

In Turner's syndrome, one of the X chromosomes (or part of the second X chromosome) may be lost from either the ovum or sperm through nondisjunction or chromosome lag. Mixed aneuploidy may result from mitotic nondisjunction.

This disorder occurs in 1 in 3,000 births; up to 95% of affected fetuses are spontaneously aborted. Maternal age isn't a risk factor in this disorder.

Signs and symptoms

In utero, the fetus may have a cystic hygroma seen on ultrasound; however, these may also be seen in fetuses that don't have Turner's syndrome. The mother may have elevated or low levels of serum alpha-fetoprotein.

At birth, 50% of infants with this syndrome measure below the third percentile in length. Many have swollen hands and feet, a wide chest with laterally displaced nipples, and a low hairline that becomes more obvious as they grow. They may have webbing of the neck and coarse, enlarged, prominent ears. Gonadal dysgenesis is seen at birth and typically causes sterility in adult females (unless they have the mosaic form).

Cardiovascular defects, such as bicuspid aortic valve and coarctation of the aorta, occur in 10% to 40% of patients. Short stature (usually under 59″ [150 cm]) is the most common adult sign.

Most patients have average or slightly below-average intelligence; they commonly exhibit spatial defects, right-left disorientation for extrapersonal space, and defective figure drawing.

Diagnosis and treatment

Turner's syndrome can be diagnosed by chromosome analysis. Differential diagnoses should rule out mixed gonadal dysgenesis, Noonan's syndrome, and other similar disorders.

Treatment should begin in early childhood and may include hormonal therapy (androgens, human growth hormone and, possibly, small doses of estrogen). Later, progesterone and estrogen can induce sexual maturation, but most patients remain sterile.

Causes
◆ Autosomal dominant mutation
◆ In patients with a negative family history (15% of patients), possibly advanced paternal age

Pathophysiology

Marfan syndrome is caused by a mutation in a single allele of a gene located on chromosome 15; the gene codes for fibrillin, a glycoprotein component of connective tissue. These small fibers are abundant in large blood vessels and the suspensory ligaments of the ocular lenses. The effect on connective tissue is varied and includes excessive bone growth, ocular disorders, and cardiac defects.

Signs and symptoms
◆ Increased height, long extremities, and arachnodactyly (long spiderlike fingers) due to effects on long bones and joints and excessive bone growth
◆ Defects of sternum (funnel chest or pigeon breast, for example), chest asymmetry, scoliosis, and kyphosis caused by effects on bone
◆ Hypermobile joints due to effects on connective tissue
◆ Nearsightedness due to elongated ocular globe
◆ Lens displacement due to altered connective tissue (the ocular hallmark of the syndrome)
◆ Valvular abnormalities (redundancy of leaflets, stretching of chordae tendineae, and dilation of valvulae annulus) from effects on cardiac connective tissue
◆ Mitral valve prolapse due to weakened connective tissue
◆ Aortic insufficiency due to dilation of aortic root and ascending aorta

Complications
◆ Weak joints and ligaments, predisposing to injury
◆ Cataracts due to lens displacement
◆ Retinal detachments and retinal tears
◆ Severe mitral valve regurgitation due to mitral valve prolapse
◆ Spontaneous pneumothorax due to chest wall instability
◆ Inguinal and incisional hernias
◆ Dilation of the dural sac (portion of the dura mater beyond caudal end of the spinal cord)

Diagnosis
◆ Positive family history in one parent (85% of patients) and typical clinical features

◆ Presence of lens displacement and aneurysm of the ascending aorta without other symptoms or familial tendency
◆ Detection of fibrillin defects in cultured skin
◆ X-rays confirming skeletal abnormalities
◆ Echocardiogram showing dilation of the aortic root
◆ Deoxyribonucleic acid analysis of the gene

Treatment

Typical treatment for Marfan syndrome is aimed at relieving symptoms and may involve:
◆ surgical repair of aneurysms to prevent rupture
◆ surgical correction of ocular deformities to improve vision
◆ steroid and sex hormone therapy to induce early epiphyseal closure and limit adult height
◆ a beta-adrenergic blocker to delay or prevent aortic dilation
◆ surgical replacement of aortic valve and mitral valve for extreme dilation
◆ mechanical bracing and physical therapy for mild scoliosis if curvature is greater than 20 degrees
◆ surgery for scoliosis if curvature is greater than 45 degrees.

Special considerations

◆ High school and college athletes (particularly basketball players) who fit the criteria for Marfan syndrome should undergo a careful clinical and cardiac examination before being allowed to play to avoid sudden death due to dissecting aortic aneurysm or other cardiac complications.
◆ Provide the patient with supportive care, as appropriate for his clinical status.
◆ Educate the patient and his family about the course of the disease and its potential complications.
◆ Stress the need for frequent checkups to detect and treat degenerative changes early.
◆ Emphasize the importance of taking prescribed medications as ordered and avoiding contact sports and isometric exercise.
◆ If recommended by the physician, encourage hormonal therapy to induce early epiphyseal closure, thus preventing abnormal adult height.
◆ To encourage normal adolescent development, advise the parents to avoid unrealistic expectations for their child simply because he's tall and looks older than his years.
◆ Refer the patient and family to the National Marfan Foundation for additional information.

NEURAL TUBE DEFECTS

Neural tube defects (NTDs) are serious birth defects that involve the spine or skull; they result from failure of the neural tube to close at approximately 28 days after conception. The most common forms of NTD are spina bifida (50% of cases), anencephaly (40%), and encephalocele (10%). Spina bifida occulta is the most common and least severe spinal cord defect.

The incidence of NTDs varies greatly among countries and by region in the United States. For example, the incidence is significantly higher in the British Isles and low in southern China and Japan. In the United States, North and South Carolina have at least twice the incidence of NTDs as most other parts of the country. These birth defects are also less common in Blacks than in Whites.

Causes

◆ Exposure to a teratogen
◆ Part of a multiple malformation syndrome (for example, chromosomal abnormalities such as trisomy 18 or 13 syndrome)
◆ In isolated birth defects, a combination of genetic and environmental factors (mostly unknown, though possibly a lack of folic acid in the mother's diet)

Pathophysiology

Neural tube closure normally occurs at 24 days' gestation in the cranial region and continues distally, with closure of the lumbar regions by 28 days.

Spina bifida occulta is characterized by incomplete closure of one or more vertebrae without protrusion of the spinal cord or meninges.

However, in more severe forms of spina bifida, incomplete closure of one or more vertebrae causes protrusion of the spinal contents in an external sac or cystic lesion (spina bifida cystica). Spina bifida cystica has two classifications: myelomeningocele (meningomyelocele) and meningocele. In myelomeningocele, the external sac contains meninges, cerebrospinal fluid (CSF), and a portion of the spinal cord or nerve roots distal to the conus medullaris. When the spinal nerve roots end at the sac, motor and sensory functions below the sac are terminated. In meningocele, less severe than myelomeningocele, the sac contains only meninges and CSF. Meningocele may produce no neurologic symptoms.

In encephalocele, a saclike portion of the meninges and brain protrudes through a defective opening in the skull. Usually, it occurs in the occipital area, but it may also occur in the parietal, nasopharyngeal, or frontal area.

In anencephaly, the most severe form of NTD, the closure defect occurs at the cranial end of the neuroaxis and, as a result, part or the entire top of the skull is missing, severely damaging the brain. Portions of the brain stem and spinal cord may also be missing. No diagnostic or therapeutic efforts are helpful; this condition is invariably fatal.

Signs and symptoms

Signs and symptoms depend on the type and severity of NTD:
◆ possibly, a depression or dimple, tuft of hair, soft fatty deposits, port wine nevi, or a combination of these abnormalities on the skin over the spinal defect (spina bifida occulta) due to incomplete closure
◆ foot weakness or bowel and bladder disturbances, especially likely during rapid growth phases (spina bifida occulta) related to effect on spinal nerve roots
◆ saclike structure that protrudes over the spine (myelomeningocele, meningocele) caused by incomplete closure
◆ depending on the level of the defect, permanent neurologic dysfunction, such as flaccid or spastic paralysis and bowel and bladder incontinence (myelomeningocele) caused by effect on spinal nerve roots.

Associated disorders include:
◆ trophic skin disturbances (ulcerations, cyanosis)
◆ clubfoot
◆ knee contractures
◆ hydrocephalus (in about 90% of patients)
◆ mental retardation
◆ Arnold-Chiari syndrome (part of the brain protrudes into the spinal canal)
◆ curvature of the spine.

Clinical effects of encephalocele vary with the degree of tissue involvement and location of the defect. Paralysis and hydrocephalus are common. Infants with this defect have a better chance of survival than anencephalic infants and usually suffer less paralysis; however, surviving infants are usually severely mentally retarded.

Complications
◆ Paralysis below the level of the defect
◆ Infection such as meningitis

Diagnosis
◆ Amniocentesis to detect elevated alpha-fetoprotein (AFP) levels in amniotic fluid, which indicates the presence of an open NTD
◆ Acetylcholinesterase levels (not usually effective for closed NTDs)
◆ Fetal karyotype to detect chromosomal abnormalities (present in 5% to 7% of NTDs)
◆ Maternal serum AFP screening in combination with other serum markers, such as human chorionic gonadotropin (HCG), free beta-HCG,

or unconjugated estriol (for patients with a lower risk of NTDs and those who will be younger than age 34½ at the time of delivery) to estimate a fetus's risk of NTD as well as possible increased risk for perinatal complications, such as premature rupture of the membranes, abruptio placentae, or fetal death
◆ Ultrasound when increased risk of open NTD exists, based on family history or abnormal serum screening results (not conclusive for open NTDs or ventral wall defects)

If the NTD isn't diagnosed before birth, other tests are used to make the diagnosis:
◆ palpation and spinal X-ray for spina bifida occulta
◆ myelography to differentiate spina bifida occulta from other spinal abnormalities, especially spinal cord tumors
◆ transillumination of the protruding sac to distinguish between myelomeningocele (typically doesn't transilluminate) and meningocele (typically does transilluminate)
◆ pinprick examination of the legs and trunk to show the level of sensory and motor involvement in myelomeningocele
◆ skull X-rays, cephalic measurements, and computed tomography (CT) scan demonstrate associated hydrocephalus.

Other appropriate laboratory tests in patients with myelomeningocele include urinalysis, urine cultures, and tests for renal function starting in the neonatal period and continuing at regular intervals.

In encephalocele, X-rays show a basilar bony skull defect. CT scan and ultrasonography further define the defect.

Treatment

Spina bifida occulta usually requires no treatment. Prompt neurosurgical repair and aggressive management may improve the condition of children with some NTDs. However, surgery doesn't reverse neurologic deficits and serious and permanent disabilities are likely. Fetal surgery has been successful at repairing some open defects, thereby reducing damage. Treatment may include:
◆ surgical closure of the protruding sac and continual assessment of growth and development (meningocele)
◆ repair of the sac and supportive measures to promote independence and prevent further complications (myelomeningocele)
◆ shunt to relieve associated hydrocephalus
◆ surgery during infancy to place protruding tissues back in the skull, excise the sac, and correct associated craniofacial abnormalities (encephalocele).

PREVENTION
Folic acid supplement recommendations

The following recommendations for folic acid supplement dosages have been endorsed by the Centers for Disease Control and Prevention, the U.S. Public Health Service, the March of Dimes Birth Defects Foundation, and the Spina Bifida Association of America, among other groups.

All women of childbearing age
All women who are capable of becoming pregnant should:
♦ consume 0.4 mg of folic acid daily to reduce their risk of having a child with spina bifida or another neural tube defect (NTD)
♦ continue to consume 0.4 mg of folic acid daily when pregnant until their physician prescribes other prenatal vitamins.

Women at high risk
Women with a previous pregnancy affected by an NTD should:
♦ receive genetic counseling before their next pregnancy
♦ consume 0.4 mg of folic acid daily
♦ when actively trying to become pregnant (at least 1 month before conception), increase their dosage of folic acid to 4 mg daily (by taking a separate folic acid supplement, not by increasing their intake of multivitamins)
♦ continue to take 4 mg of folic acid daily through the first 3 months of pregnancy.

Special considerations
♦ When an NTD has been diagnosed prenatally, refer the prospective parents to a genetic counselor, who can provide information and support the couple's decisions on how to manage the pregnancy.
♦ Recent research sponsored by the March of Dimes and others has indicated that the risk of an open NTD may be reduced 50% to 70% in pregnant women who take a daily multivitamin with folic acid. Urge all women of childbearing age to take such a vitamin supplement until menopause or the end of childbearing potential. (See *Folic acid supplement recommendations*.)
♦ The parents of a child with an NTD will need assistance from physicians, nurses, surgeons, rehabilitation providers, and social workers.

Help to coordinate such assistance as needed. Obviously, care is most complex when the neurologic deficit is severe. Immediate goals include psychological support to help parents accept the diagnosis and preoperative and postoperative care. Long-term goals include patient and family teaching and measures to prevent contractures, pressure ulcers, urinary tract infections (UTIs), and other complications.

Before surgery:
♦ Prevent local infection by cleaning the defect gently with sterile saline solution or other solutions as ordered. Inspect the defect often for signs of infection and cover it with sterile dressings moistened with warmed sterile saline solution. Prevent skin breakdown by placing sheepskin or a foam pad under the infant. Keep skin clean and apply lotion to the infant's knees, elbows, chin, and other pressure areas. Give an antibiotic as ordered.
♦ Handle the infant carefully, and don't apply pressure to the defect. Usually the infant can't wear a diaper or a shirt until after surgical correction because it will irritate the sac, so keep him warm in an infant Isolette. Hold and cuddle the infant. Place the infant on his abdomen on your lap; teach parents to do the same.
♦ Provide adequate time for parent-child bonding, if possible.
♦ Measure head circumference daily and watch for signs of hydrocephalus and meningeal irritation, such as fever or nuchal rigidity. Be sure to mark the spot so you get accurate readings.
♦ Contractures can be minimized by passive range-of-motion exercises and casting. To prevent hip dislocation, moderately abduct hips with a pad between the knees or with sandbags and ankle rolls.
♦ Monitor intake and output. Watch for decreased skin turgor, dryness, or other signs of dehydration. Provide meticulous skin care to genitals and buttocks to prevent infection.
♦ Ensure adequate nutrition.

After surgery:
♦ Watch for hydrocephalus, which often follows surgery. Measure the infant's head circumference as ordered.
♦ Monitor vital signs often. Watch for signs of shock, infection, and increased intracranial pressure (ICP), such as projectile vomiting. Frequently assess the infant's fontanels. Remember that before age 2, infants don't show typical signs of increased ICP because suture lines aren't fully closed. In infants, the most telling sign is bulging fontanels.
♦ Change the dressing regularly as ordered, and check and report any signs of drainage, wound rupture, and infection.

◆ Place the infant in the prone position to protect and assess the site.
◆ If leg casts have been applied to treat deformities, watch for signs that the child is outgrowing the cast. Regularly check distal pulses to ensure adequate circulation.

To help parents cope with their infant's physical problems and successfully meet long-term treatment goals:
◆ Teach them to recognize early signs of complications, such as hydrocephalus, pressure ulcers, and UTIs.
◆ Provide psychological support and encourage a positive attitude. Help parents work through their feelings of guilt, anger, and helplessness.
◆ Encourage parents to begin training their child in a bladder routine by age 3 years. Emphasize the need for increased fluid intake to prevent UTIs. Teach intermittent catheterization and conduit hygiene as ordered.
◆ To prevent constipation and bowel obstruction, stress the need for increased fluid intake, a high-bulk diet, exercise, and a stool softener as ordered. If possible, teach parents to help empty their child's bowel by telling him to bear down, and giving a glycerin suppository as needed.
◆ Urge early recognition of developmental lags (a possible result of hydrocephalus). If present, stress the importance of follow-up IQ assessment to help plan realistic educational goals. The child may need to attend a school with special facilities. Also, stress the need for stimulation to ensure maximum mental development. Help parents plan activities appropriate to their child's age and abilities.
◆ Refer parents for genetic counseling and suggest that amniocentesis be performed in future pregnancies. Also refer parents to the Spina Bifida Association of America.

SICKLE CELL ANEMIA

Sickle cell anemia is a congenital hemolytic anemia resulting from defective hemoglobin molecules. It occurs most commonly in tropical Africans and in people of African descent; about 1 in 10 American Blacks carry the abnormal gene. However, sickle cell anemia also appears in other ethnic populations, including those of Mediterranean or East Indian ancestry.

Cause
◆ Mutation of hemoglobin S gene (heterozygous inheritance results in sickle cell trait, usually an asymptomatic condition)

Pathophysiology
Sickle cell anemia results from substitution of the amino acid valine for glutamic acid in the hemoglobin S gene encoding the beta chain of hemoglobin. Abnormal hemoglobin S, found in the red blood cells (RBCs) of patients, becomes insoluble during hypoxia. As a result, these cells become rigid, rough, and elongated, forming a crescent or sickle shape. (See *Characteristics of sickled cells,* page 120.) The sickling produces hemolysis. The altered cells also pile up in the capillaries and smaller blood vessels, making the blood more viscous. Normal circulation is impaired, causing pain, tissue infarctions, and swelling.

Each patient with sickle cell anemia has a different hypoxic threshold and different factors that trigger a sickle cell crisis. Illness, exposure to cold, stress, acidotic states, or a pathophysiologic process that pulls water out of the sickle cells precipitates a crisis in most patients. (See *Sickle cell crisis,* page 121.) The blockages then cause anoxic changes that lead to further sickling and obstruction.

Signs and symptoms
AGE ALERT *Signs and symptoms of sickle cell anemia don't develop until after age 6 months because fetal hemoglobin protects infants for the first few months after birth.*

Signs and symptoms may include:
◆ tachycardia, cardiomegaly, chronic fatigue, and unexplained dyspnea caused by tissue ischemia
◆ hepatomegaly caused by infarction secondary to sluggish blood flow
◆ joint swelling caused by aseptic infarction of the bones
◆ severe pain in the abdomen, thorax, muscle, or bones (characterizes painful crisis) caused by obstructed blood flow to the area and subsequent ischemia
◆ jaundice, dark urine, and low-grade fever due to blood vessel obstruction by rigid, tangled, sickle cells (leading to tissue anoxia and possibly necrosis)
◆ *Streptococcus pneumoniae* sepsis due to autosplenectomy (splenic damage and scarring in patients with long-term disease).

Suspect any of the following crises in a sickle cell anemia patient with pale lips, tongue, palms or nail beds; lethargy; listlessness; sleepiness; irritability; severe pain; and fever:
◆ aplastic crisis (megaloblastic crisis) due to bone marrow depression (associated with infection, usually viral, and characterized by pallor, lethargy, sleepiness, dyspnea, possible coma, markedly decreased bone marrow activity, and RBC hemolysis)
◆ acute sequestration crisis (rare; affects infants ages 8 months to 2 years; may cause lethargy, pallor, and hypovolemic shock) due to

Characteristics of sickled cells

Normal red blood cells (RBCs) and sickled cells vary in shape, life span, oxygen-carrying capacity, and the rate at which they're destroyed. The illustrations (below) show normal and sickled cells and list their major differences.

Normal RBCs
◆ 120-day life span
◆ Hemoglobin (Hb) has normal oxygen-carrying capacity
◆ 12 to 14 g/dl of Hb
◆ RBCs destroyed at normal rate

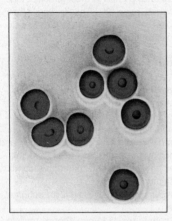

Sickled cells
◆ 10- to 20-day life span
◆ Hb has decreased oxygen-carrying capacity
◆ 6 to 9 g/dl of Hb
◆ RBCs destroyed at accelerated rate

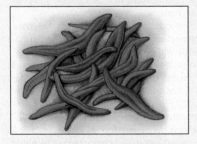

the sudden massive entrapment of cells in spleen and liver
◆ hemolytic crisis (rare; usually affects patients who also have glucose-6-phosphate dehydrogenase deficiency; degenerative changes cause liver congestion and enlargement and chronic jaundice worsens).

Complications
◆ Retinopathy, nephropathy, and cerebral vessel occlusion due to organ infarction
◆ Hypovolemic shock and death due to massive entrapment of cells
◆ Necrosis
◆ Infection and gangrene

Diagnosis
◆ Positive family history and typical clinical features
◆ Hemoglobin electrophoresis, showing hemoglobin S
◆ Electrophoresis of umbilical cord blood to provide screening for all neonates at risk
◆ Stained blood smear showing sickle cells
◆ Low RBC count, elevated white blood cell and platelet counts, decreased erythrocyte sedimentation rate, increased serum iron level, decreased RBC survival, and reticulocytosis (hemoglobin level may be low or normal)
◆ Lateral chest X-ray showing "Lincoln log" deformity in the vertebrae of many adults and some adolescents
◆ Neonate screening for hemoglobin abnormalities, including sickle cell anemia (mandated in some states)
◆ Available prenatal and preimplantation diagnosis, especially if the mutation in the family is known

Treatment
◆ Packed RBC transfusion to correct hypovolemia (if hemoglobin level decreases)
◆ Sedation and an analgesic, such as meperidine (Demerol) or morphine sulfate, for pain
◆ Oxygen administration to correct hypoxia
◆ Large amounts of oral or I.V. fluids to correct hypovolemia and prevent dehydration and vessel occlusion
◆ Prophylactic penicillin before age 4 months to prevent infection
◆ Hydroxyurea to reduce painful episodes by increasing the production of fetal hemoglobin which seems to alleviate symptoms
◆ Iron and folic acid supplements to prevent anemia

⚠ **CLINICAL ALERT** *Vaccines to prevent illness and anti-infectives, such as low-dose penicillin, should be considered to prevent complications in patients with sickle cell anemia.*

CLOSER LOOK
Sickle cell crisis

Infection, exposure to cold, high altitudes, overexertion, or other situations that cause cellular oxygen deprivation may trigger a sickle cell crisis. The deoxygenated, sickle-shaped red blood cells stick to the capillary wall and each other, blocking blood flow and causing cellular hypoxia. The crisis worsens as tissue hypoxia and acidic waste products cause more sickling and cell damage. With each new crisis, organs and tissues are slowly destroyed, especially the spleen and kidneys.

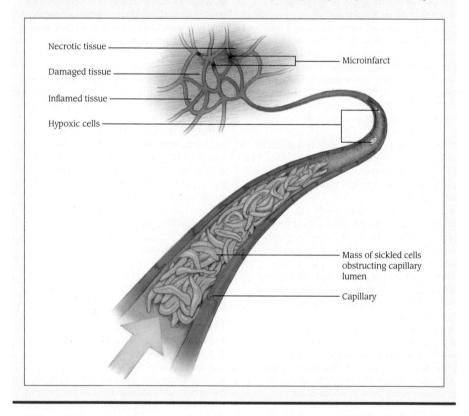

Necrotic tissue

Microinfarct

Damaged tissue

Inflamed tissue

Hypoxic cells

Mass of sickled cells obstructing capillary lumen

Capillary

Special considerations

Supportive measures during crises and precautions to avoid them are important. Here are some actions you can take during a painful crisis:

◆ Apply warm compresses to painful areas, and cover the child with a blanket. (Never use cold compresses because they aggravate the condition.)

◆ Administer an analgesic-antipyretic, such as aspirin or acetaminophen. (Additional pain relief may be required during an acute crisis.)

◆ Encourage bed rest, and place the patient in a sitting position. If dehydration or severe pain occurs, hospitalization may be necessary.

◆ When cultures indicate, give an antibiotic as ordered.

During remissions:

◆ Advise the patient to avoid tight clothing that restricts circulation.

◆ Warn against strenuous exercise, vasoconstricting medications, cold temperatures (including drinking large amounts of ice water and swimming), unpressurized aircraft, high altitude, and other conditions that provoke hypoxia.

◆ Stress the importance of normal childhood immunizations, meticulous wound care, good oral hygiene, regular dental checkups, and a balanced diet as safeguards against infection.

◆ Emphasize the need for prompt treatment of infection.

◆ Inform the patient of the need to increase fluid intake to prevent dehydration due to impaired ability to concentrate urine properly. Tell parents to encourage the child to drink more fluids, especially in the summer, by offering such fluids as milkshakes, ice pops, and eggnog.

During pregnancy or surgery:

◆ Warn women with sickle cell anemia that they may have increased obstetric risks. However, use of hormonal contraceptives may also be risky; refer them for birth control counseling to a qualified obstetric-gynecologic physician.

◆ If a woman with sickle cell anemia becomes pregnant, encourage her to maintain a balanced diet and take a folic acid supplement.

◆ During general anesthesia, a sickle cell anemia patient requires optimal ventilation to prevent hypoxic crisis. Make sure the surgeon and the anesthesiologist know that the patient has sickle cell anemia. Provide a preoperative transfusion of packed RBCs, as needed.

General tips:

◆ To encourage normal mental and social development, warn parents against being overprotective. Although the child must avoid strenuous exercise, he can enjoy most everyday activities.

◆ Refer parents of children with sickle cell anemia for genetic counseling to answer their questions about the risk to future offspring. Recommend screening of other family members to determine if they're heterozygote carriers. These parents may also need psychological counseling to cope with guilt feelings. In addition, suggest they join an appropriate community support group.

◆ Adolescents or adult males with sickle cell anemia may develop sudden, painful episodes of priapism. Such episodes are common and, if prolonged, can have serious reproductive consequences. Advise the patient to contact the physician when these episodes occur.

TAY-SACHS DISEASE

Tay-Sachs disease, also known as *GM₂ gangliosidosis*, is the most common lipid-storage disease.

AGE ALERT *Progressive mental and motor deterioration often causes death before age 5. Tay-Sachs disease appears in fewer than 100 infants born each year in the United States.*

Tay-Sachs affects persons of Eastern European Jewish (Ashkenazic) ancestry about 100 times more often than the general population, occurring in about 1 in 3,600 live births in this ethnic group. About 1 in 30 Ashkenazic Jews, French Canadians, and American Cajuns are heterozygous carriers. If two such carriers have children, each of their offspring has a 25% chance of having Tay-Sachs disease.

Cause

◆ Congenital deficiency of the enzyme hexosaminidase A

Pathophysiology

Tay-Sachs disease is an autosomal recessive disorder in which the enzyme hexosaminidase A is absent or deficient. This enzyme is necessary to metabolize gangliosides, water-soluble glycolipids found primarily in the central nervous system (CNS). Without hexosaminidase A, lipid pigments accumulate and progressively destroy and demyelinate the CNS cells.

Signs and symptoms

◆ Exaggerated Moro reflex (also called *startle reflex*) at birth and apathy (response only to loud sounds) by ages 3 to 6 months due to demyelination of CNS cells

◆ Inability to sit up, lift the head, or grasp objects; difficulty turning over; progressive vision loss due to CNS involvement

◆ Deafness, blindness, seizure activity, paralysis, spasticity, and continued neurologic deterioration (by age 18 months)

◆ Recurrent bronchopneumonia due to diminished protective reflexes

Complications

◆ Blindness

◆ Generalized paralysis

◆ Recurrent bronchopneumonia, usually fatal by age 5 years

Diagnosis

◆ Clinical features

◆ Serum analysis showing deficient hexosaminidase A

◆ Amniocentesis or chorionic villus sampling can detect hexosaminidase A deficiency in the fetus

GENETIC LINK *Diagnostic screening is recommended for all couples of Ashkenazic Jewish ancestry and for others with a familial history of the disease. A blood test can detect carriers.*

Treatment

Tay-Sachs disease has no known cure. Supportive treatment includes:

◆ tube feedings to provide nutritional supplements

◆ suctioning and postural drainage to maintain a patent airway

◆ skin care to prevent pressure ulcers in bedridden children

◆ laxatives to relieve neurogenic constipation.

Special considerations

Your most important job is to help the family deal with inevitably progressive illness and death.

◆ Offer carrier testing to all couples from high-risk ethnic groups.

◆ Refer the parents for genetic counseling, and stress the importance of amniocentesis in future pregnancies. Refer siblings for screening to determine if they're carriers. If they are carriers and are adults, refer them for genetic counseling, but stress that there's no danger of transmitting the disease to offspring if they don't marry another carrier.

◆ Some in vitro fertilization centers have recently started offering preimplantation genetics. Refer the couple to an appropriate center if they express interest in assisted reproductive technology.

◆ Because the parents of an affected child may feel excessive stress or guilt because of the child's illness and the emotional and financial burden it places on them, refer them for psychological counseling if indicated.

◆ If the parents care for their child at home, teach them how to do suctioning, postural drainage, and tube feeding. Also teach them how to provide good skin care to prevent pressure ulcers.

◆ For more information on this disease, refer parents to the National Tay-Sachs and Allied Diseases Association.

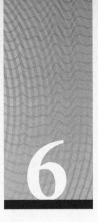

CARDIOVASCULAR SYSTEM

The cardiovascular system begins its activity when the fetus is barely 4 weeks old and is the last system to cease activity at the end of life. This body system is so vital that it helps define the presence of life.

The heart, arteries, veins, and lymphatics form the cardiovascular network that serves as the body's transport system. This system brings life-supporting oxygen and nutrients to cells, removes metabolic waste products, and carries hormones from one part of the body to another.

The cardiovascular system, commonly called the circulatory system, may be divided into two branches: pulmonary and systemic circulations. In *pulmonary circulation,* blood picks up oxygen and liberates the waste product carbon dioxide. In *systemic circulation* (which includes coronary circulation), blood carries oxygen and nutrients to all active cells and transports waste products to the kidneys, liver, and skin for excretion.

Circulation requires normal heart function, which propels blood through the system by continuous rhythmic contractions. Blood circulates through three types of vessels: arteries, veins, and capillaries. The sturdy, pliable walls of the arteries adjust to the volume of blood leaving the heart. The aorta is the major artery arching out of the left ventricle; its segments and branches ultimately divide into minute, thin-walled (one cell thick) capillaries. Capillaries pass the blood to the veins, which return it to the heart. In the veins, valves prevent blood backflow.

Pathophysiologic changes

Pathophysiologic manifestations of cardiovascular disease may stem from aneurysm, cardiac shunts, embolus, release of cardiac enzymes and proteins, stenosis, thrombus, and valve incompetence.

ANEURYSM

An aneurysm is a localized outpouching or dilation of a weakened arterial wall. This weakness can be the result of either atherosclerotic plaque formation that erodes the vessel wall or the loss of elastin and collagen in the vessel wall. Congenital abnormalities in the media of the arterial wall, trauma, and infections, such as syphilis, may lead to aneurysm formation. A ruptured aneurysm may cause massive hemorrhage and death.

Several types of aneurysms can occur:
♦ A *saccular aneurysm* occurs when increased pressure in the artery pushes out a pouch on one side of the artery, creating a bulge. (See *Types of aortic aneurysms.*)
♦ A *fusiform aneurysm* develops when the arterial wall weakens around its circumference, creating a spindle-shaped aneurysm along an extended section.
♦ A *dissecting aneurysm* occurs when blood is forced between the layers of the arterial wall, causing them to separate and creating a false lumen.
♦ A *false aneurysm* develops when there's a break in all layers of the arterial wall and blood leaks out — but is contained by surrounding structures — creating a pulsatile hematoma.

Types of aortic aneurysms

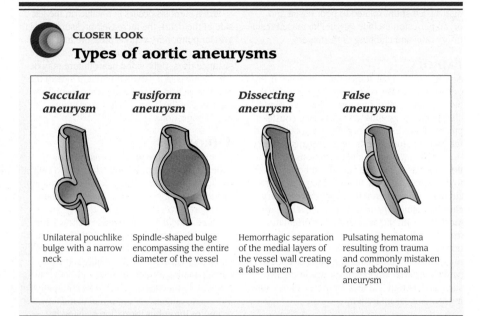

Saccular aneurysm	Fusiform aneurysm	Dissecting aneurysm	False aneurysm
Unilateral pouchlike bulge with a narrow neck	Spindle-shaped bulge encompassing the entire diameter of the vessel	Hemorrhagic separation of the medial layers of the vessel wall creating a false lumen	Pulsating hematoma resulting from trauma and commonly mistaken for an abdominal aneurysm

Common locations include:
◆ abdominal aortic aneurysm — an abnormal dilation in the arterial wall, generally occurring in the aorta between the renal arteries and iliac branches
◆ thoracic aortic aneurysm — an abnormal widening of the ascending, transverse, or descending part of the aorta
◆ cerebral aneurysm — a localized dilation of a cerebral artery that may arise at an arterial junction in the circle of Willis, the circular anastomosis forming the major cerebral arteries at the base of the brain
◆ femoral and popliteal aneurysms (sometimes called peripheral arterial aneurysms) — the end result of progressive atherosclerotic changes occurring in the walls (medial layer) of these major peripheral arteries.

CARDIAC SHUNTS

A cardiac shunt provides communication between the pulmonary and systemic circulations. Before birth, shunts between the right and left sides of the heart and between the aorta and pulmonary artery are a normal part of fetal circulation. After birth, however, the mixing of pulmonary and systemic blood or the movement of blood between the left and right sides of the heart is abnormal. Blood flows through a shunt from an area of high pressure to an area of low pressure or from an area of high resistance to an area of low resistance.

Left-to-right shunts

In a left-to-right shunt, blood flows from the left side of the heart to the right side through an atrial or ventricular defect, or from the aorta to the pulmonary circulation through a patent ductus arteriosus. Because the blood in the left side of the heart is rich in oxygen, a left-to-right shunt delivers oxygenated blood back to the right side of the heart or to the lungs. Consequently, a left-to-right shunt that occurs as a result of a congenital heart defect is called an *acyanotic defect*.

In a left-to-right shunt, pulmonary blood flow increases as blood is continually recirculated to the lungs, leading to hypertrophy of the pulmonary vessels. The increased amounts of blood circulated from the left side of the heart to the right side can result in right-sided heart failure. Eventually, left-sided heart failure may also occur.

Right-to-left shunts

A right-to-left shunt occurs when blood flows from the right side of the heart to the left side, such as in tetralogy of Fallot, or from the pulmonary artery directly into the systemic circulation through a patent ductus arteriosus. Because blood returning to the right side of the heart and the pulmonary artery is low in oxygen, a right-to-left shunt adds deoxygenated blood to the systemic circulation, causing hypoxia and cyanosis. A congenital defect that involves right-to-left shunts is therefore called a *cyanotic defect*. Common signs and symptoms of a right-to-left shunt related to poor tissue and organ perfusion include fatigue, increased respiratory rate, and clubbing of the fingers.

EMBOLUS

An embolus is a substance that circulates from one location in the body to another through the bloodstream. Although most emboli are blood clots from a thrombus, they may also consist of pieces of tissue, an air bubble, amniotic fluid, fat, bacteria, tumor cells, or a foreign substance.

Emboli that originate in the venous circulation, such as from deep vein thrombosis, travel to the right side of the heart to the pulmonary circulation and eventually lodge in a capillary, causing pulmonary infarction and even death. Most emboli in the arterial system originate from the left side of the heart from such conditions as arrhythmias, valvular heart disease, myocardial infarction, heart failure, or endocarditis. Arterial emboli may lodge in organs, such as the brain, kidneys, or extremities, causing ischemia or infarction.

RELEASE OF CARDIAC ENZYMES AND PROTEINS

When the heart muscle is damaged, the cell membrane's integrity is impaired, and intracellular contents — including cardiac enzymes and proteins — are released and can be measured in the bloodstream. The release follows a characteristic rising and falling of values. The released enzymes include creatine kinase, lactate dehydrogenase, and aspartate aminotransferase; the proteins released include troponin T, troponin I, and myoglobin. (See *Release of cardiac enzymes and proteins*.)

STENOSIS

Stenosis is the narrowing of a tubular structure— for example, a blood vessel or heart valve. When an artery is stenosed, the tissues and organs perfused by that blood vessel may become ischemic, function abnormally, or die. An occluded vein may result in venous congestion and chronic venous insufficiency.

When a heart valve is stenosed, blood flow through that valve is reduced, causing blood to accumulate in the chamber behind the valve. Pressure in that chamber increases to pump against the resistance of the stenosed valve. Consequently, the heart has to work harder, resulting in hypertrophy. Hypertrophy and an increase in workload raise the heart's oxygen demands. A heart with diseased coronary arteries may not be able to sufficiently increase oxygen supply to meet the increased demand.

When stenosis occurs in a valve on the left side of the heart, the increased pressure leads to greater pulmonary venous pressure and pulmonary congestion. As pulmonary vascular resistance rises, right-sided heart failure may occur. Stenosis in a valve on the right side of the heart causes an increase in pressures on the right side of the heart, leading to systemic venous congestion.

THROMBUS

A thrombus is a blood clot, consisting of platelets, fibrin, and red and white blood cells. It can form anywhere within the vascular system, including the arteries, veins, heart chambers, and heart valves.

Three conditions, known as Virchow's triad, promote thrombus formation: endothelial injury, sluggish blood flow, and increased coagulability. When a blood vessel wall is injured, the endothelial lining attracts platelets and other inflammatory mediators, which may stimulate clot formation. Sluggish or abnormal blood flow also promotes thrombus formation by allowing platelets and clotting factors to accumulate and adhere to the blood vessel walls. Conditions that increase the coagulability of blood also promote clot formation.

The consequences of thrombus formation include occlusion of the blood vessel or the formation of an embolus (if a portion of a thrombus breaks loose and travels through the circulatory system until it lodges in a smaller vessel).

VALVE INCOMPETENCE

Valve incompetence, also called insufficiency or regurgitation, occurs when valve leaflets don't completely close. Incompetence may affect valves of the veins or heart.

In the veins, valves keep the blood flowing in one direction, toward the heart. When valve leaflets close improperly, blood flows backward and pools above, causing that valve to weaken and become incompetent. Eventually, the veins become distended, which may result in varicose veins, chronic venous insufficiency, and venous stasis ulcers. Blood clots may form as blood flow becomes sluggish.

In the heart, incompetent valves allow blood to flow in both directions through the valve, increasing the volume of blood that must be pumped (as well as the heart's workload) and resulting in hypertrophy. As blood volume in the heart increases, the involved heart chambers dilate to accommodate the increased volume. Although incompetence may occur in any heart valve, it's more common in the mitral and aortic valves.

Release of cardiac enzymes and proteins

Because they're released by damaged tissue, serum proteins and isoenzymes (catalytic proteins that vary in concentration in specific organs) can help identify the compromised organ and assess the extent of damage. After an acute myocardial infarction, cardiac enzyme and protein levels rise and fall in a characteristic pattern, as shown in the graph below.

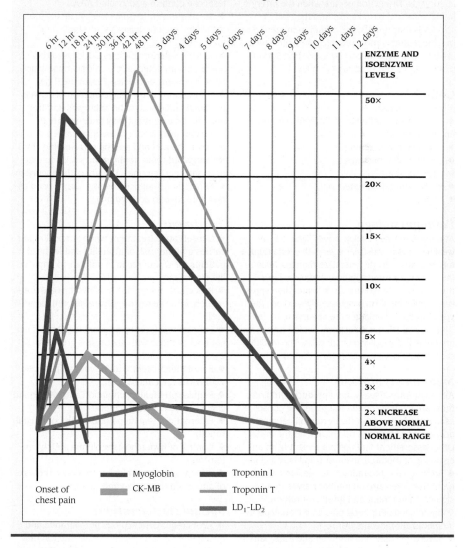

Disorders

This section discusses disorders of the cardiovascular system, some of which are life-threatening. They include abdominal aortic aneurysm, acute coronary syndromes, arterial occlusive disease, atrial septal defect, Buerger's disease, cardiac arrhythmias, cardiac tamponade, cardiomyopathy, coarctation of the aorta, coronary artery disease, endocarditis, heart failure, hypertension, myocarditis, patent ductus arteriosus, pericarditis, Raynaud's disease, rheumatic fever and rheumatic heart disease, shock, tetralogy of Fallot, thrombophlebitis, transposition of the great arteries, valvular heart disease, varicose veins, and ventricular septal defect.

ABDOMINAL AORTIC ANEURYSM

Abdominal aortic aneurysm (AAA), an abnormal dilation in the arterial wall, generally occurs in the aorta between the renal arteries and iliac branches. Rupture, in which the aneurysm breaks open, resulting in profuse bleeding, is a common complication that occurs in larger aneurysms. Dissection occurs when the artery's lining tears and blood leaks into the walls.

AAA is four times more common in men than in women and is most prevalent in whites who are between ages 40 and 70. Less than 50% of people with a ruptured AAA survive.

Causes

- Arteriosclerosis
- Blunt abdominal injury or Marfan syndrome (in children)
- Congenital weakening
- Cystic medial necrosis
- Hypertension
- Syphilis and other infections
- Trauma

Pathophysiology

Aortic aneurysms develop slowly. First, a focal weakness in the muscular layer of the aorta (tunica media), caused by degenerative changes, allows the inner layer (tunica intima) and outer layer (tunica adventitia) to stretch outward. Blood pressure within the aorta progressively weakens the vessel walls and enlarges the aneurysm.

Nearly all AAAs are fusiform, which causes the arterial walls to balloon on all sides. The resulting sac fills with necrotic debris and thrombi.

Signs and symptoms

Although AAAs usually don't produce symptoms, most are evident (unless the patient is obese) as a pulsating mass in the periumbilical area, accompanied by a systolic bruit over the aorta. Other assessment findings may result from an enlarging or ruptured aneurysm, and may include:

- lumbar pain that radiates to the flank and groin from pressure on lumbar nerves (may signify enlargement and imminent rupture)
- diminished peripheral pulses or claudication if embolization occurs (rare)
- severe, persistent abdominal and back pain if the aneurysm ruptures into the peritoneal cavity
- weakness, sweating, tachycardia, and hypotension due to hemorrhage if the aneurysm ruptures.

Complications

- Rupture
- Obstruction of blood flow to other organs
- Embolization to a peripheral artery
- Diminished blood supply to vital organs resulting in organ failure (with rupture)

Diagnosis

Because AAAs seldom produce symptoms, they're usually detected accidentally as the result of an X-ray or a routine physical examination. Several tests can confirm a suspected AAA:

- Serial ultrasound (*sonography*) can accurately determine the aneurysm's size, shape, and location.
- Anteroposterior and lateral X-rays of the abdomen can detect aortic calcification, which outlines the mass, at least 75% of the time.
- Aortography shows the condition of vessels proximal and distal to the aneurysm and the aneurysm's extent but may underestimate aneurysm diameter because it visualizes only the flow channel and not the surrounding clot.
- Computed tomography scan is used to diagnose and help determine the size of the aneurysm.
- Magnetic resonance imaging can be used as an alternative to aortography.

Treatment

- Conservative treatment when surgical repair carries a higher risk of mortality and in those patients for whom repair is unlikely to improve life expectancy
- Resection and replacement of damaged aortic section with Dacron or polytetrafluoroethylene graft
- Surgical repair or replacement for symptomatic patients or those with aneurysms greater than 2″ (5 cm) in diameter
- Endoluminal stent grafting (not all patients with AAAs are candidates)
- Regular physical examination and ultrasound checks to detect enlargement
- External grafting (in patients with poor distal runoff)
- Control of hypercholesterolemia and hypertension
- A beta-adrenergic blocker to reduce the risk of aneurysm expansion and rupture

Special considerations

- AAAs require meticulous preoperative and postoperative care, psychological support, and comprehensive patient teaching. After diagnosis, if rupture isn't imminent, elective surgery allows time for additional preoperative tests to evaluate the patient's clinical status.
- Monitor vital signs, and type and crossmatch blood.
- Use only gentle abdominal palpation.
- As ordered, obtain renal function tests (blood urea nitrogen, creatinine, and electrolyte levels),

blood samples (complete blood count with differential), electrocardiogram (ECG) and cardiac evaluation, baseline pulmonary function tests, and arterial blood gas (ABG) analysis.

⚠️ **CLINICAL ALERT** *Be alert for signs of rupture, which may be immediately fatal. Watch closely for signs of acute blood loss, such as decreasing blood pressure; increasing pulse and respiratory rate; cool, clammy skin; restlessness; and decreased sensorium.*

If rupture occurs, get the patient to surgery immediately. A pneumatic antishock garment may be used while transporting him there. Surgery allows direct compression of the aorta to control hemorrhage. Large amounts of blood may be needed during the resuscitative period to replace blood loss. In such a patient, renal failure caused by ischemia is a major postoperative complication, possibly requiring hemodialysis.

◆ Before elective surgery, weigh the patient, insert an indwelling urinary catheter and an I.V. line, and assist with insertion of an arterial line and pulmonary artery catheter to monitor fluid and hemodynamic balance. Give a prophylactic antibiotic as ordered.

◆ Explain the surgical procedure and the expected postoperative care in the intensive care unit (ICU) for patients undergoing complex abdominal surgery (I.V. lines, endotracheal [ET] and nasogastric [NG] intubation, and mechanical ventilation).

◆ After surgery, in the ICU, closely monitor vital signs, intake and hourly output, neurologic status (level of consciousness, pupil size, and sensation in arms and legs), and ABG values. Assess the depth, rate, and character of respirations and breath sounds at least every hour.

◆ Watch for signs of bleeding (increased pulse and respiratory rates and hypotension) and back pain, which may indicate the graft is tearing. Check abdominal dressings for excessive bleeding or drainage. Be alert for temperature elevations and other signs of infection. After NG intubation for intestinal decompression, irrigate the tube frequently to ensure patency. Record the amount and type of drainage.

◆ Suction the ET tube often. If the patient can breathe unassisted and has good breath sounds and adequate ABG values, tidal volume, and vital capacity 24 hours after surgery, he'll be extubated and require oxygen by mask.

◆ Weigh the patient daily to evaluate fluid balance.

◆ Help the patient walk as soon as he's able (generally the second day after surgery).

◆ Provide psychological support for the patient and his family. Help ease their fears about the ICU, the threat of impending rupture, and

surgery by providing appropriate explanations and answering all questions.

ACUTE CORONARY SYNDROMES

Acute myocardial infarction (MI), including ST-segment elevation MI (STEMI) and non–ST-segment elevation MI (NSTEMI), and unstable angina are now recognized as part of a group of clinical diseases called *acute coronary syndromes* (ACSs).

Rupture or erosion of plaque—an unstable and lipid-rich substance—initiates all coronary syndromes. The rupture results in platelet adhesions, fibrin clot formation, and activation of thrombin.

In cardiovascular disease—the leading cause of death in the United States and Western Europe—death usually results from cardiac damage after an MI. Each year, about 1 million people in the United States experience an MI. Incidence is higher in males younger than age 70. (Females have the protective effects of estrogen until menopause.) Mortality is high when treatment is delayed, and almost one-half of sudden deaths caused by an MI occur before hospitalization or within 1 hour of the onset of symptoms. The prognosis improves if vigorous treatment begins immediately.

Causes

Causes of ACS include atherosclerosis and embolus. In atherosclerosis, plaque (an unstable and lipid-rich substance) forms and subsequently ruptures or erodes, resulting in platelet adhesions, fibrin clot formation, and activation of thrombin.

Risk factors for ACS include:
◆ diabetes
◆ family history of heart disease
◆ high-fat, high-carbohydrate diet
◆ hyperlipoproteinemia
◆ hypertension
◆ menopause
◆ obesity
◆ sedentary lifestyle
◆ smoking
◆ stress.

Pathophysiology

ACS most commonly results when a thrombus progresses and occludes blood flow. The degree of blockage and the time that the affected vessel remains occluded determine the type of infarct that occurs. The underlying effect is an imbalance in myocardial oxygen supply and demand. (See *Stages of myocardial ischemia, injury, and infarct*, page 130.)

For patients with unstable angina, a thrombus full of platelets partially occludes a coronary

Stages of myocardial ischemia, injury, and infarct

Three stages occur when there's occlusion of a vessel: ischemia, injury, and infarct.

Ischemia

Ischemia is the first stage and indicates that blood flow and oxygen demand are out of balance. It can be resolved by improving flow or reducing oxygen needs. Electrocardiogram (ECG) changes reveal ST-segment depression or T-wave changes.

Injury

The second stage, injury, occurs when the ischemia is prolonged enough to damage the area of the heart. ECG changes usually reveal ST-segment elevation (usually in two or more leads).

Infarct

Infarct is the the third stage and occurs with actual death of myocardial cells. Scar tissue eventually replaces the dead tissue, and the damage caused is irreversible.

In the earliest stage of a myocardial infarction (MI), hyperacute or very tall and narrow T waves may be seen on the ECG. Within hours the T waves become inverted and ST-segment elevation occurs in the leads facing the area of damage. The last change to occur in the evolution of an MI is the development of the pathologic Q wave, which is the only permanent ECG evidence of myocardial necrosis. Q waves are considered pathologic when they appear greater than or equal to 0.04 second wide and their height is greater than 25% of the R wave height in that lead. Pathologic Q waves develop in over 90% of the patients with ST-segment elevation MI. About 25% of the patients with a non–ST-segment elevation MI will develop pathologic Q waves and the remaining patients will have a non–Q wave MI.

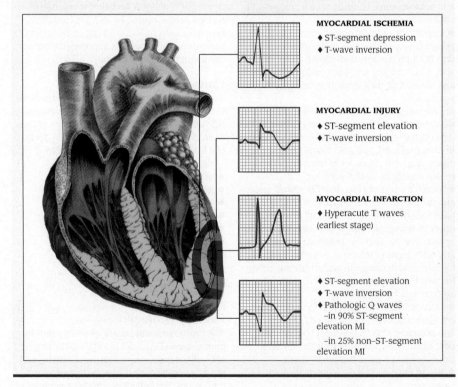

MYOCARDIAL ISCHEMIA
♦ ST-segment depression
♦ T-wave inversion

MYOCARDIAL INJURY
♦ ST-segment elevation
♦ T-wave inversion

MYOCARDIAL INFARCTION
♦ Hyperacute T waves
 (earliest stage)

♦ ST-segment elevation
♦ T-wave inversion
♦ Pathologic Q waves
 –in 90% ST-segment elevation MI
 –in 25% non–ST-segment elevation MI

vessel. The partially occluded vessel may have distal microthrombi that cause necrosis in some myocytes. The smaller vessels infarct, thus placing the patient at higher risk for a NSTEMI.

If a thrombus fully occludes the vessel for a prolonged time, it's classified as a STEMI. This type of an MI involves a greater concentration of thrombin and fibrin. (See *How ACS affects the body*.)

The location of the area of damage depends on the blood vessels involved:

MULTISYSTEM DISORDER
How ACS affects the body

Acute coronary syndrome (ACS) can have far-reaching effects and requires a multidisciplinary approach to care. Here's what happens in ACS:

Cardiovascular system

◆ An area of viable ischemic tissue surrounds the zone of injury.
◆ When the heart muscle is damaged, the integrity of the cell membrane is impaired.
◆ Intracellular contents, including cardiac enzymes (such as creatine kinase, lactate dehydrogenase, and aspartate aminotransferase) and proteins (such as troponin T, troponin I, and myoglobin) are released.
◆ Within 24 hours, the infarcted area becomes edematous and cyanotic.
◆ During the next several days, leukocytes infiltrate the necrotic area and begin to remove necrotic cells, thinning the ventricular wall.
◆ Scar formation begins by the 3rd week after a myocardial infarction (MI); by the 6th week, scar tissue is well established.
◆ The scar tissue that forms on the necrotic area inhibits contractility.
◆ Compensatory mechanisms (vascular constriction, increased heart rate, and renal retention of sodium and water) try to maintain cardiac output.
◆ Ventricular dilation may also occur in a process called *remodeling*.
◆ Functionally, an MI may cause reduced contractility with abnormal wall motion, altered left ventricular compliance, reduced stroke volume, reduced ejection fraction, and elevated left ventricular end-diastolic pressure.
◆ Cardiogenic shock is caused by failure of the heart to perform as an effective pump and can result in low cardiac output, diminished peripheral perfusion, pulmonary congestion, and elevated systemic vascular resistance and pulmonary vascular pressures.
◆ Ineffective contractility of the heart leads to accumulation of blood in the venous circulation upstream to the failing ventricle.
◆ Arrhythmias can occur in the patient with an acute MI as a result of autonomic nervous system imbalance, electrolyte disturbances, ischemia, and slowed conduction in zones of ischemic myocardium.

Neurologic system

◆ Hypoperfusion of the brain results in altered mental status, involving changes in levels of consciousness, restlessness, irritability, confusion, or disorientation.
◆ Stupor or coma may result if the decrease in cerebral perfusion continues.

Renal system

◆ Shock and hypoperfusion from an MI cause the kidney to respond by conserving salt and water.
◆ Poor perfusion results in diminished renal blood flow, and increased afferent arteriolar resistance occurs, causing a decreased glomerular filtration rate.
◆ Increased amounts of antidiuretic hormone and aldosterone are released to help maintain perfusion. Urine formation, however, is reduced.
◆ Depletion of renal adenosine triphosphate stores results from prolonged renal hypoperfusion, causing impaired renal function.

Respiratory system

◆ Cardiogenic shock with left-sided heart failure results in increased fluid in the lungs. This process can overwhelm the capacity of the pulmonary lymphatics, resulting in interstitial and alveolar edema.
◆ Lung edema occurs when pulmonary capillary pressure exceeds 18 mm Hg.
◆ Pulmonary alveolar edema develops when pressures exceed 24 mm Hg, impairing oxygen diffusion.
◆ Increased interstitial and intra-alveolar fluid causes progressive reduction in lung compliance, increasing the work of ventilation and increasing perfusion of poorly ventilated alveoli.

Collaborative management

A cardiologist is consulted for initial assessment and treatment. A cardiothoracic surgeon may also be consulted if the patient requires invasive therapy. Other specialists may be required after initial therapy and treatment, such as a physical therapist for cardiac rehabilitation and a nutritionist for dietary and lifestyle changes.

◆ *Anterior-wall MI* — occurs when the left anterior descending artery becomes occluded.

◆ *Septal-wall MI* — typically accompanies an anterior-wall MI because the ventricular septum is supplied by the left anterior descending artery as well.

◆ *Lateral-wall MI* — caused by a blockage in the left circumflex artery, and usually accompanies an anterior- or inferior-wall MI.

◆ *Inferior-wall MI* — caused by occlusion of the right coronary artery; usually occurs alone or with a lateral-wall or right-ventricular MI.

◆ *Posterior-wall MI* — caused by occlusion of the right coronary artery or the left circumflex arteries.

◆ *Right-ventricular MI* — follows occlusion of the right coronary artery; this type of an MI rarely occurs alone (in 40% of patients, a right-ventricular MI accompanies an inferior-wall MI).

Signs and symptoms

Signs and symptoms of ACS are caused by myocardial ischemia, resulting from an imbalance between supply and demand for myocardial oxygen.

These findings are typical of angina:

◆ burning, squeezing, and a crushing tightness in the substernal or precordial chest that may radiate to the left arm or shoulder blade, the neck, or the jaw

◆ pain after physical exertion, emotional excitement, exposure to cold, or consumption of a large meal.

Although other diagnoses may have chest pain as a symptom, retrosternal chest discomfort, pain, or pressure is a prime symptom of infarction. Patients typically describe these signs and symptoms of acute ischemia and an MI:

◆ uncomfortable pressure, squeezing, burning, severe persistent pain, or fullness in the center of the chest lasting several minutes (usually longer than 15 minutes)

◆ pain radiating to the shoulders, neck, arms, or jaw or pain in the back between the shoulder blades

◆ accompanying signs and symptoms of lightheadedness, fainting, sweating, nausea, shortness of breath, anxiety, or a feeling of impending doom.

⚠ **CLINICAL ALERT** *Females may experience typical chest pain with acute ischemia and an MI; however, females — and occasionally males, elderly patients, and those patients with diabetes — may also experience atypical chest pain. Signs and symptoms include upper back discomfort between the shoulder blades, palpitations, a feeling of fullness in the neck, nausea, abdominal discomfort, dizziness, unexplained fatigue, and exhaustion or shortness of breath.*

Complications

◆ Arrhythmias
◆ Ventricular irritability
◆ Heart failure
◆ Sudden death

Diagnosis

An electrocardiogram (ECG) helps to determine which area of the heart and which coronary arteries are involved. By recognizing danger early, you may be able to prevent an MI or even death. (See *ECG characteristics in acute coronary syndromes*.)

Other diagnostic tests may include:

◆ Serial cardiac enzyme and protein levels may show a characteristic rise and fall of cardiac enzymes, specifically CK-MB, the proteins troponin T and I, and myoglobin.

◆ Laboratory testing may reveal elevated white blood cell count and erythrocyte sedimentation rate and changes in electrolyte levels.

◆ Echocardiography may show ventricular wall motion abnormalities and may detect septal or papillary muscle rupture or identify pericardial effusions.

◆ Transesophageal echocardiography may reveal areas of decreased heart muscle wall movement, indicating ischemia.

◆ Chest X-rays may show left-sided heart failure, cardiomegaly, or other noncardiac causes of dyspnea or chest pain.

◆ Nuclear imaging scanning using thallium 201 and technetium 99 m can be used to identify areas of infarction and areas of viable muscle cells.

◆ Multiple-gated acquisition scanning is used to determine left ventricular function and identify aneurysms, problems with wall motion, and intracardiac shunting.

◆ Cardiac catheterization may be used to identify the involved coronary artery as well as to provide information on ventricular function and pressures and volumes within the heart.

Treatment

Treatment goals for patients experiencing ACS include:

◆ reducing the amount of myocardial necrosis in those with ongoing infarction

◆ decreasing cardiac workload and increasing oxygen supply to the myocardium

◆ preventing major adverse cardiac events

◆ providing for rapid defibrillation when ventricular fibrillation or pulseless ventricular tachycardia is present. (See *Treating an MI*, pages 134 and 135.)

ECG characteristics in acute coronary syndromes

The initial step in assessing a patient complaining of chest pain is to obtain an electrocardiogram (ECG). This should be done within 10 minutes of being seen by a physician. It's crucial in determining the presence of myocardial ischemia, and the findings will direct the treatment plan.

Angina

Most patients with angina show ischemic changes on an ECG only during the attack. Because these changes may be fleeting, always obtain an order for and perform a 12-lead ECG as soon as the patient reports chest pain.

MI

According to the American Heart Association, patients should be classified as having ST-segment elevation or new left bundle-branch block (LBBB), ST-segment depression or dynamic T-wave inversion, or nondiagnostic or normal ECG.

ST-segment elevation or new LBBB

◆ Patients with an ST-segment elevation greater than or equal to 1 mm in two or more contiguous leads or with new LBBB need to be treated for an acute MI.
◆ More than 90% of patients with this presentation will develop new Q waves and have positive serum cardiac markers.

◆ Repeating the ECG may be helpful for patients who present with hyperacute T waves.

ST-segment depression or dynamic T-wave inversion

◆ Patients with ST-segment depression indicating a posterior MI benefit most when an acute MI is diagnosed.
◆ Ischemia should be suspected with findings of ST-segment depression greater than or equal to 0.5 mm, marked symmetrical T-wave inversion in multiple precordial leads, and dynamic ST-T changes with pain.
◆ Patients who display persistent symptoms and recurrent ischemia, diffuse or widespread ECG abnormalities, heart failure, and positive serum markers are considered high risk.

Nondiagnostic or normal ECG

◆ A normal ECG won't show ST-segment changes or arrhythmias.
◆ If the ECG is nondiagnostic, it may show an ST-segment depression of less than 0.5 mm or a T-wave inversion or flattening in leads with dominant R waves.
◆ Continue assessment of myocardial changes through use of serial ECGs, ST-segment monitoring, and serum cardiac markers.
◆ If further assessment is warranted, perform perfusion radionuclide imaging and stress echocardiography.

Initial treatment

Obtain a 12-lead ECG and serum cardiac markers to help confirm the diagnosis of an acute MI. Serum cardiac markers (especially troponin I and CK-MB) are used to distinguish unstable angina and NSTEMI.

Use the memory aid MONA, which stands for morphine, oxygen, nitroglycerin, and aspirin, to institute treatment of any patient experiencing ischemic chest pain or suspected ACS. Also, give:
◆ oxygen to increase oxygenation of blood
◆ nitroglycerin sublingually to relieve chest pain (unless systolic blood pressure is less than 90 mm Hg or heart rate is less than 50 beats/minute or greater than 100 beats/minute)
◆ morphine to relieve pain
◆ aspirin to inhibit platelet aggregation
◆ oral antiplatelet agent such as clopidogrel (Plavix) to help prevent clot formation.

For the patient with unstable angina and NSTEMI, treatment includes the above initial measures as well as:

◆ a beta-adrenergic blocker to reduce the heart's workload and oxygen demands
◆ heparin and a glycoprotein IIb/IIIa inhibitor to minimize platelet aggregation and the danger of coronary occlusion with high-risk patients (patients with planned cardiac catheterization and positive troponin)
◆ nitroglycerin I.V. to dilate coronary arteries and relieve chest pain (unless systolic blood pressure is less than 90 mm Hg or heart rate is less than 50 beats/minute or more than 100 beats/minute)
◆ an antiarrhythmic, transcutaneous pacing (or transvenous pacemaker), or defibrillation, if the patient has ventricular fibrillation or pulseless ventricular tachycardia (VT)
◆ percutaneous coronary interventions (PCI) or coronary artery bypass graft surgery for obstructive lesions

(Text continues on page 136.)

DISEASE BLOCK

Treating an MI

This flowchart shows how treatments can be applied to a myocardial infarction (MI) at various stages of its development.

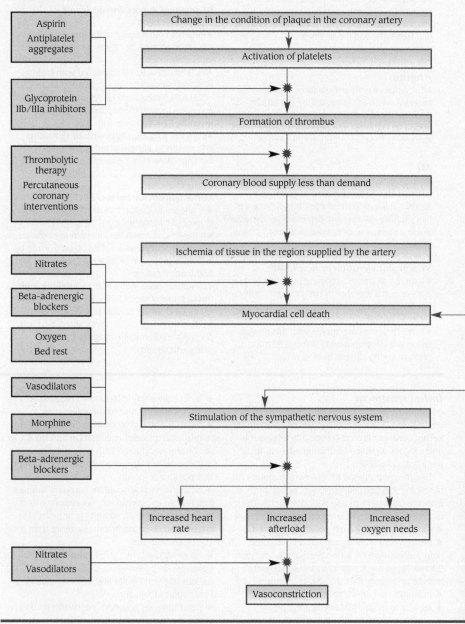

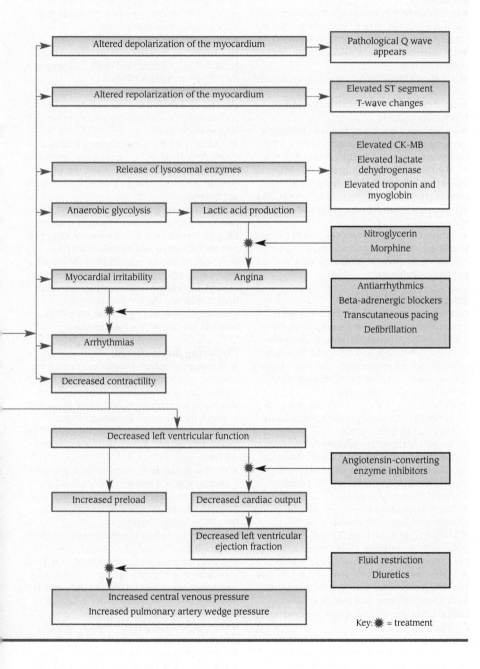

Key: ✳ = treatment

◆ an antilipemic to reduce elevated serum cholesterol or triglyceride levels.

For the patient with STEMI, treatment includes the above initial measures and these additional measures:

◆ thrombolytic therapy (unless contraindicated) within 12 hours of onset of symptoms to restore vessel patency and minimize necrosis in STEMI

◆ I.V. heparin to promote patency in the affected coronary artery

◆ a beta-adrenergic blocker to reduce myocardial workload

◆ a glycoprotein IIb/IIIa inhibitor to reduce platelet aggregation

◆ an antiarrhythmic, transcutaneous pacing (or transvenous pacemaker), or defibrillation, if the patient has ventricular fibrillation or pulseless VT

◆ an angiotensin-converting enzyme (ACE) inhibitor to reduce afterload and preload and prevent remodeling (begin in STEMI 6 hours after admission or when the patient's condition is stable)

◆ interventional procedures (such as PCI, stent placement, or surgical procedures, such as coronary artery bypass graft) may open blocked or narrowed arteries.

Special considerations

Care for patients who have suffered an MI is directed toward detecting complications, preventing further myocardial damage, and promoting comfort, rest, and emotional well-being. Most MI patients receive treatment in the intensive care unit (ICU), where they're under constant observation for complications.

◆ On admission to the ICU, monitor and record the patient's ECG, blood pressure, temperature, and heart and breath sounds.

◆ Assess and record the severity and duration of pain, and administer an analgesic. Avoid I.M. injections; absorption from the muscle is unpredictable and bleeding is likely if the patient is receiving thrombolytic therapy.

◆ Check the patient's blood pressure after giving nitroglycerin, especially the first dose.

◆ Frequently monitor the ECG to detect rate changes or arrhythmias. Place rhythm strips in the patient's chart periodically for evaluation.

◆ During episodes of chest pain, obtain a 12-lead ECG (before and after nitroglycerin therapy as well), blood pressure, and pulmonary artery catheter measurements and monitor them for changes.

◆ Watch for signs and symptoms of fluid retention (crackles, cough, tachypnea, and edema), which may indicate impending heart failure. Carefully monitor daily weight, intake and output, respirations, serum enzyme levels, and blood pressure. Auscultate for adventitious breath sounds periodically (patients on bed rest commonly have atelectatic crackles, which disappear after coughing), for S_3 or S_4 gallops, and for new-onset heart murmurs.

◆ Organize patient care and activities to maximize periods of uninterrupted rest.

◆ Initiate a cardiac rehabilitation program, which typically includes education regarding heart disease, exercise, and emotional support for the patient and his family.

◆ Ask the dietary department to provide a clear liquid diet until nausea subsides. A low-cholesterol, low-sodium, low-fat, high-fiber diet may be prescribed.

◆ Provide a stool softener to prevent straining during defecation, which causes vagal stimulation and may slow the heart rate. Allow use of a bedside commode, and provide as much privacy as possible.

◆ Assist with range-of-motion exercises. If the patient is completely immobilized by a severe MI, turn him often. Antiembolism stockings help prevent venostasis and thrombophlebitis.

◆ Provide emotional support and help reduce stress and anxiety; administer a tranquilizer as needed. Explain procedures and answer questions. Explaining the ICU environment and routine can ease anxiety. Involve the patient's family in his care as much as possible.

Preparing for discharge

◆ Thoroughly explain dosages and therapy to promote compliance with the prescribed drug regimen and other treatment measures. Warn about drug adverse effects, and advise the patient to watch for and report signs and symptoms of toxicity (anorexia, nausea, vomiting, and yellow vision, for example, if the patient is receiving digoxin).

◆ Review dietary restrictions with the patient. If he must follow a low-sodium or a low-fat, low-cholesterol diet, provide a list of foods that he should avoid. Ask the dietitian to speak to the patient and his family.

◆ Counsel the patient to resume sexual activity progressively.

◆ Advise the patient to report typical or atypical chest pain. Postinfarction syndrome may develop, producing chest pain that must be differentiated from a recurrent MI, a pulmonary infarct, or heart failure.

◆ If the patient has a Holter monitor in place, explain its purpose and use.

◆ Stress the need to stop smoking.

◆ Encourage participation in a cardiac rehabilitation program.

◆ Review follow-up procedures, such as office visits and treadmill testing, with the patient.

ARTERIAL OCCLUSIVE DISEASE

Arterial occlusive disease, also called peripheral artery disease, is the obstruction or narrowing of the lumen of the aorta and its major branches, causing an interruption of blood flow, usually to the legs and feet. This disorder may affect the carotid, vertebral, innominate, subclavian, mesenteric, iliac, and femoral arteries.

Arterial occlusive disease is more common in males than in females. The prognosis depends on the occlusion's location, the development of collateral circulation to counteract reduced blood flow and, in acute disease, the time elapsed between occlusion and its removal.

Causes

Arterial occlusive disease is a common complication of atherosclerosis. The occlusive mechanism may be endogenous, due to emboli formation or thrombosis, or exogenous, due to trauma or fracture.

Other predisposing factors include:
◆ aging
◆ diabetes
◆ family history of vascular disorders, an MI, or a stroke
◆ hyperlipidemia
◆ hypertension
◆ smoking.

Pathophysiology

Arterial occlusive disease is almost always the result of atherosclerosis, in which fatty, fibrous plaques narrow the lumen of blood vessels. This occlusion can occur acutely or progressively over 20 to 40 years, with areas of vessel branching, or bifurcation, being the most common sites. The narrowing of the lumens reduces the blood volume that can flow through them, causing arterial insufficiency to the affected area. Ischemia usually occurs after the vessel lumens have narrowed by at least 50%, reducing blood flow to a level at which it no longer meets the needs of tissue and nerves.

AGE ALERT *Aging causes sclerotic changes in blood vessels, which leads to decreased elasticity and narrowing of the lumen, further contributing to the development of arterial occlusive disease. In people older than age 70, the prevalence of the disease is estimated to be 10% to 18%.*

Signs and symptoms

Signs and symptoms of arterial occlusive disease depend on the site of the occlusion. (See *Types of arterial occlusive disease,* page 138.)

Complications

◆ Severe ischemia and necrosis
◆ Skin ulceration
◆ Gangrene, which can lead to limb amputation
◆ Impaired nail and hair growth
◆ Stroke or transient ischemic attack
◆ Peripheral or systemic embolism

Diagnosis

Diagnosis of arterial occlusive disease is usually indicated by patient history and physical examination. These pertinent tests support the diagnosis:

◆ Arteriography demonstrates the type (thrombus or embolus), location, and degree of obstruction and the collateral circulation. Arteriography is particularly useful in chronic disease or for evaluating candidates for reconstructive surgery.

◆ Doppler ultrasonography and plethysmography are noninvasive tests that show decreased blood flow distal to the occlusion in acute disease.

◆ Ankle-branchial index (ABI) (the ratio of systolic blood pressure at the ankle to that at the arm) decreases with worsening arterial occlusive disease. An ABI less than 0.9 indicates some degree of arterial occlusive disease.

◆ Ophthalmodynamometry helps determine the degree of obstruction in the internal carotid artery by comparing ophthalmic artery pressure to brachial artery pressure on the affected side. More than a 20% difference between pressures suggests insufficiency.

◆ EEG and computed tomography scan may be necessary to rule out brain lesions.

Treatment

Treatment of arterial occlusive disease depends on the cause, location, and size of the obstruction. For mild chronic disease, supportive measures include smoking cessation, hypertension control, hyperlipidemia control, and mild exercise, such as walking. For carotid artery occlusion, the patient should begin life-long aspirin therapy. For chronic occlusive disease, antiplatelet therapy should begin with aspirin (first-line agent), clopidogrel, or ticlopidine. Cilostazol is recommended for patients with disabling intermittent claudication who are poor candidates for surgery.

Acute arterial occlusive disease usually requires immediate anticoagulation therapy with heparin and surgery to restore circulation to the affected area, for example:

◆ *Embolectomy* — A balloon-tipped Fogarty catheter is used to remove thrombotic material from the artery. Embolectomy is used mainly for mesenteric, femoral, or popliteal artery occlusion.

Types of arterial occlusive disease

Site of occlusion	Signs and symptoms
Carotid arterial system ♦ Internal carotids ♦ External carotids	Neurologic dysfunction: transient ischemic attacks (TIAs) due to reduced cerebral circulation produce unilateral sensory or motor dysfunction (transient monocular blindness, hemiparesis), possible aphasia or dysarthria, confusion, decreased mentation, and headache; recurrent clinical features usually lasting 5 to 10 minutes, but may persist up to 24 hours and may herald a stroke; absent or decreased pulsation with an auscultatory bruit over the affected vessels
Vertebrobasilar system ♦ Vertebral arteries ♦ Basilar arteries	Neurologic dysfunction: TIAs of brain stem and cerebellum produce binocular visual disturbances, vertigo, dysarthria, and "drop attacks" (falling down without loss of consciousness); less common than carotid TIA
Innominate artery	Neurologic dysfunction: signs and symptoms of vertebrobasilar occlusion; indications of ischemia (claudication) of right arm; possible bruit over right side of neck
Subclavian artery	Subclavian steal syndrome (characterized by blood backflow from the brain through the vertebral artery on the same side as the occlusion, into the subclavian artery distal to the occlusion); clinical effects of vertebrobasilar occlusion and exercise-induced arm claudication; possible gangrene, usually limited to the digits
Mesenteric artery ♦ Superior (most commonly affected) ♦ Celiac axis ♦ Inferior	Bowel ischemia, infarct necrosis, and gangrene; sudden, acute abdominal pain; nausea and vomiting; diarrhea; leukocytosis; and shock due to massive intraluminal fluid and plasma loss
Aortic bifurcation (saddle-block occlusion, a medical emergency associated with cardiac embolization)	Sensory and motor deficits (muscle weakness, numbness, paresthesia, paralysis) and signs and symptoms of ischemia (sudden pain; cold, pale legs with decreased or absent peripheral pulses) in both legs
Iliac artery (Leriche's syndrome)	Intermittent claudication of lower back, buttocks, and thighs, relieved by rest; absent or reduced femoral or distal pulses; possible bruit over femoral arteries; impotence in males
Femoral and popliteal arteries (associated with aneurysm formation)	Intermittent claudication of the calves on exertion; ischemic pain in feet; pretrophic pain (heralds necrosis and ulceration); leg pallor and coolness; blanching of feet on elevation; gangrene; no palpable pulses in ankles and feet

♦ *Thromboendarterectomy*—Opening of the occluded artery and direct removal of the obstructing thrombus and the medial layer of the arterial wall; usually performed after angiography and commonly used with autogenous vein or Dacron bypass surgery (femoral-popliteal or aortofemoral).

♦ *Patch grafting*—The thrombosed arterial segment is removed and replaced with an autogenous vein or Dacron graft.
♦ *Bypass graft*—Blood flow is diverted through an anastomosed autogenous or Dacron graft past the thrombosed segment.

◆ *Thrombolytic therapy*—Urokinase, streptokinase, or alteplase causes lysis of clot around or in the plaque.
◆ *Atherectomy*—Plaque is excised using a drill or slicing mechanism.
◆ *Balloon angioplasty*—Balloon inflation compresses the obstruction.
◆ *Laser angioplasty*—Obstruction is excised and vaporized using hot-tip lasers.
◆ *Stents*—A mesh of wires that stretch and mold to the arterial wall is inserted to prevent reocclusion. This new adjunct follows laser angioplasty or atherectomy.

Combined therapy, which is simply the concomitant use of any surgical treatment listed above, may be appropriate. Also, lumbar sympathectomy is a possible adjunct to surgery, depending on the condition of the sympathetic nervous system.

Amputation becomes necessary if arterial reconstructive surgery fails or if gangrene, persistent infection, or intractable pain develops.

Other therapy may include bowel resection after restoration of blood flow (for mesenteric artery occlusion).

Special considerations
◆ Provide comprehensive patient teaching, such as proper foot care.
◆ Explain all diagnostic tests and procedures.
◆ Advise the patient to stop smoking and to follow the prescribed medical regimen.

Preoperatively
During an acute episode:
◆ Assess the patient's circulatory status by checking for the most distal pulses and by inspecting his skin color and temperature.
◆ Provide pain relief as needed.
◆ Administer heparin by continuous I.V. drip, as ordered, using an infusion pump to ensure the proper flow rate.
◆ Wrap the patient's affected foot in soft cotton batting, and reposition it frequently to prevent pressure on any one area.
◆ Strictly avoid elevating or applying heat to the affected leg.
◆ Watch for signs of fluid and electrolyte imbalance, and monitor intake and output for signs of renal failure (urine output less than 30 ml/hour).
◆ If the patient has carotid, innominate, vertebral, or subclavian artery occlusion, monitor him for signs and symptoms of stroke, such as numbness in his arm or leg and intermittent blindness.

Postoperatively
During postoperative management:
◆ Monitor the patient's vital signs. Continuously assess his circulatory function by inspecting skin color and temperature and by checking for distal pulses. In charting, compare earlier assessments and observations. Watch closely for signs of hemorrhage (tachycardia and hypotension), and check dressings for excessive bleeding.
◆ In carotid, innominate, vertebral, or subclavian artery occlusion, assess the patient's neurologic status frequently for changes in level of consciousness or muscle strength and pupil size.
◆ In mesenteric artery occlusion, connect a nasogastric tube to low intermittent suction. Monitor the patient's intake and output (low urine output may indicate damage to renal arteries during surgery). Check bowel sounds for return of peristalsis. Increased abdominal distention and tenderness may indicate extension of bowel ischemia with resulting gangrene, necessitating further excision, or it may indicate peritonitis.
◆ In saddle block occlusion, check distal pulses for adequate circulation. Watch for signs of renal failure and mesenteric artery occlusion (severe abdominal pain) as well as cardiac arrhythmias, which may precipitate embolus formation.
◆ In iliac artery occlusion, monitor urine output for signs of renal failure from decreased perfusion to the kidneys as a result of surgery. Provide meticulous catheter care.
◆ In femoral and popliteal artery occlusions, assist the patient with early ambulation, but discourage prolonged sitting.
◆ After amputation, check the patient's stump carefully for drainage and record its color and amount and the time. Elevate the stump, as ordered, and administer an adequate amount of analgesic. Because phantom limb pain is common, explain this phenomenon to the patient.
◆ When preparing the patient for discharge, instruct him to watch for signs and symptoms of recurrence (pain, pallor, numbness, paralysis, and absence of pulse), which can result from graft occlusion or occlusion at another site. Warn him against wearing constrictive clothing.

ATRIAL SEPTAL DEFECT
In atrial septal defect (ASD)—a congenital heart defect that increases pulmonary blood flow—an opening between the left and right atria allows blood to flow from left to right, resulting in ineffective pumping of the heart, thus increasing the risk of heart failure.

The three types of ASDs include:
◆ an *ostium secundum defect,* the most common type, which occurs in the region of the fossa ovalis and, occasionally, extends inferiorly, close to the vena cava
◆ a *sinus venosus defect,* which occurs in the superior-posterior portion of the atrial septum, sometimes extending into the vena cava, and is almost always associated with abnormal drainage of pulmonary veins into the right atrium
◆ an *ostium primum defect,* which occurs in the inferior portion of the septum primum and is usually associated with atrioventricular valve abnormalities (cleft mitral valve) and conduction defects.

ASD accounts for about 10% of congenital heart defects and is almost twice as common in females as in males, with a strong familial tendency. Although an ASD is usually a benign defect during infancy and childhood, delayed development of symptoms and complications makes it one of the most common congenital heart defects diagnosed in adults.

The prognosis is excellent in asymptomatic patients and in those with uncomplicated surgical repair, but poor in patients with cyanosis caused by large, untreated defects.

Causes
◆ Unknown
◆ Ostium primum defects commonly occurring in patients with Down syndrome

Pathophysiology
In an ASD, blood shunts from the left atrium to the right atrium because the left atrial pressure is normally slightly higher than the right atrial pressure. This pressure difference forces large amounts of blood through a defect. This shunt results in right heart volume overload, affecting the right atrium, right ventricle, and pulmonary arteries. Eventually, the right atrium enlarges, and the right ventricle dilates to accommodate the increased blood volume. If pulmonary artery hypertension develops, increased pulmonary vascular resistance and right ventricular hypertrophy follow. In some adults, irreversible pulmonary artery hypertension causes reversal of the shunt direction, which results in unoxygenated blood entering the systemic circulation, causing cyanosis.

Signs and symptoms
◆ Fatigue after exertion caused by decreased cardiac output from the left ventricle
◆ Early systolic to midsystolic murmur at the second or third left intercostal space, caused by extra blood passing through the pulmonic valve
◆ Low-pitched diastolic murmur at the lower left sternal border, more pronounced on inspiration, resulting from increased tricuspid valve flow in patients with large shunts
◆ Fixed, widely split S_2 due to delayed closure of the pulmonic valve, resulting from an increased volume of blood
◆ Systolic click or late systolic murmur at the apex, resulting from mitral valve prolapse in older children with an ASD
◆ Clubbing and cyanosis, if a right-to-left shunt develops

AGE ALERT *An infant may be cyanotic because he has a cardiac or pulmonary disorder. Cyanosis that worsens with crying is most likely associated with cardiac causes because crying increases pulmonary resistance to blood flow, resulting in an increased right-to-left shunt. Cyanosis that improves with crying is most likely associated with pulmonary causes because deep breathing improves tidal volume.*

Complications
◆ Physical underdevelopment
◆ Respiratory tract infections
◆ Heart failure
◆ Atrial arrhythmias
◆ Mitral valve prolapse

Diagnosis
A history of increasing fatigue and characteristic physical features suggest an ASD. These tests confirm the diagnosis:
◆ Chest X-ray shows an enlarged right atrium and right ventricle, a prominent pulmonary artery, and increased pulmonary vascular markings.
◆ Electrocardiography results may be normal, but they commonly show right-axis deviation, a prolonged PR interval, varying degrees of right bundle-branch block, right ventricular hypertrophy, atrial fibrillation (particularly in severe cases in patients older than age 30) and, in ostium primum defect, left-axis deviation.
◆ Echocardiography measures right ventricular enlargement, may locate the defect, and shows volume overload in the right side of the heart. It may reveal right ventricular and pulmonary artery dilation.
◆ Two-dimensional echocardiography with color Doppler flow, contrast echocardiography, or both have supplanted cardiac catheterization as the confirming tests for an ASD. Cardiac catheterization is used if inconsistencies exist in the clinical data or if significant pulmonary hypertension is suspected.

Treatment
Operative repair is advised for the patient with an uncomplicated ASD with evidence of significant

left-to-right shunting. Ideally, this is performed when the patient is between ages 2 and 4. Operative treatment shouldn't be performed on a patient with small defects and trivial left-to-right shunts. Because an ASD seldom produces complications in an infant or a toddler, surgery can be delayed until preschool or early school age. A large defect may need immediate surgical closure with sutures or a patch graft. Alternatively, placement of a wire mesh septal occluder device during cardiac catheterization is becoming a more common intervention than open-heart surgery. Patients recover more quickly from this procedure than from surgery.

Special considerations
◆ Before cardiac catheterization, explain pretest and posttest procedures to the child and parents. If possible, use drawings or other visual aids to explain it to the child.
◆ As needed, teach the patient about antibiotic prophylaxis to prevent infective endocarditis.
◆ If surgery is scheduled, teach the child and parents about the intensive care unit and introduce them to the staff. Show parents where they can wait during the operation. Explain postoperative procedures, tubes, dressings, and monitoring equipment.
◆ After surgery, closely monitor the patient's vital signs, central venous and intra-arterial pressures, and intake and output. Watch for atrial arrhythmias, which may remain uncorrected.

BUERGER'S DISEASE
Buerger's disease (sometimes called *thromboangiitis obliterans*) — an inflammatory, nonatheromatous occlusive condition — impairs circulation to the legs, feet and, occasionally, hands. It affects 6 out of every 10,000 people, most commonly occuring in men ages 20 to 40 who have a history of smoking or chewing tobacco.

Causes
◆ Unknown
◆ Definite link to smoking has been found, suggesting a hypersensitivity reaction to nicotine

Pathophysiology
In Buerger's disease, polymorphonuclear leukocytes infiltrate the walls of small and medium-sized arteries and veins. Thrombus develops in the vascular lumen, eventually occluding and obliterating portions of the small vessels, resulting in decreased blood flow to the feet and legs. This diminished blood flow may produce ulceration and, eventually, gangrene.

Signs and symptoms
◆ Intermittent claudication of the instep, which is aggravated by exercise and relieved by rest, resulting from tissue ischemia
◆ Initially, coldness, cyanosis, and numbness in feet during exposure to low temperature, resulting from diminished blood flow; later, redness, heat, and tingling
◆ Impaired peripheral pulses and migratory superficial thrombophlebitis caused by inflammatory changes in the vessel walls

Complications
◆ Ulceration, muscle atrophy, and gangrene due to impaired blood flow
◆ Painful fingertip ulcerations if the hands are affected

Diagnosis
Patient history and physical examination strongly suggest Buerger's disease. Supportive diagnostic tests include:
◆ Doppler ultrasonography to show diminished circulation in the peripheral vessels
◆ plethysmography to help detect decreased circulation in the peripheral vessels
◆ arteriography to locate lesions and rule out atherosclerosis.

Treatment
The primary goals of treatment are to relieve symptoms and prevent complications. Such therapy may include:
◆ an exercise program that uses gravity to fill and drain the blood vessels
◆ in severe disease, a lumbar sympathectomy to increase blood supply to the skin
◆ possibly amputation for nonhealing ulcers, intractable pain, or gangrene.

Special considerations
◆ Strongly urge the patient to permanently discontinue smoking to enhance the effectiveness of treatment. If necessary, refer him to a self-help group to stop smoking.
◆ Warn the patient to avoid such precipitating factors as emotional stress, exposure to extreme temperatures, and trauma.
◆ Teach proper foot care, especially the importance of wearing well-fitting shoes and cotton or wool socks. Show the patient how to inspect his feet daily for cuts, abrasions, and signs of skin breakdown, such as redness and soreness. Remind him to seek medical attention at once after trauma.
◆ If the patient has ulcers and gangrene, enforce bed rest and use a padded footboard or bed cradle to prevent pressure from bed

linens. Protect the feet with soft padding. Wash them gently with a mild soap and tepid water, rinse thoroughly, and pat dry with a soft towel.

◆ Provide emotional support. If necessary, refer the patient for psychological counseling to help him cope with restrictions imposed by this chronic disease. If he has undergone amputation, assess rehabilitative needs, especially regarding changes in body image. Refer him to a physical therapist, an occupational therapist, or a social service agency, as needed.

CARDIAC ARRHYTHMIAS

In arrhythmias, abnormal electrical conduction or automaticity changes the heart's rate and rhythm. Arrhythmias vary in severity, from those that are mild, asymptomatic, and require no treatment (such as sinus arrhythmia, in which heart rate increases and decreases with respiration) to catastrophic ventricular fibrillation, which requires immediate resuscitation. Arrhythmias are generally classified according to their origin (ventricular or supraventricular). Their effect on cardiac output and blood pressure, partially influenced by the site of origin, determines their clinical significance.

Causes
◆ Acid-base imbalances
◆ Cellular hypoxia
◆ Congenital defects
◆ Connective tissue disorders
◆ Degeneration of the conductive tissue
◆ Drug toxicity
◆ Electrolyte imbalances
◆ Emotional stress
◆ Hypertrophy of the heart muscle
◆ Myocardial ischemia or infarction
◆ Organic heart disease
   Keep in mind that each arrhythmia may have its own specific causes. (See *Types of cardiac arrhythmias*, pages 144 to 151.)

Pathophysiology
Arrhythmias may result from enhanced automaticity, reentry, escape beats, or abnormal electrical conduction. (See *Comparing normal and abnormal conduction*, pages 150 and 151.)

Signs and symptoms
Signs and symptoms of arrhythmias result from reduced cardiac output and altered perfusion to the organs, and may include:
◆ dyspnea
◆ hypotension
◆ dizziness, syncope, and weakness

◆ chest pain
◆ cool, clammy skin
◆ altered level of consciousness
◆ reduced urine output.

Complications
◆ Sudden cardiac death
◆ Myocardial infarction
◆ Heart failure
◆ Thromboembolism

Diagnosis
◆ Electrocardiography detects arrhythmias as well as ischemia and infarction that may result in arrhythmias.
◆ Laboratory testing may reveal electrolyte abnormalities, acid-base abnormalities, or drug toxicities that may cause arrhythmias.
◆ Holter monitoring, event monitoring, and loop recording can detect arrhythmias and the effectiveness of drug therapy during a patient's daily activities.
◆ Exercise testing may detect exercise-induced arrhythmias.
◆ Electrophysiologic testing identifies the mechanism of an arrhythmia and the location of accessory pathways; it also assesses the effectiveness of antiarrhythmics, radiofrequency ablation, and implanted cardioverter-defibrillators.

Treatment
Follow the specific treatment guidelines for each arrhythmia. (See *Types of cardiac arrhythmias*, pages 144 to 151.)

Special considerations
◆ Assess an unmonitored patient for rhythm disturbances.
◆ If the patient's pulse is abnormally rapid, slow, or irregular, watch for signs of hypoperfusion, such as hypotension and diminished urine output.
◆ Document arrhythmias in a monitored patient, and assess him for possible causes and effects.
◆ When life-threatening arrhythmias develop, rapidly assess level of consciousness, respirations, and pulse rate.
◆ Initiate cardiopulmonary resuscitation, if indicated.
◆ Evaluate the patient for altered cardiac output resulting from arrhythmias.
◆ Administer medications as ordered, and prepare to assist with medical procedures, if indicated (for example, cardioversion).
◆ Monitor the patient for predisposing factors—such as fluid and electrolyte imbalances—and signs of drug toxicity, especially with digoxin. If you suspect drug toxicity, report such signs to

the physician immediately and withhold the next dose.

♦ To prevent arrhythmias in a postoperative cardiac patient, provide adequate oxygen and reduce the heart's workload while carefully maintaining metabolic, neurologic, respiratory, and hemodynamic status.

♦ As appropriate, explain to the patient that he may undergo transcutaneous pacing as a non-invasive therapy for emergency use before he receives a temporary wire or permanent pacing wire.

♦ To avoid temporary pacemaker malfunction, install a fresh battery before each insertion. Carefully secure the external catheter wires and the pacemaker box. Assess the threshold daily. Watch closely for premature contractions, a sign of myocardial irritation.

♦ To avert permanent pacemaker malfunction, restrict the patient's activity after insertion, as ordered. Monitor the pulse rate regularly, and watch for signs of decreased cardiac output.

♦ If the patient has a permanent pacemaker, warn him about environmental hazards, as indicated by the pacemaker's manufacturer. Although hazards may not present a problem, 24-hour Holter monitoring may be helpful. Tell the patient to report light-headedness or syncope, and stress the importance of regular checkups.

▌▌▌ **LIFE-THREATENING DISORDER**

CARDIAC TAMPONADE

Cardiac tamponade is a rapid, unchecked increase in pressure in the pericardial sac that compresses the heart, impairs diastolic filling, and reduces cardiac output. The pressure increase usually results from blood or fluid accumulation in the pericardial sac. Even a small amount of fluid (50 to 100 ml) can cause a serious tamponade if it accumulates rapidly.

Prognosis depends on the rate of fluid accumulation. If it accumulates rapidly, cardiac tamponade requires emergency lifesaving measures to prevent death. A slow accumulation and increase in pressure, as in pericardial effusion associated with malignant tumors, may not produce immediate symptoms because the fibrous wall of the pericardial sac can gradually stretch to accommodate as much as 1 to 2 L of fluid.

Causes

♦ Acute myocardial infarction
♦ Chronic renal failure requiring dialysis
♦ Connective tissue disorders (such as rheumatoid arthritis, systemic lupus erythematosus, rheumatic fever, vasculitis, and scleroderma)

♦ Drug reaction from procainamide, hydralazine, minoxidil, isoniazid, penicillin, methysergide maleate, or daunorubicin
♦ Effusion (from cancer, bacterial infections, tuberculosis and, rarely, acute rheumatic fever)
♦ Hemorrhage from nontraumatic causes (such as anticoagulant therapy in patients with pericarditis or rupture of the heart or great vessels)
♦ Hemorrhage from trauma (such as gunshot or stab wounds to the chest or perforation by the catheter during cardiac or central venous catheterization or postcardiac surgery)
♦ Idiopathic causes (Dressler's syndrome)
♦ Viral or postirradiation pericarditis

Pathophysiology

In cardiac tamponade, the accumulation of pericardial fluid causes increased stiffness of the ventricle, requiring higher filling pressures. The progressive accumulation of fluid in the pericardial sac causes pericardial pressure increases above the ventricular filling pressure, resulting in reduced cardiac output. This compression obstructs blood flow into the ventricles and reduces the amount of blood that can be pumped out of the heart with each contraction. (See *Understanding cardiac tamponade,* page 152.)

Each time the ventricles contract, more fluid accumulates in the pericardial sac. This further limits the amount of blood that can fill the ventricular chambers — especially the left ventricle — during the next cardiac cycle. A further decrease in cardiac output occurs due to equilibration of pericardial and left ventricular filling pressures.

⚠ **CLINICAL ALERT** *Cardiac tamponade may cause a cardiac condition called pulseless electrical activity (PEA). In PEA, isolated electrical activity occurs sporadically without evidence of myocardial contraction. Unless the underlying cardiac tamponade is identified and treated quickly, PEA results in death.*

The amount of fluid necessary to cause cardiac tamponade varies greatly; it may be as little as 50 ml when the fluid accumulates rapidly or more than 2 L when the fluid accumulates slowly and the pericardium stretches to adapt.

Signs and symptoms

♦ Elevated central venous pressure (CVP) with neck vein distention due to increased jugular venous pressure
♦ Muffled heart sounds caused by fluid in the pericardial sac

(Text continues on page 153.)

Types of cardiac arrhythmias

This chart reviews many common cardiac arrhythmias and outlines their features, causes, and treatment. Use a normal electrocardiogram strip, if available, to compare normal cardiac rhythm configurations with the rhythm strips below. Characteristics of normal sinus rhythm include:
♦ ventricular and atrial rates of 60 to 100 beats/minute
♦ regular and uniform QRS complexes and P waves
♦ PR interval of 0.12 to 0.20 second
♦ QRS duration of 0.06 to 0.10 second
♦ identical atrial and ventricular rates, with constant PR intervals.

Arrhythmia	Features
Sinus tachycardia 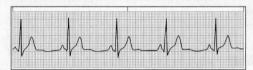	♦ Atrial and ventricular rhythms regular ♦ Rate > 100 beats/minute; rarely, > 160 beats/minute ♦ Normal P wave preceding each QRS complex
Sinus bradycardia 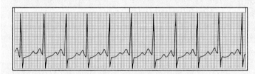	♦ Atrial and ventricular rhythms regular ♦ Rate < 60 beats/minute ♦ Normal P waves preceding each QRS complex
Paroxysmal supraventricular tachycardia 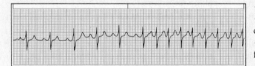	♦ Atrial and ventricular rhythms regular ♦ Heart rate > 160 beats/minute; rarely exceeds 250 beats/minute ♦ P waves regular but aberrant; difficult to differentiate from preceding T wave ♦ P wave preceding each QRS complex ♦ Sudden onset and termination of arrhythmia
Atrial flutter	♦ Atrial rhythm regular; rate 250 to 400 beats/minute ♦ Ventricular rate variable, depending on degree of AV block (usually 60 to 100 beats/minute) ♦ No P waves, atrial activity appears as flutter waves; sawtooth configuration common in lead II ♦ QRS complexes uniform in shape, but commonly irregular in rate

Causes	Treatment

♦ Normal physiologic response to fever, exercise, anxiety, pain, dehydration; may also accompany shock, left-sided heart failure, cardiac tamponade, hyperthyroidism, anemia, hypovolemia, pulmonary embolism, and an anterior-wall myocardial infarction (MI)
♦ May also occur with atropine, epinephrine, isoproterenol, quinidine, caffeine, alcohol, cocaine, amphetamine, and nicotine use

♦ Correction of underlying cause
♦ Beta-adrenergic blocker or calcium channel blocker for symptomatic patients

---

♦ Normal in a well-conditioned heart, as in an athlete
♦ Increased intracranial pressure; increased vagal tone due to straining during defecation, vomiting, intubation, or mechanical ventilation; sick sinus syndrome; hypothyroidism; and an inferior-wall MI
♦ May also occur with anticholinesterase, beta-adrenergic blocker, digoxin, or morphine use

♦ Correction of underlying cause
♦ For low cardiac output, dizziness, weakness, altered level of consciousness, or low blood pressure; advanced cardiac life support (ACLS) protocol for administration of atropine
♦ Temporary or permanent pacemaker
♦ Dopamine or epinephrine infusion

♦ Intrinsic abnormality of atrioventricular (AV) conduction system
♦ Physical or psychological stress, hypoxia, hypokalemia, cardiomyopathy, congenital heart disease, an MI, valvular disease, Wolff-Parkinson-White syndrome, cor pulmonale, hyperthyroidism, and systemic hypertension
♦ Digoxin toxicity; use of caffeine, marijuana, or central nervous system stimulants

♦ If patient's condition is unstable, immediate cardioversion
♦ If patient's condition is stable, vagal stimulation, Valsalva's maneuver, and carotid sinus massage
♦ Adenosine I.V. to rapidly convert arrhythmia
♦ If patient has normal ejection fraction, possibly a calcium channel blocker, a beta-adrenergic blocker or amiodarone
♦ If the ejection fraction is less than 40%, possibly amiodarone

---

♦ Heart failure, tricuspid or mitral valve disease, pulmonary embolism, cor pulmonale, an inferior-wall MI, and pericarditis
♦ Digoxin toxicity

♦ If patient's condition is unstable with a ventricular rate > 150 beats/minute, immediate cardioversion
♦ If patient's condition is stable, drug therapy may include a calcium channel blocker, a beta-adrenergic blocker, or an antiarrhythmic
♦ Possibly, anticoagulation therapy

(continued)

Types of cardiac arrhythmias *(continued)*

Arrhythmia	**Features**

Atrial fibrillation

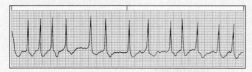

♦ Atrial rhythm grossly irregular; rate > 400 beats/minute
♦ Ventricular rhythm grossly irregular
♦ QRS complexes of uniform configuration and duration
♦ PR interval indiscernible
♦ No P waves, atrial activity appears as erratic, irregular, baseline fibrillatory waves

Junctional rhythm

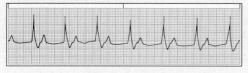

♦ Atrial and ventricular rhythms regular; atrial rate 40 to 60 beats/minute; ventricular rate usually 40 to 60 beats/minute (60 to 100 beats/minute is accelerated junctional rhythm)
♦ P waves preceding, hidden within (absent), or after QRS complex; usually inverted if visible
♦ PR interval (when present) < 0.12 second
♦ QRS complex configuration and duration normal, except in aberrant conduction

First-degree AV block

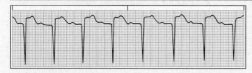

♦ Atrial and ventricular rhythms regular
♦ PR interval > 0.20 second
♦ P wave precedes QRS complex
♦ QRS complex normal

Second-degree AV block

Mobitz I (Wenckebach)

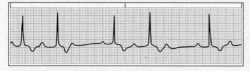

♦ Atrial rhythm regular
♦ Ventricular rhythm irregular
♦ Atrial rate exceeds ventricular rate
♦ PR interval progressively, but only slightly, longer with each cycle until QRS complex disappears (dropped beat); PR interval shorter after dropped beat

Causes	Treatment
♦ Heart failure, chronic obstructive pulmonary disease, thyrotoxicosis, constrictive pericarditis, ischemic heart disease, sepsis, pulmonary embolus, rheumatic heart disease, hypertension, mitral stenosis, atrial irritation, or complication of coronary bypass or valve replacement surgery	♦ If patient's condition is unstable with a ventricular rate > 150 beats/minute, immediate cardioversion ♦ If patient's condition is stable, drug therapy may include a calcium channel blocker, a beta-adrenergic blocker, digoxin, procainamide, quinidine, ibutilide, or amiodarone ♦ Possibly, anticoagulation therapy ♦ Possibly, dual-chamber atrial pacing, placement of an implantable atrial pacemaker, or surgical maze procedure
♦ An inferior-wall MI or ischemia, hypoxia, vagal stimulation, and sick sinus syndrome ♦ Acute rheumatic fever ♦ Valve surgery ♦ Digoxin toxicity	♦ Correction of underlying cause ♦ Atropine for symptomatic slow rate ♦ Pacemaker insertion if patient doesn't respond to drugs ♦ Discontinuation of digoxin if appropriate
♦ May be seen in healthy persons ♦ An inferior-wall MI or ischemia, hypothyroidism, hypokalemia, and hyperkalemia ♦ Digoxin toxicity; quinidine, procainamide, beta-adrenergic blocker, calcium channel blocker, or amiodarone use	♦ Correction of underlying cause ♦ Possibly atropine if PR interval exceeds 0.26 second or symptomatic bradycardia develops ♦ Cautious use of digoxin, a calcium channel blocker, and a beta-adrenergic blocker
♦ An inferior-wall MI, cardiac surgery, acute rheumatic fever, and vagal stimulation ♦ Digoxin toxicity; propranolol, quinidine, or procainamide use	♦ Treatment of underlying cause ♦ Atropine or temporary pacemaker for symptomatic bradycardia ♦ Discontinuation of digoxin if appropriate

(continued)

Types of cardiac arrhythmias (continued)

Arrhythmia	Features

Second-degree AV block

Mobitz II

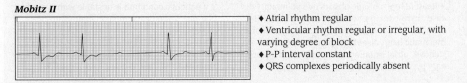

♦ Atrial rhythm regular
♦ Ventricular rhythm regular or irregular, with varying degree of block
♦ P-P interval constant
♦ QRS complexes periodically absent

Third-degree AV block

Complete heart block

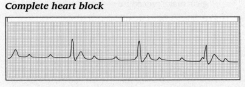

♦ Atrial rhythm regular
♦ Ventricular rhythm regular and rate slower than atrial rate
♦ No relation between P waves and QRS complexes
♦ No constant PR interval
♦ QRS complex normal (nodal pacemaker) or wide and bizarre (ventricular pacemaker)

Premature ventricular contraction (PVC)

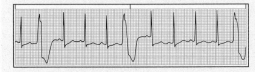

♦ Atrial rhythm regular
♦ Ventricular rhythm irregular
♦ QRS complex premature, usually followed by a complete compensatory pause
♦ QRS complex wide and distorted, usually > 0.14 second
♦ Premature QRS complexes occurring alone, in pairs, or in threes, alternating with normal beats; focus from one (uniform) or more (multiform) sites
♦ Ominous when clustered, multifocal, with R wave on T pattern

Ventricular tachycardia

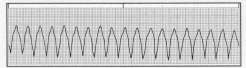

♦ Ventricular rate 140 to 220 beats/minute, rhythm usually regular
♦ QRS complexes wide, bizarre, and independent of P waves
♦ P waves not discernible
♦ May start and stop suddenly

Causes	Treatment
♦ Severe coronary artery disease, an anterior-wall MI, and acute myocarditis ♦ Digoxin toxicity	♦ Atropine, dopamine, or epinephrine for symptomatic bradycardia ♦ Temporary or permanent pacemaker for symptomatic bradycardia ♦ Discontinuation of digoxin if appropriate
♦ An inferior- or anterior-wall MI, congenital abnormality, rheumatic fever, hypoxia, postoperative complication of mitral valve replacement, postprocedure complication of radiofrequency ablation in or near AV nodal tissue, Lev's disease (fibrosis and calcification that spreads from cardiac structures to the conductive tissue), and Lenègre's disease (conductive tissue fibrosis) ♦ Digoxin toxicity	♦ Atropine, dopamine, or epinephrine for symptomatic bradycardia ♦ Temporary or permanent pacemaker for symptomatic bradycardia
♦ Heart failure; a previous or acute MI, ischemia, or contusion; myocardial irritation by ventricular catheter or a pacemaker; hypercapnia; hypokalemia; hypocalcemia; and hypomagnesemia ♦ Drug toxicity (digoxin, aminophylline, tricyclic antidepressant, beta-adrenergic blocker, isoproterenol, or dopamine) ♦ Caffeine, tobacco, or alcohol use ♦ Psychological stress, anxiety, pain, or exercise	♦ If warranted, procainamide, amiodarone, or lidocaine I.V. ♦ Treatment of underlying cause ♦ Discontinuation of drug causing toxicity ♦ Potassium chloride I.V. infusion if PVC induced by hypokalemia ♦ Magnesium sulfate I.V. if PVC induced by hypomagnesemia
♦ Myocardial ischemia, an MI, or aneurysm; coronary artery disease; rheumatic heart disease; mitral valve prolapse; heart failure; cardiomyopathy; ventricular catheters; hypokalemia; hypercalcemia; hypomagnesemia; and pulmonary embolism ♦ Digoxin, procainamide, epinephrine, or quinidine toxicity ♦ Anxiety	♦ With pulse: If hemodynamically stable, ACLS protocol for administration of amiodarone; if drug is ineffective, synchronized cardioversion ♦ If polymorphic VT complexes, consultation with an expert in arrhythmia management ♦ Pulseless: CPR; ACLS protocol for defibrillation, endotracheal (ET) intubation, and administration of epinephrine or vasopressin, followed by amiodarone or lidocaine and, if ineffective, magnesium sulfate

(continued)

Types of cardiac arrhythmias *(continued)*

Arrhythmia	Features

Ventricular fibrillation

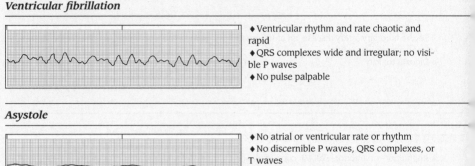

♦ Ventricular rhythm and rate chaotic and rapid
♦ QRS complexes wide and irregular; no visible P waves
♦ No pulse palpable

Asystole

♦ No atrial or ventricular rate or rhythm
♦ No discernible P waves, QRS complexes, or T waves
♦ No pulse palpable

CLOSER LOOK

Comparing normal and abnormal conduction

Normal cardiac conduction

The heart's conduction system, shown below, begins at the sinoatrial (SA) node—the heart's pacemaker. When an impulse leaves the SA node, it travels through the atria along Bachmann's bundle and the internodal pathways to the atrioventricular (AV) node, and then down the bundle of His, along the bundle branches and, finally, down the Purkinje fibers to the ventricles.

Bachmann's bundle

SA node

Internodal tracts:
    Posterior (Thorel's)
    Middle (Wenckebach's)
    Anterior

AV node

Bundle of His

Right bundle branch

Left bundle branch

Purkinje fibers

Causes	Treatment

♦ Myocardial ischemia, an MI, untreated ventricular tachycardia, R-on-T phenomenon, hypokalemia, hyperkalemia, hypercalcemia, hypoxemia, alkalosis, electric shock, and hypothermia
♦ Digoxin, epinephrine, or quinidine toxicity

♦ Pulseless: CPR; ACLS protocol for defibrillation, ET intubation, and administration of epinephrine or vasopressin, amiodarone, or lidocaine and, if ineffective, magnesium sulfate or procainamide
♦ ICD if risk for recurrent ventricular fibrillation

♦ Myocardial ischemia, an MI, aortic valve disease, heart failure, hypoxia, hypokalemia, severe acidosis, electric shock, ventricular arrhythmia, AV block, pulmonary embolism, heart rupture, cardiac tamponade, hyperkalemia, and electromechanical dissociation
♦ Cocaine overdose

♦ CPR, ACLS protocol for ET intubation, transcutaneous pacing, and administration of epinephrine or vasopressin; and consider atropine.

Abnormal cardiac conduction
Altered automaticity, reentry, or conduction disturbances may cause cardiac arrhythmias.

Altered automaticity
Altered automaticity is the result of partial depolarization, which may increase the intrinsic rate of the SA node or latent pacemakers or may induce ectopic pacemakers to reach threshold and depolarize.

Automaticity may be altered by drugs, such as epinephrine, atropine, and digoxin, and by such conditions as acidosis, alkalosis, hypoxia, a myocardial infarction (MI), hypokalemia, and hypocalcemia. Examples of arrhythmias caused by altered automaticity include atrial fibrillation and flutter; supraventricular tachycardia; premature atrial, junctional, and ventricular complexes; ventricular tachycardia and fibrillation; and accelerated idioventricular and junctional rhythms.

Reentry
Ischemia or a deformity causes an abnormal circuit to develop within conductive fibers. Although current flow is blocked in one direction within the circuit, the descending impulse can travel in the other direction. By the time the impulse completes the circuit, the previously depolarized tissue within the circuit is no longer refractory to stimulation, allowing reentry of the impulse and repetition of this cycle.

Conditions that increase the likelihood of reentry include hyperkalemia, myocardial ischemia, and the use of certain antiarrhythmics. Reentry may be responsible for such arrhythmias as paroxysmal supraventricular tachycardia; premature atrial, junctional, and ventricular complexes; and ventricular tachycardia.

An alternative reentry mechanism depends on the presence of a congenital accessory pathway linking the atria and the ventricles outside the AV junction; for example, Wolff-Parkinson-White syndrome.

Conduction disturbances
Conduction disturbances occur when impulses are conducted too quickly or too slowly. Possible causes include trauma, drug toxicity, myocardial ischemia, MI, and electrolyte abnormalities. The AV blocks occur as a result of conduction disturbances.

CLOSER LOOK

Understanding cardiac tamponade

The pericardial sac, which surrounds and protects the heart, is composed of several layers. The *fibrous pericardium* is the tough outermost membrane; the inner membrane, called the *serous membrane,* consists of the visceral and parietal layers. The visceral layer clings to the heart and is also known as the *epicardial layer* of the heart. The *parietal layer* lies between the visceral layer and the fibrous pericardium. The pericardial space — between the visceral and parietal layers — contains 10 to 30 ml of pericardial fluid. This fluid lubricates the layers and minimizes friction when the heart contracts.

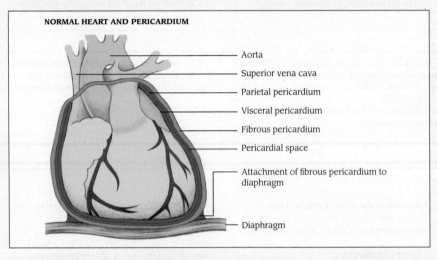

NORMAL HEART AND PERICARDIUM

- Aorta
- Superior vena cava
- Parietal pericardium
- Visceral pericardium
- Fibrous pericardium
- Pericardial space
- Attachment of fibrous pericardium to diaphragm
- Diaphragm

In cardiac tamponade, blood or fluid fills the pericardial space, compressing the heart chambers, increasing intracardiac pressure, and obstructing venous return. As blood flow into the ventricles falls, so does cardiac output. Without prompt treatment, low cardiac output can be fatal.

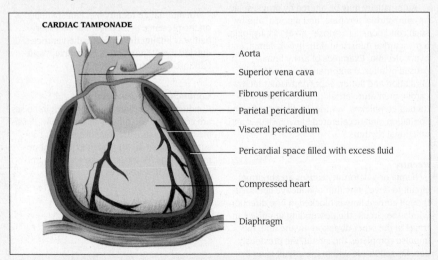

CARDIAC TAMPONADE

- Aorta
- Superior vena cava
- Fibrous pericardium
- Parietal pericardium
- Visceral pericardium
- Pericardial space filled with excess fluid
- Compressed heart
- Diaphragm

◆ Paradoxical pulse (an inspiratory decrease in systemic blood pressure greater than 15 mm Hg) due to impaired diastolic filling
◆ Diaphoresis and cool, clammy skin caused by a decrease in cardiac output
◆ Anxiety, restlessness, and syncope due to a drop in cardiac output
◆ Cyanosis due to reduced oxygenation of the tissues
◆ Weak, rapid pulse in response to a drop in cardiac output
◆ Cough, dyspnea, orthopnea, and tachypnea due to lung compression by an expanding pericardial sac and the inability to move blood from the pulmonary vasculature into the compromised left ventricle

Complications
Reduced cardiac output (fatal without prompt treatment)

Diagnosis
◆ Chest X-rays show a slightly widened mediastinum and possible cardiomegaly. The cardiac silhouette may have a goblet-shaped appearance.
◆ Electrocardiography (ECG) may show a low-amplitude QRS complex and electrical alternans, an alternating beat-to-beat change in amplitude of the P wave, QRS complex, and T wave. Generalized ST-segment elevation is noted in all leads. An ECG is used to rule out other cardiac disorders; it may reveal changes produced by acute pericarditis.
◆ Pulmonary artery catheterization detects increased right atrial pressure, right ventricular diastolic pressure, and CVP.
◆ Echocardiography may reveal pericardial effusion with signs of right ventricular and atrial compression.

Treatment
◆ Supplemental oxygen to improve oxygenation
◆ Continuous ECG and hemodynamic monitoring in an intensive care unit to detect complications and monitor effects of therapy
◆ Pericardiocentesis (needle aspiration of the pericardial cavity) to reduce fluid in the pericardial sac and improve systemic arterial pressure and cardiac output (A catheter may be left in the pericardial space attached to a drainage container to allow for continuous fluid drainage.)
◆ Pericardial window (surgical creation of an opening) to remove accumulated fluid from the pericardial sac
◆ Pericardectomy (resection of a portion or all of the pericardium) to allow full communication with the pleura, if repeated pericardiocentesis fails to prevent recurrence

◆ Trial volume loading with crystalloids, such as I.V. normal saline solution, to maintain systolic blood pressure
◆ An inotropic drug, such as isoproterenol or dopamine, to improve myocardial contractility until fluid in the pericardial sac can be removed
◆ Blood transfusion or a thoracotomy to drain reaccumulating fluid or to repair bleeding sites may be necessary in traumatic injury
◆ The heparin antagonist protamine sulfate to stop bleeding in heparin-induced tamponade
◆ Vitamin K to stop bleeding in warfarin-induced tamponade

Special considerations
Pericardiocentesis
◆ Explain the procedure to the patient. Keep at the bedside a pericardial aspiration needle attached to a 50-ml syringe by a three-way stopcock, an ECG machine, and an emergency cart with a defibrillator. Make sure the equipment is turned on and ready for immediate use. Position the patient at a 45- to 60-degree angle. Connect the precordial ECG lead to the hub of the aspiration needle with an alligator clamp and connecting wire, and assist with fluid aspiration. When the needle touches the myocardium, you'll see an ST-segment elevation or premature ventricular contractions.
◆ Monitor blood pressure and CVP during and after pericardiocentesis. Infuse I.V. solutions, as prescribed, to maintain blood pressure. Watch for a decrease in CVP and a concomitant increase in blood pressure, which indicate relief of cardiac compression.
◆ Watch for complications of pericardiocentesis, such as ventricular fibrillation, vasovagal response, or coronary artery or cardiac chamber puncture. Closely monitor ECG changes, blood pressure, pulse rate, level of consciousness, and urine output.

Thoracotomy
◆ Explain the procedure to the patient. Tell him what to expect postoperatively (chest tubes, drainage bottles, and administration of oxygen). Teach him how to turn, deep breathe, and cough.
◆ Give an antibiotic, protamine sulfate, or vitamin K, as ordered.
◆ Postoperatively, monitor critical parameters, such as vital signs and arterial blood gas values, and assess heart and respiratory rates. Give pain medication, as ordered. Maintain the chest drainage system, and be alert for complications, such as hemorrhage and arrhythmias.

||| **LIFE-THREATENING DISORDER**

CARDIOMYOPATHY

Cardiomyopathy generally applies to disease of the heart muscle fibers, and it occurs in three main forms: dilated, hypertrophic, and restrictive (extremely rare). Cardiomyopathy is the second most common direct cause of sudden death; coronary artery disease (CAD) is the first. About 5 to 8 per 100,000 Americans have *dilated cardiomyopathy,* the most common type. At greatest risk for dilated cardiomyopathy are males and blacks; other risk factors include CAD, hypertension, pregnancy, viral infections, and alcohol or illegal drug use. Because dilated cardiomyopathy usually isn't diagnosed until its advanced stages, the prognosis is generally poor.

There are two types of hypertrophic cardiomyopathy. The more common form—nonobstructive hypertrophic cardiomyopathy—is caused by pressure overload–hypertension or aortic valve stenosis. Hypertrophic obstructive cardiomyopathy (HOCM) is due to a genetic abnormality. The course of *hypertrophic cardiomyopathy* varies. Some patients progressively deteriorate, whereas others remain stable for years. It's estimated that almost 50% of all sudden deaths in competitive athletes age 35 or younger are due to HOCM. If severe, *restrictive cardiomyopathy* is irreversible.

Causes

Most patients with dilated cardiomyopathy have idiopathic, or primary, disease but some are secondary to identifiable causes. (See *Comparing cardiomyopathies,* pages 156 and 157.) HOCM is almost always inherited as a non-sex-linked autosomal dominant trait.

Pathophysiology

Dilated cardiomyopathy results from extensively damaged myocardial muscle fibers. Consequently, there's reduced contractility in the left ventricle. As systolic function declines, stroke volume, ejection fraction, and cardiac output fall. As end-diastolic volumes rise, pulmonary congestion may occur. The elevated end-diastolic volume is a compensatory response to preserve stroke volume, despite a reduced ejection fraction. The sympathetic nervous system is also stimulated to increase heart rate and contractility. The kidneys are stimulated to retain sodium and water to maintain cardiac output, and vasoconstriction also occurs as the renin-angiotensin-aldosterone system is stimulated. When these compensatory mechanisms can no longer maintain cardiac output, the heart begins to fail. Left ventricular dilation occurs as venous return and systemic vascular resistance rise. Eventually, the atria also dilate as more work is required to pump blood into the full ventricles. Cardiomegaly occurs as a consequence of dilation of the atria and ventricles. Blood pooling in the ventricles increases the risk of emboli.

▟ **AGE ALERT** *Barth syndrome is a rare genetic disorder that can cause dilated cardiomyopathy in boys. This syndrome may be associated with skeletal muscle changes, short stature, neutropenia, and increased susceptibility to bacterial infections. Evidence of dilated cardiomyopathy may appear as early as the first few days or months of life.*

Unlike dilated cardiomyopathy, which affects systolic function, hypertrophic cardiomyopathy primarily affects diastolic function. The hypertrophied ventricle becomes stiff, noncompliant, and unable to relax during ventricular filling. Consequently, ventricular filling is reduced and left ventricular filling pressure rises, causing a rise in left atrial and pulmonary venous pressures and leading to venous congestion and dyspnea. Ventricular filling time is further reduced as a compensatory response to tachycardia leading to low cardiac output. If papillary muscles become hypertrophied and don't close completely during contraction, mitral insufficiency occurs. The features of HOCM include asymmetrical left ventricular hypertrophy; hypertrophy of the intraventricular septum; rapid, forceful contractions of the left ventricle; impaired relaxation; and obstruction to left ventricular outflow. The forceful ejection of blood draws the anterior leaflet of the mitral valve to the intraventricular septum. This causes early closure of the outflow tract, decreasing ejection fraction. Moreover, intramural coronary arteries are abnormally small and may not be sufficient to supply the hypertrophied muscle with enough blood and oxygen to meet the increased needs of the hyperdynamic muscle.

Restrictive cardiomyopathy is characterized by stiffness of the ventricle caused by left ventricular hypertrophy and endocardial fibrosis and thickening, thus reducing the ability of the ventricle to relax and fill during diastole. Moreover, the rigid myocardium fails to contract completely during systole. As a result, cardiac output falls.

Signs and symptoms
Dilated cardiomyopathy

◆ Shortness of breath, orthopnea, exertional dyspnea, paroxysmal nocturnal dyspnea, fatigue, and a dry cough at night due to left-sided heart failure

◆ Peripheral edema, hepatomegaly, jugular venous distention, and weight gain caused by right-sided heart failure
◆ Peripheral cyanosis associated with a low cardiac output
◆ Tachycardia as a compensatory response to low cardiac output
◆ Pansystolic murmur associated with mitral and tricuspid insufficiency secondary to cardiomegaly and weak papillary muscles
◆ S_3 and S_4 gallop rhythms associated with heart failure
◆ Irregular pulse if atrial fibrillation exists
◆ Worsening renal function as decreased cardiac output produces decreased renal perfusion

Hypertrophic cardiomyopathy
◆ Dyspnea due to elevated left ventricular filling pressure
◆ Fatigue associated with a reduced cardiac output
◆ Angina caused by the inability of the intramural coronary arteries to supply enough blood to meet the increased oxygen demands of the hypertrophied heart
◆ Peripheral pulse with a characteristic double impulse (pulsus biferiens) caused by powerful left ventricular contractions and rapid ejection of blood during systole
◆ Abrupt arterial pulse secondary to vigorous left ventricular contractions
◆ Irregular pulse if an enlarged atrium causes atrial fibrillation

HOCM
◆ Systolic ejection murmur along the left sternal border and at the apex caused by mitral insufficiency
◆ Angina caused by the inability of the intramural coronary arteries to supply enough blood to meet the increased oxygen demands of the hypertrophied heart
◆ Syncope resulting from arrhythmias or reduced ventricular filling leading to a reduced cardiac output
◆ Activity intolerance due to worsening of outflow tract obstruction from exercise-induced catecholamine release
◆ Abrupt arterial pulse secondary to vigorous left ventricular contractions and early termination of left ventricular ejection
◆ Irregular pulse if an enlarged atrium causes atrial fibrillation

Restrictive cardiomyopathy
◆ Fatigue, dyspnea, orthopnea, chest pain, edema, liver engorgement, peripheral cyanosis, pallor, and S_3 or S_4 gallop rhythms due to heart failure

◆ Systolic murmurs caused by mitral and tricuspid insufficiency

Complications
◆ Heart failure
◆ Arrhythmias
◆ Systemic or pulmonary embolization
◆ Sudden death

Diagnosis
◆ Echocardiography confirms dilated cardiomyopathy.
◆ Chest X-ray may reveal cardiomegaly associated with any of the cardiomyopathies.
◆ Cardiac catheterization with possible heart biopsy can be definitive with HOCM.
◆ Diagnosis requires elimination of other possible causes of heart failure and arrhythmias. (See *Comparing diagnostic tests in cardiomyopathy,* pages 158 and 159.)

Treatment
Dilated cardiomyopathy
◆ Treatment of the underlying cause, if identifiable
◆ An angiotensin-converting enzyme (ACE) inhibitor, as first-line therapy, to reduce afterload through vasodilation
◆ A diuretic, taken with an ACE inhibitor, to reduce fluid retention
◆ Digoxin, for the patient who doesn't respond to ACE inhibitor and diuretic therapy, to improve myocardial contractility
◆ Hydralazine and isosorbide dinitrate in combination, to produce vasodilation
◆ A beta-adrenergic blocker or angiotensin-receptor blocker for the patient with New York Heart Association (NYHA) class II or III heart failure (See *Classifying heart failure,* page 160.)
◆ An antiarrhythmic, such as amiodarone, used cautiously to control arrhythmias
◆ Implantable cardioverter-defibrillator (ICD) to treat ventricular arrhythmias and for prophylaxis (because of the high incidence of sudden death in the patient with NYHA class III or IV heart failure)
◆ Cardioversion to convert atrial fibrillation to sinus rhythm
◆ Pacemaker insertion to correct arrhythmias
◆ An anticoagulant (controversial) to reduce the risk of emboli
◆ Biventricular pacemaker for cardiac resynchronization therapy if symptoms continue despite optimal drug therapy if the patient is classified as NYHA class III or IV heart failure, if duration of the QRS complex is 0.13 second or more, or if the ejection fraction is 35% or less

Comparing cardiomyopathies

Cardiomyopathies include various structural or functional abnormalities of the ventricles. They're grouped into three main pathophysiologic types—dilated, hypertrophic, and restrictive. These conditions may lead to heart failure by impairing myocardial structure and function.

Normal heart	**Dilated cardiomyopathy**

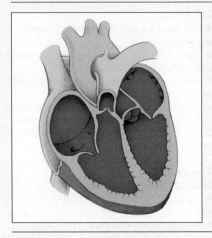

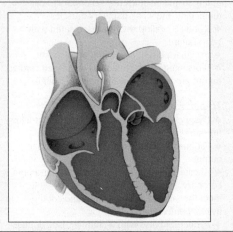

Ventricles	♦ Greatly increased chamber size ♦ Thinning of left ventricular muscle
Atrial chamber size	♦ Increased
Myocardial mass	♦ Increased
Ventricular inflow resistance	♦ Normal
Contractility	♦ Decreased
Possible causes	♦ Cardiotoxic effects of drugs or alcohol ♦ Chemotherapy ♦ Drug hypersensitivity ♦ Hypertension ♦ Ischemic heart disease ♦ Peripartum syndrome related to toxemia ♦ Valvular disease ♦ Viral or bacterial infection

♦ Revascularization, such as coronary artery bypass graft surgery, if dilated cardiomyopathy is due to ischemia
♦ Valvular repair or replacement, if dilated cardiomyopathy is due to valve dysfunction
♦ Heart transplantation if the patient unresponsive to medical therapy
♦ Lifestyle modifications, such as smoking cessation; low-fat, low-sodium diet; physical activity; and abstinence from alcohol

Hypertrophic cardiomyopathy
♦ Optimal control of hypertension
♦ Aortic valve replacement if valve is stenotic
♦ Verapamil or diltiazem to reduce ventricular stiffness and elevated diastolic pressures
♦ Cardioversion to treat atrial fibrillation
♦ Anticoagulation to reduce the risk of systemic embolism with atrial fibrillation

Hypertrophic cardiomyopathy

Restrictive cardiomyopathy

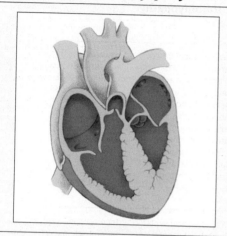

- ◆ Normal right and decreased left chamber size
- ◆ Left ventricular hypertrophy
- ◆ Thickened interventricular septum (hypertrophic obstructive cardiomyopathy [HOCM])

- ◆ Decreased ventricular chamber size
- ◆ Left ventricular hypertrophy

◆ Increased on left	◆ Increased
◆ Increased	◆ Normal
◆ Increased	◆ Increased
◆ Increased or decreased	◆ Decreased

- ◆ Autosomal dominant trait (HOCM)
- ◆ Hypertension
- ◆ Obstructive valvular disease
- ◆ Thyroid disease

- ◆ Amyloidosis
- ◆ Hemochromatosis
- ◆ Infiltrative neoplastic disease
- ◆ Sarcoidosis

HOCM

◆ A beta-adrenergic blocker to slow the heart rate, reduce myocardial oxygen demands, and increase ventricular filling by relaxing the obstructing muscle, thereby increasing cardiac output

◆ An antiarrhythmic, such as amiodarone, to reduce arrhythmias

◆ Cardioversion to treat atrial fibrillation

◆ Anticoagulation to reduce the risk of systemic embolism with atrial fibrillation

◆ Verapamil or diltiazem to reduce septal stiffness and elevated diastolic pressures

◆ Ablation of the atrioventricular node and implantation of a dual-chamber pacemaker (controversial), in the patient with HOCM and ventricular tachycardia, to reduce the outflow gradient by altering the pattern of ventricular contractions

Comparing diagnostic tests in cardiomyopathy

The four main forms of cardiomyopathy—dilated, hypertrophic, hypertrophic obstructive and restrictive—each have unique diagnostic test findings.

Dilated cardiomyopathy	Hypertrophic cardiomyopathy	Hypertrophic obstructive cardiomyopathy	Restrictive cardiomyopathy
Electrocardiography			
Biventricular hypertrophy, sinus tachycardia, atrial enlargement, atrial and ventricular arrhythmias, bundle-branch block, and ST-segment and T-wave abnormalities	Left ventricular hypertrophy, ST-segment and T-wave abnormalities, left anterior hemiblock, Q waves in precordial and inferior leads, ventricular arrhythmias and, possibly, atrial fibrillation	Left ventricular hypertrophy with QRS complexes tallest across midprecordium, ST segment and T-wave abnormalities, left-axis deviation, left-atrial abnormality, supraventricular tachycardia, and ventricular tachycardia	Low voltage, hypertrophy, atrioventricular conduction defects, and arrhythmias
Echocardiography			
Left ventricular thrombi, global hypokinesia, enlarged atria, left ventricular dilation and, possibly, valvular abnormalities	Symmetrical thickening of the left ventricular wall and intraventricular septum and left atrial dilation	Asymmetrical septal hypertrophy; anterior movement of the anterior mitral leaflet during systole, early termination of left ventricular ejection that worsens with dobutamine or nitrate provocation, mitral insufficiency, and atrial dilation	Increased left ventricular muscle mass, normal or reduced left ventricular cavity size, and decreased systolic function; rules out constrictive pericarditis
Chest X-ray			
Cardiomegaly, pulmonary congestion, pulmonary venous hypertension, and pleural or pericardial effusions	Cardiomegaly	Normal or mild cardiomegaly	Cardiomegaly, pericardial effusion, and pulmonary congestion

♦ ICD to treat ventricular arrhythmias
♦ Ventricular myotomy or myectomy (resection of the hypertrophied septum) to ease outflow tract obstruction and relieve symptoms
♦ Mitral valve replacement to treat mitral insufficiency (controversial)
♦ Heart transplantation for intractable symptoms

Restrictive cardiomyopathy
♦ Treatment of the underlying cause, such as administering deferoxamine to bind iron in restrictive cardiomyopathy due to hemochromatosis

♦ Although no therapy exists for restricted ventricular filling, digoxin, diuretics, and a restricted sodium diet to ease the symptoms of heart failure
♦ Oral vasodilators to decrease afterload and facilitate ventricular ejection

Special considerations
Dilated cardiomyopathy in acute failure
♦ Monitor the patient for signs of progressive failure (increasing crackles and dyspnea and increased neck vein distention) and compromised renal perfusion (oliguria, elevated blood urea

Comparing diagnostic tests in cardiomyopathy *(continued)*

Dilated cardiomyopathy	Hypertrophic cardiomyopathy	Hypertrophic obstructive cardiomyopathy	Restrictive cardiomyopathy
Cardiac catheterization			
Elevated left atrial and left ventricular end-diastolic pressures, left ventricular enlargement, and mitral and tricuspid incompetence; may identify coronary artery disease as a cause	Elevated ventricular end-diastolic pressure and, possibly, mitral insufficiency, hyperdynamic systolic function, and aortic valve pressure gradient if aortic valve is stenotic	Asymetrical septal hypertrophy, early termination of systole with decreased ejection fraction, outflow tract pressure gradient increasing from the apex to just below the aortic valve, and mitral insufficiency	Reduced systolic function and myocardial infiltration; increased left ventricular end-diastolic pressure; rules out constrictive pericarditis
Radionuclide studies			
Left ventricular dilation and hypokinesia, reduced ejection fraction	Reduced left ventricular volume, increased muscle mass, and ischemia	Reduced left ventricular volume, increased septal muscle mass, septal ischemia	Left ventricular hypertrophy with restricted ventricular filling and reduced ejection fraction

nitrogen and creatinine levels, and electrolyte imbalances). Weigh the patient daily.

◆ If the patient is receiving a vasodilator, check blood pressure and heart rate. If he becomes hypotensive, stop the infusion and place him in a supine position, with legs elevated to increase venous return and to ensure cerebral blood flow.

◆ If the patient is receiving a diuretic, monitor him for signs of resolving congestion (decreased crackles and dyspnea) or too vigorous diuresis. Check serum potassium level for hypokalemia, especially if therapy includes digoxin.

◆ Therapeutic restrictions and an uncertain prognosis usually cause profound anxiety and depression, so offer support and let the patient express his feelings. Be flexible with visiting hours.

◆ Before discharge, teach the patient about his illness and its treatment. Emphasize the need to avoid alcohol, to restrict sodium intake, to watch for weight gain, and to take digoxin as prescribed and watch for adverse reactions to it (anorexia, nausea, vomiting, and yellow vision).

◆ Encourage family members to learn cardiopulmonary resuscitation (CPR).

Hypertrophic cardiomyopathy
◆ Warn the patient against strenuous physical activity, such as running, because syncope or sudden death may follow well-tolerated exercise.

◆ Administer medications as prescribed. Avoid nitroglycerin, digoxin, and diuretics because they can worsen obstruction. Warn the patient not to stop taking propranolol abruptly because doing so may increase myocardial demands. To determine the patient's tolerance for an increased dosage of propranolol, take his pulse to check for bradycardia. Also take his blood pressure while he's in a supine position and standing (a drop in blood pressure [more than 10 mm Hg] when standing may indicate orthostatic hypotension).

◆ Administer prophylaxis for subacute infective endocarditis before dental work or surgery.

◆ Provide psychological support. If the patient is hospitalized for a long time, be flexible with visiting hours, and encourage occasional weekends away from the hospital, if possible. Refer the patient for psychosocial counseling to help him and his family accept his restricted lifestyle and poor prognosis.

◆ If the patient is a child, have his parents arrange for him to continue his studies in the health care facility.

◆ Urge the patient's family to learn CPR because sudden cardiac arrest is possible.

Restrictive cardiomyopathy
◆ In the acute phase, monitor heart rate and rhythm, blood pressure, urine output, and

Classifying heart failure

The New York Heart Association classification is a standard gauge of heart failure severity based on physical limitations.

Class I: Minimal
♦ No limitations
♦ Ordinary physical activity doesn't cause undue fatigue, dyspnea, palpitations, or angina

Class II: Mild
♦ Slightly limited physical activity
♦ Comfortable at rest
♦ Ordinary physical activity results in fatigue, palpitations, dyspnea, or angina

Class III: Moderate
♦ Markedly limited physical activity
♦ Comfortable at rest
♦ Less than ordinary activity produces symptoms

Class IV: Severe
♦ Unable to perform physical activity without discomfort
♦ Angina or symptoms of cardiac inefficiency may develop at rest

---

pulmonary artery pressure readings to help guide treatment.
♦ Give psychological support. Provide appropriate diversionary activities for the patient restricted to prolonged bed rest. Because a poor prognosis may cause profound anxiety and depression, be especially supportive and understanding and encourage the patient to express his fears. Refer him for psychosocial counseling, as necessary, for assistance in coping with his restricted lifestyle. Be flexible with visiting hours whenever possible.
♦ Before discharge, teach the patient to watch for and report signs and symptoms of digoxin toxicity (anorexia, nausea, vomiting, and yellow vision); to record and report weight gain; and, if sodium restriction is ordered, to avoid canned foods, pickles, smoked meats, and use of table salt.

COARCTATION OF THE AORTA
Coarctation is a narrowing of the aorta, usually just below the left subclavian artery, near the site where the ligamentum arteriosum (the remnant of the ductus arteriosus, a fetal blood vessel) joins the pulmonary artery to the aorta.

Coarctation may occur with aortic valve stenosis (usually of a bicuspid aortic valve) and with severe cases of hypoplasia of the aortic arch, patent ductus arteriosus (PDA), and ventricular septal defect (VSD). The obstruction of blood flow results in ineffective pumping of the heart and increases the risk for heart failure.

This obstructive condition accounts for about 7% of all congenital heart defects in children and is twice as common in males as in females. When coarctation of the aorta occurs in females, it's commonly associated with Turner's syndrome, a chromosomal disorder that causes ovarian dysgenesis.

The prognosis depends on the severity of associated cardiac anomalies. If corrective surgery is performed before isolated coarctation induces severe systemic hypertension or degenerative changes in the aorta, the prognosis is good.

Causes
♦ Unknown
♦ May be associated with Turner's syndrome

Pathophysiology
Coarctation of the aorta may develop as a result of spasm and constriction of the smooth muscle in the ductus arteriosus as it closes. Possibly, this contractile tissue extends into the aortic wall, causing narrowing. The obstructive process causes hypertension in the aortic branches above the constriction (arteries that supply the arms, neck, and head) and diminished pressure in the vessel below the constriction.

Restricted blood flow through the narrowed aorta increases the pressure load on the left ventricle and causes dilation of the proximal aorta and ventricular hypertrophy.

As oxygenated blood leaves the left ventricle, a portion travels through the arteries that branch off the aorta proximal to the coarctation. If PDA is present, the rest of the blood travels through the coarctation, mixes with deoxygenated blood from the PDA, and travels to the legs. If the PDA is closed, the legs and lower portion of the body must rely solely on the blood that gets through the coarctation.

Untreated, this condition may lead to left-sided heart failure and, rarely, to cerebral hemorrhage and aortic rupture. If VSD accompanies coarctation, blood shunts from left to right, straining the right side of the heart. This leads to pulmonary hypertension and, eventually, right-sided heart hypertrophy and failure.

If coarctation is asymptomatic in infancy, it usually remains so throughout adolescence as collateral circulation develops to bypass the narrowed segment.

Signs and symptoms

♦ Tachypnea, dyspnea, pulmonary edema, pallor, tachycardia, failure to thrive, cardiomegaly, and hepatomegaly due to heart failure during an infant's first year of life
♦ Claudication due to reduced blood flow to the legs
♦ Hypertension in the upper body due to increased pressure in the arteries proximal to the coarctation
♦ Headache, vertigo, and epistaxis secondary to hypertension
♦ Upper-extremity blood pressure greater than lower-extremity blood pressure because blood flow through the coarctation is greater to the upper body than to the lower body
♦ Pink upper extremities and cyanotic lower extremities resulting from reduced oxygenated blood reaching the legs
♦ Absent or diminished femoral pulses resulting from restricted blood flow to the lower extremities through the constricted aorta
♦ In most cases, normal heart sounds unless a coexisting cardiac defect is present
♦ Chest and arms may be more developed than the legs because circulation to the legs is restricted

Complications

♦ Heart failure
♦ Severe hypertension
♦ Cerebral aneurysms and hemorrhage
♦ Rupture of the aorta
♦ Aortic aneurysm
♦ Infective endocarditis

Diagnosis

♦ Physical examination reveals the cardinal signs — resting systolic hypertension in the upper body, absent or diminished femoral pulses, and a wide pulse pressure.
♦ Chest X-rays may demonstrate left ventricular hypertrophy, heart failure, a wide ascending and descending aorta, and notching of the undersurfaces of the ribs owing to erosion by collateral circulation.
♦ Electrocardiography may reveal left ventricular hypertrophy.
♦ Echocardiography may show increased left ventricular muscle thickness, coexisting aortic valve abnormalities, and the coarctation site.
♦ Cardiac catheterization evaluates collateral circulation and measures pressure in the right and left ventricles and in the ascending and descending aortas (on both sides of the obstruction). Aortography locates the site and extent of coarctation.

Treatment

♦ Digoxin, a diuretic, oxygen, and a sedative in infants with heart failure
♦ Prostaglandin infusion to keep the ductus open
♦ Antibiotic prophylaxis against infective endocarditis before and after surgery
♦ Antihypertensive therapy for children with previous undetected coarctation until surgery
♦ Preparation of the infant with heart failure or hypertension for early surgery; otherwise surgery is delayed until the preschool years (Options include end-to-end anastomosis, in which the area of coarctation is resected and the distal and proximal aorta are anastomosed end to end; patch aortoplasty, in which the area of coarctation is incised and an elliptical Dacron patch is sutured in place to widen the diameter; and subclavian flap aortoplasty, in which the distal subclavian artery is divided and the flap of the proximal portion of this vessel is used to expand the coarcted area. The ductus arteriosus is always ligated with each of these surgical techniques. Balloon angioplasty may be performed if recoarctation occurs.)

Special considerations

♦ When coarctation in an infant requires rapid digitalization, monitor vital signs closely and watch for digoxin toxicity (poor feeding and vomiting).
♦ Balance intake and output carefully, especially if the infant is receiving a diuretic and fluids are restricted.
♦ Because the infant may not be able to maintain proper body temperature, regulate environmental temperature with an overbed warmer, if needed.
♦ Monitor blood glucose levels to detect possible hypoglycemia, which may occur as glycogen stores become depleted.
♦ Offer the parents emotional support and an explanation of the disorder. Also explain diagnostic procedures, surgery, and drug therapy. Tell parents what to expect postoperatively.
♦ For an older child, assess the blood pressure in his extremities regularly, explain exercise restrictions, stress the need to take medications properly and to watch for adverse reactions, and teach him about tests and other procedures.

After corrective surgery

♦ Monitor blood pressure closely, using an intra-arterial line. Take blood pressure in all extremities. Monitor intake and output.
♦ If the patient develops hypertension and requires nitroprusside, administer as ordered by continuous I.V. infusion, using an infusion pump. Watch for severe hypotension, and regulate the dosage carefully.

♦ Provide pain relief, and encourage a gradual increase in activity.
♦ Promote adequate respiratory functioning through turning, coughing, and deep breathing.
♦ Watch for abdominal pain or rigidity and signs of GI or urinary bleeding.
♦ If an older child needs to continue antihypertensive therapy after surgery, teach him and his parents about them.
♦ Stress the importance of continued endocarditis prophylaxis.

CORONARY ARTERY DISEASE

Coronary artery disease (CAD) results from the narrowing of the coronary arteries over time resulting from atherosclerosis. The primary effect of CAD is the loss of oxygen and nutrients to myocardial tissue because of diminished coronary blood flow. As the population ages, the prevalence of CAD is increasing. It's more common in males over age 40, but as women age, the risk increases until it's almost as high as the risk for men. With proper care, the prognosis for CAD is favorable.

Causes

CAD is commonly caused by atherosclerosis. Modifiable and nonmodifiable risk factors are associated with the development of atherosclerosis and CAD. Modifiable risk factors include:
♦ diabetes mellitus, especially in females
♦ elevated homocysteine levels
♦ inactivity
♦ increased low-density and decreased high-density lipoprotein levels
♦ obesity, which increases the risk of diabetes mellitus, hypertension, and high cholesterol
♦ smoking (risk dramatically drops within 1 year of quitting)
♦ stress
♦ systolic blood pressure greater than 119 mm Hg or diastolic blood pressure greater than 79 mm Hg.
 Other modifiable risk factors include:
♦ elevated hematocrit
♦ high resting heart rate
♦ hormonal contraceptive use
♦ increased levels of serum fibrinogen and uric acid
♦ reduced vital capacity
♦ thyrotoxicosis.
 Nonmodifiable risk factors include:
♦ age older than 40
♦ family history of CAD
♦ male
♦ white.

 GENETIC LINK *Researchers have identified more than 250 genes that may play a role in CAD. It commonly results from the combined effects of multiple genes, making it difficult to determine the impact of specific genes that can influence a person's risk for the disease.*
 Some of the best understood genes linked to CAD include:
♦ *low-density lipoprotein (LDL) receptor—a protein that removes LDL from the bloodstream; a mutation in this gene is responsible for familial hypercholesterolemia*
♦ *apolipoprotein E—mutations in this gene, commonly called apo E, also affect blood levels of LDL*
♦ *apolipoprotein B-100—commonly called apo B-11, it's a component of LDL; mutations of this gene cause LDL to stay in the blood longer than normal, leading to high LDL levels*
♦ *apolipoprotein A—a glycoprotein that combines with LDL to form a particle called Lp(a); it appears as part of plaque on blood vessels*
♦ *MTHFR—an enzyme that clears homocysteine from the blood; mutations in MTHFR genes may cause higher homocysteine levels*
♦ *cystathionine B–synthase—also known as CBS, it's another enzyme involved in homocysteine metabolism; CBS mutations cause a condition known as homocystinuria (homocysteine levels are so high that homocysteine can be detected in the urine).*

Less common causes of reduced coronary artery blood flow include:
♦ congenital defects
♦ dissecting aneurysm
♦ infectious vasculitis
♦ syphilis.

Pathophysiology

Fatty, fibrous plaques progressively narrow the coronary artery lumina, reducing the volume of blood that can flow through them and leading to myocardial ischemia.
 As atherosclerosis progresses, luminal narrowing is accompanied by vascular changes that impair the ability of the diseased vessel to dilate. This causes a precarious balance between myocardial oxygen supply and demand, threatening the myocardium beyond the lesion. When oxygen demand exceeds what the diseased vessel can supply, localized myocardial ischemia results. (See *The progression of coronary artery disease in atherosclerosis,* pages 164 and 165.)
 Myocardial cells become ischemic within 10 seconds of a coronary artery occlusion. Transient ischemia causes reversible changes at the cellular and tissue levels, depressing myocardial function. Untreated, this can lead to tissue injury or necrosis. Within several minutes, oxygen deprivation forces the myocardium to shift from aerobic to anaerobic metabolism, leading to

accumulation of lactic acid and reduction of cellular pH.

The combination of hypoxia, reduced energy availability, and acidosis rapidly impairs left ventricular function. The strength of contractions in the affected myocardial region is reduced as the fibers shorten inadequately, resulting in less force and velocity. Moreover, wall motion is abnormal in the ischemic area, resulting in less blood being ejected from the heart with each contraction. Restoring blood flow through the coronary arteries restores aerobic metabolism and contractility. However, if blood flow isn't restored, myocardial infarction (MI) results.

Signs and symptoms

◆ Angina, the classic sign of CAD, results from a reduced supply of oxygen to the myocardium. It may be described as burning, squeezing, or tightness in the chest that may radiate to the left arm or shoulder blade, the neck, or the jaw. (See *Types of angina,* page 166.)

⚠ **CLINICAL ALERT** *Not all patients experience angina in the same way. Some, particularly females, may not experience chest discomfort. Their symptoms may be primarily dyspnea and fatigue, which is called an anginal equivalent. This presentation is also seen in Black and Hispanic patients. Patients with diabetes may develop central neuropathies and therefore not experience chest pain. Signs of sympathetic stimulation may be their primary anginal symptom.*

◆ Nausea and vomiting as a result of reflex stimulation of the vomiting centers by pain
◆ Cool extremities and pallor caused by sympathetic stimulation
◆ Diaphoresis due to sympathetic stimulation
◆ Xanthelasma (fat deposits on the eyelids) occurring secondary to hyperlipidemia and atherosclerosis

🔳 **AGE ALERT** *In the older adult, CAD may be asymptomatic because of a decrease in sympathetic response. Dyspnea and fatigue are two key signals of ischemia in an active, older adult.*

Complications
◆ Arrhythmias
◆ MI
◆ Ischemic cardiomyopathy

Diagnosis
◆ Electrocardiography (ECG) may be normal between anginal episodes. During angina, it may show ischemic changes, such as T-wave inversion, ST-segment depression and, possibly, arrhythmias. ST-segment elevation suggests either MI or Prinzmetal's angina.

◆ Electron-beam computed tomography scan may be used to identify calcium deposits in coronary arteries. Calcium scoring correlates with the degree of CAD.
◆ Stress testing may be performed to detect ST-segment changes during exercise or pharmacologic stress, indicating ischemia, and to determine a safe exercise prescription.
◆ Coronary angiography reveals the location and degree of coronary artery stenosis or obstruction, collateral circulation, and the condition of the artery beyond the narrowing.
◆ Intravascular ultrasound may be used to further define coronary anatomy and luminal narrowing.
◆ Myocardial perfusion imaging with thallium-201 may be performed during treadmill exercise to detect ischemic areas of the myocardium; they appear as "cold spots," which normalize during rest, indicating viable tissue.
◆ Stress echocardiography may show abnormal wall motion in ischemic areas.
◆ Rest perfusion imaging with sestamibi can be used to rule out myocardial ischemia in the patient with a chest pain syndrome that isn't clearly cardiac in nature.

Treatment
◆ A nitrate, such as nitroglycerin (given sublingually, orally, transdermally, or topically in ointment form), isosorbide dinitrate (given sublingually or orally), or isosorbide mononitrate (given orally) to reduce myocardial oxygen consumption
◆ A beta-adrenergic blocker to reduce the heart's workload and oxygen demands by reducing heart rate and peripheral resistance to blood flow
◆ A calcium channel blocker to prevent coronary artery spasm
◆ An antiplatelet drug to minimize platelet aggregation and the risk of coronary occlusion
◆ A glycoprotein IIb to IIIa inhibitor, such as abciximab, eptifibatide, or tirofiban, to reduce the risk of blood clots
◆ An antilipemic to reduce serum cholesterol or triglyceride levels
◆ An antihypertensive to control hypertension
◆ Coronary artery bypass graft (CABG) surgery to restore blood flow by bypassing an occluded artery using another vessel
◆ "Key-hole" (or minimally invasive) surgery, an alternative to traditional CABG using fiber-optic cameras inserted through small cuts in the chest, to correct blockages in one or two accessible arteries (may not be appropriate for more complicated cases)

(Text continues on page 166.)

The progression of coronary artery disease in atherosclerosis

Coronary artery disease (CAD) results as atherosclerotic plaque fills the lumens of the coronary arteries and obstructs blood flow. The primary effect of CAD is a diminished supply of oxygen and nutrients to myocardial tissue.

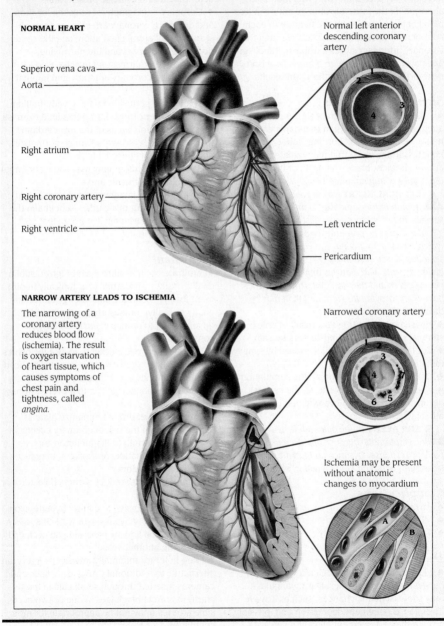

NORMAL HEART

Normal left anterior descending coronary artery

Superior vena cava

Aorta

Right atrium

Right coronary artery

Right ventricle

Left ventricle

Pericardium

NARROW ARTERY LEADS TO ISCHEMIA

The narrowing of a coronary artery reduces blood flow (ischemia). The result is oxygen starvation of heart tissue, which causes symptoms of chest pain and tightness, called *angina*.

Narrowed coronary artery

Ischemia may be present without anatomic changes to myocardium

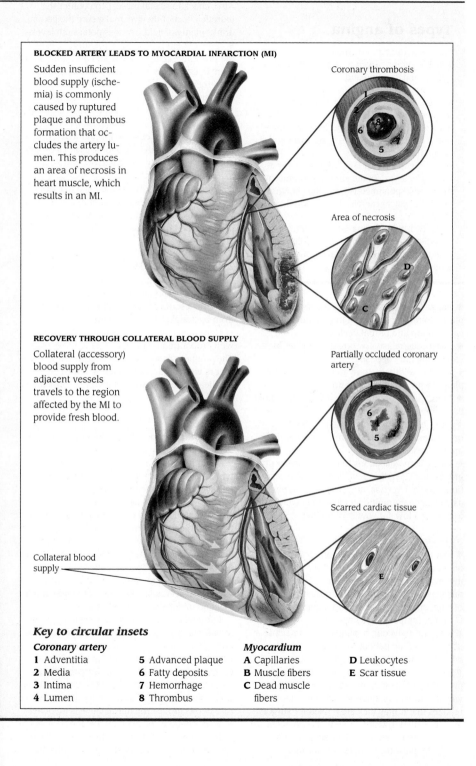

BLOCKED ARTERY LEADS TO MYOCARDIAL INFARCTION (MI)

Sudden insufficient blood supply (ischemia) is commonly caused by ruptured plaque and thrombus formation that occludes the artery lumen. This produces an area of necrosis in heart muscle, which results in an MI.

Coronary thrombosis

Area of necrosis

RECOVERY THROUGH COLLATERAL BLOOD SUPPLY

Collateral (accessory) blood supply from adjacent vessels travels to the region affected by the MI to provide fresh blood.

Partially occluded coronary artery

Scarred cardiac tissue

Collateral blood supply

Key to circular insets

Coronary artery

1 Adventitia	**5** Advanced plaque
2 Media	**6** Fatty deposits
3 Intima	**7** Hemorrhage
4 Lumen	**8** Thrombus

Myocardium

A Capillaries	**D** Leukocytes
B Muscle fibers	**E** Scar tissue
C Dead muscle fibers	

Types of angina

There are four types of angina:
◆ Stable angina—pain is predictable in frequency and duration and is relieved by rest and nitroglycerin.
◆ Unstable angina—pain increases in frequency and duration and is more easily induced; it indicates a worsening of coronary artery disease that may progress to a myocardial infarction.
◆ Prinzmetal's, or variant, angina—pain is caused by spasm of the coronary arteries; it may occur spontaneously and may be unrelated to physical exercise or emotional stress.
◆ Microvascular angina—impairment of vasodilator reserve causes angina-like chest pain in a person with normal coronary arteries.

◆ Percutaneous transluminal coronary angioplasty, to relieve occlusion in patients without calcification and partial occlusion
◆ Laser angioplasty to correct occlusion by vaporizing fatty deposits
◆ Rotational atherectomy to remove arterial plaque with a high-speed burr
◆ Stent placement in a reopened artery to hold the artery open
◆ Drug-eluting stent placement to hold a reopened artery open and to minimize the risk of in-stent restenosis
◆ Lifestyle modifications to reduce further progression of CAD; these include smoking cessation, regular exercise, and stress management, as well as maintaining an ideal body weight and following a low-fat, low-sodium diet.

Special considerations
◆ During anginal episodes, monitor the patient's blood pressure and heart rate. Take an ECG during anginal episodes and before administering nitroglycerin or other nitrates. Record duration of pain, amount of medication required to relieve it, and accompanying symptoms.
◆ Keep nitroglycerin available for immediate use. Instruct the patient to call immediately whenever he feels chest, arm, or neck pain.
◆ Before cardiac catheterization, explain the procedure to the patient. Make sure he knows why it's necessary, understands the risks, and realizes that it may indicate a need for surgery.
◆ After catheterization, review the expected course of treatment with the patient and his family. Monitor the catheter site for bleeding.

Also, check for distal pulses. To counter the diuretic effect of the dye, make sure the patient drinks plenty of fluids. Assess potassium levels.
◆ If the patient is scheduled for surgery, explain the procedure to the patient and his family. Give them a tour of the intensive care unit, and introduce them to the staff.
◆ After surgery, monitor blood pressure, intake and output, breath sounds, chest tube drainage, and ECG, watching for signs of ischemia and arrhythmias. Also, observe for and treat chest pain and possible dye reactions. Give vigorous chest physiotherapy and guide the patient in expelling secretions.
◆ Before discharge, stress the need to follow the prescribed drug regimen (antihypertensives, nitrates, and antilipemics, for example), exercise program, and diet. (See *Preventing coronary artery disease.*)

ENDOCARDITIS

Endocarditis (also known as *infective* or *bacterial endocarditis*) is an infection of the endocardium, heart valves, or cardiac prosthesis resulting from bacterial or fungal invasion.

Untreated endocarditis is usually fatal, but with proper treatment 70% of patients recover. The prognosis is worst when endocarditis causes severe valvular damage, leading to insufficiency and heart failure, or when it involves a prosthetic valve.

Causes
Most cases of endocarditis occur in patients who:
◆ are I.V. drug abusers
◆ have mitral valve prolapse (especially males with a systolic murmur)
◆ have prosthetic heart valves
◆ have rheumatic heart disease.

Other predisposing conditions include coarctation of the aorta; tetralogy of Fallot; subaortic and valvular aortic stenosis; ventricular septal defects; pulmonary stenosis; Marfan syndrome; degenerative heart disease, especially calcific aortic stenosis; and, rarely, a syphilitic aortic valve. However, some patients with endocarditis have no underlying heart disease.

Infecting organisms differ among these groups. In patients with native valve endocarditis who aren't I.V. drug abusers, causative organisms usually include (in order of frequency) streptococci, especially *Streptococcus viridans;* staphylococci; or enterococci. Although other bacteria occasionally cause the disorder, fungal causes are rare in this group. The mitral valve is involved most commonly, followed by the aortic valve.

In patients who are I.V. drug abusers, *Staphylococcus aureus* is the most common infecting

PREVENTION
Preventing coronary artery disease

Because coronary artery disease (CAD) is so widespread, prevention plays a crucial role. Follow these steps to help your patient reduce the risk of developing CAD:
◆ Encourage the patient to maintain a diet low in salt, saturated fats, and cholesterol.
◆ Explain the importance of regular exercise.
◆ Recommend that an overweight patient follow a low-calorie diet.
◆ Suggest enrolling in a smoking-cessation program to a patient who smokes.
◆ Teach the patient ways to reduce stress.
◆ Explain other ways to control risk factors, including taking antihypertensives to control hypertension, antilipemics to control elevated serum cholesterol or triglyceride levels, and aspirin or other antiplatelets drugs to minimize platelet aggregation and reduce the risk of developing blood clots.

Degenerative changes in endocarditis

This illustration shows typical growths on the endocardium produced by fibrin and platelet deposits on infection sites.

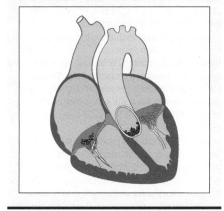

---

organism. Less commonly, streptococci, enterococci, gram-negative bacilli, or fungi cause the disorder. The tricuspid valve is involved most commonly, followed by the aortic and then the mitral valve.

In patients with prosthetic valve endocarditis, early cases (those that develop within 60 days of valve insertion) are usually caused by staphylococcal infection. However, gram-negative aerobic organisms, fungi, streptococci, enterococci, or diphtheroids may also cause the disorder. The course is usually fulminant and is associated with a high mortality rate. Late cases (occurring after 60 days) show signs and symptoms similar to native valve endocarditis.

Pathophysiology
In endocarditis, bacteremia — even transient bacteremia after dental or urogenital procedures — introduces the pathogen into the bloodstream. This infection causes fibrin and platelets to aggregate on the valve tissue and engulf circulating bacteria or fungi that flourish and form friable wartlike vegetative growths on the heart valves, the endocardial lining of a heart chamber, or the epithelium of a blood vessel. (See *Degenerative changes in endocarditis*.) Such growths may cover the valve surfaces, causing ulceration and necrosis; they may also extend to the chordae tendineae, leading to rupture and subsequent valvular insufficiency. Ultimately,

they may embolize to the spleen, kidneys, central nervous system, and lungs.

Signs and symptoms
Early clinical features of endocarditis are usually nonspecific and include:
◆ malaise
◆ weakness
◆ fatigue
◆ weight loss
◆ anorexia
◆ arthralgia
◆ night sweats
◆ chills
◆ valvular insufficiency
◆ an intermittent fever that may recur for weeks (in 90% of patients).

A more acute onset is associated with organisms of high pathogenicity, such as *S. aureus.* Endocarditis commonly causes a loud, regurgitant murmur typical of the underlying heart lesion from the vegetative growths on the valves. A suddenly changing murmur or the discovery of a new murmur in the presence of fever is a classic physical sign of endocarditis.

In about 30% of patients, embolization from growing lesions or diseased valvular tissue may produce:
◆ *splenic infarction* — pain in the left upper quadrant, radiating to the left shoulder, and abdominal rigidity
◆ *renal infarction* — hematuria, pyuria, flank pain, and decreased urine output

◆ *cerebral infarction* — hemiparesis, aphasia, or other neurologic deficits
◆ *pulmonary infarction* — (most common in right-sided endocarditis, which commonly occurs in I.V. drug abusers and after cardiac surgery) cough, pleuritic pain, pleural friction rub, dyspnea, and hemoptysis
◆ *peripheral vascular occlusion* — numbness and tingling in an arm, leg, finger, or toe or signs of impending peripheral gangrene.

Other signs may include splenomegaly; petechiae of the skin (especially common on the upper anterior trunk) and buccal, pharyngeal, or conjunctival mucosa caused by small emboli lodging in the small vessels; and splinter hemorrhages under the nails secondary to bleeding in the small vessels of the nail beds from lodging emboli.

Rarely, endocarditis produces Osler's nodes (tender, raised, subcutaneous lesions on the fingers or toes), Roth's spots (hemorrhagic areas with white centers on the retina from emboli in the nerve fiber layer of the eye), and Janeway lesions (purplish macules on the palms or soles from emboli).

Complications
◆ Heart failure
◆ Death
◆ Aortic root abscesses
◆ Myocardial abscesses
◆ Pericarditis
◆ Cardiac arrhythmia
◆ Meningitis
◆ Cerebral emboli
◆ Brain abscesses
◆ Septic pulmonary infarcts
◆ Arthritis
◆ Glomerulonephritis
◆ Acute renal failure

Diagnosis
Three or more blood cultures in a 24- to 48-hour period (each from a separate venipuncture) identify the causative organism in up to 90% of patients. Blood cultures should be drawn from three different sites, with 1 hour between each venipuncture.

The remaining 10% of patients may have negative blood cultures, possibly suggesting fungal infection or infections that are difficult to diagnose, such as *Haemophilus parainfluenzae*.

Other abnormal but nonspecific laboratory test results include:
◆ normal or elevated white blood cell count
◆ abnormal histiocytes (macrophages)
◆ elevated erythrocyte sedimentation rate

◆ normocytic, normochromic anemia (in 70% to 90% of patients)
◆ proteinuria and microscopic hematuria (in about 50% of patients)
◆ positive serum rheumatoid factor (in about one-half of all patients after endocarditis is present for 3 to 6 weeks)
◆ valvular damage, identified by echocardiography (ECG), particularly transesophageal
◆ atrial fibrillation and other arrhythmias that accompany valvular disease, identified by ECG.

Treatment
The goal of treatment is to eradicate the infecting organism. First-line therapy is usually a combination of penicillin and an aminoglycoside, usually gentamicin. Antimicrobial therapy should start promptly and continue over 4 to 6 weeks. Selection of an antibiotic is based on identification of the infecting organism and on sensitivity studies. While awaiting results — or if blood cultures are negative — empiric antimicrobial therapy is based on the likely infecting organism.

Supportive treatment includes bed rest, aspirin for fever and aches, and sufficient fluid intake. Severe valvular damage, especially aortic or mitral insufficiency, may require corrective surgery if refractory heart failure develops or if an infected prosthetic valve must be replaced.

Special considerations
◆ Before giving an antibiotic, obtain a patient history of allergies. Administer the antibiotic on time to maintain consistent blood antibiotic levels.
◆ Observe the venipuncture site for signs of infiltration or inflammation, possible complications of long-term I.V. drug administration. To reduce the risk of these complications, rotate venous access sites.
◆ Watch for signs of embolization (hematuria, pleuritic chest pain, left upper quadrant pain, or paresis), a common occurrence during the first 3 months of treatment. Tell the patient to watch for and report these signs, which may indicate impending peripheral vascular occlusion or splenic, renal, cerebral, or pulmonary infarction.
◆ Monitor the patient's renal status (blood urea nitrogen levels, creatinine clearance, and urine output) to check for signs of renal emboli or evidence of drug toxicity.
◆ Observe the patient for signs of heart failure, such as dyspnea, tachypnea, tachycardia, crackles, neck vein distention, edema, and weight gain.
◆ Teach the patient about antibiotic prophylaxis against endocarditis.

◆ Provide reassurance by teaching the patient and his family about this disease and the need for prolonged treatment. Tell them to watch closely for fever, anorexia, and other signs and symptoms of relapse about 2 weeks after treatment stops. Suggest quiet diversionary activities to prevent excessive physical exertion.
◆ If the patient is susceptible to endocarditis, make sure that he understands the need for prophylactic a antibiotic before, during, and after dental work, childbirth, and genitourinary, GI, or gynecologic procedures.
◆ Teach the patient how to recognize symptoms of endocarditis, and tell him to notify the physician immediately if such symptoms occur. (See *Preventing endocarditis.*)

||| LIFE-THREATENING DISORDER

HEART FAILURE

A syndrome rather than a disease, heart failure occurs when the heart can't pump enough blood to meet the body's metabolic needs. Heart failure results in intravascular and interstitial volume overload and poor tissue perfusion. An individual with heart failure experiences reduced exercise tolerance, a reduced quality of life, and a shortened life span.

Although the most common cause of heart failure is coronary artery disease, it also occurs in infants, children, and adults with congenital and acquired heart defects. The incidence of heart failure increases with age. Mortality from heart failure is greater for males, blacks, and elderly people.

Although advances in diagnostic and therapeutic techniques have greatly improved the outlook for patients with heart failure, the prognosis still depends on the underlying cause and its response to treatment.

Causes
Causes of heart failure may be divided into four general categories. (See *Causes of heart failure,* page 170.)

Pathophysiology
Heart failure may be classified according to the side of the heart affected (left- or right-sided heart failure) or by the cardiac cycle involved (systolic or diastolic dysfunction).

Left-sided heart failure
Left-sided heart failure occurs as a result of ineffective left ventricular contractile function. As the pumping ability of the left ventricle fails, cardiac output falls. Blood is no longer effectively

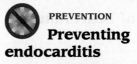

pumped out into the body; it backs up into the left atrium and then into the lungs, causing pulmonary congestion, dyspnea, and activity intolerance. If the condition persists, pulmonary edema and right-sided heart failure may result. Common causes include left ventricular infarction, hypertension, and aortic and mitral valve stenosis.

Right-sided heart failure
Right-sided heart failure results from ineffective right ventricular contractile function. Consequently, blood isn't pumped effectively through the right ventricle to the lungs, causing blood to back up into the right atrium and the peripheral circulation. The patient gains weight and develops peripheral edema and engorgement of the kidney and other organs. It may result from an acute right ventricular infarction, pulmonary hypertension, or a pulmonary embolus. However, the most common cause is profound backward blood flow due to left-sided heart failure.

Systolic dysfunction
Systolic dysfunction occurs when the left ventricle can't pump enough blood out to the systemic circulation during systole and the ejection fraction falls. Consequently, blood backs up into the pulmonary circulation and pressure increases in the pulmonary venous system. Cardiac output falls; weakness, fatigue, and shortness of breath may occur. Causes of systolic dysfunction include a myocardial infarction and dilated cardiomyopathy.

Causes of heart failure

Cause	Examples
Abnormal cardiac muscle function	♦ Cardiomyopathy ♦ Myocardial infarction

Abnormal left ventricular filling	♦ Atrial fibrillation
	♦ Atrial myxoma
	♦ Constrictive pericarditis
	♦ Impaired ventricular relaxation:
	  – Hypertension
	  – Myocardial hibernation
	  – Myocardial stunning
	♦ Mitral valve stenosis
	♦ Tricuspid valve stenosis

Abnormal left ventricular pressure	♦ Aortic or pulmonic valve stenosis ♦ Chronic obstructive pulmonary disease ♦ Hypertension ♦ Pulmonary hypertension

Abnormal left ventricular volume	♦ High-output states:
	  – Arteriovenous fistula
	  – Beriberi
	  – Chronic anemia
	  – Infusion of a large volume of I.V. fluids in a short period
	  – Pregnancy
	  – Septicemia
	  – Thyrotoxicosis
	♦ Valvular insufficiency

Diastolic dysfunction

Diastolic dysfunction occurs when the ability of the left ventricle to relax and fill during diastole is reduced and the stroke volume falls. Therefore, higher volumes are needed in the ventricles to maintain cardiac output. Consequently, pulmonary congestion and peripheral edema develop. Diastolic dysfunction may occur as a result of left ventricular hypertrophy, hypertension, or restrictive cardiomyopathy. This type of heart failure is less common than systolic dysfunction, and its treatment isn't as clear.

All causes of heart failure eventually lead to reduced cardiac output, which triggers compensatory mechanisms, such as increased sympathetic activity, activation of the renin-angiotensin-aldosterone system, ventricular dilation, and hypertrophy. These mechanisms improve cardiac output at the expense of increased ventricular work.

Increased sympathetic activity—a response to decreased cardiac output and blood pressure—enhances peripheral vascular resistance, contractility, heart rate, and venous return. Signs of increased sympathetic activity, such as cool extremities and clamminess, may indicate impending heart failure.

Increased sympathetic activity also restricts blood flow to the kidneys, causing them to secrete rennin, which in turn converts angiotensinogen to angiotensin I, which then becomes angiotensin II—a potent vasoconstrictor. Angiotensin causes the adrenal cortex to release aldosterone, leading to sodium and water retention and an increase in circulating blood volume. This renal mechanism is initially helpful; however, if it persists unchecked, it can aggravate heart failure as the heart struggles to pump against the increased volume.

In ventricular dilation, an increase in end-diastolic ventricular volume (preload) causes increased stroke work and stroke volume during contraction, stretching cardiac muscle fibers so that the ventricle can accept the increased intravascular volume. Eventually, the muscle becomes stretched beyond optimum limits and contractility declines.

In ventricular hypertrophy, an increase in ventricular muscle mass allows the heart to pump against increased resistance to the outflow of blood, improving cardiac output. However, this increased muscle mass also increases myocardial oxygen requirements. An increase in the ventricular diastolic pressure necessary to fill the enlarged ventricle may compromise diastolic coronary blood flow, limiting the oxygen supply to the ventricle, and causing ischemia and impaired muscle contractility.

In heart failure, counterregulatory substances —prostaglandins and atrial natriuretic factor— are produced in an attempt to reduce the negative effects of volume overload and vasoconstriction caused by the compensatory mechanisms.

The kidneys release the prostaglandins, prostacyclin and prostaglandin E_2, which are potent vasodilators. These vasodilators also act to reduce volume overload produced by the renin-angiotensin-aldosterone system by inhibiting sodium and water reabsorption by the kidneys.

Atrial natriuretic factor is a hormone secreted mainly by the atria in response to stimulation of the stretch receptors in the atria caused by excess fluid volume. B-type natriuretic factor is secreted by the ventricles because of fluid volume overload. These natriuretic factors work to counteract the negative effects of sympathetic nervous system stimulation and the renin-angiotensin-aldosterone system by producing vasodilation and diuresis. (See *How heart failure affects the body,* page 172.)

Signs and symptoms
Left-sided heart failure (early stages)
◆ Dyspnea caused by pulmonary congestion
◆ Orthopnea as blood is redistributed from the legs to the central circulation when the patient lies down at night
◆ Paroxysmal nocturnal dyspnea due to the reabsorption of interstitial fluid when lying down and reduced sympathetic stimulation while sleeping
◆ Fatigue associated with reduced oxygenation and an inability to increase cardiac output in response to physical activity
◆ Nonproductive cough associated with pulmonary congestion

Left-sided heart failure (late stages)
◆ Crackles due to pulmonary congestion
◆ Hemoptysis resulting from bleeding veins in the bronchial system caused by venous distention
◆ Point of maximal impulse displaced toward the left anterior axillary line caused by left ventricular hypertrophy
◆ Tachycardia due to sympathetic stimulation
◆ S_3 caused by rapid ventricular filling

◆ S_4 resulting from atrial contraction against a noncompliant ventricle
◆ Cool, pale skin resulting from peripheral vasoconstriction
◆ Restlessness and confusion due to reduced cardiac output

Right-sided heart failure
◆ Elevated jugular vein distention due to venous congestion
◆ Positive hepatojugular reflux and hepatomegaly secondary to venous congestion
◆ Right upper quadrant pain caused by liver engorgement
◆ Anorexia, fullness, and nausea, which may be due to congestion of the liver and intestines
◆ Nocturia as fluid is redistributed at night and reabsorbed
◆ Weight gain due to sodium and water retention
◆ Edema associated with fluid volume excess
◆ Ascites or anasarca caused by fluid retention

Complications
Acute
◆ Pulmonary edema
◆ Acute renal failure
◆ Arrhythmias

Chronic
◆ Activity intolerance
◆ Renal impairment
◆ Cardiac cachexia
◆ Metabolic impairment
◆ Thromboembolism

Diagnosis
◆ Chest X-rays show increased pulmonary vascular markings, interstitial edema, or pleural effusion and cardiomegaly.
◆ Electrocardiography may indicate hypertrophy, ischemic changes, or infarction and may also reveal tachycardia and extrasystoles.
◆ Laboratory testing may reveal abnormal liver function test results and elevated blood urea nitrogen (BUN) and creatinine levels. Prothrombin time may be prolonged as congestion impairs the liver's ability to synthesize procoagulants.
◆ Brain natriuretic peptide (BNP) assay, a blood test, may show elevated levels. Along with such clinical signs as edematous ankles, elevated BNP levels strongly indicate heart failure.
◆ Echocardiography may reveal left ventricular hypertrophy, dilation, and abnormal contractility.
◆ Pulmonary artery monitoring typically demonstrates elevated pulmonary artery and pulmonary artery wedge pressures, left ventricular end-diastolic pressure in left-sided heart

MULTISYSTEM DISORDER
How heart failure affects the body

This summary highlights how heart failure affects the major body systems and the multidisciplinary care required.

Cardiovascular system
♦ In left-sided heart failure, the pumping ability of the left ventricle fails and cardiac output falls. Blood backs up into the right atrium.
♦ In right-sided heart failure, the right ventricle becomes stressed and hypertrophies, leading to increased conduction time and arrhythmias.

Respiratory system
♦ As blood backs up into the left atrium (because the heart's pumping ability has failed), blood backs into the lungs, causing pulmonary congestion.

GI system
♦ Congestion of the peripheral tissues leads to GI tract congestion and anorexia, GI distress, and weight loss.

♦ Liver failure can occur as a result of blood backing up into the peripheral circulation and subsequent engorgement of organs.

Renal system
♦ With right-sided heart failure, blood backs up into the right atrium and the peripheral circulation. The patient gains weight and develops peripheral edema and engorgement of the kidney and other organs.

Collaborative management
Multidisciplinary care is needed to determine the underlying cause and precipitating factors of heart failure, and may include the expertise of a respiratory therapist, dietitian, and physical therapist. Surgery may be indicated if the patient has coronary artery disease or is experiencing severe limitations or recurrent hospitalizations despite maximal medical treatment. Social services may be necessary to help the patient's transition to his home setting after the acute situation is resolved.

---

failure, and elevated right atrial pressure or central venous pressure in right-sided heart failure.
♦ Radionuclide ventriculography may reveal an ejection fraction less than 40%; in diastolic dysfunction, the ejection fraction may be normal.

Treatment
♦ Treatment of the underlying cause, if known
♦ An angiotensin-converting enzyme (ACE) inhibitor for left ventricle dysfunction to reduce production of angiotensin II, resulting in preload and afterload reduction

AGE ALERT *An elderly patient may require lower doses of an ACE inhibitor because of impaired renal clearance. Monitor him for severe hypotension, signifying a toxic effect.*

♦ Digoxin for heart failure due to left ventricular systolic dysfunction, to increase myocardial contractility, improve cardiac output, reduce the volume of the ventricle, and decrease ventricular stretch
♦ Diuretics to reduce fluid volume overload and venous return
♦ Beta-adrenergic blockers for New York Heart Association (NYHA) class II or III heart failure caused by left ventricular systolic dysfunction, to prevent remodeling (See *Classifying heart failure,* page 160.)

♦ Inotropic therapy with dobutamine or milrinone for acute treatment of heart failure exacerbation
♦ Long-term or long-term intermittent inotropic therapy to augment ventricular contractility to avoid exacerbations of heart failure in the patient with NYHA class IV heart failure
♦ Nesiritide, a human B-type natriuretic peptide, to augment diuresis and to decrease afterload in short-term management of heart failure exacerbation
♦ Diuretics, nitrates, morphine, and oxygen to treat pulmonary edema
♦ Lifestyle modifications (to reduce symptoms of heart failure), such as weight loss (if obese), limited sodium (3 g/day) and alcohol intake, reduced fat intake, smoking cessation, stress reduction, and development of an exercise program (Heart failure is no longer a contraindication to exercise and cardiac rehabilitation.)
♦ Biventricular pacemaker to control ventricular dyssynchrony
♦ Coronary artery bypass surgery or angioplasty for heart failure due to CAD
♦ Valve surgery to reshape and support the mitral valve and improve cardiac functioning
♦ Left ventricular remodeling surgery to return the ventricle to a more normal shape and allow the heart to pump blood more efficiently

◆ Left ventricular assist device, also known as the "bridge to transplantation," to improve the pumping ability of the heart until transplantation can be performed

◆ Heart transplantation in the patient receiving aggressive medical treatment, but still experiencing limitations or repeated hospitalizations

AGE ALERT *In children, heart failure occurs mainly as a result of congenital heart defects. Therefore, treatment guidelines are directed toward the specific cause.*

Special considerations
During acute phase
◆ Place the patient in Fowler's position and give him supplemental oxygen to help him breathe more easily.

◆ Weigh the patient daily, and check for peripheral edema. Carefully monitor I.V. intake and urine output, vital signs, and mental status. Auscultate the heart for abnormal sounds (S_3 gallop) and the lungs for crackles or rhonchi. Report changes at once.

◆ Frequently monitor BUN, creatinine, and serum potassium, sodium, chloride, and magnesium levels.

◆ Make sure the patient has continuous cardiac monitoring during acute and advanced stages so that arrhythmias can promptly be identified and treated.

◆ To prevent deep vein thrombosis due to vascular congestion, assist the patient with range-of-motion exercises. Enforce bed rest, and apply antiembolism stockings. Check the patient regularly for calf pain and tenderness.

◆ Allow adequate rest periods.

Preparing for discharge
◆ Advise the patient to avoid foods high in sodium, such as canned or commercially prepared foods and dairy products, to curb fluid overload.

◆ Encourage the patient to participate in an outpatient cardiac rehabilitation program.

◆ Explain to the patient that the potassium he loses through diuretic therapy may need to be replaced by taking a prescribed potassium supplement and eating high-potassium foods, such as bananas and apricots.

◆ Stress the need for regular checkups.

◆ Stress the importance of taking digoxin exactly as prescribed. Tell the patient to watch for and immediately report signs and symptoms of toxicity, such as anorexia, vomiting, and yellow vision.

◆ Tell the patient to notify the physician promptly if his pulse is unusually irregular or measures less than 60 beats/minute; if he experiences dizziness, blurred vision, shortness of breath, a persistent dry cough, palpitations, increased fatigue, paroxysmal nocturnal dyspnea, swollen ankles, or decreased urine output; or if he notices rapid weight gain (3 to 5 lb [1.4 to 2.3 kg] in 1 week).

HYPERTENSION
Hypertension, an elevation in diastolic or systolic blood pressure, occurs as two major types: essential (primary) hypertension, which is the most common form; and secondary hypertension, which results from renal disease or another identifiable cause. Malignant hypertension is a severe, fulminant form of hypertension common to both types. Hypertension is a major cause of stroke, cardiac disease, and renal failure.

Hypertension affects about 25% of adults in the United States. The risk of hypertension increases with age and is higher for blacks than for whites and in those with less education and lower income. Males have a higher incidence of hypertension in young and early middle adulthood; thereafter, females have a higher incidence.

Essential hypertension usually begins insidiously as a benign disease, slowly progressing to a malignant state. If untreated, even mild cases can cause major complications and death. Carefully managed treatment, which may include lifestyle modifications and drug therapy, improves the prognosis. Untreated, it carries a high mortality rate. Severely elevated blood pressure (hypertensive crisis) may be fatal.

Causes
Primary hypertension
◆ Advancing age
◆ Diabetes mellitus
◆ Excessive alcohol consumption
◆ Excess renin

AGE ALERT *Elderly people may have isolated systolic hypertension (ISH), in which just the systolic blood pressure is elevated, as atherosclerosis causes a loss of elasticity in large arteries. Previously, it was believed that ISH was a normal part of the aging process and shouldn't be treated. Results of the Systolic Hypertension in the Elderly Program, however, found that treating ISH with an antihypertensive lowered the incidence of stroke, coronary artery disease (CAD), and left-sided heart failure.*

◆ Family history
◆ High saturated fat intake
◆ High sodium intake
◆ Mineral deficiencies (calcium, potassium, and magnesium)
◆ Obesity
◆ Race (most common in Blacks)

⚠️ **CLINICAL ALERT** *Blacks are at an increased risk for primary hypertension when predisposition to low plasma renin levels diminishes the ability to excrete excess sodium. Hypertension develops at an earlier age and is more severe than in Whites.*
- Sedentary lifestyle
- Sleep apnea
- Stress
- Tobacco use

Secondary hypertension
- Brain tumor, quadriplegia, and head injury
- Coarctation of the aorta
- Excessive alcohol consumption
- Hormonal contraceptives, cocaine, epoetin alfa, sympathetic stimulants, monoamine oxidase inhibitors taken with tyramine, estrogen replacement therapy, and nonsteroidal anti-inflammatory drugs
- Pheochromocytoma, Cushing's syndrome, hyperaldosteronism, and thyroid, pituitary, or parathyroid dysfunction
- Pregnancy-induced hypertension
- Renal artery stenosis and parenchymal disease

Pathophysiology
Arterial blood pressure is a product of total peripheral resistance and cardiac output. Cardiac output is increased by conditions that increase heart rate, stroke volume, or both. Peripheral resistance is increased by factors that increase blood viscosity or reduce the lumen size of vessels, especially the arterioles.

Several theories help to explain the development of hypertension, including:
- changes in the arteriolar bed, causing increased peripheral vascular resistance
- abnormally increased tone in the sympathetic nervous system that originates in the vasomotor system centers, causing increased peripheral vascular resistance
- increased blood volume resulting from renal or hormonal dysfunction
- an increase in arteriolar thickening caused by genetic factors, leading to increased peripheral vascular resistance
- abnormal renin release, resulting in the formation of angiotensin II, which constricts the arteriole and increases blood volume. (See *Understanding blood pressure regulation*.)

Prolonged hypertension increases the heart's workload as resistance to left ventricular ejection increases. To increase contractile force, the left ventricle hypertrophies, raising the heart's oxygen demands and workload. Cardiac dilation and failure may occur when hypertrophy can no longer maintain sufficient cardiac output. Because hypertension promotes coronary atherosclerosis, the heart may be further compromised by reduced blood flow to the myocardium, resulting in angina or myocardial infarction (MI). Hypertension also causes vascular damage, leading to accelerated atherosclerosis and target organ damage, such as retinal injury, renal failure, stroke, and aortic aneurysm and dissection. (See *Blood vessel damage in hypertension*.)

The pathophysiology of secondary hypertension is related to the underlying disease. For example:
- The most common cause of secondary hypertension is chronic renal disease. Insult to the kidney from chronic glomerulonephritis or renal artery stenosis interferes with sodium excretion, the renin-angiotensin-aldosterone system, or renal perfusion, causing blood pressure to increase.
- In Cushing's syndrome, increased cortisol levels raise blood pressure by increasing renal sodium retention, angiotensin II levels, and vascular response to norepinephrine.
- In primary aldosteronism, increased intravascular volume, altered sodium concentrations in vessel walls, or high aldosterone levels cause vasoconstriction and increased resistance.
- Pheochromocytoma is a chromaffin cell tumor of the adrenal medulla that secretes epinephrine and norepinephrine. Epinephrine increases cardiac contractility and rate, whereas norepinephrine increases peripheral vascular resistance.

Signs and symptoms
Although hypertension is typically asymptomatic, these signs and symptoms may occur:
- elevated blood pressure readings on at least two consecutive occasions after initial screening, caused by pathophysiologic changes in blood vessels

📊 **AGE ALERT** *Because many older adults have a wide auscultatory gap—the hiatus between the first Korotkoff sound and the next sound—failure to pump the blood pressure cuff up high enough can lead to missing the first beat and underestimating systolic blood pressure. To avoid missing the first Korotkoff sound, palpate the radial artery and inflate the cuff to a point about 20 mm beyond which the pulse beat disappears.*
- occipital headache (may worsen on rising in the morning as a result of increased intracranial pressure) resulting from vascular changes; nausea and vomiting may also occur
- epistaxis possibly due to vascular involvement
- bruits (which may be heard over the abdominal aorta or carotid, renal, and femoral arteries) caused by stenosis or aneurysm

Understanding blood pressure regulation

Hypertension may result from a disturbance in one of these intrinsic mechanisms.

Renin-angiotensin-aldosterone system

The renin-angiotensin-aldosterone system acts to increase blood pressure through these mechanisms:
♦ sodium depletion, reduced blood pressure, and dehydration stimulate renin release
♦ renin reacts with angiotensin, a liver enzyme, and converts it to angiotensin I, which increases preload and afterload
♦ angiotensin I converts to angiotensin II in the lungs; angiotensin II is a potent vasoconstrictor that targets the arterioles
♦ angiotensin II works to increase preload and afterload by stimulating the adrenal cortex to secrete aldosterone; this increases blood volume by conserving sodium and water.

Autoregulation

Several intrinsic mechanisms work to change an artery's diameter to maintain tissue and organ perfusion despite fluctuations in systemic blood pressure. These mechanisms include stress relaxation and capillary fluid shifts:
♦ in stress relaxation, blood vessels gradually dilate when blood pressure increases to reduce peripheral resistance

♦ in capillary fluid shift, plasma moves between vessels and extravascular spaces to maintain intravascular volume.

Sympathetic nervous system

When blood pressure drops, baroreceptors in the aortic arch and carotid sinuses decrease their inhibition of the medulla's vasomotor center. The consequent increases in sympathetic stimulation of the heart by norepinephrine increases cardiac output by strengthening the contractile force, raising the heart rate, and augmenting peripheral resistance by vasoconstriction. Stress can also stimulate the sympathetic nervous system to increase cardiac output and peripheral vascular resistance.

Antidiuretic hormone

The release of antidiuretic hormone can regulate hypotension by increasing reabsorption of water by the kidney. With reabsorption, blood plasma volume increases, thus raising blood pressure.

Blood vessel damage in hypertension

Sustained hypertension damages blood vessels. Vascular injury begins with alternating areas of dilation and constriction in the arterioles. The illustrations below show how damage occurs.

Increased intra-arterial pressure damages the endothelium. Angiotensin induces endothelial wall contraction, allowing plasma to leak through interendothelial spaces. Plasma constituents deposited in the vessel wall cause medial necrosis.

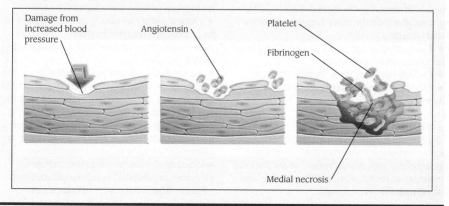

Damage from increased blood pressure

Angiotensin

Platelet

Fibrinogen

Medial necrosis

♦ dizziness, confusion, and fatigue caused by decreased tissue perfusion due to vasoconstriction of blood vessels
♦ blurry vision as a result of retinal damage
♦ nocturia caused by an increase in blood flow to the kidneys and an increase in glomerular filtration
♦ edema caused by increased capillary pressure.
   If secondary hypertension exists, other signs and symptoms may be related to the cause. For example, Cushing's syndrome may cause truncal obesity and purple striae, whereas patients with pheochromocytoma may develop headache, nausea, vomiting, palpitations, pallor, and profuse perspiration.

Complications
♦ Hypertensive crisis, peripheral arterial disease, dissecting aortic aneurysm, CAD, angina, MI, heart failure, arrhythmias, and sudden death (See *What happens in hypertensive crisis.*)
♦ Transient ischemic attacks, stroke, retinopathy, and hypertensive encephalopathy
♦ Renal failure

Diagnosis
♦ Serial blood pressure measurements may be useful. (See *Classifying blood pressure readings*, page 178.)
♦ Urinalysis may show protein, casts, red blood cells, or white blood cells, suggesting renal disease; presence of catecholamines associated with pheochromocytoma; or glucose, suggesting diabetes.
♦ Laboratory test results may reveal elevated blood urea nitrogen and serum creatinine levels (suggestive of renal disease) or hypokalemia (indicating adrenal dysfunction, or primary hyperaldosteronism).
♦ Complete blood count may reveal other causes of hypertension, such as polycythemia or anemia.
♦ Excretory urography may reveal renal atrophy, indicating chronic renal disease. One kidney smaller than the other suggests unilateral renal disease.
♦ Electrocardiography may show left ventricular hypertrophy or ischemia.
♦ Chest X-rays may show cardiomegaly.
♦ Echocardiography may reveal left ventricular hypertrophy.

Treatment
The Seventh Report of the Joint National Committee on Prevention, Detection, Evaluation, and Treatment of High Blood Pressure of the National Institutes of Health, National Heart, Lung, and Blood Institute recommends:

♦ Lifestyle modification including weight reduction, use of a Dietary Approaches to Stop Hypertension diet (involves an increased intake of fruits, vegetables, and low-fat dairy products and a decreased intake of saturated and total fat), reduction of dietary sodium intake, physical activity (regular aerobic activity, such as brisk walking), and moderation of alcohol intake.
♦ If the patient fails to achieve the desired blood pressure or make significant progress, continue lifestyle modifications and begin drug therapy.
♦ For stage 1 hypertension in the absence of compelling indications (heart failure, post–MI, high coronary disease risk, diabetes, chronic kidney disease, or recurrent stroke), give most patients a thiazide-type diuretic. Consider using an angiotensin-converting enzyme (ACE) inhibitor, an angiotensin receptor blocker, a beta-adrenergic blocker, a calcium channel blocker, or a combination.
♦ For stage 2 hypertension in the absence of compelling indications, give most patients a two-drug combination (usually a thiazide-type diuretic and an ACE inhibitor, an angiotensin receptor blocker, a beta-adrenergic blocker, or a calcium channel blocker).
♦ If the patient has one or more compelling indications, base drug treatment on benefits from outcome studies or existing clinical guidelines. Treatment may include the following, depending on indication:
♦ Heart failure—a diuretic, a beta-adrenergic blocker, an ACE inhibitor, an angiotensin receptor blocker, or an aldosterone antagonist
♦ Post–myocardial infarction—a beta-adrenergic blocker, an ACE inhibitor, or an aldosterone antagonist
♦ High coronary disease risk—a diuretic, a beta-adrenergic blocker, an ACE inhibitor, or a calcium channel blocker
♦ Diabetes—a diuretic, a beta-adrenergic blocker, an ACE inhibitor, an angiotensin receptor blocker, or a calcium channel blocker
♦ Chronic kidney disease—an ACE inhibitor or an angiotensin receptor blocker
♦ Recurrent stroke prevention—a diuretic or an ACE inhibitor.
♦ As needed—another antihypertensive.
   Treatment of secondary hypertension focuses on correcting the underlying cause and controlling hypertensive effects.
   Typically, hypertensive emergencies require parenteral administration of a vasodilator or an adrenergic inhibitor or oral administration of a selected drug, such as nifedipine, captopril, clonidine, or labetalol, to rapidly reduce blood pressure. The initial goal is to reduce mean

CLOSER LOOK
What happens in hypertensive crisis

Hypertensive crisis is a severe increase in arterial blood pressure caused by a disturbance in one or more of the regulating mechanisms. If untreated, hypertensive crisis may result in renal, cardiac, or cerebral complications and, possibly, death.

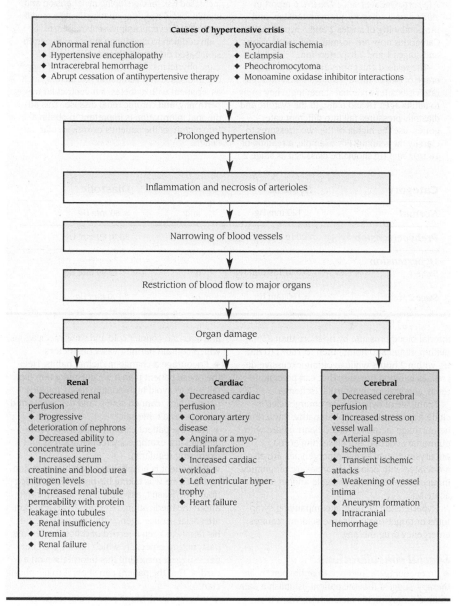

Causes of hypertensive crisis

- Abnormal renal function
- Hypertensive encephalopathy
- Intracerebral hemorrhage
- Abrupt cessation of antihypertensive therapy
- Myocardial ischemia
- Eclampsia
- Pheochromocytoma
- Monoamine oxidase inhibitor interactions

Prolonged hypertension

Inflammation and necrosis of arterioles

Narrowing of blood vessels

Restriction of blood flow to major organs

Organ damage

Renal	Cardiac	Cerebral
◆ Decreased renal perfusion	◆ Decreased cardiac perfusion	◆ Decreased cerebral perfusion
◆ Progressive deterioration of nephrons	◆ Coronary artery disease	◆ Increased stress on vessel wall
◆ Decreased ability to concentrate urine	◆ Angina or a myocardial infarction	◆ Arterial spasm
◆ Increased serum creatinine and blood urea nitrogen levels	◆ Increased cardiac workload	◆ Ischemia
◆ Increased renal tubule permeability with protein leakage into tubules	◆ Left ventricular hypertrophy	◆ Transient ischemic attacks
◆ Renal insufficiency	◆ Heart failure	◆ Weakening of vessel intima
◆ Uremia		◆ Aneurysm formation
◆ Renal failure		◆ Intracranial hemorrhage

Classifying blood pressure readings

In 2003, the National Institutes of Health issued *The Seventh Report of the Joint National Committee on Prevention, Detection, Evaluation, and Treatment of High Blood Pressure (The JNC 7 Report)*. Updates since *The JNC 6* report include a new category, prehypertension, and the combining of stages 2 and 3 hypertension. Categories now are normal, prehypertension, and stages 1 and 2 hypertension.

The revised categories are based on the average of two or more readings taken on separate visits after an initial screening. They apply to adults ages 18 and older. (If the systolic and diastolic pressures fall into different categories, use the higher of the two pressures to classify the reading. For example, a reading of 160/92 mm Hg should be classified as stage 2.)

Normal blood pressure with respect to cardiovascular risk is a systolic reading below 120 mm Hg and a diastolic reading below 80 mm Hg. Patients with prehypertension are at increased risk for developing hypertension and should follow health-promoting lifestyle modifications to prevent cardiovascular disease.

In addition to classifying stages of hypertension based on average blood pressure readings, physicians should also take note of target organ disease and additional risk factors, such as a patient with diabetes, left ventricular hypertrophy, and chronic renal disease. This additional information is important to obtain a true picture of the patient's cardiovascular health.

Category	Systolic		Diastolic
Normal	< 120 mm Hg	and	≤ 80 mm Hg
Prehypertension	120 to 139 mm Hg	or	80 to 89 mm Hg
Hypertension *Stage 1*	140 to 159 mm Hg	or	90 to 99 mm Hg
Stage 2	≥ 160 mm Hg	or	≥100 mm Hg

arterial blood pressure by no more than 25% (within minutes to hours) then to 160/110 mm Hg within 2 hours while avoiding excessive decreases in blood pressure that can precipitate renal, cerebral, or myocardial ischemia.

Examples of hypertensive emergencies include hypertensive encephalopathy, intracranial hemorrhage, acute left-sided heart failure with pulmonary edema, and dissecting aortic aneurysm. Hypertensive emergencies are also associated with eclampsia or severe pregnancy-induced hypertension, unstable angina, and an acute MI.

Hypertension without accompanying symptoms or target-organ disease seldom requires emergency drug therapy.

Special considerations

◆ To encourage adherence to antihypertensive therapy, suggest that the patient establish a daily routine for taking his medication. Warn that uncontrolled hypertension may cause stroke and heart attack. Tell him to report adverse reactions. Also, advise him to avoid high-sodium antacids

and over-the-counter cold and sinus medications, which contain harmful vasoconstrictors.
◆ Encourage a change in dietary habits. Help the obese patient plan a weight-reduction diet; tell him to avoid high-sodium foods (pickles, potato chips, canned soups, and deli meats and cheeses) and table salt.
◆ Help the patient examine and modify his lifestyle (for example, by reducing stress and exercising regularly).
◆ If a patient is hospitalized with hypertension, find out if he was taking his prescribed medication. If he wasn't, ask why. If the patient can't afford the medication, refer him to an appropriate social service agency. Tell the patient and his family to keep a record of drugs used in the past, noting especially which ones were effective. Suggest recording this information on a card so that the patient can show it to his physician.
◆ When routine blood pressure screening reveals elevated pressure, make sure the cuff size is appropriate for the patient's upper arm circumference. Take the pressure in both arms in lying, sitting, and standing positions. Ask the

PREVENTION
Preventing hypertension

Certain risk factors for hypertension can't be changed, such as family history, race, and aging, but lifestyle modifications can help prevent hypertension. Based on American Heart Association recommendations, advise your patient to do the following:

Maintain a healthy weight
Maintain a normal weight or lose weight if overweight. Weight loss lowers blood pressure.

Reduce salt
Salt intake should be reduced to about 1.5 g per day. Reducing salt intake can lower blood pressure in individuals with and without hypertension.

Increase potassium
Patients should eat 8 to 10 servings of fruits and vegetables per day to increase potassium intake. Potassium reduces blood pressure in individuals with and without hypertension. Those with kidney disease or heart failure should contact their practitioner before increasing their potassium intake.

Limit alcohol intake
Studies have shown a correlation between alcohol intake and increased blood pressure, especially in individuals who drink more than 2 drinks per day.

Include exercise
Regular physical activity is defined by the American Heart Association as moderate to vigorous exercise for 30 to 60 minutes a day on most or all days of the week. A lack of physical activity can lead to obesity and increase the risk of hypertension, heart attack, and stroke.

Manage stress
Stress can lead to increased alcohol consumption, smoking, overeating, and other activities that increase the risk of heart attack or stroke. Daily relaxation for short periods during the workday and on weekends can also lower blood pressure.

Stop smoking
Smoking even filtered and light or ultra-light cigarettes can lead to atherosclerosis. Quitting or not starting is the only way to prevent this major risk factor for heart attack and stroke.

Follow the DASH diet
The dietary approaches to stopping hypertension (DASH) diet encourages vegetables, fruits, and low-fat dairy as well as whole grains, fish, poultry, and nuts. Discourage the eating of fats, red meat, sweets, and sugar-containing beverages. However, individuals with reduced kidney function should always consult their practitioners before starting this diet; it's rich in potassium, which isn't recommended for individuals with these disorders.

---

patient if he smoked, drank a beverage containing caffeine, or was emotionally upset before the test. Advise the patient to return for blood pressure testing at frequent, regular intervals.
♦ To help identify hypertension and prevent untreated hypertension, participate in public education programs dealing with hypertension and ways to reduce risk factors. Encourage public participation in blood pressure screening programs. Routinely screen all patients, especially those at risk (blacks and people with family histories of hypertension, stroke, or heart attack). (See *Preventing hypertension.*)

MYOCARDITIS
Myocarditis is focal or diffuse inflammation of the cardiac muscle (myocardium). It may be acute or chronic and can occur at any age. In many cases, myocarditis fails to produce specific cardiovascular symptoms or electrocardiogram (ECG) abnormalities, and recovery is usually spontaneous without residual defects. Occasionally, myocarditis is complicated by heart failure; in some cases, it leads to cardiomyopathy. Rarely, it can produce fulminant fatal heart failure due to diffuse myocarditis.

Causes

♦ Bacterial infections, such as diphtheria, tuberculosis, typhoid fever, tetanus, and staphylococcal, pneumococcal, and gonococcal infections
♦ Fungal infections, including candidiasis and aspergillosis
♦ Helminthic infections such as trichinosis
♦ Hypersensitive immune reactions, including acute rheumatic fever and postcardiotomy syndrome
♦ Parasitic infections, especially South American trypanosomiasis (Chagas' disease) in infants and immunosuppressed adults; also, toxoplasmosis
♦ Radiation therapy—large doses of radiation to the chest in treating lung or breast cancer
♦ Toxins, such as lead, chemicals, and cocaine, and alcoholism
♦ Viral infections (most common cause in the United States and western Europe), such as coxsackievirus A and B strains and, possibly, poliomyelitis, influenza, Epstein-Barr virus, human immunodeficiency virus, cytomegalovirus, measles, mumps, rubeola, rubella, and adenoviruses and echoviruses

Pathophysiology

Damage to the myocardium occurs when an infectious organism triggers an autoimmune, cellular, and humoral reaction. The resulting inflammation may lead to hypertrophy, fibrosis, and inflammatory changes of the myocardium and conduction system. The heart muscle weakens and contractility is reduced. The heart muscle becomes flabby and dilated and pinpoint hemorrhages may develop.

Signs and symptoms

♦ Nonspecific signs and symptoms, such as fatigue, dyspnea, palpitations, and fever caused by systemic infection
♦ Mild, continuous pressure or soreness in the chest (occasionally) related to inflammation
♦ Tachycardia due to a compensatory sympathetic response
♦ S_3 and S_4 gallops as a result of heart failure
♦ Murmur of mitral insufficiency may be heard if papillary muscles are involved
♦ Pericardial friction rub, if pericarditis exists
♦ If myofibril degeneration occurs, it may lead to right-sided and left-sided heart failure, with cardiomegaly, neck vein distention, dyspnea, edema, pulmonary congestion, persistent fever with resting or exertional tachycardia disproportionate to the degree of fever, and supraventricular and ventricular arrhythmias

Complications

♦ Recurrence of myocarditis
♦ Chronic valvulitis (when it results from rheumatic fever)
♦ Dilated cardiomyopathy
♦ Arrhythmias and sudden death
♦ Heart failure
♦ Pericarditis
♦ Ruptured myocardial aneurysm
♦ Thromboembolism

Diagnosis

History reveals recent febrile upper respiratory tract infection. These tests help confirm the diagnosis of myocarditis:
♦ Laboratory testing may reveal elevated levels of creatine kinase (CK), CK-MB, troponin I, troponin T, aspartate aminotransferase, and lactate dehydrogenase. Also, inflammation and infection can cause elevated white blood cell count and erythrocyte sedimentation rate.
♦ Antibody titers, such as antistreptolysin-O titer in rheumatic fever, may be elevated.
♦ ECG may reveal diffuse ST-segment and T-wave abnormalities, conduction defects (prolonged PR interval, bundle-branch block, or complete heart block), supraventricular arrhythmias, and ventricular extrasystoles.
♦ Chest X-rays may show an enlarged heart and pulmonary vascular congestion.
♦ Echocardiography may demonstrate some degree of left ventricular dysfunction.
♦ Radionuclide scanning may identify inflammatory and necrotic changes characteristic of myocarditis.
♦ Laboratory cultures of stool, throat, and other body fluids may identify bacterial or viral causes of infection.
♦ Endomyocardial biopsy may confirm the diagnosis. A negative biopsy doesn't exclude the diagnosis.

Treatment

♦ An antibiotic to treat bacterial infections
♦ An antipyretic to reduce fever and decrease stress on the heart
♦ Bed rest to reduce oxygen demands and the heart's workload
♦ Restricted activity to minimize myocardial oxygen consumption, supplemental oxygen therapy, sodium restriction and a diuretic to decrease fluid retention, an angiotensin-converting enzyme inhibitor, and digoxin to increase myocardial contractility for patients with heart failure (Administer digoxin cautiously because some patients may show a paradoxical sensitivity even to small doses.)
♦ An antiarrhythmic, such as quinidine or procainamide, to treat arrhythmias (Use antiarrhythmics cautiously because these drugs may

depress myocardial contractility. A temporary pacemaker may be inserted if complete atrioventricular block occurs.)
◆ Anticoagulation to prevent thromboembolism
◆ A corticosteroid and an immunosuppressant, although controversial, to combat life-threatening complications, such as intractable heart failure
◆ Nonsteroidal anti-inflammatory drugs contraindicated during the acute phase (first 2 weeks) because they increase myocardial damage
◆ Cardiac assist devices or transplantation as a last resort in severe cases that resist treatment

Special considerations
◆ Assess the patient's cardiovascular status frequently, watching for signs of heart failure, such as dyspnea, hypotension, and tachycardia. Check for changes in cardiac rhythm or conduction.
◆ Observe patients for signs and symptoms of digoxin toxicity (anorexia, nausea, vomiting, blurred vision, and cardiac arrhythmias) and for complicating factors that may potentiate toxicity, such as electrolyte imbalance or hypoxia.
◆ Stress the importance of bed rest. Assist the patient with bathing as necessary; provide a bedside commode because this stresses the heart less than using a bedpan. Reassure the patient that activity limitations are temporary. Offer diversionary activities that are physically undemanding.
◆ During recovery, recommend that the patient resume normal activities slowly and that he avoid competitive sports.

PATENT DUCTUS ARTERIOSUS
The ductus arteriosus is a fetal blood vessel that connects the pulmonary artery to the descending aorta, just distal to the left subclavian artery. Normally, the ductus closes within days after birth. In patent ductus arteriosus (PDA), the lumen of the ductus remains open after birth. This creates a left-to-right shunt of blood from the aorta to the pulmonary artery and results in recirculation of arterial blood through the lungs. Initially, PDA may produce no clinical effects, but over time it can precipitate pulmonary vascular disease, causing symptoms to appear by age 40. PDA affects twice as many females as males.

The prognosis is good if the shunt is small or surgical repair is effective. Otherwise, PDA may advance to intractable heart failure, which may be fatal.

Causes
◆ Coarctation of the aorta
◆ Living at high altitudes
◆ Premature birth, probably as a result of abnormalities in oxygenation or the relaxant action of prostaglandin E, which prevents ductal spasm and contracture necessary for closure
◆ Pulmonary and aortic stenosis
◆ Rubella syndrome
◆ Ventricular septal defect

Pathophysiology
The ductus arteriosus normally closes as prostaglandin levels from the placenta fall and oxygen levels rise. This process should begin as soon as the neonate takes its first breath, but may take as long as 3 months in some children.

In PDA, relative resistances in pulmonary and systemic vasculature and the size of the ductus determine the quantity of blood that's shunted from left to right. Because of increased aortic pressure, oxygenated blood is shunted from the aorta through the ductus arteriosus to the pulmonary artery. The blood returns to the left side of the heart and is pumped out to the aorta once more.

The left atrium and left ventricle must accommodate the increased pulmonary venous return, increasing filling pressure and workload on the left side of the heart and causing left ventricular hypertrophy and possibly heart failure. In the final stages of untreated PDA, the left-to-right shunt leads to chronic pulmonary artery hypertension that becomes fixed and unreactive. This causes the shunt to reverse so that unoxygenated blood enters systemic circulation, causing cyanosis.

Signs and symptoms
◆ Respiratory distress with signs of heart failure in infants, especially those who are premature, resulting from the tremendous volume of blood shunted to the lungs through a patent ductus and the increased workload on the left side of the heart
◆ Classic machinery murmur (Gibson murmur), a continuous murmur heard throughout systole and diastole in older children and adults from shunting of blood from the aorta to the pulmonary artery throughout systole and diastole (It's best heard at the base of the heart, at the second left intercostal space under the left clavicle. The murmur may obscure S_2. However, in a right-to-left shunt, this murmur may be absent.)
◆ Thrill palpated at the left sternal border caused by the shunting of blood from the aorta to the pulmonary artery
◆ Prominent left ventricular impulse due to left ventricular hypertrophy

◆ Bounding peripheral pulses (Corrigan's pulse) due to the high-flow state
◆ Widened pulse pressure because of an elevated systolic blood pressure and, primarily, a drop in diastolic blood pressure as blood is shunted through the PDA, thus reducing peripheral resistance
◆ Slow motor development caused by heart failure
◆ Failure to thrive as a result of heart failure
◆ Fatigue and exertional dyspnea, which may develop in adults with undetected PDA

Complications
◆ Infective endocarditis
◆ Heart failure
◆ Recurrent pneumonia

Diagnosis
◆ Chest X-rays may show increased pulmonary vascular markings, prominent pulmonary arteries, and enlargement of the left ventricle and aorta.
◆ Electrocardiography (ECG) may be normal or may indicate left atrial or ventricular hypertrophy and, in pulmonary vascular disease, biventricular hypertrophy.
◆ Echocardiography detects and estimates the size of a PDA. It also reveals an enlarged left atrium and left ventricle, or right ventricular hypertrophy from pulmonary vascular disease.
◆ Cardiac catheterization shows higher pulmonary arterial oxygen content than right ventricular content because of the influx of aortic blood. Increased pulmonary artery pressure indicates a large shunt or, if it exceeds systemic arterial pressure, severe pulmonary vascular disease. Cardiac catheterization allows for the calculation of blood volume crossing the ductus and can aid in ruling out associated cardiac defects. Injection of a contrast agent can conclusively demonstrate PDA.

Treatment
◆ Indomethacin (a prostaglandin inhibitor) to induce ductus spasm and closure in premature infants
◆ Left thoracotomy to ligate the ductus if medical management can't control heart failure (Asymptomatic infants with PDA don't require immediate treatment. If symptoms are mild, surgical ligation of the PDA is usually delayed until age 1.)
◆ Visual assisted thoracoscopic surgery (VATS) to ligate the ductus as an alternative to surgery with a thoracotomy (VATS may be done at the bedside or in a procedure room and involves three small incisions on the left side of the chest through which a clip is placed on the ductus.)

◆ A prophylactic antibiotic to protect against infective endocarditis
◆ Treatment of heart failure with fluid restriction, a diuretic, and digoxin
◆ Other therapy, including cardiac catheterization, to deposit a plug (or "umbrella") or coils in the ductus to stop shunting

Special considerations
◆ PDA necessitates careful monitoring, patient and family teaching, and emotional support.
◆ Watch all premature infants carefully for signs of PDA.
◆ Be alert for respiratory distress symptoms resulting from heart failure, which may develop rapidly in a premature infant. Frequently assess vital signs, ECG, electrolyte levels, and intake and output. Record response to diuretic and other therapy.
◆ If the infant receives indomethacin for ductus closure, watch for possible adverse reactions, such as diarrhea, jaundice, bleeding, and renal dysfunction.
◆ Before surgery, carefully explain all treatments and tests to parents. Include the child in your explanations. Arrange for the child and parents to meet the intensive care unit staff. Tell them about expected I.V. lines, monitoring equipment, and postoperative procedures.
◆ Immediately after surgery, the child may have a central venous pressure catheter and an arterial line in place. Carefully assess vital signs, intake and output, and arterial and venous pressures. Provide pain relief, as needed.
◆ Before discharge, review instructions with the parents about activity restrictions based on the child's tolerance and energy levels. Advise parents not to become overprotective as their child's tolerance for physical activity increases.
◆ Stress the need for regular medical follow-up examinations. Advise parents to inform any physician who treats their child about his history of surgery for PDA—even if the child is being treated for an unrelated medical problem.

PERICARDITIS
Pericarditis is an inflammation of the pericardium—the fibroserous sac that envelops, supports, and protects the heart. It occurs in acute and chronic forms. Acute pericarditis can be fibrinous or effusive, with purulent, serous, or hemorrhagic exudate. Chronic constrictive pericarditis is characterized by dense fibrous pericardial thickening. Although the prognosis depends on the underlying cause, it's generally good in patients with acute pericarditis, unless constriction occurs.

Causes

◆ Aortic aneurysm with pericardial leakage (less common)
◆ Bacterial, fungal, or viral infection (infectious pericarditis)
◆ Drugs, such as hydralazine or procainamide
◆ High-dose radiation to the chest
◆ Hypersensitivity or autoimmune disease, such as acute rheumatic fever (most common cause of pericarditis in children), systemic lupus erythematosus, and rheumatoid arthritis
◆ Idiopathic factors (most common in acute pericarditis)
◆ Myxedema with cholesterol deposits in the pericardium (less common)
◆ Neoplasms (primary, or metastases from lungs, breasts, or other organs)
◆ Previous cardiac injury, such as a myocardial infarction (Dressler's syndrome), trauma, or surgery (postcardiotomy syndrome), that leaves the pericardium intact but causes blood to leak into the pericardial cavity
◆ Uremia

Pathophysiology

Pericardial tissue damaged by bacteria or other substances results in the release of chemical mediators of inflammation (prostaglandins, histamines, bradykinins, and serotonin) into the surrounding tissue, thereby initiating the inflammatory process. Friction occurs as the inflamed pericardial layers rub against each other. Histamines and other chemical mediators dilate vessels and increase vessel permeability. Vessel walls then leak fluids and protein (including fibrinogen) into tissues, causing extracellular edema. Macrophages already present in the tissue begin to phagocytize the invading bacteria and are joined by neutrophils and monocytes. After several days, the area fills with an exudate composed of necrotic tissue and dead and dying bacteria, neutrophils, and macrophages. Eventually, the contents of the cavity autolyze and are gradually reabsorbed into healthy tissue.

A pericardial effusion develops if fluid accumulates in the pericardial cavity. Cardiac tamponade results when fluid accumulates rapidly in the pericardial space, compressing the heart, preventing it from filling during diastole, and resulting in a drop in cardiac output. (See *Understanding cardiac tamponade*, page 152.)

Chronic constrictive pericarditis develops if the pericardium becomes thick and stiff from chronic or recurrent pericarditis, encasing the heart in a stiff shell and preventing it from properly filling during diastole. This causes an increase in left- and right-sided filling pressures, leading to a drop in stroke volume and cardiac output.

Signs and symptoms

◆ Pericardial friction rub caused by the roughened pericardial membranes rubbing against one another (Although rub may be heard intermittently, it's best heard when the patient leans forward and exhales.)
◆ Sharp and typically sudden pain, usually starting over the sternum and radiating to the neck (especially the left trapezius ridge), shoulders, back, and arms due to inflammation and irritation of the pericardial membranes (The pain is commonly pleuritic, increasing with deep inspiration and decreasing when the patient sits up and leans forward, pulling the heart away from the diaphragmatic pleurae of the lungs.)
◆ Shallow, rapid respirations to reduce pleuritic pain
◆ Mild fever caused by the inflammatory process
◆ Dyspnea, orthopnea, and tachycardia as well as other signs and symptoms of heart failure may occur as fluid builds up in the pericardial space, causing pericardial effusion, a major complication of acute pericarditis
◆ Muffled and distant heart sounds due to fluid buildup
◆ Pallor, clammy skin, hypotension, paradoxical pulse, jugular vein distention and, eventually, cardiovascular collapse may occur with the rapid fluid accumulation of cardiac tamponade
◆ Fluid retention, ascites, hepatomegaly, jugular vein distention, and other signs of chronic right-sided heart failure may occur with chronic constrictive pericarditis as the systemic venous pressure gradually increases
◆ Pericardial knock in early diastole along the left sternal border produced by restricted ventricular filling
◆ Kussmaul's sign, increased jugular vein distention on inspiration, due to restricted right-sided filling

Complications

◆ Pericardial effusion
◆ Cardiac tamponade

Diagnosis

◆ Electrocardiography may reveal diffuse ST-segment elevation in the limb leads and most precordial leads that reflects the inflammatory process. Downsloping PR segments and upright T waves are present in most leads. QRS complexes may be diminished when pericardial effusion exists. Arrhythmias, such as atrial fibrillation and sinus arrhythmias, may occur. In chronic constrictive pericarditis, there may be low-voltage QRS complexes, T-wave inversion or flattening, and P mitral (wide P waves) in leads I, II, and V_6.

◆ Laboratory testing may reveal an elevated erythrocyte sedimentation rate as a result of the inflammatory process or a normal or elevated white blood cell count, especially in infectious pericarditis; blood urea nitrogen level may point to uremia as a cause of pericarditis.

◆ Blood cultures may help identify an infectious cause.

◆ Antistreptolysin-O titers may be positive if pericarditis is due to rheumatic fever.

◆ Purified protein derivative skin test may be positive if pericarditis is due to tuberculosis.

◆ Echocardiography may show an echo-free space between the ventricular wall and the pericardium and reduced pumping action of the heart.

◆ Chest X-rays may be normal with acute pericarditis. The cardiac silhouette may be enlarged with a water bottle shape caused by fluid accumulation if pleural effusion is present.

Treatment

◆ Bed rest as long as fever and pain persist to reduce metabolic needs

◆ Treatment of the underlying cause if it can be identified

◆ A nonsteroidal anti-inflammatory drug (NSAID) such as aspirin or indomethacin, to relieve pain and reduce inflammation

◆ A corticosteroid if the NSAID is ineffective and no infection exists (Corticosteroids must be administered cautiously because episodes may recur when therapy is discontinued.)

◆ Antibacterial, antifungal, or antiviral therapy if an infectious cause is suspected

◆ Pericardiocentesis to remove excess fluid from the pericardial space

◆ Partial pericardectomy, for recurrent pericarditis, to create a window that allows fluid to drain into the pleural space

◆ Total pericardectomy, for constrictive pericarditis, to permit adequate filling and contraction of the heart

◆ Idiopathic pericarditis may be benign and self-limiting.

Special considerations

A patient with pericarditis needs complete bed rest. In addition, health care includes:

◆ assessing pain in relation to respiration and body position to distinguish pericardial pain from myocardial ischemic pain

◆ placing the patient in an upright position to relieve dyspnea and chest pain, providing an analgesic and oxygen, and reassuring the patient with acute pericarditis that his condition is temporary and treatable

◆ monitoring for signs of cardiac compression or cardiac tamponade and possible complications

of pericardial effusion, which include decreased blood pressure, increased central venous pressure, and paradoxical pulse (Because cardiac tamponade requires immediate treatment, keep a pericardiocentesis set handy whenever pericardial effusion is suspected.)

◆ explaining tests and treatments to the patient. If surgery is necessary, he should learn deep-breathing and coughing exercises before the procedure. Postoperative care is similar to that given after cardiothoracic surgery.

RAYNAUD'S DISEASE

Raynaud's disease is one of several primary arteriospastic disorders characterized by episodic vasospasm in the small peripheral arteries and arterioles, precipitated by exposure to cold or stress. This condition occurs bilaterally and usually affects the hands or, less commonly, the feet. Raynaud's disease is most prevalent in females, particularly between puberty and age 40. It's a benign condition, requiring no specific treatment and causing no serious aftereffects.

Raynaud's phenomenon, however, a condition usually associated with several connective tissue disorders—such as scleroderma, systemic lupus erythematosus (SLE), or polymyositis—has a progressive course, leading to ischemia, gangrene, and amputation. Distinguishing between the two disorders is difficult because some patients who experience mild symptoms of Raynaud's disease for several years may later develop overt connective tissue disease, especially scleroderma.

Causes

Although family history is a risk factor, the cause of this disorder is unknown.

Raynaud's phenomenon may develop secondary to:

◆ arterio-occlusive disease

◆ connective tissue disorders, such as scleroderma, rheumatoid arthritis, SLE, or polymyositis

◆ exposure to heavy metals

◆ long-term exposure to cold, vibrating machinery (such as operating a jackhammer), or pressure to the fingertips (such as in typists and pianists)

◆ myxedema

◆ previous damage from cold exposure

◆ pulmonary hypertension

◆ serum sickness

◆ thoracic outlet syndrome

◆ trauma.

Pathophysiology

Although the cause is unknown, several theories account for reduced digital blood flow, including:

◆ intrinsic vascular wall hyperactivity to cold

♦ increased vasomotor tone due to sympathetic stimulation
♦ antigen-antibody immune response (the most likely theory because abnormal immunologic test results accompany Raynaud's phenomenon).

Signs and symptoms
♦ Blanching of the fingers bilaterally after exposure to cold or stress as vasoconstriction or vasospasm reduces blood flow (This is followed by cyanosis due to increased oxygen extraction resulting from sluggish blood flow. As the spasm resolves, the fingers turn red as blood rushes back into the arterioles.)
♦ Cold and numbness, possibly occurring during the vasoconstrictive phase because of ischemia
♦ Throbbing, aching pain, swelling, and tingling, possibly occurring during the hyperemic phase
♦ Trophic changes, such as sclerodactyly, ulcerations, or chronic paronychia, possibly occurring as a result of ischemia in long-standing disease

Complications
Cutaneous gangrene may occur as a result of prolonged ischemia, necessitating amputation of one or more digits (although extremely rare).

Diagnosis
♦ Clinical criteria include skin color changes induced by cold or stress; bilateral involvement; absence of gangrene or, if present, minimal cutaneous gangrene; normal arterial pulses; and patient history of symptoms for at least 2 years.
♦ Antinuclear antibody (ANA) titer is used to identify autoimmune disease as an underlying cause of Raynaud's phenomenon; further tests must be performed if ANA titer is positive.
♦ Arteriography rules out arterial occlusive disease.
♦ Doppler ultrasonography may show reduced blood flow if symptoms result from arterial occlusive disease.

Treatment
♦ Teaching the patient to avoid triggers, such as cold and mechanical or chemical injury
♦ Encouraging the patient to stop smoking and avoid decongestants and caffeine to reduce vasoconstriction
♦ Teaching patient that keeping fingers and toes warm reduces vasoconstriction
♦ A calcium channel blocker, such as nifedipine, diltiazem, or nicardipine, to produce vasodilation and prevent vasospasm
♦ An adrenergic blocker, such as phenoxybenzamine or reserpine, which may improve blood flow to fingers or toes

♦ Biofeedback and relaxation exercises to reduce stress and improve circulation
♦ Sympathectomy to prevent ischemic ulcers by promoting vasodilation (necessary in less than 25% of patients)
♦ Amputation, if ischemia causes ulceration and gangrene

Special considerations
♦ Warn the patient against exposure to the cold. Tell her to wear mittens or gloves in cold weather or when handling cold items or defrosting the freezer.
♦ Advise the patient to avoid stressful situations and to stop smoking.
♦ Instruct the patient to inspect her skin frequently and to seek immediate care for signs of skin breakdown or infection.
♦ Teach the patient about drugs, their use, and their adverse effects.
♦ Provide psychological support and reassurance to allay the patient's fear of amputation and disfigurement.

RHEUMATIC FEVER AND RHEUMATIC HEART DISEASE
A systemic inflammatory disease of childhood, acute rheumatic fever develops after infection of the upper respiratory tract with group A beta-hemolytic streptococci. It mainly involves the heart, joints, central nervous system, skin, and subcutaneous tissues and commonly recurs. Rheumatic heart disease refers to the cardiac manifestations of rheumatic fever and includes pancarditis (myocarditis, pericarditis, and endocarditis) during the early acute phase and chronic valvular disease later.

Rheumatic fever tends to run in families, lending support to the existence of genetic predisposition. Environmental factors also seem to be significant in the development of the disorder. The incidence is highest in children between ages 6 and 15, probably because of malnutrition and crowded living conditions. About 3% of those with untreated streptococcal infections develop rheumatic fever.

Patients without carditis or with mild carditis have a good long-term prognosis. Severe pancarditis occasionally produces fatal heart failure during the acute phase. Antibiotic therapy has greatly reduced the mortality from rheumatic heart disease.

Causes
♦ Group A beta-hemolytic streptococcal pharyngitis

Pathophysiology

Rheumatic fever appears to be a hypersensitivity reaction to group A beta-hemolytic streptococcal infection. Because few persons (3%) with streptococcal infections contract rheumatic fever, altered host resistance must be involved in its development or recurrence. The antigens of group A streptococci bind to receptors in the heart, muscle, brain, and synovial joints, causing an autoimmune response. Because of a similarity between the antigens of the streptococcus bacteria and the antigens of the body's own cells, antibodies may attack healthy body cells by mistake.

Carditis may affect the endocardium, myocardium, or pericardium during the early acute phase. Later, the heart valves may be damaged, causing chronic valvular disease.

Pericarditis produces a serofibrinous effusion. Myocarditis produces characteristic lesions called Aschoff bodies (fibrin deposits surrounded by necrosis) in the interstitial tissue of the heart as well as cellular swelling and fragmentation of interstitial collagen. These lesions lead to progressively fibrotic nodule and interstitial scar formation.

Endocarditis causes valve leaflet swelling, erosion along the lines of leaflet closure, and blood, platelet, and fibrin deposits, which form beadlike growths. Eventually, the valve leaflets become scarred, lose their elasticity, and begin to adhere to each other. Endocarditis most commonly effects the mitral valve in females and the aortic valve in males. In both sexes, it occasionally affects the tricuspid valve and, rarely, the pulmonic valve.

Signs and symptoms

Classic signs and symptoms include:
◆ polyarthritis or migratory joint pain, caused by inflammation, occurring in most patients (Swelling, redness, and signs of effusion usually accompany such pain, which most commonly affects the knees, ankles, elbows, and hips.)
◆ erythema marginatum, a nonpruritic, macular, transient rash on the trunk or inner aspects of the upper arms or thighs, that gives rise to red lesions with blanched centers
◆ subcutaneous nodules—firm, movable, and nontender, 3 mm to 2 cm in diameter, usually near tendons or bony prominences of joints, especially the elbows, knuckles, wrists, and knees (They commonly accompany carditis and may last a few days to several weeks.)
◆ chorea—rapid, jerky movements—possibly developing up to 6 months after the original streptococcal infection. (Mild chorea may produce hyperirritability, a deterioration in hand-writing, or inability to concentrate. Severe chorea causes purposeless, nonrepetitive, involuntary muscle spasms; poor muscle coordination; and weakness.)

Other signs and symptoms include:
◆ a streptococcal infection a few days to 6 weeks earlier, occurring in 95% of those with rheumatic fever
◆ temperature of at least 100.4° F (38° C) due to infection and inflammation
◆ a new mitral or aortic heart murmur, or a worsening murmur in a person with a preexisting murmur
◆ pericardial friction rub caused by inflamed pericardial membranes rubbing against one another, if pericarditis exists
◆ chest pain, typically pleuritic, due to inflammation and irritation of the pericardial membranes (Pain may increase with deep inspiration and decrease when the patient sits up and leans forward, pulling the heart away from the diaphragmatic pleurae of the lungs.)
◆ dyspnea, tachypnea, nonproductive cough, bibasilar crackles, and edema due to heart failure in severe rheumatic carditis.

Complications
◆ Destruction of the mitral and aortic valves
◆ Pancarditis (pericarditis, myocarditis, and endocarditis)
◆ Heart failure

Diagnosis
◆ Jones criteria revealing either two major criteria or one major criterion and two minor criteria, plus evidence of a previous group A streptococcal infection, are necessary for diagnosis. (See *Jones criteria for diagnosing rheumatic fever*.)
◆ Laboratory testing may reveal an elevated white blood cell count and elevated erythrocyte sedimentation rate during the acute phase.
◆ Hemoglobin level and hematocrit may show slight anemia due to suppressed erythropoiesis during inflammation.
◆ C-reactive protein may be positive, especially during the acute phase.
◆ Cardiac enzyme levels may be increased in severe carditis.
◆ Antistreptolysin-O titer may be elevated in 95% of patients within 2 months of onset.
◆ Throat cultures may continue to show the presence of group A beta-hemolytic streptococci; however, they usually occur in small numbers.
◆ Electrocardiography may show changes that aren't diagnostic, but the PR interval is prolonged in 20% of patients.
◆ Chest X-rays may show normal heart size or cardiomegaly, pericardial effusion, or heart failure.

◆ Echocardiography can detect valvular damage and pericardial effusion and can measure chamber size and provide information on ventricular function.
◆ Cardiac catheterization provides information on valvular damage and left ventricular function.

Treatment
◆ Prompt treatment of all group A beta-hemolytic streptococcal pharyngitis with oral penicillin V or I.M. benzathine penicillin G, or erythromycin for patients with penicillin hypersensitivity
◆ A salicylate to relieve fever and pain and minimize joint swelling
◆ A corticosteroid if the patient has carditis or if the salicylate fails to relieve pain and inflammation
◆ Strict bed rest for about 5 weeks for the patient with active carditis to reduce cardiac demands
◆ Bed rest, sodium restriction, an angiotensin-converting enzyme inhibitor, angiotensin-receptor blocker, digoxin, and a diuretic to treat heart failure
◆ Corrective surgery, such as commissurotomy (separation of adherent, thickened valve leaflets of the mitral valve), valvuloplasty (inflation of a balloon within a valve), or valve replacement (with a prosthetic valve) for severe mitral or aortic valvular dysfunction that causes persistent heart failure
◆ Secondary prevention of rheumatic fever, which begins after the acute phase subsides with monthly I.M. injections of penicillin G benzathine or daily doses of oral penicillin V or sulfadiazine (Treatment usually continues for at least 5 years or until age 21, whichever is longer.)
◆ A prophylactic antibiotic for dental work and other invasive or surgical procedures to prevent endocarditis

Special considerations
◆ Because rheumatic fever and rheumatic heart disease require prolonged treatment, your care plan should include comprehensive patient teaching to promote compliance with the prescribed therapy.
◆ Before giving penicillin, ask the patient or (if the patient is a child) his parents if he has ever had a hypersensitivity reaction to it. Even if the patient has never had a reaction, warn that such a reaction is possible. Tell him to stop the drug and call the physician immediately if a rash, fever, chills, or other signs of allergy develop at any time during penicillin therapy.
◆ Instruct the patient and his family to watch for and report early signs and symptoms of

Jones criteria for diagnosing rheumatic fever

The Jones criteria are used to standardize the diagnosis of rheumatic fever. Diagnosis requires that the patient have either two major criteria *or* one major criterion and two minor criteria, plus evidence of a previous streptococcal infection.

Major criteria
◆ Carditis
◆ Migratory polyarthritis
◆ Sydenham's chorea
◆ Subcutaneous nodules
◆ Erythema marginatum

Minor criteria
◆ Fever
◆ Arthralgia
◆ Elevated acute phase reactants
◆ Prolonged PR interval

heart failure, such as dyspnea and a hacking, nonproductive cough.
◆ Stress the need for bed rest during the acute phase and suggest appropriate, physically undemanding diversions. After the acute phase, encourage family members and friends to spend as much time as possible with the patient to minimize boredom. Advise parents to secure tutorial services to help the child keep up with schoolwork during the long convalescence.
◆ Help parents overcome any guilt they may feel about their child's illness. Tell them that failure to seek treatment for streptococcal infection is common because this illness typically seems no worse than a cold. Encourage the parents and the child to vent their frustrations during the long, tedious recovery. If the child has severe carditis, help the parents prepare for permanent changes in the child's lifestyle.
◆ Teach the patient and his family about this disease and its treatment. Warn parents to watch for and immediately report signs and symptoms of recurrent streptococcal infection—sudden sore throat, diffuse throat redness and oropharyngeal exudate, swollen and tender cervical lymph glands, pain on swallowing, temperature of 101° to 104° F (38.3° to 40° C), headache, and nausea. Urge them to keep the child away from people with respiratory tract infections.
◆ Promote good dental hygiene to prevent infection. Make sure the patient and his family

understand the need to comply with prolonged antibiotic therapy and follow-up care and the need for an additional antibiotic during dental surgery or other invasive procedures. Arrange for a home health nurse to oversee care, if necessary.

◆ Teach the patient to follow current recommendations of the American Heart Association for prevention of bacterial endocarditis. Antibiotic regimens used to prevent recurrence of acute rheumatic fever are inadequate for preventing bacterial endocarditis.

||| LIFE-THREATENING DISORDER

SHOCK

Shock isn't a disease, but rather a clinical syndrome leading to reduced tissue and organ perfusion and, eventually, organ dysfunction and failure. Shock can be classified into four major categories based on the precipitating factors: distributive (neurogenic, septic, and anaphylactic), cardiogenic, hypovolemic, and obstructive. Even with treatment, shock accounts for a high mortality rate after the body's compensatory mechanisms fail. (See *Types of shock.*)

Causes
Neurogenic shock
◆ Hypoglycemia
◆ Medications
◆ Severe pain
◆ Spinal anesthesia
◆ Spinal cord injury
◆ Vasomotor center depression

Septic shock
◆ Gram-negative bacteria (most common cause)
◆ Gram-positive bacteria
◆ Viruses, fungi, *Rickettsiae*, parasites, yeast, protozoa, or mycobacteria

AGE ALERT *The immature immune system of neonates and infants and the weakened immune system of older adults, commonly accompanied by chronic illness, make these populations more susceptible to septic shock.*

Anaphylactic shock
◆ ABO-incompatible blood
◆ Contrast media
◆ Foods
◆ Medications, vaccines
◆ Venom

Cardiogenic shock
◆ Arrhythmias
◆ Cardiomyopathy
◆ Heart failure

◆ Myocardial infarction (MI) (most common cause)
◆ Obstruction
◆ Pericardial tamponade
◆ Pulmonary embolism
◆ Tension pneumothorax

Hypovolemic shock
◆ Ascites
◆ Blood loss (most common cause)
◆ Burns
◆ Fluid shifts
◆ GI fluid loss
◆ Hemothorax
◆ Peritonitis
◆ Renal loss (diabetic ketoacidosis, diabetes insipidus, adrenal insufficiency)

Obstructive shock
◆ Congenital abnormalities
◆ Pericardial tamponade
◆ Tension pneumothorax

Pathophysiology
There are three basic stages common to each type of shock: compensatory, progressive, and irreversible (or refractory) stages.

Compensatory stage
When arterial pressure and tissue perfusion are reduced, compensatory mechanisms are activated to maintain perfusion to the heart and brain. As the baroreceptors in the carotid sinus and aortic arch sense a decrease in blood pressure, epinephrine and norepinephrine are secreted to increase peripheral resistance, blood pressure, and myocardial contractility. Reduced blood flow to the kidney activates the renin-angiotensin-aldosterone system, causing vasoconstriction and sodium and water retention, leading to increased blood volume and venous return. As a result of these compensatory mechanisms, cardiac output and tissue perfusion are maintained.

Progressive stage
The progressive stage of shock begins as compensatory mechanisms fail to maintain cardiac output. Tissues become hypoxic because of poor perfusion. As cells switch to anaerobic metabolism, lactic acid builds up, producing metabolic acidosis. This acidotic state depresses myocardial function. Tissue hypoxia also promotes the release of endothelial mediators, which produce vasodilation and endothelial abnormalities, leading to venous pooling and increased capillary permeability. Sluggish blood flow increases the risk of disseminated intravascular coagulation (DIC).

Types of shock

Distributive shock

In distributive shock, vasodilation causes a state of hypovolemia. There are three types of distributive shock—neurogenic, septic, and anaphylactic.

Neurogenic shock

In neurogenic shock, a loss of sympathetic vasoconstrictor tone in the vascular smooth muscle and reduced autonomic function lead to widespread arterial and venous vasodilation. Venous return is reduced as blood pools in the venous system, leading to a drop in cardiac output and hypotension.

Septic shock

In septic shock, an immune response is triggered when bacteria release endotoxins. In response, macrophages secrete tumor necrosis factor (TNF) and interleukins. These mediators, in turn, are responsible for an increased release of platelet-activating factor (PAF), prostaglandins, leukotrienes, thromboxane A_2, kinins, and complement. The consequences are vasodilation and vasoconstriction, increased capillary permeability, reduced systemic vascular resistance, microemboli, and elevated cardiac output. Endotoxins also stimulate the release of histamine, further increasing capillary permeability. Moreover, myocardial depressant factor, TNF, PAF, and other factors depress myocardial function. Cardiac output falls, resulting in multisystem organ failure.

Anaphylactic shock

Triggered by an allergic reaction, anaphylactic shock occurs when a person is exposed to an antigen to which he has already been sensitized. Exposure results in the production of specific immunoglobulin (Ig) E antibodies by plasma cells that bind to membrane receptors on mast cells and basophils. On reexposure, the antigen binds to IgE antibodies or cross-linked IgE receptors, triggering the release of powerful chemical mediators from mast cells. IgG or IgM enters into the reaction and activates the release of complement factors. At the same time, the chemical mediators bradykinin and leukotrienes induce vascular collapse by stimulating contraction of certain groups of smooth muscles and by increasing vascular permeability, leading to decreased peripheral resistance and plasma leakage into the extravascular tissues, thereby reducing blood volume and causing hypotension, hypovolemic shock, and cardiac dysfunction. Bronchospasm and laryngeal edema also occur.

Cardiogenic shock

In cardiogenic shock, the left ventricle can't maintain adequate cardiac output. Compensatory mechanisms increase heart rate, strengthen myocardial contractions, promote sodium and water retention, and cause selective vasoconstriction. However, these mechanisms increase myocardial workload and oxygen consumption, which reduces the heart's ability to pump blood, especially if the patient has myocardial ischemia. Consequently, blood backs up, resulting in pulmonary edema. Eventually, cardiac output falls and multisystem organ failure develops as the compensatory mechanisms fail to maintain perfusion.

Hypovolemic shock

In hypovolemic shock, venous return to the heart is reduced when fluid is lost from the intravascular space through external losses or the shift of fluid from the vessels to the interstitial or intracellular spaces. This reduction in preload decreases ventricular filling, leading to a drop in stroke volume. Then, cardiac output falls, causing reduced perfusion of the tissues and organs.

Obstructive shock

In obstructive shock, inadequate circulating blood volume results from an obstruction in the great vessels, aorta, pulmonary artery, or heart. These mechanical factors interfere with filling or emptying of the heart, resulting in reduced cardiac output.

Irreversible (refractory) stage

As the shock syndrome progresses, permanent organ damage occurs as compensatory mechanisms can no longer maintain cardiac output. Reduced perfusion damages cell membranes, lysosomal enzymes are released, and energy stores are depleted, possibly leading to cell death. As cells use anaerobic metabolism, lactic acid accumulates, increasing capillary permeability and the movement of fluid out of the vascular space. This loss of intravascular fluid further contributes to hypotension. Perfusion to the coronary arteries is reduced, causing myocardial depression and a further reduction in cardiac output. Eventually, circulatory and respiratory failure occur. Death is inevitable.

Signs and symptoms
Compensatory stage
◆ Tachycardia and bounding pulse due to sympathetic stimulation
◆ Restlessness and irritability related to cerebral hypoxia
◆ Tachypnea to compensate for hypoxia
◆ Reduced urine output secondary to vasoconstriction
◆ Cool, pale skin associated with vasoconstriction; warm, dry skin in septic shock due to vasodilation

Progressive stage
◆ Hypotension as compensatory mechanisms begin to fail
◆ Narrowed pulse pressure associated with reduced stroke volume; weak, rapid, thready pulse caused by decreased cardiac output; shallow respirations as the patient weakens; reduced urine output as poor renal perfusion continues
◆ Cold, clammy skin caused by vasoconstriction
◆ Cyanosis related to hypoxia

AGE ALERT *In infants and elderly patients, hypotension, an altered level of consciousness, and hyperventilation may be the only signs of septic shock.*

Irreversible (refractory) stage
◆ Unconsciousness and absent reflexes caused by reduced cerebral perfusion, acid-base imbalance, or electrolyte abnormalities
◆ Rapidly falling blood pressure as decompensation occurs
◆ Weak pulse caused by reduced cardiac output
◆ Slow, shallow, or Cheyne-Stokes respirations secondary to respiratory center depression
◆ Anuria related to renal failure

Complications
◆ Acute respiratory distress syndrome
◆ Acute tubular necrosis
◆ DIC
◆ Cerebral hypoxia
◆ Death

Diagnosis
◆ Hematocrit may be reduced in hemorrhage or elevated in other types of shock due to hypovolemia.
◆ Blood, urine, and sputum cultures may identify the organism responsible for septic shock.
◆ Coagulation studies may detect coagulopathy from DIC.

◆ Laboratory test results may reveal increased white blood cell count and erythrocyte sedimentation rate due to injury and inflammation; elevated blood urea nitrogen and creatinine levels due to reduced renal perfusion; the serum lactate level may be increased secondary to anaerobic metabolism; and the serum glucose level may be elevated in early stages of shock as liver releases glycogen stores in response to sympathetic stimulation.
◆ Cardiac enzyme and protein levels may be elevated, indicating MI as a cause of cardiogenic shock.
◆ Arterial blood gas (ABG) analysis may reveal respiratory alkalosis in early shock associated with tachypnea, respiratory acidosis in later stages associated with respiratory depression, and metabolic acidosis in later stages secondary to anaerobic metabolism.
◆ Urine specific gravity may be high in response to effects of antidiuretic hormone.
◆ Chest X-rays may be normal in early stages; pulmonary congestion may be evident in later stages.
◆ Hemodynamic monitoring may reveal characteristic patterns of intracardiac pressures and cardiac output, which are used to guide fluid and drug management. (See *Understanding hemodynamic monitoring*.)
◆ Electrocardiography (ECG) determines the heart rate and detects arrhythmias, ischemic changes, and MI.
◆ Echocardiography determines left ventricular function and reveals valvular abnormalities.

Treatment
◆ Identification and treatment of the underlying cause, if possible
◆ Maintaining a patent airway; preparing for intubation and mechanical ventilation if the patient develops respiratory distress
◆ Supplemental oxygen to increase oxygenation
◆ Continuous cardiac monitoring to detect changes in heart rate and rhythm; administration of an antiarrhythmic, as necessary
◆ Initiating and maintaining at least two I.V. lines with large-gauge needles for fluid and drug administration
◆ I.V. fluids, crystalloids, colloids, or blood products, as necessary, to maintain intravascular volume

Hypovolemic shock
◆ Pneumatic antishock garment, which may be applied to control internal and external hemorrhage by direct pressure
◆ Fluids, such as normal saline or lactated Ringer's solution, initially, to restore filling pressures

Understanding hemodynamic monitoring

Hemodynamic monitoring provides information on intracardiac pressures and cardiac output. To understand intracardiac pressures, picture the cardiovascular system as a continuous loop with constantly changing pressure gradients that keep the blood moving.

Right atrial pressure (RAP), or central venous pressure (CVP)

RAP reflects right atrial—or right-sided heart—function and end-diastolic pressure.
◆ **Normal:** 1 to 6 mm Hg (1.34 to 8 cm H₂O). (To convert mm Hg to cm H₂O, multiply mm Hg by 1.34.)
◆ **Elevated value suggests:** right-sided heart failure, volume overload, tricuspid valve stenosis or regurgitation, constrictive pericarditis, pulmonary hypertension, cardiac tamponade, or right ventricular infarction.
◆ **Low value suggests:** reduced circulating blood volume.

Right ventricular pressure

Right ventricular systolic pressure normally equals pulmonary artery systolic pressure; right ventricular end-diastolic pressure, which equals RAP, reflects right ventricular function.
◆ **Normal:** systolic, 15 to 25 mm Hg; diastolic, 0 to 8 mm Hg.
◆ **Elevated value suggests:** mitral stenosis or insufficiency, pulmonary disease, hypoxemia, constrictive pericarditis, chronic heart failure, atrial and ventricular septal defects, and patent ductus arteriosus.

Pulmonary artery pressure

Pulmonary artery systolic pressure reflects right ventricular function and pulmonary circulation pressures. Pulmonary artery diastolic pressure reflects left ventricular pressures,

specifically left ventricular end-diastolic pressure.
◆ **Normal:** systolic, 15 to 25 mm Hg; diastolic, 8 to 15 mm Hg; mean, 10 to 20 mm Hg.
◆ **Elevated value suggests:** left-sided heart failure, increased pulmonary blood flow (left or right shunting, as in atrial or ventricular septal defects), mitral stenosis or insuffiency, and in any condition causing increased pulmonary arteriolar resistance.

Pulmonary artery wedge pressure (PAWP)

PAWP reflects left atrial and left ventricular pressures unless the patient has mitral stenosis. Changes in PAWP reflect changes in left ventricular filling pressure. The heart momentarily relaxes during diastole as it fills with blood from the pulmonary veins; this permits the pulmonary vasculature, left atrium, and left ventricle to act as a single chamber.
◆ **Normal:** mean pressure, 6 to 12 mm Hg.
◆ **Elevated value suggests:** left-sided heart failure, mitral stenosis or insufficiency, and pericardial tamponade.
◆ **Low value suggests:** hypovolemia.

Left atrial pressure

Left atrial pressure reflects left ventricular end-diastolic pressure in patients without mitral valve disease.
◆ **Normal:** 6 to 12 mm Hg.

Cardiac output

Cardiac output is the amount of blood ejected by the heart each minute.
◆ **Normal:** 4 to 8 L; varies with a patient's weight, height, and body surface area. Adjusting the cardiac output to the patient's size yields a measurement called the cardiac index.

◆ Packed red blood cells in hemorrhagic shock to restore blood loss and improve the blood's oxygen-carrying capacity

Cardiogenic shock
◆ Inotropic drug, such as dopamine, dobutamine, inamrinone, and epinephrine, to increase heart contractility and cardiac output
◆ Vasodilator, such as nitroglycerin or nitroprusside, given with a vasopressor to reduce the left ventricle's workload
◆ Diuretic to reduce preload if the patient has fluid volume overload

◆ Intra-aortic balloon pump (IABP) therapy to reduce the work of the left ventricle by decreasing systemic vascular resistance (Diastolic pressure is increased, resulting in improved coronary artery perfusion.)
◆ Thrombolytic therapy or coronary artery revascularization to restore coronary artery blood flow if cardiogenic shock is due to an acute MI
◆ Emergency surgery to repair papillary muscle rupture or ventricular septal defect if either is the cause of cardiogenic shock

♦ Ventricular assist device to assist the pumping action of the heart when IABP and drug therapy fail
♦ Heart transplantation, which may be considered when other medical and surgical therapeutic measures fail

Septic shock
♦ Antibiotic therapy to eradicate the causative organism
♦ Inotropic drug and vasopressor, such as dopamine, dobutamine, and norepinephrine, to improve perfusion and maintain blood pressure

Neurogenic shock
♦ Vasopressor to raise blood pressure by vasoconstriction
♦ Fluid replacement to maintain blood pressure and cardiac output

Obstructive shock
♦ Thrombolysis or surgical removal of the obstruction if the underlying cause is pulmonary emboli
♦ Needle thoracostomy for tension pneumothorax
♦ Pericardiocentesis for cardiac tamponade
♦ Fluid resuscitation as indicated to improve cardiac output and hemodynamic status

Special considerations
Management of shock necessitates prompt, aggressive supportive measures and careful assessment and monitoring of vital signs. Follow these priorities:

⚠️ **CLINICAL ALERT** *Check for a patent airway and adequate circulation. If blood pressure and heart rate are absent, start cardiopulmonary resuscitation.*

♦ Record the patient's blood pressure, pulse rate, peripheral pulses, respiratory rate, and other vital signs every 15 minutes and the ECG continuously. Systolic blood pressure lower than 80 mm Hg usually results in inadequate coronary artery blood flow, cardiac ischemia, arrhythmias, and further complications of low cardiac output. When blood pressure drops below 80 mm Hg, increase the oxygen flow rate, and notify the physician immediately. A progressive decrease in blood pressure accompanied by a thready pulse generally signals inadequate cardiac output from reduced intravascular volume. Notify the physician, and increase the infusion rate.
♦ Start an I.V. line with normal saline or lactated Ringer's solution, using a large-bore catheter (14G), which allows easier administration of later blood transfusions.

⚠️ **CLINICAL ALERT** *In the patient with shock who has suffered abdominal trauma, don't start I.V. administration in the legs because the infused fluid may escape through the ruptured vessel into the abdomen.*

♦ An indwelling urinary catheter may be inserted to measure hourly urine output. If output is less than 30 ml/hour in adults, increase the fluid infusion rate, but watch for signs of fluid overload, such as an increase in pulmonary artery wedge pressure (PAWP). Notify the physician if urine output doesn't improve. An osmotic diuretic, such as mannitol, may be ordered to increase renal blood flow and urine output. Determine how much fluid to give by checking blood pressure, urine output, central venous pressure (CVP), or PAWP. (To increase accuracy, CVP should be measured at the level of the right atrium, using the same reference point on the chest each time.)
♦ Draw an arterial blood sample to measure ABG levels. Administer oxygen by face mask or airway to ensure adequate tissue oxygenation. Adjust the oxygen flow rate to a higher or lower level, as ABG measurements indicate.
♦ Draw venous blood for complete blood count and electrolyte, type and crossmatch, and coagulation studies.
♦ During therapy, assess skin color and temperature, and note changes. Cold, clammy skin may be a sign of continuing peripheral vascular constriction, indicating progressive shock.
♦ Watch for signs of impending coagulopathy (petechiae, bruising, and bleeding or oozing from gums or venipuncture sites).
♦ Explain all procedures and their purpose to the patient. Throughout these emergency measures, provide emotional support to the patient and his family.

TETRALOGY OF FALLOT
Tetralogy of Fallot is a combination of four cardiac defects: ventricular septal defect (VSD), right ventricular outflow tract obstruction (pulmonic stenosis), right ventricular hypertrophy, and overriding of the aorta (positioned above the VSD). Blood shunts from right to left through the VSD, allowing unoxygenated blood to mix with oxygenated blood and resulting in cyanosis. This heart defect that decreases pulmonary blood flow sometimes coexists with other congenital heart defects, such as patent ductus arteriosus or atrial septal defect. It accounts for about 10% of all congenital defects and occurs equally in males and females. Before surgical advances made correction possible, about one-third of these children died in infancy.

Causes

The cause of tetralogy of Fallot is unknown, but it may be associated with:

- fetal alcohol syndrome
- thalidomide use during pregnancy.

Pathophysiology

In tetralogy of Fallot, unoxygenated venous blood returning to the right side of the heart may pass through the VSD to the left ventricle, bypassing the lungs, or it may enter the pulmonary artery, depending on the extent of the pulmonic stenosis. Rather than originating from the left ventricle, the aorta overrides both ventricles.

The VSD usually lies in the outflow tract of the right ventricle and is generally large enough to permit equalization of right and left ventricular pressures. However, the ratio of systemic vascular resistance to pulmonic stenosis affects the direction and magnitude of shunt flow across the VSD. Severe obstruction of right ventricular outflow produces a right-to-left shunt, causing decreased systemic arterial oxygen saturation, cyanosis, reduced pulmonary blood flow, and hypoplasia of the entire pulmonary vasculature. Right ventricular hypertrophy develops in response to the extra force needed to push blood into the stenotic pulmonary artery. Milder forms of pulmonic stenosis result in a left-to-right shunt or no shunt at all.

Signs and symptoms

- Cyanosis, the hallmark of tetralogy of Fallot, caused by a right-to-left shunt
- Cyanotic, or "blue," spells (tet spells), characterized by dyspnea; deep, sighing respirations; bradycardia; fainting; seizures; and loss of consciousness after exercise, crying, straining, infection, or fever (It may result from reduced oxygen to the brain because of increased right-to-left shunting, possibly caused by spasm of the right ventricular outflow tract, increased systemic venous return, or decreased systemic arterial resistance.)
- Clubbing, diminished exercise tolerance, increasing dyspnea on exertion, growth retardation, and eating difficulties in older children because of poor oxygenation
- Squatting with shortness of breath to reduce venous return of unoxygenated blood from the legs and to increase systemic arterial resistance
- Loud systolic murmur best heard along the left sternal border, which may diminish or obscure the pulmonic component of S_2
- Continuous murmur of the ductus in a patient with a large patent ductus, which may obscure systolic murmur

- Thrill at the left sternal border caused by abnormal blood flow through the heart
- Obvious right ventricular impulse and prominent inferior sternum associated with right ventricular hypertrophy

Complications

- Pulmonary thrombosis
- Venous thrombosis
- Cerebral embolism
- Infective endocarditis
- Risk of spontaneous abortion, premature birth, and low-birth-weight infants born to women with tetralogy of Fallot

Diagnosis

- Chest X-rays may demonstrate decreased pulmonary vascular marking (depending on the severity of the pulmonary obstruction), an enlarged right ventricle, and a boot-shaped cardiac silhouette.
- Electrocardiography shows right ventricular hypertrophy, right-axis deviation and, possibly, right atrial hypertrophy.
- Echocardiography identifies septal overriding of the aorta, the VSD, and pulmonic stenosis and detects the hypertrophied walls of the right ventricle.
- Laboratory testing reveals diminished oxygen saturation and polycythemia (hematocrit may be more than 60%) if the cyanosis is severe and long-standing, predisposing the patient to thrombosis.
- Cardiac catheterization confirms the diagnosis by providing visualization of pulmonic stenosis, the VSD, and the overriding aorta and ruling out other cyanotic heart defects. This test also measures the degree of oxygen saturation in aortic blood.

Treatment

- Knee-chest position and administration of oxygen and morphine to improve oxygenation
- Propranolol to prevent "tet" spells and a prophylactic antibiotic to prevent infective endocarditis or cerebral abscesses
- Palliative surgery with a Blalock-Taussig procedure, which joins the subclavian artery to the pulmonary artery to enhance blood flow to the lungs to reduce hypoxia
- Corrective surgery to relieve pulmonic stenosis and close the VSD, directing left ventricular outflow to the aorta

Special considerations

- Explain tetralogy of Fallot to the parents. Inform them that their child will set his own exercise limits and will know when to rest. Make sure they understand that their child can engage in physical activity, and advise them not to be overprotective.

⚠ **CLINICAL ALERT** *Teach parents to recognize serious hypoxic spells, which can cause dramatically increased cyanosis; deep, sighing respirations; and loss of consciousness. Tell them to place their child in the knee-chest position and to report such spells immediately. Emergency treatment may be necessary.*

◆ To prevent infective endocarditis and other infections, warn parents to keep their child away from people with infections. Urge them to encourage good dental hygiene, and tell them to watch for ear, nose, and throat infections and dental caries, all of which necessitate immediate treatment. When dental care, infections, or surgery requires a prophylactic antibiotic, tell parents to make sure the child completes the prescribed regimen.

◆ If the child requires medical attention for an unrelated problem, advise the parents to inform the physician immediately of the child's history of tetralogy of Fallot because any treatment must take this serious heart defect into consideration.

◆ During hospitalization, alert the staff to the child's condition. Because of the right-to-left shunt through the VSD, treat I.V. lines like arterial lines. Remember, a clot dislodged from a catheter tip in a vein can cross the VSD and cause cerebral embolism. The same thing can happen if air enters the venous lines.

After palliative surgery

◆ Monitor oxygenation and arterial blood gas (ABG) values closely in the intensive care unit.

◆ If the child has undergone the Blalock-Taussig procedure, don't use the arm on the operative side for measuring blood pressure, inserting I.V. lines, or drawing blood samples because blood perfusion on this side diminishes greatly until collateral circulation develops. Note this on the child's chart and at his bedside.

After corrective surgery

◆ Watch for right bundle-branch block or more serious disturbances of atrioventricular conduction and for ventricular ectopic beats.

◆ Be alert for other postoperative complications, such as bleeding, right-sided heart failure, and respiratory failure. After surgery, transient heart failure is common and may require treatment with digoxin and a diuretic.

◆ Monitor left atrial pressure directly. A pulmonary artery catheter may also be used to check central venous and pulmonary artery pressures.

◆ Frequently check color and vital signs. Obtain ABG measurements regularly to assess oxygena-

tion to prevent atelectasis [and mo]nitor mechanical ventilation. [Reco]rd intake and output accurately.

◆ If atrioventricular block develops with a low heart rate, a temporary external pacemaker may be necessary.

◆ If blood pressure or cardiac output is inadequate, a catecholamine may be ordered by continuous I.V. infusion. To decrease left ventricular workload, administer nitroprusside, if ordered. Provide an analgesic, as needed.

◆ Keep the parents informed about their child's progress. After discharge, the child may require digoxin, a diuretic, and other drugs. Stress the importance of complying with the prescribed regimen, and make sure the parents know how and when to administer these medications. Teach parents to watch for signs of digoxin toxicity (anorexia, nausea, and vomiting). A prophylactic antibiotic to prevent infective endocarditis will still be required. Advise the parents to avoid becoming overprotective as the child's tolerance for physical activity increases.

THROMBOPHLEBITIS

An acute condition characterized by inflammation and thrombus formation, thrombophlebitis may occur in deep (intermuscular or intramuscular) or superficial (subcutaneous) veins. Deep vein thrombosis (DVT) affects small veins such as the soleal venous sinuses or large veins, such as the vena cava and the femoral, iliac, and subclavian veins, causing venous insufficiency. Thrombophlebitis is typically progressive, leading to pulmonary embolism, a potentially life-threatening complication. Superficial thrombophlebitis is usually self-limiting and seldom leads to pulmonary embolism. Thrombophlebitis typically begins with localized inflammation alone (phlebitis), but such inflammation rapidly provokes thrombus formation. Rarely, venous thrombosis develops without associated inflammation of the vein (phlebothrombosis).

Causes
DVT

◆ Idiopathic, but usually results from endothelial damage, accelerated blood clotting, and reduced blood flow

◆ Predisposing factors include prolonged bed rest, trauma, surgery, childbirth, and use of hormonal contraceptives, such as estrogens

Superficial thrombophlebitis

◆ Chemical irritation due to extensive use of the I.V. route for medications and diagnostic tests

◆ Infection

◆ I.V. drug abuse
◆ Trauma

Pathophysiology
A thrombus occurs when an alteration in the epithelial lining causes platelet aggregation and consequent fibrin entrapment of red and white blood cells and additional platelets. Thrombus formation is more rapid in areas where blood flow is slower, resulting from greater contact between platelet and thrombin accumulation. The rapidly expanding thrombus initiates a chemical inflammatory process in the vessel epithelium, which leads to fibrosis. The enlarging clot may occlude the vessel lumen partially or totally, or it may detach and embolize to lodge elsewhere in systemic circulation.

Signs and symptoms
In both types of thrombophlebitis, clinical features vary with the site and length of the affected vein. Although DVT may occur asymptomatically, it may also produce:
◆ severe pain, fever, chills, and malaise due to inflammation
◆ possibly swelling and cyanosis of the affected arm or leg due to impaired circulation.
   Superficial thrombophlebitis produces visible and palpable signs, such as:
◆ heat, pain, swelling, rubor, tenderness, and induration along the length of the affected vein due to inflammation
◆ possibly varicose veins due to impaired venous return
◆ lymphadenitis if vein involvement is extensive.

Complications
◆ Pulmonary embolism
◆ Chronic venous insufficiency

Diagnosis
◆ Some patients may display signs of inflammation and, possibly, a positive Homans' sign (pain on dorsiflexion of the foot) during physical examination; others are asymptomatic.
◆ Duplex Doppler ultrasonography and impedance plethysmography make it possible to non-invasively examine the major veins (but not calf veins).
◆ Plethysmography shows decreased circulation distal to the affected area; this test is more sensitive than ultrasound in detecting DVT.
◆ Phlebography, which shows filling defects and diverted blood flow, usually confirms the diagnosis.
   Diagnosis must also rule out arterial occlusive disease, lymphangitis, cellulitis, and myositis.
   Diagnosis of superficial thrombophlebitis is based on physical examination (redness and

warmth over the affected area, palpable vein, and pain during palpation or compression).

Treatment
◆ Control thrombus development, prevent complications, relieve pain, and prevent recurrence

Symptomatic measures
◆ Bed rest, with elevation of the affected arm or leg
◆ Warm, moist soaks to the affected area
◆ Analgesic

After acute episode of DVT
◆ Wearing antiembolism stockings applied before getting out of bed
◆ Anticoagulants (initially, heparin; later, warfarin) to prolong clotting time
◆ Low-molecular-weight (LMW) heparin (Although LMW heparin is more expensive, it doesn't require monitoring for its anticoagulant effect. Full anticoagulant doses must be discontinued during any operative period because of the risk of hemorrhage. After some types of surgery, especially major abdominal or pelvic operations prophylactic doses of an anticoagulant may reduce the risk of DVT and pulmonary embolism.)
◆ Insertion of a vena cava filter to prevent mobilization of clots to organs

For lysis of acute, extensive DVT
◆ Streptokinase
◆ Rarely, DVT may cause complete venous occlusion, necessitating venous interruption through simple ligation to vein plication, or clipping
◆ Embolectomy and insertion of a vena caval umbrella or filter

Severe superficial thrombophlebitis
◆ Anti-inflammatory, such as indomethacin
◆ Antiembolism stockings
◆ Warm soaks
◆ Elevation of the leg

Special considerations
Patient teaching, identification of high-risk patients, and measures to prevent venostasis can prevent DVT; close monitoring of anticoagulant therapy can prevent serious complications, such as internal hemorrhage.
◆ Enforce bed rest as ordered, and elevate the patient's affected arm or leg. If you plan to use pillows for elevating the leg, place them so they support the entire length of the affected extremity to prevent possible compression of the popliteal space.

♦ Apply warm soaks to increase circulation to the affected area and to relieve pain and inflammation. Give an analgesic to relieve pain, as ordered.

♦ Measure and record the affected arm or leg's circumference daily and compare this measurement to the other arm or leg. To ensure accuracy and consistency of serial measurements, mark the skin over the area and measure at the same spot daily.

♦ Administer heparin I.V., as ordered, with an infusion monitor or pump to control the flow rate if necessary.

♦ Measure partial thromboplastin time regularly for the patient on heparin therapy; prothrombin time and international normalized ratio (INR) for the patient on warfarin (therapeutic anticoagulation values are 1½ to 2 times control values for prothrombin time and an INR of 2 to 3). Watch for signs and symptoms of bleeding, such as dark, tarry stools; coffee-ground vomitus; and ecchymoses. Encourage the patient to use an electric razor and to avoid medications that contain aspirin.

⚠ **CLINICAL ALERT** *Be alert for signs of pulmonary emboli that include crackles, dyspnea, hemoptysis, sudden changes in mental status, restlessness, and hypotension.*

Preparing for discharge

♦ Emphasize the importance of follow-up blood studies to monitor anticoagulant therapy.

♦ If the patient is being discharged on heparin therapy, teach him or his family how to give subcutaneous injections. If he requires further assistance, arrange for a home health nurse.

♦ Tell the patient to avoid prolonged sitting or standing to help prevent recurrence.

♦ Teach the patient how to properly apply and use antiembolism stockings. Tell him to report any complications, such as cold, blue toes. (See *Preventing thrombophlebitis.*)

♦ To prevent thrombophlebitis in high-risk patients, perform range-of-motion exercises while the patient is on bed rest, use intermittent pneumatic calf massage during lengthy surgical or diagnostic procedures, apply antiembolism stockings postoperatively, and encourage early ambulation.

TRANSPOSITION OF THE GREAT ARTERIES

Transposition of the great arteries is a congenital heart defect in which the great arteries are reversed such that the aorta arises from the right ventricle and the pulmonary artery from the left ventricle, producing two noncommunicating circulatory systems (pulmonic and systemic). The right-to-left shunting of blood leads to an increased risk of heart failure and anoxia. Transposition accounts for about 5% of all congenital heart defects and commonly coexists with other congenital heart defects, such as ventricular septal defect (VSD), VSD with pulmonic stenosis, atrial septal defect (ASD), and patent ductus arteriosus (PDA). It affects two to three times more males than females.

Causes
♦ Unknown

Pathophysiology
Transposition of the great arteries results from faulty embryonic development. Oxygenated blood returning to the left side of the heart is carried back to the lungs by a transposed pulmonary artery. Unoxygenated blood returning to the right side of the heart is carried to the systemic circulation by a transposed aorta.

Communication between the pulmonary and systemic circulations is necessary for survival. In infants with isolated transposition, blood mixes only at the patent foramen ovale and at the PDA, resulting in slight mixing of unoxygenated systemic blood and oxygenated pulmonary blood. In infants with concurrent cardiac defects, greater mixing of blood occurs.

Signs and symptoms
♦ Cyanosis and tachypnea that worsens with crying within the first few hours after birth, when no other heart defects exist that allow mixing of systemic and pulmonary blood (Cyanosis may be minimized with associated defects, such as ASD, VSD, or PDA.)

♦ Gallop rhythm, tachycardia, dyspnea, hepatomegaly, and cardiomegaly within days to weeks due to heart failure

♦ Loud S_2 because the anteriorly transposed aorta is directly behind the sternum

♦ Murmurs of ASD, VSD, or PDA, if these defects are present

♦ Diminished exercise tolerance, fatigability, and clubbing due to reduced oxygenation

Complications
♦ Heart failure
♦ Infective endocarditis

Diagnosis
♦ Chest X-rays are normal in the first days after birth. Within days to weeks, right atrial and right ventricular enlargement characteristically cause the heart to appear oblong. X-ray may also show increased pulmonary vascular markings, except when pulmonic stenosis exists.

◆ Although electrocardiography typically reveals right-axis deviation and right ventricular hypertrophy, results may be normal in a neonate.
◆ Echocardiography demonstrates the reversed position of the aorta and pulmonary artery and records echoes from both semilunar valves simultaneously because of aortic valve displacement. It also detects other cardiac defects.
◆ Cardiac catheterization reveals decreased oxygen saturation in left ventricular blood and aortic blood; increased right atrial, right ventricular, and pulmonary artery oxygen saturation; and right ventricular systolic pressure equal to systemic pressure. Dye injection reveals the transposed vessels and the presence of other cardiac defects.
◆ Arterial blood gas (ABG) analysis indicates hypoxia and secondary metabolic acidosis.

Treatment
◆ Prostaglandin infusion to keep the ductus arteriosus patent until surgical correction
◆ Atrial balloon septostomy (Rashkind procedure) during cardiac catheterization, if needed as a palliative measure until surgery can be performed (It enlarges the patent foramen ovale and thereby improves oxygenation and alleviates hypoxia by allowing greater mixing of blood from the pulmonary and systemic circulations.)
◆ Corrective surgery to redirect blood flow by switching the positions of the major blood vessels (typically performed in the first few weeks of life)

Special considerations
◆ Explain cardiac catheterization and all necessary procedures to the parents. Offer emotional support.
◆ Monitor vital signs, ABG values, urine output, and central venous pressure, watching for signs of heart failure. Administer I.V. fluids, being careful to avoid fluid overload.
◆ Teach parents to recognize signs of heart failure. Stress the importance of regular checkups to monitor cardiovascular status.
◆ Teach parents to protect their infant from infection and to give an antibiotic.
◆ Tell the parents to let their child develop normally. They need not restrict activities; he'll set his own limits.
◆ If the patient is scheduled for surgery, explain the procedure to the parents and child, if old enough. Teach them about the intensive care unit, and introduce them to the staff. Also, explain postoperative care.
◆ Preoperatively, monitor ABG values, acid-base balance, intake and output, and vital signs.

⊘ **PREVENTION**
Preventing thrombophlebitis

To prevent thrombophlebitis in a high-risk patient, perform range-of-motion exercise while the patient is on bedrest, use intermittent pneumatic calf massage during lengthy surgical or diagnostic procedures, apply antiembolism stockings postoperatively, and encourage early ambulation.

After some types of surgery, especially major abdominal or pelvic operations, prophylactic doses of anticoagulants may reduce the risk of deep vein thrombosis and pulmonary embolism.

After corrective surgery
◆ Monitor cardiac output by checking blood pressure, skin color, heart rate, urine output, central venous and left atrial pressures, and level of consciousness. Report abnormalities or changes.
◆ Carefully measure ABG levels.
◆ To detect supraventricular conduction blocks and arrhythmias, monitor the patient closely. Watch for signs of atrioventricular block, atrial arrhythmia, and faulty sinoatrial function.
◆ Encourage parents to help their child assume new activity levels and independence. Teach them about postoperative antibiotic prophylaxis for endocarditis.

VALVULAR HEART DISEASE
In valvular heart disease, three types of mechanical disruption can occur: stenosis, or narrowing, of the valve opening; incomplete closure of the valve; or valve prolapse. Valvular disorders in children and adolescents most commonly occur as a result of congenital heart defects. In adults, rheumatic heart disease is a common cause.

Causes
The causes of valvular heart disease are varied and are different for each type of valve disorder. (See *Types of valvular heart disease*, pages 198 and 199.)

Pathophysiology
Pathophysiology of valvular heart disease varies according to the valve and the disorder.

(Text continues on page 200.)

Types of valvular heart disease

Causes and incidence	Clinical findings

Mitral insufficiency

♦ Results from rheumatic fever, hypertrophic obstructive cardiomyopathy, mitral valve prolapse, myocardial infarction, severe left ventricular dilation or left-sided heart failure, or ruptured chordae tendineae
♦ Associated with other congenital anomalies, such as transposition of the great arteries
♦ Rare in children without other congenital anomalies

♦ Orthopnea, dyspnea, fatigue, angina, and palpitations
♦ Peripheral edema, jugular vein distention, and hepatomegaly (right-sided heart failure)
♦ Tachycardia, crackles, and pulmonary edema
♦ Auscultation revealing a holosystolic murmur at apex, a possible split S_2, and an S_3

Mitral stenosis

♦ Results from rheumatic fever (most common cause) or endocarditis
♦ Most common in females
♦ May be associated with other congenital anomalies

♦ Exertional dyspnea, paroxysmal nocturnal dyspnea, orthopnea, weakness, fatigue, and palpitations
♦ Peripheral edema, jugular vein distention, ascites, and hepatomegaly (right-sided heart failure)
♦ Crackles, atrial fibrillation, and signs of systemic emboli
♦ Auscultation revealing a loud S_1 or opening snap and a diastolic murmur at the apex

Aortic insufficiency

♦ Results from rheumatic fever, syphilis, hypertension, or endocarditis or may be idiopathic
♦ Associated with Marfan syndrome
♦ Most common in males
♦ Associated with ventricular septal defect, even after surgical closure

♦ Dyspnea, cough, fatigue, palpitations, angina, and syncope
♦ Pulmonary congestion, left-sided heart failure, and "pulsating" nail beds (Quincke's sign)
♦ Rapidly rising and collapsing pulses (pulsus biferiens), cardiac arrhythmias, and widened pulse pressure
♦ Auscultation revealing an S_3 and a diastolic blowing murmur at left sternal border
♦ Palpation and visualization of apical impulse in chronic disease

Aortic stenosis

♦ Results from congenital aortic bicuspid valve (associated with coarctation of the aorta), congenital stenosis of valve cusps, rheumatic fever, or atherosclerosis in elderly patients
♦ Most common in males

♦ Exertional dyspnea, paroxysmal nocturnal dyspnea, fatigue, syncope, angina, and palpitations
♦ Pulmonary congestion and left-sided heart failure
♦ Diminished carotid pulses, decreased cardiac output, and cardiac arrhythmias; may have alternating pulse
♦ Auscultation revealing systolic murmur heard at base or in carotids and, possibly, an S_4

Pulmonic stenosis

♦ Results from congenital stenosis of valve cusp or rheumatic heart disease (uncommon)
♦ Associated with tetralogy of Fallot

♦ Asymptomatic or symptomatic with exertional dyspnea, fatigue, chest pain, and syncope
♦ May cause jugular vein distention or right-sided heart failure
♦ Auscultation revealing a systolic murmur at the left sternal border and a split S_2 with a delayed or absent pulmonic component

Diagnostic measures

♦ *Cardiac catheterization:* mitral insufficiency with increased left ventricular end-diastolic volume and pressure, increased atrial pressure and pulmonary artery wedge pressure (PAWP), and decreased cardiac output
♦ *Chest X-rays:* left atrial and ventricular enlargement and pulmonary vein congestion
♦ *Echocardiography:* abnormal valve leaflet motion and left atrial enlargement
♦ *Electrocardiography (ECG):* may show left atrial and ventricular hypertrophy, sinus tachycardia, and atrial fibrillation

♦ *Cardiac catheterization:* diastolic pressure gradient across valve; elevated left atrial pressure and PAWP >15 mm Hg with severe pulmonary hypertension; elevated right-sided heart pressure with decreased cardiac output; and abnormal contraction of the left ventricle
♦ *Chest X-rays:* left atrial and ventricular enlargement, enlarged pulmonary arteries, and mitral valve calcification
♦ *Echocardiography:* thickened mitral valve leaflets and left atrial enlargement
♦ *ECG:* left atrial hypertrophy, atrial fibrillation, right ventricular hypertrophy, and right-axis deviation

♦ *Cardiac catheterization:* reduction in arterial diastolic pressures, aortic insufficiency, other valvular abnormalities, and increased left ventricular end-diastolic pressure
♦ *Chest X-rays:* left ventricular enlargement and pulmonary vein congestion
♦ *Echocardiography:* left ventricular enlargement, alterations in mitral valve movement (indirect indication of aortic valve disease), and mitral thickening
♦ *ECG:* sinus tachycardia, left ventricular hypertrophy, and left atrial hypertrophy in severe disease

♦ *Cardiac catheterization:* pressure gradient across valve (indicating obstruction) and increased left ventricular end-diastolic pressures
♦ *Chest X-rays:* valvular calcification, left ventricular enlargement, and pulmonary vein congestion
♦ *Echocardiography:* thickened aortic valve and left ventricular wall, possibly coexistent with mitral valve stenosis
♦ *ECG:* left ventricular hypertrophy

♦ *Cardiac catheterization:* increased right ventricular pressure, decreased pulmonary artery pressure, and abnormal valve orifice
♦ *ECG:* may show right ventricular hypertrophy, right-axis deviation, right atrial hypertrophy, and atrial fibrillation

Mitral insufficiency

An abnormality of the mitral leaflets, mitral annulus, chordae tendineae, papillary muscles, left atrium, or left ventricle can lead to mitral insufficiency. Blood from the left ventricle flows back into the left atrium during systole, causing the atrium to enlarge to accommodate the backflow. As a result, the left ventricle also dilates to accommodate the increased blood volume from the atrium and to compensate for diminishing cardiac output. Ventricular hypertrophy and increased end-diastolic pressure result in increased pulmonary artery pressure, eventually leading to left-sided and right-sided heart failure.

Mitral stenosis

Narrowing of the valve by valvular abnormalities, fibrosis, or calcification obstructs blood flow from the left atrium to the left ventricle. Consequently, left atrial volume and pressure rise and the chamber dilates. Greater resistance to blood flow causes pulmonary hypertension, right ventricular hypertrophy, and right-sided heart failure. Also, inadequate filling of the left ventricle produces low cardiac output.

Aortic insufficiency

Blood flows back into the left ventricle during diastole, causing fluid overload in the ventricle, which dilates and hypertrophies. The excess volume causes fluid overload in the left atrium and, finally, the pulmonary system. Left-sided heart failure and pulmonary edema eventually result.

Aortic stenosis

Increased left ventricular pressure tries to overcome the resistance of the narrowed valvular opening. The added workload increases the demand for oxygen, and diminished cardiac output causes poor coronary artery perfusion, ischemia of the left ventricle, and left-sided heart failure.

Pulmonic stenosis

Obstructed right ventricular outflow causes right ventricular hypertrophy, eventually resulting in right-sided heart failure.

Signs and symptoms

The clinical manifestations vary according to the type of valvular defects. (See *Types of valvular heart disease,* pages 198 and 199, for specific clinical features of each valve disorder.)

Complications

◆ Heart failure
◆ Pulmonary edema
◆ Thromboembolism

◆ Endocarditis
◆ Arrhythmias

Diagnosis

The diagnosis of valvular heart disease can be made through cardiac catheterization, chest X-rays, echocardiography, or electrocardiography. (See *Types of valvular heart disease,* pages 198 and 199.)

Treatment

◆ Digoxin, a low-sodium diet, a diuretic, a vasodilator, and especially an angiotensin-converting enzyme inhibitor to treat left-sided heart failure
◆ Oxygen in acute situations, to increase oxygenation
◆ An anticoagulant to prevent thrombus formation around diseased or replaced valves
◆ A prophylactic antibiotic before and after surgery or dental care to prevent endocarditis
◆ Nitroglycerin to relieve angina in conditions such as aortic stenosis
◆ A beta-adrenergic blocker or digoxin to slow the ventricular rate in atrial fibrillation or atrial flutter
◆ Cardioversion to convert atrial fibrillation to sinus rhythm
◆ Open or closed commissurotomy to separate thick or adherent mitral valve leaflets
◆ Balloon valvuloplasty to enlarge the orifice of a stenotic mitral, aortic, or pulmonic valve
◆ Annuloplasty or valvuloplasty to reconstruct or repair the valve in mitral insufficiency
◆ Valve replacement with a prosthetic valve for mitral and aortic valve disease

Special considerations

◆ Watch closely for signs of heart failure or pulmonary edema and for adverse reactions to drug therapy.
◆ Teach the patient about diet restrictions, medications, and the importance of consistent follow-up care.
◆ If the patient has had surgery, watch for hypotension, arrhythmias, and thrombus formation. Monitor vital signs, arterial blood gas values, intake, output, daily weight, blood chemistries, chest X-rays, and pulmonary artery catheter readings.

VARICOSE VEINS

Varicose veins are dilated, tortuous veins, engorged with blood and resulting from improper venous valve function. They can be primary, originating in the superficial veins, or secondary, occurring in the deep veins.

Primary varicose veins tend to be familial and to affect both legs; they're twice as common in females as in males. They account for about 90% of varicose veins; 10% to 20% of Americans have primary varicose veins. Usually, secondary varicose veins occur in one leg. Both types are more common in middle adulthood.

Without treatment, varicose veins continue to enlarge. Although there's no cure, certain measures, such as walking and using compression stockings, can reduce symptoms. Surgery may remove varicose veins, but the condition can occur in other veins.

Causes

Primary varicose veins

◆ Conditions that produce prolonged venous stasis or increased intra-abdominal pressure, such as pregnancy, obesity, constipation, or wearing tight clothes
◆ Congenital weakness of the valves or venous wall
◆ Family history of varicose veins
◆ Occupations that necessitate standing for an extended period

Secondary varicose veins

◆ Arteriovenous fistulas
◆ Deep vein thrombosis
◆ Occlusion
◆ Trauma to the venous system
◆ Venous malformation

Pathophysiology

Veins are thin-walled, distensible vessels with valves that keep blood flowing in one direction. Any condition that weakens, destroys, or distends these valves allows blood backflow to the previous valve. If a valve can't hold the pooling blood, it can become incompetent, allowing even more blood to flow backward. As the volume of venous blood builds, pressure in the vein increases and the vein becomes distended. As the veins are stretched, their walls weaken and they lose their elasticity. As the veins enlarge, they become lumpy and tortuous. As hydrostatic pressure increases, plasma is forced out of the veins and into the surrounding tissues, resulting in edema.

People who stand for prolonged periods may also develop venous pooling because there's no muscular contraction in the legs, forcing blood back up to the heart. If the valves in the veins are too weak to hold the pooling blood, they begin to leak, allowing blood to flow backward.

Signs and symptoms

◆ Dilated, tortuous, purplish, ropelike veins, particularly in the calves, due to venous pooling
◆ Edema of the calves and ankles due to deep vein incompetence
◆ Leg heaviness that worsens in the evening and in warm weather; caused by venous pooling
◆ Dull aching in the legs after prolonged standing or walking, which may be due to tissue breakdown
◆ Aching during menses as a result of increased fluid retention

Complications

◆ Blood clots secondary to venous stasis
◆ Venous stasis ulcers
◆ Chronic venous insufficiency

■ **AGE ALERT** *As a person ages, veins dilate and stretch, increasing susceptibility to varicose veins and chronic venous insufficiency. Because the skin is friable and can easily break down, ulcers in an older adult caused by chronic venous insufficiency may take longer to heal.*

Diagnosis

◆ A manual compression test detects a palpable impulse when the vein is firmly occluded at least 8″ (20 cm) above the point of palpation, indicating incompetent valves in the vein.
◆ Trendelenburg's test (retrograde filling test) detects incompetent deep and superficial vein valves.
◆ Photoplethysmography characterizes venous blood flow by noting changes in the skin's circulation.
◆ Doppler ultrasonography detects the presence or absence of venous backflow in deep or superficial veins.
◆ Venous outflow and reflux plethysmography detects deep venous occlusion; this test is invasive and not routinely used.
◆ Ascending and descending venography demonstrates venous occlusion and patterns of collateral flow.

Treatment

◆ Treatment of the underlying cause, such as an abdominal tumor or obesity, if possible
◆ Antiembolism stockings or elastic bandages to counteract swelling by supporting the veins and improving circulation
◆ Regular exercise to promote muscular contraction to force blood through the veins and reduce venous pooling
◆ Injection of a sclerosing agent into small to medium-sized varicosities
◆ Surgical stripping and ligation of severe varicose veins
◆ Phlebectomy, removing the varicose vein through small incisions in the skin, which may be performed in an outpatient setting

◆ Discouraging the patient from wearing constrictive clothing that interferes with venous return

◆ Encouraging the obese patient to lose weight to reduce increased intra-abdominal pressure

◆ Telling the patient to elevate her legs above her heart whenever possible to promote venous return

◆ Instructing the patient to avoid prolonged standing or sitting because these actions enhance venous pooling

Special considerations

◆ After stripping and ligation or after injection of a sclerosing agent, administer an analgesic, as ordered, to relieve pain.

◆ Frequently check circulation in toes (color and temperature), and observe elastic bandages for bleeding. When ordered, rewrap bandages at least once per shift, wrapping from toe to thigh, with the leg elevated.

⚠ **CLINICAL ALERT** *Watch for signs and symptoms of complications, such as sensory loss in the leg (which could indicate saphenous nerve damage), calf pain (which could indicate thrombophlebitis), and fever (a sign of infection).*

VENTRICULAR SEPTAL DEFECT

In a ventricular septal defect (VSD), an opening in the septum between the ventricles allows blood to shunt between the left and right ventricles. This results in ineffective pumping of the heart and increases the risk of heart failure.

VSDs account for up to 30% of all congenital heart defects. The prognosis is good for defects that close spontaneously or are correctable surgically, but poor for untreated defects, which are sometimes fatal in children by age 1, usually from secondary complications.

Causes

◆ Down syndrome and other autosomal trisomies

◆ Fetal alcohol syndrome

◆ Patent ductus arteriosus and coarctation of the aorta

◆ Prematurity

◆ Renal anomalies

Pathophysiology

In infants with a VSD, the ventricular septum fails to close completely by eight weeks' gestation. VSDs are located in the membranous or muscular portion of the ventricular septum and vary in size. Some defects close spontaneously; in other defects, the septum is entirely absent, creating a single ventricle. Small VSDs are likely to close spontaneously. Large VSDs should be surgically repaired before pulmonary vascular disease occurs or while it's still reversible.

A VSD isn't readily apparent at birth because right and left pressures are about equal and pulmonary artery resistance is elevated. Alveoli aren't yet completely opened, so blood doesn't shunt through the defect. As the pulmonary vasculature gradually relaxes, between 4 and 8 weeks after birth, right ventricular pressure decreases, allowing blood to shunt from the left to the right ventricle. Initially, large VSD shunts cause left atrial and left ventricular hypertrophy. Later, an uncorrected VSD causes right ventricular hypertrophy due to increasing pulmonary resistance. Eventually, right- and left-sided heart failure and cyanosis (from reversal of the shunt direction) occur. Fixed pulmonary hypertension may occur much later in life with right-to-left shunting (Eisenmenger's syndrome), causing cyanosis and clubbing of the nail beds.

Signs and symptoms

◆ Thin, small infants who gain weight slowly when a large VSD is present secondary to heart failure

◆ Loud, harsh, widely transmitted systolic murmur heard best along the left sternal border at the third or fourth intercostal space, caused by abnormal blood flow through the VSD

◆ Palpable thrill caused by turbulent blood flow between the ventricles through a small VSD

◆ Loud, widely split pulmonic component of S_2 caused by increased pressure gradient across the VSD

◆ Displacement of point of maximal impulse to the left due to hypertrophy of the heart

▮ **AGE ALERT** *Typically, the apical impulse in infants is palpated over the fourth intercostal space, just to the left of the midclavicular line. In children older than age 7, it's palpated over the fifth intercostal space. When the heart is enlarged, the apical beat is displaced to the left or downward.*

◆ Prominent anterior chest secondary to cardiac hypertrophy

◆ Liver, heart, and spleen enlargement because of systemic congestion

◆ Feeding difficulties associated with heart failure

◆ Diaphoresis, tachycardia, and rapid, grunting respirations secondary to heart failure

◆ Cyanosis and clubbing if right-to-left shunting occurs later in life secondary to pulmonary hypertension

Complications

◆ Pulmonary hypertension

◆ Infective endocarditis

◆ Pneumonia

◆ Heart failure
◆ Eisenmenger's syndrome
◆ Aortic insufficiency (if the aortic valve is involved)

Diagnosis

◆ Chest X-rays appear normal in small defects. In large VSDs, the X-ray may show cardiomegaly, left atrial and left ventricular enlargement, and prominent vascular markings.
◆ Electrocardiography may be normal with small VSDs, whereas in large VSDs it may show left and right ventricular hypertrophy, suggestive of pulmonary hypertension.
◆ Echocardiography can detect a VSD in the septum, estimate the size of the left-to-right shunt, suggest pulmonary hypertension, and identify associated lesions and complications.
◆ Cardiac catheterization determines the size and exact location of the VSD and the extent of pulmonary hypertension; it also detects associated defects. It calculates the degree of shunting by comparing the blood oxygen saturation in each ventricle. The oxygen saturation of the right ventricle is greater than normal because oxygenated blood is shunted from the left to the right ventricle.

Treatment

Many VSDs (20% to 60%) may close spontaneously during the first year of life, especially small VSDs. Correction involves:
◆ early surgical correction for a large VSD, usually performed using a patch graft, before heart failure and irreversible pulmonary vascular disease develop
◆ placement of a permanent pacemaker, which may be necessary after VSD repair if complete heart block develops from interference with the bundle of His during surgery
◆ surgical closure of small defects using sutures (They may not be surgically repaired if the patient has normal pulmonary artery pressure and a small shunt.)
◆ pulmonary artery banding to normalize pressures and flow distal to the band and to prevent pulmonary vascular disease if the child has other defects and will benefit from delaying surgery
◆ digoxin, sodium restriction, and a diuretic before surgery to prevent heart failure
◆ a prophylactic antibiotic before and after surgery to prevent infective endocarditis.

Special considerations

Although the parents of an infant with a VSD commonly suspect something is wrong with their child before diagnosis, they need psychological support to help them accept the reality of a serious cardiac disorder. Because surgery may take place months after diagnosis, parent teaching is vital to prevent complications until the child is scheduled for surgery or the defect closes. Thorough explanations of all tests are also essential.
◆ Instruct parents to watch for signs of heart failure, such as poor feeding, sweating, and heavy breathing.
◆ If the child is receiving digoxin or other medications, tell the parents how to give it and how to recognize adverse reactions. Caution them to keep medications out of the reach of all children.
◆ Teach parents to recognize and report early signs of infection and to avoid exposing the child to people with obvious infections.
◆ Encourage parents to let the child engage in normal activities.
◆ Stress the importance of taking a prophylactic antibiotic before and after surgery.

After surgery

◆ Monitor vital signs and intake and output. Maintain the infant's body temperature with an overbed warmer. Give a catecholamine, nitroprusside, and a diuretic, as ordered, and an analgesic as needed.
◆ Monitor central venous pressure, intra-arterial blood pressure, and left atrial or pulmonary artery pressure readings. Assess heart rate and rhythm for signs of conduction block.
◆ Check oxygenation, particularly in a child who requires mechanical ventilation. Suction as needed to maintain a patent airway and to prevent atelectasis and pneumonia.
◆ Monitor pacemaker effectiveness, if needed. Watch for signs of failure, such as bradycardia and hypotension.
◆ Reassure parents, and allow them to participate in their child's care.

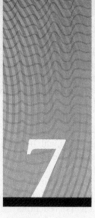

RESPIRATORY SYSTEM

The respiratory system's major function is gas exchange, in which air enters the body on inhalation (inspiration); travels throughout the respiratory passages, exchanging oxygen for carbon dioxide at the tissue level; and expels carbon dioxide on exhalation (expiration).

The upper airway—composed of the nose, mouth, pharynx, and larynx—allows airflow into the lungs. This area is responsible for warming, humidifying, and filtering the air, thereby protecting the lower airway from foreign matter.

The lower airway consists of the trachea, mainstem bronchi, secondary bronchi, bronchioles, and terminal bronchioles. These structures are anatomic dead spaces and function only as passageways for moving air into and out of the lungs. Distal to each terminal bronchiole is the acinus, which consists of respiratory bronchioles, alveolar ducts, and alveolar sacs. The bronchioles and ducts function as conduits, and the alveoli are the chief units of gas exchange. These final subdivisions of the bronchial tree make up the lobules—the functional units of the lungs. (See *Structure of the lobule*.)

In addition to warming, humidifying, and filtering inspired air, the lower airway protects the lungs with several defense mechanisms. Clearance mechanisms include the cough reflex and mucociliary system. The *mucociliary system* produces mucus, which traps foreign particles. Foreign matter is then swept to the upper airway for expectoration by specialized fingerlike projections called cilia. A breakdown in the epithelium of the lungs or the mucociliary system can cause the defense mechanisms to malfunction,

and pollutants and irritants then enter and inflame the lungs. The lower airway also provides immunologic protection and initiates pulmonary injury responses.

The external component of respiration (ventilation or breathing) delivers inspired air to the lower respiratory tract and alveoli. Contraction and relaxation of the respiratory muscles moves air into and out of the lungs.

Normal expiration is passive; the inspiratory muscles cease to contract, and the elastic recoil of the lungs and the chest wall causes them to contract again. These actions raise the pressure within the lungs to above atmospheric pressure, moving air from the lungs to the atmosphere.

An adult lung contains an estimated 300 million alveoli; each alveolus is supplied by many capillaries. To reach the capillary lumen, oxygen must cross the alveolar capillary membrane.

The pulmonary alveoli promote gas exchange by diffusion—the passage of gas molecules through respiratory membranes. In diffusion, oxygen passes to the blood, and carbon dioxide, a by-product of cellular metabolism, passes out of the blood and is channeled away.

Circulating blood delivers oxygen to the cells of the body for metabolism and transports metabolic wastes and carbon dioxide from the tissues back to the lungs. When oxygenated arterial blood reaches tissue capillaries, the oxygen diffuses from the blood into the cells because of an oxygen tension gradient. The amount of oxygen available to cells depends on the concentration of hemoglobin (the principal carrier of oxygen) in the blood, the regional blood flow, the arterial oxygen content, and cardiac output.

CLOSER LOOK
Structure of the lobule

Each lobule contains terminal bronchioles, respiratory bronchioles, and the alveolar sacs.

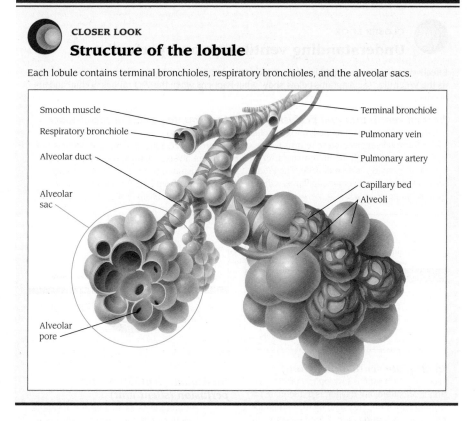

Smooth muscle

Respiratory bronchiole

Alveolar duct

Alveolar sac

Alveolar pore

Terminal bronchiole

Pulmonary vein

Pulmonary artery

Capillary bed

Alveoli

Because circulation is continuous, carbon dioxide doesn't normally accumulate in tissues. Carbon dioxide produced during cellular respiration diffuses from tissues to regional capillaries and is transported by the systemic venous circulation. When carbon dioxide reaches the alveolar capillaries, it diffuses into the alveoli, where the partial pressure of carbon dioxide ($Paco_2$) is lower. Carbon dioxide is removed from the alveoli during exhalation.

For effective gas exchange, ventilation and perfusion at the alveolar level must match closely. (See *Understanding ventilation and perfusion,* page 206.)

The ratio of ventilation to perfusion is called the $\dot{V}/\dot{Q}$ ratio. A $\dot{V}/\dot{Q}$ mismatch can result from ventilation-perfusion dysfunction or altered lung mechanics.

The amount of air carrying oxygen that reaches the lungs depends on lung volume and capacity, compliance, and resistance to airflow. Changes in compliance can occur in either the lung or the chest wall. Destruction of the lung's elastic fibers, which occurs in acute respiratory distress syndrome, decreases lung compliance. The lungs become stiff, making breathing difficult. The alveolar capillary membrane may also be affected, causing hypoxia. Chest wall compliance is affected by disorders causing thoracic deformity, muscle spasm, and abdominal distention.

Respiration is also controlled neurologically by the lateral medulla oblongata of the brain stem. Impulses travel down the phrenic nerves to the diaphragm and then down the intercostal nerves to the intercostal muscles between the ribs. The rate and depth of respiration are controlled similarly.

Apneustic and pneumotaxic centers in the pons of the midbrain influence the pattern of breathing. Stimulation of the lower pontine apneustic center (by trauma, tumor, or stroke) produces forceful inspiratory gasps alternating with weak expiration. This pattern doesn't occur if the vagi are intact. The apneustic center continually excites the medullary inspiratory center and thus facilitates inspiration. Signals from the pneumotaxic center and afferent impulses from the vagus nerve inhibit the apneustic center and "turn off" inspiration.

In addition, chemoreceptors respond to the hydrogen ion concentration of arterial blood

CLOSER LOOK
Understanding ventilation and perfusion

Effective gas exchange depends on the relationship between ventilation and perfusion, expressed as the $\dot{V}/\dot{Q}$ ratio. The diagrams below show what happens when the $\dot{V}/\dot{Q}$ ratio is normal and abnormal.

Normal ventilation and perfusion
When the $\dot{V}/\dot{Q}$ ratio is matched, unoxygenated blood from the venous system returns to the right ventricle through the pulmonary artery to the lungs, carrying carbon dioxide. The arteries branch into the alveolar capillaries, where gas exchange occurs.

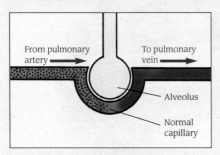

Inadequate perfusion (dead-space ventilation)
When the $\dot{V}/\dot{Q}$ ratio is high, ventilation is normal, but alveolar perfusion is reduced or absent (illustrated by the perfusion blockage). This results from a perfusion defect, such as pulmonary embolism or a disorder that decreases cardiac output.

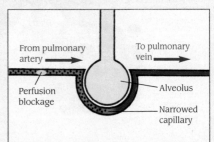

Inadequate ventilation (shunt)
When the $\dot{V}/\dot{Q}$ ratio is low, pulmonary circulation is adequate, but oxygen is inadequate for normal diffusion (illustrated by the ventilation blockage). A portion of the blood flowing through the pulmonary vessels doesn't become oxygenated.

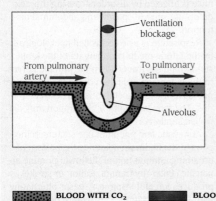

Inadequate ventilation and perfusion (silent unit)
The silent unit indicates an absence of ventilation and perfusion to the lung area (illustrated by blockages in perfusion and ventilation). The silent unit may try to compensate for this $\dot{V}/\dot{Q}$ imbalance by delivering blood flow to better-ventilated lung areas.

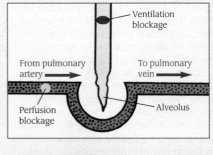

BLOOD WITH CO_2	BLOOD WITH O_2	BLOOD WITH CO_2 AND O_2

(pH), $Paco_2$, and the partial pressure of arterial oxygen (Pao_2). Central chemoreceptors respond indirectly to arterial blood by sensing changes in the pH of the cerebrospinal fluid (CSF). $Paco_2$ also helps regulate ventilation by impacting the pH of CSF. If $Paco_2$ is high, the respiratory rate increases; if $Paco_2$ is low, the respiratory rate decreases. Information from peripheral chemoreceptors in the carotid and aortic bodies also responds to decreased Pao_2 and pH. Either change results in increased respiratory drive within minutes.

Pathophysiologic changes

Pathophysiologic manifestations of respiratory disease may stem from atelectasis, bronchiectasis, cyanosis, and hypoxemia.

ATELECTASIS

Atelectasis occurs when the alveolar sacs or entire lung segments expand incompletely, producing a partial or complete lung collapse. This phenomenon removes certain regions of the lung from gas exchange, allowing unoxygenated blood to pass unchanged through these regions and resulting in hypoxia. Atelectasis may be chronic or acute, and commonly occurs in patients undergoing upper-abdominal or thoracic surgery. There are two major causes of collapse due to atelectasis: *absorption atelectasis,* secondary to bronchial or bronchiolar obstruction, and *compression atelectasis.*

Absorption atelectasis

Bronchial occlusion, which prevents air from entering the alveoli distal to the obstruction, can cause absorption atelectasis — the air present in the alveoli is absorbed gradually into the bloodstream and eventually the alveoli collapse. This may result from intrinsic or extrinsic bronchial obstruction. The most common intrinsic cause is retained secretions or exudate forming mucus plugs. Such disorders as cystic fibrosis, chronic bronchitis, and pneumonia increase the risk of absorption atelectasis. Extrinsic bronchial atelectasis usually results from occlusion caused by foreign bodies, bronchogenic carcinoma, and scar tissue.

Impaired production of surfactant can also cause absorption atelectasis. Increasing surface tension of the alveolus due to reduced surfactant leads to collapse.

Compression atelectasis

Compression atelectasis results from external compression, which drives the air out and causes the lung to collapse. This may result from upper-

Causes of bronchiectasis

Bronchiectasis results from conditions associated with repeated damage to bronchial walls and with abnormal mucociliary clearance, leading to a breakdown in the supporting tissue adjacent to the airways. Such conditions include:

◆ complications of measles, pneumonia, pertussis, or influenza
◆ congenital anomalies, such as bronchomalacia, congenital bronchiectasis, and Kartagener's syndrome (bronchiectasis, sinusitis, and dextrocardia)
◆ cystic fibrosis
◆ immune disorders (agammaglobulinemia)
◆ inhalation of corrosive gas or repeated aspiration of gastric juices into the lungs
◆ obstruction (from a foreign body, tumor, or stenosis) with recurrent infection
◆ rare disorders, such as immotile cilia syndrome
◆ recurrent bacterial respiratory tract infections that were inadequately treated (tuberculosis).

abdominal surgical incisions, rib fractures, pleuritic chest pain, tight chest dressings, and obesity (which elevates the diaphragm and reduces tidal volume). These situations inhibit full lung expansion or make deep breathing painful, thus resulting in this disorder.

BRONCHIECTASIS

Bronchiectasis is marked by chronic abnormal dilation of the bronchi and destruction of the bronchial walls and can occur throughout the tracheobronchial tree. It may also be confined to a single segment or lobe. This disorder is usually bilateral in nature and involves the basilar segments of the lower lobes.

There are three forms of bronchiectasis: cylindrical, fusiform (varicose), and saccular (cystic). It results from conditions associated with repeated damage to bronchial walls with abnormal mucociliary clearance, which causes a breakdown of supporting tissue adjacent to the airways. (See *Causes of bronchiectasis.*)

In patients with bronchiectasis, sputum stagnates in the dilated bronchi and leads to secondary infection, characterized by inflammation and leukocytic accumulations. Additional debris collects within and occludes the bronchi. Increasing pressure from the retained secretions induces mucosal injury.

Major causes of hypoxemia

This chart lists the major causes of hypoxemia and contributing factors.

Major cause	Contributing factors
Alveolar capillary diffusion abnormality	Emphysema, conditions resulting in fibrosis, or pulmonary edema
Decrease in inspired oxygen	High altitudes, inhaling poorly oxygenated gases, or breathing in an enclosed space
Hypoventilation	Respiratory center inappropriately stimulated (such as by oversedation, overdosage, or neurologic damage), chronic obstructive pulmonary disease
Shunting	Acute respiratory distress syndrome, idiopathic respiratory distress syndrome of the newborn, or atelectasis
Ventilation-perfusion mismatch	Asthma, chronic bronchitis, or pneumonia

CYANOSIS

Cyanosis is a bluish discoloration of the skin and mucous membranes. In most populations, it's readily detectable by a visible blue tinge on the nail beds and lips. *Central cyanosis* indicates decreased oxygen saturation of hemoglobin in arterial blood, which is best observed in the buccal mucous membranes and the lips. *Peripheral cyanosis* is a slowed blood circulation of the fingers and toes that's best visualized by examining the nail bed area.

⚠ **CLINICAL ALERT** *In patients with black or dark complexions, cyanosis may not be evident in the lip area or nail beds. A better indicator in these individuals is to assess the membranes of the oral mucosa (buccal mucous membranes) and of the conjunctivae of the eyes.*

Cyanosis is caused by desaturation of arterial blood with oxygen or reduced hemoglobin amounts. It develops when unsaturated hemoglobin reaches 5 g/ml, even if hemoglobin counts are adequate or reduced. Conditions that result in cyanosis include decreased arterial oxygenation (indicated by low Pao$_2$), pulmonary or cardiac right-to-left shunts, decreased cardiac output, anxiety, and a cold environment.

An individual who isn't cyanotic doesn't necessarily have adequate oxygenation. Inadequate tissue oxygenation occurs in severe anemia, resulting in inadequate hemoglobin concentration. It also occurs in carbon monoxide poisoning, in which hemoglobin binds to carbon monoxide instead of to oxygen. Although assessment doesn't reveal cyanosis, oxygenation is inadequate.

Another patient may appear cyanotic even though oxygenation is adequate — as in polycythemia, an abnormal increase in the red blood cell count. Because the hemoglobin level is increased and oxygenation occurs at a normal rate, the patient may still present with cyanosis.

Cyanosis as a presenting condition must be interpreted in relation to the patient's underlying pathophysiology. Diagnosis of inadequate oxygenation may be confirmed by analyzing arterial blood gases and measuring Pao$_2$.

HYPOXEMIA

Hypoxemia is reduced oxygenation of the arterial blood, evidenced by reduced Pao$_2$ of arterial blood. It's caused by respiratory alterations, whereas hypoxia is diminished tissue oxygenation at the cellular level that may be caused by conditions affecting other body systems that are unrelated to alterations of pulmonary function. Low cardiac output or cyanide poisoning can result in hypoxia, in addition to alterations in respiration. Hypoxia can occur anywhere in the body. If hypoxia occurs in the blood, it's termed *hypoxemia.* Hypoxemia can lead to tissue hypoxia.

Hypoxemia can be caused by decreased oxygen content of inspired gas, hypoventilation, diffusion abnormalities, abnormal $\dot{V}/\dot{Q}$ ratios, and pulmonary right-to-left shunts. The physiologic mechanism for each cause of hypoxemia varies. (See *Major causes of hypoxemia.*)

Disorders

Respiratory disorders can be acute or chronic. The disorders described here include examples from each type.

||| LIFE-THREATENING DISORDER

ACUTE RESPIRATORY DISTRESS SYNDROME

Acute respiratory distress syndrome (ARDS) is a form of pulmonary edema that can quickly lead to acute respiratory failure. Also known as *shock lung, stiff lung, white lung, wet lung,* or *Da Nang lung,* ARDS may follow direct or indirect injury to the lung. However, its diagnosis is difficult, and death can occur within 48 hours of onset if not promptly diagnosed and treated. A differential diagnosis needs to rule out cardiogenic pulmonary edema, pulmonary vasculitis, and diffuse pulmonary hemorrhage. Patients who recover may have little or no permanent lung damage.

Causes

◆ Acute miliary tuberculosis
◆ Anaphylaxis
◆ Aspiration of gastric contents
◆ Coronary artery bypass grafting
◆ Diffuse pneumonia, especially viral pneumonia
◆ Drug overdose, such as heroin, aspirin, or ethchlorvynol
◆ Hemodialysis
◆ Idiosyncratic drug reaction to ampicillin or hydrochlorothiazide
◆ Inhalation of noxious gases, such as nitrous oxide, ammonia, or chlorine
◆ Injury to the lung from trauma (most common cause) such as airway contusion
◆ Leukemia
◆ Near drowning
◆ Oxygen toxicity
◆ Pancreatitis
◆ Sepsis
◆ Thrombotic thrombocytopenic purpura
◆ Trauma-related factors, such as fat emboli, sepsis, shock, pulmonary contusions, and multiple transfusions, which increase the likelihood that microemboli will develop
◆ Uremia
◆ Venous air embolism

Pathophysiology

Injury in ARDS involves the alveolar epithelium and pulmonary capillary endothelium. (See *Looking at ARDS,* page 210.) A cascade of cellular and biochemical changes is triggered by the specific causative agent. (See *How ARDS affects the body,* pages 212 and 213.)

Signs and symptoms

◆ Rapid, shallow breathing and dyspnea, which occur hours to days after the initial injury in response to decreasing oxygen levels in the blood
◆ Increased rate of ventilation due to hypoxemia and its effects on the pneumotaxic center
◆ Intercostal and suprasternal retractions due to the increased effort required to expand the stiff lung
◆ Crackles and rhonchi, which are audible and result from fluid accumulation in the lungs
◆ Restlessness, apprehension, and mental sluggishness, which occur as the result of brain hypoxia
◆ Motor dysfunction, which occurs as hypoxia progresses
◆ Tachycardia, which signals the heart's effort to deliver more oxygen to the cells and vital organs
◆ Respiratory acidosis, which occurs as carbon dioxide accumulates in the blood and oxygen levels decrease
◆ Metabolic acidosis, which eventually results from failure of compensatory mechanisms

Complications

◆ Hypotension
◆ Decreased urine output
◆ Metabolic acidosis
◆ Respiratory acidosis
◆ Multiple organ dysfunction syndrome
◆ Ventricular fibrillation
◆ Ventricular standstill

Diagnosis

◆ Arterial blood gas (ABG) analysis with the patient breathing room air initially reveals a decreased ratio of Pao_2 to the fraction of inspired oxygen (less than or equal to 200 mm Hg), a long with a reduced Pao_2 (less than 60 mm Hg) and a decreased $Paco_2$ (less than 35 mm Hg). Hypoxemia, despite increased supplemental oxygen, is the hallmark of ARDS; the resulting blood pH reflects respiratory alkalosis. As ARDS worsens, ABG values show respiratory acidosis evident by an increasing $Paco_2$ (over 45 mm Hg), metabolic acidosis evident by a decreasing HCO_3^- less than 22 mEq/L, and a declining Pao_2 despite oxygen therapy.
◆ Pulmonary artery catheterization helps identify the cause of pulmonary edema (cardiac versus noncardiac) by measuring pulmonary artery wedge pressure (PAWP); allows collection of pulmonary artery blood, which shows decreased

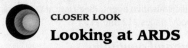

CLOSER LOOK

Looking at ARDS

These diagrams show the process and progress of acute respiratory distress syndrome (ARDS).

Phase 1. Injury reduces normal blood flow to the lungs. Platelets aggregate and release histamine (H), serotonin (S), and bradykinin (B).

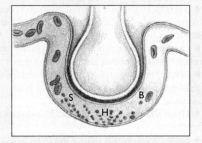

Phase 2. The released substances inflame and damage the alveolar capillary membrane, increasing capillary permeability. Fluids then shift into the interstitial space.

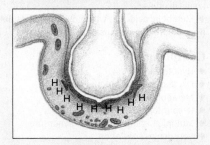

Phase 3. Capillary permeability increases and proteins and fluids leak out, increasing interstitial osmotic pressure and causing pulmonary edema.

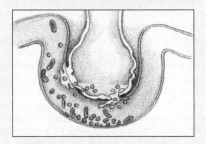

Phase 4. Decreased blood flow and fluids in the alveoli damage surfactant and impair the cell's ability to produce more. The alveoli then collapse, thus impairing gas exchange.

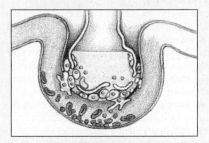

Phase 5. Oxygenation is impaired, but carbon dioxide (CO_2) easily crosses the alveolar capillary membrane and is expired. Blood oxygen (O_2) and CO_2 levels are low.

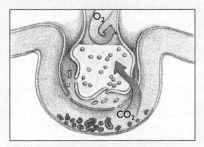

Phase 6. Pulmonary edema worsens and inflammation leads to fibrosis. Gas exchange is further impeded.

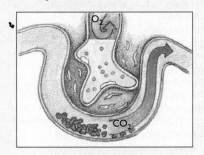

oxygen saturation, reflecting tissue hypoxia; measures pulmonary artery pressure; measures cardiac output by thermodilution techniques; and provides information to allow calculation of the percentages of blood shunted though the lungs.

◆ Serial chest X-rays in early stages show bilateral infiltrates; in later stages, lung fields with a ground-glass appearance and "whiteouts" of both lung fields (with irreversible hypoxemia) may be observed. To differentiate ARDS from heart failure, note that the normal cardiac silhouette appears diffuse; bilateral infiltrates tend to be more peripheral and patchy, as opposed to the usual perihilar "bat wing" appearance of cardiogenic pulmonary edema; and there are fewer pleural effusions.

◆ Sputum analysis, including Gram stain and culture and sensitivity, identifies causative organisms.

◆ Blood cultures aid in identifying infectious organisms.

◆ Toxicology testing screens for drug ingestion.

◆ Serum amylase rules out pancreatitis.

Treatment

Therapy is focused on correcting the causes of ARDS and preventing progression of hypoxemia and respiratory acidosis; it may involve:

◆ administration of humidified oxygen by a tight-fitting mask, which allows for the use of continuous positive airway pressure

◆ for hypoxemia that doesn't respond adequately to the above measures, ventilatory support with intubation, volume ventilation, and positive end-expiratory pressure (PEEP)

◆ pressure-controlled inverse ratio ventilation to reverse the conventional inspiration-to-expiration ratio and minimize the risk of barotrauma (Mechanical breaths are pressure-limited to prevent increased damage to the alveoli.)

◆ permissive hypercapnia to limit peak inspiratory pressure (Although carbon dioxide removal is compromised, treatment isn't given for subsequent changes in blood hydrogen and oxygen concentration.)

◆ a sedative, an opioid, or a neuromuscular blocker, such as vecuronium, which may be given during mechanical ventilation to minimize restlessness, oxygen consumption, and carbon dioxide production and to facilitate ventilation

◆ sodium bicarbonate, which may reverse severe metabolic acidosis

◆ I.V. fluid administration to maintain blood pressure by treating hypovolemia

◆ a vasopressor to maintain blood pressure

◆ an antimicrobial to treat nonviral infections and to prevent ventilator-associated infections (based on culture results)

◆ a diuretic to reduce interstitial and pulmonary edema

◆ corticosteroids, as necessary to reduce inflammation

◆ correction of electrolyte and acid-base imbalances to maintain cellular integrity, particularly the sodium-potassium pump

◆ fluid restriction to prevent increase of interstitial and alveolar edema.

Special considerations

Caring for the patient with ARDS requires careful monitoring and supportive care.

◆ Frequently assess the patient's respiratory status. Be alert for retractions on inspiration. Note the rate, rhythm, and depth of respirations; watch for dyspnea and the use of accessory muscles of respiration. On auscultation, listen for adventitious or diminished breath sounds. Check for clear, frothy sputum, which may indicate pulmonary edema.

◆ Observe and document the hypoxemic patient's neurologic status (level of consciousness and mental sluggishness).

◆ Maintain a patent airway by suctioning, using sterile, nontraumatic technique. Ensure adequate humidification to help liquefy tenacious secretions.

◆ Closely monitor the patient's heart rate and blood pressure. Watch for arrhythmias that may result from hypoxemia, acid-base disturbances, or electrolyte imbalances. With pulmonary artery catheterization, know the desired PAWP level. Check readings often, and watch for decreasing mixed venous oxygen saturation.

◆ Monitor serum electrolyte levels and correct imbalances. Measure intake and output; weigh the patient daily.

◆ Check ventilator settings frequently, and empty condensate from tubing promptly to ensure maximum oxygen delivery. Monitor ABG levels; check for metabolic and respiratory acidosis and Pao_2 changes. The patient with severe hypoxemia may need controlled mechanical ventilation with positive pressure. Give a sedative, as needed, to reduce restlessness.

◆ Because PEEP may decrease cardiac output, check for hypotension, tachycardia, and decreased urine output. Suction only as needed to maintain PEEP or use an in-line suctioning apparatus. Reposition the patient often and record an increase in secretions, temperature, or hypotension that may indicate a deteriorating condition. Monitor peak pressures during ventilation. Because of stiff, noncompliant lungs, the

MULTISYSTEM DISORDER
How ARDS affects the body

The cascade of events that occurs in acute respiratory distress syndrome (ARDS) can eventually affect every body system. Here's how the process occurs, step-by-step, and how multidiscipinary care can help.

Respiratory system
◆ Damage to alveolar and pulmonary capillary, membranes triggers neutrophils, macrophages, monocytes, and lymphocytes to produce various cytokines that promote cellular activation, chemotaxis, and adhesion.
◆ Damage can occur directly (by aspiration of gastric contents and inhalation of noxious gases) or indirectly (from chemical mediators released in response to systemic injury).
◆ The activated cells produce inflammatory mediators, including oxidants, proteases, kinins, growth factors, and neuropeptides, which initiate the complement cascade, intravascular coagulation, and fibrinolysis.
◆ Vascular permeability to proteins increases. Plasma and blood leak into the alveoli and interstitial space.
◆ Fluid accumulates in the lung interstitium, the alveolar spaces, and the small airways, causing the lungs to stiffen and thus impairing ventilation and reducing oxygenation of the pulmonary capillary blood.
◆ Pressure changes and decreased surfactant result in alveolar collapse and atelectasis.
◆ Interstitial inflammation develops, and epithelial cells proliferate.
◆ Fluid in the alveoli and alveolar cell damage reduce surfactant production. Without surfactant, surface tension in the alveoli increases.
◆ Lung surface area is decreased as the lungs become less compliant and the alveoli collapse.
◆ Gas exchange is impaired, and respirations increase to address hypoxia.

◆ Initially, oxygenation is affected and carbon dioxide (CO_2) levels decrease because CO_2 is more easily diffused across the impaired alveolar-capillary membrane. As gas exchange worsens, hypercapnia develops.
◆ Hyaline membranes form because of the lack of surfactant and the collection of tissue debris and white blood cells in the airway.
◆ Inflammation leads to fibrosis, further impeding gas exchange. Fibrosis progressively obliterates alveoli, respiratory bronchioles, and the interstitium. Functional residual capacity decreases, and shunting becomes more serious.
◆ Increasing partial pressure of arterial carbon dioxide leads to respiratory acidosis.
◆ Hypoxia further increases acidosis; pH decreases.
◆ Hypoxia and acidosis result in changes in mental status.

Immune system
◆ The lung injury causes an inflammatory response, which continues as ARDS progresses.
◆ Platelets aggregate at the lung injury site and release substances — such as serotonin, bradykinin, and histamine — that attract and activate neutrophils. These substances inflame and damage the alveolar membrane and increase capillary permeability.
◆ Additional chemotactic factors are released, including endotoxins (such as those present in septic states), tumor necrosis factor, and interleukin-1. The activated neutrophils also release several inflammatory mediators and platelet aggravating factors that damage the alveolar capillary membrane and increase capillary permeability.
◆ Histamines and other inflammatory substances increase capillary permeability, allowing fluids to move into the interstitial space. As capillary permeability increases, proteins,

patient is at high risk for barotrauma (pneumothorax), evidenced by increased peak pressures, decreased breath sounds on one side, and restlessness.
◆ Monitor nutrition, maintain joint mobility, and prevent skin breakdown. Accurately record caloric intake. Give tube feedings and parenteral nutrition, as ordered. Perform passive range-of-motion exercises or help the patient perform active exercises, if possible. Provide meticulous

skin care. Plan patient care to allow periods of uninterrupted sleep.
◆ Provide emotional support. Warn the patient who's recovering from ARDS that recovery will take some time and that he'll feel weak for a while.
◆ Watch for and immediately report all respiratory changes in the patient with injuries that may adversely affect the lungs (especially during the 2- to 3-day period after the injury, when the patient may appear to be improving).

blood cells, and more fluid leak out, increasing interstitial osmotic pressure and causing pulmonary edema.
♦ Mediators released by neutrophils and macrophages cause varying degrees of pulmonary vasoconstriction, resulting in pulmonary hypertension and causing a ventilation-perfusion mismatch.
♦ Systemically, neutrophils and inflammatory mediators cause generalized endothelial damage and increased capillary permeability throughout the body.
♦ Multiple organ dysfunction syndrome (MODS) occurs as the cascade of mediators affects each body system.
♦ Death may occur from the influence of ARDS and MODS.

Collaborative management
A pulmonary specialist can help evaluate and treat the patient's respiratory system. If infectious agents are involved, an infectious disease specialist may be called in; if cardiac involvement is suspected, a cardiologist may be consulted. If the patient progresses through the later stages of ARDS and a prolonged course is expected, a nutritional consult for total parenteral nutrition may be needed as well as specialists in physical and occupational therapy to assist with rehabilitation. If this patient develops a prolonged dependency on mechanical ventilation, he may require an extended care facility that can accommodate this treatment (after his condition is stabilized). If a prolonged stay in the health care facility is expected and the patient requires long-term care, social services should be consulted. Alternatively, if ARDS is successfully treated in the initial stages, the patient may be discharged to home with instructions to follow up with his physician.

||| **LIFE-THREATENING DISORDER**

ACUTE RESPIRATORY FAILURE
When the lungs can't adequately maintain arterial oxygenation or eliminate carbon dioxide, acute respiratory failure (ARF) results, which can lead to tissue hypoxia. In patients with essentially normal lung tissue, ARF usually means partial pressure of arterial carbon dioxide ($Paco_2$) above 60 mm Hg or partial pressure of

arterial oxygen (Pao_2) below 50 mm Hg. These limits, however, don't apply to patients with chronic obstructive pulmonary disease (COPD), who often have a consistently high $Paco_2$ and low Pao_2. In patients with COPD, only acute deterioration in arterial blood gas (ABG) values, with corresponding clinical deterioration, indicates ARF.

Causes
Conditions that can result in alveolar hypoventilation, ventilation-perfusion ($\dot{V}/\dot{Q}$) mismatch, or right-to-left shunting can lead to respiratory failure; these include:
♦ atelectasis
♦ bronchitis
♦ bronchospasm
♦ central nervous system (CNS) depression — head trauma or injudicious use of sedatives, opioids, tranquilizers, or oxygen
♦ CNS disease
♦ COPD
♦ cor pulmonale
♦ cystic fibrosis
♦ heart failure
♦ pneumonia
♦ pneumothorax
♦ pulmonary edema
♦ pulmonary emboli
♦ ventilatory failure.

Pathophysiology
Respiratory failure results from impaired gas exchange. Conditions associated with alveolar hypoventilation, $\dot{V}/\dot{Q}$ mismatch, and intrapulmonary (right-to-left) shunting can cause ARF if left untreated. (See *How ARF affects the body*, page 214.)

Signs and symptoms
Specific signs and symptoms vary with the underlying cause of ARF, but may include these systems:
♦ *Respiratory* — Rate may be increased, decreased, or normal depending on the cause; respirations may be shallow, deep, or alternate between the two; air hunger may occur. Cyanosis may or may not be present, depending on the hemoglobin level and arterial oxygenation. Auscultation of the chest may reveal crackles, rhonchi, wheezing, or diminished breath sounds secondary to possible airway obstruction and subsequent hypoventilation.
♦ *CNS* — When hypoxemia and hypercapnia occur, the patient may show evidence of restlessness, confusion, loss of concentration, irritability, tremulousness, diminished tendon reflexes, papilledema, and coma.

MULTISYSTEM DISORDER
How ARF affects the body

Hypoxemia and hypercapnia that result from acute respiratory failure (ARF) stimulate strong compensatory responses by all body systems.

Rapid detection of the condition and a multidisciplinary approach to care allow for the best outcome.

Respiratory system
♦ Decreased oxygen saturation may result from alveolar hypoventilation, in which chronic airway obstruction reduces alveolar minute ventilation. Partial pressure of arterial oxygen (Pao$_2$) levels fall and partial pressure of arterial carbon dioxide levels rise, resulting in hypoxemia. The most common cause of alveolar hypoventilation is airway obstruction, commonly seen with chronic obstructive pulmonary disease (emphysema or bronchitis).
♦ Most commonly, hypoxemia — ventilation-perfusion ($\dot{V}/\dot{Q}$) imbalance — occurs when such conditions as pulmonary embolism or acute respiratory distress syndrome interrupt normal gas exchange in a specific lung region. Too little ventilation with normal blood flow or too little blood flow with normal ventilation may cause the imbalance, resulting in decreased Pao$_2$ levels and, thus, hypoxemia.
♦ Although uncommon, a decreased fraction of inspired oxygen may lead to respiratory failure. Inspired air doesn't contain adequate oxygen to establish an adequate gradient for diffusion into the blood — for example, at high altitudes or in confined, enclosed spaces. As a result, hypoxemia occurs.
♦ Tissue hypoxemia results in anaerobic metabolism and lactic acidosis. Respiratory acidosis occurs from hypercapnia. Cyanosis occurs because of increased amounts of unoxygenated blood. As respiratory failure worsens, intercostal, supraclavicular, and suprasternal retractions may also occur.

Cardiovascular system
♦ Untreated $\dot{V}/\dot{Q}$ imbalances can lead to right-to-left shunting, in which blood passes from the heart's right side to its left without being oxygenated. This results in unoxygenated blood reaching the arterial system to be distributed to the rest of the body.
♦ Heart rate and stroke volume increases; heart failure may occur.
♦ Hypoxemia deprives the myocardial tissue of oxygen and nutrients, possibly resulting in ischemia or a myocardial infarction.

Neurologic system
♦ In response to hypoxemia, the sympathetic nervous system triggers vasoconstriction, increases peripheral resistance, and increases the heart rate.
♦ Hypoxemia or hypercapnia (or both) causes the brain's respiratory control center to increase respiratory depth (tidal volume) and then to increase the respiratory rate.

Hematologic system
♦ Hypoxia of the kidneys results in release of erythropoietin from renal cells, causing the bone marrow to increase production of red blood cells — an attempt by the body to increase the blood's oxygen-carrying capacity.

Collaborative management
A pulmonary specialist can help evaluate and treat the patient's respiratory conditions. A respiratory therapy team member can assist with oxygen therapy and ventilatory support. If infectious agents are involved, an infectious disease specialist may be required; if cardiac involvement is suspected, a cardiologist may be consulted. The patient may require nutritional support to maintain and improve overall nutrition, strengthen the immune system, and meet metabolic needs. Initially, the patient may require total parenteral nutrition, depending on the severity of the condition and the patient's status. If the patient is able to eat, a registered dietitian can provide planning to meet the patient's needs.

Physical and occupational therapy may be necessary to help with energy conservation and rehabilitation, depending on the patient's condition and length of stay. If a prolonged stay in the health care facility is expected and the patient requires long-term care, social services should be contacted early.

◆ *Cardiovascular* — Tachycardia, with increased cardiac output and mildly elevated blood pressure secondary to adrenal release of catecholamine, occurs early in response to low Pao_2. With myocardial hypoxia, arrhythmias may develop. Pulmonary hypertension, secondary to pulmonary capillary vasoconstriction, may cause increased pressures on the right side of the heart, neck vein distention, an enlarged liver, and peripheral edema.

Complications
◆ Tissue hypoxia
◆ Metabolic acidosis
◆ Multiple organ failure
◆ Cardiac arrest

Diagnosis
◆ ABG analysis indicates respiratory failure by deteriorating values and a pH below 7.3. Patients with COPD may have a lower than normal pH compared with previous levels.
◆ Chest X-rays identify pulmonary diseases or conditions, such as emphysema, atelectasis, lesions, pneumothorax, infiltrates, and effusions.
◆ Electrocardiography can demonstrate ventricular arrhythmias (indicating myocardial hypoxia) or right ventricular hypertrophy (indicating cor pulmonale).
◆ Pulse oximetry reveals decreasing arterial oxygen saturation.
◆ White blood cell count detects the underlying infection.
◆ Abnormally low hemoglobin levels and hematocrit signal blood loss, which indicates decreased oxygen-carrying capacity.
◆ Hypokalemia may result from compensatory hyperventilation, the body's attempt to correct acidosis.
◆ Hypochloremia usually occurs in metabolic alkalosis.
◆ Blood cultures may aid in identifying pathogens.
◆ Pulmonary artery catheterization helps to distinguish pulmonary and cardiovascular causes of ARF and monitors hemodynamic pressures.

Treatment
◆ Oxygen therapy to promote oxygenation and raise Pao_2
◆ Bidirectional positive-pressure airway mask over the oronasal region or mechanical ventilation with an endotracheal or a tracheostomy tube, if needed, to provide adequate oxygenation and reverse acidosis
◆ High-frequency ventilation, if the patient doesn't respond to treatment, to force the air-ways open, promoting oxygenation and preventing alveoli collapse
◆ An antibiotic to treat infection
◆ A bronchodilator to maintain airway patency
◆ A corticosteroid to decrease inflammation
◆ Fluid restrictions in cor pulmonale to reduce volume and cardiac workload
◆ A positive inotropic agent to increase cardiac output
◆ A vasopressor to maintain blood pressure
◆ A diuretic to reduce edema and fluid overload
◆ Deep breathing with pursed lips if patient isn't intubated and mechanically ventilated to help keep airway patent
◆ Incentive spirometry to increase lung volume

Special considerations
◆ Because the patient with ARF is usually treated in an intensive care unit (ICU), orient him to the environment, procedures, and routines to minimize his anxiety.
◆ To reverse hypoxemia, administer oxygen at appropriate concentrations to maintain Pao_2 at a minimum of 50 to 60 mm Hg. Patients with COPD usually require only small amounts of supplemental oxygen. Watch for a positive response, such as improvement in the patient's breathing, color, and ABG results.
◆ Maintain a patent airway. If the patient is retaining carbon dioxide, encourage him to cough and to breathe deeply. Teach him to use pursed-lip and diaphragmatic breathing to control dyspnea. If the patient is alert, have him use an incentive spirometer; if he's intubated and lethargic, turn him every 1 to 2 hours. Use postural drainage and chest physiotherapy to help clear secretions.
◆ In an intubated patient, suction the trachea as needed after hyperoxygenation. Observe for change in quantity, consistency, and color of sputum. Provide humidification to liquefy secretions.
◆ Observe the patient closely for respiratory arrest. Auscultate for chest sounds. Monitor ABG levels and report changes immediately.
◆ Monitor and record serum electrolyte levels carefully, and correct imbalances; monitor fluid balance by recording intake and output or daily weight.
◆ Check the cardiac monitor for arrhythmias.

For mechanical ventilation
◆ Check ventilator settings, cuff pressures, and ABG values often because the fraction of inspired oxygen (Fio_2) setting depends on ABG levels. Draw specimens for ABG analysis 20 to 30 minutes after every Fio_2 change or check with oximetry.

◆ Prevent infection by using sterile technique while suctioning.

◆ Stress ulcers are common in intubated ICU patients. Check gastric secretions for evidence of bleeding if the patient has a nasogastric tube or complains of epigastric tenderness, nausea, or vomiting. Monitor hemoglobin level and hematocrit; check stool for occult blood. Administer an antacid, a histamine₂-receptor antagonist, or sucralfate, as ordered.

◆ Prevent tracheal erosion, which can result from artificial airway cuff overinflation. Use the minimal leak technique and a cuffed tube with high residual volume (low-pressure cuff), a foam cuff, or a pressure-regulating valve on the cuff.

◆ To prevent oral or vocal cord trauma, make sure the endotracheal tube is positioned midline.

◆ To prevent nasal necrosis, keep the nasotracheal tube midline within the nostrils and provide good hygiene. Loosen the tape periodically to prevent skin breakdown. Avoid excessive movement of any tubes; make sure the ventilator tubing is adequately supported.

ASBESTOSIS

Considered a form of pneumoconiosis, asbestosis is characterized by diffuse interstitial pulmonary fibrosis. Prolonged exposure to airborne particles causes pleural plaques and tumors of the pleura and peritoneum. Asbestosis may develop 15 to 20 years after regular exposure to asbestos has ended. It's a potent co-carcinogen and increases the smoker's risk of lung cancer. An asbestos worker who smokes is 90 times more likely to develop lung cancer than a smoker who has never worked with asbestos.

Causes

◆ Exposure to asbestos used in paints, plastics, and brake and clutch linings

◆ Exposure to fibrous asbestos dust in deteriorating buildings or in waste piles from asbestos manufacturing plants

◆ Family members of asbestos workers, who may be exposed to stray fibers from the worker's clothing

◆ Prolonged inhalation of asbestos fibers; people at high risk include workers in the mining, milling, construction, fireproofing, and textile industries

Pathophysiology

Asbestosis occurs when lung spaces become filled with asbestos fibers. The inhaled asbestos fibers (50 microns or more in length and 0.5 microns or less in diameter) travel down the air-

way and penetrate respiratory bronchioles and alveolar walls. Coughing attempts to expel the foreign matter. Mucus production and goblet cells are stimulated to protect the airway from the debris and aid in expectoration. Fibers then become encased in a brown, iron-rich protein-like sheath in sputum or lung tissue, called asbestosis bodies. Chronic irritation by the fibers continues to affect the lower bronchioles and alveoli. The foreign material and inflammation swell airways, and fibrosis develops in response to the chronic irritation. Interstitial fibrosis may develop in lower lung zones, affecting lung parenchyma and the pleurae. Raised hyaline plaques may form in the parietal pleura, the diaphragm, and the pleura adjacent to the pericardium. Hypoxia develops as more alveoli and lower airways are affected.

Signs and symptoms

◆ Exertional dyspnea as a result of increased mucus production and airway narrowing

◆ Dyspnea at rest with extensive fibrosis

◆ Severe, nonproductive cough in nonsmokers or productive cough in smokers from chronic irritation of bronchial tree and mucus production

◆ Clubbed fingers due to chronic hypoxia

◆ Chest pain (commonly pleuritic) due to pleural irritation

◆ Recurrent respiratory tract infections as pulmonary defense mechanisms begin to fail

◆ Pleural friction rub due to fibrosis

◆ Crackles on auscultation attributed to air moving through thickened sputum

◆ Decreased lung inflation due to lung stiffness

◆ Recurrent pleural effusions due to fibrosis

◆ Decreased forced expiratory volume due to diminished alveoli

◆ Decreased vital capacity due to fibrotic changes

Complications

◆ Pulmonary fibrosis due to progression of asbestosis

◆ Respiratory failure

◆ Pulmonary hypertension

◆ Cor pulmonale

Diagnosis

◆ Chest X-rays may show fine, irregular, linear, and diffuse infiltrates. Extensive fibrosis is revealed by a honeycomb or ground-glass appearance. Chest X-rays may also show pleural thickening and calcification, bilateral obliteration of the costophrenic angles and, in later stages, an enlarged heart with a classic "shaggy" border.

◆ Pulmonary function studies may identify decreased vital capacity, forced vital capacity

(FVC), and total lung capacity; decreased or normal forced expiratory volume in 1 second (FEV_1); a normal FEV_1-to-FVC ratio; and reduced diffusing capacity for carbon monoxide when fibrosis destroys alveolar walls and thickens the alveolar capillary membrane.

♦ Arterial blood gas analysis may reveal decreased partial pressure of arterial oxygen and partial pressure of arterial carbon dioxide from hyperventilation.

Treatment

The goal of treatment is to relieve symptoms and control complications; it may involve:

♦ chest physiotherapy (controlled coughing and postural drainage with chest percussion and vibration) to help relieve respiratory signs and symptoms and manage hypoxia and cor pulmonale

♦ aerosol therapy to liquefy mucus

♦ an inhaled mucolytic to liquefy and mobilize secretions

♦ increased fluid intake to 3 qt (3 L) daily

♦ an antibiotic to treat respiratory tract infections

♦ oxygen administration to relieve hypoxia

♦ possibly a diuretic to decrease edema, digoxin to enhance cardiac output, and salt restriction to prevent fluid retention for patients with cor pulmonale.

Special considerations

♦ Teach the patient to prevent infections by avoiding crowds and persons with infections and by receiving influenza and pneumococcal vaccines.

♦ Improve the patient's ventilatory efficiency by encouraging physical reconditioning, energy conservation in daily activities, and relaxation techniques.

ASTHMA

Asthma is a chronic inflammatory airway disorder characterized by airflow obstruction and airway hyperresponsiveness to a multiplicity of stimuli. This widespread but variable airflow obstruction is caused by bronchospasm, edema of the airway mucosa, and increased mucus production with plugging and airway remodeling. It's a type of chronic obstructive pulmonary disease (COPD), a long-term pulmonary disease characterized by increased airflow resistance; other types of COPD include chronic bronchitis and emphysema.

AGE ALERT *Although asthma strikes at any age, about 50% of patients are younger than age 10; twice as many boys as girls are affected in this age-group. One-third of patients develop*

asthma between ages 10 and 30, and the incidence is the same in both sexes in this age-group. Moreover, about one-third of all patients share the disease with at least one immediate family member.

Asthma may result from sensitivity to extrinsic or intrinsic allergens. Extrinsic, or atopic, asthma begins in childhood; typically, patients are sensitive to specific external allergens.

CLINICAL ALERT *Extrinsic asthma is commonly accompanied by other hereditary allergies, such as eczema and allergic rhinitis, in children.*

Intrinsic, or *nonatopic*, patients with asthma react to internal, nonallergenic factors; external substances can't be implicated in patients with intrinsic asthma. Most episodes occur after a severe respiratory tract infection, especially in adults. However, many patients with asthma, especially children, have intrinsic and extrinsic asthma.

GENETIC LINK *Asthma is a complex inheritable disease, meaning there are several genes that make a person susceptible to the disease, including genes on chromosomes 5, 6, 11, 12, and 14.*

The role of these genes in the development of asthma isn't clear, but one of the most promising sites of study is chromosome 5. Even though researchers haven't specifically identified a gene from this site, they do know that the area is rich in genes coding for molecules that play a key role in the inflammatory response seen in asthma. Scientists continue to search for specific asthma genes.

A significant number of adults acquire an allergic form of asthma or exacerbation of existing asthma from exposure to agents in the workplace. Irritants, such as chemicals in flour, acid anhydrides, toluene di-isocyanates, screw flies, river flies, and excreta of dust mites in carpet, have been identified as agents that trigger asthma.

Causes
Extrinsic allergens

♦ Animal dander

♦ Food additives containing sulfites

♦ House dust or mold

♦ Kapok or feather pillows

♦ Other sensitizing substances

♦ Pollen

Intrinsic allergens

♦ Anxiety

♦ Coughing or laughing

♦ Emotional stress

♦ Endocrine changes

♦ Exposure to noxious fumes

- Fatigue
- Genetic factors (see below)
- Humidity variations
- Irritants
- Strenuous exercise
- Temperature variations

Pathophysiology

There are two genetic influences identified with asthma, namely the ability of an individual to develop asthma (atopy) and the tendency to develop hyperresponsiveness of the airways independent of atopy. A locus of chromosome 11 associated with atopy contains an abnormal gene that encodes a part of the immunoglobulin (Ig) E receptor. Environmental factors interact with inherited factors to cause asthmatic reactions with associated bronchospasms.

In asthma, bronchial linings overreact to various stimuli, causing episodic smooth-muscle spasms that severely constrict the airways. (See *Pathophysiology of asthma*.) IgE antibodies, attached to histamine-containing mast cells and receptors on cell membranes, initiate intrinsic asthma attacks. When exposed to an antigen, such as pollen, the IgE antibody combines with the antigen.

On subsequent exposure to the antigen, mast cells degranulate and release mediators. Mast cells in the lung interstitium are stimulated to release histamine and leukotrienes. Histamine attaches to receptor sites in the larger bronchi, where it causes swelling in smooth muscles. Mucous membranes become inflamed, irritated, and swollen. The patient may experience dyspnea, prolonged expiration, and an increased respiratory rate.

Leukotrienes attach to receptor sites in the smaller bronchi and cause local swelling of the smooth muscle. Leukotrienes also cause prostaglandins to travel through the bloodstream to the lungs, where they enhance histamine's effect. A wheeze may be audible during coughing — the higher the pitch, the narrower the bronchial lumen. Histamine stimulates the mucous membranes to secrete excessive mucus, further narrowing the bronchial lumen. Goblet cells secrete viscous mucus that's difficult to cough up, resulting in coughing, rhonchi, increased-pitch wheezing, and increased respiratory distress. Mucosal edema and thickened secretions further block the airways. (See *Looking at a bronchiole in asthma*, page 220.)

On inhalation, the narrowed bronchial lumen can still expand slightly, allowing air to reach the alveoli. On exhalation, increased intrathoracic pressure closes the bronchial lumen completely. Air enters but can't escape. The patient develops a barrel chest and hyperresonance to percussion.

Mucus fills the lung bases, inhibiting alveolar ventilation. Blood is shunted to alveoli in other lung parts, but still can't compensate for diminished ventilation.

Hyperventilation is triggered by lung receptors to increase lung volume because of trapped air and obstructions. Intrapleural and alveolar gas pressures rise, causing a decreased perfusion of alveoli. Increased alveolar gas pressure, decreased ventilation, and decreased perfusion result in uneven ventilation-perfusion ratios and mismatching within different lung segments.

Hypoxia triggers hyperventilation by respiratory center stimulation, which in turn decreases partial pressure of arterial carbon dioxide ($Paco_2$) and increases pH, resulting in a respiratory alkalosis. As the airway obstruction increases in severity, more alveoli are affected. Ventilation and perfusion remain inadequate, and carbon dioxide retention develops. Respiratory acidosis results, and respiratory failure occurs.

If status asthmaticus occurs, hypoxia worsens and expiratory flows and volumes decrease even further. If treatment isn't initiated, the patient begins to tire out. (See *Averting an asthma attack*, page 221.) Acidosis develops as arterial carbon dioxide increases. The situation becomes life-threatening as no air becomes audible upon auscultation (a silent chest) and $Paco_2$ rises to over 70 mm Hg.

Signs and symptoms

Extrinsic asthma is usually accompanied by signs and symptoms of atopy (type I IgE-mediated allergy), such as eczema and allergic rhinitis. It commonly follows a severe respiratory tract infection, especially in adults.

An acute asthma attack begins dramatically, with simultaneous onset of severe multiple symptoms, or insidiously, with gradually increasing respiratory distress. Asthma that occurs with cyanosis, confusion, and lethargy indicates the onset of life-threatening status asthmaticus and respiratory failure.

Signs and symptoms of asthma include:
- sudden dyspnea, wheezing, and tightness in the chest from bronchoconstriction
- coughing that produces thick, clear, or yellow sputum resulting from excess mucus production
- tachypnea, along with use of accessory respiratory muscles due to increasing air trapping and respiratory distress
- rapid pulse from increased workload of the heart due to the effects of hypoxemia and hyperinflation on the pulmonary vasculature

CLOSER LOOK
Pathophysiology of asthma

In asthma, hyperresponsiveness of the airways and bronchospasms occur. These illustrations show the progression of an asthma attack.

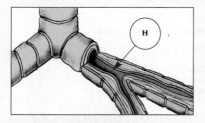

♦ Histamine (H) attaches to receptor sites in larger bronchi, causing swelling of the smooth muscles.

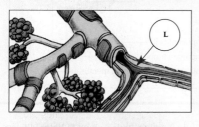

♦ Leukotrienes (L) attach to receptor sites in the smaller bronchi and cause swelling of smooth muscle there. Leukotrienes and prostaglandins travel through the bloodstream to the lungs, where they enhance histamine's effects.

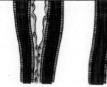

Bronchial lumen on inhalation   Bronchial lumen on exhalation

♦ Histamine stimulates the mucous membranes to secrete excessive mucus, further narrowing the bronchial lumen. On inhalation, the narrowed bronchial lumen can still expand slightly; however, on exhalation, the increased intrathoracic pressure closes the bronchial lumen completely.

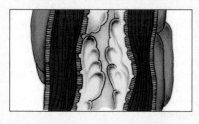

♦ Mucus fills lung bases, inhibiting alveolar ventilation. Blood is shunted to alveoli in other parts of the lungs, but it still can't compensate for diminished ventilation.

♦ hyperresonant lung fields from air trapping
♦ diminished breath sounds from obstruction and air trapping.

In 1997, the National Heart, Lung, and Blood Institute of the National Institutes of Health identified four levels of asthma severity based on the frequency of symptoms and exacerbations, effects on activity level, and lung function study results: *mild intermittent, mild persistent, moderate persistent,* and *severe persistent.*

Mild intermittent asthma
♦ Symptoms occur less than two times per week.
♦ The patient is asymptomatic with normal peak expiratory flow (PEF) between exacerbations.
♦ Brief exacerbations (from a few hours to a few days) vary in intensity.
♦ Nighttime symptoms occur less than two times per month.

CLOSER LOOK
Looking at a bronchiole in asthma

Asthma is characterized by bronchospasms, increased mucus secretion, and mucosal edema, which contribute to airway narrowing and obstruction. Shown here is a normal bronchiole in cross section and an obstructed bronchiole, as it occurs in asthma.

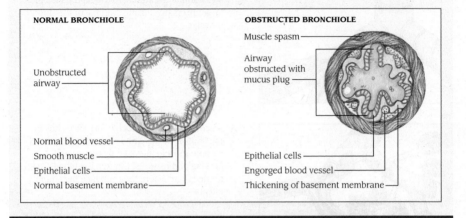

NORMAL BRONCHIOLE

Unobstructed airway

Normal blood vessel
Smooth muscle
Epithelial cells
Normal basement membrane

OBSTRUCTED BRONCHIOLE

Muscle spasm

Airway obstructed with mucus plug

Epithelial cells
Engorged blood vessel
Thickening of basement membrane

◆ Lung function studies show forced expiratory volume in 1 second (FEV_1) or PEF more than 80% of normal values; PEF may vary by less than 20%.

Mild persistent asthma
◆ Symptoms occur more than two times per week, but less than once per day; exacerbations may affect activity.
◆ Nighttime symptoms occur more than two times per month.
◆ Lung function studies show FEV_1 or PEF more than 80% of normal values; PEF may vary by 20% to 30%.

Moderate persistent asthma
◆ Symptoms occur daily.
◆ Exacerbations occur more than two times per week and may last for days; exacerbations affect activity.
◆ Bronchodilator therapy is used daily.
◆ Nighttime symptoms occur more than once per week.
◆ Lung function studies show FEV_1 or PEF 60% to 80% of normal values; PEF may vary by more than 30%.

Severe persistent asthma
◆ Symptoms occur on a continuous basis.
◆ Exacerbations occur frequently and limit physical activity.
◆ Nighttime symptoms occur frequently.

◆ Lung function studies show FEV_1 or PEF less than 60% of normal values; PEF may vary by more than 30%.

Complications
◆ Status asthmaticus
◆ Respiratory failure

Diagnosis
◆ Pulmonary function studies reveal signs of airway obstructive disease, low-normal or decreased vital capacity, and increased total lung and residual capacities. Pulmonary function may be normal between attacks. Partial pressure of arterial oxygen (PaO_2) and $PaCO_2$ are usually decreased, except in severe asthma, when $PaCO_2$ may be normal or increased, indicating severe bronchial obstruction.
◆ Serum IgE levels may increase from an allergic reaction.
◆ Sputum analysis may indicate the presence of Curschmann's spirals (casts of airways), Charcot-Leyden crystals, and eosinophils.
◆ Complete blood count with differential reveals an increased eosinophil count.
◆ Chest X-rays can be used to diagnose or monitor the progress of asthma and may show hyperinflation with areas of atelectasis.
◆ Arterial blood gas (ABG) analysis detects hypoxemia (decreased PaO_2; decreased, normal, or increasing $PaCO_2$) and guides treatment.

◆ Skin testing may identify specific allergens. Results read in 1 to 2 days detect an early reaction; after 4 to 5 days, a late reaction.
◆ Bronchial challenge testing evaluates the clinical significance of allergens identified by skin testing.
◆ Electrocardiography shows sinus tachycardia during an attack; a severe attack may show signs of cor pulmonale (right-axis deviation, peaked P wave) that resolve after the attack.

Treatment

Drug therapy for asthma is typically based on the severity of disease. Correcting asthma usually involves:
◆ prevention, by identifying and avoiding precipitating factors, such as environmental allergens or irritants, which is the best treatment
◆ desensitization to specific antigens — helpful if the stimuli can't be removed entirely — which decreases the severity of attacks of asthma with future exposure
◆ treatment of underlying conditions or diseases
◆ a bronchodilator — including a methylxanthine (theophylline or aminophylline) and perhaps a beta$_2$-adrenergic agonist (albuterol or terbutaline) — to decrease bronchoconstriction, reduce bronchial airway edema, and increase pulmonary ventilation
◆ a corticosteroid (such as hydrocortisone sodium succinate, prednisone, methylprednisolone, or beclomethasone) for its anti-inflammatory and immunosuppressive effects, which decrease inflammation and edema of the airways
◆ a mast cell stabilizer (cromolyn sodium or nedocromil sodium), effective in patients with atopic asthma who have seasonal disease (When given prophylactically, it blocks the acute obstructive effects of antigen exposure by inhibiting the degranulation of mast cells, thereby preventing the release of chemical mediators responsible for anaphylaxis.)
◆ a leukotriene modifier, such as zileuton (Zyflo), or a leukotriene receptor antagonist (LTRA), such as montelukast (Singulair) or zafirlukast (Accolate), to inhibit the potent bronchoconstriction and inflammatory effects of the cysteinyl leukotrienes (An LTRA can be used as adjunctive therapy to avoid a high-dose inhaled corticosteroid. Although this class of medications doesn't replace inhaled corticosteroids as first-line anti-inflammatory treatment, it can be used successfully in cases where poor compliance with corticosteroid inhalation therapy is suspected.)
◆ an anticholinergic bronchodilator, such as ipratropium, which blocks acetylcholine, another chemical mediator

DISEASE BLOCK

Averting an asthma attack

The flowchart below shows pathophysiologic changes that occur with asthma. Treatments and interventions show where the physiologic cascade would be altered to stop an asthma attack.

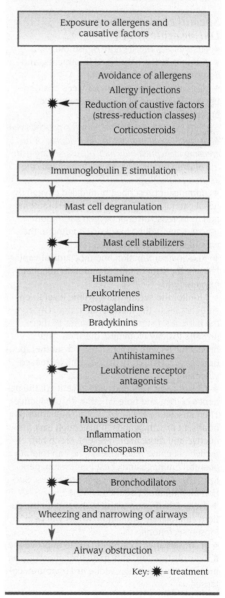

Exposure to allergens and causative factors

↓

Avoidance of allergens
Allergy injections
Reduction of caustive factors
(stress-reduction classes)
Corticosteroids

↓

Immunoglobulin E stimulation

↓

Mast cell degranulation

↓

Mast cell stabilizers

↓

Histamine
Leukotrienes
Prostaglandins
Bradykinins

↓

Antihistamines
Leukotriene receptor antagonists

↓

Mucus secretion
Inflammation
Bronchospasm

↓

Bronchodilators

↓

Wheezing and narrowing of airways

↓

Airway obstruction

Key: ✳ = treatment

♦ low-flow humidified oxygen, which may be needed to treat dyspnea, cyanosis, and hypoxemia (However, the amount delivered should maintain Pao_2 between 65 and 85 mm Hg, as determined by ABG analysis.)
♦ mechanical ventilation—necessary if the patient doesn't respond to initial ventilatory support and drugs, or develops respiratory failure
♦ relaxation exercises, such as yoga, to help increase circulation and to help a patient recover from an asthma attack.

Special considerations
During acute attack
♦ First, assess the severity of asthma.
♦ Administer the prescribed treatments, and assess the patient's response.
♦ Place the patient in high Fowler's position. Encourage pursed-lip and diaphragmatic breathing. Help him to relax.

⚠ **CLINICAL ALERT** *Monitor the patient's vital signs. Keep in mind that developing or increasing tachypnea may indicate worsening asthma or drug toxicity. Hypertension may indicate asthma-related hypoxemia.*

♦ Administer prescribed humidified oxygen by nasal cannula at 2 L/minute to ease breathing and to increase arterial oxygen saturation (Sao_2). Later, adjust oxygen according to the patient's vital signs and ABG levels.
♦ Anticipate intubation and mechanical ventilation if the patient fails to maintain adequate oxygenation.
♦ Monitor the serum theophylline level to ensure that it's in the therapeutic range. Observe the patient for signs and symptoms of theophylline toxicity (vomiting, diarrhea, and headache) as well as for signs of a subtherapeutic dosage (respiratory distress and increased wheezing).
♦ Observe the frequency and severity of the patient's cough, and note whether it's productive. Then auscultate his lungs, noting adventitious or absent breath sounds. If his cough isn't productive and rhonchi are present, teach him effective coughing techniques. If he can tolerate postural drainage and chest percussion, perform these procedures to clear secretions. Suction an intubated patient as needed.
♦ Treat dehydration with I.V. fluids until the patient can tolerate oral fluids, which will help loosen secretions.
♦ If conservative treatment fails to improve the airway obstruction, anticipate bronchoscopy or bronchial lavage when a lobe or larger area collapses.

During long-term care
♦ Monitor the patient's respiratory status to detect baseline changes, to assess response to treatment, and to prevent or detect complications.
♦ Auscultate the lungs frequently, noting the degree of wheezing and quality of air movement.
♦ Review ABG levels, pulmonary function test results, and Sao_2 readings.
♦ If the patient is taking a systemic corticosteroid, observe for complications, such as an elevated blood glucose level and friable skin and bruising. Cushingoid effects resulting from long-term use of corticosteroids may be minimized by alternate-day dosing or use of a prescribed inhaled corticosteroid.
♦ If the patient is taking a corticosteroid by inhaler, watch for signs of candidal infection in the mouth and pharynx. Using an extender device and rinsing the mouth afterward may prevent this.
♦ Observe the patient's anxiety level. Keep in mind that measures that reduce hypoxemia and breathlessness should help relieve anxiety.
♦ Keep the room temperature comfortable and use an air conditioner or a fan in hot, humid weather.
♦ Instruct the patient to use a bronchodilator or cromolyn 30 minutes before exercise to help control exercise-induced asthma. Also instruct him to use pursed-lip breathing while exercising. (See *Preventing asthma attacks*.)

During patient education
♦ Describe prescribed drugs, including their names, dosages, actions, adverse effects, and special instructions.
♦ Tell the patient to notify the physician if he develops a fever above 100° F (37.8° C), chest pain, shortness of breath without coughing or exercising, or uncontrollable coughing. An uncontrollable asthma attack requires immediate attention.
♦ Teach the patient diaphragmatic and pursed-lip breathing as well as effective coughing techniques.
♦ Urge the patient to drink at least 3 qt (3 L) of fluids daily to help loosen secretions and maintain hydration.

CHRONIC BRONCHITIS
Chronic bronchitis is inflammation of the bronchi caused by irritants or infection. A form of chronic obstructive pulmonary disease (COPD), bronchitis may be classified as acute or chronic. In chronic bronchitis, hypersecretion of mucus and chronic productive cough last for

3 months of the year and occur for at least 2 consecutive years. The distinguishing characteristic of bronchitis is airflow obstruction.

⚠️ **CLINICAL ALERT** *COPD is more prevalent in urban environments than in rural ones and is also related to occupational factors (mineral or organic dusts).*

🔲 **AGE ALERT** *Children of parents who smoke are at higher risk for respiratory tract infection that can lead to chronic bronchitis.*

Causes
♦ Cigarette smoking
♦ Exposure to irritants
♦ Exposure to noxious gases
♦ Exposure to organic or inorganic dusts
♦ Genetic predisposition
♦ Respiratory tract infection

Pathophysiology
Chronic bronchitis occurs when irritants are inhaled for a prolonged time. The irritants inflame the tracheobronchial tree, leading to increased mucus production and a narrowed or blocked airway. As the inflammation continues, changes in the cells lining the respiratory tract result in resistance of the small airways and severe ventilation-perfusion ($\dot{V}/\dot{Q}$) imbalance, which decreases arterial oxygenation.

Chronic bronchitis results in hypertrophy and hyperplasia of the mucous glands, increased goblet cells, ciliary damage, squamous metaplasia of the columnar epithelium, and chronic leukocytic infiltration of bronchial walls. (See *Changes in chronic bronchitis,* page 224.) Hypersecretion of the goblet cells blocks the free movement of the cilia, which normally sweep dust, irritants, and mucus away from the airways. With mucus and debris accumulating in the airway, the defenses are altered, and the individual is prone to respiratory tract infections.

Additional effects include widespread inflammation, airway narrowing, and mucus within the airways. Bronchial walls become inflamed and thickened from edema and accumulation of inflammatory cells, and the effects of smooth-muscle bronchospasm further narrow the lumen. Initially, only large bronchi are involved but, eventually, all airways are affected. Airways become obstructed and closure occurs, especially on expiration. The gas is then trapped in the distal portion of the lung. Hypoventilation occurs, leading to a $\dot{V}/\dot{Q}$ mismatch and resultant hypoxemia.

Hypoxemia and hypercapnia occur secondary to hypoventilation. Pulmonary vascular resistance (PVR) increases as inflammatory and compensatory vasoconstriction in hypoventilated areas narrows the pulmonary arteries. Increased

Preventing asthma attacks

Take the following steps to help prevent asthma attacks:
♦ Tell the patient to avoid possible triggers, such as pollens, mold, smoke, and cold air, and emphasize the importance of using inhaled corticosteroids, antihistamines, decongestants, cromolyn powder by inhalation, leukotriene modifiers, and oral or aerosol bronchodilators as ordered.
♦ Explain the role stress and anxiety can play in asthma attacks.
♦ Describe the frequent association of asthma attacks with exercise—especially running—and cold air, and explain nighttime flare-ups of asthma.
♦ Teach the patient how to use a metered-dose inhaler and peak flow meter. If he has difficulty using an inhaler, he may need an extender device to optimize drug delivery and to lower the risk of *Candida* infection associated with orally inhaled corticosteroids.
♦ Tell him to keep a record of peak flow readings and to bring his peak flow meter to medical appointments. Explain that if the peak flow drops suddenly, he should call his physician at once because the drop may signal severe respiratory problems.
♦ Provide the patient and his family with an individualized, written action plan developed by the physician that allows the patient to manage his asthma based on either peak flow monitoring or his symptoms.

PVR leads to increased afterload of the right ventricle. With repeated inflammatory episodes, scarring of the airways occurs, and permanent structural changes develop. Respiratory tract infections can trigger acute exacerbations, and respiratory failure can occur.

Patients with chronic bronchitis have a diminished respiratory drive. The resulting chronic hypoxia causes the kidneys to produce erythropoietin, which stimulates excessive red blood cell production and leads to polycythemia. Although hemoglobin levels are high, the amount of reduced (not fully oxygenated) hemoglobin in contact with oxygen is low; therefore, cyanosis occurs.

⬤ CLOSER LOOK
Changes in chronic bronchitis

In chronic bronchitis, irritants inflame the tracheobronchial tree over time, leading to increased mucus production and a narrowed or blocked airway. As the inflammation continues, goblet and epithelial cells hypertrophy. Because the natural defense mechanisms are blocked, the airways accumulate debris in the respiratory tract. The illllustrations here show these changes.

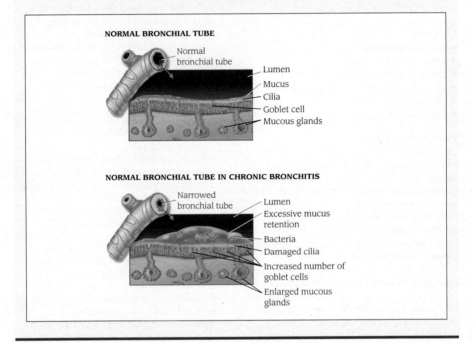

NORMAL BRONCHIAL TUBE

Normal bronchial tube

Lumen
Mucus
Cilia
Goblet cell
Mucous glands

NORMAL BRONCHIAL TUBE IN CHRONIC BRONCHITIS

Narrowed bronchial tube

Lumen
Excessive mucus retention
Bacteria
Damaged cilia
Increased number of goblet cells
Enlarged mucous glands

Signs and symptoms
◆ Copious gray, white, or yellow sputum due to hypersecretion of goblet cells
◆ Productive cough to expectorate mucus produced by the lungs
◆ Dyspnea due to airflow obstruction to the lower tracheobronchial tree
◆ Cyanosis related to diminished oxygenation and cellular hypoxia; reduced oxygen is supplied to the tissues
◆ Use of accessory muscles for breathing due to compensated attempts to supply the cells with increased oxygen
◆ Tachypnea due to hypoxia
◆ Pedal edema due to right-sided heart failure
◆ Neck vein distention due to right-sided heart failure
◆ Weight gain due to edema
◆ Wheezing due to air moving through narrowed respiratory passages
◆ Prolonged expiratory time due to the body's attempt to keep airways patent
◆ Rhonchi due to air moving through narrow, mucus-filled passages
◆ Pulmonary hypertension caused by involvement of small pulmonary arteries, due to inflammation in the bronchial walls and spasms of pulmonary blood vessels from hypoxia

Complications
◆ Recurrent respiratory tract infections
◆ Cor pulmonale (right ventricular hypertrophy with right-sided heart failure) due to increased right ventricular end-diastolic pressure
◆ Pulmonary hypertension
◆ Heart failure, resulting in increased venous pressure, liver engorgement, and dependent edema
◆ Acute respiratory failure

Diagnosis
◆ Chest X-rays may show hyperinflation and increased bronchovascular markings.
◆ Pulmonary function studies indicate increased residual volume, decreased vital capacity and

forced expiratory flow, and normal static compliance and diffusing capacity.
◆ Arterial blood gas analysis reveals decreased partial pressure of arterial oxygen and normal or increased partial pressure of arterial carbon dioxide.
◆ Sputum analysis may reveal many microorganisms and neutrophils.
◆ Electrocardiography may show atrial arrhythmias; peaked P waves in leads II, III, and aV$_F$; and, occasionally, right ventricular hypertrophy.

Treatment
◆ Avoidance of air pollutants (most effective)
◆ Smoking cessation and avoidance of second-hand smoke
◆ An antibiotic to treat recurring infections
◆ A bronchodilator to relieve bronchospasms and facilitate mucociliary clearance
◆ Adequate hydration to liquefy secretions
◆ Chest physiotherapy to mobilize secretions
◆ An ultrasonic or mechanical nebulizer to loosen and mobilize secretions
◆ A corticosteroid to combat inflammation
◆ A diuretic to reduce edema
◆ Oxygen to treat hypoxia

Special considerations
◆ If the patient smokes, encourage him to stop. Provide him with smoking-cessation resources or counseling if necessary.
◆ Assess the patient for changes in baseline respiratory function. Evaluate sputum quality and quantity, restlessness, increased tachypnea, and altered breath sounds. Report changes immediately.
◆ As needed, perform chest physiotherapy, including postural drainage as well as chest percussion and vibration for involved lobes, several times daily.
◆ Weigh the patient three times weekly, and assess for edema.
◆ Provide the patient with a high-calorie, protein-rich diet. Offer small, frequent meals to conserve the patient's energy and prevent fatigue.
◆ Make sure the patient receives adequate fluids (at least 3 qt [3 L] per day) to loosen secretions.
◆ Schedule respiratory therapy at least 1 hour before or after meals. Provide mouth care after bronchodilator inhalation therapy.
◆ Advise the patient to avoid crowds and people with known infections and to obtain influenza and pneumococcal immunizations.
◆ Urge the patient to avoid inhaled irritants, such as automobile exhaust fumes, aerosol sprays, and industrial pollutants.
◆ Warn the patient that exposures to blasts of cold air may precipitate bronchospasm. Suggest that he avoid cold, windy weather or that he cover his mouth and nose with a scarf or mask if he must go outside.

COR PULMONALE
Cor pulmonale (also called *right-sided heart failure*) is a condition in which hypertrophy and dilation of the right ventricle develop secondary to disease affecting the structure or function of the lungs or their vasculature. It can occur at the end stage of various chronic disorders of the lungs, pulmonary vessels, chest wall, and respiratory control center. Cor pulmonale doesn't occur with disorders stemming from congenital heart disease or with those affecting the left side of the heart.

About 85% of patients with cor pulmonale also have chronic obstructive pulmonary disease (COPD), and about 25% of patients with bronchial COPD eventually develop cor pulmonale. The disorder is most common in smokers and in middle-aged and elderly males; however, its incidence in females is increasing. Because cor pulmonale occurs late in the course of the individual's underlying condition and with other irreversible diseases, the prognosis is poor.

AGE ALERT *In children, cor pulmonale may be a complication of cystic fibrosis, hemosiderosis, upper-airway obstruction, scleroderma, extensive bronchiectasis, neuromuscular diseases that affect respiratory muscles, or abnormalities of the respiratory control area.*

Causes
◆ Bronchial asthma
◆ COPD
◆ Disorders that affect the pulmonary parenchyma
◆ External vascular obstruction resulting from a tumor or aneurysm
◆ High altitude
◆ Kyphoscoliosis
◆ Muscular dystrophy
◆ Obesity
◆ Pectus excavatum (funnel chest)
◆ Poliomyelitis
◆ Primary pulmonary hypertension
◆ Pulmonary emboli
◆ Vasculitis

Pathophysiology
In cor pulmonale, pulmonary hypertension increases the heart's workload. To compensate, the right ventricle hypertrophies to force blood through the lungs. As long as the heart can compensate for the increased pulmonary vascular resistance, signs and symptoms reflect only the underlying disorder.

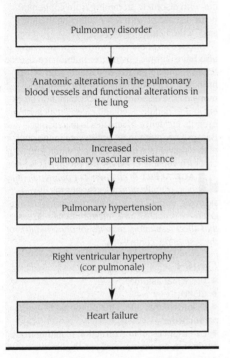

Cor pulmonale: An overview

Although pulmonary restrictive disorders (such as fibrosis or obesity), obstructive disorders (such as bronchitis), or primary vascular disorders (such as recurrent pulmonary emboli) may cause cor pulmonale, these disorders share this common pathway.

Pulmonary disorder

↓

Anatomic alterations in the pulmonary blood vessels and functional alterations in the lung

↓

Increased pulmonary vascular resistance

↓

Pulmonary hypertension

↓

Right ventricular hypertrophy (cor pulmonale)

↓

Heart failure

Severity of right ventricular enlargement in cor pulmonale is due to increased afterload. An occluded vessel impairs the heart's ability to generate enough pressure. Pulmonary hypertension results from the increased blood flow needed to oxygenate the tissues.

In response to hypoxia, the bone marrow produces more red blood cells (RBCs), causing polycythemia. The blood's viscosity increases, which further aggravates pulmonary hypertension. This increases the right ventricle's workload, causing heart failure. (See *Cor pulmonale: An overview.*)

In COPD, increased airway obstruction makes airflow worse. The resulting hypoxia and hypercarbia can have vasodilatory effects on systemic arterioles. However, hypoxia increases pulmonary vasoconstriction. The liver becomes palpable and tender because it's engorged and

displaced downward by the low diaphragm. Hepatojugular reflux may occur.

Compensatory mechanisms begin to fail, and larger amounts of blood remain in the right ventricle at the end of diastole, causing ventricular dilation. Increasing intrathoracic pressures impede venous return and raise pressure within the jugular vein. Peripheral edema can occur, and right ventricular hypertrophy increases progressively. The main pulmonary arteries enlarge, pulmonary hypertension increases, and heart failure occurs.

Signs and symptoms
Early stages
◆ Chronic productive cough to clear secretions from the lungs
◆ Exertional dyspnea due to hypoxia
◆ Wheezing respirations as airways narrow
◆ Fatigue and weakness due to hypoxemia

Progressive cor pulmonale
◆ Dyspnea at rest due to hypoxemia
◆ Tachypnea due to decreased oxygenation to the tissues
◆ Orthopnea due to pulmonary edema
◆ Dependent edema due to right-sided heart failure
◆ Neck vein distention due to pulmonary hypertension
◆ Enlarged, tender liver related to polycythemia and decreased cardiac output
◆ Hepatojugular reflux (jugular vein distention induced by pressing over the liver) due to right-sided heart failure
◆ Right upper quadrant discomfort due to liver involvement
◆ Tachycardia due to decreased cardiac output and increasing hypoxia
◆ Weakened pulses due to decreased cardiac output
◆ Pansystolic murmur at the lower left sternal border with tricuspid insufficiency, which increases in intensity when the patient inhales

Complications
◆ Right- and left-sided heart failure as the heart hypertrophies in an attempt to circulate the blood
◆ Hepatomegaly
◆ Edema
◆ Ascites
◆ Pleural effusions
◆ Thromboembolism due to polycythemia

Diagnosis
◆ Pulmonary artery catheterization shows increased right ventricular and pulmonary artery pressures, resulting from increased pulmonary

vascular resistance. Right ventricular systolic and pulmonary artery systolic pressures are more than 30 mm Hg, and pulmonary artery diastolic pressure is more than 15 mm Hg.

◆ Echocardiography demonstrates right ventricular enlargement.

◆ Angiography shows right ventricular enlargement.

◆ Chest X-rays reveal large central pulmonary arteries and right ventricular enlargement.

◆ Arterial blood gas (ABG) analysis detects decreased partial pressure of arterial oxygen (usually less than 70 mm Hg and rarely more than 90 mm Hg).

◆ Electrocardiography shows arrhythmias, such as premature atrial and ventricular contractions and atrial fibrillation during severe hypoxia, and also right bundle-branch block, right-axis deviation, prominent P waves, and an inverted T wave in right precordial leads.

◆ Pulmonary function studies reflect underlying pulmonary disease.

◆ Magnetic resonance imaging measures the right ventricular mass, wall thickness, and ejection fraction.

◆ Cardiac catheterization measures pulmonary vascular pressures.

◆ Laboratory testing may reveal hematocrit typically over 50%; serum hepatic test results may show an elevated aspartate aminotransferase level with hepatic congestion and decreased liver function, and the serum bilirubin level may be elevated if liver dysfunction and hepatomegaly exist.

Treatment

Therapy for cor pulmonale has three aims: reducing hypoxemia and pulmonary vasoconstriction, increasing exercise tolerance, and correcting the underlying condition when possible. Treatment may involve:

◆ bed rest to reduce myocardial oxygen demands

◆ digoxin to increase the strength of contraction of the myocardium

◆ an antibiotic to treat an underlying respiratory tract infection

◆ a potent pulmonary artery vasodilator, such as diazoxide, nitroprusside, hydralazine, an angiotensin-converting enzyme inhibitor, or a calcium channel blocker to reduce primary pulmonary hypertension

◆ I.V. prostacyclin therapy to dilate blood vessels and reduce clotting by stopping platelet aggregation

◆ an endothelin receptor antagonist, such as bosentan, to reduce vasoconstriction

◆ continuous administration of low concentrations of oxygen to decrease pulmonary hypertension, polycythemia, and tachypnea

◆ mechanical ventilation to reduce the workload of breathing in acute disease

◆ a low-sodium diet with restricted fluid to reduce edema

◆ diuretics as indicated to reduce edema

◆ phlebotomy to decrease excess RBC mass that occurs with polycythemia

◆ small doses of heparin to decrease the risk of thromboembolism

◆ tracheotomy, which may be required if the patient has an upper airway obstruction

◆ a corticosteroid to treat vasculitis or an underlying autoimmune disorder.

Special considerations

◆ Plan the patient's diet carefully with the patient and the staff dietitian. Because the patient may lack energy and tire easily when eating, provide small, frequent feedings rather than three heavy meals.

◆ Prevent fluid retention by limiting the patient's fluid intake to 1 to 2 qt (1 to 2 L)/day and providing a low-sodium diet.

◆ Monitor the serum potassium level closely if the patient is receiving a diuretic. A low serum potassium level can increase the risk of arrhythmias associated with cardiac glycosides.

◆ Monitor the patient for signs and symptoms of digoxin toxicity, such as anorexia, nausea, vomiting, and yellow halos around visual images; also monitor him for cardiac arrhythmias. Teach the patient to check his radial pulse before taking digoxin or a cardiac glycoside. He should be instructed to notify the physician if he detects changes in his pulse rate.

◆ Reposition the bedridden patient often to prevent atelectasis.

◆ Provide meticulous respiratory care, including oxygen therapy and, for the patient with COPD, pursed-lip breathing exercises. Periodically measure ABG levels, watching for such signs of respiratory failure as change in pulse rate; deep, labored respirations; and increased fatigue after exertion.

Before discharge, maintain this protocol:

◆ Make sure the patient understands the importance of maintaining a low-salt diet, weighing himself daily, and watching for and immediately reporting edema. Teach him to detect edema by pressing the skin over his shins with one finger, holding it for a second or two, then checking for a finger impression.

◆ Instruct the patient to allow himself frequent rest periods and to do his breathing exercises regularly.

◆ If the patient needs supplemental oxygen therapy at home, refer him to an agency that can

How croup affects the upper airway

In croup, inflammatory swelling and spasms constrict the larynx, reducing airflow. This cross section (from chin to chest) shows the upper-airway changes caused by croup. Inflammatory changes obstruct the larynx (which includes the epiglottis) and almost completely and significantly narrow the trachea.

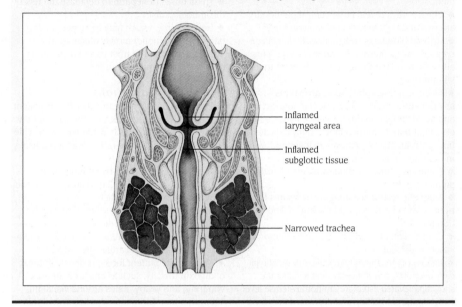

Inflamed laryngeal area

Inflamed subglottic tissue

Narrowed trachea

help him obtain the necessary equipment and, as necessary, arrange for follow-up examinations.

◆ If the patient has been placed on anticoagulant therapy, emphasize the need to watch for bleeding (epistaxis, hematuria, bruising) and to report signs to the physician. Also, encourage him to return for periodic laboratory tests to monitor partial thromboplastin time, fibrinogen level, platelet count, hematocrit, hemoglobin level, and prothrombin time.

◆ Because pulmonary infection commonly exacerbates COPD and cor pulmonale, tell the patient to watch for and immediately report early signs of infection, such as increased sputum production, change in sputum color, increased coughing or wheezing, chest pain, fever, and tightness in the chest. Tell the patient to avoid crowds and persons known to have pulmonary infections, especially during the flu season.

◆ Warn the patient to avoid nonprescribed medications that may depress the ventilatory drive, such as sedatives.

CROUP

Croup is a severe inflammation and obstruction of the upper airway, occurring as acute laryngo-tracheobronchitis (most common), laryngitis, and acute spasmodic laryngitis; it must always be distinguished from epiglottiditis. It's derived from a German word for *voice box* and refers to swelling around the larynx or vocal cords. Recovery is usually complete.

Croup is a childhood disease affecting more boys than girls (typically between ages 3 months and 5 years) that usually occurs during winter months. Up to 15% of patients have a strong family history of croup.

Causes

Croup usually results from a viral infection. Causative viruses may include:
◆ adenoviruses
◆ influenza
◆ measles
◆ parainfluenza viruses (75% of cases)
◆ respiratory syncytial virus (RSV).

Pathophysiology

Croup is usually preceded by an upper-airway infection that proceeds to laryngitis and then descends into the trachea (and sometimes the bronchi), causing inflammation of the mucosal lining and subsequent narrowing of the airway. Profound airway edema may lead to obstruction and seriously compromised ventilation. (See *How croup affects the upper airway*.)

The flexible larynx of a young child is particularly susceptible to spasm, which may cause complete airway obstruction. When the child's airway is significantly narrowed, he struggles to inhale air past the obstruction and into the lungs, producing the characteristic inspiratory stridor and suprasternal retractions, and the classic barking or seal-like cough.

Croup is characterized by gradual onset of a low-grade fever. Worsening of symptoms at night and a cough are common. The airway obstruction increases, leading to retractions, restlessness, anxiety, tachycardia, and tachypnea. Severe obstruction leads to respiratory exhaustion, hypoxemia, carbon dioxide accumulation, and respiratory acidosis.

Signs and symptoms
◆ Inspiratory stridor, hoarse or muffled vocal sounds, and a characteristic sharp, barking, seal-like cough related to the degree of laryngeal obstruction and respiratory distress (these signs and symptoms may last only a few hours or persist up to a few days)
◆ Pallor or cyanosis due to hypoxemia
◆ Tachycardia and tachypnea due to increasing airway obstruction
◆ Restlessness and anxiety related to worsening respiratory distress
◆ Severely compromised ventilation caused by inflammatory edema, and possibly spasm, of the upper airways

Complications
If the child experiences obstruction that's severe enough to prevent adequate exhalation of carbon dioxide, respiratory acidosis results and the child eventually experiences respiratory failure.

Diagnosis
Croup is easily identified and can be diagnosed almost immediately because of its characteristic signs and symptoms. When evaluating the patient with croup, assess for foreign body obstruction (a common cause of crouplike cough in young children) as well as masses and cysts to rule out other causes of the child's symptoms. Tests that may help diagnosis the disorder include:
◆ When bacterial infection is the cause, throat cultures may identify the organisms and their sensitivity to antibiotics as well as rule out diphtheria.
◆ Posterior-anterior X-ray of the chest shows narrowing of the upper airway ("steeple sign").

◆ Laryngoscopy may reveal inflammation and obstruction in epiglottal and laryngeal areas.

Treatment
◆ For most children with croup, home care with rest, cool humidification during sleep, and an antipyretic, such as acetaminophen, relieve symptoms.
◆ With respiratory distress that's severe or interferes with oral hydration, hospitalization is required and parenteral fluid replacement is needed to prevent dehydration.
◆ If bacterial infection is the cause, antibiotic therapy is necessary.
◆ Oxygen therapy may also be required.
◆ Increasing obstruction of the airway requires intubation and mechanical ventilation.
◆ Inhaled racemic epinephrine and a corticosteroid may be used to alleviate respiratory distress.

Special considerations
Monitor and support the patient's respiration, and control fever. Because croup is frightening to the child and his family, you must also provide support and reassurance.
◆ Carefully monitor cough and breath sounds, hoarseness, severity of retractions, inspiratory stridor, cyanosis, respiratory rate and character (especially prolonged and labored respirations), restlessness, fever, and cardiac rate.
◆ Keep the child as quiet as possible. However, avoid sedation because it may depress respiration. If the patient is an infant, position him in an infant seat or prop him up with a pillow; place an older child in Fowler's position. If an older child requires a cool mist tent to help him breathe, explain why it's needed.
◆ Isolate patients suspected of having RSV and parainfluenza infections if possible. Wash your hands carefully before leaving the room, to avoid transmission to other children, particularly infants. Instruct parents and others involved in the care of these children to take similar precautions.
◆ Control fever with sponge baths and an antipyretic. Keep a hypothermia blanket on hand for temperatures above 102° F (38.9° C). Watch for seizures in infants and young children with high fevers. Give an I.V. antibiotic as ordered.
◆ Relieve sore throat with soothing, water-based ices, such as fruit sherbet and popsicles. Avoid thicker, milk-based fluids if the child is producing heavy mucus or has great difficulty in swallowing. Apply petroleum jelly or another ointment around the nose and lips to soothe irritation from nasal discharge and mouth breathing.
◆ Maintain a calm, quiet environment and offer reassurance. Explain all procedures and answer any questions.

CLOSER LOOK

Lung changes in emphysema

In the patient with emphysema, recurrent pulmonary inflammation damages and eventually destroys the alveolar walls, creating large air spaces. The damaged alveoli can't recoil normally after expanding; therefore, bronchioles collapse on expiration, trapping air in the lungs and causing overdistention. As the alveolar walls are destroyed, the lungs become enlarged, and the total lung capacity and residual volume then increase. Shown here are changes that occur during emphysema.

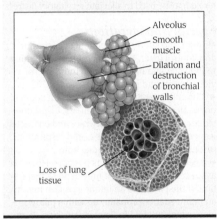

Alveolus

Smooth muscle

Dilation and destruction of bronchial walls

Loss of lung tissue

When croup doesn't require hospitalization:
◆ Teach the parents effective home care. Suggest the use of a cool humidifier (vaporizer). To relieve croupy spells, tell parents to carry the child into the bathroom, shut the door, and turn on hot water in the sink, shower, or bathtub. Breathing in warm, moist air quickly eases an acute spell of croup.
◆ Warn parents that ear infections and pneumonia are complications of croup, which may appear about 5 days after recovery. Stress the importance of immediately reporting earache, productive cough, high fever, or increased shortness of breath.

EMPHYSEMA

Emphysema, a form of chronic obstructive pulmonary disease, is the abnormal, permanent enlargement of the acini accompanied by destruction of alveolar walls. Obstruction results from tissue changes rather than mucus production, which occurs with asthma and chronic bronchitis. The distinguishing characteristic of emphysema is airflow limitation caused by lack of elastic recoil in the lungs.

Emphysema appears to be more prevalent in males than in females; about 57% of patients with well-defined emphysema are males and 43% are females.

AGE ALERT *Aging is a risk factor for emphysema. Senile emphysema results from degenerative changes; stretching occurs without destruction in the smooth muscle. Connective tissue isn't usually affected.*

Causes
◆ Alpha₁-antitrypsin (AAT) deficiency
◆ Cigarette smoking

Pathophysiology

GENETIC LINK *Primary emphysema has been linked to an inherited deficiency of the enzyme AAT, a major component of alpha₁-globulin. AAT inhibits the activation of several proteolytic enzymes; deficiency of this enzyme is an autosomal recessive trait that predisposes an individual to develop emphysema because proteolysis in lung tissues isn't inhibited. Homozygous individuals have up to an 80% chance of developing lung disease; people who smoke have a greater chance of developing emphysema. Patients who develop emphysema before or during their early 40s and those who are nonsmokers are believed to have an AAT deficiency. Potential treatments for patients with AAT deficiency are currently under study and include AAT replacement therapy and gene therapy.*

In emphysema, recurrent inflammation is associated with the release of proteolytic enzymes from lung cells. This causes irreversible enlargement of the air spaces distal to the terminal bronchioles. Enlargement of air spaces destroys the alveolar walls, which results in a breakdown of elasticity and loss of fibrous and muscle tissue, thus making the lungs less compliant.

In normal breathing, the air moves into and out of the lungs to meet metabolic needs. A change in airway size compromises the lungs' ability to circulate sufficient air. In patients with emphysema, recurrent pulmonary inflammation damages and eventually destroys the alveolar walls, creating large air spaces. (See *Lung changes in emphysema*.) The alveolar septa are initially destroyed, eliminating a portion of the capillary bed and increasing air volume in the acinus. This breakdown leaves the alveoli unable to recoil normally after expanding and results in bronchiolar collapse on expiration. The damaged or destroyed alveolar walls can't support the airways to keep them open. (See *Air trapping in emphysema*.) The amount of air that can be

CLOSER LOOK
Air trapping in emphysema

After alveolar walls are damaged or destroyed, they can't support and keep the airways open. The alveolar walls then lose their capability of elastic recoil. Collapse then occurs on expiration, as shown here.

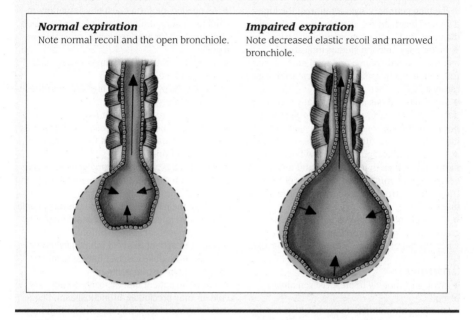

Normal expiration
Note normal recoil and the open bronchiole.

Impaired expiration
Note decreased elastic recoil and narrowed bronchiole.

expired passively is diminished, thus trapping air in the lungs and leading to overdistention. Hyperinflation of the alveoli produces bullae (air spaces) adjacent to the pleura (blebs). Septal destruction also decreases airway calibration. Part of each inspiration is trapped because of increased residual volume and decreased calibration. Septal destruction may affect only the respiratory bronchioles and alveolar ducts, leaving alveolar sacs intact (centriacinar emphysema), or it may involve the entire acinus (panacinar emphysema), with damage more random and involving the lower lobes of the lungs.

⚠ **CLINICAL ALERT** *Panacinar emphysema tends to occur in elderly people with an AAT deficiency, whereas centriacinar emphysema occurs in smokers with chronic bronchitis.*

Associated pulmonary capillary destruction usually allows a patient with severe emphysema to match ventilation to perfusion. This process prevents the development of cyanosis. The lungs are usually enlarged; therefore, the total lung capacity and residual volume increase.

Signs and symptoms
◆ Tachypnea related to decreased oxygenation
◆ Exertional dyspnea, commonly the initial symptom from changes in airway size
◆ Barrel-shaped chest due to the lungs overdistending and overinflating
◆ Prolonged expiration and grunting, which occur because the accessory muscles are used for inspiration and abdominal muscles are used for expiration
◆ Decreased breath sounds caused by air trapping in the alveoli and alveolar wall destruction
◆ Clubbed fingers and toes related to chronic hypoxic changes
◆ Decreased tactile fremitus on palpation as air moves through poorly functioning alveoli
◆ Decreased chest expansion due to hypoventilation
◆ Hyperresonance on chest percussion due to overinflated air spaces
◆ Crackles and wheezing on inspiration as bronchioles collapse

Complications
◆ Right ventricular hypertrophy (cor pulmonale)
◆ Respiratory failure
◆ Recurrent respiratory tract infections

Diagnosis
◆ Chest X-rays in advanced disease may show a flattened diaphragm, reduced vascular markings at the lung periphery, overaeration of the lungs, a vertical heart, enlarged anteroposterior chest diameter, and a large retrosternal air space.
◆ Pulmonary function studies indicate increased residual volume and total lung capacity, reduced diffusing capacity, and increased inspiratory flow.
◆ Arterial blood gas analysis usually reveals reduced partial pressure or arterial oxygen and a normal partial pressure of arterial carbon dioxide until late in the disease process.
◆ Electrocardiography may show tall, symmetrical P waves in leads II, III, and aV$_F$; a vertical QRS complex and signs of right ventricular hypertrophy are seen late in the disease.
◆ Complete blood count usually reveals an increased hemoglobin level late in the disease when the patient has persistent, severe hypoxia.

Treatment
◆ Avoiding smoking to preserve remaining alveoli
◆ Avoiding air pollution to preserve remaining alveoli
◆ A bronchodilator, such as a beta-adrenergic blocker, albuterol, or ipratropium bromide, to reverse bronchospasms and promote mucociliary clearance
◆ An antibiotic to treat respiratory tract infections
◆ Immunizations to prevent influenza and pneumococcal pneumonia
◆ Adequate hydration to liquefy and mobilize secretions
◆ Chest physiotherapy to mobilize secretions
◆ Oxygen therapy at low settings to correct hypoxia
◆ A mucolytic to thin secretions and aid in mucus expectoration
◆ An aerosolized or systemic corticosteroid
◆ Transtracheal catheterization to enable the patient to receive oxygen therapy at home
◆ Lung volume reduction surgery for selected patients (Nonfunctional parts of the lung [tissue filled with disease providing little ventilation or perfusion] are surgically removed; removal allows more functional lung tissue to expand and the diaphragm to return to its normally elevated position.)

Special considerations
◆ If the patient smokes, encourage him to stop. Provide him with smoking-cessation resources or counseling if necessary.
◆ Assess respiratory function for changes. Evaluate sputum quality and quantity, restlessness, increased tachypnea, and altered breath sounds. Report changes immediately.
◆ As needed, perform chest physiotherapy, including postural drainage and chest percussion and vibration for involved lobes, several times daily.
◆ Weigh the patient three times weekly, and assess him for edema.
◆ Provide the patient with a high-calorie, protein-rich diet. Offer small, frequent meals to conserve his energy and prevent fatigue.
◆ Make sure the patient receives an adequate amount of fluids (at least 3 qt [3 L] per day) to loosen secretions.
◆ Schedule respiratory therapy at least 1 hour before or after meals. Provide mouth care after bronchodilator inhalation therapy.
◆ Advise the patient to avoid crowds and people with known infections and to obtain influenza and pneumococcal immunizations.
◆ Urge the patient to avoid inhaled irritants, such as automobile exhaust fumes, aerosol sprays, and industrial pollutants.
◆ Warn the patient that exposure to blasts of cold air may precipitate bronchospasm. Suggest that he avoid cold, windy weather or that he cover his mouth and nose with a scarf or mask if he must go outside.

⚠ **CLINICAL ALERT** *Inform the patient about signs and symptoms that suggest ruptured alveolar blebs and bullae. Explain the seriousness of possible spontaneous pneumothorax. Urge him to notify the physician if he feels sudden, sharp pleuritic pain exacerbated by chest movement, breathing, or coughing.*
◆ For family members of the patient with familial emphysema, recommend a blood test for AAT deficiency. If a deficiency is found, stress the importance of not smoking and avoiding areas (if possible) where smoking is permitted.

PLEURAL EFFUSION AND EMPYEMA
Pleural effusion is excess fluid in the pleural space. Normally, this space contains a small amount of extracellular fluid that lubricates the pleural surfaces. Increased production or inadequate removal of this fluid results in pleural effusion. Empyema is the accumulation of pus and necrotic tissue in the pleural space. Blood (hemothorax) and chyle (chylothorax) may also collect in this space.

Causes

Transudative pleural effusions commonly result from heart failure, hepatic disease with ascites, peritoneal dialysis, hypoalbuminemia, and disorders resulting in overexpanded intravascular volume.

Exudative pleural effusions occur with tuberculosis (TB), subphrenic abscess, pancreatitis, bacterial or fungal pneumonitis or empyema, malignancy, pulmonary embolism with or without infarction, connective tissue disease (lupus erythematosus [LE] and rheumatoid arthritis), myxedema, and chest trauma.

Empyema may result from idiopathic infection or may be related to pneumonitis, carcinoma, perforation, or esophageal rupture.

Pathophysiology

The balance of osmotic and hydrostatic pressures in parietal pleural capillaries normally results in fluid movement into the pleural space. Balanced pressures in visceral pleural capillaries promote reabsorption of this fluid. Excessive hydrostatic pressure or decreased osmotic pressure can cause excess fluid to pass across intact capillaries. The result is a transudative pleural effusion, an ultrafiltrate of plasma containing low concentrations of protein.

Exudative pleural effusions result when capillaries exhibit increased permeability with or without changes in hydrostatic and colloid osmotic pressures, allowing protein-rich fluid to leak into the pleural space.

Empyema is usually associated with an infection in the pleural space, which results from an extension of an infection of nearby structures.

Signs and symptoms

Patients with pleural effusion characteristically display symptoms relating to the underlying pathologic condition. Most patients with large effusions, particularly those with underlying pulmonary disease, report dyspnea. Those with effusions associated with pleurisy report pleuritic chest pain. Other clinical features depend on the cause of the effusion. Patients with empyema also develop fever and malaise.

Complications
Pleural effusion
◆ Impaired ventilation
◆ Pleurisy

Empyema
◆ Pleurisy
◆ Pericarditis
◆ Septicemia

Diagnosis

Auscultation of the chest reveals decreased breath sounds; percussion detects dullness over the effused area, which doesn't change with breathing. Chest X-ray shows radiopaque fluid in dependent regions. However, diagnosis also requires other tests to distinguish transudative from exudative effusions and to help pinpoint the underlying disorder.

The most useful test is thoracentesis, in which analysis of aspirated pleural fluid shows:
◆ *transudative effusions* — lactate dehydrogenase (LD) level less than 200 IU and protein level less than 3 g/dl
◆ *exudative effusions* — ratio of protein in pleural fluid to serum of 0.5 or more, LD in pleural fluid of 200 IU or more, and ratio of LD in pleural fluid to LD in serum of 0.6 or more
◆ *empyema* — acute inflammatory white blood cells and microorganisms
◆ *empyema* or *rheumatoid arthritis* — extremely decreased pleural fluid glucose level.

In addition, if a pleural effusion results from esophageal rupture or pancreatitis, the fluid amylase level is usually higher than the serum level. Aspirated fluid may be tested for LE cells, antinuclear antibodies, and neoplastic cells. It may also be analyzed for color and consistency; acid-fast bacillus, fungal, and bacterial cultures; and triglycerides (in chylothorax). Cell analysis shows leukocytosis in empyema. A negative tuberculin skin test strongly rules against TB as the cause. In exudative pleural effusions in which thoracentesis isn't definitive, pleural biopsy may be done. It's particularly useful for confirming TB or malignancy.

Treatment

Depending on the amount of fluid present, symptomatic effusion may require thoracentesis to remove fluid or careful monitoring of the patient's own reabsorption of the fluid. Hemothorax requires drainage to prevent fibrothorax formation. Pleural effusions associated with lung cancer typically reaccumulate quickly. If a chest tube is inserted to drain the fluid, a sclerosing agent, such as talc, may be injected through the tube to cause adhesions between the parietal and visceral pleura, thereby obliterating the potential space for fluid to recollect.

Treatment of empyema requires insertion of one or more chest tubes after thoracentesis, to allow drainage of purulent material, and possibly decortication (surgical removal of the thick coating over the lung) or rib resection to allow open drainage and lung expansion. Empyema also requires a parenteral antibiotic. Associated hypoxia requires oxygen administration.

Special considerations

◆ Explain thoracentesis to the patient. Before the procedure, tell the patient to expect a stinging sensation from the local anesthetic and a feeling of pressure when the needle is inserted. Instruct him to tell you immediately if he feels uncomfortable or has trouble breathing during the procedure.

◆ Reassure the patient during thoracentesis. Remind him to breathe normally and avoid sudden movements, such as coughing or sighing. Monitor vital signs, and watch for syncope.

⚠ **CLINICAL ALERT** *If fluid is removed too quickly during thoracentesis, the patient may experience bradycardia, hypotension, pain, pulmonary edema, or even cardiac arrest. Watch for respiratory distress or pneumothorax (sudden onset of dyspnea and cyanosis) after thoracentesis.*

◆ Administer oxygen and, in empyema, an antibiotic, as ordered.

◆ Encourage the patient to perform deep-breathing exercises to promote lung expansion. Use an incentive spirometer to promote deep breathing.

◆ Provide meticulous chest tube care, and use aseptic technique for changing dressings around the tube insertion site in empyema. Ensure tube patency by watching for fluctuations of fluid in the underwater-seal chamber. Watch for bubbling in the water-seal chamber, indicating the presence of air in the pleural spaces. Record the amount, color, and consistency of tube drainage.

◆ If the patient has open drainage through a rib resection or intercostal tube, use hand and dressing precautions. Because weeks of such drainage are usually necessary to obliterate the space, make visiting nurse referrals for the patient who'll be discharged with the tube in place.

◆ If pleural effusion is a complication of pneumonia or influenza, advise prompt medical attention for chest colds.

||||| LIFE-THREATENING DISORDER

PNEUMOTHORAX

Pneumothorax is an accumulation of air in the pleural cavity that leads to partial or complete lung collapse. When the air between the visceral and parietal pleurae collects and accumulates, increasing tension in the pleural cavity can cause the lung to progressively collapse. Air is trapped in the intrapleural space and determines the degree of lung collapse. Venous return to the heart may be impeded to cause a life-threatening condition called tension pneumothorax.

The most common types of pneumothorax are open, closed, and tension.

Causes

Open pneumothorax

◆ Chest surgery
◆ Insertion of a central venous catheter
◆ Penetrating chest injury (gunshot or stab wound)
◆ Thoracentesis or closed pleural biopsy
◆ Transbronchial biopsy

Closed pneumothorax

◆ Air leakage from ruptured blebs
◆ Blunt chest trauma
◆ Interstitial lung disease, such as eosinophilic granuloma
◆ Rupture resulting from barotrauma caused by high intrathoracic pressures during mechanical ventilation
◆ Tubercular or cancerous lesions that erode into the pleural space

Tension pneumothorax

◆ Chest tube occlusion or malfunction
◆ Fractured ribs
◆ High-level positive end-expiratory pressure that causes alveolar blebs to rupture
◆ Mechanical ventilation
◆ Penetrating chest wound treated with an airtight dressing

Pathophysiology

A rupture in the visceral or parietal pleura and chest wall causes air to accumulate and separate the visceral and parietal pleurae. Negative pressure is destroyed, and the elastic recoil forces are affected. The lung recoils by collapsing toward the hilus.

Open pneumothorax (also called a *sucking chest wound* or *communicating pneumothorax*) results when atmospheric air (positive pressure) flows directly into the pleural cavity (negative pressure). As the air pressure in the pleural cavity becomes positive, the lung collapses on the affected side, resulting in decreased total lung capacity, vital capacity, and lung compliance. Ventilation-perfusion imbalances lead to hypoxia.

Closed pneumothorax occurs when air enters the pleural space from within the lung, causing increased pleural pressure, which prevents lung expansion during normal inspiration. Spontaneous pneumothorax is another type of closed pneumothorax.

▲ **AGE ALERT** *Spontaneous pneumothorax is common in older patients with chronic pulmonary disease, but it may also occur in healthy, tall, young adults.*

Both types of closed pneumothorax can result in a collapsed lung with hypoxia and decreased total lung capacity, vital capacity, and lung compliance. The range of lung collapse is between 5% and 95%.

Tension pneumothorax results when air in the pleural space is under higher pressure than air in the adjacent lung. The air enters the pleural space from the site of pleural rupture, which acts as a one-way valve. Air is allowed to enter into the pleural space on inspiration, but can't escape as the rupture site closes on expiration. More air enters on inspiration, and air pressure begins to exceed barometric pressure. Increasing air pressure pushes against the recoiled lung, causing compression atelectasis. Air also presses against the mediastinum, compressing and displacing the heart and great vessels. The air can't escape, and the accumulating pressure causes the lung to collapse. As air continues to accumulate and intrapleural pressures increase, the mediastinum shifts away from the affected side and decreases venous return. This forces the heart, trachea, esophagus, and great vessels to the unaffected side, compressing the heart and the contra-lateral lung. Without immediate treatment, this emergency can rapidly become fatal. (See *Understanding tension pneumothorax.*)

Signs and symptoms
◆ Sudden, sharp pleuritic pain exacerbated by chest movement, breathing, and coughing
◆ Asymmetrical chest wall movement due to lung collapse
◆ Shortness of breath due to hypoxia
◆ Cyanosis due to hypoxia
◆ Respiratory distress due to moderate or severe pneumothorax
◆ Decreased vocal fremitus related to lung collapse
◆ Absent breath sounds on the affected side due to lung collapse
◆ Chest rigidity on the affected side due to decreased expansion
◆ Tachycardia due to hypoxia
◆ Crackling beneath the skin on palpation (subcutaneous emphysema), which is due to air leaking into the tissues

Tension pneumothorax
◆ Hypotension and compensatory tachycardia due to decreased cardiac output
◆ Tachypnea due to hypoxia
◆ Lung collapse due to air or blood in the intrapleural space
◆ Mediastinal shift and tracheal deviation to the opposite side due to increasing tension
◆ Neck vein distention due to intrapleural pressure, mediastinal shift, and increased cardiovascular pressure
◆ Pallor related to decreased cardiac output

CLOSER LOOK

Understanding tension pneumothorax

In tension pneumothorax, air accumulates intrapleurally and can't escape. As intrapleural pressure increases, the ipsilateral lung is affected and also collapses.

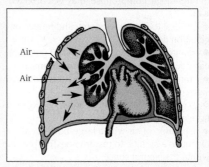

On inspiration, the mediastinum shifts toward the unaffected lung, impairing ventilation.

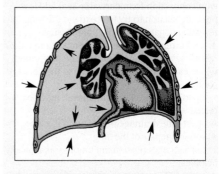

◆ Anxiety related to hypoxia
◆ Weak and rapid pulse due to decreased cardiac output

Complications
◆ Decreased cardiac output
◆ Hypoxemia
◆ Cardiac arrest

Diagnosis
◆ Chest X-rays confirm the diagnosis by revealing air in the pleural space and, possibly, a mediastinal shift.
◆ Arterial blood gas analysis may reveal hypoxemia, possibly with respiratory acidosis and

hypercapnia. Partial pressure of arterial oxygen levels may decrease at first, but typically return to normal within 24 hours.
◆ Pulse oximetry reveals hypoxemia.

Treatment

Treatment depends on the type of pneumothorax.

Spontaneous pneumothorax with less than 30% of lung collapse, no signs of increased pleural pressure, and no dyspnea or indications of physiologic compromise, may be corrected with:
◆ bed rest to conserve energy and reduce oxygenation demands
◆ monitoring of blood pressure and pulse for early detection of physiologic compromise
◆ monitoring of respiratory rate to detect early signs of respiratory compromise
◆ oxygen administration to enhance oxygenation and improve hypoxia
◆ aspiration of air with a large-bore needle attached to a syringe to restore negative pressure within the pleural space.

Correction of pneumothorax with more than 30% of lung collapse may include:
◆ thoracostomy tube placed in the second or third intercostal space in the midclavicular line with connection to underwater-seal and low-pressure suction to try to reexpand the lung by restoring negative intrapleural pressure
◆ if recurrent spontaneous pneumothorax, thoracotomy and pleurectomy may be performed, which causes the lung to adhere to the parietal pleura.

Open (traumatic) pneumothorax may be corrected with:
◆ chest tube drainage to reexpand the lung
◆ surgical repair of the lung.

Correction of tension pneumothorax typically involves:
◆ immediate treatment with large-bore needle insertion into the pleural space through the second intercostal space to reexpand the lung
◆ insertion of a thoracostomy tube
◆ an analgesic to promote comfort and encourage deep breathing and coughing.

Special considerations

⚠ **CLINICAL ALERT** *Watch for pallor, gasping respirations, and sudden chest pain. Carefully monitor vital signs at least every hour for indications of shock, increasing respiratory distress, or mediastinal shift. Listen for breath sounds over both lungs. Falling blood pressure and rising pulse and respiratory rates may indicate tension pneumothorax, which could be fatal without prompt treatment.*

◆ Urge the patient to control coughing and gasping during thoracotomy. However, after the chest tube is in place, encourage him to cough and breathe deeply (at least once per hour) to facilitate lung expansion.
◆ If the patient is undergoing chest tube drainage, watch for continuing air leakage (bubbling), indicating the lung defect has failed to close; this may require surgery. Also watch for increasing subcutaneous emphysema by checking around the neck or at the tube insertion site for crackling beneath the skin. If the patient is on a ventilator, watch for difficulty in breathing in time with the ventilator as well as pressure changes on ventilator gauges.
◆ Change dressings around the chest tube insertion site, as necessary. Be careful not to reposition or dislodge the tube. If the tube dislodges, place a petroleum gauze dressing over the opening immediately to prevent rapid lung collapse.
◆ Monitor vital signs frequently after thoracotomy. Also, for the first 24 hours, assess respiratory status by checking breath sounds hourly. Observe the chest tube site for leakage, noting the amount and color of drainage. Help the patient walk, as ordered (usually on the first postoperative day), to facilitate deep inspiration and lung expansion.
◆ To reassure the patient, explain what pneumothorax is, what causes it, and all diagnostic tests and procedures. Make him as comfortable as possible. (The patient with pneumothorax is usually most comfortable sitting upright.)

||| **LIFE-THREATENING DISORDER**

PULMONARY EDEMA

Pulmonary edema is an accumulation of fluid in the extravascular spaces of the lungs. It's a common complication of cardiac disorders and may occur as a chronic condition or may develop quickly and rapidly become fatal.

Causes

Pulmonary edema is caused by left-sided heart failure due to:
◆ arteriosclerosis
◆ cardiomyopathy
◆ hypertension
◆ valvular heart disease.

Factors that predispose the patient to pulmonary edema include:
◆ barbiturate or opiate poisoning
◆ cancer
◆ cardiac failure
◆ excess infusion of I.V. fluids or overly rapid infusion

CLOSER LOOK
Understanding pulmonary edema

In pulmonary edema, diminished function of the left ventricle causes blood to back up into pulmonary veins and capillaries. The increasing capillary hydrostatic pressure pushes fluid into the interstitial spaces and alveoli. These illustrations show how pulmonary edema develops.

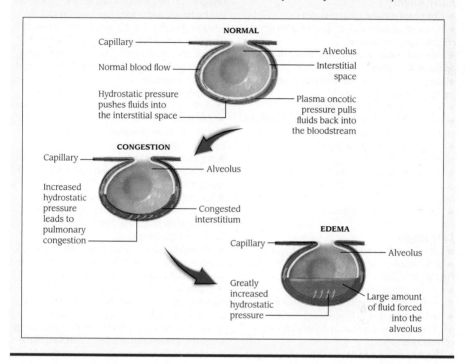

NORMAL

Capillary

Normal blood flow

Hydrostatic pressure pushes fluids into the interstitial space

Alveolus

Interstitial space

Plasma oncotic pressure pulls fluids back into the bloodstream

CONGESTION

Capillary

Increased hydrostatic pressure leads to pulmonary congestion

Alveolus

Congested interstitium

EDEMA

Capillary

Greatly increased hydrostatic pressure

Alveolus

Large amount of fluid forced into the alveolus

♦ impaired pulmonary lymphatic drainage (from Hodgkin's disease or obliterative lymphangitis after radiation)
♦ inhalation of irritating gases
♦ infectious disease
♦ mitral stenosis and left atrial myxoma (which impairs left atrial emptying)
♦ pneumonia
♦ pulmonary venoocclusive disease.
♦ sepsis

Pathophysiology

Normally, pulmonary capillary hydrostatic pressure, capillary oncotic pressure, capillary permeability, and lymphatic drainage are in balance. When this balance changes or the lymphatic drainage system is obstructed, fluid infiltrates into the lung and pulmonary edema results. If pulmonary capillary hydrostatic pressure increases, the compromised left ventricle requires increased filling pressures to maintain adequate cardiac output. These pressures are transmitted to the left atrium, pulmonary veins, and pulmonary capillary bed, forcing fluids and solutes from the intravascular compartment into the interstitium of the lungs. As the interstitium overloads with fluid, fluid floods the peripheral alveoli and impairs gas exchange. (See *Understanding pulmonary edema.*)

A blockage of the lymph vessels can result from compression by edema or tumor fibrotic tissue and by increased systemic venous pressure. Hydrostatic pressure in the large pulmonary veins increases, the pulmonary lymphatic system can't drain correctly into the pulmonary veins, and excess fluid moves into the interstitial space. Pulmonary edema then results from fluid accumulation.

Capillary injury, such as occurs in acute respiratory distress syndrome (ARDS) or with inhalation of toxic gases, increases capillary permeability. The injury causes plasma proteins and water to leak out of the capillary and move into the interstitium, increasing the interstitial oncotic pressure, which is normally low. As interstitial oncotic pressure begins to equal capillary oncotic pressure, the water begins to move out of the capillary and into the lungs, resulting in pulmonary edema.

Signs and symptoms
Early stages
♦ Exertional dyspnea due to hypoxia
♦ Paroxysmal nocturnal dyspnea due to decreased lung expansion
♦ Orthopnea due to decreased ability of the diaphragm to expand
♦ Cough due to stimulation of cough reflex by excessive fluid
♦ Mild tachypnea due to hypoxia
♦ Increased blood pressure due to increased pulmonary pressures and decreased oxygenation
♦ Dependent crackles as air moves through fluid in the lungs
♦ Neck vein distention due to decreased cardiac output and increased pulmonary vascular resistance
♦ Tachycardia due to hypoxia

Late stages
♦ Labored, rapid respiration due to hypoxia
♦ More diffuse crackles as air moves through fluid in the lungs
♦ Cough, producing frothy, bloody sputum
♦ Increased tachycardia due to hypoxemia
♦ Arrhythmias due to hypoxic myocardium
♦ Cold, clammy skin due to peripheral vasoconstriction
♦ Diaphoresis due to decreased cardiac output and shock
♦ Cyanosis due to hypoxia
♦ Decreased blood pressure due to decreased cardiac output and shock
♦ Thready pulse due to decreased cardiac output and shock

Complications
♦ Respiratory failure
♦ Respiratory acidosis
♦ Cardiac arrest

Diagnosis
♦ Arterial blood gas (ABG) analysis usually reveals hypoxia with variable partial pressure of arterial carbon dioxide, depending on the patient's degree of fatigue. Respiratory acidosis may occur.
♦ Chest X-rays show diffuse haziness of the lung fields and, usually, cardiomegaly and pleural effusion.
♦ Pulse oximetry may reveal decreasing arterial oxygen saturation levels.

♦ Pulmonary artery catheterization identifies left-sided heart failure and helps rule out ARDS.
♦ Electrocardiography may show a previous or current myocardial infarction.

Treatment
Treatment measures for pulmonary edema are designed to reduce extravascular fluid, to improve gas exchange and myocardial function and, if possible, to correct underlying pathologic conditions. Correcting this disorder typically involves:
♦ high concentrations of oxygen administered by nasal cannula to enhance gas exchange and improve oxygenation
♦ assisted ventilation to improve oxygen delivery to the tissues and promote acid-base balance
♦ a diuretic, such as furosemide, and bumetanide, to increase urination, which helps mobilize extravascular fluid
♦ a positive inotropic agent, such as digoxin or inamrinone, to enhance contractility in myocardial dysfunction
♦ a vasopressor to enhance contractility and promote vasoconstriction in peripheral vessels
♦ an antiarrhythmic for arrhythmias related to decreased cardiac output
♦ an arterial vasodilator, such as nitroprusside, to decrease peripheral vascular resistance, preload, and afterload
♦ a human B–type natriuretic peptide, such as nesiritide, to reduce pulmonary artery wedge pressure and systemic arterial pressure
♦ morphine to reduce anxiety and dyspnea and to dilate the systemic venous bed, promoting blood flow from pulmonary circulation to the periphery.

Special considerations
♦ Carefully monitor the vulnerable patient for early signs and symptoms of pulmonary edema, especially tachypnea, tachycardia, and abnormal breath sounds. Report abnormalities. Check for peripheral edema, which may also indicate that fluid level is accumulating in pulmonary tissue.
♦ Administer oxygen as ordered.
♦ Monitor vital signs every 15 to 30 minutes while administering nitroprusside in dextrose 5% in water by I.V. drip. Protect the nitroprusside solution from light by wrapping the bottle or bag with aluminum foil, and discard unused solution after 4 hours. Watch for arrhythmias in the patient receiving a cardiac glycoside and for marked respiratory depression in the patient receiving morphine.
♦ Assess the patient's condition frequently, and record his response to treatment. Monitor ABG levels, oral and I.V. fluid intake, urine output and, in the patient with a pulmonary artery catheter, pulmonary end-diastolic and wedge

pressures. Check cardiac monitoring often. Report changes immediately.

◆ Carefully record the time and amount of morphine given.

◆ Reassure the patient in a calm voice, and explain all procedures. Provide emotional support to his family as well.

||| LIFE-THREATENING DISORDER

PULMONARY EMBOLISM

The most common pulmonary complication in hospitalized patients, pulmonary embolism is an obstruction of the pulmonary arterial bed by a dislodged thrombus, heart valve growths, or a foreign substance. It affects an estimated 600,000 adults each year in the United States, resulting in 60,000 deaths. Although pulmonary infarction that results from embolism may be so mild as to be asymptomatic, massive embolism (more than 50% obstruction of pulmonary arterial circulation) and the accompanying infarction can be rapidly fatal.

Causes

Pulmonary embolism generally results from dislodged thrombi originating in the leg veins or pelvis. More than one-half of such thrombi arise in the deep veins of the legs. Other less common sources of thrombi are the pelvic veins, renal veins, hepatic vein, right side of the heart, and upper extremities.

Predisposing factors for pulmonary embolism include:

◆ advanced age
◆ autoimmune hemolytic anemia
◆ burns
◆ cancer
◆ chronic pulmonary disease
◆ heart failure or atrial fibrillation
◆ hormonal contraceptives
◆ I.V. drug abuse
◆ long-term immobility
◆ lower-extremity fractures or surgery
◆ obesity
◆ polycythemia vera
◆ pregnancy
◆ recent surgery
◆ sickle cell disease
◆ thrombocytosis
◆ thrombophlebitis
◆ varicose veins
◆ vascular injury.

Pathophysiology

Thrombus formation results directly from vascular wall damage, venostasis, or hypercoagulability

of the blood. Trauma, clot dissolution, sudden muscle spasm, intravascular pressure changes, or a change in peripheral blood flow can cause the thrombus to loosen or fragment. Then the thrombus—now called an embolus—floats to the heart's right side and enters the lung through the pulmonary artery. There, the embolus may dissolve, continue to fragment, or grow.

By occluding the pulmonary artery, the embolus prevents alveoli from producing enough surfactant to maintain alveolar integrity. As a result, alveoli collapse and atelectasis develops. If the embolus enlarges, it may clog most or all of the pulmonary vessels and cause death. (See *Looking at pulmonary emboli*, page 240.)

Rarely, the emboli contain air, fat, bacteria, amniotic fluid, talc (from drugs intended for oral administration, which are injected I.V. by addicts), or tumor cells.

Signs and symptoms

Total occlusion of the main pulmonary artery is rapidly fatal; smaller or fragmented emboli produce symptoms that vary with the size, number, and location. Usually, the first symptom of pulmonary embolism is dyspnea, which may be accompanied by angina or pleuritic chest pain, from pulmonary infarction. Other clinical features include tachycardia (related to hypoxemia), productive cough (sputum may be blood-tinged [related to mucus production from obstruction from embolus]), and pleural effusion (related to changes in intrapulmonary pressures secondary to embolus). Less common signs include massive hemoptysis, splinting of the chest, leg edema and, with a large embolus, cyanosis, syncope, and neck vein distention.

In addition, pulmonary embolism may cause pleural friction rub and signs and symptoms of circulatory collapse (weak, rapid pulse and hypotension) and of hypoxia (restlessness and anxiety).

Complications

◆ Pulmonary infarction
◆ Acute respiratory failure
◆ Acute cor pulmonale
◆ Death

Diagnosis

The patient history should reveal predisposing conditions for pulmonary embolism. A triad of deep vein thrombosis (DVT) formation is stasis, endothelial injury, and hypercoagulability. Risk factors include long car or plane trips, cancer, pregnancy, hypercoagulability, previous DVTs, and pulmonary emboli.

Looking at pulmonary emboli

This illustration shows multiple emboli in pulmonary artery branches and a larger embolus that has resulted in an infarcted area in the lung.

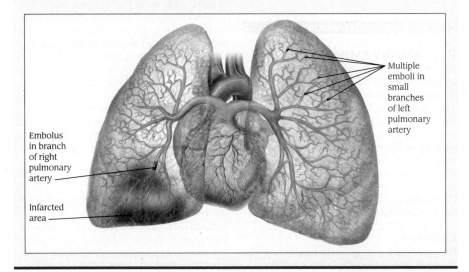

Multiple emboli in small branches of left pulmonary artery

Embolus in branch of right pulmonary artery

Infarcted area

These tests support the diagnosis of pulmonary embolism:

◆ Chest X-ray helps to rule out other pulmonary diseases; areas of atelectasis, elevated diaphragm and pleural effusion, prominent pulmonary artery and, occasionally, the characteristic wedge-shaped infiltrate suggestive of pulmonary infarction, or focal oligemia of blood vessels, are apparent.

◆ Lung scan shows perfusion defects in areas beyond occluded vessels; however, it doesn't rule out microemboli.

◆ Pulmonary angiography is the most definitive test, but requires a skilled angiographer and radiologic equipment; it also poses some risk to the patient. Its use depends on the uncertainty of the diagnosis and the need to avoid unnecessary anticoagulant therapy in a high-risk patient.

◆ Electrocardiography (ECG) is inconclusive, but helps distinguish pulmonary embolism from a myocardial infarction. In extensive embolism, the ECG may show right-axis deviation; right bundle-branch block; tall, peaked P waves; depression of ST segments and T-wave inversions (indicative of right-sided heart strain); and supraventricular tachyarrhythmias. A pattern sometimes observed is S_1, Q_3, and T_3 (S wave in lead I, Q wave in lead III, and inverted T wave in lead III).

◆ Auscultation occasionally reveals a right ventricular S_3 gallop and increased intensity of a pulmonic component of S_2. Also, crackles and a pleural rub may be heard at the embolism site.

◆ Arterial blood gas (ABG) measurements showing decreased partial pressure of arterial oxygen and partial pressure of arterial carbon dioxide are characteristic, but they don't always occur.

◆ If pleural effusion is present, thoracentesis may rule out empyema, which indicates pneumonia.

Treatment

Treatment is designed to maintain adequate cardiovascular and pulmonary function during resolution of the obstruction and to prevent embolus recurrence. Because most emboli resolve within 10 to 14 days, treatment consists of:

◆ oxygen therapy, as needed

◆ anticoagulation with heparin to inhibit new thrombus formation. (Heparin therapy is monitored by daily coagulation studies [partial thromboplastin time (PTT)].)

Depending on the type of embolism the patient has, treatment may include:

◆ thrombolytic therapy with urokinase, streptokinase, or tissue plasminogen activator to enhance fibrinolysis of the pulmonary emboli and remaining thrombi for massive pulmonary embolism and shock

◆ a vasopressor for emboli that cause hypotension
◆ an antibiotic and evaluation for the infection's source, particularly endocarditis for septic emboli.
   In patients who can't take anticoagulants (because of recent surgery or blood dyscrasia) or who have recurrent emboli during anticoagulant therapy, pulmonary embolism is treated with:
◆ surgery (which shouldn't be performed without angiographic evidence of pulmonary embolism), consisting of vena caval ligation, plication, or insertion of a device (umbrella filter) to filter blood returning to the heart and lungs
◆ a combination of heparin and dihydroergotamine to prevent postoperative venous thromboembolism.

Special considerations
◆ Give oxygen by nasal cannula or mask. Check ABG levels if the patient develops fresh emboli or worsening dyspnea. Be prepared to provide endotracheal intubation with assisted ventilation if breathing is severely compromised.
◆ Administer heparin, as ordered, through I.V. push or continuous drip. Monitor coagulation studies daily. Effective heparin therapy raises the PTT to more than 1½ times normal. Watch closely for nosebleed, petechiae, and other signs of abnormal bleeding; check stools for occult blood. Tell the patient to prevent bleeding by shaving with an electric razor and by brushing his teeth with a soft toothbrush.
◆ After the patient's condition is stable, encourage him to move about often, and assist with isometric and range-of-motion exercises. Check pedal pulses, temperature, and color of his feet for venostasis. Never vigorously massage the patient's legs. Offer diversionary activities to promote rest and relieve restlessness. (See *preventing pulmonary embolism.*)
◆ Report frequent pleuritic chest pain so that an analgesic can be prescribed. Also, incentive spirometry can assist in deep breathing.
◆ To relieve anxiety, explain procedures and treatments. Encourage the patient's family to participate in his care.
◆ The patient usually takes an oral anticoagulant (warfarin) for 3 to 6 months after a pulmonary embolism. Advise him to watch for signs of bleeding (bloody stools, blood in urine, and large ecchymoses), to take the prescribed medication exactly as ordered, not to change his dosage without consulting his physician, and to avoid taking additional medication (even for headaches or colds). Stress the importance of follow-up laboratory tests (prothrombin time) to monitor anticoagulant therapy.

PREVENTION
Preventing pulmonary embolism
Several interventions can help prevent a pulmonary embolism from developing. For instance, encouraging a patient to walk as soon as possible after surgery can prevent venostasis, and maintaining adequate nutrition and fluid balance promotes healing. Prophylactic treatment with low-dose heparin under close medical supervision can also help prevent pulmonary embolisms; high-risk patients may benefit from treatment with low-molecular-weight heparin. To help prevent thrombus formation, warn the patient not to cross his legs or sit with his legs in a dependent position for prolonged periods.

||| LIFE-THREATENING DISORDER

PULMONARY HYPERTENSION
Pulmonary hypertension occurs when pulmonary artery pressure (PAP) rises above normal for reasons other than aging or altitude. No definitive set of values is used to diagnose pulmonary hypertension, but the National Institutes of Health requires a mean PAP of 25 mm Hg or more. Primary or *idiopathic pulmonary hypertension* is characterized by increased PAP and increased pulmonary vascular resistance. This form is most common in women ages 20 to 40 and is usually fatal within 3 to 4 years.
   CLINICAL ALERT *Mortality is highest in pregnant women.*
   Secondary pulmonary hypertension results from existing cardiac or pulmonary disease or both. The prognosis in secondary pulmonary hypertension depends on the severity of the underlying disorder.
   The patient may have no signs or symptoms of the disorder until lung damage becomes severe. In fact, it may not be diagnosed until an autopsy is performed.

Causes
Causes of primary pulmonary hypertension are unknown, but may include:
◆ altered immune mechanisms
◆ hereditary factors.
   Secondary pulmonary hypertension results from hypoxemia caused by various conditions, including:

♦ acquired cardiac disease resulting from:
– mitral stenosis
– rheumatic valvular disease.
♦ alveolar hypoventilation resulting from:
– chronic obstructive pulmonary disease
– diffuse interstitial pneumonia
– kyphoscoliosis
– malignant metastases
– obesity
– sarcoidosis
– scleroderma.
♦ primary cardiac disease resulting from:
– atrial septal defect
– patent ductus arteriosus (PDA)
– ventricular septal defect (VSD).
♦ vascular obstruction resulting from:
– fibrosing mediastinitis
– idiopathic veno-occlusive disease
– left atrial myxoma
– mediastinal neoplasm
– pulmonary embolism
– vasculitis.

Pathophysiology

In primary pulmonary hypertension, the smooth muscle in the pulmonary artery wall hypertrophies, narrowing the small pulmonary artery (arterioles) or obliterating it completely. Fibrous lesions also form around the vessels, impairing distensibility and increasing vascular resistance. Pressures in the left ventricle, which receives blood from the lungs, remain normal. However, the increased pressures generated in the lungs are transmitted to the right ventricle, which supplies the pulmonary artery. Eventually, the right ventricle fails (cor pulmonale). Although oxygenation isn't severely affected initially, hypoxia and cyanosis eventually occur. Death results from cor pulmonale.

Alveolar hypoventilation can result from diseases caused by alveolar destruction or from disorders that prevent the chest wall from expanding sufficiently to allow air into the alveoli. The resulting decreased ventilation increases pulmonary vascular resistance. Hypoxemia resulting from this ventilation-perfusion mismatch also causes vasoconstriction, further increasing vascular resistance and resulting in pulmonary hypertension.

Coronary artery disease or mitral valvular disease causing increased left ventricular filling pressures may cause secondary pulmonary hypertension. VSD and PDA cause secondary pulmonary hypertension by increasing blood flow through the pulmonary circulation through left-to-right shunting. Pulmonary emboli and chronic destruction of alveolar walls, as in emphysema, cause secondary pulmonary hypertension by obliterating or obstructing the pulmonary vascular bed. Secondary pulmonary hypertension can also occur by vasoconstriction of the vascular bed, such as through hypoxemia, acidosis, or both. Conditions resulting in vascular obstruction can also cause pulmonary hypertension because blood isn't allowed to flow appropriately through the vessels.

Secondary pulmonary hypertension can be reversed if the disorder is resolved. If hypertension persists, hypertrophy occurs in the medial smooth-muscle layer of the arterioles. The larger arteries stiffen, and hypertension progresses. Pulmonary pressures begin to equal systemic blood pressure, causing right ventricular hypertrophy and, eventually, cor pulmonale.

Primary cardiac diseases may be congenital or acquired. Congenital defects cause a left-to-right shunt, rerouting blood through the lungs twice and causing pulmonary hypertension. Acquired cardiac diseases, such as rheumatic valvular disease and mitral stenosis, result in left-sided heart failure that diminishes the flow of oxygenated blood from the lungs. This increases pulmonary vascular resistance and right ventricular pressure.

Signs and symptoms

♦ Increasing exertional dyspnea from left-sided heart failure
♦ Fatigue and weakness from diminished tissue oxygenation
♦ Syncope due to diminished oxygenation to brain cells
♦ Difficulty breathing due to left-sided heart failure
♦ Shortness of breath due to left-sided heart failure
♦ Pain with breathing due to lactic acid buildup in the tissues
♦ Ascites due to right-sided heart failure
♦ Neck vein distention due to right-sided heart failure
♦ Restlessness and agitation due to hypoxia
♦ Decreased level of consciousness, confusion, and memory loss because of hypoxia
♦ Decreased diaphragmatic excursion and respiration because of hypoventilation
♦ Possible displacement of point of maximal impulse beyond the midclavicular line due to fluid accumulation
♦ Peripheral edema due to right-sided heart failure
♦ Easily palpable right ventricular lift due to altered cardiac output and pulmonary hypertension

◆ Palpable and tender liver due to pulmonary hypertension
◆ Tachycardia because of hypoxia
◆ Systolic ejection murmur due to pulmonary hypertension and altered cardiac output
◆ Split S_2, S_3, and S_4 due to pulmonary hypertension and altered cardiac output
◆ Decreased breath sounds because of fluid accumulation in the lungs
◆ Loud, tubular breath sounds because of fluid accumulation in the lungs

Complications
◆ Cor pulmonale
◆ Cardiac failure
◆ Cardiac arrest

Diagnosis
◆ Arterial blood gas (ABG) analysis reveals hypoxemia.
◆ Electrocardiography in right ventricular hypertrophy shows right-axis deviation and tall or peaked P waves in inferior leads.
◆ Cardiac catheterization reveals a mean pulmonary artery pressure greater than 25 mm Hg at rest or greater than 30 mm Hg during exercise. It may also show an increased pulmonary artery wedge pressure (PAWP) if the underlying cause is left atrial myxoma, mitral stenosis, or left-sided heart failure; otherwise, PAWP is normal.
◆ Pulmonary angiography detects filling defects in pulmonary vasculature such as those that develop with pulmonary emboli.
◆ Pulmonary function studies may show decreased flow rates and increased residual volume in underlying obstructive disease; in underlying restrictive disease, they may show reduced total lung capacity.
◆ Radionuclide imaging detects abnormalities in right and left ventricular functioning.
◆ Open lung biopsy may determine the type of disorder.
◆ Echocardiography allows the assessment of ventricular wall motion and possible valvular dysfunction. It can also demonstrate right ventricular enlargement, abnormal septal configuration consistent with right ventricular pressure overload, and reduction in left ventricular cavity size.
◆ Perfusion lung scanning may produce normal or abnormal results, with multiple patchy and diffuse filling defects that don't suggest pulmonary embolism.

Treatment
◆ Oxygen therapy to correct hypoxemia and resulting increased pulmonary vascular resistance
◆ Fluid restriction in right-sided heart failure to decrease the heart's workload

◆ Digoxin to increase cardiac output
◆ A diuretic to decrease intravascular volume and extravascular fluid accumulation
◆ A vasodilator to reduce myocardial workload and oxygen consumption
◆ A calcium channel blocker to reduce myocardial workload and oxygen consumption
◆ A bronchodilator to relax smooth muscles and increase airway patency
◆ A beta-adrenergic blocker to improve oxygenation
◆ Oral anticoagulants to prevent pulmonary arterial embolism and cerebral thrombosis
◆ Treatment of the underlying cause to correct pulmonary edema
◆ Heart-lung transplantation in severe cases

Special considerations
Pulmonary hypertension requires keen observation and careful monitoring as well as skilled supportive care.
◆ Administer oxygen therapy as ordered, and observe the patient's response. Report signs of increasing dyspnea to the physician so he can adjust treatment accordingly.
◆ Monitor ABG levels for acidosis and hypoxemia. Report changes in level of consciousness at once.
◆ When caring for a patient with right-sided heart failure, especially one receiving a diuretic, record weight daily, carefully measure intake and output, and explain all medications and diet restrictions. Check for worsening neck vein distention, which may indicate fluid overload.
◆ Monitor vital signs, especially blood pressure and heart rate. Watch for hypotension and tachycardia. If the patient has a pulmonary artery catheter, check PAP and PAWP as ordered. Report changes.
◆ Before discharge, help the patient adjust to the limitations imposed by this disorder. Advise against overexertion, and suggest frequent rest periods between activities. Refer her to the social services department if she needs special equipment, such as oxygen equipment, for home use. Make sure she understands the prescribed medications and diet and the need to weigh herself daily.

||| LIFE-THREATENING DISORDER

RESPIRATORY DISTRESS SYNDROME OF THE NEWBORN
Respiratory distress syndrome (RDS) of the newborn, also known as *hyaline membrane disease,* is the most common cause of neonatal death; in the United States alone, it kills about 40,000 neonates every year.

⚠️ **CLINICAL ALERT** *RDS of the newborn occurs most exclusively in neonates born before 37 weeks' gestation; it occurs in about 60% of those born before 28 weeks' gestation.*

RDS of the newborn is marked by widespread alveolar collapse. Occurring mainly in premature neonates and in sudden infant death syndrome, it strikes apparently healthy neonates. It's most common in neonates of mothers who have diabetes and in those delivered by cesarean birth, or it may occur suddenly after antepartum hemorrhage.

In RDS of the newborn, premature neonates develop a widespread alveolar collapse due to surfactant deficiency. If untreated, the syndrome causes death within 72 hours of birth in up to 14% of neonates weighing under 5.5 lb (2,500 g). Aggressive management and mechanical ventilation can improve the prognosis, although some surviving neonates are left with bronchopulmonary dysplasia. Mild cases of the syndrome subside after about 3 days.

Causes

◆ Lack of surfactant
◆ Premature birth

Pathophysiology

Surfactant, a lipoprotein present in alveoli and respiratory bronchioles, helps to lower surface tension, maintain alveolar patency, and prevent alveolar collapse, particularly at the end of expiration.

Although the neonatal airways are developed by 27 weeks' gestation, the intercostal muscles are weak and the alveoli and capillary blood supply are immature. Surfactant deficiency causes a higher surface tension. The alveoli aren't able to maintain patency and begin to collapse.

With alveolar collapse, ventilation is decreased and hypoxia develops. The resulting pulmonary injury and inflammatory reaction lead to edema and swelling of the interstitial space, thus impeding gas exchange between the capillaries and the functional alveoli. The inflammation also stimulates production of hyaline membranes composed of white fibrin accumulation in the alveoli. These deposits further reduce gas exchange in the lung and decrease lung compliance, resulting in increased work of breathing.

Decreased alveolar ventilation results in decreased ventilation-perfusion ratio and pulmonary arteriolar vasoconstriction. The pulmonary vasoconstriction can result in increased right cardiac volume and pressure, causing blood to be shunted from the right atrium through a patent foramen ovale to the left atrium. Increased pulmonary resistance also results in deoxygenated blood passing through the ductus arteriosus, totally bypassing the lungs, and causing a right-to-left shunt. The shunt further increases hypoxia.

Because of immature lungs and an already increased metabolic rate, the infant must expend more energy to ventilate collapsed alveoli. This further increases oxygen demand and contributes to cyanosis. The infant attempts to compensate with rapid shallow breathing, causing an initial respiratory alkalosis as carbon dioxide is expelled. The increased effort at lung expansion causes respirations to slow and respiratory acidosis to occur, leading to respiratory failure.

Signs and symptoms

⚠️ **CLINICAL ALERT** *Suspect RDS of the newborn in a patient with a history that includes preterm birth (before 28 weeks' gestation), cesarean delivery, maternal history of diabetes, or antepartum hemorrhage.*

◆ Rapid, shallow respirations due to hypoxia
◆ Intercostal, subcostal, or sternal retractions due to hypoxia
◆ Nasal flaring due to hypoxia
◆ Audible expiratory grunting (The grunting is a natural compensatory mechanism that produces positive end-expiratory pressure [PEEP] to prevent further alveolar collapse.)
◆ Hypotension due to cardiac failure
◆ Peripheral edema due to cardiac failure
◆ Oliguria because of vasoconstriction of the kidneys

In severe cases

◆ Apnea due to respiratory failure
◆ Bradycardia due to cardiac failure
◆ Cyanosis from hypoxemia, right-to-left shunting through the foramen ovale, or right-to-left shunting through the atelectatic lung areas
◆ Pallor due to decreased circulation
◆ Frothy sputum due to pulmonary edema and atelectasis
◆ Low body temperature, resulting from an immature nervous system and inadequate subcutaneous fat
◆ Diminished air entry and crackles on auscultation because of atelectasis

Complications

◆ Respiratory failure
◆ Cardiac failure
◆ Bronchopulmonary dysplasia

Diagnosis

◆ Chest X-rays may be normal for the first 6 to 12 hours in 50% of patients, although later films

show a fine reticulonodular pattern and dark streaks, indicating air-filled, dilated bronchioles.
◆ Arterial blood gas (ABG) analysis reveals a diminished partial pressure of arterial oxygen level; a normal, decreased, or increased partial pressure of arterial carbon dioxide level; and a reduced pH, indicating a combination of respiratory and metabolic acidosis.
◆ Lecithin/sphingomyelin ratio helps to assess prenatal lung development and infants at risk for this syndrome; this test is usually ordered if a cesarean delivery will be performed before 36 weeks' gestation.

Treatment
◆ Warm, humidified, oxygen-enriched gases administered by oxygen hood or, if such treatment fails, by mechanical ventilation to promote adequate oxygenation and reverse hypoxia
◆ Administration of surfactant by an endotracheal tube to prevent atelectasis
◆ Mechanical ventilation with PEEP or continuous positive airway pressure (CPAP) administered by nasal prongs or a small, triangular nasal mask (This forces the alveoli to remain open on expiration and promotes increased surface area for exchange of oxygen and carbon dioxide.)
◆ High-frequency oscillation ventilation if the neonate can't maintain adequate gas exchange (This provides satisfactory minute volume [the total air breathed in 1 minute] with lower airway pressures.)
◆ Radiant warmer or an Isolette to help maintain thermoregulation and reduce metabolic demands
◆ I.V. fluids to promote adequate hydration and maintain circulation with capillary refill time of less than 2 seconds (Fluid and electrolyte balance is also maintained.)
◆ Sodium bicarbonate to control acidosis
◆ Tube feedings or total parenteral nutrition
◆ A prophylactic antibiotic for underlying infections
◆ A diuretic to reduce pulmonary edema
⚠ **CLINICAL ALERT** *A corticosteroid may be administered to the mother to stimulate surfactant production in a fetus at high risk for preterm birth.*
◆ Delayed delivery of an infant (if premature labor) to possibly prevent RDS

Special considerations
Infants with RDS require continual assessment and monitoring in a neonatal intensive care unit.
◆ Closely monitor blood gases as well as fluid intake and output. If the infant has an umbilical catheter (arterial or venous), check for arterial hypotension or abnormal central venous pressure. Watch for complications, such as infec-

tion, thrombosis, or decreased circulation to the legs. If the infant has a transcutaneous oxygen monitor, change the site of the lead placement every 2 to 4 hours to avoid burning the skin.
◆ Weigh the infant once daily. To evaluate his progress, assess skin color, rate and depth of respirations, severity of retractions, nostril flaring, frequency of expiratory grunting, frothing at the lips, and restlessness.
◆ Regularly assess the effectiveness of oxygen or ventilator therapy. Evaluate every change in fraction of inspired oxygen and PEEP or CPAP by monitoring arterial oxygen saturation or ABG levels. Be sure to adjust PEEP or CPAP as indicated, based on findings.
◆ Mechanical ventilation in infants is usually done in a pressure-limited mode rather than the volume-limited mode used in adults.
◆ When the infant is on mechanical ventilation, watch carefully for signs of barotrauma (increase in respiratory distress and subcutaneous emphysema) and accidental disconnection from the ventilator. Check ventilator settings frequently. Be alert for signs of complications of PEEP or CPAP therapy, such as decreased cardiac output, pneumothorax, and pneumomediastinum. Mechanical ventilation increases the risk of infection in premature infants, so preventive measures are essential.
◆ If the infant requires CPAP delivered via nasal prongs, take steps to prevent skin breakdown in and around the nares. Apply strips of a colloidal dressing such as Duoderm around the nares and under the ties of the hat that helps hold the nasal prongs in place. Avoid applying the ties too tight to reduce pressure on the nares and face.
◆ As needed, arrange for follow-up care with a neonatal ophthalmologist to check for retinal damage. Premature infants in an oxygen-rich environment are at increased risk for developing retinopathy of prematurity.
◆ Teach the parents about their infant's condition and, if possible, let them participate in his care, to encourage normal parent-infant bonding. Advise parents that full recovery may take up to 12 months. When the prognosis is poor, prepare the parents for the infant's impending death, and offer emotional support.
◆ Help reduce mortality from RDS by detecting respiratory distress early. Recognize intercostal retractions and grunting, especially in a premature infant, as signs of RDS; make sure the infant receives immediate treatment.

SEVERE ACUTE RESPIRATORY SYNDROME
Severe acute respiratory syndrome (SARS) is a viral respiratory tract infection that can progress

PREVENTION

Preventing the spread of SARS

To help prevent the spread of severe acute respiratory syndrome (SARS), provide appropriate patient and family teaching. Emphasize the importance of frequent hand washing, covering the mouth and nose when coughing or sneezing, and avoiding close personal contact while infected or potentially infected with SARS. Explain to the patient and his family that they shouldn't share such items as eating utensils, towels, and bedding until the items have been washed with soap and hot water; recommend wearing disposable gloves and using household disinfectant to clean any surface that may have been exposed to the patient's body fluids. Tell the patient that he shouldn't go to work, school, or other public places until instructed to by his physician.

---

to pneumonia and, eventually, death. The disease was first recognized in 2003 with outbreaks in China, Canada, Singapore, Taiwan, and Vietnam; other countries—including the United States—reported smaller numbers of cases. According to the World Health Organization, a total of 8,098 people worldwide became ill with SARS during the 2003 outbreak. Of those cases, 774 died.

Causes

SARS is caused by the SARS-associated coronavirus (SARS-CoV). *Coronaviruses* are a common cause of mild respiratory illnesses in humans, but researchers believe that a virus may have mutated, allowing it to cause this potentially life-threatening disease.

Pathophysiology

The method of SARS transmission involves close contact with a person who's infected with the viral infection, including contact with infectious aerosolized droplets or body secretions. Most people who contracted SARS during the 2003 outbreak contracted it during travel to endemic areas. However, the virus has been found to live on hands, paper tissues, and other surfaces (such as countertops, telephones, and doorknobs) for up to 6 hours in its droplet form. It has also been found to live in the stool of people with SARS for up to 4 days. The virus may be able to live for months or years in below-

freezing temperatures. The incubation period for SARS is typically 3 to 5 days but may last as long as 14 days.

Signs and symptoms
◆ Fever
◆ General discomfort
◆ Minor respiratory signs and symptoms (such as cough, shortness of breath, and difficulty breathing)
◆ Headache
◆ Rigor
◆ Chills
◆ Myalgia
◆ Sore throat
◆ Diarrhea
◆ Rash

■ **AGE ALERT** *In elderly patients who may have no fever, SARS may present atypically. During the 2003 outbreak, SARS was found to be less common among children and to be in milder form when it did occur.*

Complications
◆ Respiratory failure
◆ Liver failure
◆ Heart failure
◆ Myelodysplastic syndromes
◆ Death

Diagnosis
◆ Diagnosis of severe respiratory illness is made when the patient has a fever greater than 100.4° F (38° C) or upon clinical findings of lower respiratory tract illness and a chest X-ray demonstrating pneumonia or acute respiratory distress syndrome.
◆ Laboratory tests for the virus include cell culture of SARS-CoV, detection of SARS-CoV ribonucleic acid by the reverse transcription polymerase chain reaction (PCR) test, or detection of serum antibodies to SARS-CoV. Detectable levels of antibodies may not be present until 21 days after the onset of illness, but some patients develop antibodies within 14 days. A negative PCR, antibody test, or cell culture doesn't rule out the diagnosis.

Treatment

The Centers for Disease Control and Prevention recommends using the same treatment for patients with SARS as for patients with serious community-acquired pneumonia, including oxygen support, as needed. Some experts advocate the use of antiviral agents, such as oseltamivir or ribavirin. Steroid use is highly controversial.

Other treatments under study include:
◆ interferon beta to block the virus from entering the cell; however, stopping the virus may require 10 times the normal dose

◆ a cysteine protease inhibitor to inhibit SARS virus replication; however, this has been effective in only 30% of cases
◆ Surfaxin, a liquid surfactant.

Special considerations
◆ Report suspected cases of SARS to local and national health organizations.
◆ Frequently monitor the patient's vital signs and respiratory status.
◆ Maintain isolation as recommended. The patient will need emotional support to deal with anxiety and fear related to the diagnosis of SARS and as a result of isolation. (See *Preventing the spread of SARS*.)

||| **LIFE-THREATENING DISORDER**

SUDDEN INFANT DEATH SYNDROME
Sudden infant death syndrome (SIDS) is the third leading cause of death among apparently healthy infants, ages 1 month to 1 year. The incidence has declined dramatically with the practice of placing infants on their backs to sleep.

⚠️ **CLINICAL ALERT** *The incidence of SIDS is slightly higher in preterm infants, males, and those who sleep on their stomachs on soft bedding. Incidence is also higher in neonates born in poverty, in those who were one of a single multiple birth (such as twins and triplets), in those who live in an environment where someone smokes, in those whose mothers failed to seek prenatal care until late in pregnancy or who smoked or took drugs during pregnancy.*

Causes
◆ Hypoxemia, possibly due to apnea or an immature respiratory system
◆ Rebreathing of carbon dioxide, as occurs when an infant is face down on the mattress

Pathophysiology
Current theories focus on neurologic immaturity related to the infant's inability to sense and regulate oxygenation status. The infant may also have periods of sleep apnea and eventually dies during an episode.

Normally, increased carbon dioxide levels stimulate the respiratory center to initiate breathing until high levels actually depress the ventilatory effort. In infants who experience SIDS or near-miss episodes of SIDS, the child may not respond to increasing carbon dioxide levels, showing only depressed ventilation. In these infants, an episode of apnea may occur and carbon dioxide levels increase; however,

the child isn't stimulated to breathe. Apnea continues until high levels of carbon dioxide completely suppress the ventilatory effort and the child ceases to breathe.

🔗 **GENETIC LINK** *Although no single gene has been found to be a direct cause of SIDS, researchers are investigating the possibility of "SIDS genes" that predispose and infant to SIDS, especially when combined with other factors, such as a slight infection, warm environment, or prone sleeping position.*

Signs and symptoms
◆ History indicating that the infant was found not breathing
◆ Mottling of the skin due to cyanosis
◆ Apnea and absence of a pulse due to severe hypoxemia

Complications
◆ Brain damage from near-miss episodes
◆ Death

Diagnosis
An autopsy is performed to rule out other causes of death.

Treatment
◆ Resuscitation to restore circulation and oxygenation (usually futile)
◆ Emotional support to the family
◆ Prevention of SIDS in high-risk infants or those who have had near-miss episodes

⚠️ **CLINICAL ALERT** *Infants at risk for SIDS should be monitored at home on an apnea monitor until the age of vulnerability has passed. Also, parents should be educated in prompt emergency treatment of detected apnea.*

Special considerations
◆ Make sure the parents are present when the child's death is announced. The parents may lash out at emergency department personnel, the babysitter, or anyone else involved in the child's care — even each other. Stay calm and let them express their feelings. Reassure them that they weren't to blame.
◆ Let the parents see the baby in a private room. Allow them to express their grief in their own way. Offer to call clergy, friends, or relatives.
◆ After the parents and family have recovered from their initial shock, explain the need for an autopsy to confirm the diagnosis of SIDS (in some states, this is mandatory). At this time, provide the family with some basic facts about SIDS and encourage them to give their consent for the autopsy. Make sure they receive the autopsy report promptly.

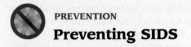

PREVENTION

Preventing SIDS

To help prevent sudden infant death syndrome (SIDS), make sure parents understand the importance of following the latest guidelines from the American Academy of Pediatrics:

♦ Place the baby on his back to sleep, and make sure he's placed to sleep on his back when staying with relatives or at child care.

♦ Provide a smoke-free environment during pregnancy and during the first year of life.

♦ Select bedding carefully; choose a firm mattress rather than a softer surface, such as waterbed or beanbag.

♦ Don't place the baby on thick, fluffy padding, such as lambskin or a thick quilt.

♦ Remove all fluffy toys or stuffed animals from the baby's crib.

♦ Use a sleep sack or other sleep clothing that doesn't require additional covers to keep the baby warm. If you do use a blanket, make sure it's lightweight and tucked securely at the foot of the crib, with just enough length to cover the baby's shoulders. Place the baby in the crib, near the foot, covered loosely with the blanket.

♦ Place the baby to sleep in a crib or bassinet, not in the parents' bed. Adult beds aren't safe for infants. A baby can become trapped and suffocate between the headboard slats, the space between the mattress and the bed frame, or the space between the mattress and the wall. A baby can also suffocate if a sleeping parent accidentally rolls over and covers the baby's nose and mouth.

♦ Keep the baby close by. Babies who sleep in the same room—though not in the same bed—as their parents have a lower risk of SIDS.

♦ Offer a pacifier at naptime and bedtime. Using of a pacifier may reduce the risk of SIDS.

♦ Keep the temperature in the baby's room at a comfortable level, not warmer than normal.

♦ Find out whether your community has a local counseling and information program for parents. Participants in such a program will contact the parents, ensure that they receive the autopsy report promptly, put them in touch with a professional counselor, and maintain supportive telephone contact. Also, find out whether there's a local parents' group; such a group can provide significant emotional support. Contact the National SIDS/Infant Death Resource Center for information about such local groups.

♦ If your facility's policy is to assign a public health nurse to the family, she will provide the continuing reassurance and assistance the parents will need.

♦ If the parents decide to have another child, they'll need information and counseling to help them through the pregnancy and the first year of the new infant's life.

♦ Infants at high risk for SIDS may be placed on apnea monitoring at home.

♦ All new parents should be informed of the American Academy of Pediatrics' recommendation that infants be positioned on their back, not on their stomach or side, for sleeping. (See *Preventing SIDS*.)

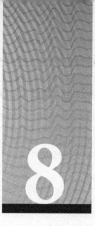

NERVOUS SYSTEM

The nervous system coordinates and organizes the functions of all body systems. This intricate network of interlocking receptors and transmitters is a dynamic system that controls and regulates every mental and physical function. It has three main divisions:

◆ central nervous system (CNS)—the brain and spinal cord (See Reviewing the central nervous system, page 250.)

◆ peripheral nervous system—the motor and sensory nerves, which carry messages between the CNS and remote parts of the body (See Reviewing the peripheral nervous system, pages 251 and 252.)

◆ autonomic nervous system—actually part of the peripheral nervous system, regulates involuntary functions of the internal organs.

The fundamental unit that participates in all nervous system activity is the neuron, a highly specialized cell that receives and transmits electrochemical nerve impulses through delicate, threadlike fibers that extend from the central cell body. Axons carry impulses away from the cell body; dendrites carry impulses to it. Most neurons have several dendrites but only one axon.

◆ Sensory (or afferent) neurons transmit impulses from receptors to the spinal cord or the brain.

◆ Motor (or efferent) neurons, or motoneurons, transmit impulses from the CNS to regulate the activity of muscles or glands.

◆ Interneurons, also known as connecting or association neurons, carry signals through complex pathways between sensory and motoneurons. Interneurons account for 99% of all the neurons in the nervous system.

From birth to death, the nervous system efficiently organizes and controls the smallest actions, thoughts, or feelings; monitors communication and the instinct for survival; and allows introspection, wonder, abstract thought, and self-awareness. Together, the CNS and peripheral nervous system keep a person alert, awake, oriented, and able to move about freely without discomfort and with all body systems working to maintain homeostasis.

Thus, any disorder affecting the nervous system can cause signs and symptoms in any and all body systems. Patients with nervous system disorders commonly have signs and symptoms that are elusive, subtle, and sometimes latent.

Pathophysiologic changes

Typically, disorders of the nervous system involve some alteration in arousal, cognition, movement, muscle tone, homeostatic mechanisms, or pain. Most disorders cause more than one alteration, and the close intercommunication between the CNS and peripheral nervous system means that one alteration may lead to another.

AROUSAL

Arousal refers to the level of consciousness or state of awareness. A person who is aware of himself and the environment and can respond in specific ways is said to be fully conscious. Full consciousness requires that the reticular activating system (RAS), higher systems in the cerebral cortex, and thalamic connections are intact

(Text continues on page 252.)

Reviewing the central nervous system

The central nervous system includes the brain and spinal cord. The brain consists of the cerebrum, cerebellum, brain stem, and primitive structures that lie below the cerebrum: the diencephalon, limbic system, and reticular activating system (RAS). The spinal cord is the primary pathway for messages between peripheral areas of the body and the brain. It also mediates spinal reflexes.

Cerebrum

The left and right cerebral hemispheres are joined by the corpus callosum, a mass of nerve fibers that allows communication between corresponding centers in the right and left hemispheres. Each hemisphere is divided into four lobes, based on anatomic landmarks and functional differences. The lobes are named for the cranial bones that lie over them (frontal, temporal, parietal, and occipital):

♦ *frontal lobe* — influences personality, judgment, abstract reasoning, social behavior, language expression, and movement (in the motor portion)

♦ *temporal lobe* — controls hearing, language comprehension, and storage and recall of memories (although memories are stored throughout the brain)

♦ *parietal lobe* — interprets and integrates sensations, including pain, temperature, and touch; also interprets size, shape, distance, and texture (The parietal lobe of the nondominant hemisphere, usually the right, is especially important for awareness of body schema [shape].)

♦ *occipital lobe* — functions primarily in interpreting visual stimuli.

The cerebral cortex, the thin surface layer of the cerebrum, is composed of gray matter (unmyelinated cell bodies). The surface of the cerebrum has convolutions (gyri) and creases or fissures (sulci).

Cerebellum

The cerebellum, which also has two hemispheres, maintains muscle tone, coordinates muscle movement, and controls balance.

Brain stem

Composed of the pons, midbrain, and medulla oblongata, the brain stem relays messages between upper and lower levels of the nervous system. The cranial nerves originate from the pons, midbrain, and medulla oblongata:

♦ *pons* — connects the cerebellum with the cerebrum and the midbrain to the medulla oblongata, and contains one of the respiratory centers

♦ *midbrain* — mediates the auditory and visual reflexes

♦ *medulla oblongata* — regulates respiratory, vasomotor, and cardiac function.

Primitive structures

The diencephalon contains the thalamus and hypothalamus, which lie beneath the cerebral hemispheres. The thalamus relays all sensory stimuli (except olfactory) as they ascend to the cerebral cortex. Thalamic functions include primitive awareness of pain, screening of incoming stimuli, and focusing of attention. The hypothalamus controls or affects body temperature, appetite, water balance, pituitary secretions, emotions, and autonomic functions, including sleep and wake cycles.

The limbic system lies deep within the temporal lobe. It initiates primitive drives (hunger, aggression, and sexual and emotional arousal) and screens all sensory messages traveling to the cerebral cortex.

The RAS, a diffuse network of hyperexcitable neurons fanning out from the brain stem through the cerebral cortex, screens all incoming sensory information and channels it to appropriate areas of the brain for interpretation. RAS activity also stimulates wakefulness.

Spinal cord

The spinal cord joins the brain stem at the level of the foramen magnum and terminates near the second lumbar vertebra.

A cross section of the spinal cord reveals a central H-shaped mass of gray matter divided into dorsal (posterior) and ventral (anterior) horns. Gray matter in the dorsal horns relays sensory (afferent) impulses; in the ventral horns, motor (efferent) impulses. White matter (myelinated axons of sensory and motor nerves) surrounds these horns and forms the ascending and descending tracts.

Reviewing the peripheral nervous system

The peripheral nervous system consists of the cranial nerves (CN), the spinal nerves, and the autonomic nervous system (ANS).

Cranial nerves

The 12 pairs of cranial nerves transmit motor or sensory messages, or both, primarily between the brain or brain stem and the head and neck. All cranial nerves, except for the olfactory and optic nerves, originate from the midbrain, pons, or medulla oblongata. The cranial nerves are sensory, motor, or mixed (both sensory and motor) as follows:

♦ olfactory (CN I) — Sensory: smell
♦ optic (CN II) — Sensory: vision
♦ oculomotor (CN III) — Motor: extraocular eye movement (superior, medial, and inferior lateral), pupillary constriction, and upper eyelid elevation
♦ trochlear (CN IV) — Motor: extraocular eye movement (inferior medial)
♦ trigeminal (CN V) — Sensory: transmitting stimuli from face and head, corneal reflex; Motor: chewing, biting, and lateral jaw movements
♦ abducens (CN VI) — Motor: extraocular eye movement (lateral)
♦ facial (CN VII) — Sensory: taste receptors (anterior two-thirds of tongue); Motor: facial muscle movement, including muscles of expression (those in the forehead and around the eyes and mouth)
♦ acoustic (CN VIII) — Sensory: hearing, sense of balance
♦ glossopharyngeal (CN IX) — Motor: swallowing movements; Sensory: sensations of throat; taste receptors (posterior one-third of tongue)
♦ vagus (CN X) — Motor: movement of palate, swallowing, gag reflex; activity of the thoracic and abdominal viscera, such as heart rate and peristalsis; Sensory: sensations of throat, larynx, and thoracic and abdominal viscera (heart, lungs, bronchi, and GI tract)
♦ spinal accessory (CN XI) — Motor: shoulder movement, head rotation
♦ hypoglossal (CN XII) — Motor: tongue movement.

Spinal nerves

The 31 pairs of spinal nerves are named according to the vertebra immediately below their exit point from the spinal cord. Each spinal nerve consists of afferent (sensory) and efferent (motor) neurons, which carry messages to and from particular body regions, called dermatomes.

Autonomic nervous system

The ANS innervates all internal organs. Sometimes known as the visceral efferent nerves, autonomic nerves carry messages to the viscera from the brain stem and neuroendocrine system. The ANS has two major divisions: the sympathetic (thoracolumbar) nervous system and the parasympathetic (craniosacral) nervous system.

Sympathetic nervous system

Sympathetic nerves exit the spinal cord between the levels of the 1st thoracic and 2nd lumbar vertebrae — hence the name thoracolumbar. These preganglionic neurons enter small relay stations (ganglia) near the cord. The ganglia form a chain that disseminates the impulse to postganglionic neurons, which reach many organs and glands, and can produce widespread, generalized responses.

The physiologic effects of sympathetic activity include:

♦ vasoconstriction
♦ elevated blood pressure
♦ enhanced blood flow to skeletal muscles
♦ increased heart rate and contractility
♦ heightened respiratory rate
♦ smooth-muscle relaxation of the bronchioles, GI tract, and urinary tract
♦ sphincter contraction
♦ pupillary dilation and ciliary muscle relaxation
♦ increased sweat gland secretion
♦ reduced pancreatic secretion.

Parasympathetic nervous system

The fibers of the parasympathetic, or craniosacral, nervous system leave the central nervous system (CNS) by way of the cranial nerves from the midbrain and medulla and with the spinal nerves between the 2nd and 4th sacral vertebrae (S2 to S4).

After leaving the CNS, the long preganglionic fiber of each parasympathetic nerve travels to a ganglion near a particular organ or gland, and the short postganglionic fiber enters the organ or gland. Parasympathetic nerves have a specific response involving only one organ or gland.

The physiologic effects of parasympathetic system activity include:

♦ reduced heart rate, contractility, and conduction velocity
♦ bronchial smooth-muscle constriction

(continued)

Reviewing the peripheral nervous system *(continued)*

♦ increased GI tract tone and peristalsis with sphincter relaxation
♦ urinary system sphincter relaxation and increased bladder tone
♦ vasodilation of external genitalia, causing erection

♦ pupillary constriction
♦ increased pancreatic, salivary, and lacrimal secretions.
The parasympathetic system has little effect on mental or metabolic activity.

---

and functioning properly. Several mechanisms can alter arousal:
♦ direct destruction of the reticular activating system and its pathways
♦ destruction of the entire brain stem, either directly by invasion or indirectly by impairment of its blood supply
♦ compression of the RAS by disease, either from direct pressure or compression as structures expand or herniate.

Those mechanisms may result from structural, metabolic, or psychogenic disturbances:
♦ Structural changes include infections, vascular problems, neoplasms, trauma, and developmental and degenerative conditions. They usually are identified by their location relative to the tentorial plate, the double fold of dura that supports the temporal and occipital lobes and separates the cerebral hemispheres from the brain stem and cerebellum. Those above the tentorial plate are called supratentorial, whereas those below are called infratentorial.
♦ Metabolic changes that affect the nervous system include hypoxia, electrolyte disturbances, hypoglycemia, drugs, and toxins (endogenous and exogenous). Essentially, any systemic disease can affect the nervous system.
♦ Psychogenic changes are commonly associated with mental and psychiatric illnesses. Ongoing research has linked neuroanatomy and neurophysiology of the CNS and supporting structures, including neurotransmitters, with certain psychiatric illnesses. For example, dysfunction of the limbic system has been associated with schizophrenia, depression, and anxiety disorders.

Decreased arousal may be a result of diffuse or localized dysfunction in supratentorial areas:
♦ Diffuse dysfunction reflects damage to the cerebral cortex or underlying subcortical white matter. Disease is the most common cause of diffuse dysfunction; other causes include neoplasms, closed trauma with subsequent bleeding, and pus accumulation.
♦ Localized dysfunction reflects mechanical forces on the thalamus or hypothalamus. Masses

(such as bleeding, infarction, emboli, and tumors) may directly impinge on the deep diencephalic structures or herniation may compress them.

Stages of altered arousal

An alteration in arousal usually begins with some interruption or disruption in the diencephalon. When this occurs, the patient shows evidence of dullness, confusion, lethargy, and stupor. Continued decreases in arousal result from midbrain dysfunction and are evidenced by a deepening of the stupor. Eventually, if the medulla and pons are affected, coma results.

A patient may move back and forth between stages or levels of arousal, depending on the cause of the altered arousal state, initiation of treatment, and response to the treatment. Typically, if the underlying problem isn't or can't be corrected, then the patient will progress through the various stages of decreased consciousness, termed *rostral-caudal progression.* Six levels of altered arousal or consciousness have been identified. (See *Stages of altered arousal.*)

Typically, five areas of neurologic function are evaluated to help identify the cause of altered arousal:
♦ level of consciousness (includes awareness and cognitive functioning, which reflect cerebral status)
♦ pattern of breathing (helps to localize the cause to the cerebral hemisphere or brain stem)
♦ pupillary changes (reflects the level of brain stem function; the brain stem areas that control arousal are anatomically next to the areas that control the pupils)
♦ eye movement and reflex responses (help identify the level of brain stem dysfunction and its mechanism, such as destruction or compression)
♦ motor responses (help identify the level, side, and severity of brain dysfunction).

COGNITION

Cognition is the ability to be aware, to use intuition, and to perceive, reason, judge, and remember. It reflects higher functioning of the cerebral cortex, including the frontal, parietal,

Stages of altered arousal

This chart highlights the six levels or stages of altered arousal and their manifestations.

Stage	Manifestations
Confusion	◆ Loss of ability to think rapidly and clearly ◆ Impaired judgment and decision making
Disorientation	◆ Beginning of loss of consciousness ◆ Disorientation to time progresses to include disorientation to place ◆ Impaired memory ◆ Lack of recognition of self (last to go)
Lethargy	◆ Limited spontaneous movement or speech ◆ Easy to arouse by normal speech or touch ◆ Possible disorientation to time, place, or person
Obtundation	◆ Mild to moderate reduction in arousal ◆ Limited responsiveness to environment ◆ Ability to fall asleep easily without verbal or tactile stimulation from others ◆ Ability to answer questions with minimum response
Stupor	◆ State of deep sleep or unresponsiveness ◆ Arousable (motor or verbal response only to vigorous and repeated stimulation) ◆ Withdrawal or grabbing response to stimulation
Coma	◆ Lack of motor or verbal response to external environment or any stimuli ◆ No response to noxious stimuli, such as deep pain ◆ Unable to be aroused by any stimulus

and temporal lobes, and portions of the brain stem. Typically, an alteration in cognition results from direct destruction by ischemia and hypoxia or from indirect destruction by compression or the effects of toxins and chemicals.

Altered cognition may manifest as agnosia, aphasia, or dysphasia:
◆ Agnosia is a defect in the ability to recognize the form or nature of objects. Usually, agnosia involves only one sense — hearing, vision, or touch.
◆ Aphasia is loss of the ability to comprehend or produce language.
◆ Dysphasia is impairment of the ability to comprehend or use symbols in either verbal or written language, or to produce language.

Dysphasia typically arises from the left cerebral hemisphere, usually the frontotemporal region. However, different types of dysphasia occur, depending on the specific area of the brain involved. For example, a dysfunction in the posteroinferior frontal lobe (Broca's area) causes a motor dysphasia in which the patient can't find the words to speak and has difficulty writing and repeating words. Dysfunction in the pathways connecting the primary auditory area to the auditory association areas in the middle third of the left superior temporal gyrus causes a form of dysphasia called word deafness: The patient has fluent speech, but comprehension of the spoken word and ability to repeat speech are impaired. Rather than words, the patient hears only noise that has no meaning, yet reading comprehension and writing ability are intact.

Dementia

Dementia is the loss of more than one intellectual or cognitive function, which interferes with the ability to function in daily life. The patient may experience a problem with orientation, general knowledge and information, vigilance (attentiveness, alertness, and watchfulness), recent memory, remote memory, concept formulation, abstraction (ability to generalize about nonconcrete thoughts and ideas), reasoning, or language use.

The underlying mechanism is a defect in the neuronal circuitry of the brain. The extent of dysfunction reflects the total quantity of neurons lost and the area where this loss occurred.

Factors that have been associated with dementia include:

◆ degeneration
◆ cerebrovascular disorders
◆ compression
◆ effects of toxins
◆ metabolic conditions
◆ biochemical imbalances
◆ demyelinization
◆ infection.

Three major types of dementia have been identified: amnestic, intentional, and cognitive. Each type affects a specific area of the brain, resulting in characteristic impairments:

◆ Amnestic dementia typically results from defective neuronal circuitry in the temporal lobe. Characteristically, the patient exhibits difficulty in naming things, loss of recent memory, and loss of language comprehension.

◆ Intentional dementia results from a defect in the frontal lobe. The patient is easily distracted and, although able to follow simple commands, can't carry out such sequential functions as planning, initiating, and regulating behavior or achieving specific goals. The patient may exhibit personality changes and a flat affect. Possibly appearing accident prone, he may lose motor function, as evidenced by a wide shuffling gait, small steps, muscle rigidity, abnormal reflexes, incontinence of bowel and bladder and, possibly, total immobility.

◆ Cognitive dementia reflects dysfunctional neuronal circuitry in the cerebral cortex. Typically, the patient loses remote memory, language comprehension, and mathematical skills, and has difficulty with visual-spatial relationships.

MOVEMENT

Movement involves a complex array of activities controlled by the cerebral cortex, the pyramidal system, the extrapyramidal system, and the motor units (the axon of the lower motoneuron from the anterior horn cell of the spinal cord and the muscles innervated by it). A problem in any one of these areas can affect movement. (See *Reviewing motor impulse transmission*.)

For movement to occur, the muscles must change their state from one of contraction to relaxation or vice versa. A change in muscle innervation anywhere along the motor pathway affects movement. Certain neurotransmitters, such as dopamine, play a role in altered movement.

Alterations in movement typically include excessive movement (hyperkinesia) or decreased movement (hypokinesia). Hyperkinesia is a broad category that includes many different types of abnormal movements. Each type of hyperkine-

sia is associated with a specific underlying pathophysiologic mechanism affecting the brain or motor pathway. (See *Types of hyperkinesia,* pages 256 and 257.) Hypokinesia usually involves loss of voluntary control, even though peripheral nerve and muscle functions are intact. The types of hypokinesia include paresis, akinesia, bradykinesia, and loss of associated neurons.

Paresis

Paresis is a partial loss of motor function (paralysis) and muscle power, which the patient will commonly describe as weakness. Paresis can result from the dysfunction of the:

◆ upper motoneurons in the cerebral cortex, subcortical white matter, internal capsule, brain stem, or spinal cord
◆ lower motoneurons in the brain stem motor nuclei and anterior horn of the spinal cord, or problems with their axons as they travel to the skeletal muscle
◆ motor units affecting the muscle fibers or the neuromuscular junction.

Upper motoneurons

Upper motoneuron dysfunction reflects an interruption in the pyramidal tract and consequent decreased activation of the lower motoneurons innervating one or more areas of the body. Upper motoneuron dysfunction usually affects more than one muscle group and generally affects distal muscle groups more severely than proximal groups. Onset of spastic muscle tone over several days to weeks commonly accompanies upper motoneuron paresis, unless the dysfunction is acute. In acute dysfunction, flaccid tone and loss of deep tendon reflexes indicates spinal shock, caused by a severe, acute lesion below the foramen magnum. Incoordination associated with upper motoneuron paresis manifests as slow, coarse movement with abnormal rhythm.

Lower motoneurons

Lower motoneurons are of two basic types: large (alpha) and small (gamma). Dysfunction of the large motoneurons of the anterior horn of the spinal cord, the motor nuclei of the brain stem, and their axons causes impairment of voluntary and involuntary movement. The extent of paresis is directly correlated to the number of large lower motoneurons affected. If only a small portion of the large motoneurons are involved, paresis occurs; if all motor units are affected, paralysis.

The small motoneurons play two necessary roles in movement: maintaining muscle tone and protecting the muscle from injury. Usually,

Reviewing motor impulse transmission

Motor impulses that originate in the motor cortex of the frontal lobe travel through upper motoneurons of the pyramidal or extrapyramidal tract to the lower motoneurons of the peripheral nervous system.

In the pyramidal tract, most impulses from the motor cortex travel through the internal capsule to the medulla, where they cross (decussate) to the opposite side and continue down the spinal cord as the lateral corticospinal tract, ending in the anterior (or ventral) horn of the gray matter at a specific spinal cord level. Some fibers don't cross in the medulla but continue down the anterior corticospinal tract and cross near the level of termination in the anterior horn. The fibers of the pyramidal tract are considered upper motoneurons. In the anterior horn of the spinal cord, upper motoneurons relay impulses to the lower motoneurons, which carry them via the spinal and peripheral nerves to the muscles, producing a motor response.

Motor impulses that regulate involuntary muscle tone and muscle control travel along the extrapyramidal tract from the premotor area of the frontal lobe to the pons of the brain stem, where they cross to the opposite side. The impulses then travel down the spinal cord to the anterior horn, where they're relayed to lower motoneurons for ultimate delivery to the muscles.

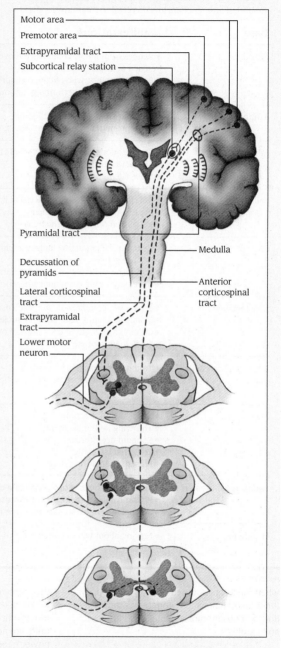

Motor area
Premotor area
Extrapyramidal tract
Subcortical relay station

Pyramidal tract
Medulla
Decussation of pyramids
Anterior corticospinal tract
Lateral corticospinal tract
Extrapyramidal tract
Lower motor neuron

Types of hyperkinesia

This chart summarizes some of the most common types of hyperkinesia, their manifestations, and the underlying mechanisms involved in their development.

Type	Manifestations
Akathisia	♦ Ranges from mildly compulsive movement (usually the legs) to severely frenzied motion ♦ Partly voluntary, with ability to suppress for short periods ♦ Relief obtained by performing motion
Asterixis	♦ Irregular flapping-hand movement ♦ More prominent when arms are outstretched
Athetosis	♦ Slow, sinuous, irregular movements in the distal extremities ♦ Characteristic hand posture ♦ Slow, flucutating grimaces
Ballism	♦ Severe, wild, flinging, stereotypical limb movements ♦ Present when awake or asleep ♦ Usually on one side of the body
Chorea	♦ Random, irregular, involuntary, rapid contractions of muscle groups ♦ Nonrepetetive ♦ Diminishes with rest; disappears during sleep ♦ Increases during emotional stress or attempts at voluntary movement
Hyperactivity	♦ Prolonged, generalized, increased activity ♦ Mainly involuntary but possibly subject to voluntary control ♦ Continual changes in body posture or excessive performance of a simple activity at inappropriate times
Intentional cerebellar tremor	♦ Tremor secondary to movement ♦ Most severe when nearing end of the movement
Myoclonus	♦ Shocklike contractions ♦ Throwing limb movements ♦ Random occurrence ♦ Triggered by startle ♦ Present even during sleep
Parkinsonian tremor	♦ Regular, rhythmic, slow flexion and extension contraction ♦ Primarily affects metacarpophalangeal and wrist joints ♦ Disappears with voluntary movement
Wandering	♦ Moving about without attention to environment

when the large motoneurons are affected, dysfunction of the small motoneurons causes reduced or absent muscle tone, flaccid paresis, and paralysis.

Motor units

The muscles innervated by motoneurons in the anterior horn of the spinal cord may also be affected. Paresis results from a decrease in the number or force of activated muscle fibers in the motor unit. The action potential of each motor unit decreases so that additional motor units are needed more quickly to produce the power necessary to move the muscle. Dysfunction of the neuromuscular junction causes paresis in a similar fashion; however, the capability of the motor units to function is lost, not the actual number of units.

Mechanisms

Possibly associated with impaired dopaminergic transmission

Believed to result from buildup of toxins not broken down by the liver (such as ammonia)

Believed to result from injury to the putamen of the basal ganglion

Injury to subthalamus nucleus, causing inhibition of the nucleus

Excess concentration or heightened sensitivity to dopamine in the basal ganglia

Possibly due to injury to frontal lobe and reticular activating system (RAS)

Errors in the feedback from the periphery and goal-directed movement due to disease of dentate nucleus and superior cerebellar peduncle

Irritability of nervous system and spontaneous discharge of neurons in the cerebral cortex, cerebellum, RAS, and spinal cord

Loss of inhibitory effects of dopamine in basal ganglia

Possibly due to bilateral injury to globus pallidus or putamen

Akinesia

Akinesia is a partial or complete loss of voluntary and associated movements, as well as a disturbance in the time needed to perform a movement. Commonly caused by dysfunction of the extrapyramidal tract, akinesia is associated with dopamine deficiency at the synapse or a defect in the postsynaptic receptors for dopamine.

Bradykinesia

Bradykinesia refers to slow voluntary movements that are labored, deliberate, and hard to initiate. The patient has difficulty performing movements consecutively and at the same time. Like akinesia, bradykinesia involves a disturbance in the time needed to perform a movement.

Loss of associated neurons

Movement involves not only the innervation of specific muscles to accomplish an action but also the work of other innervated muscles that enhance the action. Loss of associated neurons involves alterations in movement that accompany the usual habitual voluntary movements for skill, grace, and balance. For example, when a person expresses emotion, the muscles of the face change and the posture relaxes. Loss of associated neurons involving emotional expression results in a flat, blank expression and a stiff posture. Loss of associated neurons necessary for locomotion results in a decrease in arm and shoulder movement, hip swinging, and rotation of the cervical spine.

MUSCLE TONE

Like movement, muscle tone involves complex activities controlled by the cerebral cortex, pyramidal system, extrapyramidal system, and motor units. Normal muscle tone is the slight resistance that occurs in response to passive movement. When one muscle contracts, reciprocal muscles relax to permit movement with only minimal resistance. For example, when the elbow is flexed, the biceps contracts and feels firm and the triceps is somewhat relaxed and soft; with continued flexion, the biceps relaxes and the triceps contracts. Thus, when a joint is moved through range of motion, the resistance is normally smooth, even, and constant.

The two major types of altered muscle tone are hypotonia (decreased muscle tone) and hypertonia (increased muscle tone).

Hypotonia

Hypotonia (also referred to as *muscle flaccidity*) typically reflects cerebellar damage, but rarely it may result from pure pyramidal tract damage.

Hypotonia is thought to involve a decrease in muscle spindle activity as a result of a decrease in neuron excitability. Flaccidity generally occurs with loss of nerve impulses from the motor unit responsible for maintaining muscle tone.

It may be localized to a limb or muscle group, or it may be generalized, affecting the entire body. Flaccid muscles can be moved rapidly with little or no resistance; eventually they become limp and atrophy.

Hypertonia

Hypertonia is increased resistance to passive movement. There are four types of hypertonia:
◆ Spasticity is hyperexcitability of stretch reflexes caused by damage to the lateral corticospinal tract and the motor, premotor, and supplementary motor areas. (See *How spasticity develops*.)
◆ Paratonia (gegenhalten) is variance in resistance to passive movement in direct proportion to the force applied; the cause is frontal lobe injury.
◆ Dystonia is sustained, involuntary twisting movements resulting from slow muscle contraction; the cause is lack of appropriate inhibition of reciprocal muscles.
◆ Rigidity, or constant, involuntary muscle contraction, is resistance in both flexion and extension; the causes are damage to basal ganglion (cogwheel or lead-pipe rigidity) or loss of cerebral cortex inhibition or cerebellar control (gamma and alpha rigidity).

Hypertonia usually leads to atrophy of unused muscles. However, in some cases, if the motor reflex arc remains functional but isn't inhibited by the higher centers, the overstimulated muscles may hypertrophy.

HOMEOSTATIC MECHANISMS

For proper function, the brain must maintain and regulate pressure inside the skull (intracranial pressure [ICP]) as it also maintains the flow of oxygen (O_2) and nutrients to its tissues. Both of these are accomplished by balancing changes in blood flow and cerebrospinal fluid (CSF) volume.

Constriction and dilation of the cerebral blood vessels help to regulate ICP and delivery of nutrients to the brain. These vessels respond to changes in concentrations of carbon dioxide (CO_2), O_2, and hydrogen ions (H^+). For example, if the CO_2 concentration in blood increases, the gas combines with body fluids to form carbonic acid, which eventually releases H^+. An increase in H^+ concentration causes the cerebral vessels to dilate, increasing blood flow to the brain, increasing cerebral perfusion and, subsequently, causing a drop in H^+ concentration. A decrease in O_2 concentration also stimulates cerebral vasodilation, increasing blood flow and O_2 delivery to the brain.

Should these normal autoregulatory mechanisms fail, the abnormal blood chemistry stimulates the sympathetic nervous system to cause vasoconstriction of the large and medium-sized cerebral arteries. This helps to prevent increases

in blood pressure from reaching the smaller cerebral vessels.

CSF volume remains relatively constant. However, if ICP rises—even as little as 5 mm Hg—the arachnoid villi open and excess CSF drains into the venous system.

The blood-brain barrier also helps to maintain homeostasis in the brain. This barrier is composed of tight junctions between the endothelial cells of the cerebral vessels and neuroglial cells and is relatively impermeable to most substances. However, some substances required for metabolism pass through the blood-brain barrier, depending on their size, solubility, and electrical charge. This barrier also regulates water flow from the blood, thereby helping to maintain the volume within the skull.

Increased ICP

ICP is the pressure that the brain tissue, CSF, and cerebral blood (intracranial components) exert against the skull. The skull is a rigid structure; therefore, a change in the volume of the intracranial contents triggers a reciprocal change in one or more of the intracranial components to maintain a consistent pressure. Any condition that alters the normal balance of the intracranial components—including increased brain volume, increased blood volume, or increased CSF volume—can increase ICP.

Initially, the body uses its compensatory mechanisms (described above) to attempt to maintain homeostasis and lower ICP. However, if these mechanisms become overwhelmed and are no longer effective, ICP continues to rise. Cerebral perfusion pressure falls and cerebral blood flow decreases. Ischemia leads to cellular hypoxia, which initiates vasodilation of cerebral blood vessels in an attempt to increase cerebral blood flow. Unfortunately, this only causes the ICP to increase further. As the pressure continues to rise, compression of brain tissue and cerebral vessels further impairs cerebral blood flow.

If ICP continues to rise, the brain begins to shift under the extreme pressure and may herniate to an area of lesser pressure. When the herniating brain tissue's blood supply is compromised, cerebral ischemia and hypoxia worsen. The herniation increases pressure in the area where the pressure was lower, thus impairing its blood supply. As ICP approaches systemic blood pressure, cerebral perfusion slows even more, ceasing when ICP equals systemic blood pressure. (See *What happens when ICP rises*, page 260.)

How spasticity develops

Motor activity is controlled by pyramidal and extrapyramidal tracts that originate in the motor cortex, basal ganglia, brain stem, and spinal cord. Nerve fibers from the various tracts converge and synapse at the anterior (or ventral) horn of the spinal cord. Together they maintain segmental muscle tone by modulating the stretch reflex arc. This arc, shown in a simplified version below, is basically a negative feedback loop in which muscle stretch (stimulation) causes reflexive contraction (inhibition), thus maintaining muscle length and tone.

Damage to certain tracts results in loss of inhibition and disruption of the stretch reflex arc. Uninhibited muscle stretch produces exaggerated, uncontrolled muscle activity, accentuating the reflex arc, and eventually resulting in spasticity.

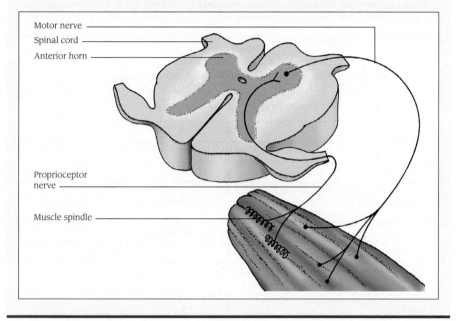

Motor nerve

Spinal cord

Anterior horn

Proprioceptor nerve

Muscle spindle

Cerebral edema

Cerebral edema is an increase in the fluid content of brain tissue that leads to an increase in the intracellular or extracellular fluid volume. Cerebral edema may result from an initial injury to the brain tissue, or it may develop in response to cerebral ischemia, hypoxia, and hypercapnia.

Cerebral edema is classified in four types — vasogenic, cytotoxic, ischemic, or interstitial — depending on the underlying mechanism responsible for the increased fluid content.

◆ *Vasogenic* — Injury to the vasculature increases capillary permeability and disruption of blood brain barrier; leakage of plasma proteins into the extracellular spaces pulls water into the brain parenchyma.

◆ *Cytotoxic (metabolic)* — Toxins cause failure of the active transport mechanisms; loss of intra-cellular potassium and influx of sodium (and water) cause cells in the brain to swell.

◆ *Ischemic* — It's caused by cerebral infarction and initially confined to intracellular compartment; after several days, released lysosomes from necrosed cells disrupt blood brain barrier.

◆ *Interstitial* — Movement of CSF from ventricles to extracellular spaces increases brain volume.

Commonly, patients simultaneously experience more than one type of cerebral edema. Regardless of the type, blood vessels become distorted and brain tissue is displaced, ultimately leading to herniation.

PAIN

Pain is the result of a complex series of steps from a site of injury to the brain, which interprets the stimuli as pain. Pain that originates outside the

CLOSER LOOK
What happens when ICP rises

Intracranial pressure (ICP) is the pressure exerted within the intact skull by the intracranial volume—about 10% blood, 10% cerebrospinal fluid (CSF), and 80% brain tissue. The rigid skull has little space for expansion of these substances.

The brain compensates for increases in ICP by regulating the volume of the three substances in the following ways:
◆ limiting blood flow to the head
◆ displacing CSF into the spinal canal
◆ increasing absorption or decreasing production of CSF—withdrawing water from brain tissue and excreting it through the kidneys.

When compensatory mechanisms become overworked, small changes in volume lead to large changes in pressure. The following chart will help you to understand increased ICP's pathophysiology.

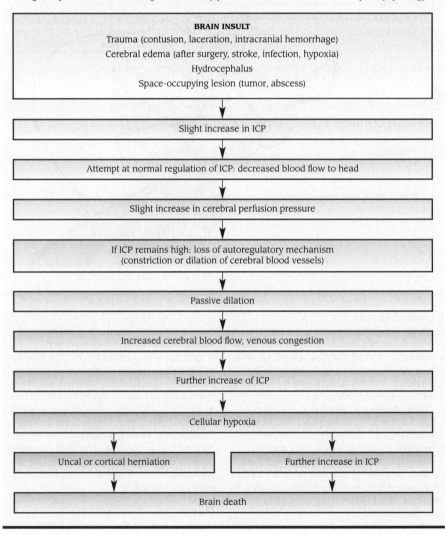

BRAIN INSULT
Trauma (contusion, laceration, intracranial hemorrhage)
Cerebral edema (after surgery, stroke, infection, hypoxia)
Hydrocephalus
Space-occupying lesion (tumor, abscess)

↓

Slight increase in ICP

↓

Attempt at normal regulation of ICP: decreased blood flow to head

↓

Slight increase in cerebral perfusion pressure

↓

If ICP remains high: loss of autoregulatory mechanism
(constriction or dilation of cerebral blood vessels)

↓

Passive dilation

↓

Increased cerebral blood flow, venous congestion

↓

Further increase of ICP

↓

Cellular hypoxia

↓   ↓

Uncal or cortical herniation   Further increase in ICP

↓   ↓

Brain death

nervous system is termed *nociceptive pain*; pain that originates from within the nervous system, *neurogenic* or *neuropathic pain*.

Nociception

Nociception begins when noxious stimuli reach pain fibers. Sensory receptors called nociceptors —which are free nerve endings in the tissues— are stimulated by various agents, such as chemicals, temperature, or mechanical pressure. If a stimulus is sufficiently strong, impulses travel via the afferent nerve fibers along sensory pathways to the spinal cord, where they initiate autonomic and motor reflexes. The information also continues to travel to the brain, which perceives it as pain. Several theories have been developed to explain pain. (See *Theories of pain*, pages 262 and 263.)

Nociception consists of four steps: transduction, transmission, modulation, and perception.

Transduction

Transduction is the conversion of noxious stimuli into electrical impulses and subsequent depolarization of the nerve membrane. These electrical impulses are created by algesic substances that sensitize the nociceptors and are released at the site of injury or inflammation. Examples include H^+ and potassium ions, serotonin, histamine, prostaglandins, bradykinin, and substance P.

Transmission

A delta fibers and C fibers transmit pain sensations from the tissues to the CNS.

A delta fibers are lightly myelinated fibers with a small diameter. Mechanical or thermal stimuli elicit a rapid or fast response. These fibers transmit localized, sharp, stinging, or pinprick-type pain sensations. A delta fibers connect with secondary neuron groupings on the dorsal horn of the spinal cord.

C fibers are smaller and unmyelinated. They connect with second order neurons in lamina I and II (the latter includes the sub-stantia gelatinosa, an area in which pain is modulated). C fibers respond to chemical stimuli, rather than heat or pressure, triggering a slow pain response, usually within 1 second. This dull ache or burning sensation isn't localized and leads to two responses: an acute response transmitted immediately through fast pain pathways, which prompts the person to evade the stimulus, and lingering pain transmitted through slow pain pathways, which persists or worsens.

The A delta and C fibers carry the pain signal from the peripheral tissues to the dorsal horn of the spinal cord. Excitatory and inhibitory interneurons and projection cells (neurons that connect pathways in the cerebral cortex of the CNS and peripheral nervous system) carry the signal to the brain by way of crossed and uncrossed pathways. An example of a crossed pathway is the spinothalamic tract, which enters the brain stem and ends in the thalamus. Sensory impulses travel from the medial and lateral lemniscus (tract) to the thalamus and brain stem. From the thalamus, other neurons carry the information to the sensory cortex, where pain is perceived and understood.

Another example of a crossed pathway is the ascending spinoreticulothalamic tract, which is responsible for the psychological components of pain and arousal. At this site, neurons synapse with interneurons before they cross to the opposite side of the cord and make their way to the medulla and, eventually, the reticular activating system, mesencephalon, and thalamus. Impulses then are transmitted to the cerebral cortex, limbic system, and basal ganglia.

After stimuli are delivered, responses from the brain must be relayed back to the original site. Several pathways carry the information in the dorsolateral white columns to the dorsal horn of the spinal cord. Some corticospinal tract neurons end in the dorsal horn and allow the brain to pay selective attention to certain stimuli while ignoring others. This allows transmission of the primary signal while suppressing the tendency for signals to spread to adjacent neurons.

Modulation

Modulation refers to modifications in pain transmission. Some neurons from the cerebral cortex and brain stem activate inhibitory processes, thus modifying the transmission. Substances—such as serotonin from the mesencephalon, norepinephrine from the pons, and endorphins from the brain and spinal cord— inhibit pain transmission by decreasing the release of nociceptive neurotransmitters. Spinal reflexes involving motoneurons may initiate a protective action, such as withdrawal from a pinprick, or may enhance the pain, such as when trauma causes a muscle spasm in the injured area.

Perception

Perception is the end result of pain transduction, transmission, and modulation. It encompasses the emotional, sensory, and subjective aspects of the pain experience. Pain perception is thought to occur in the cortical structures of the somatosensory cortex and limbic system. Alertness, arousal, and motivation are believed to result from the action of the reticular activating system and limbic system. Cardiovascular

Theories of pain

Over the years numerous theories have attempted to explain the sensation of pain and describe how it occurs. This chart highlights some major theories about pain.

Theory	Major assumptions
Specificity	◆ Four types of cutaneous sensation (touch, warmth, cold, pain); each results from stimulation of specific skin receptor sites and neural pathways. ◆ Specific pain neurons transmit pain sensation along specific pain fibers. ◆ At synapses in the *substantia gelatinosa*, pain impulses cross to the opposite side of the cord and ascend the specific pain pathways of the spinothalamic tract to the thalamus and the pain receptor areas of the cerebral cortex.
Intensity	◆ Pain results from excessive stimulation of sensory receptors. Disorders or processes causing pain create an intense summation of nonnoxious stimuli.
Pattern	◆ Nonspecific receptors transmit specific patterns (characterized by the length of the pain sensation, the amount of involved tissue, and the summation of impulses) from the skin to the spinal cord, leading to pain perception.
Neuromatrix	◆ A pattern theory. Sensations imprinted in the brain. Sensory inputs may trigger a pattern of sensation from the neuromatrix (a proposed network of neurons looping between the thalamus and the cortex, and the cortex and the limbic system). ◆ Sensation pattern is possible without the sensory trigger.
Gate control	◆ Pain is transmitted from skin via the small diameter A delta and C fibers to cells of the *substantia gelatinosa* in the dorsal horn, where interconnections between other sensory pathways exist. Stimulation of the large-diameter fast, myelinated A beta and A alpha fibers closes gate, which restricts transmission of the impulse to the CNS and diminishes pain perception. ◆ Large fiber stimulation is possible through massage, scratching or rubbing the skin, or through electrical stimulation. Concurrent firing of pain and touch paths reduces transmission and perception of the pain impulses but not of touch impulses. ◆ An increase in small-fiber activity inhibits the *substantia gelatinosa* cells, "opening the gate" and increasing pain transmission and perception. ◆ *Substantia gelatinosa* acts as a gate-control system to inhibit the flow of nerve impulses from peripheral fibers to the CNS. ◆ Central T cells act as a CNS control to stimulate selective brain processes that influence the gate-control system. Inhibition of T cells closes the gate, pain impulses aren't transmitted to the brain. ◆ T-cell activation of neural mechanisms in the brain is responsible for pain perception and response; transmitters partly regulate the release of substance P, the peptide that conveys pain information. Pain modulation is also partly controlled by the neurotransmitters, enkephalin and serotonin. ◆ Persistent pain initiates a gradual decline in the fraction of impulses that pass through the various gates. ◆ Descending efferent impulses from the brain may be responsible for closing, partially opening, or completely opening the gate.
Melzack-Casey Conceptual Model	◆ Three major psychological dimensions of pain: sensory-discriminative from thalamus and somatosensory cortex, motivational-affective from the reticular formation, and cognitive-evaluative. ◆ Interactions among the three produce descending inhibitory influences that alter pain input to the dorsal horn and ultimately modify the sensory pain experience and motivational-affective dimensions. ◆ Pain is localized and identified by its characteristics, evaluated by past experiences, and undergoes further cognitive processing. The complex sensory, motivational, and cognitive interactions determine motor activities and behaviors associated with the pain experience.

Comment

♦ Focuses on the direct relationship between the pain stimulus and perception; doesn't account for adaptation to pain and the psychosocial factors modulating it.

♦ Doesn't explain existence of intense stimuli not perceived as pain.

♦ Includes some components of the intensity theory; pain possibly a response to intense stimulation of the sensory receptors regardless of receptor type or pathway.

♦ Explains existence of phantom pain.

♦ Provides the basis for use of massage and electrical stimulation in pain management; being used to develop additional theories and models.

♦ Takes into account the powerful role of psychological functioning in determining the quality and intensity of pain.

responses and typical fight or flight responses are thought to involve the medulla and hypothalamus.

The following three variables contribute to the wide variety of individual pain experiences:

♦ *pain threshold* — level of intensity at which a stimulus is perceived as pain

♦ *perceptual dominance* — existence of pain at another location that's given more attention

♦ *pain tolerance* — duration or intensity of pain to be endured before a response is initiated.

Neurogenic pain

Neurogenic pain is associated with neural injury. Pain results from spontaneous discharges from the damaged nerves, spontaneous dorsal root activity, or degeneration of modulating mechanisms. Neurogenic pain doesn't activate nociceptors, and there's no typical pathway for transmission.

Disorders

This section discusses disorders of the nervous system, some of which can have far-reaching effects in all body systems. They include Alzheimer's disease, amyotrophic lateral sclerosis, arteriovenous malformations, Bell's palsy, cerebral palsy, complex regional pain syndrome, Creutzfeldt-Jakob disease, Guillain-Barré syndrome, headache, head trauma, Huntington's disease, hydrocephalus, intracranial aneurysm, meningitis, multiple sclerosis, myasthenia gravis, Parkinson's disease, Reye's syndrome, seizure disorder, spinal cord trauma, and stroke.

ALZHEIMER'S DISEASE

Alzheimer's disease is a degenerative disorder of the cerebral cortex, especially the frontal lobe, which accounts for more than half of all cases of dementia.

AGE ALERT *Although primarily found in the elderly population, 1% to 10% of cases have their onset in middle age.*

Because this is a primary progressive dementia, the prognosis for a patient with this disease is poor.

Causes

The exact cause of Alzheimer's disease is unknown. Factors that have been associated with its development include:

♦ *neurochemical factors,* such as deficiencies in the neurotransmitters acetylcholine, somatostatin, substance P, and norepinephrine

◆ *environmental factors,* such as repeated head trauma or exposure to aluminum or manganese
◆ *genetic factors.*

GENETIC LINK *Genetic studies show that an autosomal dominant form of Alzheimer's disease is associated with early onset and early death. A family history of Alzheimer's disease and the presence of Down syndrome are two established risk factors.*

Pathophysiology

The brain tissue of patients with Alzheimer's disease has three distinct and characteristic features:
◆ neurofibrillatory tangles (fibrous proteins)
◆ beta-amyloid plaques (composed of degenerating axons and dendrites)
◆ granulovascular degeneration of neurons.

Additional structural changes include cortical atrophy, ventricular dilation, deposition of amyloid (a glycoprotein) around the cortical blood vessels, and reduced brain volume. Also found is a selective loss of cholinergic neurons in the pathways to the frontal lobes and hippocampus, areas that are important for memory and cognitive functions. Examination of the brain after death commonly reveals an atrophic brain, in many cases weighing less than 1,000 g (normal: 1,380 g). (See *Abnormal cellular structures in Alzheimer's disease,* pages 266 and 267.)

Signs and symptoms

The typical signs and symptoms reflect neurologic abnormalities associated with pathophysiologic changes of the disease:
◆ gradual loss of recent and remote memory, loss of sense of smell, and flattening of affect and personality
◆ difficulty with learning new information
◆ deterioration in personal hygiene
◆ inability to concentrate
◆ increasing difficulty with abstraction and judgment
◆ impaired communication
◆ severe deterioration in memory, language, and motor function
◆ loss of coordination
◆ inability to write or speak
◆ personality changes
◆ tendency to wander
◆ nocturnal awakenings
◆ loss of eye contact and fearful look
◆ signs of anxiety, such as wringing of hands
◆ acute confusion, agitation, compulsiveness, or fearfulness when overwhelmed with anxiety
◆ disorientation and emotional lability
◆ progressive deterioration of physical and intellectual ability.

Complications
◆ Injury secondary to violent behavior or wandering
◆ Pneumonia and other infections
◆ Malnutrition
◆ Dehydration
◆ Aspiration
◆ Death

Diagnosis

Alzheimer's disease is diagnosed by exclusion—that is, by ruling out other disorders as the cause for the patient's signs and symptoms. The only true way to confirm Alzheimer's disease is by finding pathologic changes in the brain at autopsy. However, these diagnostic tests may be useful:
◆ Positron emission tomography shows changes in the metabolism of the cerebral cortex.
◆ Computed tomography scan shows evidence of early brain atrophy in excess of that which occurs in normal aging.
◆ Magnetic resonance imaging shows no lesion as the cause of the dementia.
◆ EEG shows evidence of slowed brain waves in the later stages of the disease.
◆ Cerebral blood flow studies show abnormalities in blood flow.

Treatment

No cure or definitive treatment exists for Alzheimer's disease. Therapy may include:
◆ a cholinesterase inhibitor, such as donepezil, rivastigmine, and galantamine, to prevent the breakdown of acetylcholine (involved in the brain's memory and thinking skills)
◆ memantine, an uncompetitive low-to-moderate affinity N-methyl-D-aspartate receptor antagonist, to regulate the activity of glutamate (involved in the brain's information processing, storing, and retrieval)
◆ a vitamin E supplement to help defend the brain against damage.

Many clinical trials are under way for the treatment of Alzheimer's disease, including a vaccine that would stimulate the immune system to recognize and attack the beta-amyloid plaques that occur with the disease.

Special considerations

Overall care is focused on supporting the patient's remaining abilities and compensating for those he has lost.
◆ Provide the patient with a safe environment. Encourage him to exercise, as ordered, to help maintain mobility.

◆ Establish an effective communication system with the patient and family to help them adjust to the patient's altered cognitive abilities.
◆ Anxiety may cause the patient to become agitated or fearful. Intervene by helping him focus on another activity.
◆ Establish a routine for the patient to help him maintain a sense of control over his environment.
◆ Offer emotional support to the patient and family members. Behavior problems may be worsened by excess stimulation or change in established routine. Teach them about the disease, and refer them to social service and community resources for legal and financial advice and support.

AMYOTROPHIC LATERAL SCLEROSIS

Commonly called *Lou Gehrig disease,* after the New York Yankees first baseman that died of this disorder, amyotrophic lateral sclerosis (ALS) is the most common of the motoneuron diseases causing muscular atrophy. Other motoneuron diseases include progressive muscular atrophy and progressive bulbar palsy. Onset usually occurs between ages 40 and 70. A chronic, progressively debilitating disease, ALS may be fatal in less than 1 year or continue for 10 years or more, depending on the muscles affected. More than 30,000 Americans have ALS; about 5,000 new cases are diagnosed each year; and the disease affects three times as many men as women.

Causes

The exact cause of ALS is unknown, but 5% to 10% of cases have a genetic component — an autosomal dominant trait that affects men and women equally.

GENETIC LINK The first and most important breakthrough so far in ALS genetic research was the discovery of mutations in the SOD1 gene. This mutation is seen in about 20% of patients with familial ALS. However, this mutation is quite complex. Researchers understand how the gene functions, but the mutation is an acquisition of a toxic property, meaning that the gene gains a function, rather than losing its normal function. Researchers are perplexed about what that gain of function is, so genetic studies continue.

Several mechanisms have been considered, including:
◆ a slow-acting virus
◆ a nutritional deficiency related to a disturbance in enzyme metabolism
◆ a metabolic interference in nucleic acid production by the nerve fibers

◆ an autoimmune disorder that affects immune complexes in the renal glomerulus and basement membrane.

Precipitating factors for acute deterioration include any severe stress, such as a myocardial infarction, trauma, a viral infection, and physical exhaustion.

Pathophysiology

ALS progressively destroys the upper and lower motoneurons. It doesn't affect cranial nerves III, IV, and VI and, therefore, some facial movements, such as blinking, persist. Intellectual and sensory functions aren't affected.

Some believe that glutamate — the primary excitatory neurotransmitter of the CNS — accumulates to toxic levels at the synapses. The affected motor units are no longer innervated, and progressive degeneration of axons causes loss of myelin. Some nearby motor nerves may sprout axons in an attempt to maintain function but, ultimately, nonfunctional scar tissue replaces normal neuronal tissue.

Signs and symptoms

Typical signs and symptoms of ALS include:
◆ fasciculations accompanied by spasticity, atrophy, and weakness due to degeneration of the upper and lower motoneurons, and loss of functioning motor units, especially in the muscles of the forearms and the hands
◆ impaired speech, difficulty chewing and swallowing, choking, and excessive drooling from degeneration of cranial nerves V, IX, X, and XII
◆ difficulty breathing, especially if the brain stem is affected
◆ muscle atrophy due to loss of innervation.

Mental deterioration doesn't usually occur, but patients may become depressed because of the disease. Progressive bulbar palsy may cause crying spells or inappropriate laughter.

Complications
◆ Respiratory tract infections
◆ Respiratory failure
◆ Aspiration

Diagnosis

Although no diagnostic tests are specific to ALS, the following may aid in the diagnosis:
◆ Electromyography shows abnormalities of electrical activity in involved muscles.
◆ Muscle biopsy shows atrophic fibers interspersed between normal fibers.
◆ Nerve conduction studies show normal results.
◆ Computed tomography scan and EEG show normal results and thus rule out multiple

(Text continues on page 268.)

Abnormal cellular structures in Alzheimer's disease

How and why neurons die in Alzheimer's disease is largely unknown. However, several characteristic abnormal cellular structures, which scientists believe cause cell malfunction or cell death, are found in the brain of every patient with Alzheimer's disease. These structures include excessive granulovacuoles, neurofibrillary tangles, and amyloid plaques.

Granulovacuolar degeneration

Granulovacuolar degeneration is found inside the neurons of the hippocampus. An abnormally high number of fluid-filled spaces, called *vacuoles*, enlarge the cell's body, possibly causing the cell to malfunction or die.

Neurofibrillary tangles

Neurofibrillary tangles are bundles of filaments inside the neuron that abnormally twist around one another. Numerous neurofibrillary tangles are found in areas of the brain associated with memory and learning (hippocampus), fear and aggression (amygdala), and thinking (cerebral cortex). Scientists believe the neurofibrillary tangles play a role in the memory loss and personality changes that the patient with Alzheimer's disease suffers.

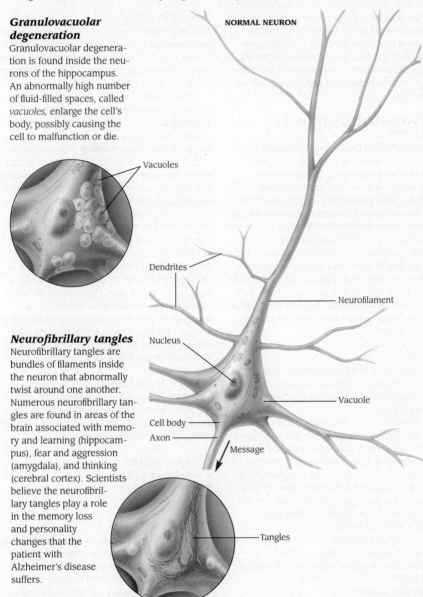

NORMAL NEURON

Vacuoles

Dendrites

Neurofilament

Nucleus

Vacuole

Cell body

Axon

Message

Tangles

Amyloid plaques

Amyloid plaques (senile plaques) are found outside neurons in the extracellular space of the cerebral cortex and hippocampus. They contain a core of beta amyloid protein that's surrounded by abnormal nerve endings, or neurites. Amyloid plaques also occur in the walls of cerebral blood vessels, causing the condition called *amyloid angiopathy.*

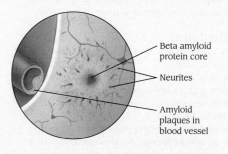

Beta amyloid protein core

Neurites

Amyloid plaques in blood vessel

Neurotransmitters: The messengers

Alzheimer's disease also destroys the way some neurons talk to each other. Neurons communicate via a chemical message that passes between two cells across a tiny gap called a *synapse.* A neuron receives messages from its dendrites and passes the information to the cell body, where the message is received. The message can then be sent to the end of the axon, where sacs containing chemicals called *neurotransmitters* are released. The sacs empty the neurotransmitter into the synapse between the two cells. The chemical message is picked up by the other cell and the process continues.

Groups of neurons that use the same neurotransmitter form specialized network systems. Several of these systems are damaged in Alzheimer's disease. One in particular, the cholinergic system, uses the neurotransmitter acetylcholine to send its messages. The relay center for this system, the nucleus basalis of Meynert, suffers severe neuron loss and decreased production of acetylcholine. This is believed to play a role in memory loss.

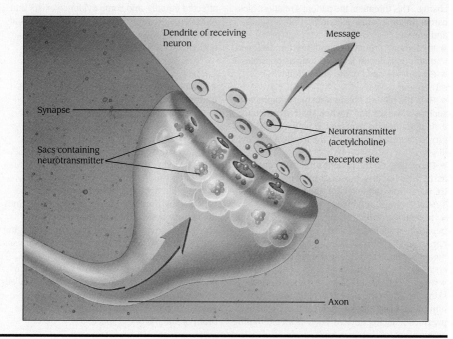

Dendrite of receiving neuron

Message

Synapse

Sacs containing neurotransmitter

Neurotransmitter (acetylcholine)

Receptor site

Axon

sclerosis, spinal cord neoplasm, polyarteritis, syringomyelia, myasthenia gravis, progressive muscular dystrophy, and progressive stroke.

Treatment

ALS has no cure. Treatment is supportive and may include:
♦ riluzole, a neuroprotector, to modulate glutamate activity and slow disease progression
♦ diazepam, dantrolene, or baclofen to decrease spasticity
♦ quinidine to relieve painful muscle cramps
♦ an anticholinergic, such as glycopyrolate or transdermal scopalamine, to decrease oral secretions
♦ thyrotropin-releasing hormone (I.V. or intrathecally) to temporarily improve motor function (successful only in some patients)
♦ mechanical ventilation to support pulmonary function
♦ respiratory, speech, and physical therapy to maintain function as much as possible
♦ psychological support to assist with coping with this progressive, fatal illness.

Special considerations

Remember that because mental status remains intact while progressive physical degeneration takes place, the patient acutely perceives every change. This threatens the patient's relationships, career, income, muscle coordination, sexuality, and energy.
♦ Implement a rehabilitation program designed to maintain independence as long as possible.
♦ Elevate the head of the bed to relieve orthopnea.
♦ Help the patient obtain assistive equipment, such as a walker and a wheelchair. Arrange for a visiting nurse to oversee the patient's status, provide support, and teach the family about the illness.
♦ Depending on the patient's muscular capacity, assist with bathing, personal hygiene, and transfers from wheelchair to bed. Help establish a regular bowel and bladder routine.
♦ To help the patient handle an increased accumulation of secretions and dysphagia, teach him to suction himself. He should have a suction machine handy at home to reduce the fear of choking.
♦ To prevent skin breakdown, provide good skin care when the patient is bedridden. Turn him often, keep his skin clean and dry, and use pressure-reducing devices, such as an alternating air mattress.
♦ If the patient has trouble swallowing, give him soft, solid foods and position him upright during meals. Gastrostomy, percutaneous jejunostomy, or nasogastric tube feedings may be necessary if he can no longer swallow. Teach the family (or the patient if he's still able to feed himself) how to administer gastrostomy feedings.
♦ Provide emotional support. A discussion of directives regarding health care decisions should be instituted before the patient becomes unable to communicate his wishes. Prepare the patient and family members for his eventual death, and encourage the start of the grieving process. Patients with ALS may benefit from a hospice program or the local ALS support group chapter.

ARTERIOVENOUS MALFORMATIONS

Arteriovenous malformations (AVMs) are tangled masses of thin-walled, dilated blood vessels between arteries and veins that don't connect by capillaries. AVMs are common in the brain, primarily in the posterior portion of the cerebral hemispheres. Abnormal channels between the arterial and venous system mix oxygenated and unoxygenated blood and, thereby, prevent adequate perfusion of brain tissue.

AVMs range in size from a few millimeters to large malformations extending from the cerebral cortex to the ventricles. Commonly, more than one AVM is present. Males and females are affected equally, and some evidence exists that AVMs are hereditary. Most AVMs are present at birth; however, symptoms typically don't occur until the person is between ages 10 and 20.

Causes

♦ Acquired from penetrating injuries such as trauma
♦ Congenital, due to a hereditary defect

Pathophysiology

AVMs lack the typical structural characteristics of the blood vessels. The vessels of an AVM are thin; one or more arteries feed into the AVM, causing it to appear dilated and tortuous. The typically high-pressured arterial flow moves into the venous system through the connecting channels to increase venous pressure, engorging and dilating the venous structures. An aneurysm may develop. If the AVM is large enough, the shunting can deprive the surrounding tissue of adequate blood flow. Additionally, the thin-walled vessels may ooze small amounts of blood or actually rupture, causing hemorrhage into the brain or subarachnoid space.

Signs and symptoms

Typically, the patient experiences few, if any, signs and symptoms unless the AVM is large,

leaks, or ruptures. Possible signs and symptoms include:
◆ chronic mild headache and confusion from AVM dilation, vessel engorgement, and increased intracranial pressure (ICP)
◆ seizures secondary to compression of the surrounding tissues by the engorged vessels
◆ systolic bruit over carotid artery, mastoid process, or orbit, indicating turbulent blood flow
◆ focal neurologic deficits (depending on the location of the AVM) resulting from compression and diminished perfusion
◆ signs and symptoms of intracranial (intracerebral, subarachnoid, or subdural) hemorrhage, including sudden severe headache, seizures, confusion, lethargy, and meningeal irritation from bleeding into the brain tissue or subarachnoid space
◆ hydrocephalus from AVM extension into the ventricular lining.

Complications
Complications depend on the severity (location and size) of the AVM and may include:
◆ aneurysm development and subsequent rupture
◆ hemorrhage (intracerebral, subarachnoid, or subdural, depending on the location of the AVM)
◆ hydrocephalus.

Diagnosis
◆ Cerebral arteriogram confirms the presence of AVMs and evaluates blood flow.
◆ Doppler ultrasonography of cerebrovascular system indicates abnormal, turbulent blood flow.

Treatment
Treatment can be supportive, corrective, or both, and includes:
◆ support measures, including aneurysm precautions to prevent possible rupture
◆ surgery—block dissection, laser, or ligation—to repair the communicating channels and remove the feeding vessels
◆ embolization or stereotactic radiosurgery if surgery isn't possible, to close the communicating channels and feeder vessels and thus reduce the blood flow to the AVM.

Special considerations
◆ Monitor vital signs frequently.
◆ Control hypertension, seizure activity, and other activity or stress that could elevate the patient's systemic blood pressure by administering drug therapy as ordered, conducting ongoing neurologic assessments, and maintaining a quiet, therapeutic environment.

◆ If the AVM has ruptured, intervene to control elevated ICP and intracranial hemorrhage. The patient with a ruptured AVM may have intracerebral or intraventricular bleeding; bleeding into the subarachnoid, subdural, or epidural space; or bleeding into the brain itself, usually causing a concurrent elevation in ICP.

BELL'S PALSY
Bell's palsy is a disease of the seventh cranial nerve (facial) that produces unilateral or bilateral facial weakness or paralysis, although bilateral involvement occurs in less than 10% of cases. The onset of symptoms is rapid. Although it affects all age-groups, Bell's palsy occurs most commonly in people younger than age 60. In 80% to 90% of patients, it subsides spontaneously, with complete recovery in 1 to 8 weeks; however, recovery may be delayed in elderly patients. If recovery is partial, contractures may develop on the paralyzed side of the face. Bell's palsy may recur on the same or opposite side of the face.

Causes
◆ Hemorrhage
◆ Infection
◆ Local trauma
◆ Meningitis
◆ Tumor

Pathophysiology
Bell's palsy reflects an inflammatory reaction around the seventh cranial nerve, usually at the internal auditory meatus where the nerve leaves bony tissue. This inflammatory reaction produces a conduction block that inhibits appropriate neural stimulation to the muscle by the motor fibers of the facial nerve, resulting in the characteristic unilateral or bilateral facial weakness.

Signs and symptoms
The signs and symptoms exhibited by the patient typically reflect interference in motor function associated with the seventh cranial nerve. Bell's palsy usually produces unilateral facial weakness, occasionally with aching pain around the angle of the jaw or behind the ear. On the weak side, the mouth droops (causing the patient to drool saliva from the corner of his mouth), and taste perception is distorted over the affected anterior portion of the tongue. The forehead appears smooth, and the patient's ability to close his eye on the weak side is markedly impaired. When he tries to close this eye, it rolls upward (Bell's phenomenon) and shows excessive tearing. Although Bell's phenomenon also occurs in people who are otherwise healthy, it isn't apparent because the eyelids close completely and cover

this eye motion. In Bell's palsy, incomplete eye closure makes this upward motion obvious. Other symptoms include loss of taste and ringing in the ear.

Complications
◆ Corneal abrasion
◆ Infection (masked by steroid use)
◆ Poor functional recovery

Diagnosis
Diagnosis is based on clinical presentation: distorted facial appearance and inability to raise the eyebrow, close the eyelid, smile, show the teeth, or puff out the cheek on the affected side. After 10 days, electromyography helps predict the level of expected recovery by distinguishing temporary conduction defects from a pathologic interruption of nerve fibers.

Treatment
Treatment consists of prednisone, an oral corticosteroid that reduces facial nerve edema and improves nerve conduction and blood flow. After the 14th day of prednisone therapy, electrotherapy may help prevent atrophy of facial muscles. Persistent paralysis may require surgical treatment.

Special considerations
Patient care includes observation for adverse reactions to prednisone, pain relief, and emotional support.
◆ During treatment with prednisone, watch for adverse reactions, especially GI distress and fluid retention. If GI distress is troublesome, a concomitant antacid usually provides relief. If the patient has diabetes, prednisone must be used with caution, which necessitates frequent monitoring of the serum glucose level.
◆ To reduce pain, apply moist heat to the affected side of the face, taking care not to burn the skin.
◆ To help maintain muscle tone, massage the patient's face with a gentle upward motion two or three times daily for 5 to 10 minutes, or have him massage his face himself. When he's ready for active exercises, teach him to exercise by grimacing in front of a mirror.
◆ Advise the patient to protect his eye by covering it with an eye patch, especially when outdoors and at night (when sleeping). Tell him to keep warm and avoid exposure to dust and wind. When exposure is unavoidable, instruct him to cover his face.
◆ To prevent excessive weight loss, help the patient cope with difficulty in eating and drinking. Instruct him to chew on the unaffected side

of his mouth. Provide a soft, nutritionally balanced diet, eliminating hot foods and fluids. Arrange for privacy at mealtimes to reduce embarrassment. Give the patient frequent and complete mouth care, being particularly careful to remove residual food that collects between the cheeks and gums.
◆ Offer psychological support.

CEREBRAL PALSY
The most common cause of crippling in children, cerebral palsy (CP) is a group of neuromuscular disorders caused by prenatal, perinatal, or postnatal damage to the upper motoneurons. Although nonprogressive, these disorders may become more obvious as an affected infant grows.

The three major types of CP—spastic, athetoid, and ataxic—may occur alone or in combination. Motor impairment may be minimal (sometimes apparent only during physical activities, such as running) or severely disabling. Common associated defects are seizures, speech disorders, and mental retardation.

Cerebral palsy occurs in an estimated 2 to 3 per 1,000 live births in the United States every year. Incidence is highest in premature infants (anoxia plays the greatest role in contributing to cerebral palsy) and in those who are small for gestational age. Almost one-half of the children with CP are mentally retarded, approximately one-fourth have seizure disorders, and more than three-fourths have impaired speech. Additionally, many children with CP have dental abnormalities, vision and hearing defects, and reading disabilities.

CP is more common in whites than in other ethnicities. The prognosis varies. Treatment may make a near-normal life possible for children with mild impairment. Those with severe impairment require special services and schooling.

Causes
The exact cause of CP is unknown; however, conditions resulting in cerebral anoxia, hemorrhage, or other CNS damage are probably responsible. Potential causes vary with time of damage.

Prenatal causes include:
◆ abnormal placental attachment
◆ anoxia
◆ exposure to radiation
◆ isoimmunization
◆ malnutrition
◆ maternal diabetes
◆ maternal infection (especially rubella)
◆ toxemia.

Perinatal and birth factors may include:
◆ abruptio placentae

- breech presentation
- depressed maternal vital signs from general or spinal anesthesia
- forceps delivery
- infection or trauma during infancy
- multiple births (especially infants born last)
- placenta previa
- premature birth
- prolapsed cord with delay in blood delivery to the head
- prolonged or unusually rapid labor.
Postnatal causes include:
- brain infection or tumor
- cerebral circulatory anomalies causing blood vessel rupture
- head trauma
- kernicterus resulting from erythroblastosis fetalis
- prolonged anoxia
- systemic disease resulting in cerebral thrombosis or embolus.

Pathophysiology

In the early stages of brain development, a lesion or abnormality causes structural and functional defects that in turn cause impaired motor function or cognition. Even though the defects are present at birth, problems may not be apparent until months later, when the axons have become myelinated and the basal ganglia are mature.

Signs and symptoms

Shortly after birth, the infant with CP may exhibit some typical signs and symptoms, including:
- excessive lethargy or irritability
- high-pitched cry
- poor head control
- weak sucking reflex.

Additional physical findings that may suggest CP results from impaired development or damage to the motor areas of the brain and may include:
- delayed motor development (inability to meet major developmental milestones)
- abnormal head circumference, typically smaller than normal for age (because the head grows as the brain grows)
- abnormal postures, such as straightening the legs when the patient is lying on his back, toes down; holding the head higher than normal when in a prone position due to arching of the back
- abnormal reflexes (neonatal reflexes lasting longer than expected, extreme reflexes, or clonus)
- abnormal muscle tone and performance (scooting on the back to crawl, toe-first walking).

Each type of CP typically produces a distinctive set of clinical features, although some children display a mixed form of the disease. (See *Assessing signs of cerebral palsy*, page 272.)

Complications

Complications depend on the type of CP and the severity of the involvement. Possible complications include:
- contractures
- skin breakdown and ulcer formation
- muscle atrophy
- malnutrition
- seizure disorders
- speech, hearing, and vision problems
- language and perceptual deficits
- mental retardation
- dental problems
- respiratory difficulties, including aspiration from poor gag and swallowing reflexes.

Diagnosis

No diagnostic tests are specific to CP. However, neurologic screening will exclude other possible conditions, such as infection, spina bifida, or muscular dystrophy. Diagnostic tests that may be performed include:
- Developmental screening reveals delay in achieving milestones.
- Vision and hearing screening demonstrates degree of impairment.
- EEG identifies the source of seizure activity.

AGE ALERT *Suspect CP whenever an infant exhibits an alteration in neurologic function during clinical observation. This may include difficulty in sucking or moving voluntarily. Infants particularly at risk include those with a low birth weight, low Apgar score at 5 minutes, seizures, and metabolic disturbances. However, all infants should have a screening test for CP as a regular part of their 6-month checkup.*

Treatment

CP can't be cured, but treatment can help affected children reach their full potential within the limits set by this disorder. Such treatment requires a comprehensive and cooperative effort, involving physicians, nurses, teachers, psychologists, the child's family, and occupational, physical, and speech therapists. Home care is usually possible. Treatment typically includes:
- braces, casts, or splints and special appliances, such as adapted eating utensils and a low toilet seat with arms, to help the child perform activities of daily living independently
- an artificial urinary sphincter for the incontinent child

Assessing signs of cerebral palsy

Each type of cerebral palsy (CP) is manifested by specific findings. This chart highlights the major signs and symptoms associated with each type of CP. The manifestations reflect impaired upper motoneuron function and disruption of the normal stretch reflex.

Type of CP	Signs and symptoms
Spastic CP (due to impairment of the pyramidal tract [most common type])	◆ Hyperactive deep tendon reflexes ◆ Increased stretch reflexes ◆ Rapid alternating muscle contraction and relaxation ◆ Muscle weakness ◆ Underdevelopment of affected limbs ◆ Muscle contraction in response to manipulation ◆ Tendency toward contractures ◆ Typical walking on toes with a scissors gait, crossing one foot in front of the other
Athetoid CP (due to impairment of the extrapyramidal tract)	◆ Involuntary movements usually affecting arms more severely than legs, including: –grimacing –wormlike writhing –dystonia –sharp jerks ◆ Difficulty with speech due to involuntary facial movements ◆ Increasing severity of movements during stress; decreased with relaxation and disappearing entirely during sleep
Ataxic CP (due to impairment of the extrapyramidal tract)	◆ Disturbed balance ◆ Incoordination (especially of the arms) ◆ Hypoactive reflexes ◆ Nystagmus ◆ Muscle weakness ◆ Tremor ◆ Lack of leg movement during infancy ◆ Wide gait as the child begins to walk ◆ Sudden or fine movements impossible (due to ataxia)
Mixed CP	◆ Spasticity and athetoid movements ◆ Ataxic and athetoid movements (resulting in severe impairment)

◆ range-of-motion exercises to minimize contractures
◆ an anticonvulsant to control seizures
◆ a muscle relaxant (sometimes) to reduce spasticity
◆ surgery to decrease spasticity or correct contractures
◆ muscle transfer or tendon lengthening surgery to improve function of joints
◆ rehabilitation, including occupational, physical, and speech therapy, to maintain or improve functional abilities.

Special considerations

A child with CP may be hospitalized for orthopedic surgery or for treatment of other complications.

◆ Speak slowly and distinctly. Encourage the child to ask for items he wants. Listen patiently and don't rush him.
◆ Plan a high-calorie diet that's adequate to meet the child's high energy needs.
◆ During meals, maintain a quiet, unhurried atmosphere with as few distractions as possible. The child should be encouraged to feed himself and may need special utensils and a chair with a solid footrest. Teach him to place food far back in his mouth to facilitate swallowing.
◆ Encourage the child to chew food thoroughly, drink through a straw, and suck on lollipops to develop the muscle control needed to minimize drooling.

◆ Allow the child to wash and dress independently, assisting only as needed. The child may need clothing modifications.
◆ Give all care in an unhurried manner; otherwise, muscle spasticity may increase.
◆ Encourage the child and his family to participate in the care plan so they can continue it at home.
◆ Care for associated hearing or vision disturbances, as necessary.
◆ Give frequent mouth and dental care, as necessary.
◆ Reduce muscle spasms that increase postoperative pain by moving and turning the child carefully after surgery; provide an analgesic as needed.
◆ After orthopedic surgery, provide good cast care. Wash and dry the skin at the edge of the cast frequently. Reposition the child often, check for foul odor, and ventilate under the cast with a cool air blow-dryer. Use a flashlight to check for skin breakdown beneath the cast. Help the child relax, perhaps by giving a warm bath, before reapplying a bivalved cast.
To help the parents:
◆ Encourage them to set realistic individualized goals for their child.
◆ Assist in planning crafts and other activities.
◆ Stress the child's need to develop peer relationships; warn the parents against being overprotective.
◆ Identify and deal with family stress. The parents may feel unreasonable guilt about their child's disability and may need psychological counseling.
◆ Refer the parents to supportive community organizations. For more information, suggest that they contact the United Cerebral Palsy Association or their local chapter.

COMPLEX REGIONAL PAIN SYNDROME

Complex regional pain syndrome (CRPS), also known as *reflex sympathetic dystrophy* (CRPS1) or *causalgia* (CRPS2), is a chronic pain disorder that results from abnormal healing after an injury—either minor or major—to a bone, muscle, or nerve. One or more extremities and other parts of the body may be affected.

CRPS is more common in people between ages 40 and 60, but has been seen in younger people as well. This disorder also may be seen in postoperative patients and in patients with diseases that can cause chronic pain, such as cancer and arthritis. Annual incidence is unknown because CRPS is commonly misdiagnosed. However, it has been reported in 1% to 2% of patients with various fractures and in 2% to 5% of patients with peripheral nerve injury.

Causes

Although the exact cause of CRPS is unknown, it can sometimes appear without obvious injury to the affected limb. Other causes include:
◆ infection or injury to an arm or leg
◆ myocardial infarction or stroke.

Pathophysiology

Impaired communication between the damaged nerves of the sympathetic nervous system and the brain may cause interference with normal signals for sensations, temperature, and blood flow. This leads to problems in the nerves, blood vessels, skin, bones, and muscles.

Signs and symptoms

The development of symptoms is commonly disproportionate to the severity of the injury and seems to result from abnormal functioning of the sympathetic nervous system, the part of the nervous system that controls the diameter of blood vessels.
Patients usually report:
◆ constant pain
◆ severe pain (common with CRPS2)
◆ altered blood flow in the affected area with feelings of either warmth or coolness to the touch, with discoloration, sweating, or swelling
◆ skin, hair, and nail changes along with impaired mobility and muscle wasting (if adequate treatment is delayed).

Complications

◆ Chronic progression (if not diagnosed and treated early)
◆ Depression and drug dependence (due to chronic pain)

Diagnosis

There's no specific laboratory test for CRPS, so the diagnosis is based on the patient's history and clinical findings. A history of injury to an extremity may point to CRPS.
◆ Bone X-rays may aid in ruling out other conditions, such as osteomyelitis and stress fractures, which cause similar signs and symptoms.
◆ Additional tests may include bone scans, nerve conduction studies, and thermography (a test to show temperature changes and lack of blood supply in the painful area of the affected limb).
With early diagnosis, prognosis improves.

Treatment

♦ Drug therapy with an anti-inflammatory, an antidepressant, a vasodilator, and an analgesic, used alone or in varying combinations (depending on the severity of the patient's symptoms)
♦ A steroid or an anti–bone loss medication, such as Actonel
♦ Physical therapy to the injured area, including application of heat and cold, the use of a transcutaneous electrical nerve stimulator (TENS) unit, and biofeedback
♦ Psychological support
♦ Nerve or regional blocks (for interrupting the hyperactivity of the sympathetic nervous system)
♦ Surgical sympathectomy, radical surgery that involves cutting the nerves to destroy the pain (in severe cases; however, this method is rarely used because other sensation may be destroyed in the process)

Special considerations

♦ Monitor the patient for adverse reactions to the prescribed medications.
♦ In addition to attending physical therapy sessions, the patient may need a home therapy regimen that includes stretching, active and passive exercises, strengthening exercises, compressive stockings or gloves to control edema, and heat or cold pack applications.
♦ Consult a pain care specialist to provide additional options for the patient, and help manage discomfort.
♦ Offer emotional support to the patient and his family. Teach them about the disease.
♦ Advise the patient to resist the temptation to keep the affected extremity immobile. Encourage him to mobilize and use the affected extremity to prevent any functional loss.
♦ Teach the patient methods to reduce pain, including how to perform a home therapy regimen, as well as how to use a TENS unit.
♦ Because chronic pain can be an emotional burden to the patient and his family, provide information on resources, such as counseling, support groups, stress-reduction methods, meditation, relaxation training, and hypnosis.

CREUTZFELDT-JAKOB DISEASE

Creutzfeldt-Jakob disease (CJD) is a rare, rapidly progressive viral disease that attacks the central nervous system, causing dementia and neurologic signs and symptoms, such as myoclonic jerking, ataxia, aphasia, visual disturbances, and paralysis. CJD is always fatal. A new variant of CJD (nvCJD) emerged in Europe in 1996. (See *Understanding nvCJD.*)

CJD generally affects adults between ages 40 and 65 and occurs in more than 50 countries.

Males and females are affected equally. In people younger than age 30, incidence is 5 in 1 million; in all other age-groups, incidence is 1 in 100 million. Most cases are sporadic; 5% to 15% are familial, with an autosomal dominant pattern of inheritance.

Causes

The causative organism of CJD is difficult to identify because no foreign ribonucleic acid or deoxyribonucleic acid has been linked to the disease. It's believed to be caused by a specific protein called a *prion,* which lacks nucleic acids, resists proteolytic digestion, and spontaneously aggregates in the brain.

Pathophysiology

Although CJD isn't transmitted by normal casual contact, human-to-human transmission can occur as a result of certain medical procedures, such as corneal and cadaveric dura mater grafts. Isolated cases are attributed to treatment during childhood with human growth hormone and to improperly decontaminated neurosurgical instruments and brain electrodes.

Signs and symptoms

Duration of the typical illness is 4 months. Signs and symptoms may include:
♦ slowness in thinking, difficulty concentrating, impaired judgment, memory loss, and dementia as the disease progresses due to mental impairment
♦ involuntary movements (such as muscle twitching, trembling, and peculiar body movements), visual disturbances, and hallucinations due to disease progression and advancing mental deterioration.

Complications

♦ Compromised neurologic functions ranging from impaired gait, to incontinence, to an akinetic mute state
♦ Death (typically resulting from bronchopneumonia that develops after the patient has become immobile and, eventually, bedridden)

Diagnosis

♦ Consider CJD in anyone experiencing signs of progressive dementia.
♦ Neurologic examination is the most effective tool in diagnosing CJD as difficulty with rapid alternating movements and point-to-point movements are typically evident early in the disease.
♦ EEG may be performed to assess for typical changes in brain wave activity.

◆ Computed tomography scan, magnetic resonance imaging of the brain, and lumbar puncture can help rule out other disorders that cause dementia.

◆ Though not diagnostic, presence of the 14-3-3 protein in the spinal fluid is highly suggestive of the disease when it's accompanied by other characteristic symptoms.

◆ Definitive diagnosis usually isn't obtained until an autopsy is done and brain tissue is examined.

Treatment

There's no cure for CJD, and its progress can't be slowed.

◆ Palliative care includes making the patient comfortable to ease symptoms.

◆ A sedative and an antipsychotic may be given to control aggressive behaviors.

◆ Monitoring and assistance in the home or institutionalized setting provide a safe environment, control aggressive or agitated behavior, and meet the patient's physiologic needs.

◆ Family counseling may help in coping with the changes required for home care.

◆ Behavior modification may be helpful, in some cases, for controlling unacceptable or dangerous behaviors.

◆ Reality orientation, with repeated reinforcement of environmental and other cues, may help reduce disorientation.

◆ Legal advice may be appropriate early in the course of the disorder to form advance directives, power of attorney, and other legal actions that may make it easier to make ethical decisions regarding the care of an individual with CJD.

Special considerations

◆ Offer emotional support to the patient and his family.

◆ Contact social services and hospice, as appropriate, to assist the family with their needs.

◆ Encourage the patient and his family to discuss and complete advance directives.

◆ To prevent disease transmission, use caution when handling body fluids and other materials from patients suspected of having CJD.

◆ Teach the patient and his family about the disease, and assist them through the grieving process.

◆ Refer the patient and his family to CJD support groups, and encourage participation.

||| **LIFE-THREATENING DISORDER**

GUILLAIN-BARRÉ SYNDROME

Also known as *infectious polyneuritis, Landry-Guillain-Barré syndrome,* and *acute idiopathic*

Understanding nvCJD

Like conventional Creutzfeldt-Jakob disease (CJD), the new variant of the disease (nvCJD) is a rare, fatal neurodegenerative disease. Most cases have been reported in the United Kingdom. Researchers believe nvCJD is most likely caused by exposure to *bovine spongiform encephalopathy* (BSE) — a fatal brain disease in cattle also known as *mad cow disease* — via ingestion of beef products from cattle with BSE.

The disease affects patients at a much younger age (younger than 55) than conventional CJD, and the duration of the illness is much longer (14 months).

Regulations have been established in Europe to control outbreaks of BSE in cattle and to prevent contaminated meat from entering the food supply. The Centers for Disease Control and Prevention and the World Health Organization are still exploring nvCJD and its relationship to BSE.

polyneuritis, Guillain-Barré syndrome is an acute, rapidly progressive, and potentially fatal form of polyneuritis that causes muscle weakness and mild distal sensory loss.

This syndrome can occur at any age but is most common between ages 30 and 50. It affects both sexes equally. Recovery is spontaneous and complete in about 95% of patients, although mild motor or reflex deficits may persist in the feet and legs. The prognosis is best when symptoms clear before 20 days after onset.

This syndrome occurs in three phases:

◆ *Acute phase* — begins with the onset of the first definitive symptom and ends 1 to 3 weeks later. Further deterioration doesn't occur after the acute phase.

◆ *Plateau phase* — lasts several days to 2 weeks.

◆ *Recovery phase* — is believed to coincide with remyelinization and regrowth of axonal processes. It extends over 4 to 6 months, but may last up to 2 to 3 years if the disease is severe.

Causes

The precise cause of Guillain-Barré syndrome is unknown, but it may be a cell-mediated immune response to a virus.

About 50% of patients with Guillain-Barré syndrome have a recent history of minor febrile illness, usually an upper respiratory tract infection or, less commonly, gastroenteritis. When infection precedes the onset of Guillain-Barré syndrome, signs of infection subside before neurologic features appear.

Other possible precipitating factors include:
◆ Hodgkin's or other malignant disease
◆ rabies or swine influenza vaccination
◆ surgery
◆ systemic lupus erythematosus.

Pathophysiology

The major pathologic manifestation is segmental demyelination of the peripheral nerves. This prevents normal transmission of electrical impulses along the sensorimotor nerve roots. Because this syndrome causes inflammation and degenerative changes in both the posterior (sensory) and the anterior (motor) nerve roots, signs of sensory and motor losses occur simultaneously. (See *Understanding sensorimotor nerve degeneration*.) Additionally, autonomic nerve transmission may be impaired.

Signs and symptoms

Signs and symptoms are progressive and include:
◆ symmetrical muscle weakness (major neurologic sign) appearing in the legs (ascending type) and then extending to the arms and facial nerves within 24 to 72 hours, from impaired anterior nerve root transmission
◆ muscle weakness developing in the arms first (descending type) or in the arms and legs simultaneously, from impaired anterior nerve root transmission
◆ muscle weakness absent or affecting only the cranial nerves (in mild forms)
◆ paresthesia, sometimes preceding muscle weakness but vanishing quickly, from impairment of the dorsal nerve root transmission
◆ diplegia, possibly with ophthalmoplegia (ocular paralysis), from impaired motor nerve root transmission and involvement of cranial nerves III, IV, and VI
◆ dysphagia or dysarthria and, less commonly, weakness of the muscles supplied by cranial nerve XI (spinal accessory nerve)
◆ hypotonia and areflexia from interruption of the reflex arc.

Complications

◆ Thrombophlebitis
◆ Pressure ulcers
◆ Muscle wasting
◆ Sepsis
◆ Joint contractures
◆ Aspiration
◆ Respiratory tract infections
◆ Mechanical respiratory failure
◆ Sinus tachycardia or bradycardia

◆ Hypertension and orthostatic hypotension
◆ Loss of bladder and bowel sphincter control

Diagnosis

◆ Cerebrospinal fluid (CSF) analysis by lumbar puncture reveals elevated protein levels, peaking in 4 to 6 weeks, probably as a result of widespread inflammation of the nerve roots; the CSF white blood cell count remains normal, but in severe disease, CSF pressure may rise above normal.
◆ Complete blood count shows leukocytosis with immature forms early in the illness, and then quickly returns to normal.
◆ Electromyography possibly shows repeated firing of the same motor unit, instead of widespread sectional stimulation.
◆ Nerve conduction velocities show slowing soon after paralysis develops.
◆ Serum immunoglobulin levels reveal elevated levels from inflammatory response.

Treatment

◆ Primarily supportive, treatments include endotracheal intubation or tracheotomy if respiratory muscle involvement causes difficulty in clearing secretions.
◆ A trial dose (7 days) of prednisone is given to reduce inflammatory response if the disease is relentlessly progressive; if prednisone produces no noticeable improvement, the drug is discontinued.
◆ Plasmapheresis is useful during the initial phase, but it's of no benefit if begun 2 weeks after onset.
◆ High doses of immunoglobulins may be administered I.V. to decrease the autoimmune response but must be started as soon as possible to have an effect.
◆ Continuous electrocardiogram monitoring alerts for possible arrhythmias from autonomic dysfunction; propranolol treats tachycardia and hypertension, or atropine is given for bradycardia; volume replacement is given for severe hypotension.

Special considerations

Monitoring the patient for escalation of symptoms is of special concern.
◆ Watch for ascending sensory loss, which precedes motor loss. Also, monitor vital signs and level of consciousness.
◆ Assess and treat respiratory dysfunction. If respiratory muscles are weak, take serial vital capacity recordings. Use a respirometer with a mouthpiece or a face mask for bedside testing.
◆ Obtain arterial blood gas measurements. Because neuromuscular disease results in primary

CLOSER LOOK
Understanding sensorimotor nerve degeneration

Guillain-Barré syndrome attacks the peripheral nerves and, thus, they can't transmit messages to the brain correctly. Here's what goes wrong.

The myelin sheath degenerates for unknown reasons. This sheath covers the nerve axons and conducts electrical impulses along the nerve pathways. Degeneration brings inflammation, swelling, and patchy demyelination. As this disorder destroys myelin, the nodes of Ranvier (at the junction of the myelin sheaths) widen. This delays and impairs impulse transmission along the dorsal and anterior nerve roots.

Because the dorsal nerve roots handle sensory function, the patient may experience tingling and numbness. Similarly, because the anterior nerve roots are responsible for motor function, impairment causes varying weakness, immobility, and paralysis.

---

hypoventilation with hypoxemia and hypercapnia, watch for partial pressure of arterial oxygen (Pao_2) below 70 mm Hg, which signals respiratory failure. Be alert for signs and symptoms of rising partial pressure of arterial carbon dioxide (confusion, tachypnea).

◆ Auscultate breath sounds, turn and position the patient, and encourage coughing, deep breathing, and incentive spirometry. Begin respiratory support at the first sign of dyspnea (in adults, vital capacity less than 800 ml; in children, less than 12 ml/kg of body weight) or with decreasing Pao_2.

◆ If respiratory failure is imminent, establish an emergency airway with an endotracheal tube.

◆ Give meticulous skin care to prevent skin breakdown and contractures. Establish a strict turning schedule; inspect the skin (especially sacrum, heels, and ankles) for breakdown, and reposition the patient every 2 hours. After each position change, stimulate circulation by carefully massaging pressure points. Also, use foam, gel, or alternating pressure pads at points of contact.

◆ Perform passive range-of-motion exercises within the patient's pain limits. (Although this disease doesn't produce pain, exercising little-used muscles will.) Remember that the proximal muscle groups of the thighs, shoulders, and trunk will be the most tender and will cause the most pain on passive movement and turning. When the patient's condition stabilizes, change to gentle stretching and active assistance exercises.

◆ To prevent aspiration, test the gag reflex, and elevate the head of the bed before giving the patient anything to eat. If the gag reflex is absent, give enteral tube feedings until this reflex returns.

◆ As the patient regains strength and can tolerate a vertical position, be alert for postural hypotension. Monitor his blood pressure and pulse during tilting periods and, if necessary, apply

toe-to-groin elastic bandages or an abdominal binder to minimize postural hypotension.

◆ If the patient has severe paralysis and is expected to have a long recovery period, a gastrostomy tube may be necessary to provide adequate nourishment.

◆ Inspect the patient's legs regularly for signs and symptoms of thrombophlebitis (localized pain, tenderness, erythema, edema, and positive Homans' sign), a common complication of Guillain-Barré syndrome. To prevent thrombophlebitis, apply antiembolism stockings and give a prophylactic anticoagulant, as ordered.

◆ If the patient has facial paralysis, give eye and mouth care every 4 hours. Protect the corneas with isotonic eyedrops and conical eye shields.

◆ Watch for urine retention. Measure and record intake and output every 8 hours, and offer the bedpan every 3 to 4 hours. Encourage adequate fluid intake of 2 qt (2 L)/day, unless contraindicated. If urine retention develops, begin intermittent catheterization, as ordered. Because the abdominal muscles are weak, the patient may need manual pressure on the bladder (Credé's method) before he can urinate.

◆ To prevent and relieve constipation, offer prune juice and a high-bulk diet. If necessary, give a stool softener, such as docusate, as ordered.

◆ Before discharge, prepare a home care plan. Teach the patient how to transfer from bed to wheelchair and from wheelchair to toilet or tub, and how to walk short distances with a walker or a cane. Teach the family how to help him eat, compensating for facial weakness, and how to help him avoid skin breakdown. Stress the need for a regular bowel and bladder routine. Refer the patient for physical therapy, as needed.

HEADACHE
The most common patient complaint, headache usually occurs as a symptom of an underlying

disorder. Some 90% of all headaches are vascular, muscle contraction, or a combination; 10% are due to an underlying intracranial, systemic, or psychological disorder. Migraine headaches, probably the most intensely studied, are throbbing, vascular headaches that usually begin to appear in childhood or adolescence and recur throughout adulthood. Affecting up to 10% of Americans, they're more common in females and have a strong familial incidence.

Causes

Most chronic headaches result from tension (muscle contraction), which may be caused by:
◆ emotional stress or fatigue
◆ environmental stimuli (noise, crowds, or bright lights)
◆ menstruation.
Other possible causes include:
◆ diseases of the scalp, teeth, extracranial arteries, or external or middle ear
◆ glaucoma
◆ head trauma or tumor
◆ hypertension
◆ increased intracranial pressure
◆ inflammation of the eyes or mucosa of the nasal or paranasal sinuses
◆ intracranial bleeding, abscess, or aneurysm
◆ systemic disease
◆ vasodilators (nitrates, alcohol, and histamine).

Pathophysiology

Headaches are believed to be associated with constriction and dilation of intracranial and extracranial arteries. During a migraine attack, certain biochemical abnormalities, including local leakage of a vasodilator polypeptide called neurokinin through the dilated arteries and a decrease in the plasma level of serotonins, are thought to occur.

Headache pain may emanate from the pain-sensitive structures of the skin, scalp, muscles, arteries, and veins; cranial nerves V, VII, IX, and X; or cervical nerves 1, 2, and 3. Intracranial mechanisms of headaches include traction or displacement of arteries, venous sinuses, or venous tributaries and inflammation or direct pressure on the cranial nerves with afferent pain fibers.

Four headache phases

The evolution of a headache has four distinct phases:
◆ *Normal* — Cerebral and temporal arteries are innervated extracranially; parenchymal arteries are noninnervated.
◆ *Vasoconstriction (aura)* — Stress-related neurogenic local vasoconstriction of innervated

cerebral arteries reduces cerebral blood flow (localized ischemia). Systematically, the prostaglandin thromboxane causes increased platelet aggregation and release of serotonin, a potent vasoconstrictor and, possibly, other vasoactive substances.
◆ *Parenchymal artery dilation* — Noninnervated parenchymal vessels dilate in response to local acidosis and anoxia (ischemia). Neurogenic or biologic factors may cause preformed arteriovenous shunts to open. Increased blood flow, increased internal pressure, and enhanced pulsations short-circuit the normal nutritive capillaries and cause pain.
◆ *Vasodilation (headache)* — Compensatory mechanisms cause marked vasodilation of the innervated arteries resulting in a headache. Systemic platelet aggregation decreases, and falling serotonin levels result in vasodilation. A painful, sterile perivascular inflammation develops and persists into a postheadache phase.

Signs and symptoms

Initially, migraine headaches usually produce unilateral, pulsating pain, which later becomes more generalized. They're commonly preceded by a scintillating scotoma, hemianopsia, unilateral paresthesia, or speech disorders. The patient may experience irritability, anorexia, nausea, vomiting, and photophobia. (See *Clinical features of migraine headaches*.)

Both muscle contraction and traction-inflammatory vascular headaches produce a dull, persistent ache; tender spots on the head and neck; and a feeling of tightness around the head, with a characteristic "hat-band" distribution. The pain is typically severe and unrelenting. If caused by intracranial bleeding, headache may result in neurologic deficits, such as paresthesia and muscle weakness; a narcotic may fail to relieve pain in these cases. If caused by a tumor, pain is most severe when the patient awakens.

Complications
◆ Misdiagnosis
◆ Status migraines
◆ Drug addiction
◆ Disruption of lifestyle

Diagnosis

Diagnosis requires a history of recurrent headaches and physical examination of the head and neck. Such examination includes percussion, auscultation for bruits, inspection for signs of infection, and palpation for defects, crepitus, or tender spots (especially after trauma). Definitive diagnosis also requires a complete

Clinical features of migraine headaches

Type	Signs and symptoms
Common migraine (most prevalent)	
Usually occurs on weekends and holidays	◆ Prodromal signs and symptoms, including fatigue, nausea, vomiting, and fluid imbalance, that precede headache by about 1 day ◆ Sensitivity to light and noise (most prominent feature) ◆ Headache pain (unilateral or bilateral, aching or throbbing)
Classic migraine	
Usually occurs in compulsive personalities and within families	◆ Prodromal signs and symptoms, including vision disturbances, (such as zigzag lines and bright lights [most common]), sensory disturbances (tingling of face, lips, and hands), or motor disturbances (staggering gait) ◆ Recurrent, periodic headaches
Hemiplegic and ophthalmoplegic migraine (rare)	
Usually occurs in young adults	◆ Severe, unilateral pain ◆ Extraocular muscle palsies (involving third cranial nerve) and ptosis ◆ With repeated headaches, possible permanent third cranial nerve injury ◆ In hemiplegic migraine, neurologic deficits (hemiparesis, hemiplegia) that may persist after headache subsides
Basilar artery migraine	
Usually occurs in young women before their menstrual periods	◆ Prodromal symptoms, including partial vision loss followed by vertigo, ataxia, dysarthria, tinnitus and, sometimes, tingling of fingers and toes that lasts from several minutes to almost an hour ◆ Headache pain, severe occipital throbbing, vomiting

neurologic examination, assessment for other systemic diseases, and a psychosocial evaluation when such factors are suspected.

Diagnostic tests include computed tomography scan — performed before lumbar puncture to rule out increased intracranial pressure (ICP) — or magnetic resonance imaging. Cervical spine and sinus X-rays and an EEG may also be performed. A lumbar puncture isn't done if there's evidence of increased ICP or if a brain tumor is suspected because rapidly reducing pressure, by removing spinal fluid, can cause brain herniation.

Treatment

Depending on the type of headache, an analgesic — for example, aspirin or codeine — may provide symptomatic relief. Other measures include identification and elimination of causative factors and, possibly, stress reduction techniques. Chronic tension headaches may also require a muscle relaxant.

For migraine headaches, ergotamine alone or with caffeine may be an effective treatment. The Food and Drug Administration allows labeling of various analgesic preparations that include caffeine to state that they're for the treatment of migraine headaches. Remember that these medications can't be taken by pregnant women because they stimulate uterine contractions. These drugs and others, such as metoclopramide or naproxen, work best when taken early in the course of an attack. If nausea and vomiting make oral administration impossible, these drugs may be given as rectal suppositories.

Drugs in the class of sumatriptan are considered by many clinicians to be the drug of choice for acute migraine attacks or cluster headaches. Drugs that can help prevent migraine headaches include antidepressants (such as nortriptyline or fluoxetine), beta-adrenergic blockers (propranolol), and calcium-channel blockers (verapamil). Corticosteroids provide short-term relief for some patients with cluster headaches.

Special considerations

Headaches seldom require hospitalization unless caused by a serious disorder. If that's the case, direct your care to the underlying problem.

◆ Obtain a complete patient history, including duration and location of the headache; time of day it usually begins; nature of the pain; concurrence with other symptoms, such as blurred vision; medications taken, such as hormonal contraceptives; prolonged fasting and diet history; and precipitating factors, such as tension, menstruation, loud noises, menopause, or alcohol. Exacerbating factors can also be assessed through ongoing observation of the patient's personality, habits, activities of daily living, family relationships, coping mechanisms, and relaxation activities.

◆ Using the history as a guide, help the patient avoid exacerbating factors. Advise her to lie down in a dark, quiet room during an attack and to place ice packs on her forehead or a cold cloth over her eyes.

◆ Instruct the patient to take the prescribed medication at the onset of migraine symptoms, to prevent dehydration by drinking plenty of fluids after nausea and vomiting subside, and to use other headache relief measures.

◆ The patient with a migraine headache usually needs to be hospitalized only if nausea and vomiting are severe enough to induce dehydration and possible shock.

◆ Instruct the patient to follow-up with a neurologist or a pain clinic to establish an effective pain control regimen.

||| **LIFE-THREATENING DISORDER**

HEAD TRAUMA

Head trauma, also known as *traumatic brain injury,* describes any traumatic insult to the brain that results in physical, intellectual, emotional, social, or vocational changes. Young children between ages 6 months and 2 years, people between ages 15 and 24, and elderly people are at highest risk for head trauma. The risk for men is double the risk for women.

Head trauma is generally categorized as closed or open trauma. Closed trauma, or *blunt trauma* as it's sometimes called, is more common. It typically occurs when the head strikes a hard surface or a rapidly moving object strikes the head. The dura is intact, and no brain tissue is exposed to the external environment. In *open trauma,* as the name suggests, an opening in the scalp, skull, meninges, or brain tissue, including the dura, exposes the cranial contents to the environment, and the risk of infection is high.

Mortality from head trauma has declined with advances in preventive measures, such as seat belts and airbags in automobiles, quicker emergency medical service response and transport times, and improved treatment, including the development of regional trauma centers. Advances in technology have increased the effectiveness of rehabilitative services, even for patients with severe head injuries.

Causes

◆ Falls
◆ Interpersonal altercations
◆ Motor vehicle collisions
◆ Sports-related incidents

Pathophysiology

The brain is shielded by the cranial vault (hair, skin, bone, meninges, and cerebrospinal fluid [CSF]), which intercepts the force of a physical blow. Below a certain level of force (the absorption capacity), the cranial vault prevents energy from affecting the brain. The degree of traumatic head injury is proportional to the amount of force reaching the cranial tissues. (See *Understanding types of head trauma,* pages 282 to 285.) Furthermore, unless ruled out, neck injuries should be presumed present in patients with traumatic head injury.

Closed trauma is typically a sudden acceleration deceleration event, resulting in a coup-contrecoup injury. In an acceleration-deceleration event, the head hits a relatively stationary object, injuring cranial tissues near the point of impact (coup); then the remaining force pushes the brain against the opposite side of the skull, causing a second impact and injury (contre-coup). Contusions and lacerations may also occur as the brain's soft tissues slide over the rough bone of the cranial cavity. In addition, the cerebrum may endure rotational shear, damaging the upper midbrain and areas of the frontal, temporal, and occipital lobes.

Open trauma may penetrate the skull, meninges, or brain. Such trauma is usually associated with skull fractures, and bone fragments commonly cause hematomas and meningeal tears with consequent loss of CSF.

Signs and symptoms

Types of head trauma include concussion, contusion, epidural hematoma, subdural hematoma, intracerebral hematoma, and skull fractures. Each is associated with specific signs and symptoms. (See *Understanding types of head trauma,* pages 282 to 285.)

Complications
◆ Increased intracranial pressure (ICP)
◆ Infection (open trauma)
◆ Respiratory depression and failure
◆ Permanent neurologic deficits
◆ Brain herniation

Diagnosis
Each type of head trauma is associated with specific diagnostic findings. (See *Understanding types of head trauma,* pages 282 to 285.)

Treatment
Surgical
◆ Evacuation of the hematoma or a craniotomy to elevate or remove fragments that have been driven into the brain, and to extract foreign bodies and necrotic tissue, thereby reducing the risk of infection and further brain damage

Supportive
◆ Close observation to detect changes in neurologic status suggesting further damage or expanding hematoma
◆ Cleaning and debridement of any wounds associated with skull fractures
◆ An osmotic diuretic, such as mannitol, to reduce cerebral edema
◆ An analgesic, such as acetaminophen or morphine (for severe headache), to relieve headache
◆ An anticonvulsant, such as phenytoin or lorazepam, to prevent and treat seizures
◆ Respiratory support, including endotracheal intubation and mechanical ventilation, as indicated, for airway protection and respiratory failure
◆ Possibly a prophylactic antibiotic to prevent the onset of meningitis from CSF leakage associated with skull fractures

Special considerations
◆ Obtain a thorough history of the injury from the patient (if he isn't suffering from amnesia), family members, eyewitnesses, or emergency medical services personnel. Ask whether the patient lost consciousness.
◆ Monitor vital signs and check for additional injuries, especially facial fractures. Palpate the skull for tenderness or hematomas.
◆ If the patient has an altered level of consciousness (LOC) or if a neurologic examination reveals abnormalities, observe the patient in the emergency department. Check vital signs, LOC, and pupil size regularly. The patient whose neurologic status has rapidly stabilized after a period of observation can be discharged (with a head injury instruction sheet) in the care of a responsible adult.

◆ After the patient's condition has been stabilized, clean and dress any superficial scalp wounds. (If the skin has been broken, tetanus prophylaxis may be in order.) Assist with suturing if necessary.
◆ If it's determined that the patient can be discharged, instruct the patient and caregiver to be alert for worsening of headache, vomiting, and signs of an ear bleed or CSF leak. Be sure to also include instructions for waking the patient every few hours during the night for observation of mental state and administration of medication.
◆ Teach the patient and his family ways to prevent future episodes of head trauma. (See *Preventing head trauma,* page 286.)
For the patient with more serious head injuries, such as a cerebral contusion or skull fracture:
◆ Establish and maintain a patent airway; nasal airways are contraindicated in patients who may have a basilar skull fracture. Intubation may be necessary. Suction the patient through the mouth, not the nose, to prevent introducing bacteria if a CSF leak is present.
◆ Assist with diagnostic tests, including a complete neurologic examination, a computed tomography scan, and other studies.
◆ Look for CSF draining from the patient's ears, nose, or mouth. Check pillowcases and linens for CSF leaks, and look for a halo sign. If the patient's nose is draining CSF, wipe it — don't let him blow it. If his ear is draining, cover it lightly with sterile gauze — don't pack it.
◆ If spinal injury is ruled out, position the patient with a head injury so that secretions can drain. Elevate the head of the bed 30 degrees if intracerebral injury is suspected.
◆ Institute seizure precautions, as indicated. Agitated behavior may be due to hypoxia or increased ICP, so check for these signs and symptoms. Speak in a calm, reassuring voice, and touch the patient gently. Don't make any sudden, unexpected moves.
◆ Use caution when giving the patient an opioid or a sedative because either drug can depress respirations, increase the carbon dioxide level, lead to increased ICP, and mask changes in neurologic status, especially LOC.
◆ Hypoxia and hypotension, even for brief periods, are associated with a poor outcome in patients with head trauma. Intervene to avoid or aggressively treat these conditions.
◆ Type and crossmatch blood for a patient suspected of having an intracerebral hemorrhage. Such a patient may need a blood transfusion and, possibly, a craniotomy to control bleeding and to aspirate blood.

(Text continues on page 284.)

Understanding types of head trauma

This chart summarizes the signs and symptoms and diagnostic test findings for the different types of head trauma.

Type	Description
Concussion (closed head injury)	◆ A blow to the head hard enough to make the brain hit or twist within the skull but not hard enough to cause a cerebral contusion; causes temporary neural dysfunction by disrupting the reticular activating system (RAS). ◆ Recovery is usually complete within 24 to 48 hours. ◆ Repeated injuries exact a cumulative toll on the brain.
Contusion (bruising of brain tissue; more serious than concussion)	◆ Coup-contrecoup injuries caused by acceleration-deceleration events disrupt normal nerve functions in bruised area. ◆ Injury is directly beneath the site of impact when the brain rebounds against the skull from the force of a blow (a beating with a blunt instrument, for example), when the force of the blow drives the brain against the opposite side of the skull, or when the head is hurled forward and stopped abruptly (as in an automobile accident when a driver's head strikes the windshield). ◆ The brain may strike bony prominences inside the skull (especially the sphenoidal ridges), causing intracranial hemorrhage or hematoma.
Epidural hematoma	◆ Most common in people ages 20 to 40. ◆ Most result from arterial bleeding. ◆ Blood commonly accumulates between skull and dura. Injury to middle meningeal artery in parietotemporal area is most common and is commonly accompanied by linear skull fractures in temporal region over middle meningeal artery. ◆ Less commonly arises from dural venous sinuses.

Signs and symptoms	Diagnostic test findings
◆ Short-term loss of consciousness (less than 6 hours, in many patients only minutes) secondary to disruption of RAS, possibly due to abrupt pressure changes in the areas responsible for consciousness, changes in polarity of the neurons, ischemia, or structural distortion of neurons ◆ Vomiting from localized injury and compression ◆ Anterograde and retrograde amnesia (patient can't recall events immediately after the injury or events that led up to the traumatic incident) correlating with severity of injury; all related to disruption of RAS ◆ Irritability or lethargy from localized injury and compression ◆ Behavior out of character due to focal injury ◆ Complaints of dizziness, nausea, or severe headache due to focal injury and compression	◆ Computed tomography (CT) scan reveals no sign of fracture, bleeding, or other nervous system lesion.
◆ Severe scalp wounds from direct injury ◆ Labored respiration and loss of consciousness secondary to increased pressure from bruising ◆ Drowsiness, confusion, disorientation, agitation, or violent behaviors from increased intracranial pressure (ICP) associated with trauma ◆ Hemiparesis related to interrupted blood flow to the site of injury ◆ Decorticate or decerebrate posturing from cortical damage or hemispheric dysfunction ◆ Unequal pupillary response from brain stem involvement	◆ CT scan shows changes in tissue density, possible displacement of the surrounding structures, and evidence of ischemic tissue, hematomas, and fractures. ◆ EEG recordings directly over area of contusion reveal progressive abnormalities by appearance of high-amplitude theta and delta waves.
◆ Brief period of unconsciousness after injury reflecting the concussive effects of head trauma, followed by a lucid interval varying from 10 to 15 minutes to hours or, rarely, days ◆ Severe headache ◆ Progressive loss of consciousness and deterioration in neurologic signs resulting from expanding lesion and extrusion of medial portion of temporal lobe through tentorial opening ◆ Compression of brain stem by temporal lobe causing clinical manifestations of intracranial hypertension ◆ Deterioration in level of consciousness resulting from compression of brain stem reticular formation as temporal lobe herniates on its upper portion ◆ Respirations, initially deep and labored, becoming shallow and irregular as brain stem is impacted ◆ Contralateral motor deficits reflecting compression of corticospinal tracts that pass through the brain stem ◆ Ipsilateral (same-side) pupillary dilation due to compression of third cranial nerve ◆ Seizures possible from high ICP ◆ Continued bleeding leading to progressive neurologic deterioration, evidenced by bilateral pupillary dilation, bilateral decerebrate posturing, increased systemic blood pressure, decreased pulse, and profound coma with irregular respiratory patterns	◆ CT scan or magnetic resonance imaging (MRI) identifies abnormal masses or structural shifts within the cranium.

(continued)

Understanding types of head trauma *(continued)*

Type	Description
Subdural hematoma	◆ Results from accumulation of blood in subdural space (between dura mater and arachnoid mater) ◆ May be acute, subacute, or chronic: unilateral or bilateral. ◆ Usually associated with torn bridging veins that connect the cerebrum to the dura. ◆ May also result from cerebral or venous sinus tears. ◆ Acute hematomas are a surgical emergency.
Intracerebral hematoma	◆ Shear forces from brain movement commonly cause vessel laceration and hemorrhage into the parenchyma. ◆ Traumatic or spontaneous disruption of cerebral vessels in brain parenchyma cause neurologic deficits, depending on site and amount of bleeding. ◆ Frontal and temporal lobes are common sites. Trauma is commonly associated with intracerebral hematomas; this condition may also be the result of hypertension.
Skull fractures	◆ There are four types of skull fractures: linear, comminuted, depressed, and basilar. ◆ Blow to the head causes one or more of the types. May not be problematic unless brain is exposed or bone fragments are driven into neural tissue. ◆ Fractures of anterior or middle fossae are associated with severe head trauma and are more common than those of posterior fossa.

HUNTINGTON'S DISEASE

Also called *Huntington's chorea, hereditary chorea, chronic progressive chorea,* and *adult chorea,* Huntington's disease is a hereditary disorder in which degeneration of the cerebral cortex and basal ganglia causes chronic progressive chorea (involuntary and irregular movements) and cognitive deterioration, ending in dementia.

Huntington's disease usually strikes people between ages 35 and 55, affecting men and women equally. However, 2% of cases occur in children, and 5% occur as late as age 60. Death usually results 10 to 15 years after onset from suicide, heart failure, or pneumonia.

Causes

The actual cause of this disorder is unknown. However, it's transmitted as an autosomal dom-

inant trait, which either sex can transmit and inherit. Each child of an affected parent has a 50% chance of inheriting it; the child who doesn't inherit it can't transmit it. Huntington's disease is prevalent in areas where affected families have lived for several generations because of hereditary transmission and delayed expression. Genetic testing is now available to families with a known history of the disease.

Pathophysiology

Huntington's disease involves a disturbance in neurotransmitter substances, primarily gamma-aminobutyric acid (GABA) and dopamine. In the basal ganglia, frontal cortex, and cerebellum, GABA neurons are destroyed and replaced by glial cells. The consequent deficiency of GABA

Signs and symptoms	Diagnostic test findings
◆ Similar to epidural hematoma but significantly slower in onset because bleeding is typically of venous origin ◆ However, prognosis worse than epidural hematoma due to direct blood-brain contact	◆ CT scan or MRI reveals mass, tissue shifting, and altered blood flow in the area, confirming hematoma.
◆ Unresponsive immediately or may experience a lucid period before lapsing into a coma from increasing ICP, neuronal disruption, and mass effect of hemorrhage ◆ Possible motor deficits and decorticate or decerebrate responses from compression of corticospinal tracts and brain stem	◆ CT scan or MRI identifes bleeding site.
◆ Possibly asymptomatic, depending on underlying brain trauma ◆ Discontinuity and displacement of bone structure occurring with severe fracture ◆ Motor sensory and cranial nerve dysfunction occurring with associated facial fractures ◆ Persons with anterior fossa basilar skull fractures may have periorbital ecchymosis (raccoon eyes), anosmia (loss of smell due to first cranial nerve involvement) and pupil abnormalities (second and third cranial nerve involvement) ◆ CSF rhinorrhea (leakage through nose), CSF otorrhea (leakage from the ear), hemotympanium (blood accumulation behind the tympanic membrane), ecchymosis over the mastoid bone (battle sign) or orbits (raccoon eyes), and facial paralysis (seventh cranial nerve injury) accompany middle fossa basilar skull fractures ◆ Signs of medullary dysfunction, such as cardiovascular and respiratory failure, accompany posterior fossa basilar skull fracture	◆ CT scan reveals fracture type, location, and underlying brain injuries.

(an inhibitory neurotransmitter) results in a relative excess of dopamine and abnormal neurotransmission along the affected pathways.

Signs and symptoms
The onset of this disease is insidious. The patient eventually becomes totally dependent — emotionally and physically — through loss of musculoskeletal control.

Neurologic
◆ Progressively severe choreic movements that are rapid, typically violent, and purposeless and caused by the relative excess of dopamine
◆ Choreic movements initially unilateral and more prominent in the face and arms than in the legs, progressing from mild fidgeting to gri-

macing, tongue smacking, dysarthria (indistinct speech), emotion-related athetoid (slow, twisting, snakelike) movements (especially of the hands) from injury to the basal ganglion, and torticollis due to shortening of neck muscles
◆ Bradykinesia (slow movement), commonly accompanied by rigidity
◆ Impairment of both voluntary and involuntary movement due to the combination of chorea, bradykinesia, and normal muscle strength
◆ Dysphagia (difficulty swallowing), occurring in most patients in the advanced stages because of impaired reflexes
◆ Dysarthria, which may be complicated by perseveration (persistent repetition of a reply), oral apraxia (difficulty coordinating movement of

Preventing head trauma

When you give the patient and his family their discharge instructions, teach them how they can help prevent future incidents of head trauma. Talk to them about wearing appropriate head protection for sports, such as protective helmets for bicycle riding, football, baseball, skate boarding, and skiing. Explain the importance of making sure children follow playground safety rules, and remind them to use seatbelts and childsafety seats. You can refer them to local and state trauma prevention agencies and appropriate Internet sites for further information.

the mouth), and aprosody (inability to accurately reproduce or interpret the tone of language)

Cognitive

◆ Dementia, an early indication of the disease, from dysfunction of the subcortex without significant impairment of immediate memory
◆ Problems with recent memory due to retrieval rather than encoding problems
◆ Deficits of executive function (planning, organizing, regulating, and programming) from frontal lobe involvement
◆ Impaired impulse control

Psychiatric

These signs and symptoms commonly occur before movement problems:
◆ depression and possible mania (earliest symptom) related to altered levels of dopamine and GABA
◆ personality changes, including irritability, lability, impulsiveness, and aggressive behavior

Complications

◆ Choking
◆ Aspiration
◆ Pneumonia
◆ Heart failure
◆ Infections

Diagnosis

◆ Genetic testing reveals autosomal dominant trait.
◆ Positron emission tomography confirms the disorder.
◆ Computed tomography scan and magnetic resonance imaging show brain atrophy in

caudate nuclei and putamen and ventricular enlargement.

Treatment

No known cure exists for Huntington's disease. Treatment is symptom based, supportive, and protective. It may include:
◆ dopamine blockers, such phenothiazine or haloperidol, to modify choreic movements and control behavioral manifestations
◆ drugs such as reserpine to control choreic movements and reduce abnormal behavior (used with varying success)
◆ tetrabenazine, amantadine, and related drugs to control chorea
◆ coenzyme Q10 to possibly minimally decrease progression of the disease
◆ psychotherapy to decrease anxiety and stress and manage psychiatric symptoms
◆ institutionalization to manage progressive mental deterioration and self-care deficits.

Special considerations

Patient comfort and support are the primary considerations.
◆ Provide physical support by attending to the patient's basic needs, such as hygiene, skin care, bowel and bladder care, and nutrition. Increase this support as mental and physical deterioration make the patient increasingly immobile.
◆ Offer emotional support to the patient and his family. Teach them about the disease, and listen to their concerns and special problems. Keep in mind the patient's dysarthria, and allow him extra time to express himself, thereby decreasing frustration. Teach the family to participate in the patient's care.
◆ Stay alert for possible suicide attempts. Control the patient's environment to protect him from suicide or other self-inflicted injury. Pad the side rails of the bed but avoid restraints, which may cause the patient to injure himself with violent, uncontrolled movements.
◆ If the patient has difficulty walking, provide a walker to help him maintain his balance.
◆ Encourage affected families to receive genetic counseling. All affected family members should realize that each of their offspring has a 50% chance of inheriting this disease.
◆ Refer people at risk who desire genetic testing to centers specializing in care of patients with Huntington's disease, where psychosocial support is available.
◆ Refer the patient and family to appropriate community organizations.
◆ For more information about this degenerative disease, refer the patient and family to the Huntington's Disease Society of America.

HYDROCEPHALUS

An excessive accumulation of cerebrospinal fluid (CSF) within the ventricular spaces of the brain, hydrocephalus is common in neonates. It can also occur in adults as a result of injury or disease. In infants, hydrocephalus enlarges the head and, in both infants and adults, the resulting compression can damage brain tissue.

With early detection and surgical intervention, the prognosis improves but remains guarded. Even after surgery, complications may persist, such as developmental delay, impaired motor function, and vision loss. Without surgery, the prognosis is poor. Mortality may result from increased intracranial pressure (ICP) in people of all ages; infants may die of infection and malnutrition.

Causes

Hydrocephalus may result from:
◆ faulty absorption of CSF (communicating hydrocephalus
◆ obstruction in CSF flow (noncommunicating hydrocephalus).

Risk factors associated with the development of hydrocephalus in infants may include:
◆ intracranial hemorrhage from birth trauma or prematurity
◆ intrauterine infection.

In older children and adults, risk factors may include:
◆ brain tumors or intracranial hemorrhage
◆ chronic otitis media
◆ mastoiditis
◆ meningitis
◆ traumatic brain injury.

Pathophysiology

In *noncommunicating hydrocephalus,* the obstruction typically occurs between the third and fourth ventricles, at the aqueduct of Sylvius, but it can also occur at the outlets of the fourth ventricle (foramina of Luschka and Magendie) or, rarely, at the foramen of Monro. This obstruction may result from faulty fetal development, infection (syphilis, granulomatous diseases, meningitis), a tumor, a cerebral aneurysm, or a blood clot (after intracranial hemorrhage).

In *communicating hydrocephalus,* faulty absorption of CSF may result from surgery to repair a myelomeningocele, adhesions between meninges at the base of the brain, or meningeal hemorrhage. Rarely, a tumor in the choroid plexus causes overproduction of CSF and consequent hydrocephalus.

In either type, both CSF pressure and volume increase. Obstruction in the ventricles causes dilation, stretching, and disruption of the lining.

Underlying white matter atrophies. Compression of brain tissue and cerebral blood vessels leads to ischemia and, eventually, cell death.

Signs and symptoms
In infants

◆ Enlargement of the head clearly disproportionate to the infant's growth (most characteristic sign) from the increased CSF volume
◆ Distended scalp veins from increased CSF pressure
◆ Thin, shiny, fragile-looking scalp skin from the increase in CSF pressure
◆ Underdeveloped neck muscles from increased weight of the head
◆ Depressed orbital roof with downward displacement of the eyes and prominent sclerae from increased pressure
◆ High-pitched, shrill cry, irritability, and abnormal muscle tone in the legs from neurologic compression
◆ Projectile vomiting from increased ICP
◆ Skull widening to accommodate increased pressure

In adults and older children

◆ Drowsiness, lethargy, irritability, or loss of consciousness from increasing ICP
◆ Ataxia from compression of the motor areas
◆ Incontinence
◆ Impaired intellect

Complications

◆ Mental retardation
◆ Impaired motor function
◆ Vision loss
◆ Brain herniation
◆ Infection
◆ Malnutrition
◆ Shunt infection (after surgery)
◆ Septicemia (after shunt insertion)
◆ Paralytic ileus, adhesions, peritonitis, and intestinal perforation (after shunt insertion)
◆ Death from increased ICP

Diagnosis

◆ Computed tomography scan and magnetic resonance imaging reveal variations in tissue density and fluid in the ventricular system.
◆ Lumbar puncture reveals increased fluid pressure from communicating hydrocephalus.
◆ Ventriculography shows ventricular dilation with excess fluid.

AGE ALERT *In infants, abnormally large head size for the patient's age strongly suggests hydrocephalus. Measurement of the head circumference is the most important diagnostic technique.*

Treatment

The only treatment for hydrocephalus is surgical correction, by insertion of:

◆ ventriculoperitoneal shunt, which transports excess fluid from the lateral ventricle into the peritoneal cavity

◆ ventriculoatrial shunt (less common), which drains fluid from the brain's lateral ventricle into the right atrium of the heart, where the fluid makes its way into the venous circulation.

Temporary hydrocephalus from head trauma or intracranial bleeding can be treated with an external ventricular drain or a lumbar drain.

Supportive care is also warranted.

Special considerations

On initial assessment, obtain a complete history from the patient or the family. Note general behavior, especially irritability, apathy, or decreased LOC. Perform a neurologic assessment. Examine the eyes; pupils should be equal and reactive to light. In adults and older children, evaluate movements and motor strength in the extremities. Watch especially for ataxia, confusion, and incontinence. Ask the patient if he has headaches, and watch for projectile vomiting; both signal increased ICP. Also watch for seizures. Note changes in vital signs.

Before surgery (shunt insertion)

◆ Encourage maternal-infant bonding when possible. When caring for the infant yourself, hold him on your lap for feeding; stroke and cuddle him, and speak soothingly.

◆ Check fontanels for tension or fullness, and measure and record head circumference. On the patient's chart, draw a picture showing where to measure the head so that other staff members measure it in the same place, or mark the forehead with ink.

◆ To prevent postfeeding aspiration and hypostatic pneumonia, place the infant on his side and reposition every 2 hours, or prop him up in an infant seat.

◆ To prevent skin breakdown, make sure that his earlobe is flat, and place a sheepskin or rubber foam under his head.

◆ When turning the infant, move his head, neck, and shoulders with his body to reduce strain on his neck.

◆ Feed the infant slowly. To lessen strain from the weight of the infant's head on your arm while holding him during feeding, place his head, neck, and shoulders on a pillow.

After surgery

◆ Place the infant on the side opposite the operative site with his head level with his body, unless the physician's orders specify otherwise.

◆ Check temperature, pulse rate, blood pressure, and LOC. Also check fontanels for fullness daily. Watch for vomiting, which may be an early sign of increased ICP and shunt malfunction.

◆ Watch for signs and symptoms of infection, especially meningitis (fever, stiff neck, irritability, tense fontanels). Also watch for redness, swelling, or other signs of local infection over the shunt tract. Check dressing often for drainage.

◆ Listen for bowel sounds after ventriculoperitoneal shunt.

◆ Check the infant's growth and development periodically, and help the parents set goals consistent with the child's ability and potential. Help the parents focus on their child's strengths, not his weaknesses. Discuss special education programs, and emphasize the infant's need for sensory stimulation appropriate for his age. Teach parents to watch for signs of shunt malfunction, infection, and paralytic ileus. Tell them that surgery for lengthening the shunt will be required periodically as the child grows older. Surgery may also be required to correct shunt malfunctioning or to treat infection. Emphasize that hydrocephalus is a lifelong problem and that the child will require regular, continuing evaluation.

||| **LIFE-THREATENING DISORDER**

INTRACRANIAL ANEURYSM

An intracranial aneurysm is a weakness in the wall of an intracranial artery that causes localized dilation. Its most common form is the berry aneurysm, a saclike outpouching in a cerebral artery. Intracranial aneurysms usually arise at an arterial junction in the Circle of Willis, the circular anastomosis forming the major cerebral arteries at the base of the brain. (See *Most common sites of intracranial aneurysm.*) Intracranial aneurysms may rupture and cause subarachnoid hemorrhage.

The incidence is slightly higher in women than in men, especially those in their late 40s or early to mid-50s, but an intracranial aneurysm may occur at any age in either sex. The prognosis is guarded. About one-half of all patients who suffer a subarachnoid hemorrhage die immediately. Of those who survive untreated, 40% die of the effects of hemorrhage and another 20% die later of recurring hemorrhage. New treatments are improving the prognosis.

Most common sites of intracranial aneurysm

Intracranial aneurysms usually arise at the arterial bifurcation in the Circle of Willis and its branches. This illustration shows the most common sites around this circle.

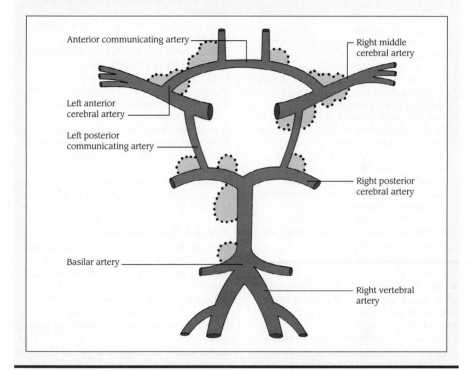

Causes
◆ Combination of congenital defect and degenerative process
◆ Congenital defect (most common)
◆ Degenerative process
◆ Trauma

Pathophysiology
Blood flow exerts pressure against a congenitally weak arterial wall, stretching it like an overblown balloon and making it likely to rupture. Such a rupture is followed by a subarachnoid hemorrhage, in which blood spills into the space normally occupied by cerebrospinal fluid. Sometimes, blood also spills into brain tissue, where a large clot can cause potentially fatal increased intracranial pressure (ICP) and brain tissue damage.

Signs and symptoms
Occasionally, the patient may exhibit premonitory symptoms resulting from oozing of blood into the subarachnoid space. These symptoms include:

◆ headache
◆ intermittent nausea
◆ nuchal rigidity
◆ stiff back and legs.
    Usually, however, the rupture occurs abruptly and without warning, causing:
◆ sudden severe headache caused by profound meningeal irritation
◆ nausea and projectile vomiting related to increased pressure
◆ altered level of consciousness (LOC), including deep coma, depending on the severity and location of bleeding, from increased pressure caused by increased cerebral blood volume
◆ meningeal irritation, resulting in nuchal rigidity, back and leg pain, fever, restlessness, irritability, occasional seizures, photophobia, and blurred vision, secondary to bleeding into the subarachnoid space
◆ hemiparesis, hemisensory defects, dysphagia, and visual defects from bleeding into the brain tissues

Determining severity of an intracranial aneurysm rupture

The severity of symptoms varies from patient to patient, depending on the site and amount of bleeding. Five grades characterize a ruptured cerebral aneurysm:

♦ Grade I (minimal bleeding) — The patient is alert with no neurologic deficit; he may have a slight headache and nuchal rigidity.

♦ Grade II (mild bleeding) — The patient is alert with a mild to severe headache and nuchal rigidity; he may have third-nerve palsy.

♦ Grade III (moderate bleeding) — The patient is confused or drowsy with nuchal rigidity and, possibly, a mild focal deficit.

♦ Grade IV (severe bleeding) — The patient is stuporous with nuchal rigidity and, possibly, mild to severe hemiparesis.

♦ Grade V (moribund; usually fatal) — If the rupture is nonfatal, the patient is in a deep coma or decerebrate.

♦ diplopia, ptosis, dilated pupil, and inability to rotate the eye caused by compression of the oculomotor nerve if the aneurysm is near the internal carotid artery.

Typically, the severity of a ruptured intracranial aneurysm is graded according to the patient's signs and symptoms. (See *Determining severity of an intracranial aneurysm rupture*.)

Complications
♦ Death from increased ICP and brain herniation
♦ Rebleeding
♦ Vasospasm

Diagnosis
♦ Cerebral angiography, computed tomography (CT), angiography, and magnetic resonance angiography reveal altered cerebral blood flow, vessel lumen dilation, and differences in arterial filling.
♦ CT scan reveals subarachnoid or ventricular bleeding with blood in subarachnoid space and displaced midline structures.
♦ Magnetic resonance imaging shows a cerebral blood flow void.

Treatment
Treatment to reduce the risk of rupture if it hasn't occurred may include:

♦ bed rest in a quiet, darkened room with minimal stimulation
♦ avoidance of coffee and other stimulants to reduce the risk of blood pressure elevation
♦ codeine or another analgesic, as needed, to maintain rest and minimize risk of pressure changes
♦ an antihypertensive agent if the patient is hypertensive
♦ phenobarbital or another sedative to prevent agitation leading to hypertension.

Other treatment may include:
♦ early surgical repair or interventional radiologic repair by clipping, ligation, coiling, or wrapping (before or after rupture)
♦ a calcium channel blocker, such as nimodipine, to decrease spasm and subsequent rebleeding
♦ a corticosteroid to manage headache and reduce edema
♦ phenytoin or another anticonvulsant to prevent seizures secondary to pressure and tissue irritation from bleeding.

Special considerations
An accurate neurologic assessment, good patient care, patient and family teaching, and psychological support can speed recovery and reduce complications.

♦ During initial treatment after hemorrhage, establish and maintain a patent airway. Position the patient to promote pulmonary drainage and prevent upper airway obstruction. If he's intubated, administering 100% oxygen before suctioning to remove secretions will prevent hypoxia and vasodilation from carbon dioxide accumulation. Suction no longer than 20 seconds to avoid increased ICP. Give frequent nose and mouth care.

♦ Until the aneurysm can be repaired, implement aneurysm precautions to minimize the risk of rebleed and to avoid increased ICP. Such precautions include bed rest in a quiet, darkened room and avoidance of strenuous physical activity and straining with bowel movements. Be sure to explain why these restrictive measures are necessary.

Preventive measures and good patient care can minimize other complications:
♦ Turn the patient often. Encourage occasional deep breathing and leg movement. Assist with active range-of-motion (ROM) exercises; if the patient is paralyzed, perform regular passive ROM exercises.

♦ Monitor arterial blood gases, LOC, and vital signs often, and measure intake and output. Avoid taking the patient's temperature rectally because vagus nerve stimulation may cause cardiac arrest.

◆ Watch for danger signs, such as decreased LOC, unilateral enlarged pupil, onset or worsening of hemiparesis or motor deficit, increased blood pressure, slowed pulse, worsening of headache or sudden onset of a headache, renewed or worsened nuchal rigidity, and renewed or persistent vomiting, which may indicate an enlarging aneurysm, rebleeding, intracranial clot, vasospasm, or other complications. Intermittent signs such as restlessness, extremity weakness, and speech alterations can also indicate increasing ICP or vasospasm.

◆ Give fluids, as ordered, and monitor I.V. infusions to avoid increased ICP.

◆ If the patient has facial weakness, assess the gag reflex and assist him during meals, placing food in the unaffected side of his mouth. If he can't swallow, insert a nasogastric tube, as ordered, and give all tube feedings slowly. Prevent skin breakdown by taping the tube so it doesn't press against the nostril. If the patient can eat, provide a high-fiber diet to prevent straining at stool, which can increase ICP. Get an order for a stool softener, such as dioctyl sodium sulfosuccinate, or a mild laxative, and administer as ordered. Implement a bowel-retraining program based on previous habits. If the patient is receiving a steroid, check the stool for blood.

◆ With oculomotor (III) or facial (VII) cranial nerve palsy, administer artificial tears or ointment to the affected eye and tape the eye shut during sleeping hours to prevent corneal damage.

◆ To minimize stress, encourage relaxation techniques. If possible, avoid using restraints because they can cause agitation and raise ICP.

◆ Administer an antihypertensive, as ordered. Carefully monitor blood pressure and immediately report any significant change, but especially a rise in systolic pressure.

◆ If the patient can't speak, establish a simple means of communication or use cards or a notepad. Try to limit conversation to topics that won't frustrate the patient. Encourage his family to speak to him in a normal tone, even if he doesn't seem to respond.

◆ Provide emotional support, and include the patient's family in his care as much as possible. Encourage family members to adopt a realistic attitude, but don't discourage hope.

◆ Before discharge, make a referral to a visiting nurse or a rehabilitation center when necessary, and teach the patient and his family how to recognize signs of rebleeding.

MENINGITIS

In meningitis, the brain and the spinal cord meninges become inflamed, usually as a result of bacterial or viral infection. Such inflammation may involve all three meningeal membranes — the dura mater, arachnoid, and pia mater.

If the disease is recognized early and the infecting organism responds to treatment, the prognosis is good and complications are rare. However, mortality in untreated meningitis is 70% to 100%. The prognosis is poorer for infants and elderly patients.

Causes

Meningitis is almost always a complication of bacteremia, especially from:

◆ empyema
◆ endocarditis
◆ osteomyelitis
◆ pneumonia.

Other infections associated with the development of meningitis include:

◆ brain abscess, usually caused by *Neisseria meningitidis, Haemophilus influenzae, Streptococcus pneumoniae,* or *Escherichia coli*
◆ encephalitis
◆ myelitis
◆ otitis media
◆ sinusitis.

Meningitis may follow trauma or invasive procedures, including:

◆ craniotomy
◆ lumbar puncture
◆ penetrating head wound
◆ skull fracture
◆ ventricular shunting.

Aseptic meningitis may result from a virus or other organism. Sometimes no causative organism can be found.

Pathophysiology

Meningitis commonly begins as an inflammation of the pia-arachnoid, which may progress to congestion of adjacent tissues and destroy some nerve cells. (See *Meningeal inflammation in meningitis,* page 292.)

The microorganism typically enters the central nervous system (CNS) by one of four routes:

◆ the blood (most common)
◆ a direct opening between the cerebrospinal fluid (CSF) and the environment as a result of trauma or surgery
◆ along the cranial and peripheral nerves
◆ through the mouth or nose.

Microorganisms can be transmitted to an infant via the intrauterine environment.

The invading organism triggers an inflammatory response in the meninges. In an attempt to ward off the invasion, neutrophils gather in the area and produce an exudate in the subarachnoid space, causing the CSF to thicken. The thickened CSF flows less readily around the

CLOSER LOOK
Meningeal inflammation in meningitis

The illustration below shows normal meninges and how the meninges become inflamed in meningitis.

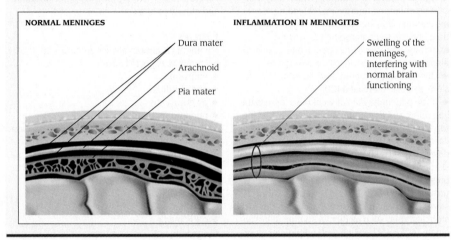

NORMAL MENINGES

Dura mater

Arachnoid

Pia mater

INFLAMMATION IN MENINGITIS

Swelling of the meninges, interfering with normal brain functioning

---

brain and spinal cord, and it can block the arachnoid villi, obstructing absorption of CSF and causing hydrocephalus.

The exudate also:
◆ exacerbates the inflammatory response, increasing the pressure in the brain
◆ can extend to the cranial and peripheral nerves, triggering additional inflammation
◆ irritates the meninges, disrupting their cell membranes and causing edema.

The consequences are elevated intracranial pressure (ICP), engorged blood vessels, disrupted cerebral blood supply, possible thrombosis or rupture and, if ICP isn't reduced, cerebral infarction. Encephalitis may also ensue as a secondary infection of the brain tissue.

In aseptic viral meningitis, lymphocytes infiltrate the pia-arachnoid layers, but usually not as severely as in bacterial meningitis, and no exudate is formed. Thus, this type of meningitis is self-limiting.

Signs and symptoms

Signs and symptoms of meningitis typically include:
◆ fever, chills, and malaise resulting from infection and inflammation
◆ headache, vomiting and, rarely, papilledema (inflammation and edema of the optic nerve) from increased ICP.

Signs of meningeal irritation include:
◆ nuchal rigidity

◆ positive Brudzinski's and Kernig's signs
◆ exaggerated and symmetrical deep tendon reflexes
◆ opisthotonos (a spasm in which the back and extremities arch backward so that the body rests on the head and heels).

Other features of meningitis may include:
◆ sinus arrhythmias from irritation of the nerves of the autonomic nervous system
◆ irritability from increasing ICP
◆ photophobia, diplopia, and other vision problems from cranial nerve irritation
◆ delirium, deep stupor, and coma from increased ICP and cerebral edema.

AGE ALERT *An infant with meningitis may show signs of infection, but most are simply fretful and refuse to eat. In an infant, vomiting can lead to dehydration, which prevents formation of a bulging fontanel, an important sign of increased ICP.*

As the illness progresses, twitching, seizures (in 30% of infants), or coma may develop. Most older children have the same symptoms as adults. In subacute meningitis, onset may be insidious.

Complications
◆ Increased ICP
◆ Hydrocephalus
◆ Cerebral infarction
◆ Cranial nerve deficits including optic neuritis and deafness
◆ Encephalitis

◆ Paresis or paralysis
◆ Endocarditis
◆ Brain abscess
◆ Syndrome of inappropriate antidiuretic hormone
◆ Seizures
◆ Shock
◆ Coma
◆ Death

In children
◆ Mental retardation
◆ Epilepsy
◆ Unilateral or bilateral sensory hearing loss
◆ Subdural effusions

Diagnosis
◆ Lumbar puncture shows elevated CSF pressure (from obstructed CSF outflow at the arachnoid villi), cloudy or milky-white CSF, high protein level, positive Gram stain and culture (unless a virus is responsible), and decreased glucose concentration.
◆ Positive Brudzinski's and Kernig's signs indicate meningeal irritation.
◆ Cultures of blood, urine, and nose and throat secretions reveal the offending organism.
◆ Chest X-ray may reveal pneumonitis or lung abscess, tubercular lesions, or granulomas secondary to a fungal infection.
◆ Computed tomography scan may identify cranial osteomyelitis or paranasal sinusitis as the underlying infectious process, or skull fracture as the entryway for the microorganism; it may also reveal hydrocephalus and can rule out cerebral hematoma, hemorrhage, or tumor as the underlying cause.
◆ White blood cell count reveals leukocytosis.

Treatment
◆ An appropriate I.V. antibiotic, followed by an oral antibiotic selected by culture and sensitivity testing (usual treatment)
◆ Mannitol to decrease cerebral edema
◆ An anticonvulsant (usually given I.V.) or a sedative to reduce restlessness and prevent or control seizure activity
◆ Acetaminophen and other analgesics to relieve headache and fever

Supportive measures
◆ Bed rest to prevent increases in ICP
◆ Fever reduction to decrease metabolic demands that may increase ICP
◆ Fluid therapy (given cautiously if cerebral edema and increased ICP are present) to prevent dehydration
◆ Appropriate therapy for any coexisting conditions, such as endocarditis or pneumonia

◆ Possibly a prophylactic antibiotic after a ventricular shunting procedure, skull fracture, or penetrating head wound, to prevent infection (use is controversial)
Staff should take droplet precautions (in addition to standard precautions) for meningitis caused by *H. influenzae* and *N. meningitidis,* until 24 hours after the start of effective therapy.

Special considerations
Patients must be watched carefully for changes in neurologic function or other signs of worsening condition.
◆ Assess neurologic function often. Observe level of consciousness (LOC) and signs of increased ICP (plucking at the bedcovers, vomiting, seizures, and a change in motor function and vital signs). Also, watch for signs of cranial nerve involvement (ptosis, strabismus, and diplopia).

⚠ **CLINICAL ALERT** *Be especially alert for a temperature increase up to 102° F (38.9° C), deteriorating LOC, onset of seizures, and altered respirations, all of which may signal an impending crisis.*
◆ Monitor fluid balance. Maintain adequate fluid intake to avoid dehydration, but avoid fluid overload because of the danger of cerebral edema. Measure central venous pressure and intake and output accurately.
◆ Watch for adverse reactions to the I.V. antibiotic and other drugs. To avoid infiltration and phlebitis, check the I.V. site often, and change the site according to facility policy.
◆ Position the patient carefully to prevent joint stiffness and neck pain. Turn him often, according to a planned positioning schedule. Assist with range-of-motion exercises.
◆ Maintain adequate nutrition and elimination. It may be necessary to provide small, frequent meals or to supplement meals with nasogastric tube or parenteral feedings. To prevent constipation and minimize the risk of increased ICP resulting from straining at stool, give the patient a mild laxative or stool softener.
◆ Ensure the patient's comfort. Provide mouth care regularly. Maintain a quiet environment. Darkening the room may decrease photophobia. Relieve headache with acetaminophen or another analgesic, as ordered.
◆ Provide reassurance and support. The patient may be frightened by his illness and frequent lumbar punctures. If he's delirious or confused, attempt to reorient him often. Reassure the family that the delirium and behavior changes caused by meningitis usually disappear. However, if a severe neurologic deficit appears permanent, refer the patient to a rehabilitation program as

soon as the acute phase of this illness has passed.

◆ To help prevent development of meningitis, teach patients with chronic sinusitis or other chronic infections the importance of proper medical treatment. Follow strict sterile technique when treating patients with head wounds or skull fractures.

MULTIPLE SCLEROSIS

Multiple sclerosis (MS) causes demyelination of the white matter of the brain and spinal cord and damage to nerve fibers and their targets. Characterized by exacerbations and remissions, MS is a major cause of chronic disability in young adults. It usually becomes symptomatic between ages 20 and 40. MS affects three women for every two men and five whites for every nonwhite. Incidence is generally higher among urban populations and upper socioeconomic groups. A family history of MS and living in a cold, damp climate increase the risk.

The prognosis varies. MS may progress rapidly, disabling the patient by early adulthood or causing death within months of onset. However, 70% of patients lead active, productive lives with prolonged remissions.

Several types of MS have been identified. Terms to describe MS types include:

◆ *elapsing-remitting* — clear relapses (or acute attacks or exacerbations) with full recovery or partial recovery and lasting disability (The disease doesn't worsen between the attacks.)

◆ *primary progressive* — steady progression from the onset with minor recovery or plateaus (This form is uncommon and may involve different brain and spinal cord damage than other forms.)

◆ *secondary progressive* — begins as a pattern of clear-cut relapses and recovery (This form becomes steadily progressive and worsens between acute attacks.)

◆ *progressive relapsing* — steadily progressive from the onset, but also has clear acute attacks. (This form is rare.)

Causes

The exact cause of MS is unknown, but current theories suggest that a slow-acting or latent viral infection triggers an autoimmune response. Other theories suggest that environmental and genetic factors may also be linked to MS.

Certain conditions appear to precede onset or exacerbation, including:

◆ acute respiratory tract infections
◆ emotional stress
◆ fatigue (physical or emotional)
◆ pregnancy.

Pathophysiology

In MS, sporadic patches of axon demyelination and nerve fiber loss occur throughout the central nervous system, producing widely disseminated and varied neurologic dysfunction. (See *How myelin breaks down*.)

New evidence of nerve fiber loss may provide an explanation for the invisible neurologic deficits experienced by many patients with MS. The axons determine the presence or absence of function; loss of myelin doesn't correlate with loss of function.

Signs and symptoms

Signs and symptoms depend on the extent and site of myelin destruction, the extent of remyelination, and the adequacy of subsequent restored synaptic transmission. Flares may be transient, or they may last for hours or weeks, waxing and waning with no predictable pattern, varying from day to day, and being bizarre and difficult for the patient to describe. Clinical effects may be so mild that the patient is unaware of them or so intense that they're debilitating. Typical first signs and symptoms related to conduction deficits and impaired impulse transmission along the nerve fiber include:

◆ vision problems
◆ sensory impairment, such as burning, pins and needles, and electrical sensations
◆ fatigue.

Other characteristic changes include:

◆ *ocular disturbances* — optic neuritis, diplopia, ophthalmoplegia, blurred vision, and nystagmus from impaired cranial nerve dysfunction and conduction deficits to the optic nerve

◆ *muscle dysfunction* — weakness, paralysis ranging from monoplegia to quadriplegia, spasticity, hyperreflexia, intention tremor, and gait ataxia from impaired motor reflex

◆ *urinary disturbances* — incontinence, frequency, urgency, and frequent infections from impaired transmission involving sphincter innervation

◆ *bowel disturbances* — involuntary evacuation or constipation from altered impulse transmission to internal sphincter

◆ *fatigue* — commonly the most debilitating symptom

◆ *speech problems* — poorly articulated or scanning speech and dysphagia from impaired transmission to the cranial nerves and sensory cortex.

Complications

◆ Injuries from falls
◆ Urinary tract infection
◆ Constipation

How myelin breaks down

Myelin speeds electrical impulses to the brain for interpretation. This lipoprotein complex formed of glial cells or oligodendrocytes protects the neuron's axon much like the insulation on an electrical wire. Its high electrical resistance and low capacitance allow the myelin to conduct nerve impulses from one node of Ranvier to the next.

Myelin is susceptible to injury— for example, by hypoxemia, toxic chemicals, vascular insufficiencies, or autoimmune responses. The sheath becomes inflamed, and the membrane layers break down into smaller components that become well-circumscribed plaques (filled with microglial elements, macroglia, and lymphocytes). This process is called demyelination.

The damaged myelin sheath can't conduct normally. The partial loss or dispersion of the action potential causes neurologic dysfunction.

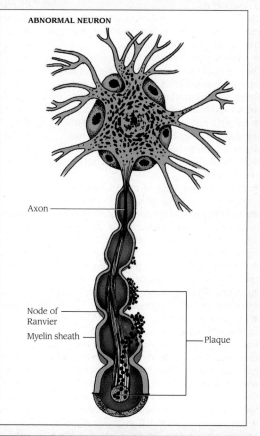

ABNORMAL NEURON

Axon

Node of Ranvier

Myelin sheath

Plaque

◆ Joint contractures
◆ Pressure ulcers
◆ Rectal distention
◆ Pneumonia
◆ Depression

Diagnosis

Because early symptoms may be mild, years may elapse between onset and diagnosis. Diagnosis of MS requires evidence of two or more neurologic attacks. Periodic testing and close observation are necessary, perhaps for years, depending on the course of the disease. Spinal cord compression, foramen magnum tumor (which may mimic the exacerbations and remissions of MS), multiple small strokes, syphilis or another infection, thyroid disease, and chronic fatigue syndrome must be ruled out.

These tests may be useful:
◆ Magnetic resonance imaging reveals multifocal white matter lesions.
◆ EEG reveals abnormalities in brain waves in one-third of patients.
◆ Lumbar puncture shows normal total cerebrospinal fluid (CSF) protein but elevated immunoglobulin (Ig) G (gamma globulin); IgG reflects hyperactivity of the immune system caused by chronic demyelination. An elevated CSF IgG is significant only when serum IgG is normal. CSF white blood cell count may be elevated.
◆ CSF electrophoresis detects bands of IgG in most patients, even when the percentage of IgG in CSF is normal. Presence of kappa light chains provide additional support to the diagnosis.

◆ Evoked potential studies (visual, brain stem, auditory, and somatosensory) reveal slowed conduction of nerve impulses in most patients.

Treatment

The aim of treatment is threefold: Treat the acute exacerbation, treat the disease process, and treat the related signs and symptoms.

◆ I.V. methylprednisolone followed by oral therapy reduces edema of the myelin sheath (speeds recovery from acute attacks). Other drugs, such as azathioprine (Imuran) or methotrexate and cytoxin, may be used.

◆ Immune system therapy consisting of interferon and glatiramer (a combination of four amino acids) reduces frequency and severity of relapses, and may possibly slow central nervous system damage.

◆ Stretching and range-of-motion exercises, coupled with correct positioning, may relieve the spasticity resulting from opposing muscle groups relaxing and contracting at the same time; such exercises help relax muscles and maintain function.

◆ Baclofen and tizanidine may be used to treat spasticity. For severe spasticity, botulinum toxin injections, intrathecal injections, nerve blocks, and surgery may be necessary.

◆ Frequent rest periods, aerobic exercise, and cooling techniques (air conditioning, breezes, water sprays) may minimize fatigue. Fatigue is characterized by an overwhelming feeling of exhaustion that can occur at any time of the day without warning. The cause is unknown. Changes in environmental conditions, such as heat and humidity, can aggravate fatigue.

◆ Amantidine (Symmetrel), pemoline (Cylert), and methylphenidate (Ritalin) have proved beneficial, as have antidepressants to manage fatigue.

◆ Bladder problems (failure to store urine, failure to empty the bladder or, more commonly, both) are managed by such strategies as drinking cranberry juice or inserting an indwelling catheter and suprapubic tubes. Intermittent self-catheterization and postvoid catheterization programs are helpful, as are anticholinergics in some patients.

◆ Bowel problems (constipation and involuntary evacuation) are managed by such measures as increasing fiber intake and using a bulking agent, and bowel-retraining strategies, such as daily suppositories and rectal stimulation.

◆ A low-dose tricyclic antidepressant, phenytoin, or carbamazepine may manage sensory symptoms, such as pain, numbness, burning, and tingling sensations.

◆ Adaptive devices and physical therapy assist with motor dysfunction, such as problems with balance, strength, and muscle coordination.

◆ A beta-adrenergic blocker, a sedative, or a diuretic may be used to alleviate tremors.

◆ Speech therapy may manage dysarthria.

◆ An antihistamine, vision therapy, or exercises may minimize vertigo.

◆ Vision therapy or adaptive lenses may help manage vision problems.

Special considerations

Management considerations focus on educating the patient and family.

◆ Assist with physical therapy. Increase patient comfort with massages and relaxing baths. Make sure the bath water isn't too hot because it may temporarily intensify otherwise subtle symptoms. Assist with active, resistive, and stretching exercises to maintain muscle tone and joint mobility, decrease spasticity, improve coordination, and boost morale.

◆ Educate the patient and his family about the chronic course of MS. Emphasize the need to avoid stress, infections, and fatigue and to maintain independence by developing new ways of performing daily activities. Be sure to tell the patient to avoid exposure to infections.

◆ Stress the importance of eating a nutritious, well-balanced diet that contains sufficient roughage and adequate fluids to prevent constipation.

◆ Evaluate the need for bowel and bladder training during hospitalization. Encourage adequate fluid intake and regular urination. Eventually, the patient may require urinary drainage by self-catheterization or, in men, condom drainage. Teach the correct use of suppositories to help establish a regular bowel schedule.

◆ Watch for adverse reactions to drug therapy. For instance, dantrolene may cause muscle weakness and decreased muscle tone.

◆ Promote emotional stability. Help the patient establish a daily routine to maintain optimal functioning. Activity level is regulated by tolerance level. Encourage regular rest periods to prevent fatigue and daily physical exercise.

◆ Inform the patient that exacerbations are unpredictable, necessitating physical and emotional adjustments in lifestyle.

◆ For more information, refer the patient to the National Multiple Sclerosis Society.

MYASTHENIA GRAVIS

Myasthenia gravis causes sporadic but progressive weakness and abnormal fatigability of striated (skeletal) muscles; symptoms are exacerbated by exercise and repeated movement and relieved by anticholinesterase drugs. Usually, this disorder affects muscles innervated by the cranial nerves (face, lips, tongue, neck, and throat), but it can affect any muscle group.

Myasthenia gravis follows an unpredictable course of periodic exacerbations and remissions. There's no known cure. Drug treatment has improved the prognosis and allows patients to lead relatively normal lives, except during exacerbations. When the disease involves the respiratory system, it may be life-threatening.

Myasthenia gravis affects 3 in 10,000 people at any age but it's more common in young women and older men.

About 20% of infants born to women with myasthenia gravis have transient (or occasionally persistent) myasthenia. This disease may coexist with immune and thyroid disorders; 15% of patients with myasthenia gravis have thymomas. Remissions occur in about 25% of patients.

Causes
The exact cause of myasthenia gravis is unknown. However, it's believed to be the result of:
◆ autoimmune response
◆ inadequate muscle fiber response to acetylcholine
◆ ineffective acetylcholine release.

Pathophysiology
Myasthenia gravis causes a failure in transmission of nerve impulses at the neuromuscular junction. The site of action is the postsynaptic membrane. Theoretically, antireceptor antibodies block, weaken, or reduce the number of acetylcholine receptors available at each neuromuscular junction and thereby impair muscle depolarization necessary for movement. (See *Impaired transmission in myasthenia gravis.*)

Signs and symptoms
Myasthenia gravis may occur gradually or suddenly. Signs and symptoms include:
◆ weak eye closure, ptosis, and diplopia from impaired neuromuscular transmission to the cranial nerves supplying the eye muscles (may be the only symptom present)
◆ skeletal muscle weakness and fatigue, increasing through the day but decreasing with rest (In the early stages, easy fatigability of certain muscles may appear with no other findings. Later, it may be severe enough to cause paralysis.)
◆ progressive muscle weakness and accompanying loss of function depending on muscle group affected; becoming more intense during menses and after emotional stress, prolonged exposure to sunlight or cold, or infections

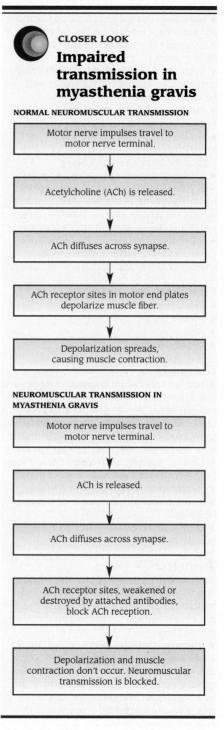

CLOSER LOOK

Impaired transmission in myasthenia gravis

NORMAL NEUROMUSCULAR TRANSMISSION

Motor nerve impulses travel to motor nerve terminal.

↓

Acetylcholine (ACh) is released.

↓

ACh diffuses across synapse.

↓

ACh receptor sites in motor end plates depolarize muscle fiber.

↓

Depolarization spreads, causing muscle contraction.

NEUROMUSCULAR TRANSMISSION IN MYASTHENIA GRAVIS

Motor nerve impulses travel to motor nerve terminal.

↓

ACh is released.

↓

ACh diffuses across synapse.

↓

ACh receptor sites, weakened or destroyed by attached antibodies, block ACh reception.

↓

Depolarization and muscle contraction don't occur. Neuromuscular transmission is blocked.

◆ blank and expressionless facial appearance and nasal vocal tones secondary to impaired transmission of cranial nerves innervating the facial muscles
◆ frequent nasal regurgitation of fluids and difficulty chewing and swallowing from cranial nerve involvement
◆ drooping eyelids from weakness of facial and extraocular muscles
◆ weakened neck muscles with head tilting back to see (Neck muscles may become too weak to support the head without bobbing.)
◆ weakened respiratory muscles, decreased tidal volume and vital capacity from impaired transmission to the diaphragm, making breathing difficult and predisposing the patient to pneumonia and other respiratory tract infections
◆ respiratory muscle weakness (myasthenic crisis) possibly severe enough to require an emergency airway and mechanical ventilation.

Complications
◆ Respiratory distress
◆ Pneumonia
◆ Aspiration
◆ Myasthenic crisis

Diagnosis
◆ Tensilon test confirms diagnosis of myasthenia gravis, revealing temporarily improved muscle function within 30 to 60 seconds after I.V. injection of edrophonium or neostigmine and lasting up to 30 minutes; this test helps in differentiating a myasthenic crisis from a cholinergic crisis.
◆ Electromyography with repeated neural stimulation shows progressive decrease in muscle fiber contraction.
◆ Serum antiacetylcholine antibody titer may be elevated.
◆ Chest X-ray reveals thymoma (in about 15% of patients).

Treatment
◆ An anticholinesterase, such as neostigmine or pyridostigmine, to counteract fatigue and muscle weakness and allow about 80% of normal muscle function (drugs less effective as disease worsens)
◆ Immunosuppressant therapy with a corticosteroid, azathioprine, cyclosporine, and cyclophosphamide used in a progressive fashion (when the previous drug response is poor, the next one is used) to decrease the immune response toward acetylcholine receptors at the neuromuscular junction
◆ Immunoglobulin G during acute relapses or plasmapheresis in severe exacerbations to suppress the immune system

◆ Thymectomy to remove thymomas and possibly induce remission in some cases of adult-onset myasthenia
◆ Tracheotomy, positive-pressure ventilation, and vigorous suctioning to remove secretions for treatment of acute exacerbations that cause severe respiratory distress
◆ Discontinuation of anticholinesterase therapy in myasthenic crisis, until respiratory function improves; requires immediate hospitalization and vigorous respiratory support

Special considerations
Careful baseline assessment, early recognition and treatment of potential crises, supportive measures, and thorough patient teaching can minimize exacerbations and complications. Continuity of care is essential.
◆ Establish an accurate neurologic and respiratory baseline. Thereafter, monitor tidal volume and vital capacity regularly. The patient may need a ventilator and frequent suctioning to remove accumulating secretions.
◆ Be alert for signs and symptoms of an impending crisis (increased muscle weakness, respiratory distress, and difficulty in talking or chewing).
◆ To prevent relapses, adhere closely to the ordered drug administration schedule. Be prepared to give atropine for anti-cholinesterase overdose or toxicity.
◆ Plan exercise, meals, patient care, and activities to make the most of energy peaks. For example, give medication 20 to 30 minutes before meals to facilitate chewing or swallowing. Allow the patient to participate in his care.
◆ When swallowing is difficult, give soft, solid foods instead of liquids to lessen the risk of choking.
◆ After a severe exacerbation, encourage the patient to increase social activity as soon as possible.
◆ Patient teaching is essential because myasthenia gravis is usually a lifelong condition. Stress the need for frequent rest periods throughout the day. Emphasize that periodic remissions, exacerbations, and day-to-day fluctuations are common.
◆ Teach the patient how to recognize the adverse reactions to and signs and symptoms of toxicity of anticholinesterases (headaches, weakness, sweating, abdominal cramps, nausea, vomiting, diarrhea, excessive salivation, and bronchospasm) and corticosteroids (euphoria, insomnia, edema, and increased appetite).
◆ Warn the patient to avoid strenuous exercise, stress, infection, and needless exposure to the sun or cold. All of these factors may worsen

signs and symptoms. Wearing an eye patch or glasses with one frosted lens may help the patient with diplopia.
◆ For more information and an opportunity to meet other myasthenia gravis patients who lead full, productive lives, refer the patient to the Myasthenia Gravis Foundation of America.

PARKINSON'S DISEASE
Named for James Parkinson, the English physician who wrote the first accurate description of the disease in 1817, Parkinson's disease (also known as *shaking palsy*) characteristically produces progressive muscle rigidity, akinesia, and involuntary tremor. Deterioration is a progressive process. Death may result from complications, such as aspiration pneumonia or some other infection.

Parkinson's disease is one of the most common crippling diseases in the United States. It strikes 2 in every 1,000 people, mostly affecting those over age 50. Roughly 60,000 new cases are diagnosed annually in the United States alone, and incidence is predicted to increase as the population ages.

Causes
The cause of Parkinson's disease is unknown. However, study of the extrapyramidal brain nuclei (corpus striatum, globus pallidus, substantia nigra) has established the following:
◆ Dopamine deficiency prevents affected brain cells from performing their normal inhibitory function in the central nervous system.
◆ Some cases are caused by exposure to toxins, such as manganese dust or carbon monoxide.

Pathophysiology
Parkinson's disease is a degenerative process involving the dopaminergic neurons in the substantia nigra (the area of the basal ganglia that produces and stores the neurotransmitter dopamine). This area plays an important role in the extrapyramidal system, which controls posture and coordination of voluntary motor movements.

Normally, stimulation of the basal ganglia results in refined motor movement because acetylcholine (excitatory) and dopamine (inhibitory) release are balanced. Degeneration of the dopaminergic neurons and loss of available dopamine leads to an excess of excitatory acetylcholine at the synapse and consequent rigidity, tremors, and bradykinesia. (See *Neurotransmitter action in Parkinson's disease*, page 300.)

Other nondopaminergic neurons may be affected, possibly contributing to depression and the other nonmotor symptoms associated with this disease. Also, the basal ganglia is interconnected to the hypothalamus, potentially affecting autonomic and endocrine function as well.

Current research on the pathogenesis of Parkinson's disease focuses on damage to the substantia nigra from oxidative stress. Oxidative stress is believed to diminish brain iron content, impair mitochondrial function, inhibit antioxidant and protective systems, reduce glutathione secretion, and damage lipids, proteins, and deoxyribonucleic acid. Brain cells are less capable of repairing oxidative damage than are other tissues.

Signs and symptoms
◆ Muscle rigidity, akinesia (loss of muscle movement), and an insidious tremor beginning in the fingers (unilateral pill-roll tremor) that increases during stress or anxiety and decreases with purposeful movement and sleep; secondary to loss of inhibitory dopamine activity at the synapse
◆ Muscle rigidity with resistance to passive muscle stretching, which may be uniform (lead-pipe rigidity) or jerky (cogwheel rigidity); secondary to depletion of dopamine
◆ Akinesia causing difficulty walking (gait that lacks normal parallel motion and may be retropulsive or propulsive) from impaired dopamine action
◆ High-pitched, monotone voice from dopamine depletion
◆ Drooling secondary to impaired regulation of motor function
◆ Masklike facial expression from depletion of dopamine
◆ Loss of posture control (the patient walks with body bent forward) from loss of motor control due to dopamine depletion
◆ Dysarthria (impaired speech due to a disturbance in muscle control), dysphagia (difficulty swallowing), or both
◆ Oculogyric crises (eyes are fixed upward, with involuntary tonic movements) or blepharospasm (eyelids are completely closed)
◆ Excessive sweating from impaired autonomic dysfunction
◆ Decreased motility of GI and genitourinary smooth muscle from impaired autonomic transmission
◆ Orthostatic hypotension from impaired vascular smooth-muscle response
◆ Oily skin secondary to inappropriate androgen production controlled by the hypothalamic-pituitary axis

Neurotransmitter action in Parkinson's disease

Degeneration of the dopaminergic neurons and loss of available dopamine lead to rigidity, tremors, and bradykinesia.

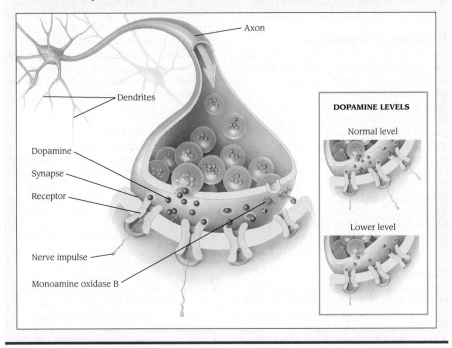

Labels: Axon, Dendrites, Dopamine, Synapse, Receptor, Nerve impulse, Monoamine oxidase B

DOPAMINE LEVELS

Normal level

Lower level

Complications
◆ Injury from falls
◆ Aspiration
◆ Urinary tract infections
◆ Pressure ulcers

Diagnosis
Generally, diagnostic tests are of little value in identifying Parkinson's disease. Diagnosis is based on the patient's age and history and on the characteristic clinical picture. However, urinalysis may support the diagnosis by revealing a decreased dopamine level.

A conclusive diagnosis is possible only after ruling out other causes of tremor, involutional depression, cerebral arteriosclerosis and, in patients younger than age 30, intracranial tumors, Wilson's disease, and phenothiazine or other drug toxicity.

Treatment
The aim of treatment is to relieve symptoms and keep the patient functional as long as possible. Treatment includes:

◆ levodopa, a dopamine replacement most effective during early stages and given in increasing doses until symptoms are relieved or adverse reactions appear (Because adverse reactions can be serious, levodopa is usually given in combination with carbidopa to halt peripheral dopamine synthesis.); a dopamine agonist (such as pramipexole, ropinirole, pergolide, bromocriptine) may be used early in the disease or in combination with levodopa to enhance response or minimize adverse reactions
◆ alternative drug therapy, including an anticholinergic, such as trihexyphenidyl; an antihistamine, such as diphenhydramine; and amantadine, an antiviral agent, or Selegiline, an enzyme-inhibitor, when levodopa is ineffective to conserve dopamine and enhance the therapeutic effect of levodopa
◆ L-deprenyl, for patients with mild disease to slow disease progression and ease symptoms
◆ deep brain stimulation, a surgical option, in which neurostimulator and electrodes are implanted that stimulate the globus pallidus subthalamic nucleus to decrease tremors and allow normal function; or fetal cell transplantation

(controversial), in which fetal brain tissue is injected into the patient's brain, in the hope that injected cells will grow, allowing the brain to process dopamine and, thereby, halting or slowing disease progression
◆ physical therapy, including active and passive range-of-motion exercises, routine daily activities, walking, and baths and massage to help relax muscles; complement drug treatment and neurosurgery attempting to maintain normal muscle tone and function.

Special considerations

Effectively caring for the patient with Parkinson's disease requires careful monitoring of drug treatment, emphasis on teaching self-reliance, and generous psychological (and sometimes physical) support.
◆ Monitor drug treatment and adjust dosage, if necessary, to minimize adverse reactions.
◆ If the patient has surgery, watch for signs of hemorrhage and increased intracranial pressure by frequently checking level of consciousness and vital signs.
◆ Encourage independence. The patient with excessive tremor may achieve partial control of his body by sitting on a chair and using its arms to steady himself. Advise the patient to change position slowly and dangle his legs before getting out of bed. Remember that fatigue may cause him to depend more on others.
◆ Help the patient overcome problems related to eating and elimination. For example, if he has difficulty eating, offer supplementary or small, frequent meals to increase caloric intake. Help establish a regular bowel routine by encouraging him to drink at least 2 qt (2 L) of liquids daily and eat high-fiber foods. He may need an elevated toilet seat to assist him from a standing to a sitting position.
◆ Give the patient and family emotional support. Teach them about the disease, its progressive stages, and adverse drug effects. Show the family how to prevent pressure ulcers and contractures by proper positioning. Inform them of the dietary restrictions levodopa imposes, and explain household safety measures to prevent injury. Help the patient and his family express their feelings and frustrations about the progressively debilitating effects of the disease. Establish long- and short-term treatment goals, and be aware of the patient's need for intellectual stimulation and diversion. Refer the patient and family to the National Parkinson Foundation or the United Parkinson Foundation for more information.

REYE'S SYNDROME

Reye's syndrome is an acute childhood illness that causes fatty infiltration of the liver with concurrent hyperammonemia, encephalopathy, and increased intracranial pressure (ICP). In addition, fatty infiltration of the kidneys, brain, and myocardium may occur. Reye's syndrome affects children from infancy to adolescence and occurs equally in boys and girls.

Prognosis depends on the severity of central nervous system depression. Until recently, mortality from Reye's syndrome was as high as 90%. Today, ICP monitoring and, consequently, early treatment of increased ICP, along with other treatment measures, have reduced that percentage to about 20%. Death is usually a result of cerebral edema or respiratory arrest. Comatose patients who survive may have residual brain damage.

Incidence commonly rises during influenza outbreaks and may be linked to aspirin use. For this reason, use of aspirin for children younger than age 15 isn't recommended.

Causes

Reye's syndrome typically begins within 1 to 3 days of an acute viral infection, such as an upper respiratory tract infection, type B influenza, or varicella (chickenpox).

Pathophysiology

In Reye's syndrome, damaged hepatic mitochondria disrupt the urea cycle, which normally changes ammonia to urea for its excretion from the body. This results in hyperammonemia, hypoglycemia (in 15% of cases), and an increase in serum short-chain fatty acids, leading to encephalopathy. Simultaneously, fatty infiltration occurs in renal tubular cells, neuronal tissue, and muscle tissue, including the heart.

Signs and symptoms

The severity of the child's signs and symptoms varies with the degree of encephalopathy and cerebral edema. In any case, Reye's syndrome develops in five stages. After the initial viral infection, a brief recovery period follows when the child doesn't seem seriously ill. A few days later, he develops intractable vomiting; lethargy; rapidly changing mental status (mild to severe agitation, confusion, irritability, and delirium); rising blood pressure, respiratory rate, and pulse rate; and hyperactive reflexes.

Reye's syndrome commonly progresses to coma. As coma deepens, seizures develop, followed by decreased tendon reflexes and, usually, respiratory failure.

Complications
♦ Increased ICP (due to increased cerebral blood volume causing intracranial hypertension developing as a result of acidosis, increased cerebral metabolic rate, and impaired autoregulatory mechanism)
♦ Respiratory failure
♦ Death

Diagnosis
A history of a recent viral disorder with typical clinical features strongly suggests Reye's syndrome. An increased serum ammonia level, abnormal clotting studies, and hepatic dysfunction confirm it. Testing the serum salicylate level rules out aspirin use. Absence of jaundice despite increased liver aminotransferase levels rules out acute hepatic failure and hepatic encephalopathy.

Abnormal test results may include:
♦ *liver function studies*—aspartate aminotransferase and alanine aminotransferase elevated to twice normal levels; bilirubin level usually normal
♦ *liver biopsy*—fatty droplets uniformly distributed throughout cells
♦ *cerebrospinal fluid (CSF) analysis*—white blood cell count less than 10/μl; with coma and increased CSF pressure
♦ *coagulation studies*—prolonged prothrombin time and partial thromboplastin time
♦ *blood values*—an elevated serum ammonia level; a normal or low (in 15% of cases) serum glucose level; increased serum fatty acid and lactate levels.

Treatment
For treatment guidelines, see *Stages of treatment for Reye's syndrome.*

Special considerations
♦ Advise parents to give a nonsalicylate analgesic and an antipyretic, such as acetaminophen.
♦ Refer the parents to the National Reye's Syndrome Foundation for more information.

SEIZURE DISORDER
Seizure disorder, or *epilepsy,* is a condition of the brain characterized by susceptibility to recurrent seizures (paroxysmal events associated with abnormal electrical discharges of neurons in the brain). Primary seizure disorder or epilepsy is idiopathic without apparent structural changes in the brain. Secondary epilepsy, characterized by structural changes or metabolic alterations of the neuronal membranes, causes increased automaticity.

⚠ **CLINICAL ALERT** *Not all seizures are associated with a seizure disorder. Childhood febrile seizures, postconcussion seizures, and toxin-induced seizures are usually one-time events.*

Epilepsy is believed to affect people of all ages, races, and ethnic backgrounds; about 2.5 million people have been diagnosed with epilepsy. The incidence is highest in childhood and old age. The prognosis is good if the patient adheres strictly to prescribed treatment.

Causes
About one-half of all seizure disorder cases are idiopathic; possible causes of other cases include:
♦ alcohol withdrawal
♦ anoxia
♦ birth trauma (inadequate oxygen supply to the brain, blood incompatibility, or hemorrhage)
♦ brain tumors
♦ head injury or trauma
♦ infectious diseases (meningitis, encephalitis, or brain abscess)
♦ ingestion of toxins (mercury, lead, or carbon monoxide)
♦ inherited disorders or degenerative disease, such as phenylketonuria or tuberous sclerosis
♦ metabolic disorders, such as hypoglycemia and hypoparathyroidism
♦ perinatal infection
♦ stroke (hemorrhage, thrombosis, or embolism).

Pathophysiology
Some neurons in the brain may depolarize easily or be hyperexcitable; this epileptogenic focus fires more readily than normal when stimulated. In these neurons, the membrane potential at rest is less negative or inhibitory connections are missing, possibly as a result of decreased gamma-aminobutyric acid activity or localized shifts in electrolytes.

On stimulation, the epileptogenic focus fires and spreads electrical current to surrounding cells. These cells fire in turn and the impulse cascades to one side of the brain (a partial seizure), both sides of the brain (a generalized seizure), or cortical, subcortical, and brain stem areas.

The brain's metabolic demand for oxygen increases dramatically during a seizure. If this demand isn't met, hypoxia and brain damage ensue. Firing of inhibitory neurons causes the excitatory neurons to slow their firing and eventually stop. If this inhibitory action doesn't occur, the result is status epilepticus: one seizure occurring right after another; without treatment the anoxia can be fatal.

Stages of treatment for Reye's syndrome

Signs and symptoms	Baseline treatment	Baseline intervention
Stage I		
Vomiting, lethargy, hepatic dysfunction	◆ To decrease intracranial pressure (ICP) and brain edema, give I.V. fluids at two-thirds maintenance. Also give an osmotic diuretic or furosemide. ◆ To treat hypoprothrombinemia, give vitamin K; if vitamin K is unsuccessful, give fresh frozen plasma. ◆ Monitor serum ammonia and blood glucose levels and plasma osmolality every 4 to 8 hours to check progress.	◆ Monitor vital signs and check level of consciousness for increasing lethargy. Take vital signs more often as the patient's condition deteriorates. ◆ Monitor fluid intake and output to prevent fluid overload. Maintain urine output at 1 ml/kg/hr; plasma osmolality, 290 mOsm; and blood glucose, 150 mg/ml. (Goal: Keep glucose level high, osmolality normal to high, and ammonia level low.) Also, restrict protein.
Stage II		
Hyperventilation, delirium, hepatic dysfunction, hyperactive reflexes	◆ Continue baseline treatment from stage I.	◆ Maintain seizure precautions. ◆ Immediately report any signs of coma that require invasive, supportive therapy, such as endotracheal intubation. ◆ Keep head of bed at 30-degree angle.
Stage III		
Coma, hyperventilation, decorticate rigidity, hepatic dysfunction	◆ Continue baseline treatment from stage I and seizure treatment. ◆ Monitor ICP with a subarachnoid screw or other invasive device. ◆ Provide endotracheal intubation and mechanical ventilation to control partial pressure of arterial carbon dioxide ($Paco_2$) levels. A paralyzing agent, such as vecuronium I.V., may help maintain ventilation. ◆ Give mannitol I.V.	◆ Monitor ICP (should be < 20 mm Hg before suctioning); keep the patient sedated. ◆ When ventilating the patient, maintain $Paco_2$ between 30 and 40 mm Hg and partial pressure of arterial oxygen between 80 and 100 mm Hg. ◆ Closely monitor cardiovascular status with a pulmonary artery catheter or central venous pressure line. ◆ Give good skin and mouth care and range-of-motion
Stage IV		
Deepening coma; decerebrate rigidity; large, fixed pupils; minimal hepatic dysfunction	◆ Continue baseline treatment from stage I and supportive care. ◆ If all previous measures fail, some pediatric centers use barbiturate coma, decompressive craniotomy, hypothermia, or exchange transfusion.	◆ Check patient for loss of reflexes and signs of flaccidity. ◆ Give the family the extra support they need, considering their child's poor prognosis.

(continued)

Stages of treatment for Reye's syndrome *(continued)*

Signs and symptoms	Baseline treatment	Baseline intervention
Stage V		
Seizures, loss of deep tendon reflexes, flaccidity, respiratory arrest, ammonia level above 300 mg/dl	◆ Continue baseline treatment from stage I and supportive care.	◆ Help the family to face the patient's impending death.

Signs and symptoms

The hallmark of epilepsy is recurring seizures, which can be classified as partial, generalized, status epilepticus, or unclassified (some patients may be affected by more than one type). (See *Types of seizures.*)

Complications

◆ Hypoxia or anoxia from airway occlusion or aspiration
◆ Traumatic injury
◆ Brain damage
◆ Depression and anxiety

Diagnosis

Clinically, the diagnosis of epilepsy is based on the occurrence of one or more seizures and proof or the assumption that the condition that caused them is still present. Various diagnostic tests help support the findings.
◆ Computed tomography scan or magnetic resonance imaging reveal abnormalities.
◆ EEG reveals paroxysmal abnormalities to confirm the diagnosis and provide evidence of the continuing tendency to have seizures. In tonic-clonic seizures, high, fast voltage spikes are present in all leads; in absence seizures, rounded spike wave complexes are diagnostic. A negative EEG doesn't rule out epilepsy because the abnormalities occur intermittently.
◆ Serum chemistry blood studies may reveal hypoglycemia, electrolyte imbalances and elevated liver enzyme and alcohol levels, providing clues to underlying conditions that increase the risk of seizure activity.

Treatment

◆ Drug therapy specific to the type of seizure, including phenytoin, carbamazepine, phenobarbital, gabapentin (Neurontin), and primidone for generalized tonic clonic seizures and complex partial seizures—I.V. fosphenytoin (Cerebyx) is an alternative to phenytoin (Dilantin) that's just as effective, with a long half-life and minimal central nervous system depression (stable for 120 days at room temperature and compatible with many commonly used I.V. solutions; can be administered rapidly without the adverse cardiovascular effects that occur with phenytoin)
◆ Valproic acid, clonazepam, and ethosuximide for absence seizures
◆ Gabapentin (Neurontin) and felbamate as other anticonvulsants
◆ Surgical removal of a demonstrated focal lesion, if drug therapy is ineffective
◆ Surgery to remove the underlying cause, such as a tumor, abscess, or vascular problem
◆ Vagus nerve stimulator implantation to help reduce the incidence of focal seizure
◆ I.V. diazepam, lorazepam, or midazolam for status epilepticus
◆ Administration of dextrose (when seizures are secondary to hypoglycemia) or thiamine (in chronic alcoholism or withdrawal)

Special considerations

A key to support is a true understanding of the nature of epilepsy and of the misconceptions that surround it.
◆ Encourage the patient and family to express their feelings about the patient's condition. Answer their questions, and help them cope by dispelling some of the myths about epilepsy—for example, the myth that it's contagious. Assure them that epilepsy is controllable for most patients who follow a prescribed drug regimen and that most patients maintain a normal lifestyle.

Because drug therapy is the treatment of choice for most people with epilepsy, information about medications is invaluable.
◆ Stress the need for compliance with the prescribed drug regimen. Reinforce dosage instructions and stress the importance of taking medication regularly and at scheduled times.

Types of seizures

The various types of seizures—partial, generalized, status epilepticus, and unclassified—have distinct signs and symptoms.

Partial seizures

Arising from a localized area of the brain, partial seizures cause focal symptoms. These seizures are classified by their effect on consciousness and whether they spread throughout the motor pathway, causing a generalized seizure.

♦ A *simple partial seizure* begins locally and generally doesn't cause an alteration in consciousness. It may present with sensory symptoms (lights flashing, smells, auditory hallucinations), autonomic signs and symptoms (sweating, flushing, pupil dilation), and psychic symptoms (dream states, anger, fear). The seizure lasts for a few seconds and occurs without preceding or provoking events. This type can be motor or sensory.

♦ A *complex partial seizure* alters consciousness. Amnesia for events that occur during and immediately after the seizure is a differentiating characteristic. During the seizure, the patient may follow simple commands. This type of seizure generally lasts for 1 to 3 minutes.

Generalized seizures

As the term suggests, *generalized seizures* cause a generalized electrical abnormality within the brain. They can be convulsive or nonconvulsive and include several types:

♦ *Absence seizures* occur most commonly in children, although they may affect adults. They usually begin with a brief change in level of consciousness, indicated by blinking or rolling of the eyes, a blank stare, and slight mouth movements. The patient retains his posture and continues preseizure activity without difficulty. Typically, each seizure lasts from 1 to 10 seconds. If not properly treated, seizures can recur as often as 100 times a day. An absence seizure is a nonconvulsive seizure, but it may progress to a generalized tonic-clonic seizure.

♦ *Myoclonic seizures* are brief, involuntary muscular jerks of the body or extremities, commonly occurring in the morning.

♦ *Clonic seizures* are characterized by bilateral rhythmic movements.

♦ *Tonic seizures* are characterized by a sudden stiffening of muscle tone, usually of the arm, but possibly including the legs.

♦ *Generalized tonic-clonic seizures* typically begin with a loud cry, precipitated by air rushing from the lungs through the vocal cords. The patient then loses consciousness and falls to the ground. The body stiffens (tonic phase) and then alternates between episodes of muscle spasm and relaxation (clonic phase). Tongue biting, incontinence, labored breathing, apnea, and subsequent cyanosis may occur. The seizure stops in 2 to 5 minutes, when abnormal electrical conduction ceases. When the patient regains consciousness, he's confused and may have difficulty talking. If he can talk, he may complain of drowsiness, fatigue, headache, muscle soreness, and arm or leg weakness. He may fall into a deep sleep after the seizure.

♦ *Atonic seizures* are characterized by a general loss of postural tone and a temporary loss of consciousness. They occur in young children and are sometimes called "drop attacks" because they cause the child to fall.

Status epilepticus

Status epilepticus is a continuous seizure state that can occur in all seizure types. The most life-threatening example is generalized tonic-clonic status epilepticus, a continuous generalized tonic-clonic seizure. Status epilepticus is accompanied by respiratory distress leading to hypoxia or anoxia. It can result from abrupt withdrawal of anticonvulsant medications, hypoxic encephalopathy, acute head trauma, metabolic encephalopathy, or septicemia secondary to encephalitis or meningitis.

Unclassified seizures

This category is reserved for seizures that don't fit the characteristics of partial or generalized seizures or status epilepticus. Included as unclassified are events that lack the data to make a more definitive diagnosis.

Caution the patient to monitor the quantity of medication he has so he doesn't run out of it.
♦ Warn against possible adverse reactions — drowsiness, lethargy, hyperactivity, confusion, and visual and sleep disturbances — all of which indicate the need for dosage adjustment. Phenytoin therapy may lead to hyperplasia of the gums, which may be relieved by conscientious oral hygiene. Instruct the patient to report adverse reactions immediately.
♦ When administering phenytoin I.V., use a large vein, administer using an infusion pump and monitor vital signs frequently. Avoid I.M. administration and mixing with dextrose solutions.
♦ Emphasize the importance of having blood anticonvulsant levels checked at regular intervals, even if the seizures are under control.
♦ Warn the patient against drinking alcoholic beverages.
♦ Know which social agencies in your community can help epileptic patients. Refer the patient to the Epilepsy Foundation of America for general information and to the state motor vehicle department for information about a driver's license.

The primary goals of the physician and family members caring for a patient having a seizure are protection from injury, protection from aspiration, and observation of the seizure activity. Generalized tonic-clonic seizures may necessitate first aid. Show the patient's family members how to administer first aid correctly:
♦ Avoid restraining the patient during a seizure. Help the patient to a lying position, loosen any tight clothing, and place something flat and soft, such as a pillow, jacket, or hand, under his head. Clear the area of hard objects. Don't force anything into the patient's mouth if his teeth are clenched — a tongue blade or spoon could lacerate the mouth and lips or displace teeth, precipitating respiratory distress. However, if the patient's mouth is open, protect his tongue by placing a soft object, such as a folded cloth (never your fingers), between his teeth. Turn his head to provide an open airway. After the seizure subsides, reassure the patient that he's all right, orient him to time and place, and inform him that he has had a seizure.
♦ Don't restrain the patient during a complex partial seizure. Clear the area of any hard objects. Protect him from injury by gently calling his name and directing him away from the source of danger. After the seizure passes, reassure him and tell him that he has just had a seizure.

SPINAL CORD TRAUMA

Spinal injuries include fractures, contusions, and compressions of the vertebral column, usually as the result of trauma to the head or neck. The real danger lies in spinal cord damage — cutting, pulling, twisting, or compression. Damage may involve the entire cord or be restricted to one-half, and it can occur at any level. Fractures of the 5th, 6th, or 7th cervical, 12th thoracic, and 1st lumbar vertebrae are most common.

Causes

The most serious spinal cord trauma typically results from:
♦ diving into shallow water
♦ falls
♦ gunshot or stab wounds
♦ motor vehicle collisions
♦ sports injuries.
Less serious injuries commonly occur from:
♦ lifting heavy objects
♦ minor falls.
Spinal dysfunction may also result from:
♦ hyperparathyroidism
♦ neoplastic lesions.

Pathophysiology

Like head trauma, spinal cord trauma results from acceleration, deceleration, or other deforming forces usually applied from a distance. Mechanisms involved with spinal cord trauma include:
♦ hyperextension from acceleration-deceleration forces and sudden reduction in the anteroposterior diameter of the spinal cord
♦ hyperflexion from sudden and excessive force, propelling the neck forward or causing an exaggerated movement to one side
♦ vertical compression from force being applied from the top of the cranium along the vertical axis through the vertebra or from the lumbar spine upward
♦ rotational forces from twisting, which adds shearing forces.
Injury causes microscopic hemorrhages in the gray matter and pia-arachnoid mater. The hemorrhages gradually increase in size until some or all of the gray matter is filled with blood, which causes necrosis. From the gray matter, the blood enters the white matter, where it impedes the circulation within the spinal cord. Ensuing edema causes compression and decreases the blood supply. Thus, the spinal cord loses perfusion and becomes ischemic. The edema and hemorrhage are greatest at and about two segments above and below the injury. The edema temporarily adds to the patient's dysfunction by increasing pressure and compressing the nerves. Edema at or above the 3rd to 5th cervical vertebrae may

Types of spinal cord injury

Injury to the spinal cord can be classified as complete or incomplete. An incomplete spinal injury may be a central cord syndrome, anterior cord syndrome, or Brown-Sequard syndrome, depending on the area of the cord affected. This chart highlights the characteristic signs and symptoms of each.

Type	Description	Signs and symptoms
Complete transection	◆ All tracts of spinal cord completely disrupted ◆ All functions involving spinal cord below level of transection lost ◆ Complete and permanent loss	◆ Loss of motor function (quadriplegia) with cervical cord transection; paraplegia with thoracic cord transection ◆ Muscle flaccidity ◆ Loss of all reflexes and sensory function below level of injury ◆ Bladder, bowel, and sexual dysfunction with lumbar or sacral disruption ◆ Paralytic ileus ◆ Loss of vasomotor tone below level of injury with low and unstable blood pressure ◆ Loss of perspiration below level of injury ◆ Dry pale skin ◆ Respiratory impairment if injury is to cervical or upper thoracic spine
Incomplete transection: Central cord syndrome	◆ Center portion of cord affected ◆ Typically from hyperextension injury	◆ Motor deficits greater in upper than in lower extremities ◆ Variable degree of bladder dysfunction
Incomplete transection: Anterior cord syndrome	◆ Occlusion of anterior spinal artery ◆ Occlusion occurs from pressure of bone fragments	◆ Loss of motor function below level of injury ◆ Loss of pain and temperature sensations below level of injury ◆ Intact touch, pressure, position and vibration senses
Incomplete transection: Brown-Sequard syndrome	◆ Hemisection of the cord ◆ Most common in stabbing and gunshot wounds ◆ Damage to cord on only one side	◆ Ipsilateral paralysis or paresis below level of injury ◆ Ipsilateral loss of touch, pressure, vibration, and position sense below level of injury ◆ Contralateral loss of pain and temperature sensations below level of injury

interfere with phrenic nerve impulse transmission to the diaphragm and inhibit respiratory function.

In the white matter, circulation usually returns to normal in about 24 hours. However, in the gray matter, an inflammatory reaction prevents restoration of circulation. Phagocytes appear at the site within 36 to 48 hours after the injury, macrophages engulf degenerating axons, and collagen replaces the normal tissue. Scarring and meningeal thickening leaves the nerves in the area blocked or tangled.

Signs and symptoms
◆ Muscle spasm and back pain that worsens with movement (In cervical fractures, pain may cause point tenderness; in dorsal and lumbar fractures, it may radiate to other body areas such as the legs.)
◆ Mild paresthesia to quadriplegia and shock, if the injury damages the spinal cord (In milder injury, such signs and symptoms may be delayed several days or weeks. Specific signs and symptoms depend on injury type and degree.) (See *Types of spinal cord injury.*)

Complications of spinal cord injury

Complications of spinal cord injury may include spinal shock, neurogenic shock, or autonomic dysreflexia.

Spinal shock

Spinal shock is the loss of autonomic, reflex, motor, and sensory activity below the level of the cord lesion. It occurs secondary to damage of the spinal cord.

Signs of spinal shock include:
♦ flaccid paralysis
♦ loss of deep tendon and perianal reflexes
♦ loss of motor and sensory function.

Until spinal shock has resolved (usually 1 to 6 weeks after injury), the extent of actual cord damage can't be fully assessed. The earliest indicator of resolution is the return of reflex activity.

Neurogenic shock

Neurogenic shock is an abnormal vasomotor response that occurs secondary to disruption of sympathetic impulses from the brain stem to the thoracolumbar area, and is seen in patients with major cord injuries above the T6 level. This temporary loss of autonomic function below the level of injury causes profound cardiovascular changes.

Signs of neurogenic shock include:
♦ orthostatic hypotension
♦ bradycardia

♦ loss of the ability to regulate body temperature
♦ loss of the ability to sweat below the level of the lesion.

Treatment is symptomatic. Symptoms resolve when spinal cord edema resolves.

Autonomic dysreflexia

Also known as autonomic hyperreflexia, autonomic dysreflexia is a serious medical condition that occurs after resolution of spinal shock. Emergency recognition and management is a must.

Autonomic dysreflexia should be suspected in the patient with:
♦ spinal cord trauma at or above level T6
♦ bradycardia
♦ hypertension and a severe pounding headache
♦ cold or goose-fleshed skin below the lesion.

Dysreflexia is caused by noxious stimuli, most commonly a distended bladder or skin lesion.

Treatment focuses on eliminating the stimulus; rapid identification and removal may avoid the need for pharmacologic control of the headache and hypertension.

Complications
♦ Spinal shock
♦ Neurogenic shock
♦ Autonomic dysreflexia (See *Complications of spinal cord injury.*)

Diagnosis
♦ Spinal X-rays, the most important diagnostic measure, detect most fractures.
♦ Thorough neurologic evaluation locates the level of injury and detects cord damage.
♦ Computed tomography (CT) scan or magnetic resonance imaging reveals spinal cord edema and compression and may reveal a spinal mass; CT scan also provides images of the fracture.

Treatment
♦ Immediate immobilization to stabilize the spine and prevent further cord damage (primary treatment); use of lightweight head blocks on both sides of the patient's head, a hard cervical collar, or skeletal traction with skull tongs or a

halo device for cervical spine injuries; position the patient on a rigid, long board for thoracic and lumbar injuries until surgical stabilization can occur
♦ High doses of methylprednisolone (controversial) to reduce inflammation with evidence of cord injury (started prehospitalization)
♦ Bed rest on firm support (such as a bed board), an analgesic, and a muscle relaxant for treatment of stable lumbar fracture until it's repaired or healed
♦ Orthotic devices to treat stable thoracic and lumbar fractures
♦ Laminectomy and spinal fusion for severe or unstable lumbar fractures
♦ Neurosurgery to relieve the pressure when the damage results in compression of the spinal column — if the cause of compression is a metastatic lesion, chemotherapy and radiation may be indicated
♦ Treatment of surface wounds accompanying the spinal injury; tetanus prophylaxis unless the patient has had recent immunization

◆ Exercises to strengthen the back muscles and a back brace or corset to provide support while walking
◆ Rehabilitation to maintain or improve functional level

Special considerations
In all spinal injuries, suspect cord damage until proved otherwise.
◆ During the initial assessment and X-ray studies, immobilize the patient on a firm surface, with an immobilization device on both sides of his head. Tell him not to move and avoid moving him yourself because hyperflexion can damage the cord. If you must move the patient, one person should stabilize the patient's neck and give the directions as at least three other members of the staff help logroll him to avoid disturbing spinal alignment.
◆ Throughout assessment, offer comfort and reassurance. Remember, the fear of possible paralysis will be overwhelming. Talk to the patient quietly and calmly. Allow a family member who isn't too distraught to accompany him.
◆ If the injury requires surgery, administer a prophylactic antibiotic as ordered. Catheterize the patient, as ordered, to avoid urine retention, and monitor bowel elimination patterns to avoid impaction.
◆ Explain traction methods to the patient and his family. Reassure them that skeletal traction devices don't penetrate the brain. If the patient has a halo or skull-tong traction device, clean pin sites according to your facility's policy, trim hair short, and provide an analgesic for persistent headaches. During traction, turn the patient often to prevent pneumonia, embolism, and skin breakdown; perform passive range-of-motion exercises to maintain muscle tone.
◆ Turn the patient on his side during feedings to prevent aspiration. Create a relaxed atmosphere at mealtimes.
◆ Suggest appropriate diversionary activities to fill the patient's hours of immobility.
◆ Watch closely for neurologic changes. Immediately report changes in skin sensation and loss of muscle strength — either of which might indicate pressure on the spinal cord, possibly as a result of edema or shifting bone fragments.
◆ Help the patient walk as soon as the physician allows; he'll probably need to wear a back brace or a halo vest.
◆ Before discharge, instruct the patient about continuing analgesic therapy or other medication, and stress the importance of regular follow-up examinations. Refer the patient for rehabilitative services.
◆ To help prevent a spinal injury from becoming a spinal cord injury, educate firemen, policemen, paramedics, and the general public about the proper way to handle such injuries.

STROKE
A stroke, also known as a *cerebrovascular accident* or *brain attack,* is a sudden impairment of cerebral circulation in one or more blood vessels. A stroke interrupts or diminishes oxygen supply, and commonly causes serious damage or necrosis in the brain tissues. The sooner the circulation returns to normal after a stroke, the better the patient's chances are for a complete recovery. However, about one-half of the patients who survive a stroke remain permanently disabled and experience a recurrence within weeks, months, or years. It's the leading cause of admission to a long-term care facility.

Stroke is the third most common cause of death in the United States and the most common cause of neurologic disability. It strikes more than 500,000 people per year and is fatal in about one-half of these cases.

AGE ALERT *Although strokes may occur in younger persons, most patients experiencing strokes are older than age 65. In fact, the risk of stroke doubles with each passing decade after age 55.*

Causes
Stroke typically results from one of three causes:
◆ embolism from thrombus originating outside the brain, such as in the heart, aorta, or common carotid artery
◆ hemorrhage from an intracranial artery or vein, such as from hypertension, ruptured aneurysm, arteriovenous malformations, trauma, hemorrhagic disorder, or septic embolism
◆ thrombosis of the cerebral arteries supplying the brain or of the intracranial vessels occluding blood flow. (See *Types of stroke* and *Ischemic stroke,* pages 310 and 311.)

Risk factors that have been identified as predisposing a patient to stroke include:
◆ cardiac disease, including arrhythmias (especially atrial fibrillation or flutter), coronary artery disease, an acute myocardial infarction, dilated cardiomyopathy, and valvular disease
◆ cigarette smoking
◆ diabetes
◆ familial hyperlipidemia
◆ family history of stroke
◆ head trauma
◆ history of transient ischemic attacks (TIAs) (See *Understanding TIAs,* page 312.)

Types of stroke

Strokes are typically classified as ischemic or hemorrhagic, depending on the underlying cause. This chart describes the major types of stroke.

Type of stroke	Description
Ischemic	
Thrombotic	♦ Most common type of stroke ♦ Commonly the result of atherosclerosis; also associated with hypertension, smoking, diabetes (disease process is similar to myocardial infarction [MI]) ♦ Thrombus in extracranial or intracranial vessel blocks blood flow to the cerebral cortex ♦ Carotid artery most commonly affected extracranial vessel ♦ Common intracranial sites include bifurcation of carotid arteries, distal intracranial portion of vertebral arteries, and proximal basilar arteries ♦ May occur during sleep or shortly after awakening; during surgery; or after MI
Embolic	♦ Second most common type of stroke ♦ Embolus from heart or extracranial arteries floats into cerebral bloodstream and lodges in middle cerebral artery or branches ♦ Embolus commonly originates during atrial fibrillation ♦ Typically occurs during activity ♦ Develops rapidly
Lacunar	♦ Subtype of thrombotic stroke ♦ Hypertension creates cavities deep in white matter of the brain, affecting the internal capsule, basal ganglia, thalamus, and pons ♦ Lipid coating lining of the small penetrating arteries thickens and weakens wall, causing microaneurysms and dissections
Hemorrhagic	
	♦ Third most common type of stroke ♦ Typically caused by hypertension or rupture of aneurysm ♦ Blood supply to area supplied by ruptured artery diminished and surrounding tissue compressed by accumulated blood

♦ hypertension
♦ increased alcohol intake
♦ I.V. drug abuse
♦ obesity
♦ sedentary lifestyle
♦ stimulant use (such as cocaine)
♦ use of a hormonal contraceptive.

Pathophysiology

Regardless of the cause, the underlying event is deprivation of oxygen and nutrients to the tissues of the brain. Normally, if the arteries become blocked, autoregulatory mechanisms help maintain cerebral circulation until collateral circulation develops to deliver blood to the affected area. If the compensatory mechanisms become overworked or cerebral blood

flow remains impaired for more than a few minutes, oxygen deprivation leads to infarction of brain tissue. The brain cells cease to function because they can neither store glucose or glycogen for use nor engage in anaerobic metabolism. (See _How stroke affects the body,_ page 313.)

Signs and symptoms

The clinical features of stroke vary according to the affected artery and the region of the brain it supplies, the severity of the damage, and the extent of collateral circulation developed. A stroke in one hemisphere causes signs and symptoms on the opposite side of the body; a stroke that damages cranial nerves affects structures on the same side as the infarction.

Ischemic stroke

Ischemic stroke results from a blockage or reduction of blood flow to an area of the brain. This blockage may result from atherosclerosis or blood clot formation.

Atherosclerosis is the deposit of cholesterol and plaque within the walls of the arteries. These deposits may become large enough to narrow the lumen and reduce the flow of blood while also causing the artery to lose its ability to stretch.

Lumen
Thrombus
Plaque

A **thrombus**, or blood clot, forms on the roughened surface of atherosclerotic plaque that develops in the wall of the artery. The thrombus can enlarge and eventually block the artery lumen.

Part of a thrombus may break off and become an **embolus.** An embolus travels through the bloodstream and may block smaller arteries. Emboli commonly come from the heart, where different disorders can cause thrombus formation.

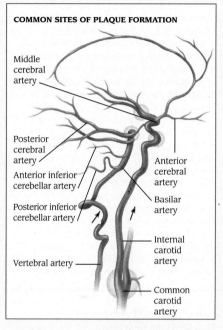

COMMON SITES OF PLAQUE FORMATION

Middle cerebral artery

Posterior cerebral artery

Anterior inferior cerebellar artery

Posterior inferior cerebellar artery

Vertebral artery

Anterior cerebral artery

Basilar artery

Internal carotid artery

Common carotid artery

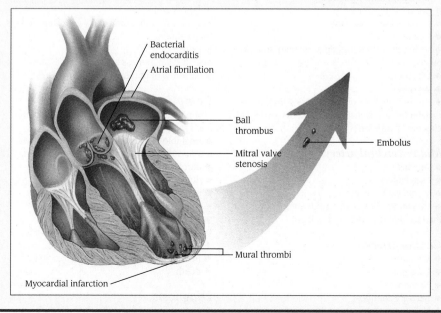

Bacterial endocarditis

Atrial fibrillation

Ball thrombus

Mitral valve stenosis

Embolus

Mural thrombi

Myocardial infarction

Understanding TIAs

A transient ischemic attack (TIA) is an episode of neurologic deficit resulting from cerebral ischemia. The recurrent attacks may last from seconds to an hour. It's usually considered a warning sign for stroke. In 14% of patients who experience a TIA, another TIA or a full stroke will occur within 1 year.

In a TIA, microemboli released from a thrombus may temporarily interrupt blood flow, especially in the small distal branches of the brain's arterial tree. Small spasms in those arterioles may impair blood flow and also precede a TIA.

The most distinctive features of TIAs are transient focal deficits with complete return of function. The deficits usually involve some degree of motor or sensory dysfunction. They may range from loss of consciousness to loss of motor or sensory function, but only for a brief time. The patient typically experiences weakness in the lower part of the face and arms, hands, fingers, and legs on the side opposite the affected region. Other manifestations include transient dysphagia, numbness or tingling of the face and lips, double vision, slurred speech, and dizziness.

General signs and symptoms
♦ Unilateral limb weakness
♦ Speech difficulties
♦ Numbness on one side
♦ Headache
♦ Vision disturbances (diplopia, hemianopsia, ptosis)
♦ Dizziness
♦ Anxiety
♦ Altered level of consciousness (LOC)

Additionally, signs and symptoms are usually classified by the artery affected.

Middle cerebral artery
♦ Aphasia
♦ Dysphasia
♦ Visual field deficits
♦ Hemiparesis of affected side (more severe in the face and arm than in the leg)

Carotid artery
♦ Weakness
♦ Paralysis
♦ Numbness
♦ Sensory changes
♦ Vision disturbances on the affected side
♦ Altered LOC
♦ Bruits
♦ Headaches
♦ Aphasia
♦ Ptosis

Vertebrobasilar artery
♦ Weakness on the affected side
♦ Numbness around lips and mouth
♦ Visual field deficits
♦ Diplopia
♦ Poor coordination
♦ Dysphagia
♦ Slurred speech
♦ Dizziness
♦ Nystagmus
♦ Amnesia
♦ Ataxia

Anterior cerebral artery
♦ Confusion
♦ Weakness
♦ Numbness, especially in the legs on the affected side
♦ Incontinence
♦ Loss of coordination
♦ Impaired motor and sensory functions
♦ Intellectual deficits
♦ Personality changes

Posterior cerebral artery
♦ Visual field deficits (homonymous hemianopsia)
♦ Sensory impairment
♦ Dyslexia
♦ Perseveration (abnormally persistent replies to questions)
♦ Coma
♦ Cortical blindness
♦ Absence of paralysis (usually)

Complications
Complications vary with the severity, location, and type of stroke, but may include:
♦ unstable blood pressure (from loss of vasomotor control)
♦ cerebral edema
♦ fluid imbalances
♦ sensory impairment
♦ infections such as pneumonia
♦ altered LOC
♦ aspiration
♦ contractures
♦ pulmonary embolism
♦ death.

Diagnosis
♦ Computed tomography scan identifies an ischemic stroke within the first 72 hours of

MULTISYSTEM DISORDER
How stroke affects the body

Stroke affects not only the brain and nervous system but other major body systems as well, which are outlined here. In addition, the patient with an acute stroke requires multidisciplinary care.

Nervous system
Pathophysiologic processes vary depending on the type of stroke.

Ischemic stroke
♦ An *ischemic stroke*, which can be *thrombotic* or *embolic*, causes ischemia. Some of the neurons served by the occluded vessel die of lack of oxygen and nutrients.
♦ Neuron death results in cerebral infarction, in which tissue injury triggers an inflammatory response that increases intracranial pressure (ICP).
♦ Injury to surrounding cells disrupts metabolism and leads to change in ionic transport, localized acidosis, and free radical formation.
♦ Calcium, sodium, and water accumulate in the injured cells, and excitatory neurotransmitters are released.
♦ Consequent continued cellular injury and swelling set up a cycle of further damage.

Hemorrhagic stroke
♦ Impaired cerebral perfusion causes infarction, and the blood itself acts as a space-occupying mass, exerting pressure on the brain tissues.
♦ The brain's regulatory mechanisms attempt to maintain equilibrium by increasing blood pressure to maintain cerebral perfusion pressure.
♦ The increased ICP forces cerebrospinal fluid out, thus restoring the balance. If the hemorrhage is small, the patient may live with only minimal neurologic deficits. If the bleeding is heavy, ICP increases rapidly and perfusion stops. Even if the pressure returns to normal, many brain cells die.
♦ Initially, the ruptured cerebral blood vessels may constrict to limit the blood loss.
♦ This vasospasm further compromises blood flow, leading to more ischemia and cellular damage.
♦ If a clot forms in the vessel, decreased blood flow promotes ischemia.
♦ If the blood enters the subarachnoid space, meningeal irritation occurs.
♦ Blood cells that pass through the vessel wall into the surrounding tissue may break down and block the arachnoid villi, causing hydrocephalus.

Cardiovascular system
♦ Cerebral ischemia and infarction can ultimately affect the autonomic nervous system, which can alter blood vessel constriction and dilation, heart rate, blood pressure, and cardiac contractility.
♦ Cardiovascular effects are increasingly problematic if the patient has an underlying disorder, such as heart disease or hypertension.

Musculoskeletal system
♦ Cerebral infarction can lead to a disturbance in impulse transmission via the cranial and peripheral nerves, altering motor and sensory function.
♦ Changes in sensation or mobility can lead to pressure areas, especially with prolonged bed rest or limited activity. In addition, the ability of the blood vessels to constrict and dilate as necessary may be altered, increasing the risk of impaired blood flow to the area. Subsequently, pressure ulcers may develop.

Respiratory system
♦ If infarction resulting from increased ICP and decreased perfusion involves the respiratory center in the medulla, respiration—including the depth and rate—can be affected because nerve impulse transmission via the phrenic nerves to the diaphragm and intercostal nerves to the intercostal muscles is interrupted.
♦ If the pons (the location for apneustic and pneumotaxic centers) is affected, breathing patterns become altered and impulse transmission via the cranial nerves (CN) may be interrupted.
♦ If the glossopharyngeal (CN IX) and vagus nerves (CN X) are affected, swallowing may be impaired and aspiration may occur.

Collaborative management
Typically, emergency services personnel are involved in confirming the signs and symptoms of an acute stroke, completing the primary survey, and transporting the patient to the health care facility. A speech therapist may assist the patient with defects in swallowing as well as speaking. A physical therapist helps the patient relearn basic activities of daily living, such as dressing, bathing, and cooking. The patient and his family may benefit from pastoral or spiritual counseling and support groups. Social services ensures continuity of care after discharge to the patient's home or to a rehabilitation facility and assists with follow-up care and financial and emotional concerns.

DISEASE BLOCK

Treating ischemic stroke

In an ischemic stroke, a thrombus occludes a cerebral vessel or one of its branches and blocks blood flow to the brain. The thrombus may either have formed in that vessel or have lodged there after traveling through the circulation from another site, such as the heart. Prompt treatment with a thrombolytic or an anticoagulant helps to minimize the effects of the occlusion. This flowchart shows how these drugs disrupt an ischemic stroke, thus minimizing the effects of cerebral ischemia and infarction. Keep in mind that thrombolytics can only be used within 3 hours after onset of the patient's symptoms.

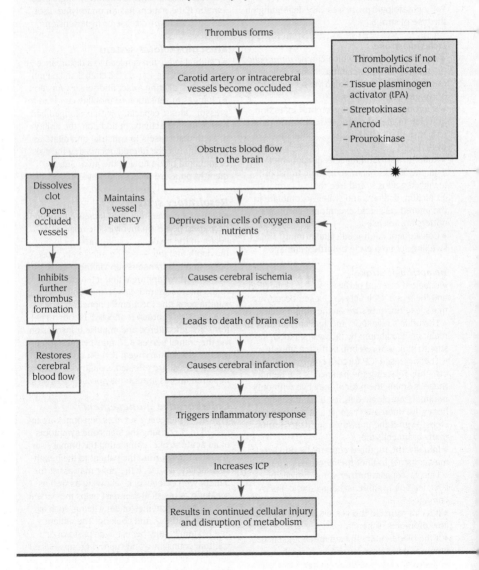

symptom onset and evidence of a hemorrhagic stroke (lesions larger than 1 cm) immediately.
◆ Magnetic resonance imaging assists in identifying areas of ischemia or infarction and cerebral swelling.
◆ Cerebral angiography reveals disruption or displacement of the cerebral circulation by occlusion, such as stenosis or acute thrombus, or hemorrhage.
◆ Digital subtraction angiography shows evidence of occlusion of cerebral vessels, lesions, or vascular abnormalities.
◆ Carotid duplex scan identifies the degree of stenosis.
◆ Brain scan shows ischemic areas but may not be conclusive for up to 2 weeks after a stroke.
◆ Single photon emission computed tomography and positron emission tomography scans identify areas of altered metabolism surrounding lesions not yet able to be detected by other diagnostic tests.
◆ Transesophageal echocardiogram reveals cardiac disorders, such as atrial thrombi, atrial septal defect, or patent foramen ovale, as causes of thrombotic stroke.
◆ Ophthalmoscopy may identify signs of hypertension and atherosclerotic changes in retinal arteries.
◆ EEG helps identify damaged areas of the brain.
◆ Electrocardiogram may detect atrial fibrillation, an arrhythmia strongly associated with embolic stroke.

Treatment

Treatment goals are to minimize and prevent further cerebral damage.

For ischemic stroke

◆ Thrombolytic therapy (alteplase, urokinase, streptokinase, reteplase) within the first 3 hours after the onset of symptoms to dissolve the clot, remove the occlusion, and restore blood flow, thus minimizing cerebral damage; these agents should be administered within 60 minutes of the patient arriving in the emergency department if criteria are met (See *Treating ischemic stroke*.)
◆ ICP management with monitoring, respiratory support (to maintain partial pressure of arterial carbon dioxide [$Paco_2$] between 30 to 35 mm Hg), and an osmotic diuretic (mannitol, to reduce cerebral edema)
◆ An antihypertensive, such as nitroglycerin paste, labetalol, or enalapril, to treat hypertension (systolic blood pressure greater than 185 mm Hg and diastolic blood pressure greater than 110 mm Hg) in stroke patients who are candidates for thrombolytic therapy or those

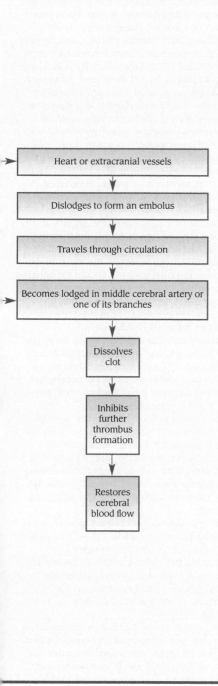

Heart or extracranial vessels

↓

Dislodges to form an embolus

↓

Travels through circulation

↓

Becomes lodged in middle cerebral artery or one of its branches

↓

Dissolves clot

↓

Inhibits further thrombus formation

↓

Restores cerebral blood flow

with specific medical conditions, such as an acute myocardial infarction, aortic dissection, hypertensive encephalopathy, or severe left ventricular function

◆ A stool softener to prevent straining, which increases ICP

◆ An anticonvulsant to treat or prevent seizures

◆ Surgery for large cerebellar infarction to remove infarcted tissue and decompress remaining live tissue

◆ Percutaneous transluminal angioplasty or stent insertion to open occluded vessels

◆ Anticoagulant therapy (heparin, warfarin) to maintain vessel patency and prevent further clot formation

◆ A histamine₂-receptor antagonist or proton pump inhibitor to protect against GI bleeding

For TIAs

◆ An antiplatelet agent (aspirin, ticlopidine, Aggrenox) to reduce the risk of platelet aggregation and subsequent clot formation

◆ Carotid endarterectomy to open partially (greater than 70%) occluded carotid arteries

For hemorrhagic stroke

◆ Vitamin K to reverse anticoagulant effects of warfarin in patients taking anticoagulant therapy

◆ Antihypertensive agents to treat hypertension in awake patients

◆ An analgesic, such as acetaminophen, to relieve headache associated with hemorrhagic stroke

◆ Aneurysm repair to prevent further hemorrhage

Special considerations

During the acute phase, efforts focus on survival needs and the prevention of further complications. Effective care emphasizes continuing neurologic assessment, respiratory support, continuous monitoring of vital signs, careful positioning to prevent aspiration and contractures, management of GI problems, and careful monitoring of fluid, electrolyte, and nutritional status. Patient care must also include measures to prevent such complications as infection.

◆ Maintain patent airway and oxygenation. Loosen constrictive clothing. Watch for ballooning of the cheek with respiration. The side that balloons is the side affected by the stroke. If the patient is unconscious he could aspirate saliva, so keep him in a lateral position to allow secretions to drain naturally or suction secretions, as needed. Insert an artificial airway, and start mechanical ventilation or supplemental oxygen, if necessary.

◆ Check vital signs and neurologic status, record observations, and report any significant changes to the physician. Monitor blood pressure, LOC, pupillary changes, motor function (voluntary and involuntary movements), sensory function, speech, skin color, temperature, signs of increased ICP, and nuchal rigidity or flaccidity.

⚠ **CLINICAL ALERT** *Remember, if a stroke is impending, blood pressure rises suddenly, the pulse is rapid and bounding, and the patient may complain of a headache. Also, watch for signs and symptoms of pulmonary emboli, such as chest pains, shortness of breath, dusky color, tachycardia, fever, and changed sensorium. If the patient is unresponsive, monitor his blood gas levels often and alert the physician to increased Paco₂ or decreased partial pressure of arterial oxygen.*

◆ Maintain fluid and electrolyte balance. If the patient can take liquids orally, offer them as often as fluid limitations permit. Administer I.V. fluids, as ordered; never give too much too fast because this can increase ICP. Offer the urinal or bedpan every 2 hours. If the patient is incontinent, he may need an indwelling urinary catheter, but this should be avoided, if possible, because of the risk of infection.

◆ Ensure adequate nutrition. Check for gag reflex before offering small oral feedings of semisolid foods. Place the food tray within the patient's visual field because loss of peripheral vision is common. If oral feedings aren't possible, insert a nasogastric tube.

◆ Manage GI problems. Be alert for signs that the patient is straining at elimination because this increases ICP. Modify diet, administer a stool softener, as ordered, and give a laxative, if necessary. If the patient vomits (usually during the first few days), keep him positioned on his side to prevent aspiration and consider gastric suction.

◆ Provide careful mouth care. Clean and irrigate the patient's mouth to remove food particles. Care for his dentures, as needed.

◆ Provide meticulous eye care. Remove secretions with a cotton ball and sterile normal saline solution. Instill eyedrops, as ordered. Patch the patient's affected eye if he can't close the lid.

◆ Position the patient and align his extremities correctly. Use high-topped sneakers or other devices to prevent footdrop and contracture and convoluted foam, flotation, or pulsating mattress or sheepskin to prevent pressure ulcers. To prevent pneumonia, turn the patient at least every 2 hours. Elevate the affected hand to control dependent edema, and place it in a functional position.

PREVENTION
Preventing stroke

Lifestyle modifications can help prevent heart attack and stroke. The American Heart Association recommends the following:

Healthy diet

Give patients the following advice:
♦ Eat five or more servings of fruits and vegetables daily.
♦ Eat six or more servings a day of grain products including whole grains.
♦ Eat fish at least twice a week, especially mackerel, lake trout, herring, sardines, albacore tuna, and salmon.
♦ Include fat-free and low-fat milk products, beans, lean meats, and skinless poultry.
♦ Choose fats and oils with 2 grams or less of saturated fat per serving (1 tablespoon).
♦ Limit your intake of foods high in calories or low in protein, such as carbonated beverages, high-sugar foods, and candy.
♦ Eat less than 6 grams of salt per day (1 teaspoon).
♦ Limit foods high in saturated fat, trans fat, or cholesterol, such as whole milk, fatty meats, tropical oils, and partially hydrogenated vegetable oils.

Exercise

Regular physical activity is defined by the American Heart Association as moderate to vigorous exercise 30 minutes a day on most or all days of the week. A lack of physical activity can lead to obesity and increase the risk of hypertension, heart attack, and stroke.

Smoking cessation

Even smoking filtered and light or ultralight cigarettes can lead to atherosclerosis. Quitting smoking will reduce this major risk factor for heart attack and stroke.

Blood pressure awareness

Individuals should know what their blood pressure is by having it checked by a practitioner. If it's high, the patient may be able to lower it by following a healthy diet and including exercise in his daily routine. If diet and exercise don't lower blood pressure, medication may be needed. Adherence to the medication regimen is foremost in reducing blood pressure and preventing stroke.

♦ Assist the patient with exercise. Perform range-of-motion exercises for both the affected and unaffected sides. Teach and encourage the patient to use his unaffected side to exercise his affected side.
♦ Give medications, as ordered, and watch for and report any adverse reactions.
♦ Establish and maintain communication with the patient. If he's aphasic, set up a simple method of communicating basic needs. Remember to phrase your questions so he'll be able to answer, using this system. Repeat yourself quietly and calmly (remember, he doesn't have hearing difficulty), and use gestures if necessary to help him understand. Even the unresponsive patient can hear, so don't say anything in his presence that you wouldn't want him to hear and remember.
♦ Provide psychological support. Set realistic short-term goals. Involve the patient's family in his care when possible, and explain his deficits and strengths.

Begin your rehabilitation of the patient with a stroke on admission. The amount of teaching you'll have to do depends on the extent of neurologic deficit.
♦ Establish rapport with the patient. Spend time with him, and provide a means of communication. Simplify your language, asking yes-or-no questions whenever possible. Don't correct his speech or treat him like a child. Remember that building rapport may be difficult because of the mood changes that may result from brain damage or as a reaction to being dependent.
♦ If necessary, teach the patient to comb his hair, dress, and wash. With the aid of a physical therapist and an occupational therapist, obtain appliances, such as walking frames, hand bars by the toilet, and ramps, as needed. The patient may fail to recognize that he has a paralyzed side (called unilateral neglect) and must be taught to inspect that side of his body for injury and to protect it from harm. If speech therapy is indicated, encourage the patient to begin as soon as possible and follow through with the

speech pathologist's suggestions. To reinforce teaching, involve the patient's family in all aspects of rehabilitation. With their cooperation and support, devise a realistic discharge plan, and let them help decide when the patient can return home.

◆ Before discharge, warn the patient or his family to report any premonitory signs or symptoms of a stroke, such as severe headache, drowsiness, confusion, or dizziness. Emphasize the importance of regular follow-up visits. (See *Preventing stroke*, page 317.)

◆ If aspirin has been prescribed to minimize the risk of thrombotic stroke, tell the patient to watch for possible GI bleeding. Make sure the patient and his family realize that acetaminophen isn't a substitute for aspirin.

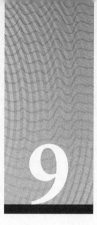

GASTROINTESTINAL SYSTEM

The GI system has the critical task of supplying essential nutrients to fuel all the physiologic and pathophysiologic activities of the body. Its functioning profoundly affects the quality of life through its impact on overall health. The GI system has two major components: the alimentary canal, or GI tract, and the accessory organs. A malfunction anywhere in the system can produce far-reaching metabolic effects, eventually threatening life itself.

The alimentary canal is a hollow muscular tube that begins in the mouth and ends at the anus. It includes the oral cavity, pharynx, esophagus, stomach, small intestine, large intestine, rectum, and anal canal. Peristalsis propels the ingested material along the tract; sphincters prevent its reflux. Accessory glands and organs include the salivary glands, liver, biliary duct system (gallbladder and bile ducts), and pancreas.

Together, the GI tract and accessory organs serve two major functions: digestion (breaking down food and fluids into simple chemicals that can be absorbed into the bloodstream and transported throughout the body) and elimination of waste products from the body through defecation.

Pathophysiologic changes

Disorders of the GI system typically manifest as vague, nonspecific complaints or problems that reflect disruption in one or more of the system's functions. For example, movement through the GI tract can be slowed, accelerated, or blocked, and secretion, absorption, or motility can be altered. As a result, one patient may present with several problems, the most common being anorexia, constipation, diarrhea, dysphagia, jaundice, nausea, and vomiting.

ANOREXIA

Anorexia is a loss of appetite or a lack of desire for food. Nausea, abdominal pain, and diarrhea may accompany it. Anorexia can result from dysfunction in the GI system or other systems, such as cancer, heart disease, renal disease, or central nervous system dysfunction.

Normally, a physiologic stimulus is responsible for the sensation of hunger. A falling blood glucose level stimulates the hunger center in the hypothalamus; rising blood fat and amino acid levels promote satiety. Hunger is also stimulated by contraction of an empty stomach and suppressed when the GI tract becomes distended, possibly as a result of stimulation of the vagus nerve. Sight, touch, and smell play subtle roles in controlling the appetite center.

In anorexia, the physiologic stimuli are present but the person has no appetite or desire to eat. Slow gastric emptying or gastric stasis can cause anorexia. High levels of neurotransmitters, such as serotonin (may contribute to satiety), and cortisol (may suppress hypothalamic control of hunger) also have been implicated as a cause of anorexia.

CONSTIPATION

Constipation is characterized by hard stools, difficult or infrequent defecation, and a decrease in the number of stools per week. It's defined individually because normal bowel habits range from two to three episodes of stool passage per day to one per week. Causes of constipation include dehydration, consumption of a low-bulk diet, a sedentary lifestyle, lack of regular exercise, and frequent repression of the urge to defecate. It's also an adverse effect of many medications.

When a person is dehydrated or delays defecation, more fluid is absorbed from the intestine, the stool becomes harder, and constipation ensues. High-fiber diets cause water to be drawn into the stool by osmosis, thereby keeping stool soft and encouraging movement through the intestine. High-fiber diets also cause intestinal dilation, which stimulates peristalsis. Conversely, a low-fiber diet contributes to constipation.

AGE ALERT *Elderly patients typically experience a decrease in intestinal motility and a slowing and dulling of neural impulses in the GI tract. Many older persons restrict fluid intake to prevent waking at night to use the bathroom or because they fear incontinence. This places them at risk for dehydration and constipation.*

A sedentary lifestyle, lack of exercise, limitations in physical activity, or inability to engage in physical activity can cause constipation because exercise stimulates the GI tract and promotes defecation. Antacids, opiates, and other drugs that inhibit bowel motility also lead to constipation.

Stress stimulates the sympathetic nervous system, and GI motility slows it. Absence or degeneration in the neural pathways of the large intestine also contributes to constipation. Other conditions, such as spinal cord trauma, multiple sclerosis, intestinal neoplasms, and hypothyroidism, can also cause constipation.

DIARRHEA

Diarrhea is an increase in the fluidity or volume of feces and the frequency of defecation. Factors that affect stool volume and consistency include water content of the colon and the presence of unabsorbed food, unabsorbable material, and intestinal secretions. Large-volume diarrhea is usually the result of an excessive amount of water, secretions, or both in the intestines. Small-volume diarrhea is usually caused by excessive intestinal motility. Diarrhea may also be caused by a parasympathetic stimulation of the intestine initiated by psychological factors, such as fear or stress.

The three major types of diarrhea are osmotic, secretory, and motility:

◆ *osmotic diarrhea* — The presence of a nonabsorbable substance such as synthetic sugar or increased numbers of osmotic particles in the intestine increases osmotic pressure and draws excess water into the intestine, thereby increasing the weight and volume of the stool.

◆ *secretory diarrhea* — A pathogen—such as a bacterial toxin (cholera, *Clostridium difficile*) or enteropathogenic virus—drugs, or presence of a tumor irritates the muscle and mucosal layers of the intestine. The consequent increase in motility and secretions (water, electrolytes, and mucus) results in diarrhea.

◆ *motility diarrhea* — Inflammation, neuropathy, or obstruction causes a reflex increase in intestinal motility that may expel the irritant or clear the obstruction.

DYSPHAGIA

Dysphagia — difficulty swallowing — can be caused by a mechanical obstruction of the esophagus or by impaired esophageal motility secondary to another disorder. Mechanical obstruction is characterized as intrinsic or extrinsic.

Intrinsic obstructions originate in the esophagus itself. Causes of intrinsic obstructions include tumors, strictures, and diverticular herniations. Extrinsic obstructions originate outside of the esophagus and narrow the lumen by exerting pressure on the esophageal wall. Most extrinsic obstructions result from a tumor.

Distention and spasm at the site of the obstruction during swallowing may cause pain. Upper esophageal obstruction causes pain 2 to 4 seconds after swallowing; lower esophageal obstructions, 10 to 15 seconds after swallowing. If a tumor is present, dysphagia begins with difficulty swallowing solids and eventually progresses to difficulty swallowing semisolids and liquids. Impaired motor function makes both liquids and solids difficult to swallow.

Neural or muscular disorders can also interfere with voluntary swallowing or peristalsis. This is known as functional dysphagia. Causes of functional dysphagia include dermatomyositis, stroke, Parkinson's disease, or achalasia. (See *What happens during swallowing*.) Malfunction of the upper esophageal striated muscles interferes with the voluntary phase of swallowing.

In achalasia, there's a complete lack of peristalsis within the body of the esophagus. Also, the lower esophageal sphincter doesn't relax to allow food to enter the stomach. Eventually, accumulated food raises the hydrostatic pressure and forces the sphincter open, and small amounts of food slowly move into the stomach.

CLOSER LOOK
What happens during swallowing

Before peristalsis can begin, the neural pattern to initiate swallowing, illustrated here, must occur:
◆ Food reaching the back of the mouth stimulates swallowing receptors that surround the pharyngeal opening.
◆ The receptors transmit impulses to the brain by way of the sensory portions of the trigeminal (V) and glossopharyngeal (IX) nerves.
◆ The brain's swallowing center relays motor impulses to the esophagus by way of the trigeminal (V), glossopharyngeal (IX), vagus (X), and hypoglossal (XII) nerves.
◆ Swallowing occurs.

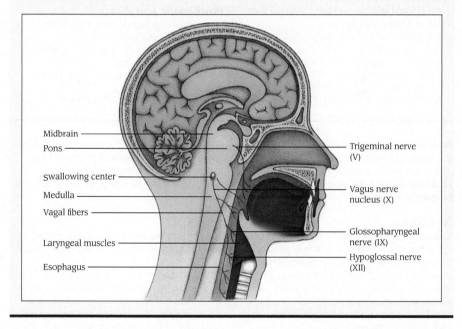

Midbrain
Pons
Swallowing center
Medulla
Vagal fibers
Laryngeal muscles
Esophagus

Trigeminal nerve (V)
Vagus nerve nucleus (X)
Glossopharyngeal nerve (IX)
Hypoglossal nerve (XII)

JAUNDICE

Jaundice—yellow pigmentation of the skin and sclera—is caused by an excess accumulation of bilirubin in the blood. Bilirubin, a product of red blood cell (RBC) breakdown, accumulates when production exceeds metabolism and excretion. This imbalance can result from excessive release of bilirubin precursors into the bloodstream or from impairment of its hepatic uptake, metabolism, or excretion. (See *Jaundice: Impaired bilirubin metabolism*, page 322.) Jaundice occurs when bilirubin levels exceed 2.0 to 2.5 mg/dl, which is about twice the upper limit of the normal range. Lower levels of bilirubin may cause detectable jaundice in patients with fair skin, and jaundice may be difficult to detect in patients with dark skin.

⚠️ **CLINICAL ALERT** *Jaundice in dark-skinned persons may appear as yellow staining in the sclera, hard palate, and palmar or plantar surfaces.*

The three main types of jaundice are hemolytic, hepatocellular, and obstructive:
◆ *hemolytic (or prehepatic) jaundice*—When RBC lysis exceeds the liver's capacity to conjugate bilirubin (binding bilirubin to a polar group makes it water soluble and able to be excreted by the kidneys), hemolytic jaundice occurs. Causes include transfusion reactions, sickle cell anemia, thalassemia, and autoimmune disease.
◆ *hepatocellular (or hepatic) jaundice*—Hepatocyte dysfunction limits uptake and conjugation of bilirubin. Liver dysfunction can occur in hepatitis, cancer, cirrhosis, or congenital disorders, and also can be caused by some drugs.
◆ *obstructive (or posthepatic) jaundice*—When the flow of bile out of the liver (through the hepatic duct) or through the common bile duct is blocked, the liver can conjugate bilirubin, but the bilirubin can't reach the small intestine.

Jaundice: Impaired bilirubin metabolism

Jaundice occurs in three forms: prehepatic, hepatic, and posthepatic. In all three, bilirubin levels in the blood increase.

Prehepatic jaundice
Certain conditions and disorders, such as transfusion reactions and sickle cell anemia, cause massive hemolysis.
◆ Red blood cells rupture faster than the liver can conjugate bilirubin.
◆ Large amounts of unconjugated bilirubin pass into the blood.
◆ Intestinal enzymes convert bilirubin to water-soluble urobilinogen for excretion in urine and stools. (Unconjugated bilirubin is insoluble in water, so it can't be directly secreted in urine.)

Hepatic jaundice
The liver becomes unable to conjugate or excrete bilirubin, leading to increased blood levels of conjugated and unconjugated bilirubin. This occurs in such disorders as hepatitis, cirrhosis, and metastatic cancer, and during prolonged use of drugs metabolized by the liver.

Posthepatic jaundice
In biliary and pancreatic disorders, bilirubin forms at its normal rate.
◆ Inflammation, scar tissue, tumor, or gallstones block the flow of bile into the intestines.
◆ Water-soluble conjugated bilirubin accumulates in the blood.
◆ The bilirubin is excreted in the urine.

Blockage of the hepatic duct by calculi or a tumor is considered an intrahepatic cause of obstructive jaundice. A blocked common bile duct is an extrahepatic cause that may be attributed to gallstones or a tumor.

NAUSEA
Nausea is feeling the urge to vomit. It may occur independently of vomiting, or it may precede or accompany it. Specific neural pathways haven't been identified, but increased salivation, diminished functional activities of the stomach, and altered small intestinal motility have been associated with nausea. Nausea may also be stimulated by high brain centers.

VOMITING
Vomiting is the forceful oral expulsion of gastric contents. The gastric musculature provides the ejection force. The gastric fundus and gastroesophageal sphincter relax, and forceful contractions of the diaphragm and abdominal wall muscles increase intra-abdominal pressure. This, combined with the annular contraction of the gastric pylorus, forces gastric contents into the esophagus. Increased intrathoracic pressure then moves the gastric content from the esophagus to the mouth.

Vomiting is controlled by two centers in the medulla: the vomiting center and the chemoreceptor trigger zone (CTZ). The vomiting center initiates the actual act of vomiting. It's stimulated by the GI tract, from higher brain stem and cortical centers, and from the CTZ. The CTZ can't induce vomiting by itself. Various stimuli or

drugs activate the zone, such as apomorphine, levodopa, digoxin, bacterial toxins, radiation, and metabolic abnormalities. The activated zone sends impulses to the medullary vomiting center, and the following sequence begins:
◆ The abdominal muscles and diaphragm contract.
◆ Reverse peristalsis begins, causing intestinal material to flow back into the stomach, distending it.
◆ The stomach pushes the diaphragm into the thoracic cavity, raising the intrathoracic pressure.
◆ The pressure forces the upper esophageal sphincter open, the glottis closes, and the soft palate blocks the nasopharynx.
◆ The pressure also forces the material up through the sphincter and out through the mouth.

Nausea and vomiting are manifestations of other disorders, such as acute abdominal emergencies, infections of the intestinal tract, central nervous system disorders, myocardial infarction, heart failure, metabolic and endocrinologic disorders, or as the adverse effect of many drugs. Nausea and vomiting can also be present in pregnancy. Vomiting may also be psychogenic, resulting from emotional or psychological disturbance.

Disorders

This section discusses disorders of the GI system, some of which are life-threatening. They include appendicitis, cholecystitis, cirrhosis, Crohn's disease, diverticular disease, gastroesophageal reflux disease, hemorrhoids, hepatitis (nonviral and viral), Hirschsprung's disease, hyperbilirubinemia, inguinal hernia, intestinal obstruction, irritable bowel syndrome, liver failure, malabsorption, pancreatitis, peptic ulcers, polyps (intestinal), and ulcerative colitis.

APPENDICITIS

The most common disease requiring emergency surgery, appendicitis is inflammation and obstruction of the vermiform appendix (a blind pouch attached to the cecum). Appendicitis may occur at any age, with peak incidence occurring from the late teens to the early 20s. It's more prevalent in men. Since the advent of antibiotics, the incidence and mortality rate from appendicitis have declined; if untreated, this disease is invariably fatal.

Causes
◆ Barium ingestion
◆ Fecal mass
◆ Mucosal ulceration
◆ Stricture
◆ Viral infection

Pathophysiology
Mucosal ulceration triggers inflammation, which temporarily obstructs the appendix. The obstruction blocks mucus outflow. Pressure in the now distended appendix increases, and the appendix contracts. Bacteria multiply, and inflammation and pressure continue to increase, restricting blood flow to the pouch and causing severe abdominal pain.

Signs and symptoms
◆ Abdominal pain, caused by inflammation of the appendix and bowel obstruction and distention, begins in the epigastric region, and then shifts to the right lower quadrant
◆ Anorexia after the onset of pain
◆ Nausea or vomiting caused by the inflammation
◆ Low-grade fever from systemic manifestation of inflammation and leukocytosis
◆ Tenderness from inflammation, positive rebound tenderness and psoas and obturator signs

Complications
◆ Wound infection
◆ Intra-abdominal abscess
◆ Fecal fistula
◆ Intestinal obstruction
◆ Incisional hernia
◆ Peritonitis

Diagnosis
◆ White blood cell count is moderately high with an increased number of immature cells.

◆ X-ray with radiographic contrast agent reveals failure of the appendix to fill with contrast.

Treatment
◆ Maintenance of nothing by mouth (NPO) status until surgery
◆ Fowler's position to aid in pain relief
◆ GI intubation for decompression
◆ Appendectomy
◆ An antibiotic to treat infection if peritonitis occurs
◆ Parental replacement of fluid and electrolytes to reverse possible dehydration resulting from surgery or nausea and vomiting

Special considerations
If appendicitis is suspected, or during preparation for appendectomy:
◆ Administer I.V. fluids to prevent dehydration. Never administer a cathartic or an enema, which may rupture the appendix. Maintain NPO status, and administer the analgesic judiciously because it may mask symptoms.
◆ To lessen pain, place the patient in Fowler's position. Never apply heat to the right lower abdomen; this may cause the appendix to rupture. An ice bag may be used for pain relief.

After appendectomy
◆ Monitor vital signs and intake and output. Give an analgesic as ordered.
◆ Encourage the patient to cough, breathe deeply, and turn frequently to prevent pulmonary complications.
◆ Document bowel sounds, passing of flatus, and bowel movements. In a patient whose nausea and abdominal rigidity have subsided, these signs indicate readiness to resume taking in oral fluids.
◆ Watch closely for possible surgical complications. Continuing pain and fever may signal an abscess. The complaint that "something gave way" may mean wound dehiscence. If an abscess or peritonitis develops, incision and drainage may be necessary. Frequently assess the dressing for wound drainage.
◆ Help the patient ambulate as soon as possible after surgery.
◆ In appendicitis complicated by peritonitis, a nasogastric tube may be needed to decompress the stomach and reduce nausea and vomiting. If so, record drainage and give good mouth and nose care.

CHOLECYSTITIS

Cholecystitis—acute or chronic inflammation causing painful distention of the gallbladder—is usually associated with a gallstone impacted in the cystic duct.

Cholecystitis accounts for 10% to 25% of all patients requiring gallbladder surgery. The acute form is most common among middle-aged women; the chronic form, among elderly people. The prognosis is good with treatment.

Causes
◆ Abnormal metabolism of cholesterol and bile salts
◆ Gallstones (the most common cause)
◆ Poor or absent blood flow to the gallbladder

Pathophysiology
In acute cholecystitis, inflammation of the gallbladder wall usually develops after a gallstone lodges in the cystic duct. (See *Understanding gallstone formation*, pages 326 and 327.) When bile flow is blocked, the gallbladder becomes inflamed and distended. Bacterial growth, usually *Escherichia coli,* may contribute to the inflammation. Edema of the gallbladder (and sometimes the cystic duct) obstructs bile flow, which chemically irritates the gallbladder. Cells in the gallbladder wall may become oxygen starved and die as the distended organ presses on vessels and impairs blood flow. The dead cells slough off, and an exudate covers ulcerated areas, causing the gallbladder to adhere to surrounding structures.

Signs and symptoms
◆ Acute abdominal pain in the right upper quadrant that may radiate to the back, between the shoulders, or to the front of the chest secondary to inflammation and irritation of nerve fibers
◆ Colic due to the passage of gallstones along the bile duct
◆ Nausea and vomiting triggered by the inflammatory response
◆ Chills related to fever
◆ Low-grade fever secondary to inflammation
◆ Jaundice from obstruction of the common bile duct by calculi
◆ Previous attack of biliary colic or cholecystitis

Complications
◆ Perforation and abscess formation
◆ Fistula formation
◆ Gangrene
◆ Empyema
◆ Cholangitis
◆ Hepatitis
◆ Pancreatitis
◆ Gallstone ileus
◆ Carcinoma

Diagnosis
◆ Ultrasonography detects gallstones as small as 2 mm and distinguishes between obstructive and nonobstructive jaundice.
◆ X-ray reveals gallstones if they contain enough calcium to be radiopaque; also helps disclose porcelain gallbladder (hard, brittle gallbladder due to calcium deposited in wall), limy bile, and gallstone ileus.
◆ Technetium-labeled scan reveals cystic duct obstruction and acute or chronic cholecystitis if ultrasound doesn't visualize the gallbladder.
◆ Percutaneous transhepatic cholangiography supports the diagnosis of obstructive jaundice and reveals calculi in the ducts.
◆ Levels of serum alkaline phosphate, lactate dehydrogenase, aspartate aminotransferase, and total bilirubin are high; the serum amylase level slightly elevated, and the icteric index is elevated.
◆ The white blood cell count is slightly elevated during a cholecystitis attack.

Treatment
◆ Cholecystectomy to surgically remove the inflamed gallbladder (laparoscopic or an "open" procedure)
◆ Choledochostomy to surgically create an opening into the common bile duct for drainage
◆ Percutaneous transhepatic cholecystostomy
◆ Endoscopic retrograde cholangiopancreatography for removal of gallstones
◆ Lithotripsy to break up gallstones and relieve obstruction
◆ Oral ursodiol or chenodiol to dissolve calculi
◆ Contact dissolution therapy using methyl terbutyl ether injected directly into the stone for dissolution in 1 to 3 days (an experimental procedure because the drug is highly flammable and toxic)
◆ Low-fat diet to prevent attacks
◆ Vitamin K to relieve itching, jaundice, and bleeding tendencies due to vitamin K deficiencies
◆ An antibiotic for use during acute attack for treatment of infection
◆ Nasogastric tube insertion during acute attack for abdominal decompression

Special considerations
Patient care for cholecystitis focuses on supportive care and close postoperative observation.
◆ Before surgery, teach the patient to deep breathe, cough, expectorate, and perform leg exercises that are necessary after surgery. Also teach splinting, repositioning, and ambulation techniques. Explain the procedures that will be performed before, during, and after surgery to

help ease the patient's anxiety and to help ensure his cooperation.
- After surgery, monitor vital signs for signs of bleeding, infection, or atelectasis.
- Evaluate the incision site for bleeding. Serosanguineous drainage is common during the first 24 to 48 hours if the patient has a wound drain. If, after a choledochostomy, a T-tube drain is placed in the duct and attached to a drainage bag, make sure the drainage tube has no kinks. Also, check that the connecting tubing from the T tube is well secured to the patient to prevent dislodgment.
- Measure and record T-tube drainage daily (200 to 300 ml is normal).
- Teach patients who will be discharged with a T tube how to perform dressing changes and routine skin care.
- Monitor intake and output. Allow the patient nothing by mouth for 24 to 48 hours or until bowel sounds return and nausea and vomiting cease (postoperative nausea may indicate a full bladder).
- If the patient doesn't void within 8 hours (or if the amount voided is inadequate based on I.V. fluid intake), percuss over the symphysis pubis for bladder distention (especially in patients receiving an anticholinergic). Patients who have had a laparoscopic cholecystectomy may be discharged the same day or within 24 hours after surgery. These patients should have minimal pain, be able to tolerate a regular diet within 24 hours after surgery, and be able to return to normal activity within 1 week.
- Encourage deep-breathing and leg exercises every hour. The patient should ambulate after surgery. Provide elastic stockings to support leg muscles and promote venous blood flow, thus preventing stasis and clot formation.
- Evaluate the location, duration, and character of pain. Administer adequate medication to relieve pain, especially before such activities as deep breathing and ambulation, which increase pain.
- At discharge, advise the patient against heavy lifting or straining for 6 weeks. Urge him to walk daily. Tell him that food restrictions are unnecessary unless he has an intolerance to a specific food or some underlying condition (such as diabetes, atherosclerosis, or obesity) that requires such restriction.
- Instruct the patient to notify the surgeon if he has pain for more than 24 hours, anorexia, nausea or vomiting, fever, or tenderness in the abdominal area or if he notices jaundice, because these may indicate a biliary tract injury from the cholestectomy, requiring immediate attention.

CIRRHOSIS

Cirrhosis is a chronic disease characterized by diffuse destruction and fibrotic regeneration of hepatic cells. As necrotic tissue yields to fibrosis, this disease damages liver tissue and normal vasculature, impairs blood and lymph flow, and ultimately causes hepatic insufficiency. It's twice as common in men as in women, and it's especially prevalent among malnourished persons older than age 50 with chronic alcoholism. Mortality is high; many patients die within 5 years of onset.

Causes

Cirrhosis may be a result of a wide range of diseases. The following clinical types of cirrhosis reflect its diverse etiology.

Hepatocellular disease

This group includes the following disorders:
- Postnecrotic cirrhosis accounts for 10% to 30% of patients and stems from various types of hepatitis (such as Types A, B, C, D viral hepatitis) or toxic exposures.
- Laënnec's cirrhosis, also called portal, nutritional, or alcoholic cirrhosis, is the most common type and is primarily caused by hepatitis C and alcoholism. Liver damage results from malnutrition (especially dietary protein) and long-term alcohol use. Fibrous tissue forms in portal areas and around central veins.
- Autoimmune disease, such as sarcoidosis or chronic inflammatory bowel disease, may cause cirrhosis.

Cholestatic diseases

This group includes diseases of the biliary tree (biliary cirrhosis resulting from bile duct diseases suppressing bile flow) and sclerosing cholangitis.

Metabolic diseases

This group includes such disorders as Wilson's disease, alpha$_1$-antitrypsin, and hemochromatosis (pigment cirrhosis).

Other types of cirrhosis

Other types of cirrhosis include Budd-Chiari syndrome (epigastric pain, liver enlargement, and ascites due to hepatic vein obstruction), cardiac cirrhosis, and cryptogenic cirrhosis. Cardiac cirrhosis is rare; the liver damage results from right-sided heart failure. Cryptogenic refers to cirrhosis of unknown etiology.

Pathophysiology

Cirrhosis begins with hepatic scarring or fibrosis. The scar begins as an increase in extracellular

CLOSER LOOK
Understanding gallstone formation

Abnormal metabolism of cholesterol and bile salts plays an important role in gallstone formation. The liver makes bile continuously. The gallbladder concentrates and stores it until the duodenum signals it needs it to help digest fat. Changes in the composition of bile may allow gallstones to form. Changes to the absorptive ability of the gallbladder lining may also contribute to gallstone formation.

Inside the liver
Certain conditions, such as age, obesity, and estrogen imbalance, cause the liver to secrete bile that's abnormally high in cholesterol or lacking the proper concentration of bile salts.

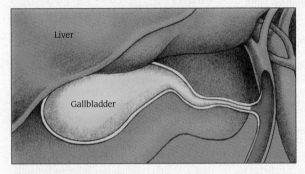

Inside the gallbladder
When the gallbladder concentrates this bile, inflammation may occur. Excessive reabsorption of water and bile salts makes the bile less soluble. Cholesterol, calcium, and bilirubin precipitate into gallstones.

Fat entering the duodenum causes the intestinal mucosa to secrete the hormone cholecystokinin, which stimulates the gallbladder to contract and empty. If a stone lodges in the cystic duct, the gallbladder contracts but can't empty.

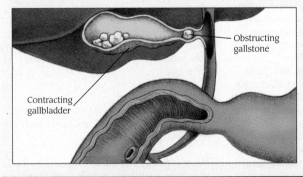

matrix components—fibril-forming collagens, proteoglycans, fibronectin, and hyaluronic acid. The site of collagen deposition varies with the cause. Hepatocyte function is eventually impaired as the matrix changes. Fat-storing cells are believed to be the source of the new matrix components. Contraction of these cells may also contribute to disruption of the lobular architecture and obstruction of the flow of blood or bile.

Cellular changes producing bands of scar tissue also disrupt the lobular structure.

Signs and symptoms
Early stages
♦ Anorexia from distaste for certain foods
♦ Nausea and vomiting from inflammatory response and systemic effects of liver inflammation

Understanding gallstone formation *(continued)*

Inside the common bile duct

If a stone lodges in the common bile duct, the bile can't flow into the duodenum. Bilirubin is absorbed into the blood and causes jaundice.

Biliary narrowing and swelling of the tissue around the stone can also cause irritation and inflammation of the common bile duct.

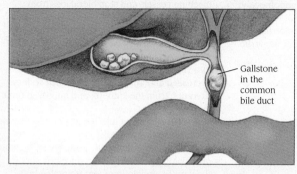

Gallstone in the common bile duct

Inside the biliary tree

Inflammation can progress up the biliary tree into any of the bile ducts. This causes scar tissue, fluid accumulation, cirrhosis, portal hypertension, and bleeding.

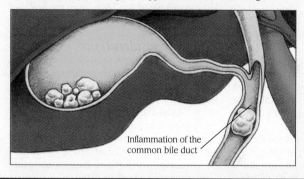

Inflammation of the common bile duct

♦ Diarrhea from malabsorption
♦ Dull abdominal ache from liver inflammation

Late stages

♦ *Respiratory*—pleural effusion, limited thoracic expansion due to abdominal ascites; interferes with efficient gas exchange, which causes hypoxia
♦ *Central nervous system*—progressive signs or symptoms of hepatic encephalopathy, including lethargy, mental changes, slurred speech, asterixis, peripheral neuritis, paranoia, hallucinations, extreme obtundation, and coma—secondary to the failure of the metabolism of ammonia into urea and consequent delivery of toxic ammonia to the brain
♦ *Hematologic*—bleeding tendencies (nosebleeds, easy bruising, bleeding gums), splenomegaly, anemia resulting from thrombocytopenia

(secondary to splenomegaly and decreased vitamin K absorption), and portal hypertension
♦ *Endocrine*—testicular atrophy, menstrual irregularities, gynecomastia, and loss of chest and axillary hair from decreased hormone metabolism
♦ *Skin*—abnormal pigmentation, spider angiomas, palmar erythema, and jaundice related to impaired hepatic function; severe pruritus secondary to jaundice from bilirubinemia; extreme dryness and poor tissue turgor related to malnutrition
♦ *Hepatic*—jaundice from decreased bilirubin metabolism; hepatomegaly secondary to liver scarring and portal hypertension; ascites and edema of the legs from portal hypertension and decreased plasma proteins; hepatic encephalopathy from ammonia toxicity; and hepatorenal

syndrome from advanced liver disease and subsequent renal failure

◆ *Miscellaneous*—musty breath secondary to ammonia buildup; enlarged superficial abdominal veins due to portal hypertension; pain in the right upper abdominal quadrant that worsens when patient sits up or leans forward, due to inflammation and irritation of area nerve fibers; palpable liver or spleen due to organomegaly; temperature of 101° to 103° F (38.3° to 39.4° C) due to inflammatory response; hemorrhage from esophageal varices resulting from portal hypertension. (See *What happens in portal hypertension*.)

Complications
◆ Respiratory compromise
◆ Ascites
◆ Portal hypertension
◆ Jaundice
◆ Coagulopathy
◆ Hepatic encephalopathy
◆ Bleeding esophageal varices; acute GI bleeding
◆ Liver failure
◆ Renal failure

Diagnosis
◆ Liver biopsy reveals tissue destruction and fibrosis.
◆ Abdominal X-ray shows enlarged liver, cysts, or gas within the biliary tract or liver, liver calcification, and massive fluid accumulation (ascites).
◆ Computed tomography and liver scans show liver size, abnormal masses, and hepatic blood flow and obstruction.
◆ Esophagogastroduodenoscopy reveals bleeding esophageal varices, stomach irritation or ulceration, or duodenal bleeding and irritation.
◆ Blood studies reveal elevated levels of liver enzymes, total serum bilirubin, and indirect bilirubin; decreased levels of total serum albumin, protein, hemoglobin, and electrolytes; prolonged prothrombin time; decreased hematocrit; and deficiency of vitamins A, C, and K.
◆ Urine studies show increased bilirubin and urobilirubinogen levels.
◆ Fecal studies show a decreased fecal urobilirubinogen level.

Treatment
◆ Vitamins and nutritional supplements to help heal damaged liver cells and improve nutritional status
◆ An antacid to reduce gastric distress and decrease the potential for GI bleeding
◆ A potassium-sparing diuretic to reduce fluid accumulation
◆ Vasopressin to treat esophageal varices

◆ Esophagogastric intubation with multilumen tubes to control bleeding from esophageal varices or other hemorrhage sites by using balloons to exert pressure on the bleeding site
◆ Gastric lavage until the contents are clear; with an antacid and a histamine antagonist if the bleeding is secondary to a gastric ulcer
◆ Esophageal balloon tamponade to compress bleeding vessels and stop blood loss from esophageal varices
◆ Paracentesis to relieve abdominal pressure and remove ascitic fluid
◆ Surgical shunt placement to divert ascites into venous circulation, leading to weight loss, decreased abdominal girth, increased sodium excretion from the kidneys, and improved urine output
◆ A sclerosing agent injected into oozing vessels to cause clotting and sclerosis
◆ Transjugular intrahepatic portosystemic shunt (a radiologic procedure) to reduce pressure in the varices, preventing them from bleeding
◆ Insertion of portosystemic shunts to control bleeding from esophageal varices and decrease portal hypertension (diverts a portion of the portal vein blood flow away from the liver; seldom performed)

Special considerations
Patients with cirrhosis need close observation, intensive supportive care, and sound nutritional counseling.
◆ Check skin, gums, stools, and vomitus regularly for bleeding. Apply pressure to injection sites to prevent bleeding. Warn the patient against taking nonsteroidal anti-inflammatory drugs, straining at stool, and blowing his nose or sneezing too vigorously. Suggest using an electric razor and soft toothbrush.
◆ Observe the patient closely for signs of behavioral or personality changes. Report increasing stupor, lethargy, hallucinations, or neuromuscular dysfunction. Awaken the patient periodically to determine level of consciousness. Watch for asterixis, a sign of developing hepatic encephalopathy.
◆ To assess fluid retention, weigh the patient and measure abdominal girth at least daily; inspect ankles and sacrum for dependent edema; and accurately record intake and output. Carefully evaluate the patient before, during, and after paracentesis; this drastic loss of fluid may induce shock.
◆ To prevent skin breakdown associated with edema and pruritus, avoid using soap when you bathe the patient; instead, use lubricating lotion or moisturizing agents. Handle the patient gently, and turn and reposition him often to keep his skin intact.

CLOSER LOOK

What happens in portal hypertension

Portal hypertension (elevated pressure in the portal vein) occurs when blood flow meets increased resistance. This common result of cirrhosis may also stem from mechanical obstruction and occlusion of the hepatic veins (Budd-Chiari syndrome).

As the pressure in the portal vein rises, blood backs up into the spleen and flows through collateral channels to the venous system, bypassing the liver. Thus, portal hypertension causes:
◆ splenomegaly with thrombocytopenia

◆ dilated collateral veins (esophageal varices, hemorrhoids, or prominent abdominal veins)
◆ ascites.

In many patients, the first sign of portal hypertension is bleeding esophageal varices (dilated tortuous veins in the submucosa of the lower esophagus).

Esophageal varices commonly cause massive hematemesis, requiring emergency care to control hemorrhage and prevent hypovolemic shock.

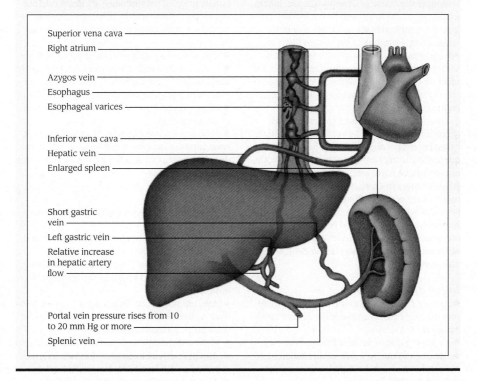

Superior vena cava
Right atrium
Azygos vein
Esophagus
Esophageal varices
Inferior vena cava
Hepatic vein
Enlarged spleen
Short gastric vein
Left gastric vein
Relative increase in hepatic artery flow
Portal vein pressure rises from 10 to 20 mm Hg or more
Splenic vein

◆ Tell the patient that rest and good nutrition will conserve energy and decrease metabolic demands on the liver. Urge him to eat frequent small meals. Stress the need to avoid infections and abstain from alcohol. Refer the patient to Alcoholics Anonymous, if necessary.

CROHN'S DISEASE

Crohn's disease, also known as *regional enteritis* or *granulomatous colitis,* is inflammation of any part of the GI tract (usually the proximal portion of the colon and less commonly the terminal ileum), extending through all layers of the intestinal wall. It may also involve regional lymph nodes and the mesentery. Crohn's disease is most prevalent in adults between ages 20 and 40.

Causes

The exact cause is unknown but conditions that may contribute include:
◆ allergies
◆ genetic predisposition

◆ immune disorders
◆ infection
◆ lymphatic obstruction.

🔗 **GENETIC LINK** *Crohn's disease sometimes occurs in identical twins, and 10% to 20% of patients with the disease have one or more affected relatives.*

Researchers recently found a mutation in the gene known as NOD2. The mutation is twice as common in patients with Crohn's disease when compared with the general population. It seems to alter the body's ability to combat bacteria. Currently, there's no practical method to screen for the presence of this genetic mutation.

Pathophysiology

Whatever the cause of Crohn's disease, inflammation spreads slowly and progressively. Enlarged lymph nodes block lymph flow in the submucosa. Lymphatic obstruction leads to edema, mucosal ulceration and fissures, abscesses, and sometimes granulomas. Mucosal ulcerations are called "skipping lesions" because they aren't continuous, as in ulcerative colitis.

Oval, elevated patches of closely packed lymph follicles in the lining of the small intestine—called Peyer's patches—become inflamed. Subsequent fibrosis thickens the bowel wall and causes stenosis, or narrowing of the lumen. (See *Bowel changes in Crohn's disease.*) The serous membrane becomes inflamed (serositis), inflamed bowel loops adhere to other diseased or normal loops, and diseased bowel segments become interspersed with healthy ones. Finally, diseased parts of the bowel become thicker, narrower, and shorter.

Signs and symptoms

◆ Steady, colicky pain in the right lower quadrant due to acute inflammation and nerve fiber irritation
◆ Cramping due to acute inflammation
◆ Tenderness due to acute inflammation
◆ Palpable mass in the right lower quadrant due to bowel thickening
◆ Weight loss secondary to diarrhea and malabsorption
◆ Diarrhea due to bile salt malabsorption, loss of healthy intestinal surface area, and bacterial growth
◆ Steatorrhea secondary to fat malabsorption
◆ Bloody stools secondary to bleeding from inflammation and ulceration

Complications

◆ Anal fistula
◆ Perineal abscess

◆ Fistulas to the bladder or vagina or to the skin in an old scar area
◆ Intestinal obstruction
◆ Nutrient deficiencies from poor digestion and malabsorption of bile salts and vitamin B_{12}
◆ Fluid imbalances

Diagnosis

◆ Fecal occult blood test reveals minute amounts of blood in stools.
◆ Small bowel X-ray with barium shows irregular mucosa, ulceration, and stiffening.
◆ Barium enema reveals the string sign (segments of stricture separated by normal bowel) and possibly fissures and narrowing of the bowel.
◆ Sigmoidoscopy and colonoscopy reveal patchy areas of inflammation (helps to rule out ulcerative colitis), with cobblestone-like mucosal surface. With colon involvement, ulcers may be seen.
◆ Computed tomography scan detects abscesses.
◆ Video capsule endoscopy identifies mild, early abnormalities from Crohn's disease and can confirm Crohn's disease during normal barium X-ray.
◆ Biopsy reveals granulomas in up to one-half of all specimens.
◆ Blood tests reveal increased white blood cell count and erythrocyte sedimentation rate and decreased potassium, calcium, magnesium, and hemoglobin levels.

Treatment

◆ Sulfasalazine or 5-aminosalicylate to reduce inflammation
◆ A corticosteroid to reduce inflammation and, subsequently, diarrhea, pain, and bleeding
◆ Immunomodulators, such as mercaptopurine and azathioprine, to suppress the response to antigens
◆ Antitumor necrosis factor agent infliximab to treat moderate to severe disease that doesn't respond to conventional therapy
◆ Metronidazole to treat perianal complications
◆ An antidiarrheal to combat diarrhea (not used in patients with significant bowel obstruction)
◆ An opioid analgesic to control pain and diarrhea
◆ Stress reduction and reduced physical activity to rest the bowel and allow it to heal
◆ Vitamin supplements to replace and compensate for the bowel's inability to absorb vitamins
◆ Dietary changes (elimination of fruits, vegetables, high-fiber foods, dairy products, spicy and fatty foods, foods that irritate the mucosa, carbonated or caffeinated beverages, and other foods or liquids that stimulate excessive intestinal activity) to decrease bowel activity while still providing adequate nutrition

Bowel changes in Crohn's disease

As Crohn's disease progresses, fibrosis thickens the bowel wall and narrows the lumen. Narrowing — or stenosis — can occur in any part of the intestine and cause varying degrees of intestinal obstruction. At first, the mucosa may appear normal, but as the disease progresses it takes on a "cobblestone" appearance as shown.

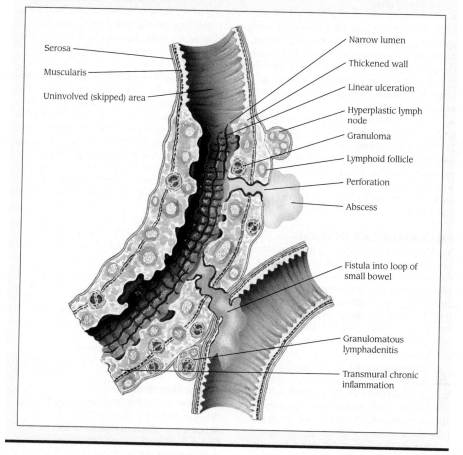

Serosa

Muscularis

Uninvolved (skipped) area

Narrow lumen

Thickened wall

Linear ulceration

Hyperplastic lymph node

Granuloma

Lymphoid follicle

Perforation

Abscess

Fistula into loop of small bowel

Granulomatous lymphadenitis

Transmural chronic inflammation

◆ Surgery, if necessary, to repair bowel perforation, drain abscesses, and correct massive hemorrhage, fistulas, or acute intestinal obstruction; colectomy with ileostomy in patients with extensive disease of the large intestine and rectum

Special considerations

Although treatment is based largely on symptoms, you should monitor the patient's status carefully for signs and symptoms of worsening.
◆ Record fluid intake and output (including the amount of stool), and weigh the patient daily. Watch for dehydration and maintain fluid and electrolyte balance. Be alert for signs of intestinal

bleeding (bloody stools); check stools daily for occult blood.
◆ If the patient is receiving a steroid, watch for adverse reactions, such as GI bleeding. Remember that steroids can mask signs of infection.
◆ Check the hemoglobin level and hematocrit regularly. Give an iron supplement and a blood transfusion, as ordered.
◆ Give an analgesic as ordered.
◆ Provide good patient hygiene and meticulous mouth care if the patient is restricted to nothing by mouth. After each bowel movement, give good skin care. Always keep a clean, covered

bedpan within the patient's reach. Ventilate the room to eliminate odors.

◆ Observe the patient for fever and pain or pneumaturia, which may signal a bladder fistula. Abdominal pain and distention and fever may indicate intestinal obstruction. Watch for stools from the vagina and an enterovaginal fistula.

◆ Before ileostomy, arrange for a visit by an enterostomal therapist.

◆ After surgery, frequently check the patient's I.V. and nasogastric tube for proper functioning. Monitor vital signs and fluid intake and output. Watch for wound infection. Provide meticulous stoma care, and teach it to the patient and family. Realize that an ileostomy changes the patient's body image, so offer reassurance and emotional support.

◆ Stress the need for a severely restricted diet and bed rest, which may be trying, particularly for the young patient. Encourage him to try to reduce tension. If stress is clearly an aggravating factor, refer him for counseling.

◆ Refer the patient to a support group such as the Crohn's and Colitis Foundation of America.

DIVERTICULAR DISEASE

In diverticular disease, bulging pouches (diverticula) in the GI wall push the mucosal lining through the surrounding muscle. Although the most common site for diverticula is in the sigmoid colon, they may develop anywhere, from the proximal end of the pharynx to the anus. Other typical sites include the duodenum, near the pancreatic border or the ampulla of Vater, and the jejunum.

⚠ **CLINICAL ALERT** *Diverticular disease is common in Western countries, suggesting that a low-fiber diet reduces stool bulk and leads to excessive colonic motility. The consequent increased intraluminal pressure causes herniation of the mucosa.*

Diverticular disease of the stomach is rare and is usually a precursor of peptic or neoplastic disease. Diverticular disease of the ileum (Meckel's diverticulum) is the most common congenital anomaly of the GI tract.

Diverticular disease has two clinical forms:

◆ *diverticulosis,* in which diverticula are present but don't cause symptoms

◆ *diverticulitis,* in which diverticula are inflamed and may cause potentially fatal obstruction, infection, or hemorrhage.

🏮 **AGE ALERT** *Diverticular disease is most prevalent in men older than age 40 and persons who eat a low-fiber diet. More than one-half of all patients older than age 50 have colonic diverticula.*

Causes

◆ Defects in colon wall strength
◆ Diminished colonic motility and increased intraluminal pressure
◆ Low-fiber diet

Pathophysiology

Diverticula probably result from high intraluminal pressure on an area of weakness in the GI wall, where blood vessels enter. Diet may be a contributing factor because insufficient fiber reduces fecal residue, narrows the bowel lumen, and leads to high intra-abdominal pressure during defecation.

In diverticulitis, retained undigested food and bacteria accumulate in the diverticular sac. This hard mass cuts off the blood supply to the thin walls of the sac, making them more susceptible to attack by colonic bacteria. Inflammation follows and may lead to perforation, abscess, peritonitis, obstruction, or hemorrhage. Occasionally, the inflamed colon segment may adhere to the bladder or other organs and cause a fistula. (See *Diverticulitis of the colon.*)

Signs and symptoms

Typically the patient with diverticulosis is asymptomatic and will remain so unless diverticulitis develops.

Mild diverticulitis

◆ Moderate left-sided lower-abdominal pain secondary to inflammation of diverticula
◆ Low-grade fever from trapping of bacteria-rich stool in the diverticula
◆ Leukocytosis from infection secondary to trapping of bacteria-rich stool in the diverticula

Severe diverticulitis

◆ Abdominal rigidity from rupture of the diverticula, abscesses, and peritonitis
◆ Left lower quadrant pain secondary to rupture of the diverticula and subsequent inflammation and infection
◆ High fever, chills, hypotension from sepsis, and shock from the release of fecal material from the rupture site
◆ Microscopic or massive hemorrhage from rupture of diverticulum near a vessel

Chronic diverticulitis

◆ Constipation, ribbon-like stools, intermittent diarrhea, and abdominal distention resulting from intestinal obstruction (possible when fibrosis and adhesions narrow the bowel's lumen)
◆ Abdominal rigidity and pain, diminishing or absent bowel sounds, nausea, and vomiting secondary to intestinal obstruction

Complications
◆ Abscess
◆ Peritonitis
◆ Intestinal obstruction
◆ Rectal hemorrhage
◆ Septicemia

Diagnosis
◆ Upper GI series confirms or rules out diverticulosis of esophagus and upper bowel.
◆ Barium enema reveals filling of diverticula, which confirms diagnosis.
◆ Sigmoidoscopy and colonoscopy help exclude diseases with similiar signs and symptoms.
◆ Biopsy reveals evidence of benign disease, ruling out cancer.
◆ Blood studies show an elevated erythrocyte sedimentation rate in diverticulitis.

Treatment
◆ Liquid or bland diet, stool softeners, and occasional doses of mineral oil for symptomatic diverticulosis to relieve symptoms, minimize irritation, and lessen the risk of progression to diverticulitis
◆ High-residue diet for treatment of diverticulosis after pain has subsided to help decrease intra-abdominal pressure during defecation
◆ Exercise to increase stool passage rate
◆ An antibiotic to treat infection of the diverticula
◆ An analgesic, such as morphine, to control pain and to relax smooth muscle
◆ An antispasmodic to control muscle spasms
◆ Colon resection with removal of involved segment to correct cases refractory to medical treatment
◆ Temporary colostomy, if necessary, to drain abscesses and rest the colon in diverticulitis accompanied by perforation, peritonitis, obstruction, or fistula
◆ Blood transfusions, if necessary, to treat blood loss from hemorrhage and fluid replacement as needed

Special considerations
Management of uncomplicated diverticulosis chiefly involves thorough patient education about fiber and dietary habits.
◆ Describe diverticula and how they form.
◆ Stress the importance of dietary fiber and the harmful effects of constipation and straining during defecation. Encourage increased intake of foods high in indigestible fiber, including fresh fruits and vegetables, whole grain bread, and wheat or bran cereals. Warn that a high-fiber diet may temporarily cause flatulence and discomfort. Advise the patient to relieve constipation with a stool softener or a bulk-forming

Diverticulitis of the colon

In diverticulitis retained undigested food and bacteria accumulate in the diverticular sac as shown below.

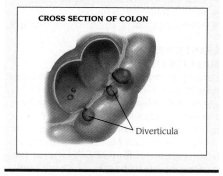

CROSS SECTION OF COLON

Diverticula

cathartic. However, caution against taking a bulk-forming cathartic without plenty of water; if swallowed dry, they may absorb enough moisture in the mouth and throat to swell and obstruct the esophagus or trachea.
◆ If the patient with diverticulosis is hospitalized, administer medications as ordered; observe his stools carefully for frequency, color, and consistency; and keep accurate pulse and temperature charts (they may signal developing inflammation or complications).
Management of diverticulitis depends on the severity of symptoms.
◆ In mild disease, give medications as ordered, explain diagnostic tests and preparations for tests, observe stools carefully, and maintain accurate records of temperature, pulse, respirations, intake, and output.
◆ If diverticular bleeding occurs, the patient may require angiography and catheter placement for vasopressin infusion. If so, inspect the insertion site frequently for bleeding, check pedal pulses often, and keep the patient from flexing his legs at the groin.
◆ Watch for vasopressin-induced fluid retention (apprehension, abdominal cramps, convulsions, oliguria, or anuria) and severe hyponatremia (hypotension; rapid, thready pulse; cold, clammy skin; and cyanosis).
After surgery to resect the colon:
◆ Watch for signs of infection.
◆ Provide meticulous wound care as perforation may already have infected the area.
◆ Check drain sites frequently for signs of infection (purulent drainage or foul odor) or fecal drainage.
◆ Change dressings as necessary.

◆ Encourage coughing and deep breathing to prevent atelectasis.
◆ Watch for signs of postoperative bleeding (hypotension and decreased hemoglobin levels and hematocrit).
◆ Record intake and output accurately.
◆ Keep the nasogastric tube patent.
◆ Teach ostomy care as needed.
◆ Arrange for a visit by an enterostomal therapist.

GASTROESOPHAGEAL REFLUX DISEASE

Popularly known as heartburn, gastroesophageal reflux disease (GERD) refers to backflow of gastric or duodenal contents or both into the esophagus and past the lower esophageal sphincter (LES), without associated belching or vomiting. The reflux of gastric contents causes acute epigastric pain, usually after a meal. The pain may radiate to the chest or arms. It commonly occurs in pregnant or obese persons. Lying down after a meal also contributes to reflux.

Causes

◆ Food, alcohol, or cigarettes that lower LES pressure
◆ Hiatal hernia
◆ Increased abdominal pressure, such as with obesity or pregnancy
◆ Medications, such as morphine, diazepam, calcium channel blockers, meperidine, and anticholinergics
◆ Nasogastric intubation for more than 4 days
◆ Weakened esophageal sphincter

Pathophysiology

Normally, the LES maintains enough pressure around the lower end of the esophagus to close it and prevent reflux. Typically the sphincter relaxes after each swallow to allow food into the stomach. In GERD, the sphincter doesn't remain closed (usually due to deficient LES pressure or pressure within the stomach exceeding LES pressure) and the pressure in the stomach pushes the stomach contents into the esophagus. The high acidity of the stomach contents causes pain and irritation when it enters the esophagus. (See *How heartburn occurs*.)

Signs and symptoms

◆ Burning pain in the epigastric area, possibly radiating to the arms and chest, from the reflux of gastric contents into the esophagus causing irritation and esophageal spasm
◆ Pain, usually after a meal or when lying down, secondary to increased abdominal pressure causing reflux

◆ Feeling of fluid accumulation in the throat without a sour or bitter taste due to hypersecretion of saliva

Complications

◆ Reflux esophagitis
◆ Esophageal stricture
◆ Esophageal ulceration
◆ Chronic pulmonary disease from aspiration of gastric contents in the throat

Diagnosis

Diagnostic tests are aimed at determining the underlying cause of GERD:
◆ Esophageal acidity test evaluates the competence of the LES and provides objective measure of reflux.
◆ Acid perfusion test confirms esophagitis and distinguishes it from cardiac disorders.
◆ Esophagoscopy allows visual examination of the lining of the esophagus to reveal the extent of the disease and confirm pathologic changes in mucosa.
◆ Barium swallow identifies hiatal hernia as the cause or esophageal stricture as a complication.
◆ Upper GI series detects hiatal hernia or motility problems.
◆ Esophageal manometry evaluates resting pressure of LES and determines sphincter competence.

Treatment

◆ Diet therapy with frequent, small meals and avoidance of eating before going to bed to reduce abdominal pressure and reduce the incidence of reflux
◆ Positioning—sitting up during and after meals and sleeping with head of bed elevated—to reduce abdominal pressure and prevent reflux
◆ Increased fluid intake to wash gastric contents out of the esophagus
◆ Antacids to neutralize acidic content of the stomach and minimize irritation
◆ A foaming agent, such as Gaviscon, to prevent reflux in patients without damage to the esophagus
◆ A histamine-2 receptor antagonist to inhibit gastric acid secretion
◆ A proton pump inhibitor to reduce gastric acidity
◆ A prokinetic agent to promote gastric emptying and increase LES
◆ A cholinergic to increase LES pressure
◆ Smoking cessation to improve LES pressure (nicotine lowers LES pressure)
◆ Surgery if hiatal hernia is the cause or patient has refractory symptoms

CLOSER LOOK
How heartburn occurs

Hormonal fluctuations, mechanical stress, and the effects of certain foods and drugs can decrease lower esophageal sphincter (LES) pressure. When LES pressure falls and intra-abdominal or intragastric pressure rises, the normally contracted LES relaxes inappropriately and allows reflux of gastric acid or bile secretions into the lower esophagus. There, the reflux irritates and inflames the esophageal mucosa, causing pyrosis (heartburn).

Persistent inflammation can cause LES pressure to decrease even more and may trigger a recurrent cycle of reflux and pyrosis.

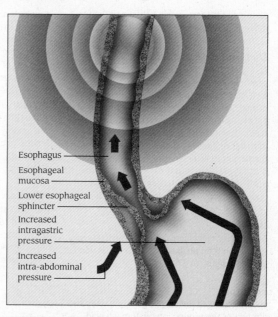

Esophagus

Esophageal mucosa

Lower esophageal sphincter

Increased intragastric pressure

Increased intra-abdominal pressure

The U.S. Food and Drug Administration has approved several devices to treat GERD, including:
◆ Bard EndoCinch system, an endoscopic device for chronic GERD, that places stitches in the LES to strengthen it
◆ Stretta system, another endoscopic device for chronic GERD, that uses electrodes to create tiny cuts on the LES; as these cuts heal, they leave scar tissue that strengthens the LES.

Special considerations
Teach the patient what causes reflux, how to avoid reflux with an antireflux regimen (medication, diet, and positional therapy), and what signs and symptoms to watch for and report.
◆ Instruct the patient to avoid circumstances that increase intra-abdominal pressure (such as bending, coughing, vigorous exercise, tight clothing, constipation, and obesity) as well as substances that reduce sphincter control (cigarettes, alcohol, fatty foods, and caffeine).
◆ Advise the patient to sit upright, particularly after meals, and to eat small, frequent meals. Tell him to avoid highly seasoned food, acidic juices, alcoholic drinks, bedtime snacks, and foods high in fat or carbohydrates, which reduce

LES pressure. He should eat meals at least 2 to 3 hours before lying down.
◆ Tell the patient to take an antacid as ordered (usually 1 and 3 hours after meals and at bedtime).
◆ Teach the patient correct preparation for diagnostic testing. For example, he shouldn't eat for 6 to 8 hours before a barium swallow or endoscopy.
◆ After surgery using a thoracic approach, carefully watch and record chest tube drainage and respiratory status. If needed, give chest physiotherapy and oxygen. Position the patient with a nasogastric tube in semi-Fowler's position to help prevent reflux. Offer reassurance and emotional support. (See *Preventing GI reflux*, page 336.)

HEMORRHOIDS
Hemorrhoids are varicosities in the superior or inferior hemorrhoidal venous plexus. Dilation and enlargement of the superior plexus of the superior hemorrhoidal veins above the dentate line cause internal hemorrhoids. Enlargement of the plexus of the inferior hemorrhoidal veins below the dentate line causes external hemorrhoids, which may protrude from the rectum.

Preventing GI reflux

Changing his lifestyle will help the patient to prevent GI reflux.

Diet and eating habits
Foods, such as caffeine, chocolate, spicy food, carbonated beverages, orange juice, liquor, wine, and tomato sauce, stimulate the production of acid. Large meals expand the stomach and put pressure on the lower esophageal sphincter (LES). Gravity helps keep the stomach juices from backing up into the esophagus: Don't allow the patient to lie down for 2 hours after eating. If nighttime heartburn is a concern, raise the head of the bed 6 to 8 inches because a flat position places pressure on the LES.

Weight
Being overweight increases abdominal pressure, which can then push stomach contents up into the esophagus.

Smoking
Nicotine relaxes the esophageal sphincter and stimulates the production of stomach acid.

Smoking also may injure the esophagus by causing irritation, making it more susceptible to damage from acid reflux. Smoking can decrease gastric motility and reduce the effectiveness of digestion because the stomach takes longer to empty.

Stress
Although stress itself doesn't cause heartburn, the anxiety that comes along with stress can lead to behaviors that increase the risk of heartburn, such as overeating, drinking, and smoking.

Alcohol
Alcohol can increase the production of stomach acid and can also lower the esophageal sphincter, which allows stomach acids to move up into the esophagus. Alcohol also makes the esophagus more sensitive to stomach acid.

Hemorrhoids occur in both sexes. Incidence is generally highest between ages 20 and 50.

Causes
◆ Constipation, low-fiber diet
◆ Obesity
◆ Pregnancy
◆ Prolonged sitting
◆ Straining at defecation

Pathophysiology
Hemorrhoids result from activities that increase intravenous pressure, causing distention and engorgement. Predisposing factors include prolonged sitting, straining at defecation, constipation, low-fiber diet, pregnancy, and obesity. Other factors include hepatic disease, such as cirrhosis, amebic abscesses, or hepatitis; alcoholism; and anorectal infections.

Hemorrhoids are classified as first, second, third, or fourth degree, depending on their severity. First-degree hemorrhoids are confined to the anal canal. Second-degree hemorrhoids prolapse during straining but reduce spontaneously. Third-degree hemorrhoids are prolapsed hemorrhoids that require manual reduction after each bowel movement. Fourth-degree

hemorrhoids are irreducible. Signs and symptoms vary accordingly.

Signs and symptoms
◆ Painless, intermittent bleeding during defecation from irritation and injury to the hemorrhoid mucosa
◆ Bright red blood on stool or toilet tissue due to injury to hemorrhoid mucosa
◆ Anal itching from poor anal hygiene
◆ Vague feeling of anal discomfort when bleeding occurs
◆ Prolapse of rectal mucosa from straining
◆ Pain from thrombosis of external hemorrhoids

Complications
◆ Constipation
◆ Local infection
◆ Thrombosis of hemorrhoids
◆ Secondary anemia from severe or recurrent bleeding

Diagnosis
◆ Physical examination confirms external hemorrhoids.
◆ Anoscopy and flexible sigmoidoscopy visualize internal hemorrhoids.

Treatment

◆ High-fiber diet, increased fluid intake, and a bulking agent to relieve constipation
◆ Avoidance of prolonged sitting on the toilet to prevent venous congestion
◆ A local anesthetic to decrease local swelling and pain
◆ Hydrocortisone cream and suppositories to reduce edematous, prolapsed hemorrhoids, and itching
◆ Warm sitz baths to relieve pain
◆ Injection sclerotherapy or rubber band ligation to reduce prolapsed hemorrhoids
◆ Hemorrhoidectomy by cauterization or excision

Special considerations

Patient care for hemorrhoids includes preoperative and postoperative support.
◆ To prepare the patient for hemorrhoidectomy, administer an enema, as ordered (usually 2 to 4 hours before surgery), and record if the enema produced feces, water, or nothing. Shave the perianal area, and clean the anus and surrounding skin.
◆ Postoperatively, check for signs of prolonged rectal bleeding, administer an analgesic, and provide sitz baths, as ordered.
◆ When the patient can resume oral feedings, administer a bulk medication, such as psyllium, about 1 hour after the evening meal, to ensure a daily stool. Warn against using stool-softening medications soon after hemorrhoidectomy because a firm stool acts as a natural dilator to prevent anal stricture from the scar tissue. (Some patients may need repeated dilation either digitally or with an anal dilator to prevent such narrowing.)
◆ Keep the wound site clean to prevent infection and irritation.
◆ Before discharge, stress the importance of regular bowel habits and good anal hygiene. Warn against too-vigorous wiping with washcloths and against using harsh soaps. Encourage the use of medicated astringent pads and white, unscented toilet paper (the fixative in colored paper and fragrances can irritate the skin).

HEPATITIS, NONVIRAL

Nonviral hepatitis is an inflammation of the liver that usually results from exposure to certain chemicals or drugs. Most patients recover from this illness, although a few develop fulminating hepatitis or cirrhosis.

Causes

◆ Hepatotoxic chemicals
◆ Hepatotoxic drugs

Pathophysiology

Various hepatotoxins—such as carbon tetrachloride, acetaminophen, trichloroethylene, poisonous mushrooms, and vinyl chloride—can cause hepatitis. After exposure to these agents, hepatic cellular necrosis, scarring, Kupffer cell hyperplasia, and infiltration by mononuclear phagocytes occur with varying severity. Alcohol, anoxia, and preexisting liver disease exacerbate the effects of some toxins.

Drug-induced (idiosyncratic) hepatitis may begin with a hypersensitivity reaction unique to the individual, unlike toxic hepatitis, which appears to affect all exposed people indiscriminately. Among possible causes are niacin, halothane, sulfonamides, isoniazid, acetaminophen, methyldopa, and phenothiazines (cholestasis-induced hepatitis). Symptoms of hepatic dysfunction may appear at any time during or after exposure to these drugs, but it usually manifests after 2 to 5 weeks of therapy.

In autoimmune hepatitis (lupoid hepatitis), the body's immune system attacks liver cells, causing them to become inflamed. A genetic factor may predispose some people to autoimmune diseases. About 70% of those with autoimmune hepatitis are women ages 15 to 40. The condition is usually chronic and can lead to cirrhosis.

Signs and symptoms

◆ Anorexia, nausea, and vomiting due to systemic effects of liver inflammation
◆ Jaundice from decreased bilirubin metabolism, leading to hyperbilirubinemia
◆ Dark urine from an elevated urobilinogen level
◆ Hepatomegaly due to inflammation
◆ Possible abdominal pain from liver inflammation
◆ Clay-colored stool secondary to decreased bile in the GI tract from liver necrosis
◆ Pruritus secondary to jaundice and hyperbilirubinemia

Complications

◆ Cirrhosis
◆ Hepatic failure

Diagnosis

◆ Liver enzyme levels, such as serum aspartate aminotransferase and alanine aminotransferase, are elevated.
◆ Total and direct bilirubin levels are elevated.
◆ The alkaline phosphatase level is elevated.
◆ White blood cell count and eosinophil count are elevated.
◆ Antibodies, including antinuclear antibodies, smooth-muscle cell antibodies, or liver and

kidney microsomes, are elevated in autoimmune hepatitis.
◆ Liver biopsy identifies underlying pathology, especially infiltration with white blood cells and eosinophils.

Treatment
◆ Lavage, catharsis, or hyperventilation, depending on the route of exposure, to remove the causative agent
◆ Acetylcysteine as an antidote for acetaminophen poisoning
◆ A corticosteroid to relieve symptoms of drug-induced and autoimmune hepatitis
◆ Azathioprine (Imuran), an immunosuppressant, in conjunction with corticosteroids to treat autoimmune hepatitis

Special considerations
Preventive measures should include instructing the patient about the proper use of drugs and the proper handling of cleaning agents and solvents.
◆ Monitor laboratory studies, and note trends.
◆ Monitor the patient's vital signs, and provide appropriate support to maintain vital functioning, depending on the severity of symptoms.

HEPATITIS, VIRAL
Viral hepatitis is a common infection of the liver, resulting in hepatic cell destruction, necrosis, and autolysis. In most patients, hepatic cells eventually regenerate with little or no residual damage. However, old age and serious underlying disorders make complications more likely. The prognosis is poor if edema and hepatic encephalopathy develop.

Five major forms of hepatitis are recognized:
◆ Type A (infectious or short-incubation hepatitis) is most common among male homosexuals and in people with human immunodeficiency virus (HIV) infection. It's commonly spread via the fecal-oral route by the ingestion of fecal contaminants.
◆ Type B (serum or long-incubation hepatitis) also is most common among HIV-positive individuals. Routine screening of donor blood for the hepatitis B surface antigen has reduced the incidence of posttransfusion cases, but transmission by needles shared by drug abusers remains a major problem.
◆ Type C accounts for about 20% of all viral hepatitis cases and for most posttransfusion cases.
◆ Type D (delta hepatitis) is responsible for about 50% of all cases of fulminant hepatitis, which has a high mortality rate. Developing in 1% of patients with viral hepatitis, fulminant hepatitis causes unremitting liver failure with encephalopathy. It progresses to coma and

commonly leads to death within 2 weeks. In the United States, type D occurs only in people who are frequently exposed to blood and blood products, such as I.V. drug users and hemophilia patients. Type D hepatitis is found only in patients with an acute or chronic episode of hepatitis B and requires the presence of hepatitis B surface antigen. The type D virus depends on the double-shelled type B virus to replicate. (For this reason, type D infection can't outlast a type B infection.)
◆ Type E (formerly grouped with types C and D under the name non-A, non-B hepatitis) occurs primarily among patients who have recently returned from an endemic area (such as India, Africa, Asia, or Central America). It's more common in young adults and more severe in pregnant woman. (See *Viral hepatitis from A to E,* pages 340 and 341.)
◆ Other types continue to be identified with growing patient populations and sophisticated laboratory identification techniques.

Causes
The five major forms of viral hepatitis result from infection with the causative viruses: A, B, C, D, or E.

Pathophysiology
Hepatic damage is usually similar in all types of viral hepatitis. Varying degrees of cell injury and necrosis occur.

On entering the body, the virus causes hepatocyte injury and death, either by directly killing the cells or by activating inflammatory and immune reactions. The inflammatory and immune reactions will, in turn, injure or destroy hepatocytes by lysing the infected or neighboring cells. Later, direct antibody attack against the viral antigens causes further destruction of the infected cells. Edema and swelling of the interstitium lead to collapse of capillaries and decreased blood flow, tissue hypoxia, and scarring and fibrosis.

Signs and symptoms
Signs and symptoms reflect the stage of the disease.

Prodromal stage
◆ Easy fatigue and generalized malaise due to systemic effects of liver inflammation
◆ Anorexia and mild weight loss due to systemic effects of liver inflammation
◆ Arthralgia and myalgia due to systemic effects of liver inflammation
◆ Nausea and vomiting from GI effects of liver inflammation

◆ Changes in the senses of taste and smell related to liver inflammation
◆ Fever secondary to inflammatory process
◆ Right upper quadrant tenderness from liver inflammation and irritation of area nerve fibers
◆ Dark-colored urine from urobilinogen
◆ Clay-colored stools from decreased bile in the GI tract

Clinical stage
◆ Worsening of all symptoms of the prodromal stage
◆ Itching from increased bilirubin in the blood
◆ Abdominal pain or tenderness from continued liver inflammation
◆ Jaundice from an elevated bilirubin level in the blood

Recovery stage
The patient's symptoms subside and appetite returns.

Complications
◆ Chronic persistent hepatitis, which may prolong recovery up to 8 months
◆ Chronic active hepatitis
◆ Cirrhosis
◆ Hepatic failure and death
◆ Primary hepatocellular carcinoma

Diagnosis
◆ Hepatitis profile study identifies antibodies specific to the causative virus, establishing the type of hepatitis.
◆ Serum aspartate aminotransferase and serum alanine aminotransferase levels are increased in the prodromal stage.
◆ Serum alkaline phosphatase level is slightly increased.
◆ Serum bilirubin level may remain high into late disease, especially in severe cases.
◆ Prothrombin time is prolonged (greater than 3 seconds longer than normal indicates severe liver damage).
◆ White blood cell count reveals transient neutropenia and lymphopenia followed by lymphocytosis.
◆ Liver biopsy confirms suspicion of chronic hepatitis.

Treatment
◆ Rest to minimize energy demands
◆ Avoidance of alcohol or other drugs to prevent further hepatic damage
◆ Diet therapy with small, high-calorie meals to combat anorexia

◆ Reduction of protein intake if signs of coma (lethargy, confusion, and mental changes) develop to help reverse the symtoms
◆ Parental nutrition if patient can't eat because of persistent vomiting
◆ Vaccination against hepatitis A and B to provide immunity to these viruses before transmission occurs

Medication
◆ All forms of hepatitis other than B and C: no specific drug therapy
◆ Chronic hepatitis B: treated successfully with a synthetic thymidine nucleoside analogue (telbivudine)
◆ Hepatitis C: treated somewhat successfully with interferon alfa-2b and peginterferon
◆ Antiemetics given 30 minutes before meals to relieve nausea and prevent vomiting.
◆ Cholestyramine for severe pruritus.

Special considerations
Use enteric precautions when caring for patients with type A or E hepatitis. Practice standard precautions for all patients.
◆ Inform visitors about isolation precautions.
◆ Provide rest periods throughout the day. Schedule treatments and tests so that the patient can rest between bouts of activity.
◆ Because inactivity may make the patient anxious, include diversionary activities as part of his care. Gradually add activities to his schedule as he begins to recover.
◆ Encourage the patient to eat. Don't overload his meal tray or overmedicate him because this will diminish his appetite.
◆ Make sure the patient drinks plenty of fluids (at least 135 oz [4 L]/day). Encourage the anorectic patient to drink fruit juices. Also, offer chipped ice and effervescent soft drinks to maintain hydration without inducing vomiting.
◆ Administer supplemental vitamins and commercial feedings, as ordered. If symptoms are severe and the patient can't tolerate oral intake, provide I.V. therapy and parenteral nutrition, as ordered by the physician.
◆ Record the patient's weight daily, and keep intake and output records. Observe stools for color, consistency, and amount, and record the frequency of bowel movements.
◆ Watch for signs of fluid shift, such as weight gain and orthostasis.
◆ Watch for signs of hepatic coma, dehydration, pneumonia, vascular problems, and pressure ulcers.
◆ In fulminant hepatitis, maintain electrolyte balance and a patent airway, prevent infections, and control bleeding. Correct hypoglycemia and

Viral hepatitis from A to E

This chart compares the features of each (characterized) type of viral hepatitis. Other types are emerging.

Feature	Hepatitis A	Hepatitis B
Incubation	15 to 45 days	30 to 180 days
Onset	Acute	Insidious
Age-group most affected	Children, young adults	Any age
Transmission	Fecal-oral, sexual (especially oral-anal contact), nonpercutaneous (sexual, maternal-neonatal), percutaneous (rare)	Blood-borne; parenteral route, sexual, maternal-neonatal; virus is shed in all body fluids
Severity	Mild	Mild to severe
Prognosis	Generally good	Worsens with age and debility
Progression to chronicity	None	Occasional

any other complications while awaiting liver regeneration and repair.
◆ Before discharge, emphasize the importance of having regular medical checkups for at least 1 year. The patient will have an increased risk of developing hepatoma. Warn the patient against using alcohol or over-the-counter drugs during this period. Teach him to recognize the signs of a recurrence. (See *Preventing the spread of hepatitis*.)

HIRSCHSPRUNG'S DISEASE

Hirschsprung's disease, also called *congenital megacolon* and *congenital aganglionic megacolon*, is a congenital disorder of the large intestine, characterized by the absence or marked reduction of parasympathetic ganglion cells in the colorectal wall.

Hirschsprung's disease appears to be a familial, congenital defect, occurring in 1 in 5,000 live births. It's up to seven times more common in males than in females (although the aganglionic segment is usually shorter in males) and is most prevalent in whites. Total aganglionosis affects

both sexes equally. Females with Hirschsprung's disease are at higher risk for having affected children. This disease usually coexists with other congenital anomalies, particularly trisomy 21 and anomalies of the urinary tract such as megaloureter.

Without prompt treatment, an infant with colonic obstruction may die within 24 hours from enterocolitis that leads to severe diarrhea and hypovolemic shock. With prompt treatment, the prognosis is good.

Causes
◆ Familial congenital defect

Pathophysiology

In Hirschsprung's disease, parasympathetic ganglion cells in the colorectal wall are absent or markedly reduced in number. The aganglionic bowel segment contracts without the reciprocal relaxation needed to propel feces forward. Impaired intestinal motility causes severe, intractable constipation. Colonic obstruction can ensue, causing bowel dilation and subsequent occlusion of surrounding blood and lymphatics. The ensuing mucosal edema, ischemia, and infarction draw large amounts of fluid into the

Hepatitis C	Hepatitis D	Hepatitis E
15 to 160 days	14 to 64 days	14 to 60 days
Insidious	Acute	Acute
More common in adults	Any age	Ages 20 to 40
Blood-borne; parenteral route	Parenteral route; most people infected with hepatitis D are also infected with hepatitis B	Primarily fecal-oral
Moderate	Can be severe and lead to fulminant hepatitis	Highly virulent with common progression to fulminant hepatitis and hepatic failure, especially in pregnant patients
Moderate	Fair, worsens in chronic cases; can lead to chronic hepatitis D and chronic liver disease	Good unless pregnant
10% to 50% of cases	Occasional	None

bowel, causing copious amounts of liquid stool. Continued infarction and destruction of the mucosa can lead to infection and sepsis.

Signs and symptoms
In the neonate
◆ Failure to pass meconium within 24 to 48 hours due to inability to propel intestinal contents forward
◆ Bile stained or fecal vomiting as a result of bowel obstruction
◆ Abdominal distention secondary to retention of intestinal contents and bowel obstruction
◆ Irritability due to resultant abdominal distention
◆ Feeding difficulties and failure to thrive related to retention of intestinal contents and abdominal distention
◆ Dehydration related to subsequent feeding difficulties and inability to ingest adequate fluids
◆ Overflow diarrhea secondary to increased water secretion into bowel with bowel obstruction

In children
◆ Intractable constipation due to decreased GI motility
◆ Abdominal distention from retention of stool

PREVENTION

Preventing the spread of hepatitis

To help prevent the spread of hepatitis, review the following guidelines with your patient:
◆ Stress the importance of frequent, through hand washing.
◆ Tell the patient not to share food, eating utensils, or toothbrushes.
◆ If the patient has hepatitis A or E, warn him not to contaminate food or water with fecal matter because the disease is transmitted by the fecal-oral route.
◆ If the patient has hepatitis B, C, D, or G, explain that transmission occurs through the exchange of blood or body fluids that contain bood. While infected, he shouldn't donate blood or have sexual contact.
◆ Advise the patient to take extra care to avoid cutting himself.

◆ Easily palpated fecal masses from retention of stool

◆ Wasted extremities (in severe cases) secondary to impaired intestinal motility and its effects on nutrition and intake

◆ Loss of subcutaneous tissue (in severe cases) secondary to malnutrition

◆ Large protuberant abdomen due to retention of stool and consequent changes in fluid and electrolyte homeostasis

In adults (occurring rarely and more prevalent in men)

◆ Abdominal distention from decreased bowel motility and constipation

◆ Chronic intermittent constipation secondary to impaired intestinal motility

Complications

◆ Bowel perforation
◆ Electrolyte imbalances
◆ Nutritional deficiencies
◆ Enterocolitis
◆ Hypovolemic shock
◆ Sepsis

Diagnosis

◆ Rectal biopsy confirms diagnosis by showing the absence of ganglion cells.

◆ Barium enema, used in older infants, reveals a narrowed segment of distal colon with a saw-toothed appearance and a funnel-shaped segment above it. This test confirms the diagnosis and assesses the extent of intestinal involvement.

◆ Rectal manometry detects failure of the internal anal sphincter to relax and contract.

◆ Upright plain abdominal X-rays show marked colonic distention.

Treatment

◆ Corrective surgery to pull the normal ganglionic segment through to the anus (usually delayed until the infant is at least age 10 months)

◆ Daily colonic lavage to empty the bowel of the infant until the time of surgery

◆ Temporary colostomy or ileostomy to compress the colon in instances of total bowel obstruction

Special considerations

Before emergency decompression surgery

◆ Maintain fluid and electrolyte balance and prevent shock.

◆ Provide adequate nutrition and hydrate with I.V. fluids, as needed. Transfusions may be necessary to correct shock or dehydration.

◆ Relieve respiratory distress by keeping the patient in an upright position. (Place an infant in an infant seat.)

After colostomy or ileostomy

◆ Place the infant in a heated incubator, with the temperature set at 98° to 99° F (36.7° to 37.2° C), or in a radiant warmer. Monitor vital signs, watching for sepsis and enterocolitis (increased respiratory rate with abdominal distention).

◆ Carefully monitor and record fluid intake and output (including drainage from ileostomy or colostomy) and electrolyte levels. Ileostomy is especially likely to cause excessive electrolyte loss. Measure and record nasogastric (NG) drainage, and replace fluids and electrolytes, as ordered. Check stools carefully for excess water — a sign of fluid loss.

◆ Check urine for specific gravity, glucose (hyperalimentation may lead to osmotic diuresis), and blood.

◆ To prevent aspiration pneumonia and skin breakdown, turn and reposition the patient often. In addition, suction the nasopharynx frequently.

◆ Keep the area around the stoma clean and dry, and cover it with dressings or a colostomy or ileostomy appliance to collect drainage. Use aseptic technique until the wound heals. Watch for prolapse, discoloration, or excessive bleeding. (Slight bleeding is common.) To prevent excoriation, use a powder, such as karaya gum, or a protective stoma disk.

◆ Oral feeding can begin when bowel sounds return. An infant may tolerate breastmilk or predigested formulas best.

◆ Teach parents to recognize the signs and symptoms of fluid loss and dehydration (decreased urine output, sunken eyes, and poor skin turgor) and of enterocolitis (sudden marked abdominal distention, vomiting, diarrhea, fever, and lethargy).

◆ Before discharge, if possible, make sure that the parents consult with an enterostomal therapist for information on ostomy care.

Before corrective surgery

◆ At least once a day, perform colonic lavage with normal saline solution to evacuate the colon; ordinary enemas and laxatives won't clean it adequately. Keep accurate records of how much lavage solution is instilled. Repeat lavage until the return solution is completely free from fecal particles.

◆ Administer an antibiotic for bowel preparation, as ordered.

After corrective surgery

◆ Keep the wound clean and dry, and check for significant inflammation (some inflammation is normal). Don't use a rectal thermometer or suppository until the wound has healed. After 3 to 4 days, the infant will have a first bowel movement, a liquid stool, which will probably create discomfort. Record the number of stools.

♦ Check urine for blood, especially in a male infant; extensive surgical manipulation may cause bladder trauma.

♦ Watch for signs of possible anastomotic leaks (sudden development of abdominal distention unrelieved by gastric aspiration, temperature spike, and extreme irritability), which may lead to pelvic abscess.

♦ Begin oral feedings when active bowel sounds begin and NG drainage decreases. As an additional check, clamp the NG tube for brief, intermittent periods, as ordered. If abdominal distention develops, the patient isn't ready to begin oral feedings. Begin oral feedings with clear fluids, increasing bulk as tolerated.

♦ Instruct parents to withhold foods that have increased the number of stools previously. Reassure them that their child will probably gain sphincter control and be able to eat a normal diet, but warn that complete continence may take several years to develop and constipation may recur at times.

♦ Because an infant with Hirschsprung's disease needs surgery and hospitalization so early in life, parents have difficulty establishing an emotional bond with their child. To promote bonding, encourage them to participate in their child's care as much as possible.

Hyperbilirubinemia

Hyperbilirubinemia, also called *neonatal jaundice,* is the result of hemolytic processes in the neonate marked by an elevated serum bilirubin level and mild jaundice. It can be physiologic (with jaundice the only symptom) or pathologic (resulting from an underlying disease).

Physiologic jaundice generally develops 24 to 48 hours after birth and disappears by day 7 in full-term neonates and by day 9 or 10 in premature infants. The serum unconjugated bilirubin level doesn't exceed 12 mg/dl. Pathologic jaundice may appear anytime after the first day of life and persist beyond 7 days. The serum bilirubin level is greater than 12 mg/dl in a term infant or 15 mg/dl in a premature infant, or it increases more than 5 mg/dl in 24 hours. Physiologic jaundice is self-limiting; pathologic jaundice varies, depending on the cause.

Causes

♦ Abnormal red blood cell (RBC) morphology
♦ Bile duct atresia
♦ Blood type incompatibility
♦ Breast-feeding
♦ Choledochal cyst
♦ Crigler-Najjar syndrome
♦ Deficiencies of RBC enzymes (glucose 6-phosphate dehydrogenase, hexokinase)
♦ Enclosed hemorrhages (bruises, subdural hematoma)
♦ Galactosemia
♦ Gilbert syndrome
♦ Heinz body anemia from drugs and toxins (vitamin K_3, sodium nitrate)
♦ Herpes simplex
♦ Hypothyroidism
♦ Infection (gram-negative bacteria)
♦ Intrauterine infection (rubella, cytomegalic inclusion body disease, toxoplasmosis, syphilis and, occasionally, bacteria such as *Escherichia coli, Staphylococcus, Pseudomonas, Klebsiella, Proteus,* and *Streptococcus)*
♦ Maternal diabetes
♦ Neonatal giant cell hepatitis
♦ Physiologic jaundice
♦ Polycythemia
♦ Pyloric stenosis
♦ Respiratory distress syndrome (hyaline membrane disease)
♦ Transient neonatal hyperbilirubinemia

Pathophysiology

As erythrocytes break down at the end of their neonatal life cycle, hemoglobin separates into globin (protein) and heme (iron) fragments. Heme fragments form unconjugated (indirect) bilirubin, which binds to albumin for transport to liver cells to conjugate with glucuronide, forming direct bilirubin. Because unconjugated bilirubin is fat soluble and can't be excreted in the urine or bile, its serum concentration increases (causing hyperbilirubinemia) and it may escape to extravascular tissue, especially fatty tissue and the brain.

Certain drugs (such as aspirin, tranquilizers, and sulfonamides) and conditions (such as hypothermia, anoxia, hypoglycemia, and hypoalbuminemia) can disrupt conjugation and usurp albumin-binding sites.

Decreased hepatic function also reduces bilirubin conjugation. Biliary obstruction or hepatitis can cause hyperbilirubinemia by blocking normal bile flow.

Increased erythrocyte production or breakdown in hemolytic disorders or in Rh or ABO incompatibility can cause hyperbilirubinemia. Lysis releases bilirubin and stimulates cell agglutination. As a result, the liver's capacity to conjugate bilirubin becomes overloaded.

Finally, maternal enzymes in breast milk inhibit the infant's glucuronyl-transferase conjugating activity.

Signs and symptoms

Signs and symptoms include jaundice from the escape of unconjugated bilirubin to extravascular tissue (primary sign of hyperbilirubinemia).

Complications

◆ Kernicterus
◆ Cerebral palsy, epilepsy, or mental retardation
◆ Perceptual-motor disabilities and learning disorders

Diagnosis

◆ Jaundice and an elevated serum bilirubin level confirm the diagnosis.
◆ A detailed patient history (including prenatal history), family history (paternal Rh factor, inherited red cell defects), present infant status (prematurity, infection), and blood testing of infant and mother (blood group incompatibilities, hemoglobin levels, direct Coomb's test, hematocrit) to identify the underlying cause.

Treatment

◆ Phototherapy (treatment of choice for physiologic jaundice and pathologic jaundice due to erythroblastosis fetalis, after the initial exchange transfusion) with fluorescent lights to decompose bilirubin in the skin by oxidation (usually discontinued after the bilirubin level falls below 10 mg/dl and continues to decrease for 24 hours)
◆ Exchange transfusion to replace the infant's blood with fresh blood (less then 48 hours old), removing some of the unconjugated bilirubin in serum; indicated for conditions such as hydrops fetalis, polycythemia, erythroblastosis fetalis; marked reticulocytosis, drug toxicity, and jaundice that develops within the first 6 hours after birth
◆ Albumin administration to provide additional albumin for binding unconjugated bilirubin

Special considerations

◆ Assess and record the infant's jaundice, and note the time it began. Report the jaundice and serum bilirubin level immediately.
◆ Reassure parents that most infants experience some degree of jaundice. Explain hyperbilirubinemia, its causes, diagnostic tests, and treatment. In addition, explain that the infant's stool contains some bile and may be greenish.

For the infant receiving phototherapy

◆ Undress the infant so that his entire body surface is exposed to the light rays. Keep him 18" to 30" (45.5 to 76 cm) from the light source. Protect his eyes with shields that filter the light.

◆ Monitor and maintain the infant's body temperature; high and low temperatures predispose him to kernicterus. Remove the infant from the light source every 3 to 4 hours, and take off the eye shields. Allow his parents to visit and feed him.
◆ The infant usually shows a decrease in serum bilirubin level 1 to 12 hours after the start of phototherapy. When the infant's bilirubin level is less than 10 mg/dl and has been decreasing for 24 hours, discontinue phototherapy, as ordered. Resume therapy, as ordered, if serum bilirubin increases several milligrams per deciliter, as it often does because of a rebound effect.

For exchange transfusions

◆ Prepare the infant warmer and tray before the transfusion. Try to keep the infant quiet. Give him nothing by mouth for 3 to 4 hours before the procedure.
◆ Check the type, Rh, and age of the blood to be used for the exchange. Keep emergency resuscitative and intubation equipment and oxygen available. During the procedure, monitor respiratory and heart rates every 15 minutes; check the infant's temperature every 30 minutes. Continue to monitor vital signs every 15 to 30 minutes for 2 hours.
◆ Measure intake and output. Observe for cord bleeding and complications, such as hemorrhage, hypocalcemia, sepsis, and shock. Report serum bilirubin and hemoglobin levels. The bilirubin level may rise, as a result of a rebound effect, within 30 minutes after transfusion, necessitating repeat transfusions.

To prevent hyperbilirubinemia

◆ Maintain oral intake. Don't skip feedings because fasting stimulates the conversion of heme to bilirubin.
◆ Administer $Rh_O(D)$ immune globulin (human), as ordered, to an Rh-negative mother after amniocentesis, or to an Rh-negative mother during the third trimester, after the birth of an Rh-positive infant, or after spontaneous or elective abortion (to prevent hemolytic disease in subsequent infants).

INGUINAL HERNIA

A hernia occurs when part of an internal organ protrudes through an abnormal opening in the wall of the cavity that surrounds it. Most hernias occur in the abdominal cavity. Although many kinds of abdominal hernias are possible, inguinal hernias (also called *ruptures*) are most common. (See *Common sites of hernia*.) Inguinal hernias may be direct or indirect. Indirect are more common; they may develop at any age,

Common sites of hernia

There are four common sites of hernia: umbilical, incisional, inguinal, and femoral. Below are descriptions of each type.

Umbilical

Umbilical hernia results from abnormal muscular structures around the umbilical cord. This hernia is quite common in neonates but also occurs in women who are obese or who have had several pregnancies. Because most umbilical hernias in infants close spontaneously, surgery is warranted only if the hernia persists for more than 4 to 5 years. Taping or binding the affected area or supporting it with a truss may relieve symptoms until the hernia closes. A severe congenital umbilical hernia allows the abdominal viscera to protrude outside the body. This condition necessitates immediate repair.

Incisional

Incisional (ventral) hernia develops at the site of previous surgery, usually along vertical incisions. This hernia may result from a weakness in the abdominal wall, perhaps as a result of an infection or impaired wound healing. Inadequate nutrition, extreme abdominal distention, or obesity also predispose a patient to incisional hernia. Palpation of an incisional hernia may reveal several defects in the surgical scar.

Effective repair requires pulling the layers of the abdominal wall together without creating tension. If this isn't possible, surgical reconstruction uses Teflon, Marlex mesh, or tantalum mesh to close the opening.

Inguinal

Inguinal hernia can be direct or indirect. An indirect inguinal hernia causes the abdominal viscera to protrude through the inguinal ring and follow the spermatic cord (in males) or round ligament (in females). A direct inguinal hernia results from a weakness in the fascial floor of the inguinal canal.

Femoral

Femoral hernia occurs where the femoral artery passes into the femoral canal. Typically, a fatty deposit within the femoral canal enlarges and eventually creates a hole big enough to accommodate part of the peritoneum and bladder. A femoral hernia appears as a swelling or bulge at the pulse point of the large femoral artery. It's usually a soft, pliable, reducible, nontender mass but commonly becomes incarcerated or strangulated.

---

are three times more common in males, and are especially prevalent in male infants.

Causes

◆ *Direct* — weakness in fascial floor of inguinal canal
◆ *Indirect* — weakness in fascial margin of internal inguinal ring
◆ *Either* — weak abdominal muscles (caused by congenital malformation, trauma, or aging) or increased intra-abdominal pressure (due to heavy lifting, pregnancy, obesity, or straining)

Pathophysiology

In an inguinal hernia, the large or small intestine, omentum, or bladder protrudes into the inguinal canal. In an indirect hernia, abdominal viscera leave the abdomen through the internal inguinal ring and follow the spermatic cord (in males) or round ligament (in females) extending down into the inguinal canal; they emerge at the external ring and extend down into the scrotum or labia.

In a direct inguinal hernia, instead of entering the canal through the internal ring, the hernia passes through the posterior inguinal wall, protrudes directly through the transverse fascia of the canal (in an area known as Hesselbach's triangle), and comes out at the external ring.

In a male infant, an inguinal hernia commonly coexists with an undescended testicle or hydrocele. During the 7th month of gestation, the testicle normally descends into the scrotum, preceded by the peritoneal sac. If the sac closes improperly, it leaves an opening through which the intestine can slip.

Hernias can be reducible (if the hernia can be manipulated back into place with relative ease), incarcerated (if the hernia can't be reduced because adhesions have formed, obstructing the intestinal flow), or strangulated (part of the herniated intestine becomes twisted or edematous, seriously interfering with normal blood flow and peristalsis and, possibly, leading to intestinal obstruction and necrosis).

Signs and symptoms
♦ Inguinal hernia usually causing a lump to appear over the herniated area when the patient stands or strains; lump disappearing when the patient is in a supine position
♦ Tension on the herniated contents may cause a sharp, steady pain in the groin, which fades when the hernia is reduced
♦ Strangulation producing severe pain and may lead to partial or complete bowel obstruction and even intestinal necrosis
♦ Partial bowel obstruction may cause anorexia, vomiting, pain and tenderness in the groin, an irreducible mass, and diminished bowel sounds
♦ Complete obstruction may cause shock, high fever, absent bowel sounds, and bloody stools
♦ In a male infant, inguinal hernia commonly coexists with an undescended testicle or a hydrocele

Complications
♦ Strangulation
♦ Intestinal obstruction
♦ Infection (after surgery)

Diagnosis
In a patient with a large hernia, physical examination reveals an obvious swelling or lump in the inguinal area. In the patient with a small hernia, the affected area may simply appear full. Palpation of the inguinal area while the patient is performing Valsalva's maneuver or coughing confirms the diagnosis. To detect a hernia in a man, the patient is asked to stand with his ipsilateral leg slightly flexed and his weight resting on the other leg. The examiner inserts an index finger into the lower part of the scrotum and invaginates the scrotal skin so the finger advances through the external inguinal ring toward the internal ring (½" to 2" [1 to 5 cm] through the inguinal canal). The patient is then told to cough. If the examiner feels pressure against the fingertip, an indirect hernia exists; if pressure is felt against the side of the finger, a direct hernia exists.

A history of sharp or "catching" pain when lifting or straining may help confirm the diagnosis. Suspected bowel obstruction requires X-rays and a white blood cell count (may be elevated).

Treatment
If the hernia is reducible, the pain may be temporarily relieved by pushing the hernia back into place. A truss may keep the abdominal contents from protruding into the hernial sac, although it won't cure the hernia. This device is especially beneficial for an elderly or debilitated patient for whom surgery might be hazardous.

For infants, adults, and otherwise healthy elderly patients, herniorrhaphy is the treatment of choice. Herniorrhaphy replaces the contents of the hernial sac into the abdominal cavity and closes the opening. In many cases, this procedure is performed under local anesthesia in a short-term unit or as a single-day admission. Another effective surgical procedure for repairing a hernia is hernioplasty, which reinforces the weakened area with steel mesh, fascia, or wire.

A strangulated or necrotic hernia necessitates bowel resection. Rarely, an extensive resection may require temporary colostomy. In either case, bowel resection lengthens postoperative recovery and requires an antibiotic, parenteral fluids, and electrolyte replacement.

Special considerations
Patient care includes managing symptoms to increase patient comfort and prevent worsening herniation.
♦ Apply a truss only after a hernia has been reduced. For best results, apply it in the morning, before the patient gets out of bed.
♦ To prevent skin irritation, tell the patient to bathe daily and apply liberal amounts of cornstarch or baby powder. Warn against applying the truss over clothing because this reduces the effectiveness of the truss and may make it slip.
♦ If incarceration and strangulation occur, don't try to reduce the hernia because this may perforate the bowel. If severe intestinal obstruction develops because of hernial strangulation, inform the physician immediately. A nasogastric tube may be inserted promptly to empty the stomach and relieve pressure on the hernial sac.
♦ Before surgery for an incarcerated hernia, closely monitor vital signs. Administer I.V. fluids and an analgesic, as ordered. Control fever with acetaminophen or tepid sponge baths, as ordered. Place the patient in Trendelenburg's position to reduce pressure on the hernia site.
♦ Give special reassurance and emotional support to a child scheduled for hernia repair. Encourage him to ask questions, and answer them as simply as possible. Offer appropriate diversions to distract him from the impending surgery.
♦ After outpatient surgery, make sure that the patient voids before he leaves the health care facility. Teach him to check his incision and dressing for drainage, inflammation, or swelling and to watch for fever. If any of these occur, he should notify the physician.
♦ To reduce scrotal swelling, have him support the scrotum with a rolled towel and apply an ice bag.

◆ Instruct the patient to drink plenty of fluids to maintain hydration and prevent constipation.
◆ Before discharge, warn the patient against lifting heavy objects or straining during bowel movements. In addition, tell him to watch for signs and symptoms of infection (oozing, tenderness, warmth, and redness) at the incision site and to keep the incision clean and covered until the sutures are removed.
◆ Advise the patient not to resume normal activity or return to work without the surgeon's permission.

‖ LIFE-THREATENING DISORDER

INTESTINAL OBSTRUCTION

Intestinal obstruction is the partial or complete blockage of the lumen in the small or large bowel. Small-bowel obstruction is far more common (90% of patients) and usually more serious. Complete obstruction in any part of the bowel, if untreated, can cause death within hours due to shock and vascular collapse. Intestinal obstruction is most likely to occur after abdominal surgery or in persons with congenital bowel deformities.

Causes
◆ Adhesions and strangulated hernias usually causing small-bowel obstruction; large-bowel obstruction typically due to carcinomas
◆ Mechanical intestinal obstruction resulting from foreign bodies (fruit pits, gallstones, or worms) or compression of the bowel wall due to stenosis, intussusception, volvulus of the sigmoid or cecum, tumors, or atresia
◆ Nonmechanical obstruction resulting from physiologic disturbances, such as paralytic ileus, electrolyte imbalances, toxicity (uremia or generalized infection), neurogenic abnormalities (spinal cord lesions), and thrombosis or embolism of mesenteric vessels. (See *Paralytic ileus,* page 348.)

Pathophysiology
Intestinal obstruction develops in three forms:
◆ *simple*—Blockage prevents intestinal contents from passing, with no other complications.
◆ *strangulated*—Blood supply to part or all of the obstructed section is cut off, in addition to blockage of the lumen.
◆ *close-looped*—Both ends of a bowel section are occluded, isolating it from the rest of the intestine.

The physiologic effects are similar in all three forms of obstruction: When intestinal obstruction occurs, fluid, air, and gas collect near the site. Peristalsis increases temporarily as the bowel tries to force its contents through the obstruction, injuring intestinal mucosa and causing distention at and above the site of the obstruction. Distention blocks the flow of venous blood and halts normal absorptive processes; as a result, the bowel wall becomes edematous and begins to secrete water, sodium, and potassium into the fluid pooled in the lumen.

Obstruction in the small intestine results in metabolic alkalosis from dehydration and loss of gastric hydrochloric acid; lower-bowel obstruction causes slower dehydration and loss of intestinal alkaline fluids, resulting in metabolic acidosis. Ultimately, intestinal obstruction may lead to ischemia, necrosis, and death. (See *Symptom progression in intestinal obstruction,* page 349.)

CLINICAL ALERT *Watch for air-fluid lock syndrome in older adults who remain recumbent for extended periods. In this syndrome, fluid collects in the dependent bowel loops. Then, peristalsis is too weak to push fluid "uphill." The resulting obstruction primarily occurs in the large bowel.*

Signs and symptoms
◆ Colicky pain, nausea, vomiting, constipation, and abdominal distention characterize small-bowel obstruction. It may also cause drowsiness, intense thirst, malaise, and aching and may dry up oral mucous membranes and the tongue.
◆ Auscultation reveals bowel sounds, borborygmi, and rushes; occasionally, these are loud enough to be heard without a stethoscope. Palpation elicits abdominal tenderness, with moderate distention; rebound tenderness occurs when obstruction has caused strangulation with ischemia. In late stages, signs of hypovolemic shock result from progressive dehydration and plasma loss.
◆ In complete small-bowel obstruction, vigorous peristaltic waves propel bowel contents toward the mouth instead of the rectum. Spasms may occur every 3 to 5 minutes and last about 1 minute each, with persistent epigastric or periumbilical pain. Passage of small amounts of mucus and blood originating from below the site of obstruction may occur. The higher the obstruction, the earlier and more severe the vomiting. Vomitus initially contains gastric juice, then bile and, finally, contents of the obstructed segments of the intestine.
◆ Signs and symptoms of large-bowel obstruction develop more slowly because the colon can absorb fluid from its contents and distend well beyond its normal size. Constipation may be the only clinical effect for days. Colicky abdominal pain may then appear suddenly, producing

Paralytic ileus

Paralytic ileus is a physiologic form of intestinal obstruction that usually develops in the small bowel after abdominal surgery. It causes decreased or absent intestinal motility that usually disappears spontaneously after 2 to 3 days. Clinical effects of paralytic ileus include severe abdominal distention, extreme distress and, possibly, vomiting. The patient may be severely constipated or may pass flatus and small liquid stools.

Causes

Paralytic ileus can develop as a response to trauma, toxemia, or peritonitis or as a result of electrolyte deficiencies (especially hypokalemia) and the use of certain drugs, such as ganglionic blockers and anticholinergics. It can also result from vascular causes, such as thrombosis and embolism involving the intestinal vasculature. Excessive air swallowing may contribute to it, but paralytic ileus brought on by this factor alone seldom lasts more than 24 hours.

Treatment

Paralytic ileus lasting longer than 48 hours requires intubation for decompression and nasogastric suctioning. Because of the absence of peristaltic activity, a long, weighted intestinal tube — called a Miller-Abbott tube — may be necessary in the patient with extraordinary abdominal distention. However, such procedures must be used with extreme caution because any additional trauma to the bowel can aggravate ileus. When paralytic ileus results from surgical manipulation of the bowel, treatment may also include a cholinergic, such as neostigmine or bethanechol.

When caring for patients with paralytic ileus, warn those receiving a cholinergic to expect certain paradoxical adverse reactions, such as intestinal cramps and diarrhea. Remember that neostigmine produces cardiovascular adverse reactions, usually bradycardia and hypotension. Check frequently for returning bowel sounds.

---

spasms that last less than 1 minute each and recur every few minutes. Continuous hypogastric pain and nausea may develop, but vomiting is usually absent at first. Large-bowel obstruction can cause dramatic abdominal distention; loops of the large bowel may become visible on the abdomen. Eventually, complete large-bowel obstruction may cause fecal vomiting, continuous pain, or localized peritonitis.

Patients with partial obstruction may display any of the above signs and symptoms in a milder form. However, leakage of liquid stool around the obstruction is common in partial obstruction.

Complications

◆ Perforation
◆ Peritonitis
◆ Septicemia
◆ Secondary infection
◆ Metabolic alkalosis or acidosis
◆ Hypovolemic or septic shock
◆ If untreated, death

Diagnosis

Progressive, colicky, abdominal pain and distention, with or without nausea and vomiting, suggest bowel obstruction. X-rays confirm the diagnosis. Abdominal films show the presence and location of intestinal gas or fluid. In small-bowel obstruction, a typical "stepladder" pattern

emerges, with alternating fluid and gas levels apparent in 3 to 4 hours. In large-bowel obstruction, barium enema reveals a distended, air-filled colon or a closed loop of sigmoid with extreme distention (in sigmoid volvulus).

Laboratory results supporting this diagnosis include:
◆ decreased sodium, chloride, and potassium levels (due to vomiting)
◆ slightly elevated white blood cell count (with necrosis, peritonitis, or strangulation)
◆ increased serum amylase level (possibly from irritation of pancreas by bowel loop).

Treatment

◆ Preoperative therapy consisting of correction of fluid and electrolyte imbalances, decompression of the bowel to relieve vomiting and distention, and treatment of shock and peritonitis
◆ Strangulated obstruction usually necessitating blood replacement as well as I.V. fluid administration
◆ Passage of a nasogastric (NG) tube, followed by use of the longer and weighted Miller-Abbott or Cantor tube, usually accomplishes decompression, especially in small-bowel obstruction
◆ Close monitoring of the patient's condition determines the duration of treatment; if the patient fails to improve or if his condition deteriorates, surgery is necessary

CLOSER LOOK

Symptom progression in intestinal obstruction

A partial or complete blockage of the small or large intestine creates an obstruction with resultant symptoms.

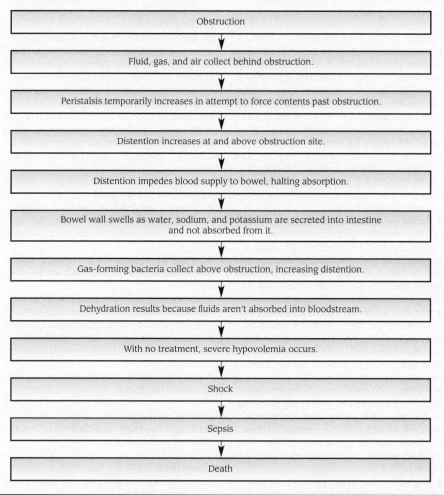

Obstruction

↓

Fluid, gas, and air collect behind obstruction.

↓

Peristalsis temporarily increases in attempt to force contents past obstruction.

↓

Distention increases at and above obstruction site.

↓

Distention impedes blood supply to bowel, halting absorption.

↓

Bowel wall swells as water, sodium, and potassium are secreted into intestine and not absorbed from it.

↓

Gas-forming bacteria collect above obstruction, increasing distention.

↓

Dehydration results because fluids aren't absorbed into bloodstream.

↓

With no treatment, severe hypovolemia occurs.

↓

Shock

↓

Sepsis

↓

Death

◆ In large-bowel obstruction, surgical resection with anastomosis, colostomy, or ileostomy commonly follows decompression with an NG tube
◆ Total parenteral nutrition, if the patient suffers a protein deficit from chronic obstruction, postoperative or paralytic ileus, or infection
◆ Drug therapy including an analgesic, a sedative, and an antibiotic for peritonitis due to bowel strangulation or infarction

Special considerations

Effective management of intestinal obstruction, a life-threatening condition that often causes overwhelming pain and distress, requires skillful supportive care and keen observation.
◆ Monitor vital signs frequently. A drop in blood pressure may indicate reduced circulating blood volume due to blood loss from a strangulated hernia. Remember, as much as 10 qt (10 L) of fluid can collect in the small bowel, drastically reducing plasma volume. Observe the patient

closely for signs of shock (pallor, rapid pulse, and hypotension).

◆ Stay alert for signs and symptoms of metabolic alkalosis (changes in sensorium; slow, shallow respirations; hypertonic muscles; and tetany) or acidosis (shortness of breath on exertion; disorientation; and, later, deep, rapid breathing, weakness, and malaise).

◆ Watch for signs and symptoms of secondary infection, such as fever and chills.

◆ Monitor urine output carefully to assess renal function, circulating blood volume, and possible urine retention caused by bladder compression by the distended intestine. If you suspect bladder compression, catheterize the patient for residual urine immediately after he has voided. In addition, measure abdominal girth frequently to detect progressive distention.

◆ Provide fastidious mouth and nose care if the patient has vomited or undergone decompression by intubation. Look for signs of dehydration (thick, swollen tongue; dry, cracked lips; and dry oral mucous membranes).

◆ Record the amount and color of drainage from the decompression tube. Irrigate the tube with normal saline solution to maintain patency. If a weighted tube has been inserted, check periodically to make sure that it's advancing. Help the patient turn from side to side (or walk around, if he can) to facilitate passage of the tube.

◆ Keep the patient in Fowler's position as much as possible to promote pulmonary ventilation and ease respiratory distress from abdominal distention. Listen for bowel sounds, and watch for signs of returning peristalsis (passage of flatus and mucus through the rectum).

◆ Explain all diagnostic and therapeutic procedures to the patient, and answer any questions he may have. Make sure that he understands that these procedures are necessary to relieve the obstruction and reduce pain. Tell him to lie on his left side for about 30 minutes before X-rays are taken.

◆ Prepare the patient and his family for the possibility of surgery, and provide emotional support and positive reinforcement afterward. Arrange for an enterostomal therapist to visit the patient who has had an ostomy.

IRRITABLE BOWEL SYNDROME

Also referred to as *spastic colon* or *spastic colitis*, irritable bowel syndrome (IBS) is marked by chronic symptoms of abdominal pain, alternating constipation and diarrhea, excess flatus, a sense of incomplete evacuation, and abdominal distention. IBS is a benign condition that has no anatomic abnormality or inflammatory component. It occurs most commonly in women ages 20 to 30.

Causes
◆ Hormonal changes (menstruation)
◆ Ingestion of irritants (coffee, raw fruit, or vegetables)
◆ Lactose intolerance
◆ Laxative abuse
◆ Psychological stress (most common)

Pathophysiology
IBS appears to reflect motor disturbances of the entire colon in response to stimuli. Some muscles of the small bowel are particularly sensitive to motor abnormalities and distention; others are particularly sensitive to certain foods and drugs. The patient may be hypersensitive to the hormones gastrin and cholecystokinin. The pain of IBS seems to be caused by abnormally strong contractions of the intestinal smooth muscle as it reacts to distention, irritants, or stress. (See *What happens in IBS.*)

Signs and symptoms
◆ Crampy lower abdominal pain secondary to muscle contraction; usually occurring during the day and relieved by defecation or passage of flatus
◆ Pain that intensifies 1 to 2 hours after a meal from irritation of nerve fibers by causative stimulus
◆ Constipation alternating with diarrhea, with one of the two being dominant; secondary to motor disturbances from causative stimulus
◆ Mucus passed through the rectum from altered secretion in intestinal lumen due to motor abnormalities
◆ Abdominal distention and bloating caused by flatus and constipation

Complications
IBS is associated with increased risk of diverticulitis and colon cancer.

Diagnosis
To establish a diagnosis of IBS, the patient must meet certain criteria:
◆ Abdominal pain or discomfort for at least 12 weeks out of the previous 12 months. (These 12 weeks don't have to be consecutive.)
◆ The abdominal pain or discomfort has two of the following three features:
– It's relieved by having a bowel movement.
– When it starts, there's a change in how often the patient has a bowel movement.
– When it starts, there's a change in the form of the stool or the way it looks.
◆ Physical examination reveals contributing psychological factors such as a recent stressful life change.

◆ Stool samples for ova, parasites, bacteria, and blood rule out infection.
◆ Lactose intolerance test rules out lactose intolerance.
◆ Barium enema may reveal colon spasm and tubular appearance of descending colon without evidence of cancers and diverticulosis.
◆ Sigmoidoscopy or colonoscopy may reveal spastic contractions without evidence of colon cancer or inflammatory bowel disease.
◆ Rectal biopsy rules out malignancy.

Treatment
◆ Stress relief measures, including counseling or a mild anxiolytic
◆ Investigation and avoidance of food irritants
◆ Increased fiber (dietary or supplemental) to relieve both constipation and diarrhea
◆ Tegaserod — for short-term treatment of women with IBS when the primary bowel symptom is constipation — to stimulate the peristaltic reflex and intestinal secretion
◆ Alosetron for women with severe IBS who haven't responded to conventional therapy and whose primary symptom is diarrhea to reduce pain, colonic transit, and GI secretions
◆ Application of heat to abdomen
◆ A bulking agent to reduce episodes of diarrhea and minimize effect of nonpropulsive colonic contractions
◆ An antispasmodic (propantheline or diphenoxylate with atropine sulfate) for pain
◆ Loperamide possibly to reduce urgency and fecal soiling in patients with persistent diarrhea
◆ Bowel training (if the cause of IBS is long-term laxative abuse) to regain muscle control

Special considerations
Because the patient with IBS isn't hospitalized, focus your care on patient teaching.
◆ Tell the patient to avoid irritating foods, and encourage him to develop regular bowel habits.
◆ Help the patient deal with stress, and warn against dependence on sedatives or antispasmodics.
◆ Encourage regular checkups because IBS is associated with a higher-than-normal incidence of diverticulitis and colon cancer. For patients older than age 40, emphasize the need for an annual sigmoidoscopy and rectal examination.

 CLOSER LOOK

What happens in IBS

Typically, the patient with irritable bowel syndrome (IBS) has a normal-appearing GI tract. However, careful examination of the colon may reveal functional irritability — an abnormality in colonic smooth-muscle function marked by excessive peristalsis and spasms, even during remission.

Intestinal function
To understand what happens in IBS, consider how smooth muscle controls bowel function. Normally, segmental muscle contractions mix intestinal contents while peristalsis propels the contents through the GI tract. Motor activity is most propulsive in the proximal (stomach) and the distal (sigmoid) portions of the intestine. Activity in the rest of the intestines is slower, permitting nutrient and water absorption.

In IBS, the autonomic nervous system, which innervates the large intestine, doesn't cause the alternating contractions and relaxations that propel stools smoothly toward the rectum.

The result is constipation or diarrhea or both.

Constipation
Some patients have spasmodic intestinal contractions that set up a partial obstruction by trapping gas and stools. This causes distention, bloating, gas pain, and constipation.

Diarrhea
Other patients have dramatically increased intestinal motility. Eating or cholinergic stimulation triggers the small intestine's contents to rush into the large intestine, dumping watery stools and irritating the mucosa. The result is diarrhea.

Mixed symptoms
If further spasms trap liquid stools, the intestinal mucosa absorbs water from the stools, leaving them dry, hard, and difficult to pass. The result is a pattern of alternating diarrhea and constipation.

Functions of the liver

The liver is one of the most essential organs of the body. To understand how liver disease affects the body, it's best to understand its main functions:

♦ detoxifies poisonous chemicals, including alcohol, beer, wine, and drugs (prescribed and over-the-counter as well as illegal substances)

♦ makes bile to help digest food

♦ stores energy by stockpiling sugar (carbohydrates, glucose, and fat) until needed

♦ stores iron reserves as well as vitamins and minerals

♦ manufactures new proteins

♦ produces important plasma proteins necessary for blood coagulation, including prothrombin and fibrinogen

♦ serves as a site for hematopoiesis during fetal development.

||| LIFE-THREATENING DISORDER

LIVER FAILURE

Liver failure can be the end result of any liver disease. The liver performs more than 100 separate functions in the body. When it fails, a complex syndrome involving the impairment of many different organs and body functions ensues. (See *Functions of the liver.*) Hepatic encephalopathy and hepatorenal syndrome are two conditions that occur with liver failure. The only cure for liver failure is a liver transplant.

Causes
♦ Cirrhosis
♦ Liver cancer
♦ Nonviral hepatitis
♦ Viral hepatitis

Pathophysiology
Manifestations of liver failure include hepatic encephalopathy and hepatorenal syndrome.

Hepatic encephalopathy, a set of central nervous system disorders, results when the liver can no longer detoxify the blood. Liver dysfunction and collateral vessels that shunt blood around the liver to the systemic circulation permit toxins absorbed from the GI tract to circulate freely to the brain. Ammonia, a by-product of protein metabolism, is one of the main toxins causing hepatic encephalopathy. The normal liver transforms ammonia to urea, which the

kidneys excrete. When the liver fails and is no longer able to transform ammonia to urea, blood ammonia levels rise and the ammonia is delivered to the brain. Short-chain fatty acids, serotonin, tryptophan, and false neurotransmitters may also accumulate in the blood and contribute to hepatic encephalopathy.

Hepatorenal syndrome is renal failure concurrent with liver disease; the kidneys appear to be normal but abruptly cease functioning. It causes expanded blood volume, accumulation of hydrogen ions, and electrolyte disturbances. It's most common in patients with alcoholic cirrhosis or fulminating hepatitis. The cause may be the accumulation of vasoactive substances that cause inappropriate constriction of renal arterioles, leading to decreased glomerular filtration and oliguria. The vasoconstriction may also be a compensatory response to portal hypertension and the pooling of blood in the splenic circulation.

Signs and symptoms
♦ Jaundice from the failure of the liver to conjugate bilirubin
♦ Abdominal pain or tenderness from liver inflammation
♦ Nausea and anorexia from systemic effects of inflammation
♦ Fatigue and weight loss from failure of hepatic metabolism
♦ Pruritus due to the accumulation of bilirubin in the skin
♦ Oliguria from intrarenal vasoconstriction
♦ Splenomegaly secondary to portal hypertension
♦ Ascites due to portal hypertension and decreased plasma proteins
♦ Peripheral edema encephalopathy, and cerebral edema from accumulation of fluid retained because of decreased plasma protein production and loss of albumin with ascites
♦ Varices of the esophagus, rectum, and abdominal wall secondary to portal hypertension
♦ Bleeding tendencies from thrombocytopenia (secondary to blood accumulation in the spleen) and prolonged prothrombin time (from the impaired production of coagulation factors)
♦ Petechia resulting from thrombocytopenia
♦ Amenorrhea secondary to altered steroid hormone production and metabolism
♦ Gynecomastia in males from estrogen buildup due to failure of hepatic biotransformation functions

Complications
♦ Variceal bleeding
♦ GI hemorrhage
♦ Coma
♦ Death

Diagnosis
◆ Liver function tests reveal elevated levels of aspartate aminotransferase, alanine aminotransferase, alkaline phosphatase, and bilirubin.
◆ Blood studies reveal anemia, impaired red blood cell production, elevated bleeding and clotting times, a low blood glucose level, and an increased serum ammonia level.
◆ Urine osmolarity is increased.

Treatment
◆ Liver transplantation
◆ Low-protein, high-carbohydrate diet to correct nutritional deficiencies and prevent overtaxing of the liver
◆ Lactulose to reduce the blood ammonia level and help alleviate some symptoms of hepatic encephalopathy

For ascites
◆ Salt restriction and a potassium-sparing diuretic to increase water excretion
◆ A potassium supplement to reverse the effects of high aldosterone
◆ Paracentesis to remove ascitic fluid and alleviate abdominal discomfort
◆ Shunt placement to aid in removal of ascitic fluid and alleviate abdominal discomfort

For portal hypertension
◆ Shunt placement between the portal vein and another systemic vein to divert blood flow and relieve pressure

For variceal bleeding
◆ A vasoconstrictor to decrease blood flow
◆ Balloon tamponade to control bleeding by exerting pressure on the varices with the use of a balloon catheter
◆ Surgery to tie off bleeding collaterals sprouting from the portal vein
◆ Vitamin K or fresh frozen plasma to control bleeding by decreasing prothrombin time
◆ Packed red blood cells to compensate for blood loss

Special considerations
Patient care for liver failure includes monitoring of symptoms and support.
◆ Frequently assess and record the patient's level of consciousness. Continually orient him to place and time. Keep a daily record of the patient's handwriting to monitor progression of neurologic involvement.
◆ Monitor intake, output, and fluid and electrolyte balance. Check daily weight and measure abdominal girth. Watch for—and immediately report—signs of anemia (decreased hemoglobin

level), infection, alkalosis (increased serum bicarbonate level), and GI bleeding (melena and hematemesis).
◆ Give drugs, as ordered, and watch for adverse reactions. Be careful of administering drugs that are hepatically metabolized.
◆ Ask the dietary department to provide the specified low-protein diet, with carbohydrates supplying most of the calories. Provide good mouth care.
◆ Promote rest, comfort, and a quiet atmosphere. Discourage stressful exercise.
◆ Use restraints, if necessary, but avoid sedatives. Protect the comatose patient's eyes from corneal injury by using artificial tears or eye patches.
◆ Provide emotional support for the patient's family in the terminal stage of encephalopathy.

MALABSORPTION
Malabsorption is failure of the intestinal mucosa to absorb single or multiple nutrients efficiently. Absorption of amino acids, fat, sugar, or vitamins may be impaired. The result is inadequate movement of nutrients from the small intestine to the bloodstream or lymphatic system. Manifestations depend primarily on what isn't being absorbed.

Causes
A wide variety of disorders result in malabsorption. (See *Causes of malabsorption*, page 354.) Causes may include:
◆ disease of the small intestine such as celiac disease
◆ drug toxicity
◆ hepatobiliary disease
◆ hereditary disorder
◆ pancreatic disorders
◆ prior gastric surgery.

Pathophysiology
The small intestine's inability to absorb nutrients efficiently may result from various diseases. The mechanism of malabsorption depends on the cause. Some common causes of malabsorption syndrome include celiac disease, lactase deficiency, gastrectomy, Zollinger-Ellison syndrome, and bacterial overgrowth in the duodenal stump.

In celiac sprue, dietary gluten—a product of wheat, barley, rye, and oats—is toxic to the patient, causing injury to the mucosal villi. The mucosa appear flat and have lost absorptive surface. Symptoms generally disappear when gluten is removed from the diet.

Lactase deficiency is a disaccharide deficiency syndrome. Lactase is an intestinal enzyme that splits nonabsorbable lactose (a disaccharide) into the absorbable monosaccharides glucose and galactose. Production may be deficient, or another intestinal disease may inhibit the enzyme.

Causes of malabsorption

Many disorders — from systemic to organ-specific diseases — may give rise to malabsorption. It may also result from drug therapy or gastric surgery.

Diseases of the small intestine
Primary small-bowel disease
◆ Bacterial overgrowth due to stasis in afferent loop after Billroth II gastrectomy
◆ Massive bowel resection
◆ Nontropical sprue (celiac disease)
◆ Regional enteritis
◆ Tropical sprue

Ischemic small-bowel disease
◆ Chronic heart failure
◆ Mesenteric atherosclerosis

Small-bowel infections and infestations
◆ Acute enteritis
◆ Giardiasis

Systemic disease involving small bowel
◆ Amyloidosis
◆ Lymphoma
◆ Sarcoidosis
◆ Scleroderma
◆ Whipple's disease

Drug-induced malabsorption
◆ Calcium carbonate
◆ Neomycin

Hepatobiliary disease
◆ Biliary fistula
◆ Biliary tract obstruction
◆ Cirrhosis and hepatitis

Hereditary disorder
◆ Primary lactase deficiency

Pancreatic disorders
◆ Chronic pancreatitis
◆ Cystic fibrosis
◆ Pancreatic cancer
◆ Pancreatic resection
◆ Zollinger-Ellison syndrome

Previous gastric surgery
◆ Billroth II gastrectomy
◆ Pyloroplasty
◆ Total gastrectomy
◆ Vagotomy

Malabsorption may occur after gastrectomy. Poor mixing of chyme with gastric secretions is the cause of postsurgical malabsorption.

In Zollinger-Ellison syndrome, increased acidity in the duodenum inhibits release of cholecystokinin, which stimulates pancreatic enzyme secretion. Pancreatic enzyme deficiency leads to decreased breakdown of nutrients and malabsorption.

Bacterial overgrowth in the duodenal stump (loop created in the Billroth II procedure) causes malabsorption of vitamin B_{12}.

Signs and symptoms
◆ Weight loss and generalized malnutrition from impaired absorption of carbohydrate, fat, and protein
◆ Diarrhea from decreased absorption of fluids, electrolytes, bile acids, and fatty acids in the colon
◆ Steatorrhea from excess fat in the stool
◆ Flatulence and abdominal distention secondary to fermentation of undigested lactose
◆ Nocturia from delayed absorption of water
◆ Weakness and fatigue from anemia and electrolyte depletion from diarrhea

◆ Edema from impaired absorption of amino acids, resulting in protein depletion and hypoproteinemia
◆ Amenorrhea from protein depletion leading to hypopituitarism
◆ Anemia from the impaired absorption of iron, folic acid, and vitamin B_{12}
◆ Glossitis, cheilosis secondary to a deficiency of iron, folic acid, vitamin B_{12}, and other vitamins
◆ Peripheral neuropathy from a deficiency of vitamin B_{12} and thiamine
◆ Bruising, bleeding tendency from vitamin K malabsorption and hypoprothrombinemia
◆ Bone pain, skeletal deformities, fractures from calcium malabsorption that leads to hypocalcemia; protein depletion leading to osteoporosis and vitamin D malabsorption causing impaired calcium absorption
◆ Tetany, paresthesia resulting from calcium malabsorption leading to hypocalcemia and magnesium malabsorption, leading to hypomagnesemia and hypokalemia

Complications
◆ Fractures
◆ Anemias

♦ Bleeding disorders
♦ Tetany
♦ Malnutrition

Diagnosis

♦ Stool specimen for fat reveals excretion of more than 6 g of fat per day.
♦ D-xylose absorption test shows less than 20% of 25 g of D-xylose in the urine after 5 hours (reflects disorders of proximal bowel).
♦ Schilling test reveals deficiency of vitamin B_{12} absorption.
♦ Culture of duodenal and jejunal contents confirms bacterial overgrowth in the proximal bowel.
♦ GI barium studies show characteristic features of the small intestine.
♦ Small intestine biopsy reveals the atrophy of mucosal villi.

Treatment

♦ Identification of cause and appropriate correction
♦ Gluten-free diet to stop progression of celiac disease and malabsorption
♦ Lactose-free diet to treat lactase deficiency
♦ Dietary supplementation to replace nutrient deficiencies
♦ Vitamin B_{12} injections to treat vitamin B_{12} deficiency

Special considerations

♦ Explain the necessity of a gluten-free diet to the patient (and to his parents, if the patient is a child). Advise elimination of wheat, barley, rye, and oats and foods made from them, such as breads and baked goods; suggest substitution of corn or rice. Advise the patient to consult a dietitian for a gluten-free diet that's high in protein but low in carbohydrates and fats. Depending on individual tolerance, the diet initially consists of proteins and gradually expands to include other foods. Assess the patient's acceptance and understanding of the disease, and encourage regular reevaluation.
♦ Observe nutritional status and progress by daily calorie counts and weight checks. Evaluate the patient's tolerance to new foods. In the early stages, offer small, frequent meals to counteract anorexia.
♦ Assess fluid status: Record intake, urine output, and number of stools (may exceed 10 per day). Watch for signs of dehydration, such as dry skin and mucous membranes and poor skin turgor.
♦ Check serum electrolyte levels. Watch for signs and symptoms of hypokalemia (weakness, lethargy, rapid pulse, nausea, and diarrhea) and

a low calcium level (impaired blood clotting, muscle twitching, and tetany).
♦ Monitor prothrombin time, hemoglobin level, and hematocrit. Protect the patient from bleeding and bruising. Administer vitamin K, iron, folic acid, and vitamin B_{12}, as ordered. Early in treatment, give hematinic supplements I.M. using a separate syringe for each. Use the Z-track method to give iron I.M. If the patient can tolerate oral iron, give it between meals, when absorption is best. Dilute oral iron preparations, and give them through a straw to prevent staining teeth.
♦ Protect patients with osteomalacia from injury by keeping the side rails up and assisting with ambulation, as necessary.
♦ Give a steroid, as ordered, and assess regularly for cushingoid adverse reactions, such as hirsutism and muscle weakness.

||| **LIFE-THREATENING DISORDER**

PANCREATITIS

Pancreatitis, inflammation of the pancreas, occurs in acute and chronic forms and may be due to edema, necrosis, or hemorrhage. In men, this disease is commonly associated with alcoholism, trauma, or peptic ulcer; in both men and women, with biliary tract disease. The prognosis is good in pancreatitis associated with biliary tract disease, but poor when associated with alcoholism. Mortality from pancreatitis is as high as 60% when associated with necrosis and hemorrhage.

Causes

♦ Abnormal organ structure
♦ Alcoholism
♦ Biliary tract disease
♦ Blunt trauma or surgical trauma
♦ Drugs, such as glucocorticoids, sulfonamides, thiazides, hormonal contraceptives, and nonsteroidal anti-inflammatory drugs
♦ Endoscopic examination of the bile ducts and pancreas
♦ Kidney failure or transplantation
♦ Metabolic or endocrine disorders, such as high cholesterol levels or overactive thyroid
♦ Pancreatic cysts or tumors
♦ Penetrating peptic ulcers

Pathophysiology

Acute pancreatitis occurs in two forms: edematous (*interstitial*) and necrotizing (*hemorrhagic*). Edematous pancreatitis causes fluid accumulation and swelling. Necrotizing pancreatitis causes cell death and tissue damage. (See *How acute pancreatitis affects the body*, page 356.)

MULTISYSTEM DISORDER

How acute pancreatitis affects the body

Acute pancreatitis can have far-reaching effects throughout the body. The summary below highlights how this disorder affects the major body systems and the multidisciplinary care required.

Gastrointestinal system

♦ Inflammation is caused by premature activation of enzymes (elastase and phospholipase A), which causes tissue damage. Enzymes back up and spill out into the pancreatic tissue, resulting in autodigestion of the pancreas.
♦ Elastase is activated by trypsin. It digests the elastic tissue of the blood vessel walls, causing hemorrhage.
♦ Phospholipase A may be activated by trypsin or bile acids. After it's activated, phospholipase A digests the phospholipids contained in the cell membranes.
♦ Large amounts of fluid shift from the intravascular space to the peritoneal and interstitial spaces.
♦ Additional fluid loss may occur because of vomiting, diarrhea, hemorrhage, and nasogastric suction.
♦ Third-space fluid shifting may occur because of hypoalbuminemia.
♦ Fluid losses eventually lead to hypovolemic shock.

Cardiovascular system

♦ Trypsin activates kallikrein, which is thought to cause local damage and systemic hypotension. In turn, kallikrein causes vasodilation and increased vascular permeability, invasion of white blood cells, and pain.
♦ Tachycardia occurs as a result of hypotension, pain, and fever.

Hematologic system

♦ Pancreatic inflammation interferes with the absorption of vitamin K, resulting in vitamin K deficiency.
♦ Vitamin K deficiency impairs clotting mechanisms, causing disseminated intravascular coagulation.

Immune system

♦ The necrosed pancreatic tissue or the tissue surrounding the pancreas may become infected; leukocytosis and fever occur in response to the inflammatory process, if infection is present.
♦ Secondary infections occur as microorganisms, typically from other body areas such as the colon, move to the necrosed pancreas.
♦ As pancreatic enzymes cause tissue necrosis, purulent drainage collects within the pancreas. This material can erode through the retroperitoneum into the bowel, pleural space, mediastinum, or pelvis, subsequently leading to sepsis.

Respiratory system

♦ Severe pain interferes with the patient's ability to breathe deeply and expand his lungs adequately, commonly resulting in pneumonia.
♦ Pancreatic enzymes released into the circulation damage the pulmonary vessels, stimulate inflammation, and cause alveolocapillary leakage, resulting in intrapulmonary shunting, hypoxemia and, possibly, pleural effusion.

Collaborative management

Respiratory therapy may be included to ensure a patent airway and improve respiratory functioning. Nutritional support is indicated to assist with tissue healing and maintain a positive nitrogen balance. A pain management team may also be called upon to assist in that area. Additionally, social services must be involved to assist with emotional support for the patient and his family and with follow-up care.

In chronic pancreatitis, persistent inflammation produces irreversible changes in the structure and function of the pancreas. It sometimes follows an episode of acute pancreatitis. Protein precipitates block the pancreatic duct and eventually harden or calcify. Structural changes lead to fibrosis and atrophy of the glands. Growths called pseudocysts contain pancreatic enzymes and tissue debris. An abscess results if pseudocysts become infected.

If pancreatitis damages the islets of Langerhans, diabetes mellitus may result. Sudden severe pancreatitis causes massive hemorrhage and total destruction of the pancreas, manifested as diabetic acidosis, shock, or coma.

Signs and symptoms

♦ Midepigastric abdominal pain, which can radiate to the back, caused by the escape of inflammatory exudate and enzymes into the back

of the peritoneum, edema and distention of the pancreatic capsule, and obstruction of the biliary tract
◆ Persistent vomiting (in a severe attack) from hypermotility or paralytic ileus secondary to pancreatitis or peritonitis
◆ Abdominal distention (in a severe attack) from bowel hypermotility and the accumulation of fluids in the abdominal cavity
◆ Diminished bowel activity (in severe attack) suggesting altered motility secondary to peritonitis
◆ Crackles at lung bases (in a severe attack) secondary to heart failure
◆ Left pleural effusion (in a severe attack) from circulating pancreatic enzymes and adjacent inflammation
◆ Mottled skin from hemorrhagic necrosis of the pancreas
◆ Tachycardia secondary to dehydration and possible hypovolemia
◆ Low-grade fever resulting from the inflammatory response
◆ Cold, sweaty extremities secondary to cardiovascular collapse
◆ Restlessness related to pain associated with acute pancreatitis
◆ Extreme malaise (in chronic pancreatitis) related to malabsorption or diabetes

Complications
◆ Massive hemorrhage and shock
◆ Pseudocysts
◆ Biliary and duodenal obstruction
◆ Portal and splenic vein thrombosis
◆ Diabetes mellitus
◆ Respiratory failure
◆ Kidney failure
◆ Destruction of pancreas
◆ Diabetic acidosis
◆ Atelectasis
◆ Pneumonia

Diagnosis
◆ Elevated serum amylase and lipase levels confirm diagnosis.
◆ Blood and urine glucose tests reveal transient glucose in urine and hyperglycemia. In chronic pancreatitis, serum glucose levels may be transiently elevated.
◆ White blood cell count is elevated.
◆ The serum bilirubin level is elevated in both acute and chronic pancreatitis.
◆ The blood calcium level may be decreased.
◆ Stool analysis shows elevated lipid and trypsin levels in chronic pancreatitis.
◆ Abdominal and chest X-rays detect pleural effusions and differentiate pancreatitis from

diseases that cause similar symptoms; may detect pancreatic calculi.
◆ Computed tomography scan and ultrasonography show enlarged pancreas with cysts and pseudocysts.
◆ Endoscopic retrograde cholangiopancreatography identifies ductal system abnormalities, such as calcification or strictures; helps differentiate pancreatitis from other disorders, such as pancreatic cancer.

Treatment
◆ I.V. replacement of fluids, protein, and electrolytes to treat shock
◆ Fluid volume replacement to help correct metabolic acidosis
◆ Blood transfusions to replace blood loss from hemorrhage
◆ Withholding of food and oral fluids to rest the pancreas and reduce pancreatic enzyme secretion
◆ Nasogastric (NG) tube suctioning to decrease stomach distention and suppress pancreatic secretions
◆ An antiemetic to alleviate nausea and vomiting
◆ An antacid to neutralize gastric secretions
◆ A histamine antagonist to decrease hydrochloric acid production
◆ An antibiotic to fight bacterial infections
◆ An anticholinergic to reduce vagal stimulation, decrease GI motility, and inhibit pancreatic enzyme secretion
◆ Calcium gluconate 10% to correct hypocalcemia
◆ Insulin to correct hyperglycemia
◆ Elemental gavage feedings or total parenteral nutrition to provide nutrition if patient can't resume oral feedings
◆ Surgical drainage to treat a pancreatic abscess or pseudocyst or to reestablish drainage of the pancreas
◆ Laparotomy (if biliary tract obstruction causes acute pancreatitis) to remove obstruction
◆ Partial pancreatectomy to relieve pain

Special considerations
Acute pancreatitis is a life-threatening emergency, requiring meticulous supportive care and continuous monitoring of vital systems.
◆ Monitor vital signs and pulmonary artery pressure closely. If the patient has a central venous pressure line instead of a pulmonary artery catheter, monitor it closely for volume expansion (it shouldn't rise above 10 cm H_2O). Give albumin, if ordered, to maintain blood pressure. Record fluid intake and output; check urine output hourly, and monitor electrolyte levels.

Assess the patient for crackles, rhonchi, or decreased breath sounds.

◆ For bowel decompression, maintain constant NG suctioning, and give nothing by mouth. Perform good mouth and nose care.

◆ Watch for signs and symptoms of calcium deficiency—tetany, cramps, carpopedal spasm, and seizures. If you suspect hypocalcemia, keep airway and suction apparatus handy and pad side rails.

◆ Administer an analgesic, as needed, to relieve the patient's pain and anxiety. *Caution:* The patient shouldn't receive morphine or codeine because of their effect on the sphincter of Oddi.

◆ Remember that anticholinergics reduce salivary and sweat gland secretions. Warn the patient that he may experience dry mouth and facial flushing. *Caution:* Narrow-angle glaucoma contraindicates the use of atropine or its derivatives.

◆ Watch for adverse reactions to the antibiotic, such as nephrotoxicity with an aminoglycoside, pseudomembranous enterocolitis with clindamycin, and blood dyscrasias with chloramphenicol.

◆ Don't confuse thirst due to hyperglycemia (indicated by a serum glucose level up to 350 mg/dl and sugar and acetone in urine) with dry mouth due to NG intubation and anticholinergic therapy.

◆ Watch for complications due to total parenteral nutrition, such as sepsis, hypokalemia, overhydration, and metabolic acidosis. Watch for fever, cardiac irregularities, changes in arterial blood gas measurements, and deep respirations. Use strict aseptic technique when caring for the catheter insertion site.

PEPTIC ULCERS

Peptic ulcers, circumscribed lesions in the mucosal membrane extending below the epithelium, can develop in the lower esophagus, stomach, pylorus, duodenum, or jejunum. (See *Common types and sites of peptic ulcers.*) Although erosions are commonly referred to as ulcers, erosions are breaks in the mucosal membranes that don't extend below the epithelium. Ulcers may be acute or chronic. Chronic ulcers are identified by scar tissue at their base. About 80% of all peptic ulcers are duodenal ulcers, which affect the proximal part of the small intestine. Duodenal ulcers usually follow a chronic course with remissions and exacerbations; 5% to 10% of patients develop complications that necessitate surgery.

Gastric ulcers are most common in elderly and middle-age men, especially in long-term users of nonsteroidal anti-inflammatory drugs (NSAIDs), alcohol, or tobacco.

Causes

◆ *Helicobacter pylori* infection
◆ Pathologic hypersecretory disorders
◆ Use of NSAIDs

Pathophysiology

Although the stomach contains acidic secretions that can digest substances, intrinsic defenses protect the gastric mucosal membrane from injury. A thick, tenacious layer of gastric mucus protects the stomach from autodigestion, mechanical trauma, and chemical trauma. Prostaglandins provide another line of defense. Gastric ulcers may be a result of destruction of the mucosal barrier.

The duodenum is protected from ulceration by the function of Brunner's glands. These glands produce a viscid, mucoid, alkaline secretion that neutralizes the acid chyme. Duodenal ulcers appear to result from excessive acid protection.

H. pylori releases a toxin that destroys the gastric and duodenal mucosa, reducing the epithelium's resistance to acid digestion and causing gastritis and ulcer disease.

Salicylates and other NSAIDs inhibit the secretion of prostaglandins (substances that block ulceration). Certain illnesses, such as pancreatitis, hepatic disease, Crohn's disease, preexisting gastritis, and Zollinger-Ellison syndrome also contribute to ulceration.

Besides peptic ulcer's main causes, several predisposing factors are acknowledged. They include blood type (gastric ulcers and type A; duodenal ulcers and type O) and other genetic factors. Exposure to irritants, such as alcohol, coffee, and tobacco, may contribute by accelerating gastric acid emptying and promoting mucosal breakdown. Emotional stress also contributes to ulcer formation because of the increased stimulation of acid and pepsin secretion and decreased mucosal defense. Physical trauma and normal aging are additional predisposing conditions.

Signs and symptoms

Signs and symptoms vary by the type of ulcer.

Gastric ulcer

◆ Pain that worsens with eating due to stretching of the mucosa by food
◆ Nausea and anorexia secondary to mucosal stretching

Duodenal ulcer

◆ Epigastric pain that's gnawing, dull, aching, or hungerlike due to excessive acid production
◆ Pain relieved by food or antacids, but usually recurring 2 to 4 hours later secondary to food acting as a buffer for acid

Common types and sites of peptic ulcers

This illustration shows common types of peptic ulcers and common sites where they can occur. The illustration also shows how an ulcer can penetrate into and through the muscle layers and muscle wall.

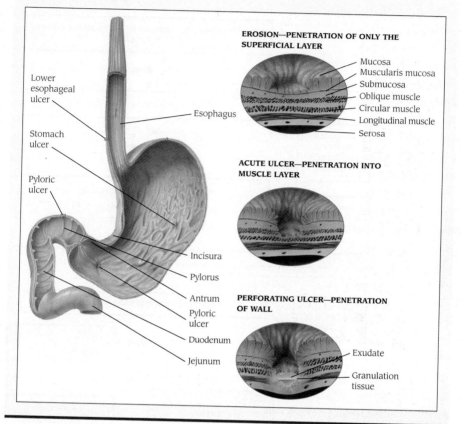

EROSION—PENETRATION OF ONLY THE SUPERFICIAL LAYER

- Mucosa
- Muscularis mucosa
- Submucosa
- Oblique muscle
- Circular muscle
- Longitudinal muscle
- Serosa

ACUTE ULCER—PENETRATION INTO MUSCLE LAYER

PERFORATING ULCER—PENETRATION OF WALL

- Exudate
- Granulation tissue

Lower esophageal ulcer

Esophagus

Stomach ulcer

Pyloric ulcer

Incisura

Pylorus

Antrum

Pyloric ulcer

Duodenum

Jejunum

Complications
- ◆ Hemorrhage
- ◆ Shock
- ◆ Gastric perforation
- ◆ Gastric outlet obstruction

Diagnosis
- ◆ Barium swallow or upper-GI and small-bowel series may reveal the presence of the ulcer. This is the first test performed on a patient when symptoms aren't severe.
- ◆ Endoscopy confirms the presence of an ulcer and permits cytologic studies and biopsy to rule out *H. pylori* or cancer.
- ◆ Upper GI tract X-rays reveal mucosal abnormalities.
- ◆ Stool analysis may reveal occult blood.

- ◆ Serologic testing may disclose clinical signs of infection, such as elevated white blood cell count.
- ◆ Gastric secretory studies show hyperchlorhydria.
- ◆ Urea breath test results reflect activity of *H. pylori*.

Treatment
- ◆ An antimicrobial, such as tetracycline, bismuth subsalicylate, or metronidazole, to eradicate *H. pylori* infection. (See *Treating peptic ulcer,* pages 360 and 361.)
- ◆ A proton gastric acid pump inhibitor, such as omeprazole, to decrease gastric acid secretion
- ◆ Misoprostol (a prostaglandin analog) to inhibit gastric acid secretion and increase carbonate

DISEASE BLOCK

Treating peptic ulcer

Peptic ulcers can result from factors that increase gastric acid production or from factors that impair mucosal barrier protection. This illustration highlights the actions of the major treatments used for peptic ulcer and where they interfere with the pathophysiologic chain of events.

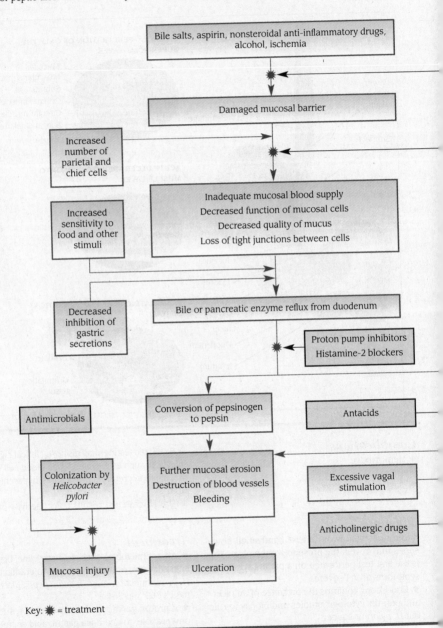

Key: ✺ = treatment

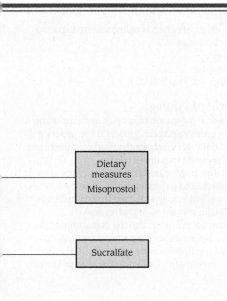

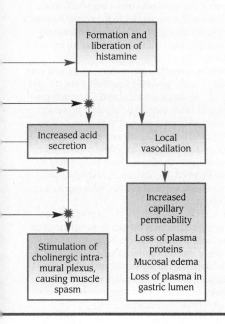

and mucus production, to protect the stomach lining
◆ An antacid to neutralize acid gastric contents by elevating the gastric pH, thus protecting the mucosa and relieving pain
◆ Avoidance of caffeine and alcohol to avoid stimulation of gastric acid secretion
◆ An anticholinergic to inhibit the effect of the vagal nerve on acid-secreting cells
◆ A histamine-2 blocker to reduce acid secretion
◆ Sucralfate, a mucosal protectant to form an acid-impermeable membrane that adheres to the mucous membrane and also accelerates mucus production
◆ Dietary therapy with small infrequent meals and avoidance of eating before bedtime to neutralize gastric contents
◆ Insertion of a nasogastric (NG) tube (in instances of GI bleeding) for gastric decompression and rest and, also, to permit iced saline lavage that may contain norepinephrine
◆ Gastroscopy to allow visualization of the bleeding site and coagulation by laser or cautery to control bleeding
◆ Surgery to repair perforation or to treat unresponsiveness to conservative treatment or suspected malignancy

Special considerations
Management of peptic ulcers requires careful administration of medications, thorough patient teaching, and skillful postoperative care.
◆ Administer prescribed medications.
◆ Watch for adverse reactions to H_2-receptor antagonists and omeprazole (dizziness, fatigue, rash, and mild diarrhea).
◆ Advise any patient who uses an antacid, has a history of cardiac disease, or follows a sodium-restricted diet to take only those antacids that contain low amounts of sodium.
◆ Warn the patient to avoid steroids and NSAIDs because they irritate the gastric mucosa. For the same reason, advise the patient to stop smoking and to avoid stressful situations, excessive intake of coffee, and any ingestion of alcoholic beverages during exacerbations of peptic ulcer disease.
◆ Inform the patient of the potential adverse effects of antibiotic therapy, for example, superinfection and diarrhea. Instruct him to notify the physician if these occur.
◆ Describe follow-up testing that the physician will order to confirm eradication of *H. pylori* infection.
◆ Tell the patient taking bismuth subsalicylate that this drug may cause constipation.

After gastric surgery

◆ Keep the NG tube patent. If the tube isn't functioning, don't reposition it; you might damage the suture line or anastomosis. Notify the surgeon promptly.

◆ Monitor intake and output, including NG tube drainage. Check for bowel sounds, and allow the patient nothing by mouth until peristalsis resumes and the NG tube is removed or clamped.

◆ Replace fluids and electrolytes. Assess the patient for signs of dehydration, sodium deficiency, and metabolic alkalosis, which may occur secondary to gastric suction.

◆ Monitor the patient for possible complications: hemorrhage; shock; iron, folate, or vitamin B_{12} deficiency anemia from malabsorption (pernicious anemia) due to lack of intrinsic factor; and dumping syndrome (a rapid gastric emptying, causing distention of the duodenum or jejunum produced by a bolus of food). Signs and symptoms of dumping syndrome include diaphoresis, weakness, nausea, flatulence, explosive diarrhea, distention, and palpitations within 30 minutes after a meal.

◆ To avoid dumping syndrome, advise the patient to lie down after meals, to drink fluids between meals rather than with meals, to avoid eating large amounts of carbohydrates, and to eat four to six small, high-protein, low-carbohydrate meals during the day.

POLYPS, INTESTINAL

A polyp is a small, tumorlike growth that projects from a mucous membrane surface. Polyps may develop in the colon or rectum, where they protrude into the GI tract. Polyps are classified according to tissue type. Common polyp types include:

◆ *adenomatous polyps,* such as tubular adenoma, tubulovillous adenoma, and villous adenoma

◆ *nonadenomatous polyps,* such as hyperplastic polyps, inflammatory polyps, and juvenile polyps.

Additionally, there are polyposis syndromes, including familial adenomatous polyposis; hamartomatous polyposis syndromes; and acquired polyposis syndromes, such as Cronkhite-Canada syndrome.

Most polyps are benign. However, villous and familial polyps show a marked inclination to become malignant. A striking feature of familial polyposis is its frequent association with rectosigmoid adenocarcinoma.

AGE ALERT *Villous adenomas are most prevalent in men older than age 55. Common polypoid adenomas are most prevalent in white women between ages 45 and 60. The incidence in both sexes increases after age 70. Juvenile polyps occur most commonly in children younger than age 10 and are characterized by rectal bleeding.*

Causes

The cause of polyps is unknown. Predisposing risk factors include:

◆ age

◆ heredity

◆ high-fat, low-fiber diet.

Pathophysiology

Intestinal polyps are masses of tissue resulting from unrestrained cell growth in the upper epithelium that rise above the mucosal membrane and protrude into the GI tract.

Polyps may be described by their appearance: pedunculated (attached by a stalk to the intestinal wall) or sessile (attached to the intestinal wall with a broad base and no stalk).

Familial polyposis and the hamartomatous polyposis syndromes are rare, autosomal dominant inherited disorders. Cronkhite-Canada syndrome is also a rare disorder with unknown etiology.

Signs and symptoms

Because intestinal polyps don't generally cause symptoms, they're usually discovered incidentally during a digital examination or rectosigmoidoscopy. Rectal bleeding is a common sign; high rectal polyps leave a streak of blood on the stool, whereas low rectal polyps bleed freely.

Polyps vary in appearance. Hyperplastic polyps are generally diminutive—less than 0.5 cm. Common polypoid adenomas are small, multiple lesions that are redder than normal mucosa. They're commonly slightly raised, pedunculated, and granular, with a red, lobular, or eroded surface.

Villous adenomas are usually sessile and vary in size, but are generally less than 2 cm. They're soft, friable, and finely lobulated. They may grow large and cause painful defecation; however, because adenomas are soft, they rarely cause bowel obstruction. Sometimes adenomas prolapse outside the anus, expelling parts of the adenoma with the feces. These polyps may cause diarrhea, bloody stools, and subsequent fluid and electrolyte depletion, with hypotension and oliguria.

In hereditary polyposis, rectal polyps resemble benign adenomas but occur as hundreds or thousands of small (0.5-cm) lesions carpeting the entire mucosal surface. Associated signs include diarrhea, bloody stools, and secondary anemia. In patients with familial polyposis, changes in bowel habits with abdominal pain usually signal rectosigmoid cancer.

Juvenile polyps appear as smooth, pedunculated cherry-red polyps and are generally large.

Mucus-filled cysts cover their usually smooth surface.

Focal polypoid hyperplasia produces small (less than 3 mm), granular, sessile lesions, similar to the colon in color, or gray or translucent. They usually occur at the rectosigmoid junction.

Complications
◆ Anemia resulting from slow-bleeding polyps
◆ Bowel obstruction resulting from large polyps
◆ Rectal bleeding
◆ Intussusception
◆ Colorectal cancer (villous adenomas and familial polyps)

Diagnosis
Firm diagnosis of rectal polyps requires identification of the polyps through sigmoidoscopy or colonoscopy and rectal biopsy. Barium enema can help identify polyps that are located high in the colon. Supportive laboratory findings include occult blood in the stools, low hemoglobin level and hematocrit (with anemia) and, possibly, serum electrolyte imbalances in patients with villous adenomas.

Treatment
Treatment varies according to the type and size of the polyps and their location in the colon. Common polypoid adenomas less than 1 cm in size require polypectomy, commonly by fulguration (destruction by high-frequency electricity) during endoscopy. For common polypoid adenomas over 4 cm and all invasive villous adenomas, treatment usually consists of abdominoperineal resection or low anterior resection.

Focal polypoid hyperplasia can be obliterated by biopsy. Depending on GI involvement, hereditary polyps necessitate total abdominoperineal resection with a permanent ileostomy, subtotal colectomy with ileoproctostomy, or ileoanal anastomosis. Juvenile polyps are prone to autoamputation, due to spontaneous sloughing of the polyp; if this doesn't occur, snare removal during colonoscopy is the treatment of choice.

Special considerations
During diagnostic evaluation
◆ Check sodium, potassium, and chloride levels daily in the patient with fluid imbalance; adjust fluid and electrolytes, as necessary. Administer normal saline solution with potassium I.V., as ordered. Weigh the patient daily, and record the amount of diarrhea. Watch for signs of dehydration (decreased urine output and an increased blood urea nitrogen level).
◆ Tell the patient to watch for and report evidence of rectal bleeding.

After biopsy and fulguration
◆ Check for signs of perforation and hemorrhage, such as sudden hypotension, decrease in the hemoglobin level or hematocrit, shock, abdominal pain, and passage of red blood through the rectum.
◆ Have the patient walk as soon as possible after the procedure.
◆ Watch for and record the first bowel movement, which may not occur for 2 to 3 days.
◆ If the patient has benign polyps, stress the need for routine follow-up studies to check for new polypoid growth.
◆ Prepare the patient with precancerous or familial lesions for abdominoperineal resection. Provide emotional support and preoperative instruction.

After ileostomy or subtotal colectomy with ileoproctostomy
◆ Properly care for abdominal dressings, I.V. lines, and indwelling urinary catheter. Record intake and output, and check vital signs for hypotension and surgical complications. Administer pain medication, as ordered.
◆ To prevent embolism, have the patient walk as soon as possible, and apply antiembolism stockings; encourage range-of-motion exercises.
◆ Provide enterostomal therapy and teach stoma care.

ULCERATIVE COLITIS
Ulcerative colitis is an inflammatory, usually chronic, disease that affects the mucosa of the colon. It invariably begins in the rectum and sigmoid colon, and commonly extends upward into the entire colon, rarely affecting the small intestine. Ulcerative colitis produces edema (leading to mucosal friability) and ulcerations. Severity ranges from a mild, localized disorder to a fulminant disease that may cause a perforated colon, progressing to potentially fatal peritonitis and toxemia. The disease cycles between exacerbation and remission.

Ulcerative colitis occurs primarily in young adults, especially women. It's more prevalent among Ashkenazim and in higher socioeconomic groups, and there seems to be a familial tendency. The prevalence is unknown; however, some studies suggest 10 to 15 out of 100,000 persons have the disease. Onset of symptoms seems to peak between ages 15 and 30 and between ages 50 and 70.

Causes
Specific causes of ulcerative colitis are unknown but may be related to abnormal immune

response in the GI tract, possibly associated with food or bacteria such as *Escherichia coli.*

Pathophysiology

Ulcerative colitis usually begins as inflammation in the base of the mucosal layer of the large intestine. The colon's mucosal surface becomes dark, red, and velvety. Inflammation leads to erosions that coalesce and form ulcers. The mucosa becomes diffusely ulcerated, with hemorrhage, congestion, edema, and exudative inflammation. Ulcerations are continuous. Abscesses in the mucosa drain purulent exudate, become necrotic, and ulcerate. Sloughing causes bloody, mucus-filled stools. As abscesses heal, scarring and thickening may appear in the bowel's inner muscle layer. As granulation tissue replaces the muscle layer, the colon narrows, shortens, and loses its characteristic pouches (haustral folds). (See *Mucosal changes in ulcerative colitis.*)

Signs and symptoms

◆ Recurrent bloody diarrhea (as many as 10 to 20 stools per day), typically containing pus and mucus (hallmark sign), from accumulated blood and mucus in the bowel
◆ Abdominal cramping and rectal urgency from accumulated blood and mucus
◆ Weight loss secondary to malabsorption
◆ Weakness related to possible malabsorption and subsequent anemia

Complications

◆ Perforation
◆ Toxic megacolon
◆ Liver disease
◆ Stricture formation
◆ Colon cancer
◆ Anemia

Diagnosis

◆ Sigmoidoscopy confirms rectal involvement: specifically, mucosal friability and flattening and thick, inflammatory exudate.
◆ Colonoscopy reveals extent of the disease, stricture areas, and pseudopolyps (not performed when the patient has active signs and symptoms).
◆ Biopsy with colonoscopy confirms the diagnosis.
◆ Barium enema reveals the extent of the disease, detects complications, and identifies cancer (not performed when the patient has active signs and symptoms).
◆ Stool specimen analysis reveals blood, pus, and mucus but no disease-causing organisms.
◆ Serology shows decreased serum potassium, magnesium, and albumin levels; decreased white blood cell count; decreased hemoglobin level; and prolonged prothrombin time. Elevated erythrocyte sedimentation rate correlates with severity of the attack.

Treatment

◆ A corticosteroid, such as prednisone and hydrocortisone
◆ An aminosalicylate such as sulfasalazine for anti-inflammatory and antimicrobial effects
◆ An antidiarrheal to relieve frequent, troublesome diarrhea in patients whose ulcerative colitis is otherwise under control
◆ An immunomodulator or 5-aminosalicylates to reduce inflammation by acting on the immune system
◆ An iron supplement to correct anemia
◆ Total parenteral nutrition (TPN) and nothing by mouth (NPO) for patients with severe disease, to rest the intestinal tract, decrease stool volume, and restore nitrogen balance
◆ Supplemental drinks to supplement nutrition in patients with moderate symptoms
◆ I.V. hydration to replace fluid loss from diarrhea
◆ Surgery to correct massive dilation of the colon and to treat patients with symptoms that are unbearable or unresponsive to drugs and supportive measures
◆ Proctocolectomy with ileostomy to remove all potentially malignant epithelia of the rectum and colon

Special considerations

Patient care includes close monitoring for changes in status.
◆ Accurately record intake and output, particularly the frequency and volume of stools. Watch for signs of dehydration and electrolyte imbalances, especially signs and symptoms of hypokalemia (muscle weakness and paresthesia) and hypernatremia (tachycardia, flushed skin, fever, and dry tongue). Monitor the patient's hemoglobin level and hematocrit, and give blood transfusions, as ordered. Provide good mouth care for the patient who's NPO.
◆ After each bowel movement, thoroughly clean the skin around the rectum. Provide an air mattress or sheepskin to help prevent skin breakdown.
◆ Administer medications as ordered. Watch for adverse reactions to prolonged corticosteroid therapy (moonface, hirsutism, edema, and gastric irritation). Be aware that corticosteroid therapy may mask infection.
◆ If the patient needs TPN, change dressings as ordered, assess the insertion site for inflammation, and check the capillary blood glucose level every 4 to 6 hours.

Mucosal changes in ulcerative colitis

In ulcerative colitis, the colon goes through inflammation and ulceration.

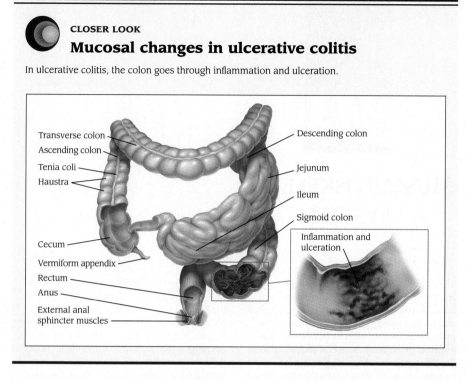

Transverse colon
Ascending colon
Tenia coli
Haustra

Descending colon
Jejunum
Ileum
Sigmoid colon

Cecum
Vermiform appendix
Rectum
Anus
External anal sphincter muscles

Inflammation and ulceration

◆ Take precautionary measures if the patient is prone to bleeding. Watch closely for signs and symptoms of complications, such as a perforated colon and peritonitis (fever, severe abdominal pain, abdominal rigidity and tenderness, and cool, clammy skin), and toxic megacolon (abdominal distention and decreased bowel sounds).

For patients requiring surgery

◆ Carefully prepare the patient for surgery, and inform him about ileostomy.
◆ Administer a bowel preparation, as ordered.
◆ After surgery, provide meticulous supportive care and continue teaching correct stoma care.
◆ Keep the nasogastric tube patent. After removal of the tube, provide a clear-liquid diet, and gradually advance to a low-residue diet, as tolerated.
◆ After a proctocolectomy and ileostomy, teach good stoma care. Wash the skin around the stoma with soapy water and dry it thoroughly. Apply karaya gum around the stoma's base to avoid irritation, and make a watertight seal. Attach the pouch over the karaya ring. Cut an opening in the ring to fit over the stoma, and secure the pouch to the skin. Empty the pouch when it's one-third full.

◆ After a pouch ileostomy, uncork the catheter every hour to allow contents to drain. After 10 to 14 days, gradually increase the length of time the catheter is left corked until it can be opened every 3 hours. Then remove the catheter and reinsert it every 3 to 4 hours for drainage. Teach the patient how to insert the catheter and how to take care of the stoma.
◆ Encourage the patient to have regular physical examinations.
◆ Refer the patient to a support group such as the Crohn's and Colitis Foundation of America.

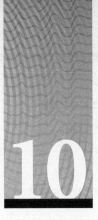

10

MUSCULOSKELETAL SYSTEM

The musculoskeletal system is a complex system of bones, joints, muscles, ligaments, tendons, and other tissues that gives the body form and shape. It also protects vital organs, makes movement possible, stores calcium and other minerals in the bony matrix for mobilization if deficiency occurs, and provides sites for hematopoiesis (blood cell production) in the marrow.

Bones

The human skeleton contains 206 bones, which are composed of inorganic salts (primarily calcium and phosphate), embedded in a framework of collagen fibers.

BONE SHAPE AND STRUCTURE
Bones are classified by shape as either long, short, flat, or irregular. Long bones are found in the extremities and include the humerus, radius, and ulna of the arm; the femur, tibia, and fibula of the leg; and the phalanges, metacarpals, and metatarsals of the hands and feet. (See *Structure of long bones*.) Short bones include the *tarsal* and *carpal* bones of the feet and hands, respectively. Flat bones include the *frontal* and *parietal* bones of the cranium, ribs, sternum, scapulae, ilium, and pubis. Irregular bones include the bones of the spine (vertebrae, sacrum, coccyx) and certain bones of the skull (the temporal, sphenoid, ethmoid, and mandible).

Classified according to structure, bone is either cortical (compact) or cancellous (spongy or trabecular). Adult cortical bone consists of networks

of interconnecting canals, or canaliculi. Each network, or haversian system, runs parallel to the bone's long axis and consists of a central haversian canal surrounded by layers (lamellae) of bone. Between adjacent lamellae are small openings called *lacunae*, which contain bone cells or osteocytes. The canaliculi, each containing one capillary or more, provide a route for tissue fluids transport; they connect all the lacunae.

Cancellous bone consists of thin plates (trabeculae) that form the interior meshwork of bone. These trabeculae are arranged in various directions to correspond with the lines of maximum stress or pressure. This gives the bone added structural strength. Chemically, inorganic salts (calcium and phosphate, with small amounts of sodium, potassium carbonate, and magnesium ions) comprise 70% of the mature bone. The salts give bone its elasticity and ability to withstand compression.

BONE GROWTH
Bone formation is ongoing and is determined by hormonal stimulation, dietary factors, and the amount of stress put on the bone. It's accomplished by the continual actions of bone-forming osteoblasts and bone-reabsorbing cells called *osteoclasts*. Osteoblasts are present on the outer surface of and within bones. They respond to various stimuli to produce the bony matrix, or osteoid. As calcium salts precipitate on the organic matrix, the bone hardens. As the bone forms, a system of microscopic canals in the bone forms around the osteocytes. Osteoclasts are phagocytic cells that digest old, weakened

Structure of long bones

Long bones are the weight-bearing bones of the body. Their structures provide maximal strength and minimal weight. Structure of a long bone in an adult is shown below.

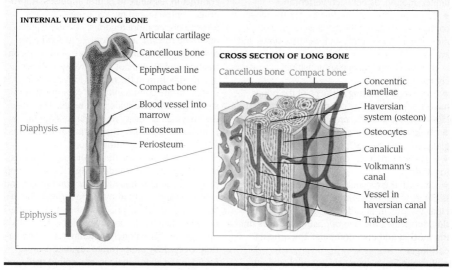

INTERNAL VIEW OF LONG BONE

Articular cartilage
Cancellous bone
Epiphyseal line
Compact bone
Blood vessel into marrow
Diaphysis
Endosteum
Periosteum
Epiphysis

CROSS SECTION OF LONG BONE

Cancellous bone Compact bone
Concentric lamellae
Haversian system (osteon)
Osteocytes
Canaliculi
Volkmann's canal
Vessel in haversian canal
Trabeculae

bone section by section. As they finish, osteoblasts simultaneously replace the cleared section with new, stronger bone.

Vitamin D supports bone calcification by stimulating osteoblast activity and calcium absorption from the gut to make it available for bone building. When the serum calcium level falls, the parathyroid gland releases parathyroid hormone, which then stimulates osteoclast activity and bone breakdown, freeing calcium into the blood. Parathyroid hormone also increases serum calcium by decreasing renal excretion of calcium and increasing renal excretion of phosphate ion.

Phosphates are essential to bone formation; about 85% of the body's phosphates are found in bone. The intestine absorbs a considerable amount of phosphates from dietary sources, but adequate levels of vitamin D are necessary for their absorption. Because calcium and phosphates interact in a reciprocal relationship, renal excretion of phosphates increases or decreases inversely proportional to the serum calcium level. Alkaline phosphatase (ALP) influences bone calcification and lipid and metabolite transport. Osteoblasts contain an abundance of ALP. A rise in the serum ALP level can indicate the presence of a skeletal disease, primarily one characterized by marked osteoblastic activity, such as bone metastases or Paget's disease. It can also point to biliary obstruction,

hyperparathyroidism, or excessive ingestion of vitamin D.

In children and young adults, bone growth occurs in the epiphyseal plate, a layer of cartilage between the diaphysis and epiphysis of long bones.

Osteoblasts deposit new bone in the area just beneath the epiphysis, making the bone longer, and osteoclasts model the new bone's shape by reabsorbing previously deposited bone. These remodeling activities promote longitudinal bone growth, which continues until the epiphyseal growth plates, located at both ends, close during adolescence. Human growth factor and sex hormones influence the rate of ossification. In adults, bone growth is complete, and cartilage is replaced by bone, becoming the epiphyseal line.

Joints

The tendons, ligaments, cartilage, and other tissues that connect two bones constitute a joint. Depending on their structures, joints either predominantly permit motion or provide stability. Joints, like bones, are classified according to structure and function.

JOINT CLASSIFICATION
The three structural types of joints are fibrous, cartilaginous, and synovial.

◆ Fibrous joints, or *synarthroses,* permit only slight movement and provide stability when tight union is necessary, as in the sutures that join the cranial bones.

◆ Cartilaginous joints, or *amphiarthroses,* allow limited motion, as between vertebrae.

◆ Synovial joints, or *diarthroses,* are the most common and permit the greatest degree of movement. These joints include the elbows and knees.

Synovial joints have distinguishing characteristics:

◆ The two articulating surfaces of the bones have a smooth hyaline covering (articular cartilage) that's resilient to pressure.

◆ Their opposing surfaces are congruous and glide smoothly on each other.

◆ A fibrous (articular) capsule holds them together.

◆ Beneath the capsule, lining the joint cavity, is the synovial membrane, which secretes a clear viscous fluid called *synovial fluid.* This fluid lubricates the two opposing surfaces during motion and also nourishes the articular cartilage.

◆ Surrounding a synovial joint are ligaments, muscles, and tendons, which strengthen and stabilize the joint but allow free movement.

JOINT MOVEMENT

The two types of synovial joint movement are *angular* and *circular.*

Angular movement

Joints of the knees, elbows, and phalanges permit the following angular movements:

◆ flexion (closing of the joint angle)

◆ extension (opening of the joint angle)

◆ hyperextension (extension of the angle beyond the usual arc).

Other joints, including the shoulders and hips, permit:

◆ abduction (movement away from the body's midline)

◆ adduction (movement toward the midline).

Circular movement

Circular movements include:

◆ rotation (motion around a central axis), as in the ball-and-socket joints of the hips and shoulders

◆ pronation (downward wrist or ankle motion)

◆ supination (upward wrist motion).

Other kinds of movement include inversion (inward turning, as of the foot), eversion (outward turning, as of the foot), protraction (as in the forward motion of the mandible), and retraction (returning protracted part into place).

Muscles

The most specialized feature of muscle tissue— contractility—makes the movement of bones and joints possible. Normal skeletal muscles contract in response to neural impulses. Appropriate contraction of muscle usually applies force to one or more tendons. The force pulls one bone toward, away from, or around a second bone, depending on the type of muscle contraction and the type of joint involved. Abnormal metabolism in the muscle may result in inappropriate contractility. For example, when stored glycogen or lipids can't be used because the enzyme necessary to convert energy for contraction is lacking, the result may be cramps, fatigue, and exercise intolerance.

Muscles permit and maintain body positions, such as sitting and standing. Muscles also pump blood through the body (cardiac contraction and vessel compression), move food through the intestines (peristalsis), and make breathing possible. Skeletal muscle activity produces heat; it's an important component in temperature regulation. Deep body temperature regulators are found in the abdominal viscera, spinal cord, and great veins. These receptors detect changes in the body core temperature and stimulate the hypothalamus to institute appropriate temperature changing responses, such as shivering in response to cold. Muscle mass accounts for about 40% of an average man's weight.

MUSCLE CLASSIFICATION

Muscles are classified according to structure, anatomic location, and function.

◆ Skeletal muscles are attached to bone and have striped (striated) appearances that reflect their cellular structures.

◆ Visceral muscles move contents through internal organs and are smooth (nonstriated).

◆ Cardiac muscles (smooth) constitute the heart wall.

When muscles are classified according to activity, they're called either *voluntary* or *involuntary.* (See chapter 8, Nervous system.) Voluntary muscles can be controlled at will and are under the influence of the somatic nervous system; these are the skeletal muscles. Involuntary muscles, controlled by the autonomic nervous system, include the cardiac and visceral muscles. Some organs contain voluntary and involuntary muscles.

MUSCLE CONTRACTION

Each skeletal muscle consists of many elongated muscle cells, called *muscle fibers,* through which run slender threads of protein, called *myofibrils.* Muscle fibers are held together in bundles by sheaths of fibrous tissues called *fascia*. Blood vessels and nerves pass into muscles through the fascia to reach the individual muscle fibers. Motoneurons synapse with the motor nerve fibers of voluntary muscles. These fibers reach the membranes of skeletal muscle cells at neuromuscular (myoneural) junctions. When an impulse reaches the myoneural junction, the junction releases the neurotransmitter, acetylcholine, which releases calcium from the sarcoplasmic reticulum, a membranous network in the muscle fiber, which, in turn, triggers muscle contraction. Muscle contraction is isometric or isotonic. Isometric contraction results in an increase in tension without change in length. Isotonic contraction occurs when the muscle shortens as weight is lifted. The energy source for this contraction is adenosine triphosphate (ATP). ATP release is also triggered by the impulse at the myoneural junction. Relaxation of a muscle is believed to take place by reversal of these mechanisms.

Muscle fatigue results when the sources of ATP in a muscle are depleted. If a muscle is deprived of oxygen, fatigue occurs rapidly. As the muscle fatigues, it switches to anaerobic metabolism of glycogen stores, in which the stored glycogen is split into glucose (glycolysis) without the use of oxygen. Lactic acid is a by-product of anaerobic glycolysis and may accumulate in the muscle and blood with intense or prolonged muscle contraction.

Tendons and ligaments

Skeletal muscles are attached to bone directly or indirectly by fibrous cords known as *tendons*. The least movable end of the muscle attachment (generally proximal) is called the *point of origin;* the most movable end (generally distal) is called the *point of insertion.*

Ligaments are fibrous connections that control joint movement between two bones or cartilages. Their purpose is to support and strengthen joints.

Pathophysiologic changes

Alterations of the normal functioning of bones and muscles are described here. Most musculoskeletal disorders are caused by or profoundly affect other body systems.

ALTERATIONS IN BONE
Disease may alter bone density, growth, or strength.

Density
In healthy young adults, the resorption and formation phases are tightly coupled to maintain bone mass in a steady state. Bone loss occurs when the two phases become uncoupled, and resorption exceeds formation. Estrogen not only regulates calcium uptake and release but also regulates osteoblastic activity. A decreased estrogen level may lead to diminished osteoblastic activity and loss of bone mass, called *osteoporosis*. In children, vitamin D deficiency prevents normal bone growth and leads to rickets.

AGE ALERT *Bone density and structural integrity decrease in women after age 30 and in men after age 45. The relatively steady loss of bone matrix can be partially offset by exercise and appropriate dietary calcium intake.*

CLINICAL ALERT *Age, race, and sex affect bone mass, structural integrity (ability to withstand stress), and bone loss. For example, blacks commonly have denser bones than whites, and men typically have denser bones than women.*

Growth
The osteochondroses are a group of disorders characterized by avascular necrosis of the epiphyseal growth plates in growing children and adolescents. In these disorders, a lack of blood supply to the femoral head leads to septic necrosis, with softening and resorption of bone. Revascularization then initiates new bone formation in the femoral head or tibial tubercle, which leads to a malformed femoral head.

Strength
Both cortical and trabecular bone contribute to skeletal strength. Any loss of the inorganic salts that constitute the chemical structure of bone will weaken bone. Cancellous bone is more sensitive to metabolic influences, so conditions that produce rapid bone loss tend to affect cancellous bone more quickly than cortical bone.

ALTERATIONS OF MUSCLE
Pathologic effects on muscle include atrophy, fatigue, weakness, myotonia, and spasticity.

Atrophy
Atrophy is a decrease in the size of a tissue or cell. In muscles, the myofibrils atrophy after prolonged inactivity from bed rest or trauma (casting), when local nerve damage makes movement impossible, or when illness removes needed nutrients from muscles. The effects of muscular deconditioning associated with lack of physical activity may be apparent in a matter of days. An individual on bed rest loses muscle

strength, as well as muscle mass, from baseline levels at a rate of 3% per day. Conditioning and stretching exercises may help prevent atrophy. If reuse isn't restored within 1 year, regeneration of muscle fibers is unlikely.

AGE ALERT *Sarcopenia, or age-related loss of skeletal muscle, is a direct cause of decrease in muscle strength. A slow decline in dynamic and isometric strength is evident in adults after age 70.*

Fatigue

Pathologic muscle fatigue may be the result of impaired neural stimulation of muscle or energy metabolism or disruption of calcium flux. See chapter 4, Fluids and electrolytes, for a detailed discussion of these events.

Weakness

AGE ALERT *Muscle mass and muscle strength may decrease in elderly patients as a result of disuse. This can be reversed with moderate, regular, weight-bearing exercise.*

Periodic paralysis is a genetic disorder that can be triggered by exercise or a process or chemical (such as medication) that alters the serum potassium level. This hyperkalemic or hypokalemic periodic paralysis may be caused by a high-carbohydrate diet, emotional stress, prolonged bed rest, or hyperthyroidism. During an attack of periodic paralysis, the muscle membrane is unresponsive to neural stimuli, and the electrical charge needed to initiate the impulse (resting membrane potential) is reduced from −90 to −45 millivolts.

Myotonia and spasticity

Myotonia is delayed relaxation after a voluntary muscle contraction — such as grip, eye closure, or muscle percussion — accompanied by prolonged depolarization of the muscle membrane. Depolarization is the reversal of the resting potential in stimulated cell membranes. It's the process by which the cell membrane "resets" its positive charge with respect to the negative charge outside the cell. Myotonia occurs in myotonic muscular dystrophy and some forms of periodic paralysis.

Stress-induced muscle tension, or spasticity, is presumably caused by increased activity in the reticular activating system and gamma loop in the muscle fiber. The reticular activating system consists of multiple diffuse pathways in the brain that control wakefulness and response to stimuli. A pathologic contracture is permanent muscle shortening caused by muscle spasticity, seen in central nervous system injury or severe muscle weakness.

Disorders

This section discusses musculoskeletal disorders, some of which have far-reaching effects in other body systems. They include bone fracture, carpal tunnel syndrome, clubfoot, developmental dysplasia of the hip, gout, herniated disk, Legg-Calvé-Perthes disease, muscular dystrophy, osteoarthritis, osteogenesis imperfecta, osteomalacia and rickets, osteomyelitis, osteoporosis, Paget's disease, rhabdomyolysis, scoliosis, and sprains and strains.

CLINICAL ALERT *Many patients with musculoskeletal disorders are elderly, have other concurrent medical conditions, or are victims of trauma. Generally, they face prolonged immobilization. (See Managing musculoskeletal pain.)*

BONE FRACTURE

When a force exceeds the compressive or tensile strength (the ability of the bone to hold together) of the bone, a fracture will occur. (For an explanation of the terms used to identify fractures, see *Classifying fractures*, page 372.)

Each year, an estimated 25% of the population has traumatic musculoskeletal injury, and a significant number of these involve fractures.

The prognosis varies with the extent of disablement or deformity, amount of tissue and vascular damage, adequacy of reduction and immobilization, and patient's age, health, and nutritional status.

AGE ALERT *Children's bones usually heal rapidly and without deformity. However, epiphyseal plate fractures in children are likely to cause deformity because they interfere with normal bone growth. In elderly people, underlying systemic illness, impaired circulation, or poor nutrition may cause slow or poor healing.*

Causes

◆ Bone tumors
◆ Falls
◆ Medications that cause iatrogenic osteoporosis such as steroids
◆ Metabolic illnesses (such as hypoparathyroidism or hyperparathyroidism)
◆ Motor vehicle crashes
◆ Sports
◆ Use of drugs that impair judgment or mobility
◆ Young age (immaturity of bone)

AGE ALERT *The highest incidence of bone fractures occurs in young males between ages 15 and 24 (tibia, clavicle, and lower humerus) and are usually the result of trauma. In elderly people, upper femur, upper humerus, forearm, wrist, vertebrae, and pelvis fractures are commonly associated with osteoporosis and falls.*

Pathophysiology

When a bone is fractured, the periosteum and blood vessels in the cortex, marrow, and surrounding soft tissue are disrupted. A hematoma forms between the broken ends of the bone and beneath the periosteum, and granulation tissue eventually replaces the hematoma.

Damage to bone tissue triggers an intense inflammatory response in which cells from surrounding soft tissue and the marrow cavity invade the fracture area, and blood flow to the entire bone is increased. Osteoblasts in the periosteum, endosteum, and marrow produce osteoid (collagenous, young bone that hasn't yet calcified, also called *callus*), which hardens along the outer surface of the shaft and over the broken ends of the bone. Osteoclasts reabsorb dead bone and osteoblasts rebuild bone. Osteoblasts then transform into osteocytes (mature bone cells). Remodeling occurs as excess callus is reabsorbed and trabecular bone is laid down.

Signs and symptoms

♦ Deformity due to unnatural alignment
♦ Swelling due to vasodilation and infiltration by inflammatory leukocytes and mast cells
♦ Muscle spasm and tenderness related to the inflammatory response
♦ Impaired sensation distal to the fracture site due to pinching or severing of neurovascular elements by the trauma or by bone fragments
♦ Limited range of motion due to misalignment, neurovascular compromise, swelling, and pain
♦ Crepitus, or "clicking" sounds on movement, caused by shifting bone fragments
♦ Bruising from blood released at the fracture site.

Complications

♦ Permanent deformity and dysfunction if bones fail to heal (nonunion) or heal improperly (malunion)
♦ Aseptic (not caused by infection) necrosis of bone segments due to impaired circulation
♦ Hypovolemic shock as a result of blood vessel damage (especially with a fractured femur)
♦ Muscle contractures
♦ Compartment syndrome (See *Recognizing compartment syndrome*, page 373.)
♦ Renal calculi from decalcification due to prolonged immobility
♦ Fat embolism due to disruption of marrow or activation of the sympathetic nervous system after the trauma (may lead to respiratory or central nervous system distress)

Diagnosis

♦ History of traumatic injury and results of the physical examination, including gentle palpation

Managing musculoskeletal pain

A patient with a musculoskeletal disorder that causes chronic, nonmalignant pain should be assessed and treated in a stepped approach. Measures include:
♦ nonpharmacologic methods, such as heat, ice, elevation, and rest
♦ acetaminophen (Tylenol)
♦ a nonsteroidal anti-inflammatory drug such as ibuprofen (Motrin)
♦ another nonopioid analgesic, such as tramadol (Ultram), topical capsaicin, (Zostrix) or lidocaine patch (Lidoderm)
♦ a tricyclic antidepressant, such as amitriptyline (Elavil), which may decrease the pain signal at the neurosynaptic junctions
♦ an opioid analgesic alone or with a tricyclic antidepressant.

and a cautious attempt by the patient to move parts distal to the injury, reveal bone fracture.
♦ X-rays of the suspected fracture and the joints above and below confirm the diagnosis. After reduction, X-rays confirm bone alignment.

Treatment

For arm or leg fracture, emergency treatment consists of:
♦ splinting the limb above and below the suspected fracture to immobilize it
♦ applying a cold pack to reduce pain and edema
♦ elevating the limb to reduce pain and edema.

⚠ **CLINICAL ALERT** *The acronym RICE is useful to help remember treatment for a fracture in the first 24 hours:*
R — *Rest*
I — *Ice*
C — *Compression*
E — *Elevation*

Treatment of severe bone fracture that causes blood loss includes:
♦ direct pressure to control bleeding
♦ fluid replacement as soon as possible to prevent or treat hypovolemic shock.

After confirming a fracture, treatment begins with a reduction. Closed reduction involves:
♦ manual manipulation
♦ a local anesthetic (such as lidocaine [Xylocaine])
♦ an analgesic (such as morphine)
♦ a muscle relaxant (such as diazepam [Valium] I.V.) or a sedative (such as midazolam [Versed]) to facilitate the muscle stretching necessary to realign the bone.

Classifying fractures

One of the best-known systems for classifying fractures uses a combination of terms that describe general classification, fragment position, and fracture line to describe fractures.

General classification of fractures
♦ Simple (closed) — Bone fragments don't penetrate the skin.
♦ Compound (open) — Bone fragments penetrate the skin.
♦ Incomplete (partial) — Bone continuity isn't completely interrupted.
♦ Complete — Bone continuity is completely interrupted.

Classification by fragment position
♦ Comminuted — The bone breaks into small pieces.
♦ Impacted — One bone fragment is forced into another.
♦ Angulated — Fragments lie at an angle to each other.
♦ Displaced — Fracture fragments separate and are deformed.
♦ Nondisplaced — The two sections of bone maintain essentially normal alignment.

♦ Overriding — Fragments overlap, shortening the total bone length.
♦ Segmental — Fractures occur in two adjacent areas with an isolated central segment.
♦ Avulsed — Fragments are pulled from the normal position by muscle contractions or ligament resistance.

Classification by fracture line
♦ Linear — The fracture line runs parallel to the bone's axis.
♦ Longitudinal — The fracture line extends in a longitudinal (but not parallel) direction along the bone's axis.
♦ Oblique — The fracture line crosses the bone at about a 45-degree angle to the bone's axis.
♦ Spiral — The fracture line crosses the bone at an oblique angle, creating a spiral pattern.
♦ Transverse — The fracture line forms a right angle with the bone's axis.

When closed reduction is impossible, open reduction by surgery involves:
♦ internal fixation, involving immobilization of the fracture by means of rods, plates, or screws and application of a plaster cast
♦ external fixation, a system of surgically placed pins and stabilizing bars to maintain bone alignment
♦ tetanus prophylaxis
♦ a prophylactic antibiotic
♦ surgery to repair soft-tissue damage
♦ thorough wound debridement
♦ physical therapy after cast removal to restore limb mobility.

When a splint or cast fails to maintain the reduction, immobilization requires skin or skeletal traction, using a series of weights and pulleys. This may involve:
♦ elastic bandages and sheepskin coverings to attach traction devices to the patient's skin (skin traction)
♦ a pin or wire inserted through the bone distal to the fracture and attached to a weight to allow more prolonged traction (skeletal traction).

Special considerations
♦ Watch for signs of shock in the patient with a severe open fracture of a large bone, such as the femur.

♦ Monitor vital signs, and be especially alert for rapid pulse, decreased blood pressure, pallor, and cool, clammy skin — all of which may indicate that the patient is in shock.
♦ Administer I.V. fluids as ordered.
♦ Offer reassurance to the patient, who is likely to be frightened and in pain.
♦ Ease pain with an analgesic as needed.
♦ Help the patient set realistic goals for recovery.
♦ If the bone fracture requires long-term immobilization with traction, reposition the patient often to increase comfort and prevent pressure ulcers. Assist with active range-of-motion exercises to prevent muscle atrophy. Encourage deep breathing and coughing to avoid hypostatic pneumonia.
♦ Urge adequate fluid intake to prevent urinary stasis and constipation. Watch for signs and symptoms of renal calculi (flank pain, nausea, and vomiting).
♦ Provide good cast care, and support the cast with pillows. Observe for skin irritation near cast edges, and check for foul odors or discharge. Tell the patient to report signs or symptoms of impaired circulation (skin coldness, numbness, tingling, or discoloration) immediately. Warn him not to get the cast wet and not to insert foreign objects under the cast.

◆ Encourage the patient to start moving around as soon as he's able. Help him to walk. (Remember, a patient who has been bedridden for some time may be dizzy at first.) Demonstrate how to use crutches properly.

◆ After cast removal, refer the patient to a physical therapist to restore limb mobility.

CARPAL TUNNEL SYNDROME
Carpal tunnel syndrome, a form of repetitive stress injury, is the most common nerve entrapment syndrome. Carpal tunnel syndrome usually occurs in women between ages 30 and 60 (posing a serious occupational health problem). However, men who are also employed as assembly-line workers and packers and who repeatedly use poorly designed tools are just as likely to develop this disorder. Any strenuous use of the hands — sustained grasping, twisting, or flexing — aggravates this condition.

Causes
Although carpal tunnel syndrome is mostly idiopathic, it may result from:
◆ acromegaly
◆ amyloidosis
◆ benign tumor
◆ conditions that increase fluid pressure in the wrist, including alterations in the endocrine or immune system
◆ diabetes mellitus
◆ flexor tenosynovitis (commonly associated with rheumatic disease)
◆ hypothyroidism
◆ multiple myeloma
◆ nerve compression
◆ obesity
◆ pregnancy
◆ repetitive stress injury
◆ rheumatoid arthritis
◆ sprain or wrist dislocation, including Colles' fracture followed by edema.

Pathophysiology
The carpal bones and the transverse carpal ligament form the carpal tunnel. Inflammation or fibrosis of the tendon sheaths that pass through the carpal tunnel usually causes edema and compression of the median nerve. (See *Cross section of the wrist with carpal tunnel syndrome,* page 374.) This compression neuropathy causes sensory and motor changes in the median distribution of the hands, initially impairing sensory transmission to the thumb, index finger, second finger, and inner aspect of the third finger.

Recognizing compartment syndrome

Compartment syndrome occurs when edema or bleeding increases pressure within a muscle compartment (a smaller section of a muscle), to the point of interfering with circulation. Crush injuries, burns, bites, and fractures requiring casts or dressings may cause this syndrome. Compartment syndrome most commonly occurs in the lower arm, hand, lower leg, or foot.

Signs and symptoms include:
◆ increased pain
◆ decreased touch sensation
◆ increased weakness of the affected part
◆ increased swelling and pallor
◆ decreased pulses and increased capillary refill time.

Treatment of compartment syndrome consists of:
◆ placing the limb at heart level
◆ removing constricting forces
◆ monitoring neurovascular status
◆ subfascial injection of hyaluronidase (Wydase)
◆ emergency fasciotomy.

Signs and symptoms
◆ Weakness, pain, burning, numbness, or tingling in one or both hands due to nerve and blood vessel compression (This paresthesia affects the thumb, forefinger, middle finger, and medial half of the fourth finger.)
◆ Inability to clench the hand into a fist; the nails may be atrophic, the skin dry and shiny
◆ Because of vasodilatation and venous stasis, symptoms that typically worsen at night and in the morning
◆ Pain spreading to the forearm and, in severe cases, as far as the shoulder
◆ Pain relief achieved by shaking or rubbing the hands vigorously or dangling the arms at the side

Complications
◆ Continued use of the affected wrist increasing tendon inflammation, compression, and neural ischemia, causing a decrease in wrist function
◆ Untreated carpal tunnel syndrome producing permanent nerve damage with loss of movement and sensation

Diagnosis
Physical examination reveals decreased sensation to light touch or pinpricks in the affected

CLOSER LOOK

Cross section of the wrist with carpal tunnel syndrome

Increased pressure on the median nerve decreases blood flow. If compression persists, the nerve begins to swell. The myelin sheath begins to thin and degenerate.

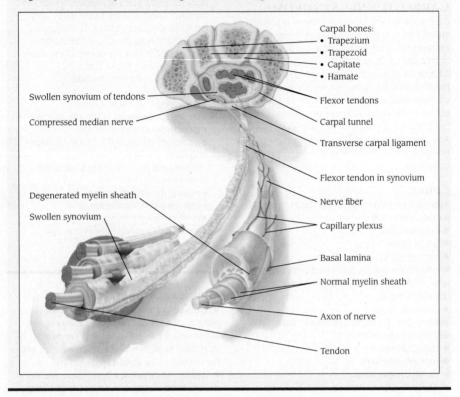

Carpal bones:
• Trapezium
• Trapezoid
• Capitate
• Hamate

Swollen synovium of tendons

Compressed median nerve

Flexor tendons

Carpal tunnel

Transverse carpal ligament

Flexor tendon in synovium

Degenerated myelin sheath

Swollen synovium

Nerve fiber

Capillary plexus

Basal lamina

Normal myelin sheath

Axon of nerve

Tendon

fingers. Thenar muscle atrophy occurs in about half of all cases of carpal tunnel syndrome but is usually a late sign.

The following tests provide rapid diagnosis of carpal tunnel syndrome:

◆ *Tinel's sign*—tingling over the median nerve on light percussion

◆ *Phalen's maneuver*—holding the forearms vertically and allowing both hands to drop into complete flexion at the wrists for 1 minute reproduces symptoms of carpal tunnel syndrome

◆ *Compression test*—blood pressure cuff inflated above systolic pressure on the forearm for 1 to 2 minutes provokes pain and paresthesia along the distribution of the median nerve.

Other tests include electromyography to detect a median nerve motor conduction delay of more than 5 milliseconds and laboratory tests to identify underlying disease.

Treatment

◆ Conservative treatment first, including resting the hands by splinting the wrist in neutral extension for 1 to 2 weeks

◆ A nonsteroidal anti-inflammatory drug for symptomatic relief

◆ Injection of the carpal tunnel with hydrocortisone and lidocaine for significant but temporary relief

◆ Seeking another occupation, if a definite link has been established between the patient's job and the development of repetitive stress injury

◆ Correction of an underlying disorder

◆ Surgical decompression of the nerve by resecting the entire transverse carpal tunnel ligament or by using endoscopic surgical techniques, when conservative treatment fails

◆ Neurolysis (freeing of the nerve fibers)

Preventing carpal tunnel syndrome

To prevent carpal tunnel syndrome, advise your patients to make these lifestyle changes.

Take frequent breaks
Gently stretching and bending the hands and wrists every 15 to 20 minutes gives the hands and wrists a break, especially when using equipment that vibrates or exerts a great amount of force. Tasks should also be alternated to avoid repetitive movements, which can contribute to tendinitis and carpal tunnel syndrome.

Watch hand and wrist positioning
When using a keyboard, bending the wrist all the way up or down should be avoided. A

relaxed middle position is best. The keyboard should be kept at elbow height or slightly lower.

Improve posture
Poor posture can cause the shoulders to roll forward, allowing the neck and shoulder muscles to shorten, which can compress the nerves in the neck. This position can affect the wrists, hands, and fingers.

Keep hands warm
Hand stiffness and pain develop more frequently in a cold environment. Using fingerless gloves may help if the temperature can't be adjusted at work.

Special considerations
♦ Administer a mild analgesic as needed. Encourage the patient to use his hands as much as possible. If his dominant hand has been impaired, you may have to help with eating and bathing.
♦ Teach the patient how to apply a splint. Tell him not to make it too tight. Show him how to remove the splint to perform gentle range-of-motion exercises, which should be done daily. Make sure the patient knows how to do these exercises before he's discharged.
♦ After surgery, monitor vital signs and regularly check the color, sensation, and motion of the affected hand.
♦ Advise the patient who is about to be discharged to exercise his hands occasionally in warm water. If the arm is in a sling, tell him to remove the sling several times per day to do exercises for his elbow and shoulder.
♦ Suggest occupational counseling for the patient who has to change jobs because of repetitive stress injury.
♦ Advise all patients on measures to prevent carpal tunnel syndrome, including using correct posture and wrist position, performing stretching exercises, and taking frequent breaks. Ergonomic workstations and tools are designed to allow a worker's wrist to maintain a natural position, preventing strain and stress to the wrist. (See *Preventing carpal tunnel syndrome*.)

CLUBFOOT
Clubfoot, also called *talipes*, is the most common congenital disorder of the lower extremities. It's marked primarily by a deformed talus and shortened Achilles tendon, which give the foot a

characteristic clublike appearance. In talipes equinovarus, the foot points downward (equinus) and turns inward (varus), and the front of the foot curls toward the heel (forefoot adduction).

Clubfoot occurs in about 1 per 1,000 live births, is bilateral in about half of all cases, and is twice as common in boys as in girls. It may be associated with other birth defects, such as myelomeningocele, spina bifida, and arthrogryposis. Clubfoot is correctable with prompt treatment.

Causes
A combination of environmental and genetic factors in utero appears to cause clubfoot, including:
♦ arrested development during the 9th and 10th weeks of embryonic life when the feet are formed (in children without a family history of clubfoot)
♦ heredity (mechanism of transmission is undetermined; the sibling of a child born with clubfoot has 1 chance in 35 of being born with the same anomaly, and a child of a parent with clubfoot has 1 chance in 10)
♦ muscle abnormalities leading to variations in length and tendon insertions
♦ secondary to cerebral palsy (older children), paralysis, or poliomyelitis, in which case treatment includes management of the underlying disease.

Pathophysiology
Abnormal development of the foot during fetal growth leads to abnormal muscles and joints and contracture of soft tissue. Clubfoot can also occur as a result of paralysis, poliomyelitis, or

cerebral palsy. The condition called *apparent clubfoot* results when a fetus maintains a position in utero that gives his feet a clubfoot appearance at birth; it can usually be corrected manually. Another form of apparent clubfoot is inversion of the feet, resulting from the denervation type of progressive muscular atrophy and progressive muscular dystrophy.

Signs and symptoms

Talipes equinovarus varies greatly in severity. Deformity may be so extreme that the toes touch the inside of the ankle, or it may be only vaguely apparent.

Every case includes:
◆ deformed talus because of abnormal development
◆ shortened Achilles tendon from contracture
◆ shortened and flattened calcaneus bone of the heel caused by abnormal development and contracture
◆ shortened, underdeveloped calf muscles and soft-tissue contractures at the site of the varus deformity (depending on degree of the varus deformity)
◆ foot tight in its deformed position, resisting manual efforts to push it back into normal position, because of shortening of muscles and contractures
◆ no pain, except in elderly patients with arthritis and secondary deformity.

Complications

Possible complications of talipes equinovarus include:
◆ chronic impairment (neglected clubfoot)
◆ incomplete correctable (when severe enough to require surgery).

Diagnosis

Early diagnosis of clubfoot is usually no problem because the deformity is obvious. In subtle deformity, however, true clubfoot must be distinguished from apparent clubfoot (metatarsus varus or pigeon toe), usually by X-rays showing superimposition of the talus and calcaneus and a ladderlike appearance of the metatarsals (true clubfoot).

Treatment

Treatment of clubfoot is done in three stages: correcting the deformity, maintaining the correction until the foot regains normal muscle balance, and observing the foot closely for several years to prevent the deformity from recurring.

Clubfoot deformities are usually corrected in sequential order: forefoot adduction first, then varus (or inversion), then equinus (or plantar flexion). Trying to correct all three deformities at once only results in a misshapen, rocker-bottomed foot.

Other essential parts of management include:
◆ stressing to parents the importance of prompt treatment and orthopedic supervision until growth is completed
◆ teaching parents cast care and how to recognize circulatory impairment before a child in a clubfoot cast is discharged
◆ explaining to an older child and his parents that surgery can improve clubfoot with good function but can't totally correct it; the affected calf muscle will remain slightly underdeveloped
◆ emphasizing the need for long-term orthopedic care to maintain correction; correcting this defect permanently takes time and patience.

Special considerations

The primary concern in clubfoot is early recognition, preferably in neonates.
◆ Look for any abnormal positioning in an infant's feet. Make sure you recognize the difference between true clubfoot and apparent clubfoot. Don't use excessive force in trying to manipulate a clubfoot. The foot with apparent clubfoot moves easily.
◆ Stress to parents the importance of prompt treatment. Clubfoot demands immediate therapy and orthopedic supervision until growth is completed.
◆ After casting, elevate the child's feet with pillows. Check the toes every 1 to 2 hours for temperature, color, sensation, motion, and capillary refill time; watch for edema. Before a child in a clubfoot cast is discharged, teach parents to recognize circulatory impairment.
◆ Keep in mind that fiberglass casting, the most commonly used kind, doesn't require petaling. Padding from the cast is turned over and used as a cushioning. (Don't rub the skin with alcohol, and don't use oils or powders, which tend to macerate the skin.)
◆ If the child is old enough to walk, caution parents not to let the foot part of the cast get soft and thin from wear. If it does, much of the correction may be lost.
◆ When the wedging method of shaping the cast is being used, check circulatory status frequently; it may be impaired by increased pressure on tissues and blood vessels. The equinus (posterior release) correction especially places considerable strain on ligaments, blood vessels, and tendons.
◆ After surgery, elevate the child's feet with pillows to decrease swelling and pain. Immediately report any signs of discomfort or pain. Try to locate the source of pain; it may result from cast pressure rather than from the incision. If bleeding

occurs under the cast, document the location and size. If bleeding spreads, report it to the physician.

◆ Explain to the older child and his parents that surgery can improve clubfoot with good function but can't totally correct it; the affected calf muscle will remain slightly underdeveloped.

◆ Emphasize the need for long-term orthopedic care to maintain correction. Teach parents the prescribed exercises that the child can do at home. Urge them to make the child wear the corrective shoes ordered and the splints during naps and at night. Make sure they understand that treatment for clubfoot continues during the entire growth period. Correcting this defect permanently takes time and patience.

DEVELOPMENTAL DYSPLASIA OF THE HIP

Developmental dysplasia of the hip (DDH), an abnormality of the hip joint present from birth, is the most common disorder affecting the hip joints in children younger than 3 years. About 85% of affected infants are females.

DDH can be unilateral or bilateral and can affect the femoral head, the acetabulum, or both. This abnormality occurs in three forms of varying severity:

◆ *Unstable dysplasia* — the hip is positioned normally but can be dislocated by manipulation.
◆ *Subluxation or incomplete dislocation* — the femoral head rides on the edge of the acetabulum.
◆ *Complete dislocation* — the femoral head is totally outside the acetabulum.

Causes

Although the causes of DDH aren't clear, many factors contribute to its development. It's more likely to occur in the following circumstances:

◆ dislocation after breech delivery (malposition in utero, 10 times more common than after cephalic delivery)
◆ elevated maternal relaxin, a hormone secreted by the corpus luteum during pregnancy that causes relaxation of pubic symphysis and cervical dilation (may promote relaxation of the joint ligaments, predisposing the infant to DDH)
◆ large neonates and twins (more common).

Pathophysiology

The precise cause of congenital dislocation is unknown. Excessive or abnormal movement of the joint during a traumatic birth may cause dislocation. Displacement of bones within the joint may damage joint structures, including articulating surfaces, blood vessels, tendons, ligaments, and nerves. This may lead to ischemic necrosis because of the disruption of blood flow to the joint.

Signs and symptoms

◆ Asymmetrical skin folds due to hip dislocation
◆ Hip riding above the acetabulum, causing the level of the knees to be uneven (Galeazzi sign)
◆ Limited abduction on the dislocated side due to a shortening of the adductor muscle on the medial aspect of the thigh while the femoral head is displaced superiorly
◆ Swaying from side to side (waddling due to uncorrected bilateral dysplasia)
◆ Limpness due to uncorrected unilateral dysplasia

Complications

If corrective treatment isn't begun until after age 2, DDH may cause:

◆ degenerative hip changes
◆ abnormal acetabular development
◆ lordosis (abnormally increased concave curvature of the lumbar and cervical spine)
◆ joint malformation
◆ sciatic nerve injury (paralysis)
◆ avascular necrosis of femoral head
◆ soft-tissue damage
◆ permanent disability.

Diagnosis

Diagnostic measures may include:

◆ X-rays (rarely used in neonates and infants) to show the location of the femur head and a shallow acetabulum (They also monitor disease or treatment progress.)
◆ sonography and magnetic resonance imaging to help with assessing reduction.

Observations during physical examination of the relaxed child that strongly suggest DDH include:

◆ the number of folds of skin over the thighs on each side when the child is placed on his back (a child in this position usually has an equal number of folds, but a child with subluxation or dislocation may have an extra fold on the affected side, which is also apparent when the child lies in a prone position)
◆ buttock fold on the affected side higher with the child lying in a prone position (also restricted abduction of the affected hip). (See *Ortolani's and Trendelenburg's signs of DDH,* page 378.)

Treatment

The earlier an infant receives treatment, the better the chances are for normal development. Treatment varies with the patient's age.

In infants younger than 6 months, treatment includes:

◆ gentle manipulation to reduce the dislocation, followed by the use of a splint or harness

Ortolani's and Trendelenburg's signs of DDH

A positive Ortolani's or Trendelenburg's sign confirms developmental dysplasia of the hip (DDH).

Ortolani's sign
♦ Place the infant on his back, with hip flexed and in abduction. Adduct the hip while pressing the femur downward. This will dislocate the hip.
♦ Then, abduct the hip while moving the femur upward. A click or a jerk (produced by the femoral head moving over the acetabular rim) indicates subluxation in an infant younger than 1 month. The sign indicates subluxation or complete dislocation in an older infant.

Trendelenburg's sign
♦ When the child rests his weight on the side of the dislocation and lifts his other knee, the pelvis drops on the normal side because abductor muscles in the affected hip are weak.
♦ However, when the child stands with his weight on the normal side and lifts the other knee, the pelvis remains horizontal.

to hold the hips in a flexed and abducted position to maintain the reduction
♦ a splint or harness worn continuously for 2 to 3 months, then a night splint for another month to tighten and stabilize the joint capsule in correct alignment.

If treatment doesn't begin until after age 6 months, it may include:
♦ bilateral skin traction (in infants) or skeletal traction (in children who have started walking) to try to reduce the dislocation by gradually abducting the hips
♦ Bryant's traction or divarication traction (both extremities placed in traction, even if only one is affected, to help maintain immobilization) for children younger than 3 years and weighing less than 35 lb (16 kg) for 2 to 3 weeks
♦ gentle closed reduction under general anesthesia to further abduct the hips, followed by a spica cast for 3 months (if traction fails)
♦ in children older than 18 months, open reduction and pelvic or femoral osteotomy to correct bony deformity followed by immobilization in a spica cast for 6 to 8 weeks

between 6 and 12 months, immobilization in a spica cast for about 3 months.

In children ages 2 to 5, treatment is difficult and includes skeletal traction and subcutaneous adductor tenotomy (surgical cutting of the tendon).

Treatment begun after age 5 rarely restores satisfactory hip function.

Special considerations
The child who must wear a splint, brace, or body cast needs special personal care that requires parent education.
♦ Teach parents how to correctly splint or brace the hips as ordered. Stress the need for frequent checkups.
♦ Listen sympathetically to the parents' expressions of anxiety and fear. Explain possible causes of developmental hip dislocation, and give reassurance that early, prompt treatment will probably result in complete correction.
♦ During the child's first few days in a cast or splint, she may be prone to irritability because of the unaccustomed restricted movement. Encourage her parents to stay with her as much as possible and to calm and reassure her.
♦ Assure the parents that the child will adjust to this restriction and return to normal sleeping, eating, and playing behavior in a few days.
♦ Instruct the parents to remove braces and splints before bathing the infant but to replace them immediately afterward. Stress good hygiene; parents should bathe and change the child frequently and wash her perineum with warm water and soap at each diaper change.

If treatment requires a spica cast:
♦ When transferring the child immediately after casting, use your palms to avoid making dents in the cast. Such dents predispose the patient to pressure sores. Remember that the cast needs 24 to 48 hours to dry naturally. Don't use heat to make it dry faster because heat also makes it more fragile.
♦ Immediately after the cast is applied, use a plastic sheet to protect it from moisture around the perineum and buttocks. Cut the sheet into strips long enough to cover the outside of the cast, and tuck them about a finger length beneath the cast edges. Using overlapping strips of tape, tack the corner of each petal to the outside of the cast. Remove the plastic under the cast every 4 hours; then wash, dry, and retuck it. Disposable diapers folded lengthwise over the perineum may also be used.
♦ Position the child either on a Bradford frame elevated on blocks, with a bedpan under the frame, or on pillows to support the child's legs.

Be sure to keep the cast dry, and change the child's diapers often.

◆ Wash and dry the skin under the cast edges every 2 to 4 hours. Don't use oils or powders; they can macerate skin.

◆ Turn the child every 2 hours during the day and every 4 hours at night. Check color, sensation, and motion of the infant's legs and feet. Be sure to examine all her toes. Notify the physician of dusky, cool, or numb toes.

◆ Shine a flashlight under the cast every 4 hours to check for objects and crumbs. Check the cast daily for odors, which may herald infection.

◆ If the child complains of itching, she may benefit from taking diphenhydramine (Benadryl) or from having a hair dryer set on cool and aimed at the cast edges. Don't scratch or probe under the cast. Investigate any persistent itching.

◆ Provide adequate nutrition and maintain adequate fluid intake to avoid renal calculi and constipation, both complications of inactivity.

◆ If the child is restless, apply a jacket restraint to keep her from falling out of bed or off the frame.

◆ Provide adequate stimuli to promote growth and development. If the child's hips are abducted in a froglike position, tell parents that she may be able to fit on a tricycle that the parent can push (if the child is unable to pedal) or in a child's electric car. Encourage parents to let the child sit at a table by seating her on pillows on a chair, to put her on the floor for short periods of play, and to let her play with other children her age.

◆ Tell parents to watch for signs and symptoms that the child is outgrowing the cast (cyanosis, cool extremities, or pain).

◆ Tell the parents that treatment may be prolonged and requires patience.

◆ Help arrange transportation for the child, or make sure the parents' vehicle has an appropriate child restraint system.

The patient in Bryant's traction may be cared for at home if the parents are taught traction application and maintenance:

◆ Encourage the parents to cuddle and hold the child and to encourage her to interact with siblings and friends.

◆ Maintain skin integrity and check circulation at least every 2 hours.

◆ Feed the child carefully to avoid aspiration and choking.

◆ If necessary, refer the child and parents to a child life specialist to ensure continued developmental progress.

GOUT

Gout, also called *gouty arthritis,* is a metabolic disease marked by urate deposits that cause painful arthritic joints. It's found mostly in the foot, especially the great toe, ankle, and midfoot, but it may affect any joint. Gout follows an intermittent course, and patients may be totally free from symptoms for years between attacks. The prognosis is good with treatment.

Causes

Although the exact cause of primary gout remains unknown, it may be caused by genetic defect in purine metabolism, causing overproduction of uric acid (hyperuricemia), retention of uric acid, or both.

In secondary gout, which develops during the course of another disease (such as diabetes mellitus, hypertension, obesity, renal disease, or sickle cell anemia), the cause may be:

◆ breakdown of nucleic acid causing hyperuricemia

◆ the result of drug therapy, especially after the use of hydrochlorothiazide or pyrazinamide, which decrease urate excretion (ionic form of uric acid); other implicated drugs include low-dose acetylsalicylic acid, cytotoxics, and ethambutol.

Pathophysiology

When uric acid becomes supersaturated in blood and other body fluids, it crystallizes and forms a precipitate of urate salts that accumulate in connective tissue throughout the body; these deposits are called *tophi.* The presence of the crystals triggers an acute inflammatory response when neutrophils begin to ingest the crystals. Tissue damage begins when the neutrophils release their lysosomes (see chapter 12, Immune system). The lysosomes not only damage the tissues but also perpetuate the inflammation.

In asymptomatic gout, the serum urate level increases, but the urate doesn't crystallize or produce symptoms. As the disease progresses, it may cause hypertension or urate kidney stones may form.

The first acute attack strikes suddenly and peaks quickly. Although it generally involves only one or a few joints, this initial attack is extremely painful. Affected joints appear hot, tender, inflamed, dusky red, or cyanotic. The metatarsophalangeal joint of the great toe usually becomes inflamed first (podagra), then the instep, ankle, heel, knee, or wrist joints. Sometimes a low-grade fever is present. Mild acute attacks typically subside quickly but tend to recur at irregular intervals. Severe attacks may persist for days or weeks.

Intercritical periods are the symptom-free intervals between gout attacks. Most patients have a second attack within 6 months to 2 years, but some attacks, common in those who are untreated, tend to be longer and more severe than initial attacks. Such attacks are also polyarticular, invariably affecting joints in the feet and legs, and sometimes accompanied by fever. A migratory attack sequentially strikes various joints and the Achilles tendon and is associated with either subdeltoid or olecranon bursitis.

Eventually, chronic polyarticular gout sets in. This final, unremitting stage of the disease is marked by persistent painful polyarthritis, with large tophi in cartilage, synovial membranes, tendons, and soft tissue. Tophi form in fingers, hands, knees, feet, ulnar sides of the forearms, helices of the ears, Achilles tendons and, rarely, in internal organs, such as the kidneys and myocardium. The skin over the tophus may ulcerate and release a chalky, white exudate that's composed primarily of uric acid crystals.

Signs and symptoms
◆ Joint pain due to uric acid deposits and inflammation
◆ Redness and swelling in joints due to uric acid deposits and irritation
◆ Tophi in the great toe, ankle, and pinna of ear due to urate deposits
◆ Elevated skin temperature and fever due to inflammation

Complications
◆ Eventual erosions, deformity, and disability due to chronic inflammation and tophi that cause secondary joint degeneration
◆ Hypertension and albuminuria (in some patients)
◆ Kidney involvement, with tubular damage from aggregates of urate crystals; progressively poorer excretion of uric acid and chronic renal dysfunction

Diagnosis
◆ Needlelike monosodium urate crystals in synovial fluid are shown by needle aspiration or in tissue sections of tophaceous deposits.
◆ Uric acid level greater than 420 μmol/mmol of creatinine reveals hyperuricemia.
◆ 24-hour urine uric acid level is usually higher in those with secondary gout than in those with primary gout.
◆ X-rays are initially normal; in those with chronic gout, they show damage of articular cartilage and subchondral bone. Outward displacement of the overhanging margin from the bone contour characterizes gout.

Treatment
The goals of treatment are to end the acute attack as quickly as possible, prevent recurring attacks,

and prevent or reverse complications. (See *Preventing gout.*)

Treatment of acute gout consists of:
◆ immobilization and protection of the inflamed, painful joints
◆ local application of heat or cold
◆ increased fluid intake (to 3 qt [3 L]/day if not contradicted by other conditions to prevent kidney stone formation)
◆ concomitant treatment with colchicine (oral or I.V.) every hour for 8 hours to inhibit phagocytosis of uric acid crystals by neutrophils, until the pain subsides or nausea, vomiting, cramping, or diarrhea develops (in acute inflammation)
◆ a nonsteroidal anti-inflammatory drug (NSAID) for pain and inflammation.

AGE ALERT *Older patients who take an NSAID are at risk for GI bleeding. Encourage such patients to take these drugs with meals, and monitor their stools for occult blood.*

Treatment of chronic gout aims to decrease the serum uric acid level, including:
◆ maintenance dosage of allopurinol (Zyloprim) to suppress uric acid formation or control the uric acid level, preventing further attacks (use cautiously in patients with renal failure)
◆ colchicine to prevent recurrent acute attacks until uric acid returns to its normal level (doesn't affect the uric acid level)
◆ a uricosuric (probenecid and sulfinpyrazone [Anturane]) to promote uric acid excretion and inhibit uric acid accumulation (of limited value in patients with renal impairment)
◆ dietary restrictions, primarily avoiding alcohol and purine-rich foods (shellfish, liver, sardines, anchovies, and kidneys) that increase the urate level (adjunctive therapy).

Special considerations
◆ Encourage bed rest during the acute phase but use a bed cradle to keep bedcovers off extremely sensitive, inflamed joints. Tell the patient that he can be out of bed but that he shouldn't put any weight on the affected joints.
◆ Give pain medication, as needed, especially during acute attacks. Apply hot or cold packs to inflamed joints according to what the patient finds effective. Administer anti-inflammatory medication and other drugs as ordered. Watch for adverse reactions. Be alert for GI disturbances with colchicine.
◆ Urge the patient to drink plenty of fluids (up to 2 qt [2 L] per day) to prevent formation of kidney stones. Record intake and output accurately. Be sure to monitor the serum uric acid level regularly. Alkalinize urine with sodium bicarbonate or other agent, if ordered.

Preventing gout

Because the cause of gout is unknown, the disease can't be prevented. However, it's important to teach your patients how to prevent acute gout attacks to reduce the risk of joint damage. Acute gout attacks can be prevented by dietary changes, weight reduction, adequate fluid intake, and drugs.

Dietary restrictions

Dietary changes include avoidance of foods high in purine , such as alcohol (especially beer and wine), organ meats, sardines, sweetbreads, peas, and lentils.

Weight reduction

Obese patients need to lose weight at a slow rate. Losing weight rapidly may temporarily increase uric acid levels.

Fluid intake

It's also important to drink adequate amounts of fluids to dilute the amount of uric acid in the blood. This will help decrease the risk of kidney stone formation. Taking the prescribed drug slows the production of uric acid and speeds its elimination from the body.

◆ Watch for acute gout attacks 24 to 96 hours after surgery. Even minor surgery can precipitate an attack. Before and after surgery, administer colchicine, as ordered, to help prevent gout attacks.

◆ Make sure the patient understands the importance of having his serum uric acid level checked periodically. Tell him to avoid high-purine foods, such as anchovies, liver, sardines, kidneys, sweetbreads, lentils, and alcoholic beverages — especially beer and wine — which raise the urate level. Explain the principles of a gradual weight reduction diet to obese patients. Such a diet features foods containing moderate amounts of protein and little fat.

◆ Advise the patient receiving allopurinol, probenecid, and other drugs to immediately report any adverse reactions, such as drowsiness, dizziness, nausea, vomiting, urinary frequency, or dermatitis. Warn the patient taking probenecid or sulfinpyrazone to avoid aspirin or any other salicylate. Their combined effect causes urate retention.

◆ Inform the patient that long-term colchicine therapy is essential during the first 3 to 6 months of treatment with a uricosuric or allopurinol.

HERNIATED DISK

Herniated disk, also called *ruptured* or *slipped disk* and *herniated nucleus pulposus*, occurs when all or part of the nucleus pulposus — the soft, gelatinous, central portion of an intervertebral disk — is forced through the disk's weakened or torn outer ring (anulus fibrosus).

Herniated disk usually occurs in adults (mostly men) younger than age 45. About 90% of herniated disks are lumbar or lumbosacral; 8%, cervical; and 1% to 2%, thoracic. Patients with a congenitally small lumbar spinal canal or with osteophyte formation along the vertebrae may be more susceptible to nerve root compression and more likely to have neurologic symptoms.

Causes

◆ Intervertebral joint degeneration
◆ Severe strain or trauma

AGE ALERT *In older patients whose disks have begun to degenerate, even minor trauma can cause herniation.*

Pathophysiology

An intervertebral disk has two parts: the soft center called the *nucleus pulposus* and the tough, fibrous surrounding ring called the *anulus fibrosus*. The nucleus pulposus acts as a shock absorber, distributing the mechanical stress applied to the spine when the body moves.

Physical stress, usually a twisting motion, can tear or rupture the anulus fibrosus so that the nucleus pulposus herniates into the spinal canal. When this happens, the extruded disk may impinge on spinal nerve roots as they exit from the spinal canal or on the spinal cord itself, resulting in back pain and other signs of nerve root irritation. The vertebrae move closer together and in turn exert pressure on the nerve roots as they exit between the vertebrae. Pain and possibly sensory and motor loss follow. A herniated disk can also follow intervertebral joint degeneration; minor trauma may cause herniation.

Herniation occurs in three steps:
◆ *protrusion* — nucleus pulposus presses against the anulus fibrosus
◆ *extrusion* — nucleus pulposus bulges forcibly through the anulus fibrosus, pushing against the nerve root

CLOSER LOOK

How a herniated disk develops

These illustrations show how herniation of an intervertebral disk develops.

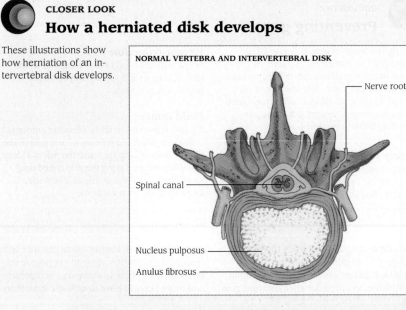

NORMAL VERTEBRA AND INTERVERTEBRAL DISK

Nerve root

Spinal canal

Nucleus pulposus

Anulus fibrosus

Physical stress, from severe trauma or strain, or intervertebral joint degeneration may cause herniation. Herniation occurs in three stages: protrusion, extrusion, and sequestration.

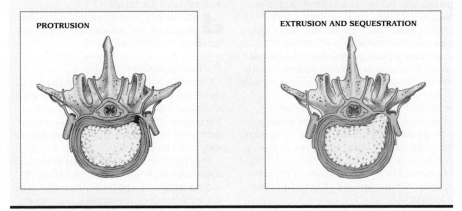

PROTRUSION

EXTRUSION AND SEQUESTRATION

◆ *sequestration*—anulus fibrosis gives way as the disk's core bursts and presses against the nerve root. (See *How a herniated disk develops*.)

Signs and symptoms
◆ In lumbar herniated disk, severe low back pain radiating to the buttocks, legs, and feet, usually unilaterally
◆ In herniation after trauma, pain may begin suddenly, subside in a few days, and then recur at shorter intervals and with progressive intensity; sciatic pain follows, beginning as a dull pain in the buttocks from pressure on the surrounding nerves

◆ Valsalva's maneuver, coughing, sneezing, or bending intensifying pain, (resulting from increased pressure on the nerve), commonly accompanied by muscle spasms
◆ Sensory and motor loss in the area innervated by the compressed spinal nerve root and, in later stages, weakness and atrophy of leg muscles in herniated disk

Complications
◆ Neurologic deficits (most common)
◆ Bowel and bladder problems (with the sacral [S_1 and S_2] nerve root area affected)

Diagnosis

◆ Obtaining a detailed patient history is vital because the events that intensify disk pain are diagnostically significant.

◆ The straight-leg-raising test and its variants are perhaps the best tests for herniated disk. For the straight-leg-raising test, the patient lies in a supine position while the examiner places one hand on the patient's ilium to stabilize the pelvis and the other hand under the ankle, then slowly raises the patient's leg. The test is positive only if the patient complains of posterior leg (sciatic) pain, not back pain. In Lasègue's sign, the patient lies flat while the thigh and knee are flexed to a 90-degree angle. Resistance and pain as well as loss of ankle or knee-jerk reflex indicate spinal root compression.

◆ X-rays of the spine are essential to rule out other abnormalities but may not help in the diagnosis of a herniated disk because marked disk prolapse can be present despite a normal X-ray.

◆ A thorough check of the patient's peripheral vascular status — including posterior tibial and dorsalis pedis pulses and skin temperature of extremities — helps rule out ischemic disease, another cause of leg pain or numbness.

◆ After physical examination and X-rays, myelography, computed tomography scans, and magnetic resonance imaging (MRI) provide the most specific diagnostic information, showing spinal canal compression by herniated disk material. MRI is the method of choice to confirm the diagnosis and determine the exact level of herniation.

Treatment

Unless neurologic impairment progresses rapidly, treatment is initially conservative and may consist of:

◆ a maximum of 3 days of bed rest (possibly with pelvic traction)

◆ administration of a nonsteroidal anti-inflammatory drug

◆ heat applications

◆ an exercise program

◆ an epidural corticosteroid, a short-term oral corticosteroid, a nerve root blocker, or physical therapy to decrease pain

◆ a muscle relaxant, such as diazepam (Valium), methocarbamol (Robaxin), or cyclobenzaprine (Flexeril), to relieve associated muscle spasms.

A herniated disk that fails to respond to conservative treatment may necessitate surgery. The most common procedure, laminectomy, involves excision of a portion of the lamina and removal of the nucleus pulposus of the protruding disk. If laminectomy doesn't alleviate pain and disability, a spinal fusion may be necessary to overcome segmental instability. Laminectomy and spinal fusion are sometimes performed concurrently to stabilize the spine. Microdiskectomy can also be used to remove fragments of nucleus pulposus.

Injection of chymopapain (Chymodiactin) into the herniated disk produces a loss of water and proteoglycans from the disk, thereby reducing both the disk's size and the pressure in the nerve root. Chymopapain is most commonly used for herniations in the lumbar region.

Special considerations

Herniated disk requires supportive care, careful patient teaching, and strong emotional support to help the patient cope with the discomfort and frustration of chronic low back discomfort.

◆ If the patient requires myelography, question him carefully about allergies to iodides, iodine-containing substances, or seafood because such allergies may indicate sensitivity to the test's radiopaque dye. Reinforce previous explanations of the need for this test, and tell the patient to expect some discomfort. Assure him that he'll receive a sedative before the test, if needed, to keep him as calm and comfortable as possible. After the test, urge the patient to remain in bed with his head elevated (especially if metrizamide was used) and to drink plenty of fluids. Monitor intake and output. Watch for seizures and allergic reaction.

◆ During conservative treatment, watch for deterioration in neurologic status (especially during the first 24 hours after admission), which may indicate an urgent need for surgery. Use antiembolism stockings as prescribed, and encourage the patient to move his legs as allowed. Provide a foam block to prevent heel cord shortening. Work closely with the physical therapy department to ensure a consistent regimen of leg- and back-strengthening exercises. Give plenty of fluids to prevent renal stasis, and remind the patient to deep-breathe and use an incentive spirometer to preclude pulmonary complications. Provide good skin care. Assess bowel function. Use a fracture bedpan for the patient on complete bed rest.

◆ After laminectomy, microdiskectomy, or spinal fusion, enforce bed rest as ordered. If a blood drainage system (Hemovac or Jackson Pratt drain) is in use, check the tubing frequently for kinks and a secure vacuum. Empty the Hemovac at the end of each shift, and record the amount and color of drainage. Report colorless moisture on dressings (possible cerebrospinal fluid leakage) or excessive drainage immediately. Observe neurovascular status of legs (color, motion, temperature, and sensation).

PREVENTION
Preventing a herniated disk

To prevent a herniated disk, tell your patient to follow these guidelines.

Exercise
Getting regular exercise can slow the degeneration of the disks related to aging. Muscle strength gained through exercising can strengthen and stabilize the spine. If the patient has previously had a herniated disk, he should remember to avoid high-impact activities, such as jogging, tennis, and high-impact aerobics, for the first few months after a herniated disk.

Maintain good posture
Good posture reduces the pressure on the spine and disks. Keeping the back straight and aligned is essential, particularly when sitting for longer periods. Also, heavy objects should be lifted properly by using the legs — not the back — to do most of the work.

Maintain a healthy weight
Excess weight puts more pressure on the spine and disks, making them more susceptible to herniation.

◆ Monitor vital signs and check for bowel sounds and abdominal distention. Use logrolling technique to turn the patient. Administer an analgesic, as ordered, especially 30 minutes before initial attempts at sitting or walking. Give the patient assistance during his first attempt to walk. Provide a straight-backed chair for limited sitting.
◆ Teach the patient who has undergone spinal fusion how to wear a brace. Assist with straightleg-raising and toe-pointing exercises as ordered. Before discharge, teach proper body mechanics—bending at the knees and hips (never at the waist), standing straight, and carrying objects close to the body. Advise the patient to lie down when tired and to sleep on his side (never on his abdomen) on an extra-firm mattress or a bed board. Urge him to maintain proper weight to prevent lordosis caused by obesity.
◆ If the patient requires chemonucleolysis, make sure he isn't allergic to meat tenderizers (chymopapain is a similar substance). Such an allergy contraindicates the use of this enzyme, which can produce severe anaphylaxis in a sensitive patient. After chemonucleolysis, enforce bed rest as ordered. Administer an analgesic and apply heat as needed. Urge the patient to cough and deep-breathe. Assist with special exercises, and tell the patient to continue these exercises after discharge.
◆ Tell the patient who must receive a muscle relaxant of possible adverse effects, especially drowsiness. Warn him to avoid activities that require alertness until he has built up a tolerance to the drug's sedative effects.
◆ Provide emotional support. Try to cheer the patient during periods of frustration and depression. Assure him of his progress, and offer encouragement. (See *Preventing a herniated disk*.)

LEGG-CALVÉ-PERTHES DISEASE
Legg-Calvé-Perthes disease (also called *coxa plana*) is avascular necrosis leading to eventual flattening of the head of the femur due to vascular interruption. This typically unilateral condition is most common in boys ages 4 to 10 and tends to occur in families. It occurs bilaterally in 20% of patients.

Although this disease usually runs its course in 3 to 4 years, it may lead to premature osteoarthritis later in life from misalignment of the acetabulum and flattening of the femoral head.

Causes
The exact vascular obstructive changes that initiate Legg-Calvé-Perthes disease are unknown. However, injury or trauma precedes the onset of Legg-Calvé-Perthes disease in about one-third of children with the disease.

Possible causes include:
◆ increased blood viscosity resulting in stasis and decreased blood flow
◆ trauma to retinacular vessels
◆ vascular irregularities (congenital or developmental)
◆ vascular occlusion secondary to increased intracapsular pressure from acute transient synovitis
◆ venous obstruction with secondary intraepiphyseal thrombosis.

Pathophysiology
The disease occurs in four stages. The first stage, synovitis, is characterized by synovial inflammation and increased joint fluid, and typically lasts 1 to 3 weeks. In the second (avascular) stage, vascular interruption causes necrosis of the ossification center of the femoral head

(usually in several months to 1 year). In the third stage (which ordinarily lasts 2 to 4 years), revascularization, a new blood supply causes bone resorption and deposition of immature bone cells. New bone replaces necrotic bone and the femoral head gradually reforms. The final, or residual, stage involves healing and regeneration. Immature bone cells are replaced by normal bone cells, thereby fixing the joint's shape. There may or may not be residual deformity, based on the degree of necrosis that occurred in stage two.

Signs and symptoms
The first indication of Legg-Calvé-Perthes disease is usually a persistent thigh pain or limp that becomes progressively severe. This symptom appears when bone resorption and deformity begin. Other signs and symptoms may include:
◆ mild pain in the hip, thigh, or knee that's aggravated by activity and relieved by rest caused by inflammation and increased joint fluid and avascular necrosis
◆ muscle spasm on rotation of the hip related to inflammation
◆ atrophy of muscles in the upper thigh caused by necrosis
◆ slight shortening of the leg
◆ severely restricted abduction and internal rotation of the hip caused by pain and necrosis.

Complications
Complications result from misalignment of the acetabulum and the flattened femoral head and may include permanent disability and premature osteoarthritis.

Diagnosis
◆ A thorough physical examination and clinical history suggest Legg-Calvé-Perthes disease.
◆ Hip X-rays taken every 3 to 4 months confirm the diagnosis, with findings that vary according to the stage of the disease.
◆ Anterior-posterior X-rays and magnetic resonance imaging enhance early diagnosis of necrosis and visualization of articular surface.
◆ Diagnostic evaluation must also differentiate between Legg-Calvé-Perthes disease (restriction of only the abduction and rotation of the hip) and infection or arthritis (restriction of all motion).
◆ Aspiration and culture of synovial fluid rule out joint sepsis.

Treatment
◆ Protection of the femoral head from further stress and damage by containing it within the acetabulum

◆ After 1 to 2 weeks of bed rest, therapy includes reduced weight bearing by means of bed rest in bilateral split counterpoised traction, then application of hip abduction splint or cast, or weight bearing while a splint, cast, or brace holds the leg in abduction
◆ Braces, remaining in place for 6 to 18 months
◆ An anti-inflammatory and an analgesic for pain relief
◆ Physical therapy with passive and active range-of-motion exercises after cast removal to help restore motion

For a young child in the early stages of the disease:
◆ osteotomy and subtrochanteric derotation providing maximum confinement of the epiphysis within the acetabulum to allow return of the femoral head to normal shape and full range of motion
◆ proper placement of the epiphysis allowing remolding with ambulation
◆ postoperatively, a spica cast for about 2 months (required).

AGE ALERT *Many older children require surgery to avoid poor congruence of the hip. Poor congruence predisposes patients to early arthritis, with nearly 50% of patients requiring hip replacement by age 40.*

Special considerations
When caring for the hospitalized child:
◆ Monitor fluid intake and output. Maintain sufficient fluid balance. Provide a diet sufficient for growth without causing excessive weight gain, which might necessitate cast change and loss of the corrective position.
◆ Provide good cast care. Turn the child every 2 to 3 hours to expose the cast to air. When the cast is still wet, turn the child with your palms because depressions in the plaster may lead to pressure ulcers. After the cast dries, petal it with pieces of adhesive tape or moleskin, changing them as they become soiled. Protect the cast with a plastic covering during toileting.
◆ Watch for complications. Check toes for color, temperature, swelling, sensation, and motion; report dusky, cool, numb toes immediately. Check the skin under the cast with a flashlight every 4 hours while the patient is awake. Follow a consistent plan of skin care to prevent skin breakdown. Never use oils or powders under the cast because they increase skin breakdown and soften the cast. Check under the cast daily for odors, particularly after surgery, to detect skin breakdown or wound problems. Report persistent soreness.

◆ Administer an analgesic as ordered.
◆ Relieve itching by using a hair dryer (set on cool) at the cast edges; this also decreases dampness from perspiration. If itching becomes excessive, get an order for an antipruritic. Never insert an object under the cast to scratch.
◆ Provide continuous emotional support. Explain all procedures and the need for bed rest, cast, or braces to the child; encourage him to verbalize his fears and anxiety. Encourage parents to participate in their child's care. Teach them proper cast care and how to recognize signs of skin breakdown. Offer tips for making home management of the bedridden child easier. Tell them what special supplies are needed: pajamas and trousers a size larger (open the side seam, and attach Velcro fasteners to close it), bedpan, adhesive tape, moleskin and, possibly, a hospital bed.
◆ When the cast is removed, debride dry, scaly skin gradually by applying lotion after bathing.
◆ Stress the need for follow-up care to monitor rehabilitation. Also stress the need for home tutoring and socialization to promote normal mental and emotional growth and development.

MUSCULAR DYSTROPHY

Muscular dystrophy is a group of congenital disorders characterized by progressive symmetric wasting of skeletal muscles without neural or sensory defects. Paradoxically, some wasted muscles tend to enlarge (pseudohypertrophy) because connective tissue and fat replace muscle tissue, giving a false impression of increased muscle strength.

The four main types of muscular dystrophy include:
◆ Duchenne's, or *pseudohypertrophic;* 50% of all cases
◆ Becker's, or *benign pseudohypertrophic*
◆ Landouzy-Dejerine, or *facioscapulohumeral*
◆ limb-girdle.

The prognosis varies with the form of disease. Duchenne's muscular dystrophy strikes during early childhood and is usually fatal during the second decade of life. Patients with Becker's muscular dystrophy can live into their 40s. Duchenn's and Becker's muscular dystrophies affect males almost exclusively. Facioscapulohumeral and limb-girdle muscular dystrophies usually don't shorten life expectancy, and they affect both sexes equally.

Causes
◆ Autosomal dominant disorder (in Landouzy-Dejerine muscular dystrophy)

◆ Autosomal recessive disorder (in limb-girdle muscular dystrophy)
◆ Various genetic mechanisms, typically involving an enzymatic or metabolic defect
◆ X-linked recessive disorders due to defects in the gene coding, mapped genetically to the Xp21 locus, for the muscle protein dystrophin, which is essential for maintaining muscle cell membrane; muscle cells deteriorating or dying without it (Duchenne's and Becker's muscular dystrophies)

Pathophysiology

Abnormally permeable cell membranes allow leakage of various muscle enzymes, particularly creatine kinase. This metabolic defect that causes the muscle cells to die is present from fetal life onward. The absence of progressive muscle wasting at birth suggests that other factors compound the effect of dystrophin deficiency. The specific trigger is unknown, but phagocytosis of the muscle cells by inflammatory cells causes scarring and loss of muscle function.

As the disease progresses, skeletal muscle becomes almost totally replaced by fat and connective tissue. The skeleton eventually becomes deformed, causing progressive immobility. Cardiac and smooth muscle of the GI tract typically become fibrotic. No consistent structural abnormalities are seen in the brain.

Signs and symptoms
Duchenne's muscular dystrophy
◆ Insidious onset between ages 3 and 5
◆ Initial effect on legs, pelvis, and shoulders
◆ Gowers' sign, in which the child must use his upper body to maneuver from a prone to an upright position, caused by weakness of the lumbar and gluteal muscles
◆ Waddling gait, toe walking, and lumbar lordosis due to muscle weakness
◆ Difficulty climbing stairs, frequent falls because of muscular weakness
◆ Enlarged, firm calf muscles from muscle replacement by fat and connective tissue
◆ Progressive immobility and skeletal deformities (use of a wheelchair is usually necessary by age 12)

Signs and symptoms of Becker's (benign pseudohypertrophic) muscular dystrophy are similar to those of Duchenne's muscular dystrophy but with slower progression.

Facioscapulohumeral (Landouzy-Dejerine) muscular dystrophy
◆ Weakened face, shoulder, and upper-arm muscles (initial sign) because of scarring and loss of muscle function

◆ Pendulous lip and absent nasolabial fold because of muscular weakness
◆ Inability to pucker mouth or whistle because of muscular weakness
◆ Abnormal facial movements and absence of facial movements when laughing or crying because of muscular weakness and scarring
◆ Diffuse facial flattening leading to a masklike expression resulting from progressive muscle scarring
◆ Inability to raise arms above the head because of extreme muscular weakness

Limb-girdle muscular dystrophy
◆ Weakness in upper arms and pelvis first
◆ Lumbar lordosis with abdominal protrusion because of loss of muscular support
◆ Winging of the scapulae due to weakened thoracic muscles
◆ Waddling gait and poor balance because of muscle weakness
◆ Inability to raise the arms caused by progressive muscle weakness

Complications
Possible complications of Duchenne's muscular dystrophy are:
◆ smooth-muscle dysfunction causing megacolon, cramping, pain, and malabsorption in the GI tract
◆ weakened cardiac and respiratory muscles leading to tachycardia, electrocardiographic abnormalities, and pulmonary complications
◆ death commonly due to sudden heart failure, respiratory failure, or infection.

Diagnosis
Diagnosis depends on typical clinical findings, family history, and diagnostic test findings. If another family member has muscular dystrophy, its clinical characteristics can suggest the type of dystrophy the patient has and how he may be affected. The following tests may help in the diagnosis:
◆ Electromyography shows short, weak bursts of electrical activity in affected muscles.
◆ Muscle biopsy shows a combination of muscle cell degeneration and regeneration. In later stages, it shows fat and connective tissue deposits.
◆ Immunologic and molecular biological techniques, now available in specialized medical centers, facilitate accurate prenatal and postnatal diagnosis of Duchenne's and Becker's muscular dystrophies. These techniques replace muscle biopsy and an elevated serum creatine kinase level in diagnosing the disorder.

Treatment
No treatment can stop the progressive muscle impairment. Supportive treatments include:
◆ a corticosteroid, such as prednisone, to improve muscle strength and slow the progression of Duchenne's muscular dystrophy
◆ coughing and deep-breathing exercises and diaphragmatic breathing
◆ teaching parents to recognize early signs of respiratory complications
◆ orthopedic appliances, exercise, physical therapy, and surgery to correct contractures (to help preserve mobility and independence)
◆ genetic counseling regarding risk or transmitting disease for family members who are carriers
◆ adequate fluid intake, increased dietary bulk, and stool softener for constipation due to inactivity
◆ low-calorie, high-protein, high-fiber diet (physical inactivity predisposes the patient to obesity)
◆ surgery to promote or maintain motility, such as tendon releases for contractures and spinal fusions for scoliosis.
◆ ventilatory support as indicated for respiratory failure

Special considerations
Comprehensive long-term care and follow-up, patient and family teaching, and psychological support can help the patient and family deal with this disorder.
◆ When respiratory involvement occurs in Duchenne's muscular dystrophy, encourage coughing, deep-breathing exercises, and diaphragmatic breathing. Teach parents how to recognize early signs of respiratory complications.
◆ Encourage and assist with active and passive range-of-motion exercises to preserve joint mobility and prevent muscle atrophy.
◆ Advise the patient to avoid long periods of bed rest and inactivity; if necessary, limit television viewing and other sedentary activities.
◆ Refer the patient for physical therapy. Splints, braces, and surgery can help correct contractures; trapeze bars, overhead slings, and a wheelchair can help preserve mobility. A footboard or high-topped sneakers and a foot cradle increase comfort and prevent footdrop.
◆ Because inactivity may cause constipation, encourage adequate fluid intake, increase dietary bulk, and obtain an order for a stool softener. The patient is prone to obesity because of reduced physical activity; help him and his family plan a low-calorie, high-protein, high-fiber diet.

◆ Always allow the patient plenty of time to perform even simple physical tasks because he's likely to be slow and awkward.

◆ Encourage communication between family members to help them deal with the emotional strain this disorder produces. Provide emotional support to help the patient cope with continual changes in body image.

◆ Help the child with Duchenne's muscular dystrophy maintain peer relationships and realize his intellectual potential by encouraging his parents to keep him in a regular school as long as possible.

◆ If necessary, refer adult patients for sexual counseling. Refer those who must acquire new job skills for vocational rehabilitation. (Contact the Department of Labor and Industry in your state for more information.) For information on social services and financial assistance, refer these patients and their families to the Muscular Dystrophy Association.

◆ Discuss end-of-life issues and patient preferences; encourage the patient to formulate advance directives and, as appropriate, make sure the family is aware of the patient's wishes.

◆ Refer family members for genetic counseling.

OSTEOARTHRITIS

Osteoarthritis (commonly referred to as *degenerative joint disease*), the most common form of arthritis, is a chronic condition causing the deterioration of joint cartilage and the formation of reactive new bone at the margins and subchondral areas of the joints. It usually affects weight-bearing joints (knees, feet, hips, lumbar vertebrae). Typically, its earliest symptoms manifest in middle age and progress from there.

Disability depends on the site and severity of involvement and can range from minor limitation of finger movement to severe disability in persons with hip or knee involvement. The rate of progression varies, and joints may remain stable for years in an early stage of deterioration.

Causes

The primary defect in both idiopathic and secondary osteoarthritis is loss of articular cartilage due to functional changes in chondrocytes (cells responsible for the formation of the proteoglycans, glycoproteins that act as cementing material in the cartilage, and collagen).

Idiopathic osteoarthritis, a normal part of aging, results from many factors, including:

◆ chemical (drugs that stimulate the collagen-digesting enzymes in the synovial membrane such as steroids)

◆ genetic (decreased collagen synthesis) and metabolic (endocrine disorders such as hyperparathyroidism)

◆ mechanical (repeated stress on the joint).

Secondary osteoarthritis usually follows an identifiable predisposing event that leads to degenerative changes, such as:

◆ congenital deformity

◆ obesity

◆ trauma (most common cause).

Pathophysiology

The major defect in primary and secondary osteoarthritis is loss of articular cartilage. Articular cartilage is probably lost through enzymatic breakdown of the cartilage matrix—the proteoglycans, glycosaminoglycans, and collagen. Other studies indicate that interleukin-1 may play a part in cartilage destruction.

Osteoarthritis occurs in synovial joints. The joint cartilage deteriorates, and reactive new bone forms at the margins and subchondral areas of the joints. The degeneration results from damage to the chondrocytes. Cartilage softens with age, narrowing the joint space. Mechanical injury erodes articular cartilage, leaving the underlying bone unprotected. This causes sclerosis, or thickening and hardening of the bone underneath the cartilage.

Articular cartilage particles within the joint irritate the synovial lining, which becomes fibrotic and limits joint movement. Synovial fluid may be forced into defects in the bone, causing cysts. New bone, called *osteophyte* (bone spur), forms at joint margins as the articular cartilage erodes, causing gross alteration of the bony contours and enlargement of the joint. The spurlike bony projections enlarge until small pieces called joint mice break off into the synovial cavity.

Signs and symptoms

Symptoms, which typically appear during the first or sixth decade of life and increase with poor posture, obesity, and occupational stress include:

◆ deep, aching joint pain due to degradation of the cartilage, inflammation, and bone stress, particularly after exercise or weight bearing (the most common symptom, usually relieved by rest)

◆ stiffness in the morning and after exercise (relieved by rest) caused by degradation of the cartilage, inflammation, and bone stress

◆ crepitus, or "grating" of the joint during motion, due to cartilage damage

◆ Heberden's nodes (bony enlargements of the distal interphalangeal joints) and Bouchard's nodes (bony enlargements of the proximal interphalangeal joints) due to repeated inflammation. (See *The effects of osteoarthritis.*)

The effects of osteoarthritis

Involvement of the interphalangeal (finger bone) joints produces irreversible changes in the distal joints (Heberden's nodes) and the proximal joints (Bouchard's nodes), as shown below. These nodes can be painless initially, with gradual progression to or sudden flare-ups of redness, swelling, tenderness, and impaired sensation and dexterity.

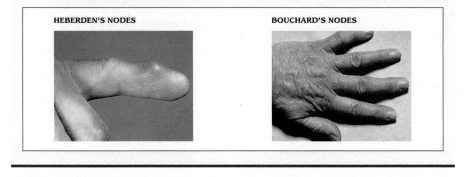

HEBERDEN'S NODES

BOUCHARD'S NODES

♦ altered gait from contractures due to over-compensation of the muscles supporting the joint
♦ decreased range of motion (ROM) due to pain and stiffness
♦ joint enlargement due to stress on the bone and disordered bone growth
♦ localized headaches (may be a direct result of cervical spine arthritis).

Complications

♦ Irreversible joint changes and node formation (nodes eventually becoming red, swollen, and tender, causing numbness and loss of finger dexterity)
♦ Subluxation of the joint
♦ Decreased joint ROM
♦ Joint contractures
♦ Pain (can be debilitating in later stages)
♦ Loss of independence in activities of daily living

Diagnosis

♦ Absence of systemic symptoms rules out inflammatory joint disorder.
♦ Magnetic resonance imaging shows bony and soft-tissue abnormalities.
♦ Increased erythrocyte sedimentation rate occurs with extensive synovitis.

X-rays of the affected joint help confirm the diagnosis but may be normal in the early stages. X-rays may require many views and typically show:
♦ narrowing of joint space or margin
♦ cystlike bony deposits in joint space and margins, sclerosis of the subchondral space

♦ joint deformity due to degeneration or articular damage
♦ bony growths at weight-bearing areas
♦ joint fusion.

Treatment

The goal of treatment is to relieve pain, maintain or improve mobility, and minimize disability. Treatment may include:
♦ weight loss to reduce stress on the joint
♦ balance of rest and exercise
♦ medications, including nonsteroidal anti-inflammatory drugs, cox-2 inhibitors and, in some cases, intra-articular injections of corticosteroids; glucosamine and chondroitin may help control symptoms and reduce functional impairment (See *Arthritic joint care*, page 390.)
♦ support or stabilization of joint with crutches, braces, a cane, a walker, or a cervical collar
♦ intra-articular injections of a corticosteroid (every 4 to 6 months) to possibly delay node development in the hands (if used too frequently, may accelerate arthritic progression by depleting the normal ground substance of the cartilage)
♦ intra-articular injection of high-molecular-weight viscose supplements, particularly hyaluronic acid, to create an artificial joint fluid (only for use in the knees).

Surgical treatment, reserved for patients with severe disability or uncontrollable pain, may include:
♦ arthroplasty (partial or total replacement of deteriorated part of joint with prosthetic appliance)

Arthritic joint care

Depending on the affected joint, such as the hand, spine, hip, or knee, specific care varies.

♦ Hand: Apply hot soaks and paraffin dips to relieve pain as ordered.
♦ Lumbar and sacral spine: Recommend a firm mattress or bed board to decrease morning pain.
♦ Cervical spine: Check cervical collar for constriction; watch for redness with prolonged use.
♦ Hip: Use moist heat pads to relieve pain, and administer an antispasmodic as ordered. Assist with range-of-motion (ROM) and strengthening exercises, always making sure the patient gets the proper rest afterward. Check crutches, cane, braces, and walker for proper fit, and teach the patient to use them correctly. For example, the patient with unilateral joint involvement should use an orthopedic appliance (such as a cane or walker) on the unaffected side. Advise use of cushions when sitting and use of an elevated toilet seat.
♦ Knee: Assist with prescribed ROM exercises, exercises to maintain muscle tone, and progressive resistance exercises to increase muscle strength. Provide elastic supports or braces, if needed.

To minimize the long-term effects of osteoarthritis, teach the patient to:
♦ plan for adequate rest during the day, after exertion, and at night
♦ take medication exactly as prescribed and report adverse reactions immediately
♦ avoid overexertion, take care to stand and walk correctly, minimize weight-bearing activities, and be especially careful when stooping or picking up objects
♦ always wear well-fitting supportive shoes and not let the heels become too worn down
♦ install safety devices at home, such as guard rails in the bathroom
♦ perform ROM exercises as gently as possible
♦ apply heat before exercising and cold after exercising
♦ maintain proper body weight to lessen strain on joints
♦ avoid percussive activities.

♦ arthrodesis (surgical fusion of bones, primarily in spine [laminectomy])
♦ osteoplasty (scraping and lavage of deteriorated bone from joint)
♦ osteotomy (change in alignment of bone to relieve stress by excision of wedge of bone or cutting of bone).

Special considerations

♦ Promote adequate rest, particularly after activity. Plan rest periods during the day, and provide for adequate sleep at night. Moderation is the key—teach the patient to pace daily activities.
♦ Assist with physical therapy, and encourage the patient to perform gentle, isometric ROM exercises.
♦ If the patient needs surgery, provide appropriate preoperative and postoperative care.
♦ Provide emotional support and reassurance to help the patient cope with limited mobility. Explain that osteoarthritis isn't a systemic disease.

OSTEOGENESIS IMPERFECTA

Osteogenesis imperfecta (also called *little bone disease*) is a genetic disease in which bones are thin, poorly developed, and fracture easily. A classification system of different types (I to VIII) is commonly used to describe the severity of the disease. Type I is the most common and mildest form. Type II is the most severe form.

Causes

♦ Dominant mutation in gene coding for type I collagen (types I, II, III, and IV)
♦ Recessive inheritance of a mutation to the cartilage-associated protein (CRTAP) gene (type VII)
♦ Mutation of the leucine proline-enriched proteoglycan (LEPRE) 1 gene (type VIII)
♦ Unknown mutation (types V and VI)

Pathophysiology

Most forms of osteogenesis imperfecta appear to be caused by mutations in the genes that determine the structure of collagen. Possible mutations in other genes may cause variations in the assembly and maintenance of bone and other connective tissues. Collectively or alone, these mutated genes lead to pathologic fractures and impaired healing.

Signs and symptoms

In the autosomal dominant disorder, the following signs and symptoms may not be apparent until the child's mobility increases:
♦ frequent fractures and poor healing due to falls as toddler begins to walk

◆ short stature due to multiple fractures caused by minor physical stress
◆ deformed cranial structure and limbs from multiple fractures
◆ thin skin and bluish sclera of the eyes; thin collagen fibers of the sclera allowing the choroid layer to be seen
◆ abnormal tooth and enamel development due to improper deposition of dentine
◆ middle ear deafness caused by bone deformity interfering with sound transmission.

Complications
◆ Deafness due to bone deformity and scarring of the middle and inner ear
◆ Stillbirth or death within the first year of life (autosomal-recessive disorder)

Diagnosis
◆ Fractures early in life, hearing loss, and blue sclerae show that mutation is expressed in more than one connective tissue.
◆ An elevated serum alkaline phosphatase level occurs during periods of rapid bone formation and cellular injury.
◆ Collagen molecular testing reveals mutation at the gene level.
◆ Skin culture shows reduced quantity of fibroblasts.
◆ Echocardiography may show mitral insufficiency or floppy mitral valves.

Treatment
◆ Prevention of fractures
◆ Internal fixation of fractures to ensure stabilization and prevent deformities
◆ Administration of bisphosphonates, growth hormones, and gene therapies (under investigation)
◆ Bone marrow transplantation and treatment to increase the density of trabecular bone formation (under investigation)

Special considerations
◆ Educate the family about the disorder. Teach the parents and child how to recognize fractures and how to correctly splint them. Also teach the parents how to protect the child during diapering, dressing, and other activities of daily living.
◆ Advise the parents to encourage their child to develop interests that don't require strenuous physical activity and to develop his fine motor skills. These actions will promote the child's self-esteem.
◆ Teach the child to assume some responsibility for precautions during physical activity—including avoiding contact sports and strenuous activity

and wearing protective devices when engaging in noncontact sports—to help foster his independence.
◆ Stress the importance of good nutrition to heal bones.
◆ Refer the parents and child for genetic counseling to assess the recurrence risk.
◆ Discuss alternatives for birth control and family planning, if appropriate.
◆ Administer an analgesic, as ordered, to relieve pain from frequent fractures, a hallmark of this disease.
◆ Monitor dental and hearing needs. Stress the need for regular dental care and immunizations.
◆ Instruct the parents to provide a medical identification bracelet for the child.

OSTEOMALACIA AND RICKETS
In vitamin D deficiency, bone can't calcify normally; the result is called *osteomalacia* in adults and *rickets* in infants and young children.

Once a common childhood disease, rickets is now rare in the United States. It does appear occasionally in breast-fed infants who don't receive a vitamin D supplement or in infants fed a formula with a nonfortified milk base. Rickets also occurs in overcrowded, urban areas where smog limits sunlight penetration.

⚠ **CLINICAL ALERT** *Incidence of rickets is highest in children with black or dark brown skin, who, because of their pigmentation, absorb less sunlight.*

With treatment, the prognosis is good. In osteomalacia, bone deformities may disappear; however, they usually persist in children with rickets.

Causes
◆ Conditions reducing the absorption of fat-soluble vitamin D (such as biliary obstruction, celiac disease, chronic pancreatitis, colitis, Crohn's disease, cystic fibrosis, fistulas, and gastric or small-bowel resections)
◆ Hepatic or renal disease (interfering with hydroxylated calciferol formation, needed to form a calcium-binding protein in intestinal absorption sites)
◆ Inadequate dietary intake of preformed vitamin D
◆ Inadequate exposure to sunlight (solar ultraviolet rays irradiate 7-dehydrocholesterol, a precursor of vitamin D, to form calciferol)
◆ Inherited impairment of renal tubular reabsorption of phosphate (from vitamin D insensitivity) in vitamin D–resistant rickets (refractory rickets, familial hypophosphatemia)
◆ Malabsorption of vitamin D

◆ Malfunctioning parathyroid gland (decreased secretion of parathyroid hormone), contributing to calcium deficiency (normally, vitamin D controls absorption of calcium and phosphorus through the intestine) and interfering with activation of vitamin D in the kidneys

Pathophysiology

Vitamin D regulates the absorption of calcium ions from the intestine. When vitamin D is lacking, a falling serum calcium level stimulates synthesis and secretion of parathyroid hormone, causing release of calcium from bone, decreasing renal calcium excretion, and increasing renal phosphate excretion. When the concentration of phosphate in the bone decreases, osteoid may be produced, but mineralization can't proceed normally. Large quantities of osteoid accumulate, coating the trabeculae and linings of the haversian canals and areas beneath the periosteum.

When mineralization of bone matrix is delayed or inadequate, bone is disorganized in structure and lacks density. The result is gross deformity of both spongy and compact bone.

Signs and symptoms

Osteomalacia may be asymptomatic until a fracture occurs. Chronic vitamin D deficiency induces numerous bone malformations due to bone softening. Possible signs and symptoms include:
◆ pain in the legs and lower back due to vertebral collapse
◆ bow legs
◆ knock knees
◆ rachitic rosary (beading of ends of ribs)
◆ enlarged wrists and ankles
◆ pigeon breast (protruding ribs and sternum)
◆ delayed closing of fontanels
◆ softening skull
◆ bulging forehead
◆ poorly developed muscles (pot belly)
◆ difficulty walking and climbing stairs caused by bone deformities
◆ kyphoscoliosis.

Complications

◆ Spontaneous multiple fractures
◆ Tetany in infants
◆ Bone deformities
◆ Cardiac and respiratory complications (kyphoscoliosis)

Diagnosis

Physical examination, dietary history, and laboratory test results help establish the diagnosis. Test results that suggest vitamin D deficiency include:
◆ a serum calcium level less than 7.5 mg/dl

◆ a serum inorganic phosphorus level less than 3 mg/dl
◆ a serum citrate level less than 2.5 mg/dl and an alkaline phosphatase level less than 4 Bodansky units/dl
◆ X-rays showing characteristic bone deformities and abnormalities, such as Looser's zones (radiolucent bands perpendicular to the surface of the bones indicating reduced bone ossification; confirms the diagnosis).

Treatment

◆ Massive oral doses of vitamin D or cod liver oil (for osteomalacia and rickets, except when caused by malabsorption)
◆ 25-hydroxycholecalciferol, 1,25-dihydroxycholecalciferol, or a synthetic analogue of active vitamin (for rickets refractory to vitamin D or rickets accompanied by hepatic or renal disease)
◆ Foods high in vitamin D (fortified milk, fish liver oils, herring, liver, and egg yolks) and sufficient sun exposure
◆ Supplemental aqueous preparations of vitamin D for chronic fat malabsorption, hydroxylated cholecalciferol for refractory rickets, and supplemental vitamin D for breast-fed infants (to prevent rickets)
◆ Possible surgical intervention for intestinal disease

Special considerations

◆ Obtain a dietary history to assess the patient's vitamin D intake.
◆ If the patient must take vitamin D for a prolonged period, tell him to watch for signs and symptoms of vitamin D toxicity (headache, nausea, constipation and, after prolonged use, renal calculi).
◆ If the patient's vitamin D deficiency appears to be linked to adverse socioeconomic conditions, refer the patient to an appropriate community agency.

OSTEOMYELITIS

Osteomyelitis is a bone infection characterized by progressive inflammatory destruction after formation of new bone. It may be chronic or acute. It commonly results from a combination of local trauma—often an open fracture with vascular injury and subsequent hematoma—and an acute infection originating elsewhere in the body. Although osteomyelitis typically remains localized, it can spread through the bone to the marrow, cortex, and periosteum. Acute osteomyelitis is usually a blood-borne disease and most commonly affects rapidly growing children. Chronic osteomyelitis is characterized by draining sinus tracts and widespread lesions.

It's seen in patients with infected total joint replacements; the risk increases proportionally to the amount of periosteal stripping during the fracture event.

■ **AGE ALERT** *Osteomyelitis is more common in children (especially boys) than in adults—usually as a complication of an acute localized infection. Typical sites in children are the lower end of the femur and the upper ends of the tibia, humerus, and radius. The most common sites in adults are the pelvis and vertebrae, generally after surgery or trauma.* (See *Stages of osteomyelitis*, page 394.)

The incidence of both chronic and acute osteomyelitis is declining, except in drug abusers.

With prompt treatment, the prognosis for acute osteomyelitis is extremely good; for chronic osteomyelitis, prognosis remains poor.

Causes

The most common pyogenic organism in osteomyelitis is *Staphylococcus aureus*. Others include:
♦ *Escherichia coli*
♦ *Hemophilus influenzae*
♦ *Mycobacterium tuberculosis*
♦ *Neisseria gonorrhoeae*
♦ *Pasteurella multocida* (part of the normal mouth flora of cats and dogs)
♦ *Proteus vulgaris*
♦ *Pseudomonas aeruginosa*
♦ *Salmonella*
♦ *Streptococcus pneumoniae*
♦ *Streptococcus pyogenes*.

Pathophysiology

Typically, these organisms find a culture site in a hematoma from recent trauma or in a weakened area, such as the site of local infection (for example, furunculosis), and travel through the bloodstream to the metaphysis, the section of a long bone that's continuous with the epiphysis plates, where the blood flows into sinusoids. (See *Avoiding osteomyelitis*, page 395.) Predisposing factors include diabetes mellitus, sickle cell disease, and being immunocompromised.

Signs and symptoms

Clinical features of chronic and acute osteomyelitis are generally the same and may include:
♦ rapid onset of acute osteomyelitis, with sudden pain in the affected bone and tenderness, heat, swelling, erythema, guarding of affected region of the limb, and restricted movement caused by inflammation and infection
♦ chronic infection persisting intermittently for years, flaring after minor trauma or persisting as

drainage of pus from an old pocket in a sinus tract
♦ accompanying fever and tachycardia resulting from the infectious process
♦ dehydration (in young children) resulting from the infectious process
♦ irritability and poor feeding (in infants).

Complications

♦ Amputation (of an arm or leg when resistant chronic osteomyelitis causes severe, unrelenting pain and decreases function)
♦ Weakened bone cortex, predisposing the bone to pathologic fracture
♦ Arrested growth of an extremity (in children with severe disease)

Diagnosis

Diagnosis must rule out septicemia, foreign bodies, poliomyelitis (rare), rheumatic fever, myositis (inflammation of voluntary muscle), and bone fracture.

History, physical examination, and laboratory test results that help confirm osteomyelitis may include:
♦ history of a urinary tract, respiratory tract, ear, or skin infection; human or animal bite; or other penetrating trauma
♦ white blood cell count showing leukocytosis
♦ elevated erythrocyte sedimentation rate
♦ blood cultures showing causative organism (however, blood cultures are positive in only 40% of patients)
♦ magnetic resonance imaging to delineate bone marrow from soft tissue (facilitates diagnosis)
♦ X-rays (may not show bone involvement until the disease has been active for 2 to 3 weeks)
♦ bone scans to detect early infection.

Treatment

Treatment of acute osteomyelitis should begin before definitive diagnosis and includes:
♦ large doses of an antibiotic I.V. (usually a penicillinase-resistant penicillin, such as nafcillin [Nafcil] or oxacillin [Bactocill] along with an aminoglycoside) after blood cultures are taken
♦ early surgical drainage to relieve pressure and abscess formation
♦ immobilization of the affected body part by cast, traction, or bed rest to prevent failure to heal or recurrence
♦ supportive measures, such as an analgesic for pain and I.V. fluids to maintain hydration
♦ incision and drainage, followed by a culture of the drainage (if an abscess or sinus tract forms).

Stages of osteomyelitis

The illustrations show the progression of osteomyelitis.

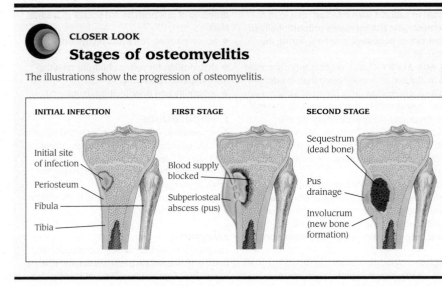

INITIAL INFECTION	FIRST STAGE	SECOND STAGE
Initial site of infection Periosteum Fibula Tibia	Blood supply blocked Subperiosteal abscess (pus)	Sequestrum (dead bone) Pus drainage Involucrum (new bone formation)

Antibiotic therapy to control infection may include:
◆ a systemic antibiotic for 6 weeks
◆ intracavitary instillation of an antibiotic through closed-system continuous irrigation with low intermittent suction
◆ limited irrigation with blood drainage system with suction (Hemovac)
◆ packed, wet, antibiotic-soaked dressings.
Chronic osteomyelitis care may include:
◆ surgery, usually required to remove dead bone and promote drainage (prognosis remains poor even after surgery)
◆ hyperbaric oxygen to stimulate normal immune mechanisms
◆ skin, bone, and muscle grafts to fill in dead space and increase blood supply.

Special considerations

Major concerns in osteomyelitis are to control infection, protect the bone from injury, and offer meticulous supportive care.
◆ Use strict aseptic technique when changing dressings and irrigating wounds. If the patient is in skeletal traction for open, comminuted fractures, cover insertion points of pin tracks with small, dry dressings, and tell him not to touch the skin around the pins and wires.
◆ Administer I.V. fluids to maintain adequate hydration as necessary. Provide a diet high in protein and vitamin C.
◆ Assess daily the vital signs, the wound appearance, and new pain, which may indicate secondary infection.

◆ Carefully monitor suctioning equipment. Monitor the amount of solution instilled and suctioned.
◆ Support the affected limb with firm pillows. Keep the limb level with the body; don't let it sag. Provide good skin care. Turn the patient gently every 2 hours and watch for signs of developing pressure ulcers. Report any signs of pressure ulcer formation immediately.
◆ Provide good cast care. Support the cast with firm pillows and smooth rough cast edges by petaling with pieces of adhesive tape or moleskin. Check circulation and drainage; if a wet spot appears on the cast, circle it with a marking pen and note the time of appearance directly on the cast. Be aware of how much drainage is expected. Check the circled spot at least every 4 hours. Report any enlargement immediately.
◆ Protect the patient from mishaps, such as jerky movements and falls, which may threaten bone integrity. Report sudden pain, crepitus, or deformity immediately. Watch for any sudden malalignment of the limb, which may indicate fracture.
◆ Provide emotional support and appropriate diversions. Before discharge, teach the patient how to protect and clean the wound and how to recognize signs and symptoms of recurring infection (increased temperature, redness, localized heat, and swelling). Stress the need for follow-up examinations. Instruct the patient to seek prompt treatment for possible sources of recurrence—blisters, boils, styes, and impetigo.

DISEASE BLOCK
Avoiding osteomyelitis

Bones are essentially isolated from the body's natural defense system once an organism gets through the periosteum. They are limited in their ability to replace necrotic tissue caused by infection, which may lead to chronic osteomyelitis.

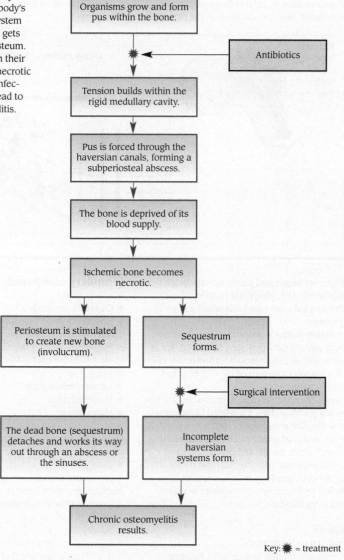

Organisms grow and form pus within the bone.

↓ ✳ ← Antibiotics

Tension builds within the rigid medullary cavity.

↓

Pus is forced through the haversian canals, forming a subperiosteal abscess.

↓

The bone is deprived of its blood supply.

↓

Ischemic bone becomes necrotic.

↓

Periosteum is stimulated to create new bone (involucrum).

Sequestrum forms.

✳ ← Surgical intervention

The dead bone (sequestrum) detaches and works its way out through an abscess or the sinuses.

Incomplete haversian systems form.

↓

Chronic osteomyelitis results.

Key: ✳ = treatment

OSTEOPOROSIS

Osteoporosis is a metabolic bone disorder in which the rate of bone resorption accelerates and the rate of bone formation slows, causing a loss of bone mass. Bones affected by this disease lose calcium and phosphate salts and become porous, brittle, and abnormally vulnerable to fractures. Osteoporosis may be primary or secondary to an underlying disease, such as Cushing's syndrome or hyperthyroidism. It primarily affects the weight-bearing vertebrae. Only when the condition is advanced or severe, as in secondary disease, do similar changes occur in the skull, ribs, and long bones. Usually,

CLOSER LOOK

What is osteoporosis?

Osteoporosis is a metabolic disease of the skeleton that reduces the amount of bone tissue. Bones weaken as local cells resorb, or take up, bone tissue. Trabecular bone at the core becomes less dense, and cortical bone on the perimeter loses thickness.

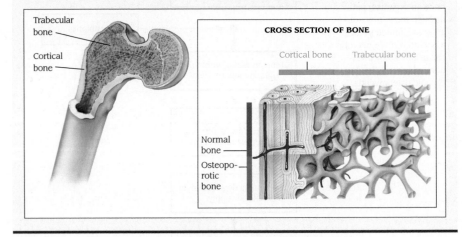

the femoral heads and pelvic acetabula are selectively affected. (See *What is osteoporosis?*)

Primary osteoporosis is classified as one of three types:

◆ *Postmenopausal osteoporosis (type I)* usually affects women between ages 51 and 75. It's related to loss of estrogen and its protective effect on bone and characterized by vertebral and wrist fractures.

◆ *Senile osteoporosis (type II)* occurs mostly between ages 70 and 85. It's related to osteoblast and osteoclast shrinkage or decreased physical activity and characterized by fractures of the humerus, tibia, femur, and pelvis.

◆ *Premenopausal osteoporosis (type III)* involves a higher estrogen level that may inhibit bone resorption by affecting the sensitivity of osteoclasts to parathyroid hormone.

Causes

Primary osteoporosis

◆ Declining adrenal and gonadal function

◆ Faulty protein metabolism due to relative or progressive estrogen deficiency (estrogen stimulates osteoblastic activity and limits the osteoclastic-stimulating effects of parathyroid hormones)

◆ Mild but prolonged negative calcium balance due to inadequate dietary intake of calcium (may be an important contributing factor)

◆ Sedentary lifestyle

Secondary osteoporosis

◆ Alcoholism

◆ Cigarette smoking

◆ Endocrine disorders, such as Cushing's syndrome, diabetes mellitus, hyperparathyroidism, or hyperthyroidism (plasma calcium and phosphate levels are maintained by the endocrine system)

◆ Lactose intolerance

◆ Malabsorption

◆ Malnutrition

◆ Medications (an antacid that contains aluminum, an anticonvulsant, or a corticosteroid)

◆ Osteogenesis imperfecta

◆ Prolonged therapy with a steroid or heparin (heparin promotes bone resorption by inhibiting collagen synthesis or enhancing collagen breakdown)

◆ Scurvy

◆ Sudeck's atrophy (localized to hands and feet, with recurring attacks)

◆ Total immobilization or disuse of a bone (as in hemiplegia)

Pathophysiology

In normal bone, the rates of bone formation and resorption are constant; replacement follows resorption immediately, and the amount of bone replaced equals the amount of bone resorbed. Osteoporosis develops when the remodeling cycle is interrupted and new bone formation falls behind resorption.

When bone is resorbed faster than it forms, the bone becomes less dense. Men have about 30% greater bone mass than women, which may explain why osteoporosis develops later in men.

Signs and symptoms

Osteoporosis is typically discovered suddenly, such as in:

◆ a postmenopausal woman who bends to lift something, hears a snapping sound, then feels a sudden pain in her lower back
◆ vertebral collapse that causes back pain that radiates around the trunk (most common presenting feature) and is aggravated by movement or jarring.

In another common pattern, osteoporosis can develop insidiously, showing:

◆ increasing deformity, kyphosis, loss of height, decreased exercise tolerance, and a markedly aged appearance
◆ spontaneous wedge fractures (compression fracture of only the anterior part of a vertebra, resulting in a wedge-shaped vertebra), pathologic fractures of the neck and femur, Colles' fractures of the distal radius after a minor fall, and hip fractures (common as bone is lost from the femoral neck)
◆ Dowager's hump, a humped back resulting from repeated vertebral fractures that increase the spinal curvature
◆ protruding abdomen to compensate for the changed center of gravity.

Complications

◆ Spontaneous fractures as the bones lose volume and become brittle and weak
◆ Shock, hemorrhage, or fat embolism (fatal complications of fractures)

Diagnosis

Differential diagnosis must exclude other causes of bone loss, especially those affecting the spine, such as metastatic cancer or advanced multiple myeloma. History is the key to identify the specific cause of osteoporosis. Diagnosis may include:

◆ dual energy X-ray absorptiometry, also known as DEXA, to measure bone mineral density of the extremities, hips, and spine
◆ X-rays showing typical degeneration in the lower thoracic and lumbar vertebrae (vertebral bodies may appear flattened and may look denser than normal; bone mineral loss is evident in only later stages)

◆ computed tomography scan to assess spinal bone loss
◆ normal serum calcium, phosphorus, and alkaline phosphatase levels, possibly elevated parathyroid hormone (PTH) level
◆ bone biopsy showing thin, porous, but otherwise normal-looking bone.

Treatment

Treatment to control bone loss, prevent fractures, and control pain may include:
◆ a diet with adequate calcium and vitamin D intake
◆ physical therapy emphasizing gentle exercise and activity and regular, low-impact weight-bearing exercise to slow bone loss and possibly reverse demineralization (the mechanical stress of exercise stimulates bone formation)
◆ a supportive device such as a back brace
◆ surgery, if indicated, for pathologic fractures
◆ an analgesic and local heat to relieve pain.

Medications

◆ Bisphosphonates (such as alendronate [Fosamax] and risedronate [Actonel]) to increase bone density and restore lost bone
◆ Calcium and vitamin D supplements to support normal bone metabolism
◆ Calcitonin (Calcimar) to reduce bone resorption and slow the decline in bone mass
◆ Hormone replacement therapy with estrogen and progesterone to slow bone loss and prevent occurrence of fractures

⚠ **CLINICAL ALERT** *Estrogen used in combination with progesterone has been shown to increase the risk of breast cancer, stroke, heart attack, and blood clots; estrogen used alone may increase the risk of stroke. Therefore, hormonal replacement therapy should be used cautiously and may not be appropriate for all patients.*
◆ A selective estrogen receptor modulator, such as raloxifene (Evista), to mimic the beneficial effects of hormone replacement therapy without increasing the associated risks
◆ Teriparatide (Forteo), a form of PTH, to stimulate bone formation (approved for postmenopausal women and men at high risk for osteoporotic fracture)

Other measures

◆ Early mobilization after surgery or trauma
◆ Decreased alcohol and tobacco consumption
◆ Careful observation for signs of malabsorption (fatty stools, chronic diarrhea)
◆ Prompt, effective treatment of the underlying disorder to prevent secondary osteoporosis (See *Preventing osteoporosis*, page 398.)

PREVENTION
Preventing osteoporosis

To help prevent osteoporosis, tell the patient to follow these guidelines.

Maintain adequate calcium and vitamin D intake

Postmenopausal women and all men and women older than age 65 should consume 1,500 mg of calcium and at least 800 international units of vitamin D daily. Getting enough vitamin D is as important as getting enough calcium because vitamin D aids in absorption of calcium and improves muscle strength.

Most people get adequate amounts of vitamin D from sunlight; however, this may not be a good source for those who live in high latitudes, are housebound, or regularly use sunscreen or avoid the sun entirely because of the risk of skin cancer. Calcium supplements with added vitamin D are a good alternative.

Exercise

Exercise can help build strong bones and slow bone loss. Strength-training exercises should be combined with weight-bearing exercises. Strength training helps strengthen muscles and bones in the arms and upper spine, and weight-bearing exercises mainly affect the bones in the legs, hips, and lower spine.

Limit alcohol intake

Consuming more than two alcoholic drinks a day may decrease bone formation and reduce the body's ability to absorb calcium.

Limit caffeine

Limit the amount of caffeinated beverages to about two to three cups of coffee a day. As long as the diet contains adequate calcium, moderate caffeine consumption won't harm you. Don't forget to count all caffeine-containing beverages, including colas and teas.

Special considerations

Your care plan should focus on the patient's fragility, stressing careful positioning, ambulation, and prescribed exercises.

◆ Check the patient's skin daily for redness, warmth, and new sites of pain, which may indicate new fractures. Encourage activity; help the patient walk several times daily. As appropriate, perform passive range-of-motion exercises or encourage the patient to perform active exercises. Make sure the patient regularly attends scheduled physical therapy sessions.

◆ Impose safety precautions. Keep side rails of patient's bed in raised position. Move the patient gently and carefully at all times. Explain to the patient's family and ancillary health care personnel how easily osteoporotic bones can fracture.

◆ Make sure the patient and family members clearly understand the prescribed drug regimen. Tell them how to recognize significant adverse reactions and to report them immediately. The patient should also report any new pain sites immediately, especially after trauma, no matter how slight. Advise the patient to sleep on a firm mattress and avoid excessive bed rest. Make sure she knows how to wear her back brace.

◆ Thoroughly explain osteoporosis to the patient and her family. If the patient and family don't understand the nature of this disease, they may feel the fractures could have been prevented if they had been more careful.

◆ Teach the patient good body mechanics — to stoop before lifting anything and to avoid twisting movements and prolonged bending.

◆ Instruct the female patient taking estrogen about the proper technique for breast self-examination. Tell her to perform this examination at least once per month and to report any lumps immediately. Emphasize the need for regular gynecologic examinations. Tell her to report abnormal bleeding promptly.

PAGET'S DISEASE

Paget's disease, also called *osteitis deformans,* is a slowly progressive metabolic bone disease characterized by accelerated patterns of bone remodeling. An initial phase of excessive bone resorption (osteoclastic phase) is followed by a reactive phase of excessive abnormal bone formation (osteoblastic phase). Chronic accelerated remodeling eventually enlarges and softens the affected bones. The new bone structure — which is chaotic, fragile, and weak — causes painful deformities of both external contour and internal structure. Paget's disease usually localizes in one or several areas of the skeleton (most commonly the lumbosacral spine, skull, pelvis, femur, and tibia are affected), but occasionally skeletal deformity is widely distributed.

Paget's disease affects those over age 40 (mostly men). It occurs worldwide, but the disease is more common in Europe, Australia, and New Zealand, where it's seen in up to 5% of the elderly population. It can be fatal, particularly when it's associated with heart failure (widespread disease creates a continuous need for high cardiac output), bone sarcoma, or giant-cell tumors.

Causes

Although the exact cause of Paget's disease is unknown, one theory is that early viral infection causes a dormant skeletal infection that erupts many years later as Paget's disease.

Other possible causes include:
◆ autoimmune disease
◆ benign or malignant bone tumors
◆ estrogen deficiency
◆ vitamin D deficiency during the bone-developing years of childhood.

Pathophysiology

Repeated episodes of accelerated osteoclastic resorption of spongy bone occur. The trabeculae diminish, and vascular fibrous tissue replaces marrow. This is followed by short periods of rapid, abnormal bone formation. The collagen fibers in this new bone are disorganized, and glycoprotein levels in the matrix decrease. The partially resorbed trabeculae thicken and enlarge because of excessive bone formation, and the bone becomes soft and weak.

Eventually, Paget's disease progresses to an inactive phase in which abnormal remodeling is minimal or absent. (See *How Paget's disease affects the body*, page 400.)

Signs and symptoms

Clinical effects of Paget's disease vary. Early stages may be asymptomatic. When signs and symptoms appear, they may include:
◆ usually severe and persistent pain intensifying with weight bearing, possibly with impaired movement due to impingement of abnormal bone on the spinal cord or sensory nerve root (pain may also result from the constant inflammation accompanying cell breakdown)
◆ characteristic cranial enlargement over frontal and occipital areas (hat size may increase) because of excessive bone formation, and possibly headaches, sensory abnormalities, and impaired motor function (with skull involvement) caused by abnormal bone impinging on the brain.

Other deformities include:
◆ kyphosis (spinal curvature due to compression fractures of vertebrae)
◆ barrel chest
◆ asymmetrical bowing of the tibia and femur (commonly reduces height)
◆ waddling gait (from softening of pelvic bones)
◆ warm and tender disease sites susceptible to pathologic fractures after minor trauma
◆ slow and, in many cases, incomplete healing of pathologic fractures.

Complications

◆ Blindness and hearing loss with tinnitus and vertigo due to bony impingement on the cranial nerves
◆ Pathologic fractures
◆ Hypertension
◆ Renal calculi
◆ Hypercalcemia
◆ Gout
◆ Heart failure due to high blood-flow demands of remodeling bones
◆ Respiratory failure due to deformed thoracic bones
◆ Malignant changes in involved bone (1% of the patients)

Diagnosis

◆ X-rays, computed tomography scan, and magnetic resonance imaging taken before overt symptoms develop showing increased bone expansion and density
◆ Radionuclide bone scan (more sensitive than X-rays) clearly showing early Paget's lesions (radioisotope concentrates in areas of active disease)
◆ Bone biopsy showing characteristic mosaic pattern

Other laboratory findings reveal:
◆ anemia
◆ an elevated serum alkaline phosphatase level (an index of osteoblastic activity and bone formation)
◆ an elevated 24-hour urine level for hydroxyproline (amino acid excreted by kidneys and an index of osteoclastic hyperactivity)
◆ a normal or elevated serum calcium level.

Treatment

Primary treatment consists of drug therapy and includes one of the following medications:
◆ a bisphosphonate (alendronate [Fosamax], etidronate [Didronel]) to inhibit osteoclast-mediated bone resorption

MULTISYSTEM DISORDER
How Paget's disease affects the body

The effects of Paget's disease can be widespread, involving multiple body systems. Treatment of this disease requires a multidisciplinary approach.

Cardiovascular system
♦ The widespread nature of Paget's disease and extreme vascularity of the newly formed bone increase metabolic demand and create a continuous need for high cardiac output.
♦ Increased metabolic demand and high cardiac output can eventually lead to heart failure.

Musculoskeletal system
♦ The trabeculae diminish, and vascular fibrous tissue replaces marrow. This activity is followed by short periods of rapid, abnormal bone formation.
♦ The collagen fibers in the new bone are disorganized, and the glycoprotein level in the matrix decreases.
♦ The partially resorbed trabeculae thicken and enlarge because of excessive bone formation, and the bone becomes soft and weak.
♦ Impingement of abnormal bone on the spinal cord or sensory nerve root leads to pain and impaired mobility. Pain may also result from the constant inflammation accompanying cell breakdown.
♦ Pelvic softening may occur, leading to a waddling gait.
♦ The legs may bow if the femurs or tibias are affected.
♦ Occasionally, malignant osteosarcoma can occur in the deformed bone.

Neurologic system
♦ In skull involvement, characteristic cranial enlargement over the frontal and occipital areas can produce headaches, sensory abnormalities, and impaired motor function, depending on the sensory areas affected.

For example, blindness and hearing loss with tinnitus and vertigo may result from bony impingement on the cranial nerves.
♦ Kyphosis, a spinal curvature, may develop as a result of compression fractures of the vertebrae.
♦ Permanent paralysis can occur if the soft bone of the vertebrae fractures and puts pressure on the spinal cord.

Renal system
♦ Because of the constant osteoclastic and osteoblastic activity, phosphates and calcium are released and reabsorbed.
♦ Phosphates and calcium may then accumulate in the renal pelvis, resulting in renal calculi.
♦ Hypercalcemia and gout may also occur.

Respiratory system
♦ Chronic accelerated remodeling eventually enlarges and softens the affected bones.
♦ Thoracic deformities may impair respiration, eventually leading to respiratory failure.

Collaborative management
Caring for the patient with Paget's disease requires a multidisciplinary approach. An orthopedic specialist can provide medical and surgical treatment of pathologic fractures, correct secondary deformities, and replace joints. A neurosurgical specialist may be involved if the head or spinal cord is affected. He may collaborate with the orthopedic surgeon to relieve pressure on the nerves, reducing sensory deficits and pain. A cardiologist may be consulted if heart failure occurs. A physical therapist and an occupational therapist may assist with optimizing range of motion of joints and bone structure. Community support resources may be needed, such as a visiting nurse or home health agency.

♦ calcitonin (Calcimar), a hormone, and etidronate (Didronel) to retard bone resorption and reduce serum alkaline phosphate and urinary hydroxyproline secretion (Calcitonin requires long-term maintenance therapy, but improvement is noticeable after the first few weeks of treatment; etidronate produces improvement after 1 to 3 months.)
♦ plicamycin (Mithracin), a cytotoxic antibiotic, to decrease serum calcium, urinary hydroxyproline,

and serum alkaline phosphatase levels; produces remission of symptoms within 2 weeks and biochemical improvement in 1 to 2 months, but may destroy platelets or compromise renal function.

Other treatment varies according to symptoms and includes:
♦ surgery to reduce or prevent pathologic fractures, correct secondary deformities, and relieve neurologic impairment; drug therapy with calcitonin and etidronate or mithramycin must

precede surgery to decrease the risk of excessive bleeding from hypervascular bone
◆ joint replacement (difficult because bonding material [methyl methacrylate] doesn't set properly on pagetic bone)
◆ analgesics or nonsteroidal anti-inflammatory drugs to control pain.

Special considerations
Incorporate the following considerations into your care of the patient with Paget's disease:
◆ To evaluate the effectiveness of the analgesic, assess pain level daily. Watch for new areas of pain or restricted movements, which may indicate new fracture sites, and sensory or motor disturbances, such as difficulty in hearing, seeing, or walking.
◆ Monitor serum calcium and alkaline phosphatase levels.
◆ If the patient is confined to prolonged bed rest, prevent pressure ulcers by providing good skin care. Reposition the patient frequently, and use a flotation mattress. Provide high-topped sneakers to prevent footdrop.
◆ Monitor intake and output. Encourage adequate fluid intake to minimize renal calculi formation.
◆ Demonstrate how to inject calcitonin properly and rotate injection sites or how to perform nasal inhalation if that's the form prescribed. Warn the patient that adverse reactions may occur (nausea, vomiting, local inflammatory reaction at injection site, facial flushing, itching of hands, and fever). Give reassurance that these adverse reactions are usually mild and infrequent.
◆ If the patient is prescribed the nasal inhalation form of calcitonin, explain proper administration to him.
◆ To help the patient adjust to the changes in lifestyle imposed by this disease, teach him how to pace activities and, if necessary, how to use assistive devices. Encourage him to follow a recommended exercise program, avoiding both immobilization and excessive activity. Suggest a firm mattress or a bed board to minimize spinal deformities. Warn against imprudent use of an analgesic because diminished sensitivity to pain resulting from analgesic use may make patient unaware of new fractures. To prevent falls at home, advise removal of throw rugs and other obstacles.
◆ Emphasize the importance of regular checkups, including the eyes and ears.
◆ Tell the patient who is receiving etidronate to take this medication with fruit juice 2 hours before or after meals (milk or other high-calcium fluids impair absorption), to divide daily dosage

to minimize adverse reactions, and to watch for and report stomach cramps, diarrhea, fractures, and new or increased bone pain.
◆ Tell the patient receiving mithramycin to watch for signs of infection, easy bruising, bleeding, and temperature elevation and to report for regular follow-up laboratory tests.
◆Help the patient and family make use of community support resources, such as a visiting nurse or home health agency. For more information, refer them to the Paget Foundation.

|||| **LIFE-THREATENING DISORDER**

RHABDOMYOLYSIS
Rhabdomyolysis, the breakdown of muscle tissue, may cause myoglobinuria, in which varying amounts of muscle protein (myoglobin) appear in the urine. Rhabdomyolysis usually follows major muscle trauma, especially a muscle crush injury. Long-distance running, certain severe infections, and exposure to electric shock can cause extensive muscle damage and excessive release of myoglobin. Prognosis is good if contributing causes are stopped or disease is checked before damage has progressed to an irreversible stage. Unchecked, it can cause renal failure.

Causes
◆ Anesthetic agents (halothane) causing intraoperative rigidity
◆ Antilipemic therapy
◆ Cardiac arrhythmias
◆ Electrolyte disturbances
◆ Excessive muscular activity associated with status epilepticus, electroconvulsive therapy, or high-voltage electrical shock
◆ Familial tendency
◆ Heat stroke
◆ Infection
◆ Strenuous exertion

Pathophysiology
Muscle trauma that compresses tissue causes ischemia and necrosis. The ensuing local edema further increases compartment pressure and tamponade; pressure from severe swelling causes blood vessels to collapse, leading to tissue hypoxia, muscle infarction, neural damage in the area of the fracture, and release of myoglobin from the necrotic muscle fibers into the circulation. Myoglobin may occlude the structures of the kidney, causing such damage as acute tubular necrosis or kidney failure. Myoglobin can also cause kidney failure because it breaks down into potentially toxic compounds.

Signs and symptoms
◆ Tenderness, swelling, and muscle weakness due to muscle trauma and pressure
◆ Dark, reddish brown urine from myoglobin

Complications
◆ Renal failure, because myoglobin is trapped in renal capillaries or tubules
◆ Amputation, if muscle necrosis is substantial

Diagnosis
Diagnosis may include:
◆ a urine myoglobin level greater than 0.5 mg/dl (evident with only 200 g of muscle damage)
◆ an elevated creatine kinase level due to muscle damage
◆ elevated serum potassium, phosphate, creatinine, and creatine levels
◆ hypocalcemia in early stages, hypercalcemia in later stages
◆ computed tomography, magnetic resonance imaging, and bone scintigraphy to detect muscle necrosis
◆ intracompartmental venous pressure measurements using a wick catheter, needle, or slit catheter inserted into the muscle.
◆ electrocardiogram changes due to hyperkalemia (intracellular potassium release from necrotic muscle cells)

Treatment
◆ Treatment of the underlying disorder
◆ Preventing renal failure by initiating I.V. hydration as early as possible
◆ Bed rest
◆ An anti-inflammatory
◆ A corticosteroid (in extreme cases)
◆ An analgesic for pain
◆ Immediate fasciotomy and debridement (if compartment venous pressure is greater than 40 mm Hg)
◆ Hemodialysis for renal failure until myoglobin is cleared

Special considerations
◆ Administer I.V. fluids and a diuretic, as ordered, to reduce nephrotoxicity.
◆ To prevent rhabdomyolysis due to physical exertion, such as long-distance running, recommend prolonged, low-intensity training as opposed to short bursts of intense exercise.
◆ Ensure adequate hydration and monitor the patient for adverse reactions to prescribed antilipemic drugs.
◆ Monitor the patient's intake and output, vital signs, electrolyte levels, daily weight, and laboratory results.

SCOLIOSIS

Scoliosis is a lateral curvature of the thoracic, lumbar, or thoracolumbar spine. The curve may be convex to the right (more common in thoracic curves) or to the left (more common in lumbar curves). Rotation of the vertebral column around its axis may cause rib cage deformity. Scoliosis is commonly associated with kyphosis (humpback) and lordosis (swayback).

Between 2% and 3% of adolescents have scoliosis. In general, the greater the magnitude of the curve and the younger the child at the time of diagnosis, the greater the risk that the spinal abnormality will progress. Favorable outcomes are usually achieved with optimal treatment.

Types of structural scoliosis are:
◆ *congenital,* such as wedge vertebrae, fused ribs or vertebrae, or hemivertebrae
◆ *Paralytic* or *musculoskeletal,* developing several months after asymmetric paralysis of the trunk muscles due to polio, cerebral palsy, or muscular dystrophy
◆ *idiopathic* (most common), may be transmitted as an autosomal dominant or multifactorial trait (appears in a previously straight spine during the growing years).

Idiopathic scoliosis can be further classified according to age at onset:
◆ *infantile* (mostly affects male infants between birth and 3 years and causes left thoracic and right lumbar curves)
◆ *juvenile* (affects both sexes between ages 4 and 10 and causes varying types of curvature)
◆ *adolescent* (generally affects girls from age 10 until skeletal maturity and causes varying types of curvature).

Causes
◆ Functional: poor posture or a discrepancy in leg lengths, not fixed deformity of the spinal column (postural scoliosis)
◆ Structural: deformity of the vertebral bodies leading to curvature

Pathophysiology
Differential stress on vertebral bone causes an imbalance of osteoblastic activity; thus the curve progresses rapidly during adolescent growth spurt. Without treatment, the imbalance continues into adulthood.

Signs and symptoms
Scoliosis rarely produces subjective symptoms until it's well established. When symptoms occur, they include:
◆ backache
◆ fatigue
◆ dyspnea.

The most common curve in functional or structural scoliosis arises in the thoracic segment, with convexity to the right and compensatory curves (S curves) in the cervical and lumbar segments, both with convexity to the left. As the spine curves laterally, compensatory curves develop to maintain body balance. Subtle signs include:

♦ uneven hemlines or pant legs that appear unequal in length
♦ one hip that appears higher than the other.
Physical examination shows:
♦ unequal shoulder heights, elbow levels, and heights of iliac crests
♦ asymmetrical thoracic cage and misalignment of the spinal vertebrae when the patient bends over
♦ asymmetrical paraspinal muscles, rounded on the convex side of the curve and flattened on the concave side
♦ asymmetrical gait.

Complications

Without treatment, curves greater than 40 degrees progress. Untreated scoliosis may result in:
♦ pulmonary insufficiency (curvature may decrease lung capacity)
♦ back pain
♦ degenerative arthritis of the spine
♦ vertebral disk disease
♦ sciatica.

Diagnosis

♦ Anterior, posterior, and lateral spinal X-rays, taken with the patient standing upright and bending, confirm scoliosis and determine the degree of curvature (Cobb method) and flexibility of the spine.
♦ Scoliometer measures the angle of trunk rotation.

Treatment

The severity of the deformity and potential spine growth determine appropriate treatment, which may include:
♦ close observation
♦ exercise
♦ brace
♦ surgery
♦ a combination of these.

To be most effective, treatment should begin early, when spinal deformity is still subtle. Bracing is less successful in paralytic and congenital curves; therefore, these conditions may more commonly require surgical intervention. For a curve less than 20 degrees, or mild scoliosis, treatment includes:

♦ X-rays to monitor curve
♦ examination every 3 months
♦ exercise program to strengthen torso muscles and prevent curve progression.
For a curve of 25 to 40 degrees:
♦ spinal exercises and a brace (may halt progression but doesn't reverse the established curvature); braces can be adjusted as the patient grows and worn until bone growth is complete)
♦ transcutaneous electrical stimulation or chiropractic manipulation (alternative therapies).
A lateral curve continues to progress at the rate of 1 degree per year even after skeletal maturity. For a curve of 40 degrees or more, treatment includes:
♦ surgery (posterior spinal fusion and instrumentation [most common surgical procedure for scoliosis]) or anterior spinal fusion
♦ periodic postoperative checkups for several months to monitor stability of the correction.

Special considerations

Scoliosis commonly affects adolescent girls, who are likely to be distressed by limitations on their activities and treatment with orthopedic appliances. Therefore, it's important to provide emotional support in addition to meticulous skin and cast care and patient teaching.
If the patient needs a brace:
♦ Enlist the help of a physical therapist, a social worker, and an orthotist. Before the patient goes home, explain what the brace does and how to care for it (how to check the screws for tightness and pad the uprights to prevent excessive wear on clothing). Suggest that loose-fitting, oversized clothes be worn for greater comfort.
♦ Tell the patient to wear the brace 23 hours per day and to remove it only for bathing and exercise. While she's still adjusting to the brace, tell her to lie down and rest several times per day.
♦ Suggest a soft mattress if a firm one is uncomfortable.
♦ To prevent skin breakdown, advise the patient not to use lotions, ointments, or powders on areas where the brace comes in contact with the skin. Tell her to keep the skin dry and clean and to wear a snug T-shirt under the brace.
♦ Advise the patient to increase activities gradually and avoid vigorous sports. Emphasize the importance of conscientiously performing prescribed exercises. Recommend swimming during the 1 hour out of the brace but strongly warn against diving.
♦ Instruct the patient to turn her whole body, instead of just her head, when looking to the side. To make reading easier, tell her to hold the book so she can look straight ahead at it instead

of down. If she finds this difficult, help her to obtain prism glasses.

If the patient needs traction or a cast before surgery:

◆ Explain these procedures to the patient and family. Remember that application of a body cast can be traumatic because it's done on a special frame and the patient's head and face are covered throughout the procedure.

◆ Check the skin around the cast edge daily. Keep the cast clean and dry and the edges of the cast petaled. Warn the patient not to insert or let anything get under the cast and to immediately report cracks in the cast, pain, burning, skin breakdown, numbness, or odor.

◆ Before surgery, assure the patient and family that she'll have adequate pain control postoperatively.

After corrective surgery:

◆ Check sensation, movement, color, and blood supply in all extremities every 2 to 4 hours for the first 48 hours and then several times per day for signs of neurovascular deficit, a serious complication after spinal surgery. Logroll the patient often.

◆ Measure intake, output, and urine specific gravity to monitor effects of blood loss, which in many patients is substantial.

◆ Monitor abdominal distention and bowel sounds.

◆ Encourage the patient to perform deep-breathing exercises to avoid pulmonary complications.

◆ Medicate for pain, especially before activity.

◆ Promote active range-of-motion (ROM) arm exercises to help maintain muscle strength. Remember that any exercise, even brushing the hair or teeth, is helpful. Encourage the patient to perform quadriceps-setting, calf-pumping, and active ROM exercises of ankles and feet.

◆ Watch for skin breakdown and signs of cast syndrome, such as nausea, abdominal pressure, and vague abdominal pain.

◆ Remove antiembolism stockings for at least 30 minutes daily.

◆ Offer emotional support to help prevent depression, which may result from altered body image and immobility. Encourage the patient to wear her own clothes, wash her hair, and use makeup.

◆ Promote activity as tolerated, and refer the patient to physical therapy as indicated.

◆ If you work in a school, screen children routinely for scoliosis during physical examinations.

SPRAINS

A sprain is a complete or incomplete tear of the supporting ligaments surrounding a joint. It usually follows a sharp twist. An immobilized sprain may heal in 2 to 3 weeks without surgical repair, after which the patient can gradually resume normal activities. A sprained ankle is the most common joint injury, followed by sprains of the wrist, elbow, and knee.

Causes

◆ Concurrent dislocations or fractures

◆ Sharply twisting with force stronger than that of the ligament, inducing joint movement beyond normal range of motion

Pathophysiology

When a ligament is torn, an inflammatory exudate develops in the hematoma between the torn ends. Granulation tissue grows inward from the surrounding soft tissue and cartilage. Collagen formation begins 4 to 5 days after the injury, eventually organizing fibers parallel to the lines of stress. With the aid of vascular fibrous tissue, the new tissue eventually fuses with surrounding tissues. As further reorganization takes place, the new ligament separates from the surrounding tissue and eventually becomes strong enough to withstand normal muscle tension.

Signs and symptoms

◆ Localized pain (especially during joint movement) caused by trauma and exudate

◆ Swelling and heat due to inflammation

◆ Loss of mobility due to pain (may not occur until several hours after the injury)

◆ Skin discoloration from blood extravasating into surrounding tissues

Complications

◆ Recurring dislocation due to torn ligaments that don't heal properly, requiring surgical repair (occasionally)

◆ Loss of function in a ligament (if a strong muscle pull occurs before it heals and stretches it, it may heal in a lengthened shape with an excessive amount of scar tissue)

Diagnosis

◆ History of recent injury or repeated overuse reveals a sprain.

◆ X-rays rule out fractures.

◆ Stress radiography visualizes the injury in motion.

◆ Arthroscopy and arthrography reveal a strain.

Treatment

Treatment to control pain and swelling includes:

◆ immobilizing the injured joint to promote healing

◆ intermittently applying ice for 12 to 48 hours to control swelling (place a towel between the ice pack and the skin to prevent a cold injury)

◆ an elastic bandage or cast, or if the sprain is severe, a soft cast or splint to immobilize the joint

◆ elevating the joint above the level of the heart for 48 to 72 hours (immediately after the injury) (Remember the "RICE" acronym — Rest, Ice, Compression, Elevation.)

◆ codeine or another analgesic (if injury is severe)

◆ crutch and gait training (sprained ankle)

◆ immediate surgical repair to hasten healing, including suturing the ligament ends in close approximation (some athletes)

◆ for prevention, taping wrists or ankles before sports activities to prevent sprains (athletes).

Special considerations

◆ If an elastic bandage has been applied, teach the patient to reapply it by wrapping from below to above the injury, forming a figure eight. For a sprained ankle, apply the bandage from the toes to midcalf. Tell the patient to remove the bandage before going to sleep and to loosen it if it causes the leg to become pale, numb, or painful.

◆ Instruct the patient to call the physician if the pain worsens or persists; if so, an additional X-ray may reveal a previously undetected fracture.

STRAINS

A strain is an injury to a muscle or tendinous attachment usually seen after trauma or a sports injury. *Strain* is a general term for muscle or tendon damage that commonly results from sudden, forced motion causing it to be stretched beyond normal capacity. Injury ranges from excessive stretch (muscle pull) to muscle rupture. (See *Muscle-tendon ruptures.*) If the muscle ruptures, the body of the muscle protrudes through the fascia. A strained muscle can usually heal without complications; regeneration may take up to 6 weeks.

AGE ALERT *Tendon rupture is more common in elderly people; muscle rupture, in younger people.*

Causes

◆ Gunshot or knife wound causing a traumatic rupture (acute strain)

Muscle-tendon ruptures

Perhaps the most serious muscle-tendon injury is a rupture of the muscle-tendon junction. This type of rupture may occur at any such junction, but it's most common at the Achilles tendon, which extends from the posterior calf muscle to the foot. An Achilles tendon rupture produces a sudden, sharp pain and, until swelling begins, a palpable defect. This rupture typically occurs in men between ages 35 and 40, especially during physical activities, such as jogging or tennis. It can also occur as a complication of fluoroquinolone antibiotic therapy.

To distinguish an Achilles tendon rupture from other ankle injuries, perform this simple test: With the patient in a prone position and his feet hanging off the foot of the table, squeeze the calf muscle. The response establishes the diagnosis:

◆ Plantar flexion — The tendon is intact.

◆ Ankle dorsiflexion — The tendon is partially intact.

◆ No flexion — The tendon is ruptured.

An Achilles tendon rupture usually requires surgical repair, followed by a long leg cast for 4 weeks, and then a short cast for an additional 4 weeks.

◆ Repeated overuse (chronic strain)

◆ Vigorous muscle overuse or overstress, causing the muscle to become stretched beyond normal capacity, especially when the muscle isn't adequately stretched before the activity (acute strain)

Pathophysiology

Bleeding into the muscle and surrounding tissue occurs if the muscle is torn. When a tendon or muscle is torn, an inflammatory exudate develops between the torn ends. Granulation tissue grows inward from the surrounding soft tissue and cartilage. Collagen formation begins 4 to 5 days after the injury, eventually organizing fibers parallel to the lines of stress. With the aid of vascular fibrous tissue, the new tissue eventually fuses with surrounding tissues. As further reorganization takes place, the new tendon or muscle separates from the surrounding tissue and eventually becomes strong enough to withstand normal muscle strain. If a muscle is chronically strained, calcium may deposit into a muscle, limiting movement by causing stiffness, and muscle fatigue.

Signs and symptoms
Acute strain
◆ Sharp, transient pain (myalgia) caused by trauma and inflammatory exudate
◆ Snapping or popping noise from tearing of the muscle
◆ Rapid swelling that may continue for 72 hours because of the inflammatory process
◆ Limited function because of pain and inflammation
◆ Tender muscle (when severe pain subsides) caused by the injury
◆ Ecchymoses (after several days) caused by bleeding into the tissue and muscle

Chronic strain
◆ Stiffness
◆ Soreness
◆ Generalized tenderness

Complications
◆ Complete muscle rupture requiring surgical repair
◆ Myositis ossificans (chronic inflammation with bony deposits) due to scar tissue calcification (late complication)

Diagnosis
◆ History of a recent injury or repeated overuse
◆ X-ray to rule out fracture
◆ Stress radiography to visualize the injury in motion
◆ Biopsy showing muscle regeneration and connective tissue repair (rarely done)

Treatment
Acute strain
◆ Compression wrap to immobilize the affected area
◆ Elevating the injured part above the level of the heart to reduce swelling
◆ An analgesic
◆ Application of ice for up to 48 hours, then application of heat to enhance blood flow, reduce cramping, and promote healing
◆ Cryokinetics (alternating applications of heat and cold) and progressive exercises based on the specific injury
◆ Surgery to suture the tendon or muscle ends in close approximation

Chronic strain
Chronic strains usually don't need treatment. Discomfort may be relieved by:
◆ heat application

◆ a nonsteroidal anti-inflammatory drug (such as ibuprofen [Motrin])
◆ an analgesic muscle relaxant.

Special considerations
◆ Tell the patient that strains can be avoided by stretching for at least 10 minutes per day.
◆ Teach the patient to warm up properly before exercise, sports, or heavy lifting to help prevent muscle strains.
◆ Know that strong, flexible muscles are less likely to experience strains.
◆ Advise the patient to rest strained muscles when pain is present. When the pain subsides, tell him that activity may be initiated slowly and in moderation.
◆ Tell the patient that strains in the leg or foot area may require the use of crutches.
◆ Advise the patient that physical therapy may be needed to speed recovery time.

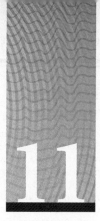

HEMATOLOGIC SYSTEM

Blood, although a fluid, is one of the body's major tissues. It continuously circulates through the heart and blood vessels, carrying vital elements to every part of the body.

Blood performs several vital functions through its special components: the liquid protein (plasma) and the formed constituents (erythrocytes, leukocytes, and thrombocytes) suspended in it. Erythrocytes (red blood cells [RBCs]) carry oxygen to the tissues and remove carbon dioxide. Leukocytes (white blood cells [WBCs]) act in inflammatory and immune responses. Plasma (a clear, straw-colored fluid) carries antibodies and nutrients to tissues and carries waste away. Plasma coagulation factors and thrombocytes (platelets) control clotting.

Hematopoiesis, the process of blood formation, occurs primarily in the marrow. There primitive blood cells (stem cells) differentiate into the precursors of erythrocytes (normoblasts), leukocytes, and thrombocytes.

The average person has 5 to 6 L of circulating blood, which constitutes 5% to 7% of body weight (as much as 10% in premature neonates). Blood is three to five times more viscous than water, has an arterial pH of 7.35 to 7.45, and is either bright red (arterial blood) or dark red (venous blood), depending on the degree of oxygen saturation and the hemoglobin level.

Pathophysiologic changes

Bone marrow cells reproduce rapidly and have a short life span, and the storage of circulating cells in the marrow is minimal. Thus, bone marrow

cells and their precursors are particularly vulnerable to physiologic changes that affect cell production. Disease can affect the structure or concentration of any hematologic cell.

HEMOGLOBIN

The protein hemoglobin is the major component of the RBC. Hemoglobin consists of an iron-containing molecule (heme) bound to the protein globulin. Oxygen binds to the heme component and is transported throughout the body and released to the cells. The hemoglobin picks up carbon dioxide and hydrogen ions from the cells and delivers them to the lungs, where they're released.

Various mutations or abnormalities in the hemoglobin protein can cause abnormal oxygen transport.

RED BLOOD CELLS

RBC disorders may be quantitative or qualitative. A deficiency of RBCs (anemia) can follow a condition that destroys or inhibits the formation of these cells. (See *Understanding erythropoiesis,* page 408.)

Common factors leading to anemia include:
◆ drugs, toxins, ionizing radiation
◆ congenital or acquired defects that cause bone marrow to stop producing new RBCs (aplasia) and generally suppress production of all blood cells (hematopoiesis, aplastic anemia)
◆ metabolic abnormalities (sideroblastic anemia)
◆ deficiency of vitamins (vitamin B_{12} deficiency, or pernicious anemia) or minerals (iron, folic acid, copper, and cobalt deficiency anemias) leading to inadequate erythropoiesis

Understanding erythropoiesis

The tissues' demand for oxygen and the blood cells' ability to deliver it regulate red blood cell (RBC) production. Lack of oxygen in the tissues (hypoxia) stimulates RBC production, which triggers the formation and release of the hormone erythropoietin. In turn, erythropoietin — 90% of which is produced by the kidneys and 10% of which is produced by the liver — activates bone marrow to produce RBCs. Androgens may also stimulate erythropoiesis, which accounts for a higher RBC count in men.

The formation of an erythrocyte (RBC) begins with an uncommitted stem cell that may eventually develop into an RBC or white blood cell. Such formation requires certain vitamins and minerals, including vitamin B_{12}, folic acid, copper, cobalt, and especially iron, which is vital to hemoglobin's oxygen-carrying capacity. Iron is obtained from various foods and is absorbed in the duodenum and jejunum. An excess of iron is temporarily stored in reticuloendothelial cells — especially those in the liver — as ferritin and hemosiderin until it's released for use in the bone marrow to form new RBCs.

♦ excessive chronic or acute blood loss (posthemorrhagic anemia)
♦ chronic illnesses, such as renal disease, cancer, and chronic infections
♦ intrinsically (sickle cell anemia) or extrinsically (hemolytic transfusion reaction) defective RBCs.

Decreased plasma volume can cause a relative excess of RBCs. The few conditions characterized by excessive production of RBCs include:
♦ abnormal proliferation of all bone marrow cells (polycythemia vera)
♦ abnormality of a single element (such as erythropoietin excess caused by hypoxemia or pulmonary disease).

LEUKOCYTOSIS

Leukocytosis is an elevation in the number of WBCs. All types — or only one type — of WBCs may be increased. (See *WBC types and functions.*) Leukocytosis is a normal physiologic response to infection or inflammation. Other factors, such as temperature changes, emotional disturbances, anesthesia, surgery, strenuous exercise, pregnancy, and some drugs, hormones, and toxins can also cause leukocytosis. Abnormal leukocytosis occurs in malignancies and bone marrow disorders.

LEUKOPENIA

Leukopenia is a deficiency of WBCs — all types or only one type. It can be caused by a number of conditions or diseases, such as human immunodeficiency virus (HIV) infection, prolonged stress, bone marrow disease or destruction, radiation or chemotherapy, lupus erythematosus, leukemia, thyroid disease, or Cushing's syndrome. Because WBCs fight infection, leukopenia increases the risk of infectious illness.

THROMBOCYTOSIS

Thrombocytosis is an excess of circulating platelets to more than 400,000/μl. Thrombocytosis may be primary or secondary.

Primary thrombocytosis

In primary thrombocytosis, the number of platelet precursor cells, called *megakaryocytes*, is increased and the platelet count is more than 1 million/μl. The condition may result from an intrinsic abnormality of platelet function and increased platelet mass. It may accompany polycythemia vera or chronic granulocytic leukemia. In the presence of thrombocytosis, both hemorrhage and thrombosis may occur. This paradox occurs because accelerated clotting results in a generalized activation of prothrombin and a consequent excess of thrombin clots in the microcirculation. This process consumes exorbitant amounts of coagulation factors and thereby increases the risk of hemorrhage.

Secondary thrombocytosis

Secondary thrombocytosis is a result of an underlying cause, such as stress, exercise, hemorrhage, or hemolytic anemia. Stress and exercise release stored platelets from the spleen. Hemorrhage or hemolytic anemia signal the bone marrow to produce more megakaryocytes.

Thrombocytosis may also occur after a splenectomy. Because the spleen is the primary site of platelet storage and destruction, platelet count may rise after its removal until the bone marrow begins producing fewer platelets.

Disorders

Specific causes of hematologic disorders include trauma, chronic disease, surgery, malnutrition, drug, exposure to toxins or radiation, and genetic or congenital defects that disrupt production or function of blood cells.

APLASTIC ANEMIA

Aplastic, or hypoplastic, anemia results from injury to or destruction of stem cells in bone marrow or the bone marrow matrix, causing pancytopenia (anemia, leukopenia, and thrombocytopenia) and bone marrow hypoplasia. Although commonly used interchangeably with other terms for bone marrow failure, *aplastic anemia* properly refers to pancytopenia resulting from the decreased functional capacity of a hypoplastic, fatty bone marrow.

⚠ **CLINICAL ALERT** *Aplastic anemias generally produce fatal bleeding or infection, especially when they're idiopathic or caused by chloramphenicol (Chloromycetin) use or infectious hepatitis. The death rate for severe aplastic anemia is 80% to 90%.*

Causes

◆ Autoimmune reactions (unconfirmed), preleukemic and neoplastic infiltration of bone marrow, or severe disease (especially hepatitis)
◆ Congenital (idiopathic anemias); two identified forms of aplastic anemia are congenital: *hypoplastic* or *Blackfan-Diamond, anemia* (develops between ages 2 and 3 months) and *Fanconi's syndrome* (develops between birth and age 10)
◆ Drugs (antibiotics, anticonvulsants) or toxic agents (such as benzene or chloramphenicol)
◆ Radiation (about half of such anemias)

Pathophysiology

Aplastic anemias usually develop when damaged or destroyed stem cells inhibit blood cell production. Less commonly, they develop when damaged bone marrow microvasculature creates an unfavorable environment for cell growth and maturation.

Signs and symptoms

Signs and symptoms of aplastic anemia vary with the severity of pancytopenia but develop insidiously in many cases. They may include:
◆ progressive weakness and fatigue, shortness of breath, bibasilar crackles, headache, pallor, and ultimately tachycardia and heart failure due to hypoxia and increased venous return
◆ ecchymosis, petechiae, and hemorrhage, especially from the mucous membranes (nose, gums, rectum, vagina) or into the retina or central nervous system due to thrombocytopenia
◆ infection (fever, oral and rectal ulcers, sore throat) without characteristic inflammation due to neutropenia (neutrophil deficiency).

WBC types and functions

White blood cells (WBCs), or leukocytes, protect the body against harmful bacteria and infection. WBCs are classified as granular leukocytes (basophils, neutrophils, and eosinophils) or nongranular leukocytes (lymphocytes, monocytes, and plasma cells). WBCs are usually produced in bone marrow; lymphocytes and plasma cells are produced in lymphoid tissue as well. Neutrophils have a circulating half-life of less than 6 hours, whereas some lymphocytes may survive for weeks or months. Normally, WBCs number between 5,000 and 10,000/μl. There are six types of WBCs:
◆ *Neutrophils* — The predominant form of granulocyte, neutrophils make up about 60% of WBCs and help devour invading organisms by phagocytosis.
◆ *Eosinophils* — Minor granulocytes that may defend against parasites and lung and skin infections and act in allergic reactions. They account for 1% to 5% of the total WBC count.
◆ *Basophils* — Minor granulocytes that may release heparin and histamine into the blood and participate in delayed hypersensitivity reactions. Basophils account for 0% to 1% of the total WBC count.
◆ *Monocytes* — Along with neutrophils, they help devour invading organisms by phagocytosis. Monocytes help process antigens for lymphocytes and form macrophages in the tissues. They account for 1% to 6% of the total WBC count.
◆ *Lymphocytes* — They occur as B cells and T cells. B cells form lymphoid follicles, produce humoral antibodies, and help T-cell mediated delayed hypersensitivity reactions and the rejection of foreign cells or cell products. Lymphocytes account for 20% to 40% of the total WBC count.
◆ *Plasma cells* — They develop from lymphoblasts, reside in the tissue, and produce antibodies.

Complications

A possible complication of aplastic anemia is life-threatening hemorrhage from the mucous membranes.

Diagnosis

The following test results help diagnose aplastic anemia:

◆ 1 million/µl or fewer red blood cells (RBCs) of normal color and size (normochromic and normocytic).

RBCs may be macrocytic (larger than normal) and anisocytotic (excessive variation in size), with:
◆ a low absolute reticulocyte count
◆ an elevated serum iron level (unless bleeding occurs), a normal or slightly reduced total iron-binding capacity, the presence of hemosiderin (a derivative of hemoglobin), and microscopically visible tissue iron storage
◆ decreased platelet, neutrophil, and lymphocyte counts
◆ abnormal coagulation test results (bleeding time) reflecting decreased platelet count
◆ "dry tap" (no cells) from bone marrow aspiration at several sites
◆ biopsy showing severely hypocellular or aplastic marrow, with varied amounts of fat, fibrous tissue, or gelatinous replacement; absence of tagged iron (because iron is deposited in the liver rather than bone marrow) and megakaryocytes (platelet precursors); and depression of RBCs and precursors (erythroid elements).

Differential diagnosis must rule out paroxysmal nocturnal hemoglobinuria and other diseases in which pancytopenia is common.

Treatment

Effective treatment must eliminate an identifiable cause and provide vigorous supportive measures, including:
◆ packed RBC or platelet transfusion; experimental histocompatibility locus antigen-matched leukocyte transfusions
◆ bone marrow transplantation (treatment of choice for anemia due to severe aplasia and for patients who need constant RBC transfusions)
◆ for patients with leukopenia, special measures to prevent infection (avoidance of exposure to communicable diseases, diligent hand washing)
◆ a specific antibiotic for infection (not given prophylactically because antibiotics encourage resistant strains of organisms)
◆ respiratory support with oxygen in addition to blood transfusions (for patients with a low hemoglobin level)
◆ a corticosteroid to stimulate erythropoiesis; a marrow-stimulating agent, such as an androgen (controversial); antilymphocyte globulin; an immunosuppressant (if the patient doesn't respond to other therapy); and a colony-stimulating factor to encourage growth of specific cellular components.

Special considerations

◆ If the platelet count is low (less than 20,000/µl), prevent bleeding by avoiding I.M. injections, suggesting the use of an electric razor and a soft toothbrush, humidifying oxygen to prevent drying of mucous membranes, avoiding enemas and rectal temperatures, and promoting regular bowel movements through the use of a stool softener and a proper diet to prevent constipation. Also, apply pressure to venipuncture sites until bleeding stops. Detect bleeding early by checking for blood in urine and stool and assessing skin for petechiae.
◆ Take safety precautions to prevent falls that could lead to prolonged bleeding or hemorrhage.
◆ Help prevent infection by washing your hands thoroughly before entering the patient's room, by making sure the patient is receiving a nutritious diet (high in vitamins and proteins) to improve his resistance, and by encouraging meticulous mouth and perianal care.
◆ Watch for life-threatening hemorrhage, infection, adverse reactions to drug therapy, or blood transfusion reaction. Make sure routine throat, urine, nose, rectal, and blood cultures are done regularly and correctly to check for infection. Teach the patient to recognize signs of infection, and tell him to report them immediately.
◆ If the patient has a low hemoglobin level, which causes fatigue, schedule frequent rest periods. Administer oxygen therapy as needed. If blood transfusions are necessary, assess for a transfusion reaction by checking the patient's temperature and watching for the development of other signs and symptoms, such as rash, hives, itching, back pain, restlessness, and shaking chills.
◆ Reassure and support the patient and family by explaining the disease and its treatment, particularly if the patient has recurring acute episodes. Explain the purpose of all prescribed drugs and their adverse effects, including which ones he should report promptly. Encourage the patient who doesn't require hospitalization to continue his normal lifestyle, with appropriate restrictions (such as regular rest periods), until remission occurs.
◆ To prevent aplastic anemia, monitor blood studies carefully in any patient receiving a drug that could cause anemia.
◆ Support efforts to educate the public about the hazards of toxic agents. Tell parents to keep toxic agents out of the reach of children. Encourage people who work with radiation to wear protective clothing and a radiation-detecting badge and to observe plant safety precautions. Those who work with benzene (solvent) should know that 10 parts per million is the highest safe environmental level and that a delayed reaction to benzene may develop.

FOLIC ACID DEFICIENCY ANEMIA

Folic acid deficiency anemia is a common, slowly progressive, megaloblastic anemia. It usually occurs in infants, adolescents, pregnant and breast-feeding females, alcoholics, elderly people, and people with malignant or intestinal diseases.

Causes

◆ Alcohol abuse (alcohol may suppress metabolic effects of folate)
◆ Bacteria competing for available folic acid
◆ Excessive cooking, which can destroy much of the folic acid in foods
◆ Impaired absorption (due to intestinal dysfunction from bowel resection and such disorders as celiac disease, tropical sprue, and regional jejunitis)
◆ Increased folic acid requirements during pregnancy, during rapid growth in infancy (common because of recent increase in survival of premature infants), during childhood and adolescence (because of general use of folate-poor cow's milk), and in patients with neoplastic diseases and some skin diseases (chronic exfoliative dermatitis)
◆ Limited capacity to store folic acid (in infants)
◆ Poor diet (common in alcoholics, elderly people living alone, and infants, especially those with infections or diarrhea)
◆ Prolonged drug therapy (with anticonvulsants or estrogens, including hormonal contraceptives)

Pathophysiology

Folic acid (pteroylglutamic acid, folacin) is found in most body tissues, where it acts as a coenzyme in metabolic processes involving one carbon transfer. It's essential for formation and maturation of red blood cells (RBCs) and for synthesis of deoxyribonucleic acid. Although its body stores are relatively small (about 70 mg), this vitamin is plentiful in most well-balanced diets.

Even so, because folic acid is water-soluble and heat-labile, it's easily destroyed by cooking. Also, about 20% of folic acid taken in through diet is excreted unabsorbed. Insufficient daily folic acid intake (less than 50 mcg/day) usually induces folic acid deficiency within 4 months, as the body stores in the liver are depleted. This deficiency inhibits cell growth, particularly of RBCs, leading to production of few, deformed RBCs. These enlarged red cells characteristic of the megaloblastic anemias have a shortened life span of weeks rather than months.

Signs and symptoms

Folic acid deficiency anemia gradually produces clinical features characteristic of other megaloblastic anemias, without the neurologic manifestations:
◆ progressive fatigue
◆ shortness of breath
◆ palpitations
◆ weakness
◆ glossitis
◆ nausea
◆ anorexia
◆ headache
◆ fainting
◆ irritability
◆ forgetfulness
◆ pallor
◆ slight jaundice.

Folic acid deficiency anemia doesn't cause neurologic impairment unless it's associated with vitamin B_{12} deficiency, as in pernicious anemia.

Complications

Folic acid deficiency anemia produces no complications.

Diagnosis

The Schilling test and a therapeutic trial of vitamin B_{12} injections help distinguish folic acid deficiency anemia from pernicious anemia. Significant findings include macrocytosis, decreased reticulocyte count, structurally abnormal platelets, and a serum folate level less than 4 mg/ml.

Treatment

◆ Primarily, a folic acid supplement (given orally or parenterally to patients who are severely ill, have malabsorption, or are unable to take oral medication) and elimination of contributing causes
◆ A well-balanced diet
If the patient has a combined vitamin B_{12} and folate deficiency, folic acid replenishment alone may aggravate neurologic dysfunction.

Special considerations

◆ Teach the patient to meet daily folic acid requirements by including a food from each food group in every meal. If the patient has a severe deficiency, explain that diet only reinforces folic acid supplementation and isn't therapeutic by itself. Urge compliance with the prescribed course of therapy. Advise the patient not to stop taking the supplements when he begins to feel better.
◆ Encourage the avoidance of alcohol, nonherbal teas, antacids, and phosphates, which impair the absorption of B vitamins and iron.
◆ If the patient has glossitis, emphasize the importance of good oral hygiene. Suggest regular

use of mild or diluted mouthwash and a soft toothbrush.

◆ Watch fluid and electrolyte balance, particularly in the patient who has severe diarrhea and is receiving parenteral fluid replacement therapy.

◆ Because anemia causes severe fatigue, schedule regular rest periods until the patient is able to resume normal activity.

◆ To prevent folic acid deficiency anemia, emphasize the importance of a well-balanced diet high in folic acid. Identify patients who are alcoholic and have poor dietary habits, and try to arrange for appropriate counseling. Tell female patients who aren't breast-feeding to use commercially prepared formulas. (See *Preventing folic acid deficiency anemia.*)

IRON DEFICIENCY ANEMIA

Iron deficiency anemia is a disorder of oxygen transport in which hemoglobin synthesis is deficient. A common disease worldwide, iron deficiency anemia affects 10% to 30% of the adult population of the United States. Iron deficiency anemia is most common in premenopausal women, infants (particularly premature or low-birth-weight infants), children, and adolescents (especially girls). The prognosis after replacement therapy is favorable.

Causes

◆ Blood loss due to drug-induced GI bleeding (from an anticoagulant, aspirin, or a steroid) or heavy menses, cancer, hemorrhage from trauma, a peptic ulcer, increased frequency of laboratory blood samples (in chronically ill patients), sequestration (in patients on dialysis), or varices

◆ Inadequate dietary intake of iron (less than 1 to 2 mg/day), as in prolonged nonsupplemented breast-feeding or bottle-feeding of infants or during periods of stress, such as rapid growth, in children and adolescents

◆ Intravascular hemolysis-induced hemoglobinuria or paroxysmal nocturnal hemoglobinuria

◆ Iron malabsorption, as in chronic diarrhea, partial or total gastrectomy, and malabsorption syndromes, such as celiac disease and pernicious anemia

◆ Mechanical trauma to red blood cells (RBCs) caused by a prosthetic heart valve or vena cava filters

◆ Pregnancy, which diverts maternal iron to the fetus for erythropoiesis

Pathophysiology

Iron deficiency anemia occurs when the supply of iron is inadequate for optimal formation of RBCs, resulting in smaller (microcytic) cells with less color (hypochromic) on staining. Body stores of iron, including plasma iron, become depleted, and the concentration of serum transferrin, which binds with and transports iron, decreases. Insufficient iron stores lead to a depleted RBC mass with a subnormal hemoglobin level and, in turn, subnormal oxygen-carrying capacity of the blood.

Signs and symptoms

Because iron deficiency anemia progresses gradually, many patients exhibit only symptoms of an underlying condition. They tend not to seek medical treatment until anemia is severe.

At advanced stages, signs and symptoms include:

◆ exertional dyspnea, fatigue, listlessness, pallor, inability to concentrate, irritability, headache, palpitations, and a susceptibility to infection due to decreased oxygen-carrying capacity of the blood caused by a decreased hemoglobin level

◆ increased cardiac output and tachycardia due to decreased oxygen perfusion

◆ coarsely ridged, spoon-shaped (koilonychia), brittle, and thin nails due to decreased capillary circulation

◆ sore, red, and burning tongue due to papillae atrophy

◆ sore, dry skin in the corners of the mouth due to epithelial changes.

Complications

◆ Infection and pneumonia

◆ Pica, compulsive eating of nonfood materials, such as soil, clay, ice, or starch

◆ Bleeding

◆ Overdose of an oral or I.M. iron supplement

Diagnosis

Blood studies (serum iron, total iron-binding capacity, and ferritin levels) and iron stores in bone marrow may confirm iron deficiency anemia. However, the results of these tests can be misleading because of complicating factors, such as infection, pneumonia, blood transfusion, or iron supplementation. Characteristic blood test results include:

◆ a low hemoglobin level (males, less than 12 g/dl; females, less than 10 g/dl)

◆ low hematocrit (males, less than 47%; females, less than 42%)

◆ a low serum iron level with high binding capacity

◆ a low serum ferritin level

◆ a low RBC count, with microcytic and hypochromic cells (in early stages, RBC count may be normal, except in infants and children)

◆ a decreased mean corpuscular hemoglobin level in severe anemia

◆ depleted or absent iron stores (by specific staining) and hyperplasia of normal precursor cells (by bone marrow studies).

Diagnosis must also include exclusion of other causes of anemia, such as thalassemia minor, cancer, and chronic inflammatory, hepatic, or renal disease.

Treatment

The first priority of treatment is to determine the underlying cause of anemia. Only then can iron replacement therapy begin. Possible treatments are:

◆ oral preparation of iron (treatment of choice) or a combination of iron and ascorbic acid (enhances iron absorption)

◆ parenteral iron (for patient noncompliant with oral dose, needing more iron than can be given orally, with malabsorption preventing adequate iron absorption, or for a maximum rate of hemoglobin regeneration).

Because total-dose I.V. infusion of supplemental iron is painless and requires fewer injections, it's usually preferred to I.M. administration. Considerations include:

◆ total-dose infusion of iron dextran in normal saline solution given over 1 to 8 hours (pregnant patients and geriatric patients with severe anemia)

◆ I.V. test dose of 0.5 ml given first (to minimize the risk of an allergic reaction).

Special considerations

◆ Monitor the patient's compliance with the prescribed iron supplement therapy. Advise the patient not to stop therapy even if he feels better because replacement of iron stores takes time.

◆ Tell the patient he may take iron supplements with a meal to decrease gastric irritation. Advise him to avoid milk, milk products, and antacids because they interfere with iron absorption; however, vitamin C can increase absorption.

◆ Warn the patient that iron supplements may result in dark green or black stools and can cause constipation.

◆ Instruct the patient to drink liquid supplemental iron through a straw to prevent staining his teeth.

◆ Tell the patient to report reactions, such as nausea, vomiting, diarrhea, constipation, fever, or severe stomach pain, which may require a dosage adjustment.

◆ If the patient receives I.V. iron, monitor the infusion rate carefully, and observe for an allergic reaction. Stop the infusion and begin supportive treatment immediately if the patient shows signs of an adverse reaction. Also, watch for dizziness and headache and for thrombophlebitis around the I.V. site.

 PREVENTION

Preventing folic acid deficiency anemia

Folic acid (pteroylglutamic acid, folacin) is found in most body tissues, where it acts as a coenzyme in metabolic processes involving one-carbon transfer. It's essential for formation and maturation of red blood cells and for synthesis of deoxyribonucleic acid. Although body stores are relatively small (about 70 mg), this vitamin is plentiful in most well-balanced diets.

However, because folic acid is water-soluble and heat-labile, it's easily destroyed by cooking. Also, approximately 20% of folic acid intake is excreted unabsorbed. Insufficient daily folic acid intake (less than 50 mcg/day) usually induces folic acid deficiency within 4 months. To prevent folic acid deficiency anemia, foods high in folic acid content should be chosen, such as those listed below:

Food	mcg/100 g
Asparagus spears	109
Beef liver	294
Broccoli spears	54
Collards (cooked)	102
Mushrooms	24
Oatmeal	33
Peanut butter	57
Red beans	180
Wheat germ	305

◆ Use the Z-track injection method when administering iron I.M. to prevent skin discoloration, scarring, and irritating iron deposits in the skin.

◆ Because an iron deficiency may recur, advise regular checkups and blood studies. (See *Preventing iron deficiency anemia*, page 414.)

PERNICIOUS ANEMIA

Pernicious anemia, the most common type of megaloblastic anemia, is caused by malabsorption of vitamin B_{12}.

AGE ALERT *Onset of pernicious anemia typically occurs between ages 50 and 60, and incidence increases with age.*

🚫 **PREVENTION**
Preventing iron deficiency anemia

Play a vital role in preventing iron deficiency anemia in your patients by encouraging the following actions:

Include iron-rich foods in diet
Teach the basics of a nutritionally balanced diet by having your patients include foods rich in iron, such as those listed below, in their diet.
◆ Meat (especially liver)
◆ Egg yolks
◆ Dried beans or peas
◆ Green leafy vegetables
◆ Dried fruits
◆ Cream of Wheat cereal
◆ Molasses

Include vitamin C–rich foods in diet
Encourage your patients to consume foods high in vitamin C (ascorbic acid) at the same time they're eating iron-rich foods. The vitamin C aids in the absorption of the iron.These foods are rich in vitamin C:
◆ Citrus fruit or juice
◆ Tomatoes
◆ Broccoli
◆ Melons
◆ Strawberries
◆ Red peppers

Include prophylactic oral iron
Emphasize the need for high-risk individuals, such as premature infants, children younger than age 2, and pregnant women, to receive prophylactic oral iron, as ordered by a physician. (Children younger than age 2 should also receive supplemental cereals and formulas high in iron.)

Assess dietary habits
Assess a family's dietary habits for iron intake and note the influence of childhood eating patterns, cultural food preferences, and family income on adequate nutrition.

Assess medication history
Carefully assess your patients' drug histories because certain drugs, such as pancreatic enzymes and vitamin E, may interfere with iron metabolism and absorption and because aspirin, steroids, and other drugs may cause GI bleeding. (Teach patients who must take medications that are gastric irritants to take these medications with meals or milk.)

If not treated, pernicious anemia is fatal. Its manifestations subside with treatment, but some neurologic deficits may be permanent.

Causes
◆ Genetic predisposition (suggested by familial incidence)
◆ Immunologically related diseases, such as Graves' disease, myxedema, and thyroiditis (significantly higher incidence in these patients)
◆ Older age (progressive loss of vitamin B_{12} absorption)
◆ Partial gastrectomy (iatrogenic induction)

🔳 **AGE ALERT** *Elderly patients commonly have a dietary deficiency of vitamin B_{12} in addition to or instead of poor absorption.*

Pathophysiology
Pernicious anemia is characterized by decreased production of hydrochloric acid in the stomach and a deficiency of intrinsic factor, which is normally secreted by the parietal cells of the gastric mucosa and is essential for vitamin B_{12} absorption in the ileum. The resulting vitamin B_{12} deficiency inhibits cell growth, particularly of red

blood cells (RBCs), leading to production of few, deformed RBCs with poor oxygen-carrying capacity. It also causes neurologic damage by impairing myelin formation.

Signs and symptoms
Characteristically, pernicious anemia has an insidious onset but eventually causes an unmistakable triad of symptoms:
◆ weakness due to tissue hypoxia
◆ sore tongue due to atrophy of the papillae
◆ numbness and tingling in the extremities as a result of interference with impulse transmission from demyelination.

Other common manifestations include:
◆ pale appearance of lips and gums due to hypoxemia
◆ faintly jaundiced sclera and pale to bright yellow skin due to hemolysis-induced hyperbilirubinemia
◆ high susceptibility to infection, especially of the genitourinary tract.

Pernicious anemia may also have GI, neurologic, and cardiovascular effects.

GI signs and symptoms include:
◆ nausea, vomiting, anorexia, weight loss, flatulence, diarrhea, and constipation from disturbed digestion due to gastric mucosal atrophy and decreased hydrochloric acid production
◆ gingival bleeding and tongue inflammation (may hinder eating and intensify anorexia).

Neurologic signs and symptoms are related to impaired myelin formation and subsequent interference with neuron transmission and may include:
◆ neuritis; weakness in the extremities
◆ peripheral numbness and paresthesia
◆ disturbed position sense
◆ lack of coordination; ataxia; impaired fine finger movement
◆ positive Babinski's and Romberg's signs
◆ light-headedness
◆ altered vision (diplopia, blurred vision), taste, and hearing (tinnitus); optic muscle atrophy
◆ loss of bowel and bladder control; and, in men, impotence, due to demyelination (initially affects peripheral nerves but gradually extends to the spinal cord) caused by vitamin B_{12} deficiency
◆ irritability, poor memory, headache, depression, and delirium (some symptoms are temporary, but irreversible central nervous system [CNS] changes may have occurred before treatment).

Cardiovascular signs and symptoms include:
◆ a low hemoglobin level due to widespread destruction of RBCs caused by increasingly fragile cell membranes
◆ palpitations, wide pulse pressure, dyspnea, orthopnea, tachycardia, premature beats and, eventually, heart failure due to compensatory increased cardiac output.

Complications
◆ Hypokalemia (first week of treatment)
◆ Permanent CNS symptoms (if the patient isn't treated within 6 months of appearance of symptoms)
◆ Gastric polyps
◆ Stomach cancer

Diagnosis
Laboratory screening must rule out other anemias with similar symptoms but different treatments, such as:
◆ folic acid deficiency anemia
◆ vitamin B_{12} deficiency resulting from malabsorption due to GI disorders, gastric surgery, radiation, or drug therapy.

A decrease in the hemoglobin level by 1 to 2 g/dl in elderly men and slightly decreased hematocrit in both men and women reflect decreased bone marrow and hematopoiesis and, in men, a decreased androgen level; these

aren't indicators of pernicious anemia. Diagnosis of pernicious anemia is established by:
◆ a positive family history
◆ a hemoglobin level of 4 to 5 g/μl
◆ a low RBC count
◆ mean corpuscular volume greater than 120/μl due to increased amounts of hemoglobin in larger-than-normal RBCs
◆ a serum vitamin B_{12} level of less than 0.1 mcg/ml
◆ bone marrow aspiration showing erythroid hyperplasia (crowded red bone marrow), with increased numbers of megaloblasts but few normally developing RBCs
◆ gastric analysis showing absence of free hydrochloric acid after histamine or pentagastrin injection
◆ Schilling test for excretion of radiolabeled vitamin B_{12} (definitive test for pernicious anemia)
◆ serologic findings including intrinsic factor antibodies and antiparietal cell antibodies.

Treatment
◆ Early parenteral vitamin B_{12} replacement (can reverse pernicious anemia, minimize complications, and possibly prevent permanent neurologic damage)
◆ Concomitant iron and folic acid replacement to prevent iron deficiency anemia (rapid cell regeneration increasing the patient's iron and folate requirements)
◆ After initial response, decreasing the vitamin B_{12} dose to a monthly self-administered maintenance dose (must be given for life)
◆ Bed rest for extreme fatigue until the hemoglobin level rises
◆ Blood transfusions for a dangerously low hemoglobin level
◆ Digoxin (Lanoxin), a diuretic, and a low-sodium diet (if patient is in heart failure)
◆ An antibiotic to combat infections

Special considerations
Supportive measures minimize the risk of complications and speed recovery. Patient and family teaching can promote compliance with lifelong vitamin B_{12} replacement.
◆ If the patient has severe anemia, plan activities, rest periods, and necessary diagnostic tests to conserve his energy. Monitor pulse rate often; tachycardia means his activities are too strenuous.
◆ To ensure accurate Schilling test results, make sure that all urine over a 24-hour period is collected and that the specimens are uncontaminated.
◆ Warn the patient to guard against infections, and tell him to report signs of infection promptly, especially respiratory and urinary tract infections,

because the patient's weakened condition may increase susceptibility.

◆ Provide a well-balanced diet, including foods high in vitamin B_{12} (meat, liver, fish, eggs, and milk). Offer between-meal snacks, and encourage the family to bring favorite foods from home.

◆ Because a sore mouth and tongue make eating painful, ask the dietitian to avoid giving the patient irritating foods. If these symptoms make talking difficult, supply a pad and pencil or some other aid to facilitate nonverbal communication; explain this problem to the family. Provide diluted mouthwash or, with severe conditions, swab the patient's mouth with tap water or warm saline solution.

◆ Warn the patient with a sensory deficit not to use a heating pad because it may cause burns.

◆ If the patient is incontinent, establish a regular bowel and bladder routine. After the patient is discharged, a home health care nurse should follow up on this schedule and make adjustments as needed.

◆ If neurologic damage causes behavioral problems, assess mental and neurologic status often; if necessary, give a tranquilizer, as ordered, and apply a jacket restraint at night.

◆ Stress that vitamin B_{12} replacement isn't a permanent cure and that these injections must be continued for life, even after symptoms subside.

◆ To prevent pernicious anemia, emphasize the importance of vitamin B_{12} supplements for patients who have had extensive gastric resections or who follow strict vegetarian diets.

SIDEROBLASTIC ANEMIAS

Sideroblastic anemias are a group of heterogenous disorders with a common defect: They fail to use iron in hemoglobin synthesis, despite the availability of adequate iron stores. These anemias may be hereditary or acquired. The acquired form can be primary or secondary. Hereditary sideroblastic anemia commonly responds to treatment with pyridoxine (vitamin B_6). The primary acquired (idiopathic) form, known as *refractory anemia with ringed sideroblasts,* resists treatment and is usually fatal within 10 years of the onset of complications or of a concomitant disease. This form is most common in elderly people. It's commonly associated with thrombocytopenia or leukopenia as part of a myelodysplastic syndrome. Correction of the secondary, acquired form depends on the cause.

Causes

Hereditary sideroblastic anemia appears to be transmitted by X-linked inheritance, occurring mostly in young males (most female carriers show no signs of this disorder).

The acquired form may be secondary to:

◆ exposure to and ingestion of toxins (such as alcohol and lead) or drugs (such as chloramphenicol [Chloromycetin] and isoniazid [Laniazid])

◆ other diseases, such as severe infections, lupus erythematosus, multiple myeloma, rheumatoid arthritis, and tuberculosis.

Pathophysiology

In sideroblastic anemia, normoblasts fail to use iron to synthesize hemoglobin. As a result, iron is deposited in the mitochondria of normoblasts, which are then termed *ringed sideroblasts.* Iron toxicity can cause organ damage; untreated, it can damage the nuclei of red blood cell (RBC) precursors. Reduced numbers of normal hemoglobin-containing red blood cells cause hypoxia. This is sensed by erythropoietin-secreting kidney cells, causing the bone marrow to become congested and increasing the production of sideroblasts (which worsens the anemia).

Signs and symptoms

◆ Anorexia, fatigue, weakness, dizziness, pale skin and mucous membranes and, occasionally, enlarged lymph nodes due to iron toxicity

◆ Dyspnea, exertional angina, slight jaundice, and hepatosplenomegaly due to heart and liver failure caused by excessive iron accumulation in these organs

◆ Increased GI absorption of iron, causing signs of hemosiderosis (hereditary sideroblastic anemia)

◆ Other symptoms depending on the underlying cause (secondary sideroblastic anemia)

Complications

◆ Heart, liver, and pancreatic disease

◆ Respiratory complications

◆ Acute myelogenous leukemia

Diagnosis

◆ Ringed sideroblasts on microscopic examination of bone marrow aspirate stained with Prussian blue or alizarin red dye

◆ Hypochromic or normochromic and slightly macrocytic RBCs on microscopic examination; RBC precursors may be megaloblastic, with anisocytosis and poikilocytosis (abnormal variation in shape)

◆ A low hemoglobin level with high serum iron, transferrin, urobilinogen, and bilirubin levels due to RBC lysis

◆ Normal platelet and leukocyte counts (occasional thrombocytopenia or leukopenia)

Treatment

Treatment of sideroblastic anemia depends on the underlying cause and includes:
♦ several weeks of treatment with high doses of pyridoxine for hereditary form
♦ removal of the causative drug or toxin or treatment of the underlying condition (symptoms usually subside in acquired secondary form)
♦ a folic acid supplement (may be beneficial when concomitant megaloblastic nuclear changes in RBC precursors are present)
♦ deferoxamine (Desferal) to treat chronic iron overload as needed
♦ blood transfusions (providing hemoglobin) or high doses of an androgen (effective palliative measures for some patients with primary acquired form)
♦ phlebotomy to prevent hemochromatosis (the accumulation of iron in body tissues) increases the rate of erythropoiesis and uses up excess iron stores, reducing serum and total-body iron levels.

Special considerations

♦ Administer medications as ordered. Teach the patient the importance of continuing prescribed therapy, even after he begins to feel better.
♦ Provide frequent rest periods if the patient becomes easily fatigued.
♦ If phlebotomy is scheduled, explain the procedure thoroughly to help reduce anxiety. If this procedure must be repeated frequently, provide a high-protein diet to help replace the protein lost during phlebotomy. Encourage the patient to follow a similar diet at home.
♦ Always inquire about the possibility of exposure to lead in the home (especially for children) or on the job.
♦ Identify patients who abuse alcohol; refer them for appropriate therapy.

ALLERGIC PURPURA

Allergic purpura, a nonthrombocytopenic purpura, is an acute or chronic vascular inflammation affecting the skin, joints, and GI and genitourinary (GU) tracts, in association with allergy symptoms. When allergic purpura primarily affects the GI tract, with accompanying joint pain, it's called *Henoch-Schönlein syndrome,* or *anaphylactoid purpura.* However, the term *allergic purpura* applies to purpura associated with many other conditions, such as erythema nodosum. An acute attack of allergic purpura can last for several weeks and is potentially fatal (usually from renal failure); however, most patients do recover.

Fully developed allergic purpura is persistent and debilitating, possibly leading to chronic glomerulonephritis (especially after a strepto-

coccal infection). Allergic purpura affects more males than females and is most prevalent in children ages 3 to 7. The prognosis is more favorable for children than adults.

Causes

♦ Allergic reactions to some drugs and vaccines, certain foods (such as chocolate, eggs, milk, and wheat), and insect bites
♦ Bacterial infection (particularly streptococcal infection)

Pathophysiology

Although the precipitating mechanism of allergic purpura isn't completely understood, it's probably an autoimmune reaction directed against vascular walls, triggered by a bacterial infection. Typically, upper respiratory tract infection occurs 1 to 3 weeks before the onset of symptoms. An inflammation of the veins and capillaries disrupts the vascular wall, resulting in loss of red blood cells and bleeding.

Signs and symptoms

Characteristic skin lesions of allergic purpura are purple, macular, ecchymotic, and of varying size and are caused by vascular leakage into the skin and mucous membranes. The lesions usually appear in symmetric patterns on the arms, legs, and buttocks and are accompanied by pruritus, paresthesia and, occasionally, angioneurotic edema.

AGE ALERT *In children, skin lesions are generally urticarial and expand and become hemorrhagic. Scattered petechiae may appear on the legs, buttocks, and perineum.*

Henoch-Schönlein syndrome commonly produces transient or severe colic, tenesmus (spasmodic contraction of the anal sphincter) and constipation, vomiting, and edema or hemorrhage of the mucous membranes of the bowel, resulting in GI bleeding, occult blood in the stool and, possibly, intussusception. Such GI abnormalities may precede overt, cutaneous signs of purpura. Musculoskeletal symptoms, such as rheumatoid pains and periarticular effusions, usually affect the legs and feet.

In 25% to 50% of patients, allergic purpura is associated with GU signs and symptoms: nephritis; renal hemorrhages that may cause microscopic hematuria and disturb renal function; bleeding from the mucosal surfaces of the ureters, bladder, or urethra; and, occasionally, glomerulonephritis. Also possible are moderate and irregular fever, headache, anorexia, and localized edema of the hands, feet, or scalp.

Complications

Complications, which may appear many years after the episode of allergic purpura, may include:
◆ renal disease (renal failure and acute glomerulonephritis), which may be fatal
◆ hypertension and resulting blood loss from renal damage.

Diagnosis

No laboratory test clearly identifies allergic purpura (although white blood cell count and erythrocyte sedimentation rate are elevated).
◆ Diagnosis therefore necessitates careful clinical observation, in many cases during the second or third attack.
◆ Except for a positive tourniquet test (a test to assess the ability of capillaries to withstand increased pressure), coagulation and platelet function tests are usually normal.
◆ Small-bowel X-rays may reveal areas of transient edema; in many cases, tests for blood in the urine and stool are positive.
◆ Increased blood urea nitrogen and creatinine levels may indicate renal involvement.
◆ Diagnosis must rule out other forms of non-thrombocytopenic purpura.

Treatment

Treatment is generally symptomatic; for example, severe allergic purpura may require a steroid to relieve edema and an analgesic to relieve joint and abdominal pain. Some patients with chronic renal disease may benefit from immunosuppression with azathioprine along with identification of the provocative allergen. An accurate allergy history is essential.

Special considerations

◆ Encourage maintenance of an elimination diet to help identify specific allergenic foods so these foods can be eliminated from the patient's diet.
◆ Monitor skin lesions and level of pain. Provide an analgesic as needed.
⚠ **CLINICAL ALERT** *Watch carefully for such complications as GI and GU tract bleeding, edema, nausea, vomiting, headache, hypertension (with nephritis), abdominal rigidity and tenderness, and absence of stool (with intussusception).*
◆ To prevent muscle atrophy in the bedridden patient, provide passive or active range-of-motion exercises.
◆ Provide emotional support and reassurance, especially if the patient is temporarily disfigured by florid skin lesions.
◆ After the acute stage, stress the need for the patient to immediately report any recurrence of symptoms (recurrence is most common about

6 weeks after initial onset) and to return for follow-up urinalysis as scheduled.

⫼ LIFE-THREATENING DISORDER

DISSEMINATED INTRAVASCULAR COAGULATION

Disseminated intravascular coagulation (DIC) occurs as a complication of diseases and conditions that accelerate clotting, causing small blood vessel occlusion, organ necrosis, depletion of circulating clotting factors and platelets, activation of the fibrinolytic system, and consequent severe hemorrhage. Clotting in the microcirculation usually affects the kidneys and extremities but may occur in the brain, lungs, pituitary and adrenal glands, and GI mucosa. DIC, also called *consumption coagulopathy* or *defibrination syndrome,* is generally an acute condition but may be chronic in cancer patients. Prognosis depends on early detection and treatment, the severity of the hemorrhage, and treatment of the underlying disease. (See *Understanding DIC and its treatment.*)

Causes

◆ Disorders that produce necrosis, including extensive burns and trauma, brain tissue destruction, hepatic necrosis, transplant rejection
◆ Infection, including gram-negative or gram-positive septicemia and fungal, protozoal, rickettsial, or viral infection
◆ Neoplastic disease, including acute leukemia, aplastic anemia, metastatic carcinoma, adenocarcinoma
◆ Obstetric complications, including abruptio placentae, amniotic fluid embolism, eclampsia, retained dead fetus, septic abortion
◆ Other conditions, including cardiac arrest, cirrhosis, fat embolism, giant hemangioma, heatstroke, incompatible blood transfusion, poisonous snakebite, purpura fulminans, severe venous thrombosis, shock, and surgery requiring cardiopulmonary bypass

Pathophysiology

It isn't clear how or why certain disorders lead to DIC. In many patients, the triggering mechanisms may be the entrance of foreign protein into the circulation and vascular endothelial injury.

Regardless of how DIC begins, the typical accelerated clotting results in generalized activation of prothrombin and a consequent excess of thrombin. The thrombin converts fibrinogen to fibrin, producing fibrin clots in the microcirculation. This process uses huge amounts of coagulation

DISEASE BLOCK

Understanding DIC and its treatment

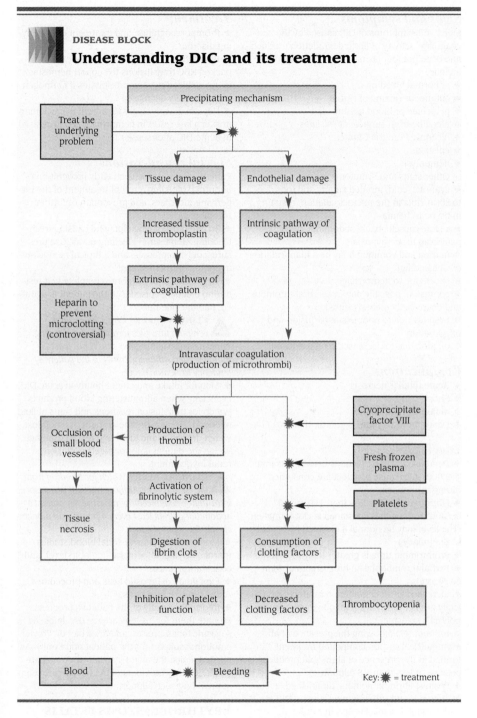

	Precipitating mechanism

Treat the underlying problem

Tissue damage → Increased tissue thromboplastin → Extrinsic pathway of coagulation

Endothelial damage → Intrinsic pathway of coagulation

Heparin to prevent microclotting (controversial)

Intravascular coagulation (production of microthrombi)

Occlusion of small blood vessels

Production of thrombi

Cryoprecipitate factor VIII

Fresh frozen plasma

Activation of fibrinolytic system

Platelets

Tissue necrosis

Digestion of fibrin clots

Consumption of clotting factors

Inhibition of platelet function

Decreased clotting factors

Thrombocytopenia

Blood → Bleeding

Key: ✳ = treatment

factors (especially fibrinogen, prothrombin, platelets, and factors V and VIII), causing hypofibrinogenemia, hypoprothrombinemia, thrombocytopenia, and deficiencies in factors V and VIII. Circulating thrombin also activates the fibrinolytic system, which dissolves fibrin clots into fibrin degradation products. Hemorrhage may be mostly the result of the anticoagulant activity of fibrin degradation products as well as depletion of plasma coagulation factors.

Signs and symptoms

Signs and symptoms of DIC caused by the anti-coagulant activity of fibrin degradation products and depletion of plasma coagulation factors include:

♦ abnormal bleeding
♦ cutaneous oozing of serum
♦ petechiae or blood blisters
♦ bleeding from surgical or I.V. sites
♦ bleeding from the GI tract
♦ epistaxis
♦ hemoptysis.

Other signs and symptoms include:
♦ cyanotic, cold, mottled fingers and toes due to fibrin clots in the microcirculation, resulting in tissue ischemia
♦ severe muscle, back, abdominal, and chest pain from tissue hypoxia
♦ nausea and vomiting (may be a manifestation of GI bleeding)
♦ shock due to hemorrhage
♦ confusion, possibly due to cerebral thrombus and decreased cerebral perfusion
♦ dyspnea due to poor tissue perfusion and oxygenation
♦ oliguria due to decreased renal perfusion.

Complications

♦ Acute tubular necrosis
♦ Shock
♦ Multiple organ failure
♦ Death (mortality rate is greater than 50%)

Diagnosis

♦ Decreased platelet count is usually less than 100,000/μl because platelets are consumed during thrombosis.
♦ Fibrinogen level is less than 150 mg/dl because fibrinogen is consumed in clot formation. (The level may be normal if elevated by hepatitis or pregnancy.)
♦ Prothrombin time is greater than 15 seconds.
♦ Partial thromboplastin time is greater than 60 seconds.
♦ Increased fibrin degradation products are typically greater than 45 μg/ml due to excess fibrinolysis by plasmin.
♦ D-dimer test (showing the presence of an asymmetrical carbon compound fragment formed in the presence of fibrin split products) is positive at less than 1:8 dilution.
♦ Positive fibrin monomers, diminished levels of factors V and VIII, fragmentation of RBCs, and hemoglobin level is less than 10 g/dl.
♦ Laboratory studies reveal reduced urine output (less than 30 ml/hour) and elevated blood urea nitrogen (greater than 25 mg/dl) and serum creatinine (greater than 1.3 mg/dl) levels.

Treatment

♦ Prompt recognition and treatment of underlying disorder
♦ Blood, fresh frozen plasma, platelet, or packed RBC transfusions to support hemostasis in active bleeding; cryoprecipitates if fibrinogen is significantly decreased
♦ Heparin in early stages to prevent microclotting and as a last resort in hemorrhage (controversial in acute DIC after sepsis)

Special considerations

Patient care must focus on early recognition of abnormal bleeding, prompt treatment of the underlying disorders, and prevention of further bleeding.

♦ To avoid dislodging clots and causing fresh bleeding, don't scrub bleeding areas. Use pressure, cold compresses, and a topical hemostatic agent to control bleeding.
♦ To prevent injury, enforce complete bed rest during bleeding episodes. If the patient is agitated, pad the side rails.

⚠ **CLINICAL ALERT** *Check all I.V. and venipuncture sites frequently for bleeding. Apply pressure to injection sites for at least 20 minutes. Alert other personnel to the patient's tendency to hemorrhage.*

♦ Monitor intake and output hourly in acute DIC, especially when administering blood products. Watch for transfusion reactions and signs of fluid overload. To measure the amount of blood lost, weigh dressings and linen and record drainage. Weigh the patient daily, particularly if there's renal involvement.

⚠ **CLINICAL ALERT** *Watch for bleeding from the GI and genitourinary tracts. If you suspect intra-abdominal bleeding, measure the patient's abdominal girth at least every 4 hours, and monitor closely for signs of shock.*

♦ Monitor the results of serial blood studies (particularly hematocrit, hemoglobin level, and coagulation times).
♦ Explain all diagnostic tests and procedures. Allow time for questions.
♦ Inform the family of the patient's progress. Prepare them for his appearance (I.V. lines, nasogastric tubes, bruises, and dried blood). Provide emotional support for the patient and family. As needed, enlist the aid of a social worker, chaplain, and other members of the health care team in providing such support.

ERYTHROBLASTOSIS FETALIS

Erythroblastosis fetalis, a hemolytic disease of the fetus and neonate, stems from an incompatibility of fetal and maternal blood—that is, mother and fetus have different ABO blood groups or the fetus is Rh-positive and the mother is Rh-negative. The mother's immune system generates antibodies against fetal red blood cells (RBCs).

The effects of hemolytic disease are more severe in Rh incompatibility than ABO incompatibility. ABO incompatibility may resolve after birth without life-threatening complications. ABO incompatibility occurs in about 25% of all pregnancies, but only 1 in 10 cases results in hemolytic disease. Rh incompatibility occurs in less than 10% of pregnancies and rarely causes hemolytic disease in the first pregnancy.

In severe, untreated erythroblastosis fetalis, the prognosis is poor, especially if brain and spinal cord become infiltrated with bilirubin (kernicterus). About 70% of these neonates die, usually within the first week of life; survivors inevitably have severe neurologic damage, including sensory impairment, mental deficiencies, and cerebral palsy. Most fetuses with hydrops fetalis (the most severe form of this disorder, associated with profound anemia and edema) are stillborn; the few who are delivered alive rarely survive longer than a few hours.

Causes
- ABO incompatibility
- Rh isoimmunization (See *What happens in Rh isoimmunization.*)

Pathophysiology
The pathophysiologies of ABO and Rh incompatibility are different.

ABO incompatibility
Each blood group has specific antigens on RBCs and specific antibodies in the serum. As in transfusion, the maternal immune system forms antibodies against fetal cells when blood groups differ. Most commonly, the mother has blood group O and the fetus has group A or B. Of course, a mother with group A or B won't form antibodies against a group O fetus, who has no fetal blood group antigens. Because the blood of most adults already contains anti-A or anti-B antibodies, ABO incompatibility can cause hemolytic disease even if fetal erythrocytes don't escape into the maternal circulation during pregnancy.

Rh incompatibility
During her first pregnancy, an Rh-negative female becomes sensitized (during delivery or abortion) by exposure to Rh-positive fetal blood antigens inherited from the father. A female may also become sensitized from blood transfusions with alien Rh antigens, from inadequate doses of

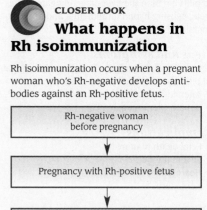

CLOSER LOOK
What happens in Rh isoimmunization

Rh isoimmunization occurs when a pregnant woman who's Rh-negative develops antibodies against an Rh-positive fetus.

Rh-negative woman before pregnancy

↓

Pregnancy with Rh-positive fetus

↓

Placental separation

↓

Maternal sensitization to Rh-positive blood

↓

Maternal development of anti-Rh antibodies

↓

Next pregnancy with Rh-positive fetus

↓

Maternal anti-Rh antibodies enter fetal circulation

↓

Anti-Rh antibodies attach to fetal Rh-positive red blood cells (RBCs)

↓

Hemolysis of fetal RBCs

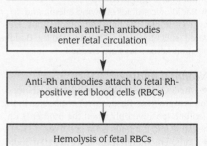

$Rh_o(D)$ (RhoGAM), or from failure to receive $Rh_o(D)$ after significant fetal-maternal leakage during abruptio placentae (premature detachment of the placenta).

A subsequent pregnancy with an Rh-positive fetus provokes maternal production of agglutinating antibodies, which cross the placental barrier, attach to Rh-positive cells in the fetus, and cause hemolysis and anemia. To compensate, the fetal blood forming organs step up the production of RBCs, and erythroblasts (immature RBCs) appear in the fetal circulation.

Extensive hemolysis releases more unconjugated bilirubin than the liver can conjugate and excrete, causing hyperbilirubinemia and hemolytic anemia.

Signs and symptoms

♦ Jaundice due to large amounts of unconjugated bilirubin released by hemolysis
♦ Anemia due to hemolysis
♦ Hepatosplenomegaly

Complications

♦ Fetal death in utero
♦ Severe anemia
♦ Heart failure
♦ Kernicterus

Diagnosis

Diagnosis considers both prenatal and neonatal findings.

Prenatal findings

♦ Maternal history (for erythroblastotic stillbirths, abortions, previously affected children, previous anti-Rh titers)
♦ Blood typing and screening (should be done frequently to determine changes in the degree of maternal immunization)
♦ Paternal blood typing for ABO and Rh
♦ History of blood transfusion
♦ Amniotic fluid analysis showing increased bilirubin and anti-Rh titers
♦ Radiologic studies showing edema and, in hydrops fetalis, the halo sign (edematous, elevated, subcutaneous fat layers) and the Buddha position (fetus's legs are crossed)

Neonatal findings

♦ Direct Coombs' test of umbilical cord blood to measure RBC (Rh-positive) antibodies in the neonate (positive only when the mother is Rh negative and the fetus is Rh positive)
♦ Cord hemoglobin level less than 10 g, indicating severe disease
♦ Many nucleated peripheral RBCs

Treatment

Treatment depends on the degree of maternal sensitization and the effects of hemolytic disease on the fetus or neonate. It may include:
♦ intrauterine-intraperitoneal transfusion (if amniotic fluid analysis suggests the fetus is severely affected and isn't mature enough to deliver)
♦ planned delivery (usually 2 to 4 weeks before term date, depending on maternal history, serologic test results, and amniocentesis)
♦ exchange transfusion to remove antibody-coated RBCs and prevent hyperbilirubinemia by replacing the infant's blood with fresh type O, Rh-negative blood
♦ albumin infusion to bind bilirubin
♦ phototherapy (exposure to ultraviolet light to reduce the bilirubin level)
♦ gamma globulin containing anti-Rh antibody ($Rh_o[D]$) to prevent Rh isoimmunization in Rh-negative females (ineffective if a previous pregnancy, abortion, or transfusion has already sensitized the mother).

Neonatal therapy for hydrops fetalis includes:
♦ intubation to maintain ventilation
♦ removal of excess fluid to relieve ascites and respiratory distress
♦ exchange transfusion
♦ maintainance of body temperature.

Special considerations

Structure the patient's care plan around close maternal and fetal observation, explanations of diagnostic tests and therapeutic measures, and emotional support.
♦ Reassure the parents that they aren't at fault in having a child with erythroblastosis fetalis. Encourage them to express their fears concerning possible complications of treatment.
♦ Before intrauterine transfusion, explain the procedure and its purpose. Before the transfusion, obtain a baseline fetal heart rate through electronic monitoring. Afterward, carefully observe the mother for uterine contractions and fluid leakage from the puncture site. Monitor fetal heart rate for tachycardia or bradycardia.
♦ During exchange transfusion, maintain the infant's body temperature by placing him under an overhead radiant warmer. Keep resuscitative and monitoring equipment handy, and warm the blood before transfusion.
♦ Watch for complications of transfusion, such as lethargy, muscular twitching, seizures, dark urine, edema, and change in vital signs. Watch for a postexchange serum bilirubin level that's usually 50% of the preexchange level (although the level may rise to 70% to 80% of the preexchange level due to rebound effect). Within 30 minutes of transfusion, bilirubin may rebound, requiring repeat exchange transfusions.
♦ Measure intake and output. Observe the patient for cord bleeding and complications, such as hemorrhage, hypocalcemia, sepsis, and shock. Report serum bilirubin and hemoglobin levels.
♦ To promote normal parental bonding, encourage parents to visit and help care for their infant as often as possible.
♦ To prevent hemolytic disease in the neonate, evaluate all pregnant women for possible Rh incompatibility. Administer $Rh_o(D)$ I.M., as ordered, to all Rh-negative, antibody-negative

women after a transfusion reaction or an ectopic pregnancy or during the second and third trimesters to patients with abruptio placentae, placenta previa, or amniocentesis.

HYPERSPLENISM

Hypersplenism is a syndrome marked by exaggerated splenic activity and, possibly, splenomegaly. This disorder results in peripheral blood cell deficiency as the spleen traps and destroys peripheral blood cells.

Causes

Hypersplenism may be idiopathic (primary) or secondary to an extrasplenic disorder:
♦ *congestive disorders* — cirrhosis, thrombosis
♦ *cystic or neoplastic disorders* — cysts, leukemia, lymphoma, myelofibrosis
♦ *hyperplastic disorders* — hemolytic anemia, polycythemia vera
♦ *infectious disorders* — acute (abscesses, subacute infective endocarditis), chronic (tuberculosis, malaria, Felty's syndrome)
♦ *infiltrative disorders* — Gaucher's disease, Niemann-Pick disease.

Pathophysiology

In hypersplenism, the spleen's normal filtering and phagocytic functions accelerate indiscriminately, automatically removing antibody-coated, aging, and abnormal cells, even though some cells may be functionally normal. The spleen may also temporarily sequester normal platelets and red blood cells (RBCs), withholding them from circulation. In this manner, the enlarged spleen may trap as much as 90% of the body's platelets and up to 45% of its RBC mass.

Signs and symptoms

♦ Anemia, leukopenia, or thrombocytopenia with splenomegaly
♦ Frequent contraction of bacterial infections (from leukopenia)
♦ Bruising easily
♦ Spontaneous hemorrhage from the mucous membranes and GI or genitourinary tract (from thrombocytopenia)
♦ Ulcerations of the mouth, legs, and feet (probably because of leukopenia)
♦ Fever, weakness, and palpitations
  Patients with secondary hypersplenism may have other clinical abnormalities, depending on the underlying disease.

Complications

♦ Anemia
♦ Leukopenia
♦ Thrombocytopenia

Diagnosis

Diagnosis requires evidence of abnormal splenic destruction or sequestration of RBCs or platelets and splenomegaly.
♦ The most definitive test measures erythrocytes in the spleen and liver after I.V. infusion of chromium-labeled RBCs or platelets. A high spleen-liver ratio of radioactivity indicates splenic destruction or sequestration.
♦ Complete blood count shows a decreased hemoglobin level (as low as 4 g/dl), white blood cell count (less than 4,000/µl), and platelet count (less than 125,000/µl) and an elevated reticulocyte count (more than 75,000/µl).
♦ Splenic biopsy, scan, and angiography may be useful, although biopsy is hazardous and should be avoided, if possible.
♦ In sequestration, the spleen is palpable. Use abdominal palpation cautiously because it may cause injury, bleeding, or rupture.

Treatment

Splenectomy is indicated only in transfusion-dependent patients who are refractory to medical therapy. Splenectomy seldom cures the patient but does correct the effects of cytopenia. Postoperative complications may include infection and thromboembolic disease. Occasionally, splenectomy may result in accelerated blood cell destruction in the bone marrow and liver. Secondary hypersplenism necessitates treatment of the underlying disease.

Special considerations

♦ If splenectomy is scheduled, administer preoperative transfusions of blood or blood products (fresh frozen plasma and platelets) to replace deficient blood elements. Also treat symptoms or complications of any underlying disorder.
♦ Postoperatively, monitor vital signs. Check for excessive drainage or apparent bleeding. Watch for infection, thromboembolism, and abdominal distention. Keep the nasogastric tube patent; listen for bowel sounds. Instruct the patient to perform deep-breathing exercises, and encourage early ambulation to prevent respiratory complications and venous stasis.

  AGE ALERT *Older adults may be at higher risk for infection because of decreased leukocyte and lymphocyte production. Fewer and weaker lymphocytes and immune system changes diminish the antigen-antibody response in older adults.*

IDIOPATHIC THROMBOCYTOPENIC PURPURA

Idiopathic thrombocytopenic purpura (ITP) is a deficiency of platelets that occurs when the immune system destroys the body's own platelets. ITP may be acute, as in postviral thrombocytopenia, or chronic, as in essential thrombocytopenia or autoimmune thrombocytopenia.

AGE ALERT *Acute ITP usually affects children between ages 2 and 6; chronic ITP mainly affects adults younger than age 50, especially women between ages 20 and 40.*

The prognosis for acute ITP is excellent; nearly four of five patients recover without treatment. The prognosis for chronic ITP is good; remissions lasting weeks or years are common, especially among women.

Causes
♦ Drug reactions
♦ Immunization with a live vaccine
♦ Immunologic disorders
♦ Viral infection

Pathophysiology
ITP occurs when circulating immunoglobulin G (IgG) molecules react with host platelets, which are then destroyed in the spleen and, to a lesser degree, in the liver. Normally, the life span of platelets in circulation is 7 to 10 days. In ITP, platelets survive 1 to 3 days or less.

Signs and symptoms
Signs and symptoms of ITP are caused by a decreased platelet count and may include:
♦ nose bleeds
♦ oral bleeding
♦ hemorrhages into the skin, mucous membranes, and other tissues causing red discoloration of skin (purpura)
♦ small purplish hemorrhagic spots on skin (petechiae)
♦ excessive menstrual bleeding.

Complications
♦ Hemorrhage
♦ Cerebral hemorrhage
♦ Purpuric lesions of vital organs (such as the brain and kidney)

Diagnosis
♦ Blood studies reveal a platelet count of less than 20,000/µl, prolonged bleeding time, abnormal size and appearance of platelets, and a decreased hemoglobin level (if bleeding occurred).
♦ Bone marrow studies show abundant megakaryocytes (platelet precursor cells) and a circulating platelet survival time of only several hours to a few days.
♦ Humoral tests measure platelet-associated IgG and may help establish the diagnosis; half the patients have an elevated IgG level.

Treatment
For acute ITP
Acute ITP may be allowed to run its course without intervention, or it may be treated with:
♦ a glucocorticoid to prevent further platelet destruction
♦ immunoglobulin to prevent platelet destruction
♦ plasmapheresis
♦ platelet pheresis.

For chronic ITP
♦ A corticosteroid to suppress phagocytic activity and enhance platelet production
♦ Splenectomy (when splenomegaly accompanies the initial thrombocytopenia)
♦ Blood and blood component transfusions and vitamin K to correct anemia and coagulation defects

Alternative treatments
♦ An immunosuppressant to help stop platelet destruction
♦ High-dose I.V. immunoglobulin
♦ Immunoabsorption apheresis using staphylococcal protein A columns

Special considerations
Patient care for ITP is essentially the same as for other types of thrombocytopenia, with emphasis on teaching the patient to watch for petechiae, ecchymoses, and other signs of recurrence. Monitor patients receiving an immunosuppressant for signs of bone marrow depression, infection, mucositis, GI ulcers, and severe diarrhea or vomiting. Tell the patient to avoid aspirin and ibuprofen.

POLYCYTHEMIA VERA
Polycythemia vera is a chronic disorder characterized by increased red blood cell (RBC) mass, erythrocytosis, leukocytosis, thrombocytosis, and an increased hemoglobin level, with normal or increased plasma volume. This disease is also known as *primary polycythemia, erythremia, polycythemia rubra vera, splenomegalic polycythemia,* or *Vaquez-Osler disease.* It usually occurs between ages 40 and 60, most commonly among Jewish men of European ancestry. It seldom affects children and doesn't appear to be familial.

The prognosis depends on age at diagnosis, the type of treatment used, and complications. Mortality is high if polycythemia is untreated, associated with leukemia, or associated with myeloid metaplasia (presence of marrow-like tissue and ectopic hematopoiesis in extramedullary sites, such as the liver and spleen, and nucleated erythrocytes in blood).

Causes

The cause of polycythemia vera is unknown, but is probably related to multipotential stem cell defect.

Pathophysiology

In polycythemia vera, uncontrolled and rapid cellular reproduction and maturation cause proliferation or hyperplasia of all bone marrow cells (panmyelosis).

Increased RBC mass makes the blood abnormally viscous and inhibits blood flow to microcirculation. Diminished blood flow and thrombocytosis set the stage for intravascular thrombosis.

Signs and symptoms

◆ Feeling of fullness in the head or headache due to altered blood volume, as in hypovolemia and hyperviscosity
◆ Dizziness due to hypervolemia and hyperviscosity
◆ Ruddy cyanosis (plethora) of the nose and clubbing of the digits due to thrombosis in smaller vessels
◆ Painful pruritus due to abnormally high concentrations of mast cells in the skin and their releases of heparin and histamine

Complications

◆ Clubbing
◆ Hemorrhage
◆ Splenomegaly
◆ Vascular thromboses
◆ Uric acid stones

Diagnosis

The following test results help diagnose the disorder:
◆ increased RBC mass
◆ normal arterial oxygen saturation in association with splenomegaly
◆ an increased uric acid level
◆ an increased blood histamine level
◆ a decreased serum iron level
◆ decreased or absent urinary erythropoietin
◆ bone marrow biopsy showing excess production of myeloid stem cells.

Treatment

◆ Phlebotomy to reduce RBC mass
◆ Myelosuppressive therapy with radioactive phosphorus (^{32}P) to suppress erythropoiesis (may increase the risk of leukemia), hydroxyurea, or other chemotherapeutic agents

Special considerations

If the patient requires phlebotomy, explain the procedure, and reassure the patient that it will relieve distressing symptoms. Check blood pressure, pulse rate, and respiratory rate. During phlebotomy, make sure the patient is lying down comfortably to prevent vertigo and syncope. Stay alert for tachycardia, clamminess, or complaints of vertigo. If any of these occur, the procedure should be stopped.

◆ Immediately after phlebotomy, check blood pressure and pulse rate. Have the patient sit up for about 5 minutes before allowing him to walk; this prevents vasovagal attack or orthostatic hypotension. Also, have the patient drink 24 oz (710 ml) of juice or water.

◆ Tell the patient to watch for and report any signs or symptoms of iron deficiency (pallor, weight loss, asthenia [weakness], and glossitis).

◆ Keep the patient active and ambulatory to prevent thrombosis. If bed rest is absolutely necessary, prescribe a daily program of both active and passive range-of-motion exercises.

⚠ **CLINICAL ALERT** *Watch for such complications as hypervolemia, thrombocytosis, and signs or symptoms of an impending stroke (decreased sensation, numbness, transitory paralysis, fleeting blindness, headache, and epistaxis).*

◆ Regularly examine the patient closely for bleeding. Tell him which are the most common bleeding sites (such as the nose, gingiva, and skin) so he can check for bleeding. Advise him to promptly report any abnormal bleeding.

◆ To compensate for increased uric acid production, give additional fluids, administer allopurinol, and alkalinize the urine to prevent uric acid calculi.

◆ If the patient has symptomatic splenomegaly, suggest or provide small, frequent meals, followed by a rest period, to prevent nausea and vomiting.

◆ Report acute abdominal pain immediately; it may signal splenic infarction, renal calculi, or abdominal organ thrombosis.

During myelosuppressive treatment

◆ Monitor complete blood count (CBC) and platelet count before and during therapy. Warn any outpatient who develops leukopenia that his resistance to infection is low; advise him to avoid crowds and watch for the symptoms of infection. If leukopenia develops in a hospitalized patient who needs reverse isolation, follow hospital guidelines. If thrombocytopenia develops, tell the patient to watch for signs of bleeding (blood in urine, nosebleeds, and black stools).

◆ Tell the patient about possible reactions (nausea, vomiting, and risk of infection) to alkylating agents. Alopecia may follow the use of busulfan, cyclophosphamide, and uracil mustard; sterile hemorrhagic cystitis may follow the use of cyclophosphamide (forcing fluids can prevent it). Watch for and report all reactions. If nausea and vomiting occur, begin antiemetic therapy and adjust the patient's diet.

During treatment with ^{32}P
◆ Explain the procedure to relieve anxiety. Tell the patient he may require repeated phlebotomies until ^{32}P takes effect. Take a blood sample for CBC and platelet count before beginning treatment. (*Note:* Use of ^{32}P requires radiation precautions to prevent contamination.)
◆ Have the patient lie down during I.V. administration (to facilitate the procedure and prevent extravasation) and for 15 to 20 minutes afterward.

SECONDARY POLYCYTHEMIA
Secondary polycythemia, also called *reactive polycythemia,* is excessive production of circulating red blood cells (RBCs) due to hypoxia, tumor, or disease. It occurs in about 2 of every 100,000 people living at or near sea level; the incidence increases among those living at high altitudes.

Causes
◆ Conditions that cause prolonged tissue hypoxia, such as compression of major blood vessels or shock
◆ Increased production of erythropoietin

Pathophysiology
Secondary polycythemia may result from increased production of the hormone erythropoietin — which stimulates bone marrow to produce RBCs — in a compensatory response to several conditions. These include hypoxemia caused by such conditions as chronic obstructive pulmonary disease, hemoglobin abnormalities (such as carboxyhemoglobinemia in heavy smokers), heart failure (causing a decreased ventilation-perfusion ratio), right-to-left shunting of blood in the heart (as in transposition of the great vessels), central or peripheral alveolar hypoventilation (as in barbiturate intoxication), and low oxygen content at high altitudes.

Increased production of erythropoietin may also be an inappropriate (pathologic) response to a renal, a central nervous system, or an endocrine disorder or to a neoplasm (such as a renal tumor, a uterine myoma, or a cerebellar hemangioma).

Signs and symptoms
◆ Ruddy cyanotic skin, emphysema, and hypoxemia without hepatomegaly or hypertension (in the hypoxic patient)
◆ Clubbing of the fingers (when the underlying cause is cardiovascular)

Complications
◆ Hemorrhage
◆ Thromboemboli secondary to hemoconcentration

Diagnosis
Diagnosis is based on the following test results:
◆ a high hemoglobin level and hematocrit
◆ high mean corpuscular volume and mean corpuscular hemoglobin
◆ a high urinary erythropoietin level
◆ a high blood histamine level
◆ normal or low arterial oxygen saturation
◆ bone marrow biopsy showing hyperplasia or erythroid precursors.

Treatment
The goal of treatment is to correct the underlying disease or environmental condition, and may include:
◆ phlebotomy or pheresis to reduce blood volume (to correct hazardous hyperviscosity or if the patient doesn't respond to treatment of the primary disease)
◆ continuous low-flow oxygen therapy to correct severe hypoxia.

Special considerations
◆ Keep the patient as active as possible to decrease the risk of thrombosis due to increased blood viscosity.
◆ Reduce calorie and sodium intake to counteract the risk of hypertension.
◆ Before and after phlebotomy, check blood pressure with the patient lying down. After the procedure, have the patient drink about 24 oz (710 ml) of water or juice. To prevent syncope, have him sit up for about 5 minutes before walking.
◆ Emphasize the importance of regular blood studies (every 2 to 3 months), even after the disease is controlled.
◆ Teach the patient and family about the underlying disorder. Help them understand its relationship to polycythemia and the measures needed to control both.
◆ Teach the patient to recognize symptoms of recurring polycythemia and the importance of reporting them promptly.

SPURIOUS POLYCYTHEMIA

Spurious polycythemia is characterized by increased hematocrit and a normal or low red blood cell (RBC) total mass. It results from diminished plasma volume and subsequent hemoconcentration. It's also known as *relative polycythemia, stress erythrocytosis, stress polycythemia, benign polycythemia, Gaisböck's disease,* or *pseudopolycythemia.* It usually affects middle-aged people and is more common in men than in women.

Causes
◆ Dehydration
◆ Elevated serum cholesterol and uric acid levels
◆ Familial tendency
◆ Hemoconcentration due to stress
◆ High-normal RBC mass and low-normal plasma volume
◆ Hypertension
◆ Thromboembolic disease

Pathophysiology
Conditions that promote severe fluid loss decrease plasma volume and lead to hemoconcentration. Such conditions include persistent vomiting or diarrhea, burns, adrenocortical insufficiency, aggressive diuretic therapy, decreased fluid intake, diabetic acidosis, and renal disease.

Nervous stress causes hemoconcentration by some unknown mechanism. This form of erythrocytosis (chronically elevated hematocrit) is particularly common in the middle-aged man who is a chronic smoker and has a type A personality (tense, hard driving, and anxious).

In many patients, an increased hematocrit merely reflects a normally high RBC mass and low plasma volume. This is particularly common in patients who don't smoke, aren't obese, and have no history of hypertension.

Signs and symptoms
◆ Headaches or dizziness due to altered circulation secondary to hypervolemia and hyperviscosity
◆ Ruddy appearance caused by cyanosis
◆ Slight hypertension from increased blood volume
◆ Tendency to hyperventilate when recumbent
◆ Cardiac or pulmonary disease

Complications
◆ Hypercholesterolemia
◆ Hyperlipidemia
◆ Hyperuricemia

Diagnosis
The following test results help to diagnose the disorder:
◆ a high hemoglobin level and hematocrit
◆ a high RBC count
◆ normal RBC mass
◆ normal arterial oxygen saturation
◆ normal bone marrow
◆ low or normal plasma volume
◆ possible hyperlipidemia
◆ possible uricosuria.

Treatment
◆ Appropriate fluids and electrolytes to correct dehydration
◆ Measures to prevent further fluid loss, such as an antidiarrheal, if needed, avoiding dietary diuretics (such as caffeine), preventing excessive perspiration, remaining hydrated

Special considerations
◆ During rehydration, carefully monitor intake and output to maintain fluid and electrolyte balance.
◆ To prevent thromboemboli in predisposed patients, suggest regular exercise and a low-cholesterol diet. An antilipemic may also be necessary. Reduced calorie intake may be required for the obese patient.
◆ Whenever appropriate, suggest counseling about the patient's work habits and lack of relaxation. If the patient is a smoker, make sure he understands how important it is that he stop smoking. Refer him to a smoking cessation program, if necessary.
◆ Emphasize the need for follow-up examinations every 3 to 4 months after leaving the health care facility.
◆ Thoroughly explain spurious polycythemia, all diagnostic measures, and therapy. The hard-driving person predisposed to spurious polycythemia is likely to be more inquisitive and anxious than the average patient. Answer questions honestly, but take care to reassure him that he can effectively control symptoms by complying with the prescribed treatment.

THALASSEMIA

Thalassemia, a hereditary group of hemolytic anemias, is characterized by defective synthesis in the polypeptide chains of the protein component of hemoglobin. Consequently, red blood cell (RBC) synthesis is also impaired.

⚠ **CLINICAL ALERT** *Thalassemia is most common in people of Mediterranean ancestry (especially Italian and Greek) but also occurs in people whose ancestors originated in Africa, southern China, southeast Asia, and India.*

In β-thalassemia, the most common form of this disorder, synthesis of the beta polypeptide chain is defective. It occurs in three clinical forms: major, intermedia, and minor. The severity of the resulting anemia depends on whether the patient is homozygous or heterozygous for the thalassemic trait. The prognosis varies:

◆ *Thalassemia major* — Patients seldom survive to adulthood.

◆ *Thalassemia intermedia* — Children develop normally into adulthood, although puberty is usually delayed.

◆ *Thalassemia minor* — Patients have normal life span.

Causes
◆ Heterozygous inheritance of the same gene (thalassemia minor)
◆ Homozygous inheritance of the partially dominant autosomal gene (thalassemia major or thalassemia intermedia)

Pathophysiology
Total or partial deficiency of beta polypeptide chain production impairs hemoglobin synthesis and results in continual production of fetal hemoglobin, lasting even past the neonatal period. Normally, immunoglobulin synthesis switches from gamma- to beta-polypeptides at the time of birth. This conversion doesn't happen in thalassemic infants. Their RBCs are hypochromic and microcytic.

Signs and symptoms
Possible signs and symptoms of thalassemia major (also known as *Cooley's anemia, Mediterranean disease,* and *erythroblastic anemia*) are related to the development of hypochromic and microcytic RBCs subsequently impairing oxygenation that lead to:

◆ development of severe anemia, bone abnormalities, failure to thrive, and life-threatening complications in a healthy infant at birth, during the second 6 months of life
◆ pallor and yellow skin and sclera in infants ages 3 to 6 months
◆ splenomegaly or hepatomegaly, with abdominal enlargement; frequent infections; bleeding tendencies (especially nose bleeds); anorexia
◆ small body, large head (characteristic features), and possible mental retardation
◆ possible features similar to Down syndrome in infants, because of thickened bone at the base of the nose from bone marrow hyperactivity.

Signs and symptoms of thalassemia intermedia are:

◆ some degree of anemia, jaundice, and splenomegaly

◆ possibly signs of hemosiderosis due to increased intestinal absorption of iron.

Signs of thalassemia minor are mild anemia (usually produces no symptoms and is commonly overlooked; it should be differentiated from iron deficiency anemia).

Complications
◆ Pathologic fractures due to expansion of the marrow cavities with thinning of the long bones
◆ Cardiac arrhythmias
◆ Heart failure

Diagnosis
Thalassemia major
◆ Blood studies reveal a low RBC count and hemoglobin level, microcytosis, and a high reticulocyte count.
◆ Laboratory studies show elevated bilirubin and urinary and fecal urobilinogen levels.
◆ A low serum folate level reflects increased folate use by hypertrophied bone marrow.
◆ Peripheral blood smear shows target cells, microcytes, pale nucleated RBCs, and marked anisocytosis.
◆ X-rays reveal thinning and widening of the marrow space on the skull and long bones due to overactive bone marrow.
◆ X-rays also show granular appearance of bones of the skull and vertebrae, areas of osteoporosis in the long bones, and deformed (rectangular or biconvex) phalanges.
◆ A significantly increased fetal hemoglobin level and a slightly increased hemoglobin A_2 level are revealed in quantitative hemoglobin studies.
◆ Laboratory studies that exclude iron deficiency anemia help to diagnose thalassemia major (also produces hypochromic microcytic RBCs).

Thalassemia intermedia
◆ Blood studies reveal hypochromic microcytic RBCs (less severe than in thalassemia major).

Thalassemia minor
◆ Blood studies reveal hypochromic microcytic RBCs.
◆ A significantly increased hemoglobin A_2 level and a moderately increased fetal hemoglobin level are revealed in quantitative hemoglobin studies.

Treatment
◆ Prompt treatment with the appropriate antibiotic for infections
◆ A folic acid supplement to help maintain the folic acid level, despite increased requirements

◆ Transfusions of packed RBCs (typically done on a schedule every 2 to 4 weeks) to increase the hemoglobin level
◆ Deferoxamine (Desferal), a chelating agent, to eliminate excess iron from the body
◆ Splenectomy and bone marrow transplantation (effectiveness hasn't been confirmed)
◆ No treatment for thalassemia intermedia and thalassemia minor
◆ No iron supplement (contraindicated in all forms of thalassemia)

Special considerations
◆ During and after RBC transfusions for thalassemia major, watch for adverse reactions—shaking chills, fever, rash, itching, and hives.
◆ Stress the importance of good nutrition, meticulous wound care, periodic dental check-ups, and other measures to prevent infection.
◆ For young patients, discuss with parents various options for healthy physical and creative outlets. Such a child must avoid strenuous athletic activity because of increased oxygen demand and the tendency toward pathologic fractures, but he may participate in less stressful activities.
◆ Teach parents to watch for signs of hepatitis and iron overload—always possible with frequent transfusions.
◆ Because parents may have questions about the vulnerability of future offspring, refer them for genetic counseling. Also, refer adult patients with thalassemia minor and thalassemia intermedia for genetic counseling; they need to recognize the risk of transmitting thalassemia major to their children if they marry another person with thalassemia. (Such children should be evaluated for thalassemia by age 1.) Be sure to tell people with thalassemia minor that their condition is benign.

THROMBOCYTOPENIA
Thrombocytopenia, the most common cause of hemorrhagic disorders, is a deficiency of circulating platelets. It may be congenital or acquired; the acquired form is more common. Because platelets are needed for coagulation, this disease poses a serious threat to hemostasis. The prognosis is excellent in drug-induced thrombocytopenia if the offending drug is withdrawn; in such cases, recovery may be immediate. In other types, the prognosis depends on the patient's response to treatment of the underlying cause.

Causes
◆ Blood loss
◆ Decreased or defective platelet production in the bone marrow (as in leukemia, aplastic anemia, or drug toxicity)

◆ Increased platelet destruction outside the marrow due to an underlying disorder (such as cirrhosis of the liver, disseminated intravascular coagulation, or severe infection)
◆ Sequestration (increased amount of blood in a limited vascular area such as the spleen)

Pathophysiology
In thrombocytopenia, lack of platelets can cause inadequate hemostasis. Four mechanisms are responsible: decreased platelet production, decreased platelet survival, pooling of blood in the spleen, and intravascular dilution of circulating platelets. Megakaryocytes, giant cells in the bone marrow, produce platelets. Platelet production decreases when the number of megakaryocytes is reduced or when platelet production becomes dysfunctional. (See *What happens in thrombocytopenia*, pages 430 and 431.)

Signs and symptoms
◆ Petechiae or blood blisters caused by bleeding into the skin
◆ Bleeding into the mucous membrane
◆ Malaise, fatigue, and general weakness related to blood loss and decreased tissue oxygenation
◆ Large blood-filled blisters in the mouth (in adults)

Complications
◆ Hemorrhage
◆ Death

Diagnosis
◆ Blood studies reveal a platelet count of less than $100,000/\mu l$ in adults and a prolonged bleeding time.
◆ Platelet antibody studies help determine why the platelet count is low (also used to select treatment).
◆ Platelet survival studies help differentiate between ineffective platelet production and platelet destruction as causes of thrombocytopenia.
◆ Bone marrow studies determine the number, size, and maturity of megakaryocytes in severe disease, helping identify ineffective platelet production as the cause and ruling out malignant disease.

Treatment
◆ Withdrawing the offending drug or treating the underlying cause
◆ A corticosteroid to increase platelet production
◆ Folate to stimulate bone marrow production
◆ I.V. gamma globulin to increase platelet production

CLOSER LOOK

What happens in thrombocytopenia

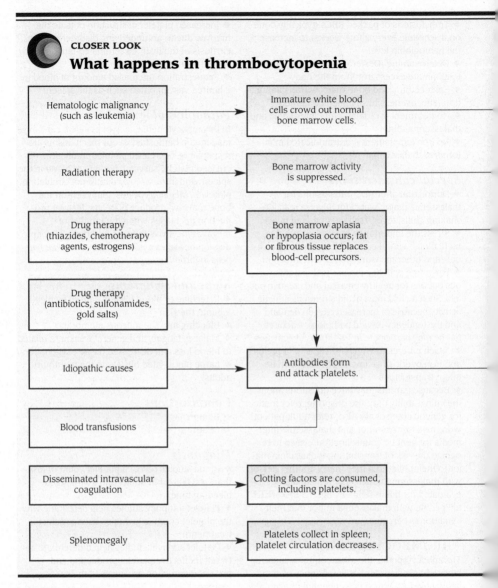

Hematologic malignancy (such as leukemia)	Immature white blood cells crowd out normal bone marrow cells.
Radiation therapy	Bone marrow activity is suppressed.
Drug therapy (thiazides, chemotherapy agents, estrogens)	Bone marrow aplasia or hypoplasia occurs; fat or fibrous tissue replaces blood-cell precursors.
Drug therapy (antibiotics, sulfonamides, gold salts)	
Idiopathic causes	Antibodies form and attack platelets.
Blood transfusions	
Disseminated intravascular coagulation	Clotting factors are consumed, including platelets.
Splenomegaly	Platelets collect in spleen; platelet circulation decreases.

◆ Platelet transfusion to treat complications of severe hemorrhage
◆ Splenectomy to correct disease caused by platelet destruction (because the spleen is the primary site of platelet removal and antibody production)

Special considerations

When caring for the patient with thrombocytopenia, take every possible precaution against bleeding.
◆ Protect the patient from trauma. Keep the side rails up and pad them, if possible. Promote the use of an electric razor and a soft toothbrush.

Avoid invasive procedures, such as venipuncture or urinary catheterization, if possible. When venipuncture is unavoidable, be sure to exert pressure on the puncture site for at least 20 minutes or until the bleeding stops.
◆ Monitor the platelet count daily. A 1- to 2-hour postplatelet count will aid assessment of response.
◆ Test stool for guaiac; dipstick urine and vomitus for blood.
◆ Watch for bleeding (petechiae, ecchymoses, surgical or GI bleeding, and menorrhagia).
◆ Warn the patient to avoid aspirin in any form and other drugs that impair coagulation. Teach

◆ During platelet transfusion, monitor for febrile reaction (flushing, chills, fever, headache, tachycardia, and hypertension). Histocompatibility locus antigen-typed platelets may be ordered to prevent febrile reaction. A patient with a history of minor reactions may benefit from acetaminophen and diphenhydramine before transfusion.
◆ If thrombocytopenia is drug-induced, stress the importance of avoiding the offending drug.
◆ If the patient must receive long-term steroid therapy, teach him to watch for and report cushingoid signs (acne, moon face, hirsutism, buffalo hump, hypertension, girdle obesity, thinning arms and legs, glycosuria, and edema). Emphasize that steroid doses must be discontinued gradually. During steroid therapy, monitor fluid and electrolyte balance, and watch for infection, pathologic fractures, and mood changes.

VON WILLEBRAND'S DISEASE

von Willebrand's disease is a hereditary bleeding disorder, characterized by prolonged bleeding time, moderate deficiency of clotting factor VIII (antihemophilic factor), and impaired platelet function; it's more common in women. The disease typically causes bleeding from the skin or mucosal surfaces and, in women, excessive uterine bleeding. Bleeding may range from mild and asymptomatic to severe, potentially fatal, hemorrhage. The prognosis is usually good.

Causes

von Willebrand's disease is caused by inherited autosomal dominant trait.

Recently, an acquired form has been identified in patients with cancer and immune disorders.

Pathophysiology

A possible mechanism is that mild to moderate deficiency of factor VIII and defective platelet adhesion prolong coagulation time. Specifically, this results from a deficiency of von Willebrand's factor (vWF), which stabilizes the factor VIII molecule and is needed for proper platelet function.

Defective platelet function is characterized in vivo by decreased agglutination and adhesion at the bleeding site and in vitro by reduced platelet retention when blood is filtered through a column of packed glass beads, and diminished ristocetin-induced platelet aggregation.

Signs and symptoms

Prolonged coagulation time may cause:
◆ easy bruising
◆ epistaxis (nose bleed)

Platelet production decreases.

Thrombocytopenic hemorrhage

Platelet destruction increases.

Platelets are distributed abnormally.

him how to recognize aspirin or ibuprofen compounds on labels of over-the-counter remedies.
◆ Advise the patient to avoid straining at stool or coughing because both can lead to increased intracranial pressure, possibly causing cerebral hemorrhage in the patient with thrombocytopenia. Provide a stool softener to avoid constipation.
◆ During periods of active bleeding, maintain the patient on strict bed rest, if necessary.
◆ When administering platelet concentrate, remember that platelets are extremely fragile, so infuse them quickly. Don't give platelets to a patient with a fever.

- bleeding from the gums
- petechiae (rarely)
- hemorrhage after laceration or surgery (in severe forms)
- menorrhagia (in severe forms)
- GI bleeding (in severe forms)
- excessive postpartum bleeding (uncommon)
- massive soft-tissue hemorrhage and bleeding into joints (rare).

Complications
A complication of von Willebrand's disease is hemorrhage.

Diagnosis
The following test results help diagnose von Willebrand's disease:
- prolonged bleeding time (greater than 6 minutes)
- slightly prolonged partial thromboplastin time (greater than 45 seconds)
- absent or low factor VIII
- absent or low factor VIII–related antigens
- low factor VIII activity
- ristocetin coagulation factor assay showing defective in vitro platelet aggregation
- a normal platelet count and clot retraction.

Treatment
- Infusion of cryoprecipitate or blood fractions rich in factor VIII to shorten bleeding time and replace factor VIII
- Parenteral or intranasal desmopressin (DDAVP) to increase the serum vWF level

Special considerations
The care plan should include local measures to control bleeding and patient teaching to prevent bleeding, unnecessary trauma, and complications.
- After surgery, monitor bleeding time for 24 to 48 hours, and watch for signs of new bleeding.
- During a bleeding episode, elevate and apply cold compresses and gentle pressure to the bleeding site.
- Refer parents of affected children for genetic counseling.
- Advise the patient to consult the physician after even minor trauma and before all surgery to determine if replacement of blood components is necessary.
- Tell the patient to watch for signs of hepatitis within 6 weeks to 6 months after transfusion.
- Warn against using aspirin and other drugs that impair platelet function.
- Advise the patient who has a severe form to avoid contact sports.

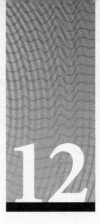

IMMUNE SYSTEM

The immune system is responsible for safeguarding the body from disease-causing microorganisms. It's part of a complex system of host defenses.

Host defenses may be *innate* or *acquired*. Innate defenses include physical and chemical barriers, the complement complex, and cells, such as phagocytes (cells programmed to destroy foreign cells, such as bacteria) and natural killer lymphocytes.

Physical barriers, such as the skin and mucous membranes, prevent invasion by most organisms. Chemical barriers include lysozymes (found in such body secretions as tears, mucus, and saliva) and hydrochloric acid in the stomach. Lysozymes destroy bacteria by removing cell walls. Hydrochloric acid breaks down foods and destroys pathogens carried by food or swallowed mucus.

Organisms that penetrate this first line of defense simultaneously trigger the inflammatory and immune responses, some innate and others acquired.

Acquired immunity comes into play when the body encounters a cell or cell product that it recognizes as foreign, such as a bacterium or a virus. The two types of immunity provided by cells are humoral (provided by B lymphocytes) and cell mediated (provided by T lymphocytes). All cells involved in the inflammatory and immune responses arrive from a single type of stem cell in the bone marrow. B cells mature in the marrow, and T cells migrate to the thymus, where they mature.

The inflammatory response is the immediate local response to tissue injury, whether from trauma or infection. It involves the action of polymorphonuclear leukocytes, basophils and mast cells, platelets and, to some extent, monocytes and macrophages. Each of these cells is described in a later section of this chapter.

Immune response

The immune response primarily involves the interaction of antigens (foreign proteins), B lymphocytes, T lymphocytes, macrophages, cytokines, complement, and polymorphonuclear leukocytes. Some immunoactive cells circulate constantly; others remain in the tissues and organs of the immune system, such as the thymus, lymph nodes, bone marrow, spleen, and tonsils. In the thymus, the T lymphocytes, which are involved in cell-mediated immunity, become able to differentiate self (host) from nonself (foreign) substances (antigens). In contrast, B lymphocytes, which are involved in humoral immunity, mature in the bone marrow. The key mechanism in humoral immunity is the production of immunoglobulin by B cells and the subsequent activation of the complement cascade. The lymph nodes, spleen, liver, and intestinal lymphoid tissue help remove and destroy circulating antigens in the blood and lymph.

AGE ALERT *The immune system's ability to fight off infections and other immune system disorders decreases with age.*

◆ *Fewer lymphocytes are present, and the ones that are there are less responsive to invasion of the body by infection and other antigens.*

433

◆ *Autoantibodies, causative factors in such diseases as rheumatoid arthritis and atherosclerosis, are more likely to occur with aging.*
◆ *Organs, such as the thymus gland, are less efficient in producing hormones related to the immune system.*

AGE ALERT *At age 2, a child's immune system is fully functioning. Infants between ages 6 and 9 months are particularly vulnerable to disease because they're no longer supported by maternal antibodies and their own immune system isn't yet established.*

ANTIGENS

An antigen is a substance that can induce an immune response. T and B lymphocytes have specific receptors that respond to specific antigen molecular shapes, called *epitopes.* In B cells, this receptor is an immunoglobulin, also called an *antibody.*

Major histocompatibility complex

The T-cell antigen receptor recognizes antigens only in association with specific cell-surface molecules known as the *major histocompatibility complex (MHC).*

The MHC, also known as the *human leukocyte antigen (HLA) locus,* is a cluster of genes on human chromosome 6 that has a pivotal role in the immune response. Every person receives one set of MHC genes from each parent, and both sets of genes are expressed on the individual's cells. These genes produce MHC molecules, which participate in:
◆ the recognition of self versus nonself
◆ the interaction of immunologically active cells by coding for cell-surface proteins.

MHC molecules differ among individuals. Slightly different antigen receptors can recognize a large number of distinct antigens, coded by distinct, variable region genes.

Groups or clones of lymphocytes that have identical receptors for a specific antigen exist. The clone of a lymphocyte rapidly proliferates when exposed to the specific antigen. Some lymphocytes further differentiate, whereas others become memory cells, which allow a more rapid response — the *memory,* or *anamnestic, response* — to subsequent challenge by the antigen.

Haptens

Most antigens are large molecules, such as proteins or polysaccharides. Smaller molecules, such as drugs, that aren't antigenic by themselves are known as *haptens.* They can bind with larger molecules, or carriers, and become antigenic or immunogenic.

Antigenicity

Many factors influence the intensity of a foreign substance's interaction with the host's immune system (antigenicity):
◆ physical and chemical characteristics of the antigen
◆ its relative foreignness — for example, little or no immune response may follow the transfusion of serum proteins between humans, but a vigorous immune response (serum sickness) commonly follows transfusion of horse serum proteins to a human
◆ the host's genetic makeup, especially the MHC molecules.

HUMORAL IMMUNITY

The humoral immune response is one of two types of immune responses that can occur when foreign substances invade the body. The other is the cell-mediated response. The humoral response is also called an *antibody-mediated response.*

B lymphocytes

B lymphocytes and their products, immunoglobulins, are the basis of humoral immunity. A soluble antigen binds with the B-cell antigen receptor, initiating the humoral immune response. The activated B cells differentiate into plasma cells, which secrete immunoglobulins, also called *antibodies.* This response is regulated by T lymphocytes and their products — lymphokines, such as interleukin-2 (IL-2), IL-4, IL-5, and interferon-8 — which determine which class of immunoglobulins a B cell will manufacture.

Immunoglobulins

The immunoglobulins that plasma cells secrete are four-chain molecules with two heavy and two light chains. Each chain has a variable (V) region and one or more constant (C) regions, which are coded by separate genes. The V regions of both light and heavy chains participate in antigen binding. The C regions of the heavy chain provide a binding site for crystallizable fragment (Fc) receptors on cells and govern other mechanisms. (See *Structure of the immunoglobulin molecule.*)

There are five known classes of immunoglobulins: IgG, IgM, IgA, IgE, and IgD. These are distinguished by the constant portions of their heavy chains. However, each class has a kappa or lambda light chain, which gives rise to many subtypes and provides almost limitless combinations of light and heavy chains that give immunoglobulins their specificity. (See *Classification of immunoglobulins,* page 436.)

Structure of the immunoglobulin molecule

The immunoglobulin molecule consists of four polypeptide chains: two heavy (H) and two light (L) chains held together by disulfide bonds. The H chain has one variable (V) and at least three constant (C) regions. The L chain has one V and one C region. Together, the V regions form a pocket known as the *antigen-binding site*. This site is located within the antigen-binding fragment (Fab) region of the molecule. Part of the C region of the H chains forms the crystallizable fragment (Fc) region of the molecule. This region mediates effector mechanisms, such as complement activation, and is the portion of the immunoglobulin molecule bound by Fc receptors on phagocytic cells, mast cells, and basophils. Each immunoglobulin (Ig) molecule also has two antibody-combining sites (except for the IgM molecule, which has 10, and IgA, which may have 2 or more).

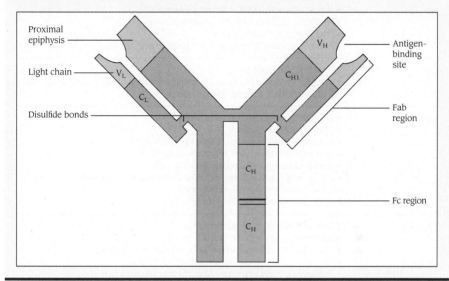

A clone of B cells is specific for only one antigen, and the V regions of its Ig light chains determines that specificity. However, the class of immunoglobulin can change if the association between the cell's V region genes and heavy chain C region genes changes through a process known as isotype switching. For example, a clone of B cells genetically programmed to recognize tetanus toxoid will first make an IgM antibody against tetanus toxoid and later an IgG or other antibody against it.

CELL-MEDIATED IMMUNITY

The cell-mediated immune response protects the body against bacterial, viral, and fungal infections and defends against transplanted cells and tumor cells. T lymphocytes and macrophages are the chief participants in the cell-mediated immune response. A macrophage processes the antigen and then presents it to T lymphocytes.

Macrophages

Macrophages influence both immune and inflammatory responses. Macrophage precursors circulate in the blood. When they collect in various tissues and organs, they differentiate into different types of macrophages. Unlike B and T lymphocytes, macrophages lack surface receptors for specific antigens. Instead, they have receptors for the C region of the heavy chain (Fc region) of immunoglobulin, for fragments of the third component of complement (C3), and for nonimmunologic substances, such as carbohydrate molecules.

One of the most important functions of macrophages is presentation of antigen to T lymphocytes. Macrophages ingest and process the antigen, then they deposit it on their own surfaces in association with HLA antigen. T lymphocytes become activated when they recognize the antigen-HLA complex. Macrophages also function in the inflammatory response by producing IL-1, which generates fever, and by

Classification of immunoglobulins

The following table shows the five classifications of immunoglobulins (Ig).

Classification	Description
IgA	♦ Secretory immunoglobulin (monomer in serum, dimer in secretory form) ♦ Found in colostrum, saliva, tears, nasal fluids, and respiratory, GI, and genitourinary secretions ♦ Accounts for 20% of total serum immunoglobulins ♦ Important role in preventing antigenic agents from attaching to epithelial surfaces
IgD	♦ Minute amounts found in serum (monomer) ♦ Predominant on surface of B lymphocytes ♦ Primarily an antigen receptor ♦ Possible function in controlling lymphocyte activation or suppression
IgE	♦ Found only in trace amounts ♦ Involved in release of vasoactive amines stored in basophils and tissue mast cell granules that cause the allergic effects
IgG	♦ Smallest immunoglobulin (monomer) ♦ Found in all body fluids ♦ Can cross membranes as a single structural unit ♦ Accounts for 75% of total serum immunoglobulins ♦ Produced mainly in secondary immune response ♦ Classic antibody reactions, including precipitation, agglutination, neutralization, and complement fixation ♦ Major antibacterial and antiviral antibody
IgM	♦ Largest immunoglobulin (pentamer) ♦ Usually found only in the vascular system ♦ Can't readily cross membrane barriers because of its size ♦ Accounts for 5% of total serum immunoglobulins ♦ Dominant activity in primary or initial immune response ♦ Classic antibody reactions, including precipitation, agglutination, neutralization, and complement fixation

synthesizing complement proteins and other mediators that have phagocytic, microbicidal, and oncolytic effects.

T lymphocytes

Immature T lymphocytes are derived from the bone marrow and migrate to the thymus, where they mature. In maturation, the products of the MCH genes "teach" T cells to distinguish between self and nonself.

Five types of T cells exist with specific functions:
♦ memory cells, sensitized cells that remain dormant until second exposure to antigen, also known as *secondary immune response*
♦ lymphokine-producing cells, delayed hypersensitivity reactions
♦ cytotoxic T cells, direct destruction of antigen or the cells carrying the antigen

♦ helper T cells, also known as *T4 cells*, facilitate the humoral and cell-mediated responses
♦ suppressor T cells, also known as *T8 cells*, inhibit humoral and cell-mediated responses.

T cells acquire specific surface molecules (markers) that identify their potential role when needed in the immune response. These markers and the T-cell antigen receptor together promote the particular activation of each type of T cell. T-cell activation requires presentation of antigens in the context of a specific HLA antigen — for example, class II HLA for helper T cells and class I HLA for cytotoxic T cells. T-cell activation also requires IL-1, produced by macrophages, and IL-2, produced by T cells.

Natural killer cells

Natural killer cells make up a discrete population of large lymphocytes, some of which resemble

T cells. They recognize surface changes on body cells infected with a virus. They bind to and, in many cases, kill the infected cells.

Cytokines

Cytokines are low-molecular-weight proteins involved in the communication among macrophages and the lymphocytes. They induce or regulate various immune or inflammatory responses. Cytokines include colony-stimulating factors, interferons, interleukins, tumor necrosis factors, and transforming growth factor.

COMPLEMENT SYSTEM

The complement system, the chief humoral effector of the inflammatory response, includes more than 20 serum proteins. When activated, these proteins interact in a cascade-like process that has profound biological effects. Complement activation takes place through one of two pathways.

Classic pathway

In the classic pathway, IgM or IgG binds with the antigen to form antigen-antibody complexes that activate the first complement component, C1. This in turn activates C4, C2, and C3.

Alternate pathway

In the alternate pathway, activating surfaces, such as bacterial cell membranes, directly amplify spontaneous cleavage of C3. Once C3 is activated in either pathway, activation of the terminal components, C5 to C9, follows.

The major biological effects of complement activation include chemotaxis (phagocyte attraction), phagocyte activation, histamine release, viral neutralization, promotion of phagocytosis by opsonization (making the bacteria susceptible to phagocytosis), and lysis of cells and bacteria. Kinins (peptides that cause vasodilation and enhance vascular permeability and smooth-muscle contraction) and other mediators of inflammation derived from the kinin and coagulation pathways interact with the complement system.

POLYMORPHONUCLEAR LEUKOCYTES

Other key factors in the inflammatory response are the polymorphonuclear leukocytes: neutrophils, eosinophils, basophils, and mast cells.

Neutrophils

Neutrophils, the most numerous of these leukocytes, derive from bone marrow and increase dramatically in number in response to infection and inflammation. They're the first to respond in

acute infection. Neutrophils are highly mobile cells attracted to areas of inflammation and are the main constituent of pus.

Neutrophils have surface receptors for immunoglobulins and complement fragments, and they avidly ingest bacteria or other particles that are coated with target-identifying antibodies (opsonins). Toxic oxygen metabolites and enzymes such as lysozyme promptly kill the ingested organisms. Unfortunately, in addition to killing invading organisms, neutrophils also damage host tissues.

Eosinophils

Eosinophils, also derived from bone marrow, multiply in allergic and parasitic disorders. Although their phagocytic function isn't clearly understood, evidence suggests that they participate in host defense against parasites. Their products may also diminish inflammatory response in allergic disorders.

Basophils and mast cells

Basophils and mast cells also function in immune disorders. Mast cells, unlike basophils, aren't blood cells. Basophils circulate in peripheral blood, whereas mast cells accumulate in connective tissue, particularly in the lungs, intestines, and skin. Both types of cells have surface receptors for IgE. When their receptors are cross-linked by an IgE antigen complex, they release mediators characteristic of the allergic response.

Pathophysiologic changes

The host defense system and the immune response are highly complex processes, subject to malfunction at any point along the sequence of events. This malfunction may involve exaggeration, misdirection, or an absence or depression of activity leading to an immune disorder.

IMMUNE RESPONSE MALFUNCTION

When the immune system responds inappropriately, three basic categories of reactions may occur: hypersensitivity, autoimmune response, and alloimmune response. The type of reaction is determined by the source of the antigen, such as environmental, self, or other person, to which the immune system is responding.

Hypersensitivity

Hypersensitivity is an exaggerated or inappropriate response that occurs on second exposure to an antigen. The result is inflammation and the destruction of healthy tissue. *Allergy* refers to the harmful effects resulting from a hypersensitivity to antigens, also called *allergens.*

Hypersensitivity reactions may be *immediate,* occurring within minutes to hours of reexposure, or *delayed,* occurring several hours after reexposure. A delayed hypersensitivity reaction typically is most severe days after the reexposure.

Generally, hypersensitivity reactions are classified as one of four types: type I (IgE mediated), type II (tissue specific), type III (immune complex mediated), type IV (cell mediated).

Type I hypersensitivity (allergic disorders)

With type I hypersensitivity, allergens activate T cells, which induce B-cell production of IgE, which binds to the Fc receptors on the surface of mast cells. Repeated exposure to relatively large doses of the allergen is usually necessary to cause this response. When enough IgE has been produced, the person is *sensitized* to the allergen. At the next exposure to the same antigen, the antigen binds with the surface IgE, cross-links the Fc receptors, and causes mast cells to degranulate and release various mediators. Degranulation also may be triggered by complement-driven anaphylatoxins—C3a and C5a—or by certain drugs, such as morphine.

Some of the mediators released are preformed, whereas others are newly synthesized on activation of the mast cells. Preformed mediators include heparin, histamine, proteolytic (protein-splitting) and other enzymes, and chemotactic factors for eosinophils and neutrophils. Newly synthesized mediators include prostaglandins and leukotrienes. Mast cells also produce various cytokines, which initiate smooth-muscle contraction, vasodilation, bronchospasm, edema, increased vascular permeability, mucus secretion, and cellular infiltration by eosinophils and neutrophils. These effects result in some of the classic associated signs and symptoms, such as hypotension, wheezing, swelling, urticaria, and rhinorrhea.

Type II hypersensitivity (antibody-dependent cytotoxicity)

A tissue-specific reaction, type II hypersensitivity, generally involves the destruction of a target cell by an antibody directed against cell-surface antigens. Alternatively, the antibody may be directed against small molecules adsorbed to cells or against cell-surface receptors, rather than against the cell constituents themselves. Tissue damage occurs through several mechanisms:
◆ binding of antigen and antibody activates complement, which ultimately disrupts cellular membranes—complement-mediated lysis

◆ various phagocytic cells with receptors for immunoglobulin (Fc region) and complement fragments envelop and destroy opsonized targets, such as red blood cells, leukocytes, and platelets
◆ cytotoxic T cells and natural killer cells, though not antigen specific, also contribute to tissue damage by releasing toxic substances that destroy the cells
◆ antibody binding causes the target cell to malfunction rather than causing its destruction.

Type III hypersensitivity (immune complex disease)

In type III hypersensitivity, circulating antigen-antibody complexes (immune complexes) accumulate and are deposited in the tissues. The most common tissues involved are the kidneys, joints, skin, and blood vessels. Normally, they clear excess immune complexes from the circulation. However, immune complexes deposited in the tissues activate the complement cascade, causing local inflammation, and trigger platelet release of vasoactive amines that increase vascular permeability, so more immune complexes accumulate in the vessel walls.

Probably the most harmful effects result from the generation of complement fragments that attract neutrophils. The neutrophils attempt to ingest the immune complexes. They're generally unsuccessful, but in the attempt, the neutrophils release lysosomal enzymes, which exacerbate the tissue damage.

The formation of immune complexes is dynamic and ever changing. The complexes that form in children may be totally different from those formed in adolescents and adults. Also, more than one type of immune complex may be present at one time.

Type IV hypersensitivity (delayed hypersensitivity)

Type IV hypersensitivity cell-mediated reactions involve the processing of the antigen by the macrophages. Once processed, the antigen is presented to the T cells. Cytotoxic T cells, if activated, attack and destroy the target cells directly. When lymphokine T cells are activated, they release lymphokines, which recruit and activate other lymphocytes, monocytes, macrophages, and polymorphonuclear leukocytes. The coagulation, kinin, and complement cascades also contribute to tissue damage in this type of reaction.

Autoimmune reactions

In autoimmune reactions, the body's normal defenses become self-destructive, recognizing self-antigens as foreign. What causes this misdirected response isn't clearly understood. For example, drugs or viruses have been implicated as causing some autoimmune reactions, but in such diseases as rheumatoid arthritis and systemic lupus erythematosus the mechanism for misdirection is unclear.

Autoimmune reactions are believed to result from a combination of factors, including genetic, hormonal, and environmental influences. Many are characterized by B-cell hyperactivity and by hypergammaglobulinemia. B-cell hyperactivity may be related to T-cell abnormalities. Hormonal and genetic factors strongly influence the onset of some autoimmune disorders.

Alloimmune reactions

Alloimmune reactions are directed at antigens from the tissues of others of the same species. These reactions commonly occur in transplant and transfusion reactions, in which the recipient reacts to antigens, primarily HLA, on the donor cells. This immune response is also seen in infants with erythroblastosis fetalis. (See chapter 11, Hematologic system.) This type of response is commonly associated with a type II hypersensitivity reaction.

Immunodeficiency

An absent or depressed immune response increases susceptibility to infection. Immunodeficiency may be primary (reflecting a defect involving T cells, B cells, or lymphoid tissues) or secondary (resulting from an underlying disease or factor that depresses or blocks the immune response). The most common forms of immunodeficiency are caused by viral infection or are iatrogenic reactions to therapeutic drugs.

Disorders

The environment contains thousands of pathogenic microorganisms. Normally, our host defense system protects us from these harmful invaders. When this network of safeguards breaks down, however, the result is an altered immune response or immune system failure. Disorders of the immune system discussed in this chapter include acquired immunodeficiency syndrome, allergic rhinitis, anaphylaxis, atopic dermatitis, latex allergy, lupus erythematosus, rheumatoid arthritis, urticaria and angioedema, and vasculitis.

ACQUIRED IMMUNODEFICIENCY SYNDROME

Human immunodeficiency virus (HIV) infection may cause acquired immunodeficiency syn-

---

Common infections and neoplasms in HIV and AIDS

This is a list of commonly seen disorders with human immunodeficiency virus (HIV) and acquired immunodeficiency syndrome (AIDS). AIDS is diagnosed when a patient diagnosed with HIV has a CD4+ T-cell count of less than 200 cells/mcl.

◆ Common infections in a patient with a CD4+ count less than 350 cells/mcl include:
– herpes simplex virus
– herpes zoster
– *Mycobacterium tuberculosis*
– non-Hodgkin's lymphoma
– oral or vaginal thrush.
◆ Common infections in a patient with a CD4+ count less than 200 cells/mcl include:
– *Candida esophagitis*
– *Pneumocystis jiroveci (carinii)* pneumonia.
◆ Common infections in a patient with a CD4+ count less than 100 cells/mcl include:
– AIDS dementia
– cryptococcal meningitis
– progressive multifocal leukoencephalopathy
– toxoplasmosis encephalitis
– wasting syndrome.
◆ Common infections in a patient with a CD4+ count less than 50 cells/mcl include:
– *Cytomegalovirus* infection
– *Mycobacterium avium.*
◆ Common neoplasms in patients with HIV and AIDS include:
– Hodgkin's lymphoma
– Kaposi's sarcoma
– malignant lymphoma.

---

drome (AIDS). Although it's characterized by gradual destruction of cell-mediated (T cell) immunity, it also affects humoral immunity and even autoimmunity because of the central role of the CD4+ (helper) T lymphocyte in immune reactions. The resulting immunodeficiency makes the patient susceptible to opportunistic infections, cancers, and other abnormalities that characterize AIDS. (See *Common infections and neoplasms in HIV and AIDS.*)

AIDS was first described by the Centers for Disease Control and Prevention (CDC) in 1981. Because transmission is similar, AIDS shares epidemiologic patterns with hepatitis B and sexually transmitted diseases.

The CDC estimates that more than 1 million people in the United States are infected with

HIV, one-quarter of whom are unaware of their infection. The AIDS epidemic is growing most rapidly among homosexual and bisexual men of all races, Blacks, and Hispanic groups in the United States. It's the leading killer of Black men ages 25 to 44, and it affects nearly seven times more Blacks and three times more Hispanics than Whites.

Depending on individual variations and the presence of cofactors that influence disease progression, the time from acute HIV infection to the appearance of symptoms (mild to severe) to the diagnosis of AIDS and, eventually, to death varies greatly. Combination drug therapy in conjunction with treatment and prophylaxis of common opportunistic infections can delay the natural progression and prolong survival.

Causes

The HIV-1 retrovirus is the primary cause. Transmission occurs by contact with infected blood or body fluids and is associated with identifiable high-risk behaviors. It's disproportionately represented in:

◆ homosexual and bisexual men
◆ I.V. drug users
◆ recipients of contaminated blood or blood products (dramatically decreased since mid-1985)
◆ heterosexual partners of persons in the former groups
◆ neonates of infected women.

Pathophysiology

The natural history of AIDS begins with infection by the HIV retrovirus, which is detectable only by laboratory tests, and ends with death. Twenty years of data strongly suggests that HIV isn't transmitted by casual household or social contact. The HIV virus may enter the body by any of several routes involving the transmission of blood or body fluids, for example:

◆ direct inoculation during intimate sexual contact, especially associated with the mucosal trauma of receptive rectal intercourse
◆ transfusion of blood or clotting factors used from 1978 to 1985
◆ sharing of contaminated needles
◆ transplacental or postpartum transmission from infected mother to fetus (by cervical or blood contact at delivery and in breast milk).

HIV strikes helper T cells bearing the CD4+ antigen. Normally a receptor for major histocompatibility complex molecules, the antigen serves as a receptor for the retrovirus and allows it to enter the cell. Viral binding also requires the presence of a coreceptor (believed to be the chemokine receptor CCR5) on the cell

surface. The virus also may infect CD4+ antigen–bearing cells of the GI tract, uterine cervix, and neuroglia.

Like other retroviruses, HIV copies its genetic material in a reverse manner compared with other viruses and cells. Through the action of reverse transcriptase, HIV produces DNA from its viral RNA. Transcription is typically poor, leading to mutations, some of which make HIV resistant to antivirals. The viral DNA enters the nucleus of the cell and is incorporated into the host cell's DNA, where it's transcribed into more viral RNA. If the host cell reproduces, it duplicates the HIV DNA along with its own and passes it on to the daughter cells. Thus, if activated, the host cell carries this information and, if activated, replicates the virus. Viral enzymes, proteases, arrange the structural components and RNA into viral particles that move out to the periphery of the host cell, where the virus buds and emerges from the host cell. Thus, the virus is now free to travel and infect other cells.

HIV replication may lead to cell death or it may become latent. HIV infection leads to profound pathology, either directly through destruction of CD4+ cells, other immune cells, and neuroglial cells, or indirectly through the secondary effects of CD4+ T-cell dysfunction and resulting immunosuppression.

The HIV infectious process takes three forms:
◆ *immunodeficiency* (opportunistic infections and unusual cancers)
◆ *autoimmunity* (lymphoid interstitial pneumonitis, arthritis, hypergammaglobulinemia, and production of autoimmune antibodies)
◆ *neurologic dysfunction* (AIDS dementia complex, HIV encephalopathy, and peripheral neuropathies).

Signs and symptoms

HIV infection manifests in many ways. After a high-risk exposure and inoculation, the infected person usually experiences a mononucleosis-like syndrome, which may be attributed to flu or another virus and then may remain asymptomatic for years. In this latent stage, the only sign of HIV infection is laboratory evidence of seroconversion.

When signs and symptoms appear, they may take many forms, including:
◆ persistent generalized lymphadenopathy secondary to impaired function of CD4+ cells
◆ nonspecific signs and symptoms, including rapid weight loss; profound, unexplained fatigue; night sweats; fevers related to altered function of CD4+ cells; immunodeficiency; infection of other CD4+ antigen–bearing cells; persistent yeast infections (oral or vaginal); dry cough;

diarrhea lasting more than a week; and pneumonia

◆ neurologic symptoms resulting from HIV encephalopathy and infection of neuroglial cells, including memory loss and depression

◆ opportunistic infection or cancer related to immunodeficiency.

AGE ALERT *In children, HIV infection has a mean incubation time of 17 months. Signs and symptoms resemble those in adults, except for findings related to sexually transmitted diseases. Children have a high incidence of opportunistic bacterial infections: otitis media, sepsis, chronic salivary gland enlargement, lymphoid interstitial pneumonia,* Mycobacterium avium-intracellulare *complex function, and pneumonias, including* Pneumocystis carinii.

Complications
◆ Opportunistic infections
◆ Certain cancers

Diagnosis

Signs and symptoms may occur at any time after infection with HIV, but AIDS is not officially diagnosed until the patient's CD4+ T cell count is less than 200 cells/µl. AIDS is the final stage of HIV infection, and it may take years for HIV infection to reach this stage, even without treatment.

The CDC recommends testing for HIV 1 month after a possible exposure—the approximate length of time before antibodies can be detected in the blood. However, because people produce detectable levels of antibodies at different rates, the time can vary from a few weeks to as long as 35 months, so an HIV-infected person can test negative for HIV antibodies. Antibody tests in neonates may also be unreliable because transferred maternal antibodies persist for up to 10 months, causing a false-positive result.

Standard HIV testing typically consists of the enzyme-linked immunoassay. If the results are positive, the test should be repeated, then confirmed by the Western blot or immunofluorescence assay.

Other blood tests support the diagnosis and are used to evaluate the severity of immunosuppression. They include CD4+ and CD8+ cell (killer T cell) subset counts, erythrocyte sedimentation rate (ESR), complete blood count, serum beta (sub 2) microglobulin, p24 antigen, neopterin levels, and anergy testing.

Many opportunistic infections in AIDS patients are reactivations of previous infections. Therefore, patients may also be tested for syphilis, hepatitis B, tuberculosis, toxoplasmosis, and histoplasmosis.

Treatment

Although no cure for AIDS exists, antiretrovirals are used to control the reproduction of HIV and slow the progression of HIV-related disease. Highly Active Antiretroviral Therapy, commonly referred to as *HAART,* is the recommended treatment for HIV infection. HAART combines three or more antiretrovirals in a daily regimen:

◆ nonnucleoside reverse transcriptase inhibitors to bind to and disable reverse transcriptase proteins

◆ nucleoside analogues or reverse transcriptase inhibitors to halt reproduction of the virus by interfering with viral reverse transcriptase, which impairs HIV's ability to turn its RNA into DNA for insertion into the host cell

◆ protease inhibitors to disable protease, a protein that HIV needs to replicate virons, the viral particles that spread the virus to other cells.

Additional treatment
◆ An immunomodulator to boost the immune system weakened by AIDS and retroviral therapy

◆ Human granulocyte colony-stimulating growth factor to stimulate neutrophil production (retroviral therapy causes anemia, so patients may receive epoetin alfa)

◆ An anti-infective and an antineoplastic to combat opportunistic infections and associated cancers (some prophylactically to help resist opportunistic infections)

◆ Supportive therapy, including nutritional support, fluid and electrolyte replacement therapy, pain relief, and psychological support

Special considerations
◆ Advise health care workers and the public to use precautions in all situations that risk exposure to blood, body fluids, and secretions. Diligent practice of standard precautions can prevent the inadvertent transmission of AIDS and other infectious diseases transmitted by similar routes.

◆ Recognize that a diagnosis of AIDS is profoundly distressing because of the disease's social impact and discouraging prognosis. The patient may lose his job and financial security as well as the support of family and friends. Do your best to help the patient cope with an altered body image, the emotional burden of serious illness, and the threat of death. Encourage and assist the patient in learning about AIDS societies and support programs. (See *Preventing AIDS transmission,* page 442.)

PREVENTION

Preventing AIDS transmission

Health care workers and the public are advised to use precautions in all situations that risk exposure to blood, body fluids, and secretions. These precautions include the following:

- Educate the patient and family, sexual partners, and friends about disease transmission and prevention of extending the disease to others.
- Inform the patient not to donate blood, blood products, organs, tissue, or sperm.
- If the patient uses I. V. drugs, caution him not to share needles.
- Inform the patient that high-risk sexual practices for AIDS transmission are those that exchange body fluids, such as vaginal or anal intercourse without a condom or oral sexual practices.
- Discuss safer sexual practices, such as hugging, petting, mutual masturbation, and protected sexual intercourse. However, emphasize that abstaining is the most protective method of not transmitting the disease.
- Advise female patients of childbearing age to avoid pregnancy. Explain that an infant may become infected before birth, during delivery, or during breast-feeding.

ALLERGIC RHINITIS

Allergic rhinitis is a reaction to airborne (inhaled) allergens. Depending on the allergen, the resulting rhinitis and conjunctivitis may occur seasonally (hay fever) or year-round (perennial allergic rhinitis). Allergic rhinitis is the most common atopic allergic reaction, affecting more than 40 million Americans. It's most prevalent in young children and adolescents but can occur in all age-groups.

AGE ALERT *Onset of allergic rhinitis is common in adolescence, with a mean onset between 8 and 11 years. In 80% of cases, it develops by age 20.*

Causes

Allergic rhinitis is caused by an immunoglobulin (Ig) E–mediated type I hypersensitivity response to an environmental antigen (allergen) in a genetically susceptible person. Common triggers include:

- perennial allergens and irritants
  - animal dander
  - cigarette smoke
  - dust mite excreta, fungal spores, molds
  - feather pillows.
- windborne pollens
  - autumn—ragweed, other weeds
  - spring—alder, birch, cottonwood, elm, maple, oak
  - summer—English plantain, grasses, and sheep sorrel.

Pathophysiology

During primary exposure to an allergen, T cells recognize the foreign allergens and release chemicals that instruct B cells to produce specific antibodies called IgE. IgE antibodies attach themselves to mast cells. Mast cells with attached IgE can remain in the body for years, ready to react when they next encounter the same allergen.

The second time the allergen enters the body, it comes into direct contact with the IgE antibodies attached to the mast cells. This stimulates the mast cells to release chemicals, such as histamine, which initiate a response that causes tightening of the smooth muscles in the airways, dilation of small blood vessels, increased mucus secretion in the nasal cavity and airways, and itching.

Signs and symptoms
Seasonal allergic rhinitis

- Paroxysmal sneezing, profuse watery rhinorrhea, nasal obstruction or congestion, and pruritus of the nose and eyes related to the effects of released chemical mediators, accompanied by:
  - pale, cyanotic, edematous nasal mucosa
  - red, edematous eyelids and conjunctivae
  - excessive lacrimation
  - headache or sinus pain
  - itching in the throat, coughing, sore throat, wheezing, and malaise.

Perennial allergic rhinitis

- Conjunctivitis and other extranasal effects (rare)
- Chronic nasal obstruction (common; in many cases, this obstruction extends to eustachian tube obstruction, particularly in children)

In both types of allergic rhinitis, dark circles may appear under the patient's eyes ("allergic shiners") because of venous congestion in the maxillary sinuses. The severity of signs and symptoms may vary from season to season and from year to year.

Complications
◆ Sinus and middle ear infections due to swelling of the turbinates and mucous membranes
◆ Nasal polyps, which may result from edema and infection and can increase nasal obstruction
◆ Adverse effects from medications, including drowsiness from antihistamines

Diagnosis
Microscopic examination of sputum and nasal secretions reveals large numbers of eosinophils. Blood chemistry shows normal or elevated IgE. A definitive diagnosis is based on the patient's personal and family history of allergies as well as physical findings during a symptomatic phase. Skin testing paired with tested responses to environmental stimuli can pinpoint the responsible allergens given the patient's history.

To distinguish between allergic rhinitis and other disorders of the nasal mucosa, remember these differences:
◆ In chronic vasomotor rhinitis, eye symptoms are absent, rhinorrhea is mucoid, and seasonal variation is absent.
◆ In infectious rhinitis (the common cold), the nasal mucosa is beet red; nasal secretions contain polymorphonuclear, not eosinophilic, exudate; and signs and symptoms include fever and sore throat. This condition isn't a recurrent seasonal phenomenon.
◆ In rhinitis medicamentosa, which results from excessive use of nasal sprays or drops, nasal drainage and mucosal redness and swelling disappear when such medication is withheld.
◆ In children, differential diagnosis should rule out a nasal foreign body, such as a bean or a button.

Treatment
Treatment aims to control symptoms by eliminating the environmental antigen, if possible, and providing drug therapy and immunotherapy.
◆ Antihistamines block histamine effects but commonly produce anticholinergic adverse reactions (sedation, dry mouth, nausea, dizziness, blurred vision, and nervousness). Newer antihistamines, such as fexofenadine (Allegra) and cetirizine (Zyrtec), produce fewer adverse reactions and are less likely to cause sedation.
◆ Inhaled intranasal steroids produce local anti-inflammatory effects with minimal systemic

adverse reactions. These drugs usually aren't effective for acute exacerbations; a nasal decongestant and an oral antihistamine may be needed instead. Advise the patient to use the intranasal steroid regularly, as prescribed, for optimal effectiveness.
◆ Cromolyn (Nasalcrom) may help prevent allergic rhinitis. But this drug may take up to 4 weeks to produce a satisfactory effect and must be taken regularly during allergy season. Leukotriene inhibitors, such as montelukast (Singulair), also help to relieve the symptoms of seasonal allergies.
◆ Long-term management includes immunotherapy, or desensitization with injections of extracted allergens, administered before or during allergy season or perennially. Seasonal allergies require particularly close dosage regulation.

Special considerations
◆ Before desensitization injections, assess the patient's symptom status. Afterward, watch for adverse reactions, including anaphylaxis and severe localized erythema.
◆ Keep epinephrine and emergency resuscitation equipment available, and observe the patient for 30 minutes after the injection. Instruct the patient to call the physician if a delayed reaction should occur.

The following protocol is recommended for allergic rhinitis:
◆ Monitor the patient's compliance with the prescribed drug regimen. Also, carefully note any changes in the control of his symptoms or any signs of drug misuse.
◆ To reduce environmental exposure to airborne allergens, suggest that the patient sleep with the windows closed, avoid the countryside during pollination seasons, use air conditioning to filter allergens and minimize moisture and dust, and eliminate dust-collecting items, such as wool blankets, deep-pile carpets, and heavy drapes, from the home. Recommend covering mattresses and pillows with impermeable casings, washing bed linens in 130° water every 2 weeks, and vacuuming carpets and draperies weekly.
◆ In severe and resistant cases, suggest that the patient consider drastic changes in lifestyle, such as relocation to a pollen-free area either seasonally or year-round.

▌▌▌ **LIFE-THREATENING DISORDER**

ANAPHYLAXIS
Anaphylaxis is an acute, potentially life-threatening type I (immediate) hypersensitivity reaction

marked by the sudden onset of rapidly progressive urticaria (vascular swelling in skin accompanied by itching) and respiratory distress. With prompt recognition and treatment, the prognosis is good. However, a severe reaction may precipitate vascular collapse, leading to systemic shock and, sometimes, death. The reaction typically occurs within minutes but can occur up to 1 hour after reexposure to the antigen.

Causes
The cause of anaphylaxis is usually the ingestion of or other systemic exposure to sensitizing drugs or other substances. Such substances may include:
♦ allergen extracts
♦ diagnostic chemicals, such as radiographic contrast media, sodium dehydrocholate, and sulfobromophthalein sodium
♦ enzymes such as L-asparaginase
♦ food additives containing sulfite
♦ food proteins, such as those in legumes, nuts, berries, seafood, and egg albumin
♦ hormones
♦ insect venom
♦ local anesthetics
♦ penicillin or other antibiotics (induce anaphylaxis in 1 to 4 of every 10,000 patients treated; most likely after parenteral administration or prolonged therapy and in patients with an inherited tendency to food or drug allergy, or atopy)
♦ polysaccharides
♦ salicylates
♦ serums (usually horse serum)
♦ sulfonamides
♦ vaccines.

Pathophysiology
Anaphylaxis requires previous sensitization or exposure to the specific antigen, resulting in immunoglobulin (Ig) E production by plasma cells in the lymph nodes and enhancement by helper T cells. IgE antibodies then bind to membrane receptors on mast cells in connective tissue and to basophils.

On reexposure, the antigen binds to adjacent IgE antibodies or cross-linked IgE receptors, activating a series of cellular reactions that trigger mast cell degranulation. With degranulation, powerful chemical mediators, such as histamine, eosinophil chemotactic factor of anaphylaxis, and platelet-activating factor, are released from the mast cells. IgG or IgM enters into the reaction and activates the complement cascade, leading to the release of the complement fractions.

At the same time, two other chemical mediators, bradykinin and leukotrienes, induce vascular collapse by stimulating contraction of certain groups of smooth muscles and increasing vascular permeability. These substances, together with the other chemical mediators, cause vasodilation, smooth-muscle contraction, enhanced vascular permeability, and increased mucus production. Continued release, along with the spread of these mediators through the body by way of the basophils in the circulation, triggers the systemic responses. Also, increased vascular permeability leads to decreased peripheral resistance and plasma leakage from the circulation to the extravascular tissues. Consequent reduction of blood volume causes hypotension, hypovolemic shock, and cardiac dysfunction. (See *Understanding anaphylaxis*, pages 446 and 447.)

Signs and symptoms
An anaphylactic reaction produces sudden physical distress within seconds or minutes after exposure to an allergen. A delayed or persistent reaction may occur up to 24 hours later. The severity of the reaction is inversely related to the interval between exposure to the allergen and the onset of symptoms. Usually, the first signs and symptoms include:
♦ a feeling of impending doom or fright due to activation of IgE and subsequent release of chemical mediators
♦ sweating due to release of histamine and vasodilation
♦ sneezing, shortness of breath, nasal pruritus, urticaria, and angioedema (swelling of nerves and blood vessels) secondary to histamine release and increased capillary permeability.

Systemic manifestations may include:
♦ hypotension, shock, and sometimes cardiac arrhythmias due to increased vascular permeability and subsequent decrease in peripheral resistance and leakage of plasma fluids
♦ nasal mucosal edema, profuse watery rhinorrhea, itching, nasal congestion, and sudden sneezing attacks due to histamine release, vasodilation, and increased capillary permeability
♦ edema of the upper respiratory tract, resulting in hypopharyngeal and laryngeal obstruction, due to increased capillary permeability and mast cell degranulation
♦ hoarseness, stridor, wheezing, and accessory muscle use secondary to bronchiole smooth-muscle contraction and increased mucus production
♦ severe stomach cramps, nausea, diarrhea, and urinary urgency and incontinence resulting from smooth-muscle contraction of the intestines and bladder.

Complications
- Respiratory obstruction
- Systemic vascular collapse
- Death

Diagnosis
No single diagnostic test can help identify anaphylaxis. Anaphylaxis can be diagnosed by the rapid onset of severe respiratory or cardiovascular symptoms after ingestion or injection of a drug, vaccine, diagnostic agent, food, or food additive, or after an insect sting. If these symptoms occur without a known allergic stimulus, other possible causes of shock (such as an acute myocardial infarction, status asthmaticus, or heart failure) must be ruled out.

These test results may provide some clues to the patient's risk for anaphylaxis:
- skin tests showing hypersensitivity to a specific allergen
- an elevated serum IgE level.

Treatment
- Immediate administration of epinephrine 1:1,000 aqueous solution to reverse bronchoconstriction and cause vasoconstriction — I.M. or subcutaneously if the patient hasn't lost consciousness and is normotensive, or I.V. if the reaction is severe (repeating dosage every 5 to 20 minutes as needed)
- Tracheostomy or endotracheal intubation and mechanical ventilation to maintain a patent airway
- Oxygen therapy to increase tissue perfusion
- A longer-acting epinephrine, a corticosteroid, and diphenhydramine (Benadryl) to reduce the allergic response (long-term management)
- Albuterol mini-nebulizer treatment
- Cimetidine or other histamine-2 blocker
- Aminophylline to reverse bronchospasm
- A volume expander to maintain and restore circulating plasma volume
- An I.V. vasopressor, such as norepinephrine (Levophed) or dopamine (Intropin), to stabilize blood pressure
- Cardiopulmonary resuscitation to treat cardiac arrest

Special considerations
- To prevent anaphylaxis, teach the patient to avoid exposure to known allergens. A person allergic to certain foods or drugs must learn to avoid the offending food or drug in all its forms. A person allergic to insect stings should avoid open fields and wooded areas during the insect season. An anaphylaxis kit (epinephrine, antihistamine, and tourniquet) should also be carried by every patient who has a known severe allergic reaction. In addition, every patient prone to anaphylaxis should wear a medical identification bracelet identifying his allergies.
- If a patient must receive a drug to which he's allergic, prevent a severe reaction by making sure he receives careful desensitization with gradually increasing doses of the antigen or advance administration of a steroid. Of course, a person with a known allergic history should receive a drug with a high anaphylactic potential only after cautious pretesting for sensitivity. Closely monitor the patient during testing, and make sure you have resuscitative equipment and epinephrine ready. When any patient needs a drug with a high anaphylactic potential (particularly a parenteral drug), make sure he receives each dose under close medical observation.
- Closely monitor a patient undergoing diagnostic tests that use radiographic contrast media, such as excretory urography, cardiac catheterization, and angiography.

ATOPIC DERMATITIS
Atopic dermatitis is a chronic skin disorder characterized by superficial skin inflammation and intense itching. Although this disorder may appear at any age, it typically begins during the first year of life, with 90% of cases developing before age 5. It may then subside spontaneously, followed by exacerbations in late childhood, adolescence, or early adulthood. Atopic dermatitis affects less than 1% of the population.

Causes
The exact cause of atopic dermatitis is unknown; however, a genetic predisposition is likely.

Possible contributing factors include:
- chemical irritants
- extremes of temperature and humidity
- food allergy (such as to eggs, milk, or peanuts)
- infection
- psychological stress or strong emotions.

Pathophysiology
The allergic mechanism of hypersensitivity results in a release of inflammatory mediators through sensitized antibodies of the immunoglobulin E (IgE) class. Histamine and other cytokines induce acute inflammation. Abnormally dry skin and a decreased threshold for itching set up the "itch-scratch-itch" cycle, which eventually causes lesions (excoriations, lichenification).

(Text continues on page 448.)

CLOSER LOOK

Understanding anaphylaxis

An anaphylactic reaction requires previous sensitization or exposure to the specific antigen. What happens in anaphylaxis is described here in detail.

1. Response to the antigen

Immunoglobulin (Ig) M and IgG recognize the antigen as a foreign substance and attach to it.

Destruction of the antigen by the complement cascade begins but remains unfinished, either because of insufficient amounts of the protein catalyst or because the antigen inhibits certain complement enzymes. The patient has no signs and symptoms at this stage.

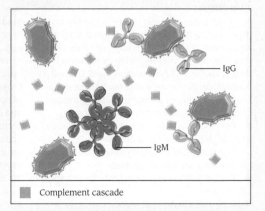

☐ Complement cascade

2. Released chemical mediators

The antigen's continued presence activates IgE on basophils. The activated IgE promotes the release of mediators, including histamine, serotonin, and leukotrienes. The sudden release of histamine causes vasodilation and increases capillary permeability. The patient begins to have signs and symptoms, including sudden nasal congestion, itchy and watery eyes, flushing, sweating, weakness, and anxiety.

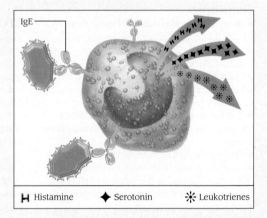

H Histamine   ◆ Serotonin   ※ Leukotrienes

3. Intensified response

The activated IgE also stimulates mast cells in connective tissue along the venule walls to release more histamine and eosinophil chemotactic factor of anaphylaxis (ECF-A). These substances produce disruptive lesions that weaken the venules. Now, red and itchy skin, wheals, and swelling appear, and signs and symptoms worsen.

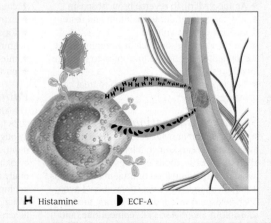

H Histamine   ▶ ECF-A

4. Distress

In the lungs, histamine causes endothelial cells to burst and endothelial tissue to tear away from surrounding tissue. Fluids leak into the alveoli, and leukotrienes prevent the alveoli from expanding, thus reducing pulmonary compliance. Tachypnea, crowing, use of accessory muscles, and cyanosis signal respiratory distress. Resulting neurologic signs and symptoms include changes in level of consciousness, severe anxiety, and, possibly, seizures.

5. Deterioration

Meanwhile, basophils and mast cells begin to release prostaglandins and bradykinin along with histamine and serotonin. These substances increase vascular permeability, causing fluids to leak from the vessels. Shock, confusion, cool and pale skin, generalized edema, tachycardia, and hypotension signal rapid vascular collapse.

6. Failed compensatory mechanisms

Damage to the endothelial cells causes basophils and mast cells to release heparin. Additional substances are also released to neutralize the other mediators. Eosinophils release arylsulfatase B to neutralize the leukotrienes, phospholipase D to neutralize heparin, and cyclic adenosine monophosphate and the prostaglandins E_1 and E_2 to increase the metabolic rate. But these events can't reverse anaphylaxis. Hemorrhage, disseminated intravascular coagulation, and cardiopulmonary arrest result.

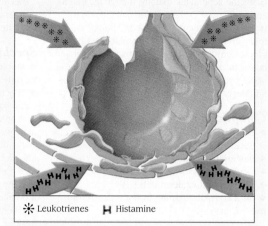

✳ Leukotrienes   H Histamine

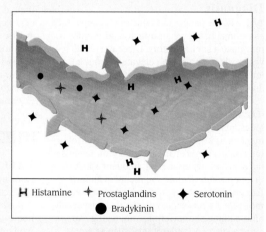

H Histamine   ✛ Prostaglandins   ✦ Serotonin   ⬤ Bradykinin

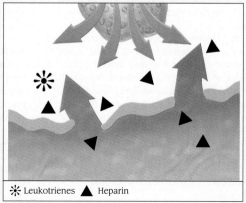

✳ Leukotrienes   ▲ Heparin

Signs and symptoms

Scratching the skin causes vasoconstriction and intensifies pruritus, resulting in erythematous, weeping lesions. Eventually, the lesions become scaly and lichenified. Usually, they're located in areas of flexion and extension, such as on the neck, in the antecubital fossa and popliteal folds, and behind the ears. In children with atopic dermatitis, severe pruritus leads to characteristic pink pigmentation and swelling of the upper eyelid and a double fold under the lower lid (Morgan's line or Dennie's sign).

Complications

◆ Scarring
◆ Severe viral infections
◆ Bacterial and fungal skin infections
◆ Ocular disorders
◆ Allergic contact dermatitis
◆ Stria and skin thinning from corticosteroid use

Diagnosis

Typically, the patient has a history of atopy, such as asthma, hay fever, or urticaria; his family may have a similar history. Laboratory tests reveal eosinophilia and an elevated serum IgE level. A skin biopsy may be performed but isn't always required to make the diagnosis.

Treatment

Measures to ease this chronic disorder include meticulous skin care, environmental control of offending allergens, and drug therapy. Because dry skin aggravates itching, frequent application of a nonirritating topical lubricant is important (creams and ointments work best to seal in moisture; lotions should be avoided), especially after bathing or showering. Minimizing exposure to allergens and irritants, such as wools and harsh detergents, also helps control symptoms.

Drug therapy for atopic dermatitis may involve:
◆ an immunomodulator, such as tacrolimus ointment (Protopic) or pimecrolimus cream (Elidel), is used to control inflammation, reduce immune system reactions, and maintain skin texture; it also can reduce the need for long-term use of a corticosteroid
◆ a topical corticosteroid, applied immediately after bathing for optimal penetration (a systemic corticosteroid should be used only if a topical corticosteroid is ineffective)
◆ an antibiotic to treat secondary skin infections
◆ an antihistamine taken at bedtime to reduce involuntary scratching during sleep and allow for more restful sleep

◆ an immunosuppressant, such as cyclosporine, methotrexate, or azathioprine, may be prescribed for adults who haven't responded to other forms of therapy.

Because this disorder may frustrate the patient and caregiver, counseling may play a role in treatment.

Special considerations

◆ Monitor the patient's compliance with drug therapy.
◆ Teach the patient when and how to apply topical corticosteroids.
◆ Emphasize the importance of regular personal hygiene using only water with little soap.
◆ Be alert for signs and symptoms of secondary infection and teach the patient how to recognize them as well.
◆ If the patient's diet is modified to exclude food allergens, monitor his nutritional status.
◆ Offer support to help the patient and his family cope with this chronic disorder. Tell them that, although treatment won't cure the disorder, it can keep it under control.
◆ Discourage use of laundry additives, such as fragrances and dyes.
◆ Dissuade the patient from scratching during urticaria to help prevent infection.
◆ Encourage the family to contact the National Eczema Association for information.

▌▌▌ LIFE-THREATENING DISORDER

LATEX ALLERGY

Latex allergy is a hypersensitivity reaction to products that contain natural latex, a substance found in an increasing number of products at home and at work, that's derived from the sap of a rubber tree, not synthetic latex. The hypersensitivity reactions can range from local dermatitis to a life-threatening anaphylactic reaction.

Causes

Exposure to latex proteins found in natural rubber products produces a true latex allergy. Those in frequent contact with latex-containing products are at risk for developing a latex allergy. More frequent exposure leads to a higher risk.

The populations at highest risk are:
◆ medical and dental professionals
◆ patients with spina bifida or any condition that requires multiple surgeries involving latex material
◆ workers in latex companies.

Other individuals at risk include patients with a history of:
◆ asthma or other allergies, especially to avocados, bananas, chestnuts, or tropical fruits
◆ frequent intermittent urinary catheterization
◆ multiple intra-abdominal or genitourinary surgeries.

Pathophysiology

A true latex allergy is an immunoglobulin E (IgE)–mediated immediate hypersensitivity reaction. Mast cells release histamine and other secretory products. Vascular permeability increases and vasodilation and bronchoconstriction occur.

Chemical sensitivity dermatitis is a type IV delayed hypersensitivity reaction to the chemicals used in processing rather than the latex itself. In a cell-mediated allergic reaction, sensitized T lymphocytes are triggered, stimulating the proliferation of other lymphocytes and mononuclear cells. This results in tissue inflammation and contact dermatitis.

Signs and symptoms

A patient may have an allergic reaction after contact with latex gloves from irritant contact dermatitis, a hypersensitivity immune system response. With a true latex allergy, the patient shows signs and symptoms of anaphylaxis, including:
◆ hypotension due to vasodilation and increased vascular permeability
◆ tachycardia secondary to hypotension
◆ urticaria and pruritus due to histamine release
◆ difficulty breathing, bronchospasm, wheezing, and stridor secondary to bronchoconstriction
◆ angioedema from increased vascular permeability and loss of water to tissues.

Complications

Like anaphylaxis, a true latex allergy may lead to:
◆ respiratory obstruction
◆ systemic vascular collapse
◆ death.

Diagnosis

Diagnosis of latex allergy is based mainly on history and physical assessment. The following tests are also useful:
◆ Radioallergosorbent test shows specific IgE antibodies to latex. (It's safest for use in patients with history of type I hypersensitivity.)
◆ The patch test results in hives with itching or redness as a positive response.

◆ IgE antibody levels in the blood measure the immune system response to latex.

Treatment

◆ Prevention of exposure, including use of latex-free products to decrease possible exacerbation of hypersensitivity
◆ Drug therapy, such as a corticosteroid, an antihistamine, and a histamine-2 receptor blocker before and after possible exposure to latex to depress immune response and block histamine release

For acute emergency

◆ Immediate administration of epinephrine 1:1,000 aqueous solution to reverse bronchoconstriction and cause vasoconstriction—I.M. or subcutaneously if the patient hasn't lost consciousness and is normotensive, or I.V. if the reaction is severe (repeating the dose every 5 to 20 minutes as needed)
◆ Tracheostomy or endotracheal intubation and mechanical ventilation to maintain a patent airway
◆ Oxygen therapy to increase tissue perfusion
◆ A volume expander to maintain and restore circulating plasma volume
◆ An I.V. vasopressor, such as norepinephrine (Levophed) or dopamine (Intropin), to stabilize blood pressure
◆ Cardiopulmonary resuscitation to treat cardiac arrest
◆ A longer-acting epinephrine, a corticosteroid, and diphenhydramine (Benadryl) to reduce the allergic response (long-term management)
◆ A drug to reverse bronchospasm, including aminophylline and albuterol

Special considerations

◆ Make sure items that aren't available latex-free, such as stethoscopes and blood pressure cuffs, are wrapped in cloth before they come in contact with a hypersensitive patient's skin.
◆ Place the patient in a private room or with another patient who requires a latex-free environment.
◆ When adding medication to an I.V. bag, inject the drug through the spike port, not the rubber latex port.
◆ Urge the patient to wear an identification tag mentioning his latex allergy.
◆ Teach the patient and family members how to use an epinephrine autoinjector.
◆ Teach the patient to be aware of all latex-containing products and to use vinyl or silicone products instead. Advise him that Mylar balloons don't contain latex.

LUPUS ERYTHEMATOSUS

Lupus erythematosus is a chronic inflammatory disorder of the connective tissues that appears in two forms: discoid lupus erythematosus, which affects only the skin, and systemic lupus erythematosus (SLE), which affects multiple organ systems as well as the skin and can be fatal. SLE is characterized by recurring remissions and exacerbations, which are especially common during spring and summer.

The prognosis improves with early detection and treatment but remains poor for patients who develop cardiovascular, renal, or neurologic complications, or severe bacterial infections.

The Lupus Foundation of America estimates that between 1.5 and 2 million Americans have a form of lupus, with women making up more than 90% of that population. It's more common in Blacks, Hispanics, Asians, and Native Americans than in Whites.

Causes

The exact cause of SLE remains a mystery, but available evidence points to interrelated immunologic, environmental, hormonal, and genetic factors. These may include:
♦ abnormal estrogen metabolism
♦ exposure to sunlight or ultraviolet light
♦ immunization
♦ physical or mental stress
♦ pregnancy
♦ streptococcal or viral infection
♦ treatment with certain drugs, such as anticonvulsants, hydralazine (Apresoline), procainamide (Pronestyl) or, less commonly, hormonal contraceptives, penicillins, and sulfa drugs.

GENETIC LINK Researchers are attempting to identify genes that play a role in the development of lupus. They suspect that a genetic defect in a cellular process called apoptosis is present in people with lupus. Apoptosis allows the body to eliminate cells that have fulfilled their function and need to be replaced. If the apoptosis process is impaired, harmful cells may linger, causing damage to the body's own tissue.

Researchers are also studying genes for complement, a series of proteins in the blood that play an important role in the immune system. Complement acts as a backup for antibodies, helping them destroy foreign substances that invade the body. A decrease in the amount of complement makes the body less able to fight or destroy foreign substances. If these substances aren't removed from the body, the immune system may become overactive and make autoantibodies.

Pathophysiology

Autoimmunity is believed to be the prime mechanism involved with SLE. The body produces antibodies, such as antinuclear antibodies (ANAs), against components of its own cells and immune complex disease follows. Patients with SLE may produce antibodies against many different tissue components, such as red blood cells (RBCs), neutrophils, platelets, lymphocytes, or almost any organ or tissue in the body. (See *How SLE affects the body*.)

Signs and symptoms

The onset of SLE may be acute or insidious and produces no characteristic clinical pattern. (See *Signs of SLE,* page 452.)

Although SLE may involve any organ system, signs and symptoms all relate to tissue injury and subsequent inflammation and necrosis resulting from the invasion by immune complexes. They commonly include:
♦ fever greater than 100° F (38° C)
♦ weight loss
♦ malaise
♦ fatigue
♦ rashes
♦ polyarthralgia.

Additional signs and symptoms may include:
♦ joint involvement, similar to rheumatoid arthritis (although the arthritis of lupus is usually nonerosive)
♦ skin lesions, most commonly an erythematous rash in areas exposed to light (the classic butterfly rash over the nose and cheeks occurs in less than 50% of the patients) or a scaly, papular rash (mimics psoriasis), especially in sun-exposed areas
♦ vasculitis (especially in the digits), possibly leading to infarctive lesions, necrotic leg ulcers, or digital gangrene
♦ Raynaud's phenomenon (about 20% of patients)
♦ patchy alopecia and painless ulcers of the mucous membranes
♦ pulmonary abnormalities, such as pleurisy, pleural effusions, pneumonitis, pulmonary hypertension and, rarely, pulmonary hemorrhage
♦ cardiac involvement, such as pericarditis, myocarditis, endocarditis, and early coronary atherosclerosis
♦ microscopic hematuria, pyuria, and urine sediment with cellular casts due to glomerulonephritis, possibly progressing to kidney failure (particularly when untreated)
♦ urinary tract infections, possibly due to heightened susceptibility to infection
♦ seizure disorders and mental dysfunction
♦ central nervous system (CNS) involvement, such as emotional instability, psychosis, and organic brain syndrome
♦ headaches, irritability, and depression (common).

MULTISYSTEM DISORDER
How SLE affects the body

In the autoimmune disorder systemic lupus erythematosus (SLE), the body produces antibodies against its own cells. The formed antigen-antibody complexes can suppress the body's normal immunity and damage tissues, affecting most major body systems. Because SLE affects multiple systems, multidisciplinary care is needed.

Cardiopulmonary system
◆ Immune complexes may be deposited in the vascular tissue (of the heart and lungs), leading to pericarditis, myocarditis, valvular disease, pleural effusions, pleuritis, pneumonitis, chronic interstitial lung disease, and pulmonary embolism.
◆ Raynaud's phenomenon may occur because of vasculitis.

Genitourinary system
◆ Immune complexes may be deposited in the renal tissue, leading to glomerulonephritis, interstitial nephritis, nephrotic syndrome and, possibly, renal failure.

Hematologic system
◆ The development of autoantibodies against blood cell components—such as the red blood cells, white blood cells, platelets, and lymphocytes—and subsequent deposition of immune complexes can affect overall blood cell function, causing anemia, leukopenia, thrombocytopenia, and lymphopenia.

Integumentary system
◆ As autoantibodies are produced and immune complexes are formed, they're deposited in the layers of the skin, causing an inflammatory response and tissue injury, resulting in the classic butterfly rash and lesions, such as hives and cyanotic discolorations.
◆ Deposition of the immune complexes may cause erythema of the nailbeds, splinter hemorrhages, and hair loss.

Musculoskeletal system
◆ Deposition of immune complexes into joint tissue may cause arthritis and arthralgias. As the disease progresses, tendons, ligaments, and joint capsules may become affected, leading to deformity and loss of function.

Neurologic system
◆ SLE may cause acute vasculitis in the cerebral blood vessels, leading to impaired cerebral blood flow and, ultimately, hemorrhage or stroke.
◆ Antibodies may be developed to specifically attack neuronal cells and phospholipids, damaging blood vessels and causing cerebral blood clots.
◆ Seizure disorders, mental dysfunction (confusion, decreased cognition, and altered levels of consciousness), and psychosis (emotional lability involving extremes of euphoria and depression) may occur.

Collaborative management
Because SLE affects multiple body systems, a multidisciplinary approach to care is essential. Immunologists typically are consulted to address the underlying problems and manage drug therapy. Cardiopulmonary and renal specialists may be involved to minimize the effects on these body systems. Orthopedic specialists may be involved to assist with joint function. Neurologists may be consulted to assist with neurologic changes. Respiratory therapy may be involved to assist with measures to improve respiratory muscle function and ventilation. Physical therapists may be consulted for assistance with exercises, muscle strengthening, and assistive devices for ambulation. Occupational therapists can help with adaptations needed for activities of daily living. Because SLE involves remissions and exacerbations, social services may be necessary to assist the patient with referrals to community support groups, financial concerns, and home care issues and equipment.

Constitutional signs and symptoms of SLE include:
◆ aching, malaise, fatigue
◆ low-grade or spiking fever and chills
◆ anorexia and weight loss
◆ lymph node enlargement (diffuse or local, and nontender)
◆ abdominal pain
◆ nausea, vomiting, diarrhea, constipation
◆ irregular menstrual periods or amenorrhea during the active phase of SLE.

Complications
◆ Concomitant infections
◆ Urinary tract infections

Signs of SLE

Diagnosing systemic lupus erythematosus (SLE) is difficult because it often mimics other diseases; symptoms may be vague and vary greatly among patients.

For these reasons, the American Rheumatism Association issued a list of criteria for classifying SLE to be used primarily for consistency in epidemiologic surveys. Usually, four or more of these signs are present at some time during the course of SLE:
- malar or discoid rash
- photosensitivity
- oral or nasopharyngeal ulcerations
- nonerosive arthritis (of two or more peripheral joints)
- pleuritis or pericarditis
- profuse proteinuria (more than 0.5 g/day) or excessive cellular casts in the urine
- seizures or psychoses
- hemolytic anemia, leukopenia, lymphopenia, or thrombocytopenia
- anti–double-stranded deoxyribonucleic acid or positive findings of antiphospholipid antibodies (elevated immunoglobulin [Ig] G or IgM anticardiolipin antibodies, positive test result for lupus anticoagulant, or false-positive serologic test results for syphilis)
- abnormal antinuclear antibody titer.

- Renal failure
- Osteonecrosis of hip from long-term steroid use

Diagnosis

Currently there's no specific laboratory test for SLE.

Test results that may indicate SLE include:
- a complete blood count with differential showing anemia and a decreased white blood cell (WBC) count
- a decreased platelet count
- an elevated erythrocyte sedimentation rate
- serum electrophoresis showing hypergammaglobulinemia.

Other diagnostic tests include:
- ANA and lupus erythematosus cell tests showing positive results in active SLE
- anti–double-stranded deoxyribonucleic acid antibody (anti-dsDNA); most specific test for SLE, correlates with disease activity, especially renal involvement, and helps monitor response to therapy; may be low or absent if the disease is in remission
- urine studies possibly showing RBCs and WBCs, urine casts and sediment, and significant protein loss (more than 0.5 g/24 hours)

- serum complement blood studies showing decreased serum complement (C3 and C4) levels indicating active disease
- chest X-ray showing pleurisy or lupus pneumonitis
- electrocardiography showing a conduction defect with cardiac involvement or pericarditis
- kidney biopsy to determine disease stage and extent of renal involvement
- lupus anticoagulant and anticardiolipin tests showing positive results in patients prone to antiphospholipid syndrome of thrombosis, abortion, and thrombocytopenia.

Treatment

- A nonsteroidal anti-inflammatory, including aspirin, to decrease inflammation and control arthritis symptoms
- An antimalarial, such as hydroxychloroquine, to treat fatigue, joint pain, skin rashes, and inflammation of the lungs by suppressing parts of the immune system
- A topical corticosteroid cream, such as hydrocortisone buteprate (Acticort) or triamcinolone (Aristocort), for acute skin lesions
- An intralesional corticosteroid to treat refractory skin lesions
- A systemic corticosteroid to reduce systemic symptoms of SLE or to treat acute generalized exacerbations or serious disease related to vital organ systems, such as pleuritis, pericarditis, lupus nephritis, vasculitis, and CNS involvement
- Dialysis or kidney transplant for renal failure
- An antihypertensive and dietary changes to minimize effects of renal involvement

Special considerations

Careful assessment, supportive measures, emotional support, and patient education are all important parts of the care plan for patients with SLE.
- Watch for such constitutional signs and symptoms as joint pain or stiffness, weakness, fever, fatigue, and chills. Observe for dyspnea, chest pain, and edema of the extremities. Note the size, type, and location of skin lesions. Check urine for hematuria, scalp for hair loss, and skin and mucous membranes for petechiae, bleeding, ulceration, pallor, and bruising.
- Provide a balanced diet. Renal involvement may mandate a low-sodium, low-protein diet.
- Urge the patient to get plenty of rest. Schedule diagnostic tests and procedures to allow adequate rest. Explain all tests and procedures. Tell the patient that several blood samples are

needed initially, then periodically, to monitor progress.

♦ Apply heat packs to relieve joint pain and stiffness. Encourage regular exercise to maintain full range of motion (ROM) and prevent contractures. Teach ROM exercises as well as body alignment and postural techniques. Arrange for physical therapy and occupational counseling as appropriate.

♦ Explain the expected benefit of prescribed medications. Watch for adverse reactions, especially when the patient is taking high doses of a corticosteroid.

♦ Advise the patient receiving cyclophosphamide to maintain adequate hydration. If prescribed, give mesna to prevent hemorrhagic cystitis and ondansetron to prevent nausea and vomiting.

♦ Monitor vital signs, intake and output, weight, and laboratory test results. Check pulse rates and observe for orthopnea. Check stools and GI secretions for blood.

♦ Observe the patient for hypertension, weight gain, and other signs of renal involvement.

♦ Assess for such signs of neurologic damage as personality change, paranoid or psychotic behavior, ptosis, or diplopia. Take seizure precautions. If Raynaud's phenomenon is present, warm and protect the patient's hands and feet.

♦ Offer cosmetic tips, such as suggesting the use of hypoallergenic makeup, and refer the patient to a hairdresser who specializes in scalp disorders.

♦ Advise the patient to purchase medications in quantity, if possible. Warn against "miracle" drugs for relief of arthritis symptoms.

♦ Teach about lupus flares, which follow a period of remission. Triggers may include sun exposure, infection, or pregnancy, but most often no specific incident can be identified. Explain that not smoking, taking medication as prescribed, reducing risks for infections, and getting plenty of rest can minimize the risk of flares occurring.

♦ Refer the patient to the Lupus Foundation of America and the Arthritis Foundation as necessary.

RHEUMATOID ARTHRITIS

Rheumatoid arthritis (RA) is a chronic, systemic inflammatory disease that primarily attacks peripheral joints and the surrounding muscles, tendons, ligaments, and blood vessels. Partial remissions and unpredictable exacerbations mark the course of this potentially crippling disease. RA strikes three times more women than men.

RA occurs worldwide, affecting more than 2.1 million people in the United States alone.

AGE ALERT *RA can occur at any age. The peak onset period for women is between ages 40 and 60.*

RA usually requires lifelong treatment and, sometimes, surgery. (See *Drug therapy for RA,* pages 454 and 455.) In most patients, it follows an intermittent course and allows normal activity between flare-ups, although 10% of affected people have total disability from severe joint deformity, associated extra-articular symptoms, such as vasculitis, or both. The prognosis worsens with the development of nodules, vasculitis, and high titers of rheumatoid factor (RF).

Causes

The cause of the chronic inflammation characteristic of RA isn't known. Possible causes include:

♦ abnormal immune activation (occurring in a genetically susceptible individual) leading to inflammation, complement activation, and cell proliferation within joints and tendon sheaths

♦ development of an immunoglobulin (Ig) M antibody against the body's own IgG (also called rheumatoid factor); RF aggregates into complexes, generates inflammation, causing eventual cartilage damage and triggering other immune responses

♦ infection (viral or bacterial), hormone action, or lifestyle factors influencing onset.

GENETIC LINK *Researchers suspect that viruses may trigger RA in some people who have an inherited tendency for the disease. Many people with RA have a genetic marker called HLA-DR4. Researchers also suspect that other genes may be implicated in RA.*

Pathophysiology

If not arrested, the inflammatory process in the joints occurs in four stages:

♦ synovitis develops from congestion and edema of the synovial membrane and joint capsule. Infiltration by lymphocytes, macrophages, and neutrophils continues the local inflammatory response. These cells, as well as fibroblast-like synovial cells, produce enzymes that help to degrade bone and cartilage

♦ pannus—thickened layers of granulation tissue—covers and invades cartilage and eventually destroys the joint capsule and bone

♦ fibrous ankylosis—fibrous invasion of the pannus and scar formation—occludes the joint space; bone atrophy and misalignment causing visible deformities and disrupting the articulation of opposing bones, which cause muscle atrophy and imbalance and, possibly, partial dislocations (subluxations)

Drug therapy for RA

This flowchart identifies the major pathophysiologic events in rheumatoid arthritis (RA) and shows where in this chain of events the major drug therapies act to control the disease.

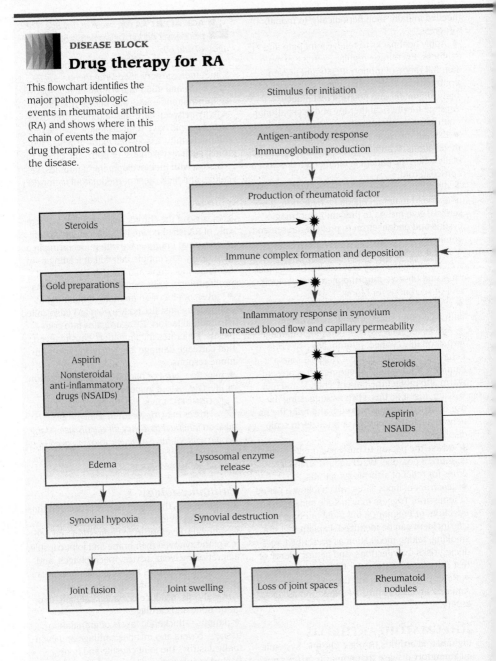

Key: ✳ = treatment

◆ fibrous tissue calcifies, resulting in bony ankylosis and total immobility (See *The effects of rheumatoid arthritis on certain joints,* page 456.)

Signs and symptoms

RA usually develops insidiously and initially causes nonspecific signs and symptoms, most likely related to the initial inflammatory reactions before the inflammation of the synovium, including:
◆ fatigue
◆ malaise
◆ loss of appetite, anorexia, and weight loss
◆ persistent low-grade fever
◆ lymphadenopathy
◆ vague articular symptoms
◆ morning stiffness that lasts more than an hour.

As the disease progresses, signs and symptoms include:
◆ specific localized, bilateral, and symmetric articular symptoms, commonly in the fingers at the proximal interphalangeal, metacarpophalangeal, and metatarsophalangeal joints, possibly extending to the wrists, knees, elbows, and ankles from inflammation of the synovium
◆ stiffening of affected joints after inactivity, especially on arising in the morning, due to progressive synovial inflammation and destruction
◆ spindle-shaped fingers from marked edema and congestion in the joints
◆ joint pain and tenderness, at first only with movement but eventually even at rest, due to prostaglandin release, edema, and synovial inflammation and destruction
◆ feeling of warmth at the joints due to inflammation
◆ diminished joint function and deformities as synovial destruction continues
◆ flexion deformities or hyperextension of metacarpophalangeal joints, subluxation of the wrist, and stretching of tendons pulling the fingers to the ulnar side (ulnar drift), or characteristic swan-neck or boutonnière deformity from joint swelling and loss of joint space
◆ carpal tunnel syndrome from synovial pressure on the median nerve causing paresthesia in the fingers.

Extra-articular findings may include:
◆ gradual appearance of rheumatoid nodules—subcutaneous, round or oval, nontender masses (20% of RF-positive patients), usually on elbows, hands, or Achilles tendon from destruction of the synovium
◆ vasculitis possibly leading to skin lesions, leg ulcers, and multiple systemic complications from infiltration of immune complexes and

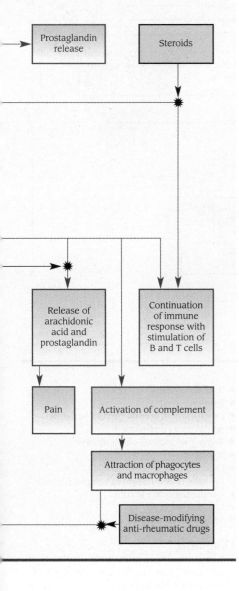

Prostaglandin release

Steroids

Release of arachidonic acid and prostaglandin

Continuation of immune response with stimulation of B and T cells

Pain

Activation of complement

Attraction of phagocytes and macrophages

Disease-modifying anti-rheumatic drugs

CLOSER LOOK

The effects of rheumatoid arthritis on certain joints

Many joints can be affected by RA, including the knee, hand and wrist, and hip.

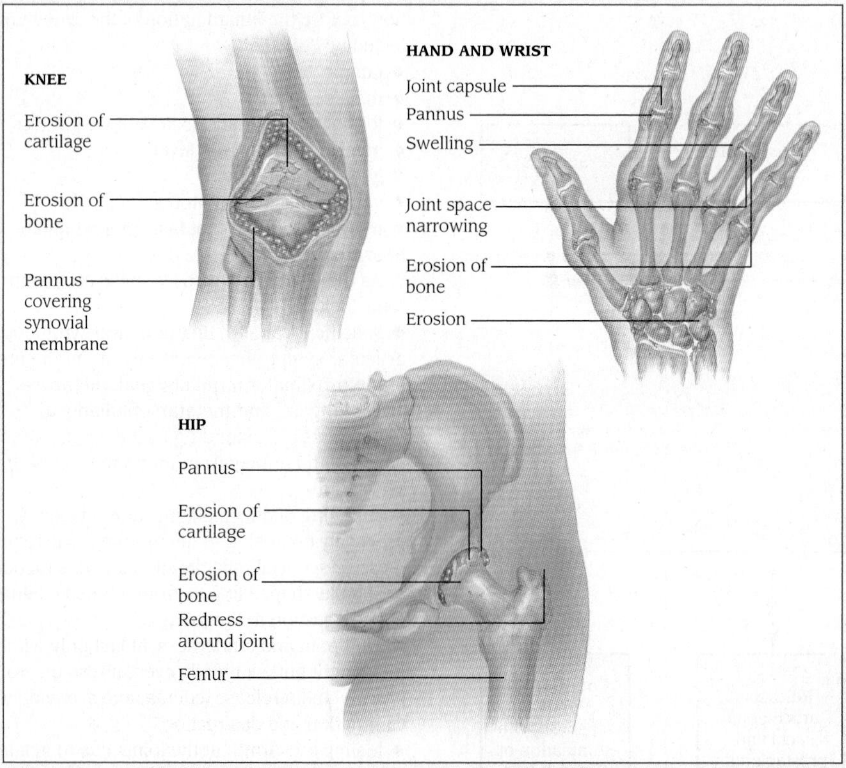

KNEE

Erosion of cartilage

Erosion of bone

Pannus covering synovial membrane

HAND AND WRIST

Joint capsule

Pannus

Swelling

Joint space narrowing

Erosion of bone

Erosion

HIP

Pannus

Erosion of cartilage

Erosion of bone

Redness around joint

Femur

subsequent tissue damage and necrosis in the vasculature
◆ pericarditis, pulmonary nodules or fibrosis, pleuritis, or inflammation of the sclera and overlying tissues of the eye from immune complex invasion and subsequent tissue damage and necrosis
◆ peripheral neuropathy with numbness or tingling in the feet or weakness and loss of sensation in the fingers from infiltration of the nerve fibers
◆ stiff, weak, or painful muscles secondary to limited mobility and decreased use.

Complications
◆ Fibrosis and ankylosis
◆ Soft tissue contractures
◆ Pain

◆ Joint deformities
◆ Sjögren's syndrome
◆ Destruction of second cervical vertebra
◆ Spinal cord compression
◆ Temporomandibular joint disease
◆ Infection
◆ Osteoporosis
◆ Myositis (inflammation of voluntary muscles)
◆ Cardiopulmonary lesions
◆ Lymphadenopathy
◆ Peripheral neuritis

Diagnosis
◆ X-rays show bone demineralization and soft-tissue swelling (in early stages), cartilage loss and narrowed joint spaces, and, finally, cartilage and bone destruction and erosion, subluxations, and deformities (in later stages).

◆ Magnetic resonance imaging (MRI) and joint ultrasounds detect early inflammation before X-rays show damage. MRI is particularly useful in identifying synovitis.

◆ RF titer is positive in 75% to 80% of patients (titer of 1:160 or higher).

◆ Synovial fluid analysis shows increased volume and turbidity but decreased viscosity and an elevated white blood cell count (usually greater than 10,000/µl).

◆ Serum protein electrophoresis may show an elevated serum globulin level.

◆ Erythrocyte sedimentation rate and C-reactive protein level show elevations in 85% to 90% of patients, which may be useful to monitor response to therapy because elevation typically parallels disease activity.

◆ Complete blood count may show moderate anemia, slight leukocytosis, and slight thrombocytosis.

Treatment

Treatment of RA involves pharmacologic therapy and supportive measures, including:

◆ a salicylate, particularly aspirin (mainstay of therapy), to decrease inflammation and relieve joint pain

◆ a nonsteroidal anti-inflammatory drug (NSAID), such as aspirin, ibuprofen (Motrin), or indomethacin (Indocin), to relieve inflammation and pain

◆ an analgesic, such as acetaminophen (Tylenol) or transdermal fentanyl (Duragesic), to relieve pain

◆ a glucocorticoid, such as prednisone, to reduce inflammation and prevent joint damage

◆ a disease-modifying anti-rheumatic drug (also known as a DMARD) — such as methotrexate (Folex), gold salts, sulfasalazine (Azulfidine), azathioprine (Imuran), or hydroxychloroquine (Plaquenil) — to promote disease remission and prevent progressive joint destruction (these drugs are used in combination with NSAIDs and prednisone)

◆ leflunomide (Arava) and a biologic response modifier (such as etanercept [Enbrel], infliximab [Remicade], adaliumumab [Humira], or anakinra [Kineret]) to intercept proteins called cytokines that contribute to inflammation

◆ protein-A immunoadsorption therapy — performed weekly for 12 weeks for patients with moderate to severe RA who haven't responded well to drug therapy — which filters blood to remove antibodies and immune complexes that promote inflammation

◆ synovectomy (removal of destructive, proliferating synovium, usually in the wrists, knees, and fingers) to possibly halt or delay the course of the disease

◆ osteotomy (cutting of bone or excision of a wedge of bone) to realign joint surfaces and redistribute stress

◆ tendon transfers to prevent deformities or relieve contractures

◆ joint reconstruction or total joint arthroplasty, including metatarsal head and distal ulnar resectional arthroplasty, insertion of a Silastic prosthesis between metacarpophalangeal and proximal interphalangeal joints (severe disease)

◆ arthrodesis (joint fusion) for stability and relief from pain (sacrifices joint mobility).

Special considerations

◆ Assess all joints carefully. Look for deformities, contractures, immobility, and inability to perform everyday activities.

◆ Monitor vital signs, and note weight changes, sensory disturbances, and level of pain. Administer an analgesic, as ordered, and watch for adverse reactions.

◆ Provide meticulous skin care. Check for rheumatoid nodules as well as pressure ulcers and breakdowns due to immobility, vascular impairment, corticosteroid treatment, or improper splinting. Use lotion or cleansing oil, not soap, for dry skin.

◆ Explain all diagnostic tests and procedures. Tell the patient to expect multiple blood samples to allow firm diagnosis and accurate monitoring of therapy.

◆ Monitor the duration, not the intensity, of morning stiffness because duration more accurately reflects the severity of the disease. Encourage the patient to take hot showers or baths at bedtime or in the morning to reduce the need for pain medication.

◆ Apply splints carefully and correctly. Observe for pressure ulcers if the patient is in traction or wearing splints.

◆ Explain the nature of the disease. Make sure the patient and his family understand that RA is a chronic disease that requires major changes in lifestyle. Emphasize that there are no miracle cures, despite claims to the contrary.

◆ Encourage a balanced diet, but make sure the patient understands that special diets won't cure RA. Stress the need for weight control because obesity adds further stress to joints.

◆ Urge the patient to perform activities of daily living, such as dressing and feeding himself (supply easy-to-open cartons, lightweight cups, and unpackaged silverware). Allow the patient enough time to calmly perform these tasks.

◆ Provide emotional support. Remember that the patient with chronic illness easily becomes depressed, discouraged, and irritable. Encourage the patient to discuss his fears concerning dependency, sexuality, body image, and self-esteem. Refer him to an appropriate social service agency as needed.

◆ Discuss sexual aids: alternative positions, pain medication, and moist heat to increase mobility.

◆ Before discharge, make sure the patient knows how and when to take prescribed medication and how to recognize adverse reactions.

◆ Teach the patient how to stand, walk, and sit correctly. Tell him to sit in chairs with high seats and armrests; he'll find it easier to get up from a chair if his knees are lower than his hips. If he doesn't own a chair with a high seat, recommend putting blocks of wood under the legs of a favorite chair. Suggest an elevated toilet seat.

◆ Instruct the patient to pace daily activities, resting for 5 to 10 minutes out of each hour and alternating sitting and standing tasks. Adequate sleep is important and so is correct sleeping posture. He should sleep on his back on a firm mattress and should avoid placing a pillow under his knees, which encourages flexion deformity.

◆ Teach him to avoid putting undue stress on joints by using the largest joint available for a given task, avoiding positions of flexion and promoting positions of extension, holding objects parallel to the knuckles as briefly as possible, always using his hands toward the center of his body, sliding — not lifting — objects whenever possible, and supporting weak or painful joints as much as possible. Enlist the aid of the occupational therapist to teach how to simplify activities and protect arthritic joints. Stress the importance of shoes with proper support.

◆ Suggest dressing aids — long-handled shoehorn, reacher, elastic shoelaces, zipper-pull, and buttonhook — and helpful household items, such as easy-to-open drawers, handheld shower nozzle, handrails, and grab bars. The patient who has trouble maneuvering fingers into gloves should wear mittens. Tell him to dress while in a sitting position as often as possible.

◆ Refer the patient to the Arthritis Foundation for more information on coping with the disease.

URTICARIA AND ANGIOEDEMA

Urticaria, commonly known as *hives*, is an episodic, usually self-limited skin reaction characterized by local dermal wheals surrounded by an erythematous flare. Angioedema is a subcutaneous and dermal eruption that produces deeper, larger wheals (usually on the hands, feet, lips, genitals, and eyelids) and a more diffuse swelling of loose subcutaneous tissue. Urticaria and angioedema can occur simultaneously, but angioedema may last longer.

Urticaria and angioedema are common allergic reactions that may occur in 20% of the general population.

Causes

◆ Allergy to drugs, foods, insect stings and, occasionally, inhalant allergens (animal dander and cosmetics) that provoke an immunoglobulin (Ig) E–mediated response to protein allergens (although certain drugs may cause urticaria without an IgE response)

◆ External physical stimuli, such as cold (usually in young adults), heat, sunlight, or water

Pathophysiology

Several mechanisms and underlying disorders may provoke urticaria and angioedema, including IgE-induced release of mediators from cutaneous mast cells; binding of IgG or IgM to an antigen, resulting in complement activation; and such disorders as localized or secondary infections (such as respiratory tract infection), neoplastic diseases (for example, Hodgkin's disease), connective tissue diseases (for example, systemic lupus erythematosus), collagen vascular diseases, and psychogenic diseases.

When urticaria and angioedema are part of an anaphylactic reaction, they almost always persist long after the systemic response has subsided. This occurs because circulation to the skin is the last to be restored after an allergic reaction, which results in slow histamine reabsorption at the reaction site.

Nonallergic urticaria and angioedema are probably also related to histamine release by some still-unknown mechanism. Dermographism urticaria, which develops after stroking or scratching the skin, occurs in as much as 20% of the population. Such urticaria develops with varying pressure, usually under tight clothing, and is aggravated by scratching.

Signs and symptoms

The characteristic features of urticaria are distinct, raised, evanescent dermal wheals surrounded by an erythematous flare. These lesions may vary in size. In cholinergic urticaria, the wheals may be tiny and blanched, surrounded by erythematous flares.

Angioedema characteristically produces nonpitted swelling of deep subcutaneous tissue, usually on the eyelids, lips, genitalia, and mucous membranes. These swellings don't usually itch but may burn and tingle.

Complications
◆ Skin abrasion and secondary infection due to scratching
◆ Life-threatening laryngeal edema, if angioedema involves the upper respiratory tract
◆ Severe abdominal colic, with possible GI involvement that can lead to surgery

Diagnosis
An accurate patient history can help determine the cause of urticaria. Such a history should include:
◆ drug history, including over-the-counter preparations (vitamins, aspirin, and antacids)
◆ frequent ingestion of highly allergenic foods (strawberries, milk products, fish, eggs, wheat, nuts)
◆ environmental influences (pets, carpet, clothing, soap, inhalants, cosmetics, hair dye, and insect bites and stings).

Diagnosis also requires physical assessment to rule out similar conditions as well as a complete blood count, urinalysis, erythrocyte sedimentation rate, and a chest X-ray to rule out inflammatory infections. Skin testing, an elimination diet, and a food diary (recording time and amount of food eaten and circumstances) can pinpoint provoking allergens. The food diary may also suggest other allergies. For instance, a patient allergic to fish may also be allergic to iodine contrast materials.

Recurrent angioedema without urticaria, along with a familial history, points to hereditary angioedema. (See *Hereditary angioedema*.) Decreased serum levels of complement 4 and complement 1 esterase inhibitors confirm this diagnosis.

Treatment
Treatment aims to prevent or limit contact with triggering factors or, if this is impossible, to desensitize the patient to them and to relieve symptoms. During desensitization, progressively larger doses of specific antigens (determined by skin testing) are injected intradermally.

Hydroxyzine or another antihistamine can ease itching and swelling in every kind of urticaria. Corticosteroid therapy may be necessary for some patients.

Special considerations
◆ Once the triggering stimulus has been removed, urticaria usually subsides in a few days — except for drug reactions, which may persist as long as the drug is in the bloodstream.
◆ Inform patients receiving an antihistamine of the possibility of drowsiness.

Hereditary angioedema

A nonallergenic type of angioedema, hereditary angioedema results from an autosomal dominant trait — a hereditary deficiency of an alpha globulin, the normal inhibitor of C1 esterase (a component of the complement system). This deficiency allows uninhibited C1 esterase release, resulting in the vascular changes common to angioedema.

The clinical effects of hereditary angioedema usually appear in childhood with recurrent episodes of subcutaneous or submucosal edema at irregular intervals of weeks, months, or years — in many cases after trauma or stress. Hereditary angioedema is unifocal, without urticarial pruritus, but associated with recurrent edema of the skin and mucosa (especially of the GI and respiratory tracts). GI tract involvement may cause nausea, vomiting, and severe abdominal pain. Laryngeal angioedema may cause fatal airway obstruction.

Treatment of acute hereditary angioedema may require an androgen, such as danazol. Tracheotomy may be necessary to relieve airway obstruction resulting from laryngeal angioedema.

◆ Inspect the skin for signs of secondary infection caused by scratching.
◆ Instruct the patient to keep his fingernails short to avoid abrading the skin when scratching.

VASCULITIS
Vasculitis includes a broad spectrum of disorders characterized by inflammation and necrosis of blood vessels. Its clinical effects depend on the vessels involved and reflect tissue ischemia caused by blood flow obstruction. The prognosis also varies. For example, hypersensitivity vasculitis is usually a benign disorder limited to the skin, but more extensive polyarteritis nodosa can be rapidly fatal. Vasculitis can occur at any age, except for mucocutaneous lymph node syndrome, which occurs only during childhood. Vasculitis may be a primary disorder or occur secondary to other disorders, such as rheumatoid arthritis or systemic lupus erythematosus.

Causes
Vasculitis has been associated with a history of serious infectious disease, such as hepatitis B or bacterial endocarditis, and high-dose antibiotic

Types of vasculitis

Type	Vessels involved	Signs and symptoms	Diagnosis
Allergic granulomatosis angiitis (Churg-Strauss syndrome)	Small to medium arteries (including arterioles, capillaries, and venules), mainly of the lungs but also other organs	Resemblance to polyarteritis nodosa with hallmark of severe pulmonary involvement; may cause fever, weight loss, fatigue, cough, shortness of breath, chest pain, diarrhea, skin nodules on extremities, numbness, weakess, and seizures and confusion (if brain is affected)	History of asthma; eosinophilia; tissue biopsy showing granulomatous inflammation with eosinophilic infiltration
Behçet's syndrome	Small vessels, primarily of the mouth and genitalia, but also of the eyes, skin, joints, GI tract, and central nervous system	Recurrent oral ulcers, eye lesions, genital lesions, cutaneous lesions, and uveitis	History of symptoms
Henoch-Schönlein purpura	Any blood vessel in the skin	Red to purple papule skin lesions, infarction, joint pain, numbness, weakness, fever, fatigue, dysmenorrhea, pyrosis, dysphonia, and dysphagia	History of symptoms; skin biopsy showing vasculitis, elevated IgA levels, and elevated erythrocyte sedimentation rate (ESR)
Hypersensitivity vasculitis	Small vessels, especially of the skin	Palpable purpura, papules, nodules, vesicles, bullae, ulcers, or chronic or recurrent urticaria	History of exposure to antigen, such as a microorganism or drug; tissue biopsy showing leukocytoclastic angiitis, usually in postcapillary venules, with infiltration of polymorphonuclear leukocytes, fibrinoid necrosis, and extravasation of erythrocytes
Mucocutaneous lymph node syndrome (Kawasaki disease)	Small to medium vessels, primarily of the lymph nodes; may progress to involve coronary arteries	Fever; nonsuppurative cervical adenitis; edema; congested conjunctivae; erythema of oral cavity, lips, and palms; and desquamation of fingertips; may progress to arthritis, myocarditis, pericarditis, myocardial infarction, and cardiomegaly	History of symptoms; elevated ESR; tissue biopsy showing intimal proliferation and infiltration of vessel walls with mononuclear cells; echocardiography necessary
Polyangiitis overlap syndrome	Small to medium arteries (including arterioles, capillaries, and venules) of the lungs and other organs	Combined symptoms of polyarteritis nodosa, allergic angiitis, and granulomatosis	Possible history of allergy; eosinophilia; tissue biopsy showing granulomatous inflammation with eosinophilic infiltration

(continued)

Types of vasculitis *(continued)*

Type	Vessels involved	Signs and symptoms	Diagnosis
Polyarteritis nodosa	Small to medium arteries throughout body, with lesions that tend to be segmental, occur at bifurcations and branchings of arteries, spread distally to arterioles and, in severe cases, circumferentially involve adjacent veins	Hypertension, abdominal pain, myalgias, headache, joint pain, and weakness	History of symptoms; elevated ESR; leukocytosis; anemia; thrombocytosis; depressed C3 complement; rheumatoid factor more than 1:60; circulating immune complexes; tissue biopsy showing necrotizing vasculitis
Takayasu's arteritis (aortic arch syndrome)	Medium to large arteries, particularly the aortic arch, its branches and, possibly, the pulmonary artery	Malaise, pallor, nausea, night sweats, arthralgias, anorexia, weight loss, pain or paresthesia distal to affected area, bruits, loss of distal pulses, syncope and, if a carotid artery is involved, diplopia and transient blindness; may progress to heart failure or stroke	Decreased hemoglobin level; leukocytosis; positive lupus erythematosus cell preparation and elevated ESR; arteriography showing calcification and obstruction of affected vessels; tissue biopsy showing inflammation of adventitia and intima of vessels, and thickening of vessel walls
Temporal arteritis	Medium to large arteries, most commonly branches of the carotid artery	Fever, myalgia, jaw claudication, visual changes, and headache (associated with polymyalgia rheumatica syndrome)	Decreased hemoglobin level; elevated ESR; tissue biopsy showing panarteritis with infiltration of mononuclear cells, giant cells within vessel wall, fragmentation of internal elastic lamina, and proliferation of intima
Wegener's granulomatosis	Small to medium vessels of the respiratory tract and kidney	Fever, pulmonary congestion, cough, malaise, anorexia, weight loss, and mild to severe hematuria	Tissue biopsy showing necrotizing vasculitis with granulomatous inflammation; leukocytosis; elevated ESR and immunoglobulin (Ig) A and IgG levels; low titer rheumatoid factor; circulating immune complexes; antineutrophil cytoplasmic antibody in more than 90% of patients

therapy. Immune system abnormality and blood vessel inflammation also play a role in the disorder.

Pathophysiology

How vascular damage develops in vasculitis isn't well understood. Current theory holds that it's initiated by excessive circulating antigen, which triggers the formation of soluble antigen–antibody complexes. These complexes can't be cleared effectively by the reticuloendothelial system, so they're deposited in blood vessel walls (type III hypersensitivity). Increased vascular permeability associated with release of vasoactive amines by platelets and basophils exacerbates this process. The deposited complexes activate the complement cascade, resulting in chemotaxis of neutrophils, which release lysosomal enzymes. In turn, these enzymes cause vessel damage and necrosis, which may precipitate thrombosis, occlusion, hemorrhage, and ischemia.

Another mechanism that may contribute to vascular damage is the cell-mediated (T-cell) immune response. In this response, circulating antigen triggers lymphocytes to release soluble mediators, which attracts macrophages. The macrophages release intracellular enzymes, which cause vascular damage. Macrophages can also transform into the epithelioid and multinucleated giant cells that typify the granulomatous vasculitides. Phagocytosis of immune complexes by macrophages enhances granuloma formation.

Signs and symptoms and diagnosis

Clinical effects of vasculitis and confirming laboratory procedures depend on the blood vessels involved. (See *Types of vasculitis*, pages 460 and 461.)

Complications

◆ Renal, cardiac, and hepatic involvement that may be fatal if vasculitis is left untreated
◆ Renal failure, renal hypertension, glomerulitis
◆ Fibrous scarring of the lung tissue
◆ Stroke
◆ GI bleeding

Treatment

Treatment of vasculitis aims to minimize irreversible tissue damage associated with ischemia.

◆ In primary vasculitis, treatment may involve removing the offending antigen or using an anti-inflammatory or an immunosuppressant. For example, antigenic drugs, food, and other environmental substances should be identified and eliminated, if possible.

◆ Drug therapy in primary vasculitis commonly involves low-dose cyclophosphamide with a daily corticosteroid. In rapidly fulminant vasculitis, cyclophosphamide dosage may be increased daily for the first 2 to 3 days, followed by the regular dose. Prednisone should be given in divided doses for 7 to 10 days, with consolidation to a single morning dose by 2 to 3 weeks. When the vasculitis appears to be in remission or when the prescribed cytotoxic drug takes full effect, the corticosteroid is tapered down to a single daily dose. Finally, an alternate-day schedule of the steroid may continue for 3 to 6 months before slow discontinuation of it.

◆ In secondary vasculitis, treatment focuses on the underlying disorder.

Special considerations

◆ Assess patients with Wegener's granulomatosis for dry nasal mucosa. Instill nose drops to lubricate the mucosa and help diminish crusting, or irrigate the nasal passages with warm normal saline solution.

◆ Monitor vital signs. Use a Doppler ultrasonic flowmeter, if available, to auscultate blood pressure in patients with Takayasu's arteritis, whose peripheral pulses are generally difficult to palpate.

◆ Monitor intake and output. Check daily for edema. Keep the patient well hydrated (3 qt [3 L] daily) to reduce the risk of hemorrhagic cystitis associated with cyclophosphamide therapy.

◆ Provide emotional support to help the patient and his family cope with an altered body image — the result of the disorder or its therapy. (For example, Wegener's granulomatosis may be associated with saddle nose, a steroid may cause weight gain, and cyclophosphamide may cause alopecia.)

◆ Teach the patient how to recognize adverse reactions to drug therapy. Monitor the patient's white blood cell count during cyclophosphamide therapy to prevent severe leukopenia.

ENDOCRINE SYSTEM

The endocrine system consists of glands, specialized cell clusters, hormones, and target tissues. The glands and cell clusters secrete hormones and chemical transmitters in response to stimulation from the nervous system and other sites. Together with the nervous system, the endocrine system regulates and integrates the body's metabolic activities and maintains internal homeostasis. Each target tissue has receptors for specific hormones. Hormones connect with the receptors, and the resulting hormone-receptor complex triggers the target cell's response.

Hormonal regulation

The hypothalamus, the main integrative center for the endocrine and autonomic nervous systems, helps control some endocrine glands by neural and hormonal pathways. Neural pathways connect the hypothalamus to the posterior pituitary gland, or neurohypophysis. Neural stimulation of the posterior pituitary causes the secretion of two effector hormones: antidiuretic hormone (ADH, also known as *vasopressin*) and oxytocin.

The hypothalamus also exerts hormonal control at the anterior pituitary gland, or adenohypophysis, by releasing and inhibiting hormones and factors, which arrive by a portal system. Hypothalamic hormones stimulate the pituitary gland to synthesize and release trophic hormones, such as corticotropin (also called *adrenocorticotropic hormone*), thyroid-stimulating hormone (TSH), and gonadotropins, such as luteinizing hormone (LH) and follicle-stimulating

hormone (FSH). Secretion of trophic hormones stimulates the adrenal cortex, thyroid gland, and gonads. Hypothalamic hormones also stimulate the pituitary gland to release or inhibit the release of effector hormones, such as growth hormone (GH) and prolactin.

In a patient with a possible endocrine disorder, this complex hormonal sequence requires careful assessment to identify the dysfunction, which may result from defects in the gland; defects of releasing, trophic, or effector hormones; or defects of the target tissue. Hyperthyroidism, for example, may result from excessive thyrotropin-releasing hormone, TSH, or thyroid hormones, or excessive response of the thyroid gland.

Besides hormonal and neural controls, a negative feedback system regulates the endocrine system. (See *Feedback mechanism of the endocrine system,* page 464.)

The feedback mechanism may be simple or complex. Simple feedback occurs when the level of one substance regulates secretion of a hormone. For example, a low serum calcium level stimulates the parathyroid glands to secrete parathyroid hormone (PTH), and a high serum calcium level inhibits PTH secretion.

One example of complex feedback occurs through the hypothalamic-pituitary target organ axis. Secretion of the hypothalamic corticotropin- releasing hormone releases pituitary corticotropin, which in turn stimulates adrenal cortisol secretion. Subsequently, an increase in the serum cortisol level inhibits corticotropin by decreasing corticotropin-releasing hormone secretion or corticotropin directly. Corticosteroid therapy disrupts the hypothalamic-

CLOSER LOOK

Feedback mechanism of the endocrine system

The hypothalamus receives regulatory information (feedback) from its own circulating hormones (simple loop) and also from target glands (complex loop).

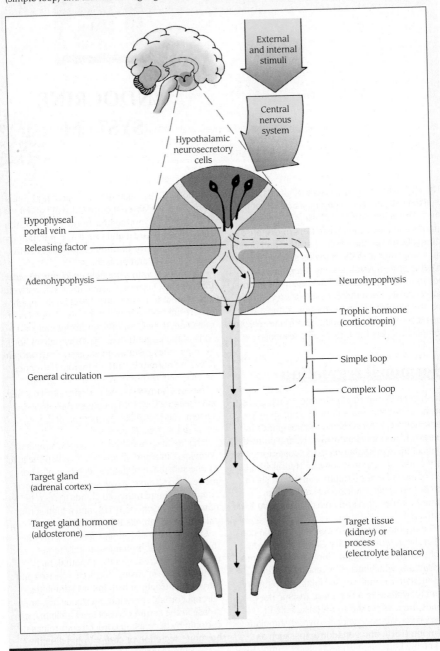

pituitary-adrenal axis by suppressing the hypothalamic-pituitary secretion mechanism. Because abrupt withdrawal of steroid therapy doesn't allow time for recovery of the hypothalamic-pituitary-adrenal axis to stimulate cortisol secretion, it can induce life-threatening adrenal crisis.

RHYTHMS

The endocrine system is also controlled by rhythms, many of which last 24 hours (*circadian*). Circadian rhythm control of corticotropin and cortisol increases levels of these hormones in the early morning hours and decreases them in the late afternoon. Stress, caused by pyrogens, surgery, hypoglycemia, exercise, severe emotional trauma, and other conditions, enhances corticotropin release and abolishes corticotropin circadian rhythmicity. High-dose glucocorticoid administration suppresses stress-related corticotropin release. An *infradian rhythm* is a biorhythm that repeats in patterns that exceed a 24-hour period. The menstrual cycle is an example of an infradian rhythm—in this case, 28 days.

HORMONAL EFFECTS

The posterior pituitary gland secretes oxytocin and ADH. Oxytocin stimulates contraction of the uterus and causes the milk-letdown reflex in breast-feeding women. ADH controls the concentration of body fluids by altering the permeability of the distal and collecting tubules of the kidneys to conserve water. ADH secretion depends on plasma osmolality, the characteristic of a solution determined by the ionic concentration of the dissolved substance and the solution, which is monitored by hypothalamic neurons. Hypovolemia and hypotension are the most powerful stimulators of ADH release. Other stimulators include trauma, nausea, morphine, tranquilizers, certain anesthetics, positive-pressure breathing, pain, and stress.

In addition to the trophic hormones, the anterior pituitary gland secretes prolactin, which stimulates milk secretion, and GH. GH affects most body tissues. It triggers growth by stimulating protein synthesis and fat mobilization, and by decreasing carbohydrate use by muscle and fat tissue. The thyroid gland synthesizes and secretes the iodinated hormones, thyroxine and triiodothyronine. Thyroid hormones are necessary for normal growth and development, and act on many tissues to increase metabolic activity and protein synthesis.

The parathyroid glands secrete PTH, which regulates calcium and phosphate metabolism. PTH elevates the serum calcium level by stimulating resorption of calcium and excretion of phosphate from bone, and enhances absorption of calcium from the GI tract by stimulating conversion of vitamin D to its most active form. Calcitonin, another hormone that the thyroid gland secretes, affects calcium metabolism, although its precise role in humans is unknown.

The pancreas produces glucagon from the alpha cells and insulin from the beta cells. Glucagon, the hormone of the fasting state, releases stored glucose from the liver to increase the blood glucose level. Insulin, the hormone of the postprandial state, facilitates glucose transport into the cells, promotes glucose storage, stimulates protein synthesis, and enhances free fatty acid uptake and storage.

The adrenal cortex secretes mineralocorticoids, glucocorticoids, and sex steroid hormones (*androgens*). Aldosterone, a mineralocorticoid, regulates the reabsorption of sodium and the excretion of potassium by the kidneys. Although affected by corticotropin, aldosterone is mainly regulated by the renin-angiotensin system. Together, aldosterone, angiotensin II, and renin may be implicated in the pathogenesis of hypertension.

Cortisol, a glucocorticoid, stimulates gluconeogenesis, increases protein breakdown and free fatty acid mobilization, suppresses the immune response, and facilitates an appropriate response to stress.

The adrenal medulla is an aggregate of nervous tissue that produces the catecholamines epinephrine and norepinephrine, which cause vasoconstriction. In addition, epinephrine stimulates the fight-or-flight response—dilation of bronchioles and increased blood pressure, blood glucose level, and heart rate. The adrenal cortex as well as the gonads secrete androgens, which are steroid sex hormones. In men and premenopausal women, the contribution of adrenal androgens is small, but in postmenopausal women, the adrenals are the major source of sex hormones.

The testes synthesize and secrete testosterone in response to gonadotropic hormones, especially LH, from the anterior pituitary gland; spermatogenesis occurs in response to FSH. The ovaries produce sex steroid hormones (primarily estrogen and progesterone) in response to anterior pituitary trophic hormones.

Pathophysiologic changes

Alterations in hormone levels, either significantly high or low, may result from various causes. Feedback systems may fail to function properly or may respond to the wrong signals. Dysfunction of an endocrine gland may manifest as either failure to produce adequate amounts of active hormone or excessive synthesis or release. After the hormones are released, they may be degraded at an altered rate or inactivated by antibodies before reaching the target cell. Abnormal target cell responses include receptor-associated alterations and intracellular alterations.

RECEPTOR-ASSOCIATED ALTERATIONS

Receptor-associated alterations have been associated with water-soluble hormones (*peptides*) and involve:
◆ fewer receptors, resulting in diminished or defective hormone-receptor binding
◆ impaired receptor function, resulting in insensitivity to the hormone
◆ presence of antibodies against specific receptors, either reducing available binding sites or mimicking hormone action and suppressing or exaggerating target cell response
◆ unusual expression of receptor function.

INTRACELLULAR ALTERATIONS

Intracellular alterations involve the inadequate synthesis of the second messenger needed to convert the hormonal signal into intracellular events. The two different mechanisms that may be involved include:
◆ faulty response of target cells for water-soluble hormones to hormone-receptor binding and failure to generate the required second messenger
◆ abnormal response of the target cell to the second messenger and failure to express the usual hormonal effect.

Pathophysiologic aberrations affecting target cells for lipid-soluble (steroid) hormones are less common or may not be as easily recognized.

Disorders

Common dysfunctions of the endocrine system are classified as hypofunction and hyperfunction, inflammation, and tumor.

ADRENAL HYPOFUNCTION

Adrenal hypofunction is classified as primary or secondary. Primary adrenal hypofunction or insufficiency (*Addison's disease*) originates within the adrenal gland and is characterized by the decreased secretion of mineralocorticoids, glucocorticoids, and androgens. Secondary adrenal hypofunction is caused by a disorder outside the gland, such as impaired pituitary secretion of corticotropin. It's characterized by decreased glucocorticoid secretion. The secretion of aldosterone, the major mineralocorticoid, is commonly unaffected.

Addison's disease is relatively uncommon and can occur at any age and in both sexes. Secondary adrenal hypofunction occurs when a patient abruptly stops long-term exogenous steroid therapy or when the pituitary is injured by a tumor or by infiltrative or autoimmune processes — these occur when circulating antibodies react specifically against adrenal tissue, causing inflammation and infiltration of the cells by lymphocytes. With early diagnosis and adequate replacement therapy, the prognosis for both primary and secondary adrenal hypofunction is good.

Adrenal crisis (*addisonian crisis*), a critical deficiency of mineralocorticoids and glucocorticoids, generally follows acute stress, sepsis, trauma, surgery, or the omission of steroid therapy in patients who have chronic adrenal insufficiency. Adrenal crisis is a medical emergency that needs immediate, vigorous treatment.

Autoimmune Addison's disease is most common in white females, and a genetic predisposition is likely. It's more common in patients with a familial predisposition to autoimmune endocrine diseases. Addison's disease affects 1 in 16,000 neonates; it also affects 8 in 100,000 adults, with males and females affected equally.

Causes

Primary and secondary adrenal hypofunction and adrenal crisis have different causes. The most common cause of primary hypofunction is Addison's disease that results in destruction of more than 90% of both adrenal glands, usually caused by an autoimmune process in which circulating antibodies react specifically against the adrenal tissue.

Other causes include:
◆ bilateral adrenalectomy
◆ family history of autoimmune disease (may predispose the patient to Addison's disease and other endocrinopathies)
◆ hemorrhage into the adrenal gland
◆ infections (human immunodeficiency virus [HIV], histoplasmosis, cytomegalovirus [CMV])
◆ neoplasms
◆ tuberculosis (once the chief cause, now responsible for less than 20% of adult cases).

Causes of secondary hypofunction (*glucocorticoid deficiency*) include:
◆ abrupt withdrawal of long-term corticosteroid therapy (long-term exogenous corticosteroid stimulation suppresses pituitary corticotropin secretion, resulting in adrenal gland atrophy)
◆ hypopituitarism (causing decreased corticotropin secretion)
◆ removal of a corticotropin-secreting tumor.

CLOSER LOOK
Understanding adrenal crisis

Adrenal crisis (*acute adrenal insufficiency*) is the most serious complication of Addison's disease. It may occur gradually or suddenly.

Risk factors
This potentially lethal condition usually develops in patients who:
◆ don't respond to hormone replacement therapy.
◆ undergo extreme stress without adequate glucocorticoid replacement.
◆ abruptly stop hormone therapy.
◆ undergo trauma.
◆ undergo bilateral adrenalectomy.

◆ develop adrenal gland thrombosis after a severe infection (Waterhouse-Friderichsen syndrome).

Pathophysiology
In adrenal crisis, destruction of the adrenal cortex leads to a rapid decline in the steroid hormones cortisol and aldosterone. This directly affects the liver, stomach, and kidneys. The flowchart below illustrates what happens in adrenal crisis.

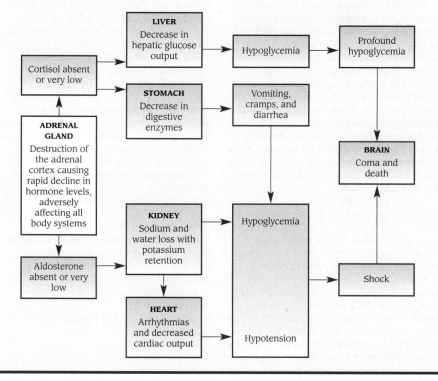

Adrenal crisis is usually caused by:
◆ exhausted body stores of glucocorticoids in a person with adrenal hypofunction after trauma, surgery, or other physiologic stress. (See *Understanding adrenal crisis.*)

Pathophysiology
Addison's disease is a chronic condition that results from the partial or complete destruction of the adrenal cortex. It manifests as a clinical syndrome in which the symptoms are associated

with deficient production of the adrenocortical hormones, cortisol, aldosterone, and androgens. High levels of corticotropin and corticotropin-releasing hormone accompany the low glucocorticoid level.

Corticotropin acts primarily to regulate the adrenal release of glucocorticoids (primarily cortisol); mineralocorticoids, including aldosterone; and sex steroids that supplement those that the gonads produce. Corticotropin secretion is controlled by corticotropin-releasing hormone from the hypothalamus and by negative feedback control by the glucocorticoids.

Addison's disease involves all zones of the cortex, causing deficiencies of the adrenocortical secretions, glucocorticoids, androgens, and mineralocorticoids.

Manifestations of adrenocortical hormone deficiency become apparent when 90% of the functional cells in both glands are lost. Usually, cellular atrophy is limited to the cortex, although medullary involvement may occur, resulting in catecholamine deficiency. Cortisol deficiency causes decreased liver gluconeogenesis (the formation of glucose from molecules that aren't carbohydrates). The resulting low blood glucose level can become dangerously low in patients who take insulin routinely.

Aldosterone deficiency causes increased renal sodium loss and enhances potassium reabsorption. Sodium excretion causes a reduction in water volume that leads to hypotension. Patients with Addison's disease may have normal blood pressure when in a supine position but show marked hypotension and tachycardia after standing for several minutes. Low plasma volume and arteriolar pressure stimulate renin release and a resulting increased production of angiotensin II.

Androgen deficiency may decrease hair growth in axillary and pubic areas as well as on the extremities of women. The metabolic effects of testicular androgens make such hair growth less noticeable in men.

Addison's disease is a decrease in the biosynthesis, storage, or release of adrenocortical hormones. In about 80% of the patients, an autoimmune process causes partial or complete destruction of both adrenal glands. Autoimmune antibodies can block the corticotropin receptor or bind with corticotropin, preventing it from stimulating adrenal cells. Infection is the second most common cause of Addison's disease, specifically tuberculosis, which causes about 20% of the cases. Other conditions that can cause Addison's disease include HIV infection, systemic fungal infections, CMV, adrenal tumor, and metastatic cancers. Infection can impair cellular function and affect corticotropin at any stage of regulation.

Signs and symptoms

Clinical features vary with the type of adrenal hypofunction.

Primary hypofunction
◆ Weakness and fatigue caused by alterations in adrenal hormone balance
◆ Weight loss, nausea, vomiting, and anorexia resulting from glucocorticoid deficiency

◆ Conspicuous bronze color of the skin, especially in the creases of the hands and over the metacarpophalangeal joints (hand and finger), elbows, and knees caused by elevated levels of corticotropin and melanocyte-stimulating hormone
◆ Darkening of scars, areas of vitiligo (absence of pigmentation), and increased pigmentation of the mucous membranes, especially the buccal mucosa, due to decreased secretion of cortisol, causing simultaneous, excessive secretion of corticotropin and melanocyte-stimulating hormone by the pituitary gland
◆ Associated cardiovascular abnormalities, including orthostatic hypotension, decreased cardiac size and output, and weak, irregular pulse caused by mineralocorticoid deficiency
◆ Decreased tolerance for even minor stress because of glucocorticoid deficiency
◆ Fasting hypoglycemia due to decreased gluconeogenesis
◆ Craving for salty food due to decreased mineralocorticoid secretion (which normally causes salt retention)

Secondary hypofunction
◆ Similar to primary hypofunction, but without hyperpigmentation due to low corticotropin and melanocyte-stimulating hormone levels
◆ Possibly no hypotension and electrolyte abnormalities due to fairly normal aldosterone secretion
◆ Usually normal androgen secretion

Addisonian crisis
Signs and symptoms are related to the severe deficiencies of adrenal hormones and may include:
◆ profound weakness and fatigue
◆ nausea, vomiting, and dehydration
◆ hypotension
◆ high fever followed by hypothermia (occasionally).

Complications
◆ Hyperpyrexia
◆ Psychotic reactions
◆ Deficient or excessive steroid treatment
◆ Shock
◆ Profound hypoglycemia
◆ Ultimate vascular collapse, renal shutdown, coma, and death (if untreated)

Diagnosis
◆ Plasma cortisol level confirming adrenal insufficiency (corticotropin stimulation test to differentiate between primary and secondary adrenal hypofunction)

◆ Metyrapone test for suspicion of secondary adrenal hypofunction (oral or I.V. metyrapone blocks cortisol production and should stimulate the release of corticotropin from the hypothalamic-pituitary system; in Addison's disease, the hypothalamic-pituitary system responds normally and the plasma corticotropin level is high, but because the adrenal glands are destroyed, the plasma level of the cortisol precursor 11-deoxycortisol increases, as does the urinary 17-hydroxycorticosteroid level)

◆ Corticotropin stimulation test by I.V. administration of corticotropin, after baseline sampling for plasma cortisol and 24-hour urine cortisol levels (in adrenal hypofunction, plasma and urine cortisol levels fail to rise normally, in response to corticotropin; in secondary hypofunction, repeated doses of corticotropin over successive days produce a gradual increase in cortisol levels until normal values are reached).

In a patient with typical addisonian symptoms, the following laboratory findings strongly suggest acute adrenal insufficiency:

◆ a decreased plasma cortisol level (less than 10 mcg/dl in the morning; less in the evening)

◆ decreased serum sodium and fasting blood glucose levels

◆ increased serum potassium, calcium, and blood urea nitrogen levels

◆ elevated hematocrit; increased lymphocyte and eosinophil counts

◆ X-rays showing adrenal calcification if the cause is infectious.

Treatment

◆ Lifelong corticosteroid replacement, usually with cortisone or hydrocortisone, both of which have a mineralocorticoid effect (primary or secondary adrenal hypofunction)

◆ Oral fludrocortisone (Florinef), a synthetic mineralocorticoid, to prevent dangerous dehydration, hypotension, hyponatremia, and hyperkalemia (Addison's disease)

◆ In adrenal crisis, I.V. bolus of hydrocortisone, then given I.M. or I.V. until the patient's condition stabilizes.

With proper treatment, adrenal crisis usually subsides quickly; blood pressure stabilizes, and water and sodium levels return to normal. After the crisis, maintenance doses of hydrocortisone preserve physiologic stability.

Special considerations

⚠ **CLINICAL ALERT** *In adrenal crisis, monitor the vital signs carefully, watching especially for hypotension, volume depletion, and other signs of shock (decreased level of consciousness and urine output). Also watch for hyperkalemia before treatment and hypokalemia after treatment (from excessive mineralocorticoid effect) and for cardiac arrhythmias (may be caused by a serum potassium disturbance).*

◆ If the patient also has diabetes, check his blood glucose level periodically because steroid replacement may require adjustment of insulin dosage.

◆ Record weight and intake and output carefully because the patient may have volume depletion. Until onset of mineralocorticoid effect, force fluids to replace excessive fluid loss.

To manage the patient receiving maintenance steroid therapy:

◆ Arrange for a diet that maintains sodium and potassium balance.

◆ If the patient is anorexic, suggest six small meals per day to increase caloric intake. Ask the dietitian to provide a diet high in protein and carbohydrates. Keep a late-morning snack available in case the patient becomes hypoglycemic.

◆ Observe the patient receiving a steroid for cushingoid signs, such as fluid retention around the eyes and face. Watch for fluid and electrolyte imbalance, especially if the patient is receiving a mineralocorticoid. Monitor weight and check blood pressure to assess body fluid status. Remember, steroids administered in the late afternoon or evening may stimulate of the central nervous system and cause insomnia in some patients. Check for petechiae because these patients bruise easily.

◆ If the patient receives only a glucocorticoid, observe for orthostatic hypotension or abnormal electrolyte levels, which may indicate a need for mineralocorticoid therapy.

◆ Explain that lifelong steroid therapy is necessary.

◆ Teach the patient the signs and symptoms of steroid overdose (swelling, weight gain) and steroid underdose (lethargy, weakness).

◆ Tell the patient that his dose may need to be increased during times of stress (when he has a cold, for example).

◆ Warn that infection, injury, or profuse sweating in hot weather may precipitate adrenal crisis.

◆ Instruct the patient to always carry a medical identification card stating that he takes a steroid and giving the name of the drug and the dosage.

◆ Teach the patient and family how to give a hydrocortisone injection.

◆ Tell the patient to keep an emergency kit available containing hydrocortisone in a prepared syringe for use in times of stress.

◆ Warn the patient that stress may necessitate additional cortisone to prevent adrenal crisis.

CONGENITAL ADRENAL HYPERPLASIA

Congenital adrenal hyperplasia (CAH) encompasses a group of genetic disorders resulting in the deficiency or absence of one of five enzymes needed for the biosynthesis of glucocorticoids and mineralocorticoids. Manifestations are usually present at birth or during early childhood, but symptoms may appear later in life in nonclassic CAH. CAH is uncommon and typically has an autosomal recessive mode of inheritance. When successfully treated, sexual functioning and fertility aren't affected.

The most common adrenal disorder in infants and children is CAH. There are two common forms: simple virilizing CAH and salt-losing CAH. Acquired adrenal virilism, usually the result of an adrenal tumor, is rare and affects twice as many females as males. With successful treatment, a normal quality of life and life span are expected. In older patients, androgen excess may be part of the syndrome of polycystic ovaries or may be secondary to an adrenal carcinoma or ovarian teratoma.

AGE ALERT *Salt-losing CAH may cause fatal adrenal crisis in neonates.*

Causes

The cause of CAH is genetic, as an autosomal recessive trait.

Pathophysiology

The cortisol level is regulated by a negative-feedback mechanism. Corticotropin in the blood stimulates the release of cortisol precursors and, consequently, of cortisol, aldosterone, and androgens. In turn, cortisol suppresses corticotropin secretion. With a deficiency of the enzyme 21-hydroxylase, cortical secretion of cortisol is impaired and pituitary secretion of corticotropin is increased. Corticotropin stimulates the adrenal cortex, which in turn stimulates aldosterone and androgen biosynthesis and release.

In salt-losing CAH, 21-hydroxylase is almost absent. Corticotropin secretion increases, causing excessive production of cortisol precursors, including salt-wasting compounds. However, cortisol and aldosterone levels—both dependent on 21-hydroxylase—fall precipitously and, combined with the excessive production of salt-wasting compounds, cause acute renal crisis. Corticotropin hypersecretion may stimulate adrenal androgens even more than in simple virilizing CAH, and produces masculinization.

Signs and symptoms

◆ Ambiguous genitalia (enlarged clitoris with urethral opening at the base and a combination of the labia and scrotum) caused by virilization from increased androgens, otherwise normal genital tract and gonads (female neonates)
◆ Pubic and axillary hair at an earlier age, a deep voice, acne, and facial hair, but no menarche (female approaching puberty), also resulting from an increased androgen level
◆ No apparent manifestations (male neonates)
◆ Accentuated masculine characteristics, including a deepened voice, acne, enlarged phallus with small testes, and frequent erections (male approaching puberty) resulting from increased androgen biosynthesis and release
◆ A high androgen level causing rapid bone and muscle growth (children)
◆ Short stature due to premature epiphyseal closure and a high androgen level (adults)
◆ More severe changes, including development of a penis in females (salt-losing CAH)

Because males have no external abnormalities, diagnosis is more difficult and commonly delayed until other signs occur. In the second week of life, signs of a salt-wasting crisis include apathy, failure to eat, diarrhea, and adrenal crisis (vomiting, dehydration from hyponatremia, and hyperkalemia). If adrenal crisis isn't treated promptly, dehydration and electrolyte imbalance cause cardiovascular collapse and cardiac arrest.

Complications

◆ Death (salt-wasting crisis) due to dehydration and hyperkalemia
◆ Precocious puberty
◆ Menstrual irregularities
◆ Sexual dysfunction, infertility, and altered external genitalia
◆ Adrenal crisis
◆ Altered growth

Diagnosis

◆ An elevated urine 17-ketosteroid level (can be suppressed by dexamethasone [Decadron])
◆ An elevated serum 17-hydroxyprogesterone level after I.V. bolus of corticotropin
◆ Serum hyperkalemia, hyponatremia, and hypochloremia (present but not diagnostic)
◆ An elevated 24-hour urine pregnanetriol level
◆ Normal or decreased 24-hour urine 17-hydroxycorticosteroid levels

Treatment

◆ Daily cortisone (Cortone) or hydrocortisone (Cortef) to stop the excessive output of corticotropin and subsequent excessive androgen production (initial and subsequent doses guided by urinary 17-ketosteroid levels) given I.M. until the infant is old enough to tolerate pills (usually about 18 months)

◆ I.V. sodium chloride and glucose to reestablish and maintain fluid and electrolyte balance, with desoxycorticosterone I.M. and hydrocortisone I.V. as needed (adrenal crisis); glucocorticoid (cortisone or hydrocortisone) and perhaps mineralocorticoids (desoxycorticosterone, fludrocortisone, or both after stabilization)
◆ Sex chromatin and karyotype studies to determine genetic sex (with ambiguous external genitalia); possible reconstructive surgery for females between ages 1 and 3

Special considerations

Suspect CAH in infants hospitalized for failure to thrive, dehydration, or diarrhea as well as in tall, sturdy-looking children with a record of numerous episodic illnesses.
◆ When caring for an infant with adrenal crisis, keep the I.V. line patent, infuse fluids, and give a steroid, as ordered. Monitor body weight, blood pressure, urine output, and serum electrolyte levels carefully, especially sodium and potassium levels.
◆ Watch for signs of shock (cyanosis, hypotension, tachycardia, and tachypnea).
◆ If the child is receiving maintenance therapy with steroid injections, rotate I.M. injection sites to prevent atrophy; tell parents to do the same. Teach them the possible adverse effects (cushingoid symptoms) of long-term therapy. Explain that lifelong maintenance therapy with hydrocortisone, cortisone, or the mineralocorticoid fludrocortisone is essential for survival. Warn parents not to stop therapy with these drugs suddenly because potentially fatal adrenal hypofunction will result. Instruct parents to report stress and infection, which require increased steroid doses.
◆ Monitor the patient receiving desoxycorticosterone or fludrocortisone for edema, weakness, and hypertension. Be alert for significant weight gain and rapid changes in height because normal growth is an important indicator of adequate therapy.
◆ Instruct the patient to wear a medical identification bracelet indicating that he's on prolonged steroid therapy and providing information about dosage.
◆ Help the parents of a female infant with male genitalia to understand that she's physiologically a female and that this abnormality can be surgically corrected. Arrange for counseling if necessary.

CUSHING'S SYNDROME

Cushing's syndrome is a cluster of clinical abnormalities caused by prolonged exposure to elevated levels of endogenous or exogenous glucocorticoids. Most cases in the United States result from exogenous glucocorticoids. Of the 13 cases per million that occur annually, 10% result from a pituitary adrenocorticotropic hormone (ACTH)-producing tumor.

Rare adrenal carcinomas are associated with a 5-year survival rate of less than 30%. Cushing's syndrome that results from an adrenal or a pituitary tumor affects women five times more frequently than men, with a peak incidence between ages 25 and 40.

Causes

◆ ACTH-producing pituitary adenoma
◆ Adrenal adenoma, carcinoma, or hyperplasia
◆ Autonomous, ectopic corticotropin secretion by a tumor outside the pituitary (usually malignant, commonly oat cell carcinoma of the lung)
◆ Excessive glucocorticoid administration, including prolonged use

Pathophysiology

Cushing's syndrome is caused by prolonged exposure to excess glucocorticoids. Cushing's syndrome can be exogenous, resulting from chronic glucocorticoid or corticotropin administration, or endogenous, resulting from increased cortisol or corticotropin secretion. Cortisol excess results in anti-inflammatory effects and excessive catabolism of protein and peripheral fat to support hepatic glucose production. The mechanism may be corticotropin dependent (an elevated plasma corticotropin level stimulates the adrenal cortex to produce excess cortisol) or corticotropin independent (excess cortisol is produced by the adrenal cortex or exogenously administered). Excess cortisol suppresses the hypothalamic-pituitary-adrenal axis, also present in ectopic corticotropin-secreting tumors.

Signs and symptoms

Like other endocrine disorders, Cushing's syndrome induces changes in many body systems. Signs and symptoms depend on the degree and duration of hypercortisolism, the presence or absence of androgen excess, and additional tumor-related effects (adrenal carcinoma or ectopic corticotropin syndrome). Specific clinical effects vary with the system affected and include:
◆ diabetes mellitus, with decreased glucose tolerance, fasting hyperglycemia, and glycosuria due to cortisol-induced insulin resistance and increased gluconeogenesis in the liver (endocrine and metabolic systems)
◆ muscle weakness due to hypokalemia or loss of muscle mass due to increased catabolism, pathologic fractures due to decreased bone mineral ionization, osteopenia, osteoporosis,

and skeletal growth retardation in children (musculoskeletal system)
◆ purple striae; facial plethora (edema and blood vessel distention); acne; fat pads above the clavicles, over the upper back (buffalo hump), on the face (moon facies), and around the trunk (truncal obesity) with slender arms and legs; little or no scar formation; poor wound healing due to decreased collagen and weakened tissues; spontaneous ecchymosis; hyperpigmentation; fungal skin infections (integumentary system)
◆ peptic ulcer due to increased gastric secretions and pepsin production and decreased gastric mucus, abdominal pain, increased appetite, weight gain (GI system)
◆ irritability and emotional lability, ranging from euphoric behavior to depression or psychosis; insomnia due to the cortisol's role in neurotransmission; headache (central nervous system [CNS])
◆ hypertension due to sodium and secondary fluid retention; heart failure; left ventricular hypertrophy; capillary weakness from protein loss, which leads to bleeding and ecchymosis; dyslipidemia; ankle edema (cardiovascular system)
◆ increased susceptibility to infection due to decreased lymphocyte production and suppressed antibody formation; decreased resistance to stress; suppressed inflammatory response masking even severe infection (immunologic system)
◆ fluid retention, increased potassium excretion, ureteral calculi from increased bone demineralization with hypercalciuria (renal and urologic systems)
◆ increased androgen production with clitoral hypertrophy, mild virilism, hirsutism, and amenorrhea or oligomenorrhea in women; sexual dysfunction; decreased libido; impotence (reproductive system).

Complications
◆ Osteoporosis
◆ Increased susceptibility to infections
◆ Hirsutism
◆ Ureteral calculi
◆ Metastasis of malignant tumors

Diagnosis
◆ Hyperglycemia, hypernatremia, glycosuria, hypokalemia, and metabolic alkalosis
◆ Urinary free-cortisol levels more than 150 mcg/24 hours
◆ Dexamethasone suppression test to confirm the diagnosis and determine the cause, possibly an adrenal tumor or a nonendocrine, corticotropin-secreting tumor

◆ Elevated serum cortisol levels when sample taken at 11 p.m. (early finding)
◆ Salivary cortisol levels greater than 1.3 ng/ml (radioimmunoassay) or greater than 1.5 ng/ml (competitive-protein binding assay)
◆ Blood levels of corticotropin-releasing hormone, corticotropin, and different glucocorticoids to diagnose and localize cause to pituitary or adrenal gland
◆ Radiologic evaluation using ultrasonography, computed tomography scan, or magnetic resonance imaging enhanced with gadolinium to locate a causative tumor in the pituitary or adrenal glands
◆ Petrosal sinus sampling to determine whether Cushing's syndrome is due to a pituitary tumor or some other cause

Treatment
Differentiation among pituitary, adrenal, and ectopic causes of hypercortisolism is essential for effective treatment, which is specific for the cause of cortisol excess and includes medication, radiation, and surgery. Possible treatments include:
◆ surgery for tumors of the adrenal and pituitary glands or other tissue (such as the lung)
◆ radiation therapy (tumor)
◆ drug therapy, which may include ketoconazole, metyrapone, and aminoglutethimide to inhibit cortisol synthesis; mitotane to destroy the adrenocortical cells that secret cortisol; and bromocriptine and cyproheptadine to inhibit corticotropin secretion.

Special considerations
Patients with Cushing's syndrome require painstaking assessment and vigorous supportive care:
◆ Frequently monitor vital signs, especially blood pressure. Carefully observe the hypertensive patient who also has cardiac disease.
◆ Check laboratory reports for hypernatremia, hypokalemia, hyperglycemia, and glycosuria.
◆ Because the cushingoid patient is likely to retain sodium and water, check for edema and monitor daily weight and intake and output carefully. To minimize weight gain, edema, and hypertension, ask the dietary department to provide a diet that's high in protein and potassium but low in calories, carbohydrates, and sodium.
◆ Watch for infection, which is a particular problem in Cushing's syndrome.
◆ If the patient has osteoporosis and is bedridden, perform passive range-of-motion exercises carefully because of the severe risk of pathologic fractures.

◆ Remember, Cushing's syndrome produces emotional lability. Record incidents that upset the patient, and try to prevent such situations from occurring, if possible. Help him get the physical and mental rest he needs—using sedation, if necessary. Offer support to the emotionally labile patient throughout the difficult testing period.

After bilateral adrenalectomy and pituitary surgery:

◆ Be sure to report wound drainage or temperature elevation to the patient's physician immediately. Use strict sterile technique in changing the patient's dressings.

◆ Administer an analgesic and a replacement steroid as ordered.

◆ Monitor urine output and check vital signs carefully, watching for signs of shock (decreased blood pressure, increased pulse rate, pallor, and cold, clammy skin). To counteract shock, give a vasopressor and increase the rate of I.V. fluids, as ordered. Because mitotane, aminoglutethimide, and metyrapone decrease mental alertness and produce physical weakness, assess neurologic and behavioral status, and warn the patient of adverse CNS effects. Also, watch for severe nausea, vomiting, and diarrhea.

◆ Check laboratory reports for hypoglycemia due to removal of the source of cortisol, a hormone that maintains the blood glucose level.

◆ Check for abdominal distention and return of bowel sounds after adrenalectomy.

◆ Check regularly for signs and symptoms of adrenal hypofunction (orthostatic hypotension, apathy, weakness, fatigue), which indicate that steroid replacement is inadequate.

◆ In the patient undergoing pituitary surgery, check for and immediately report signs and symptoms of increased intracranial pressure (confusion, agitation, changes in level of consciousness, nausea, and vomiting). Watch for hypopituitarism.

Provide comprehensive teaching to help the patient cope with lifelong treatment:

◆ Advise the patient to take the replacement steroid with an antacid or a meal, to minimize gastric irritation. (Usually, it's helpful to take two-thirds of the dose in the morning and the remaining third in the early afternoon to mimic diurnal adrenal secretion.)

◆ Tell the patient to carry a medical identification card and to immediately report physiologically stressful situations, such as infections, which necessitate an increased dose.

◆ Instruct the patient to watch closely for signs and symptoms of inadequate steroid dosing (fatigue, weakness, dizziness) and of overdosage (severe edema, weight gain). Emphatically warn against abrupt discontinuation of steroid therapy because this may produce a fatal adrenal crisis.

DIABETES INSIPIDUS

A disorder of water metabolism, diabetes insipidus results from a deficiency of circulating vasopressin (also called *antidiuretic hormone,* or *ADH*) or from renal resistance to this hormone. Pituitary diabetes insipidus is caused by a deficiency of vasopressin, and nephrogenic diabetes insipidus is caused by the resistance of renal tubules to vasopressin. Diabetes insipidus is characterized by excessive fluid intake and hypotonic polyuria. A decrease in the ADH level leads to altered intracellular and extracellular fluid control, causing renal excretion of a large amount of urine.

The disorder may start at any age and is slightly more common in men than in women. The incidence is slightly greater today than in the past.

In uncomplicated diabetes insipidus, the prognosis is good with adequate water replacement, and patients usually lead normal lives.

Causes

◆ Acquired, familial, idiopathic, neurogenic, or nephrogenic

◆ Associated with stroke, hypothalamic or pituitary tumors, and cranial trauma or surgery (neurogenic diabetes insipidus)

◆ Certain drugs, such as lithium (Duralith), phenytoin (Dilantin), or alcohol (transient diabetes insipidus)

◆ X-linked recessive trait or end-stage renal failure (nephrogenic diabetes insipidus, less common)

Pathophysiology

Diabetes insipidus is related to an insufficiency of ADH, leading to polyuria and polydipsia. The three forms of diabetes insipidus are neurogenic, nephrogenic, and psychogenic.

Neurogenic, or central, diabetes insipidus is an inadequate response of ADH to plasma osmolarity, which occurs when an organic lesion of the hypothalamus, infundibular stem, or posterior pituitary partially or completely blocks ADH synthesis, transport, or release. Many organic lesions can cause diabetes insipidus, including brain tumors, hypophysectomy, aneurysms, thrombosis, skull fractures, infections, and immunologic disorders. Neurogenic diabetes insipidus has an acute onset. A three-phase syndrome can occur, which involves:

◆ progressive loss of nerve tissue and increased diuresis

◆ normal diuresis

◆ polyuria and polydipsia, the manifestation of permanent loss of the ability to secrete adequate ADH.

Nephrogenic diabetes insipidus is caused by an inadequate renal response to ADH. The collecting duct permeability to water doesn't increase in response to ADH. Nephrogenic diabetes insipidus is generally related to disorders and drugs that damage the renal tubules or inhibit the generation of cyclic adenosine monophosphate in the tubules, preventing activation of the second messenger. Causative disorders include pyelonephritis, amyloidosis, destructive uropathies, polycystic disease, and intrinsic renal disease. Drugs include lithium (Eskalith); general anesthetics, such as methoxyflurane; and demeclocycline (Declomycin). In addition, hypokalemia or hypercalcemia impairs the renal response to ADH. A rare genetic form of nephrogenic diabetes insipidus is an X-linked recessive trait.

Psychogenic diabetes insipidus is caused by excessive fluid intake, which may be idiopathic or related to psychosis or sarcoidosis. The polydipsia and resultant polyuria wash out ADH more quickly than it can be replaced. Chronic polyuria may overwhelm the renal medullary concentration gradient, rendering patients partially or totally unable to concentrate urine.

Regardless of the cause, insufficient ADH causes the immediate excretion of large volumes of dilute urine and consequent plasma hyperosmolality. In conscious individuals, the thirst mechanism is stimulated, usually for cold liquids. With severe ADH deficiency, urine output may be greater than 12 L/day, with a low specific gravity. Dehydration develops rapidly if fluids aren't replaced.

Signs and symptoms
◆ Polydipsia (cardinal sign)—fluid intake caused by stimulation of the thirst mechanism
◆ Polyuria (cardinal sign)—urine output of 4 to 16 L/24-hour period of dilute urine caused by insufficient ADH
◆ Nocturia—caused by increased urine output leading to sleep disturbance and fatigue
◆ Low urine specific gravity—less than 1.006 caused by polyuria
◆ Changes in level of consciousness caused by central nervous system cellular dehydration
◆ Hypotension and tachycardia caused by a decrease in vascular volume related to fluid loss
◆ Headache and visual disturbance due to electrolyte disturbance and dehydration
◆ Abdominal fullness, anorexia, and weight loss due to almost continuous fluid consumption

Complications
◆ Dilation of the urinary tract
◆ Severe dehydration
◆ Shock and renal failure if dehydration is severe

Diagnosis
◆ Urinalysis showing almost colorless urine of low osmolality (50 to 200 mOsm/kg, less than that of plasma) and low specific gravity (less than 1.005)
◆ Water deprivation test to identify vasopressin deficiency, resulting in renal inability to concentrate urine

Treatment
Until the cause of diabetes insipidus can be identified and eliminated, the administration of vasopressin (Pitressin) can control fluid balance and prevent dehydration. Medications include:
◆ hydrochlorothiazide with potassium supplement for central and nephrogenic diabetes insipidus
◆ vasopressin aqueous preparation subcutaneously several times daily, effective for only 2 to 6 hours (used as a diagnostic agent and, rarely, in acute disease)
◆ desmopressin acetate (DDAVP) orally, by nasal spray absorbed through the mucous membranes, or by subcutaneous or I.V. injection, effective for 8 to 20 hours depending on the dose
◆ indomethacin and amiloride for nephrogenic diabetes insipidus.

Special considerations
◆ Patient care includes monitoring symptoms to ensure that fluid balance is restored and maintained.
◆ Record fluid intake and output carefully. Maintain adequate fluid intake to prevent severe dehydration. Watch for signs of hypovolemic shock, and monitor blood pressure and heart and respiratory rates regularly, especially during the water deprivation test. Check the patient's weight daily.
◆ If the patient is dizzy or has muscle weakness, keep the side rails up and assist him with walking.
◆ Monitor urine specific gravity between doses. Watch for a decrease in specific gravity accompanied by increased urine output, indicating the recurrence of polyuria and necessitating administration of the next dose of medication or a dosage increase.
◆ Monitor serum electrolyte levels closely. Report abnormal values, and provide treatment as ordered.

◆ If constipation develops, add more high-fiber foods and fruit juices to the patient's diet. If necessary, obtain an order for a mild laxative, such as milk of magnesia.

◆ Provide meticulous skin and mouth care; apply petroleum jelly as needed to cracked or sore lips.

◆ Before discharge, teach the patient how to monitor intake and output.

◆ Instruct the patient to administer desmopressin by nasal spray only after the onset of polyuria—not before—to prevent excess fluid retention and water intoxication.

◆ Tell the patient to report weight gain, which may indicate that his medication dose is too high. Recurrence of polyuria, as reflected on the intake and output sheet, indicates that the dose is too low.

◆ Teach the parents of a child with diabetes insipidus about normal growth and development. Discuss how their child may differ from others at his developmental stage.

◆ Advise the patient with diabetes insipidus to wear a medical identification bracelet and to carry his medication with him at all times.

DIABETES MELLITUS

Diabetes mellitus is a metabolic disorder characterized by hyperglycemia (an *elevated blood glucose level*) resulting from lack of insulin, lack of insulin effect, or both. Two general classifications are recognized:

◆ type 1, absolute insulin insufficiency

◆ type 2, insulin resistance with varying degrees of insulin secretory defects.

Several secondary forms also exist, caused by such conditions as pregnancy (gestational diabetes mellitus), pancreatic disease, hormonal or genetic problems, and certain drugs or chemicals.

Onset of type 1 (insulin-dependent) usually occurs before age 30 (although it may occur at any age); the patient is usually thin and requires exogenous insulin and dietary management to achieve control. (See *Treatment of type 1 diabetes mellitus,* pages 476 and 477.) Conversely, type 2 (non–insulin-dependent) usually occurs in obese adults after age 40 and is treated with diet and exercise in combination with various oral antidiabetics, although treatment may include insulin therapy.

Medical advances permit increased longevity and improved quality of life if the patient carefully monitors the blood glucose level, uses the data to make pharmacologic and lifestyle changes, and uses new insulin delivery systems, such as subcutaneous insulin pumps. In addition, medications now available enhance the body's own glucose metabolism and insulin sensitivity

to optimize glycemic control and prevent progression to long-term complications.

Causes

◆ Conditions that antagonize the actions of insulin (Cushing's syndrome, acromegaly, pheochromocytoma)

◆ Environment (infection, diet, toxins, stress, glucocorticoids)

◆ Heredity

◆ Lifestyle changes in genetically susceptible persons

◆ Pregnancy

Pathophysiology

In persons genetically susceptible to type 1 diabetes, a triggering event, possibly a viral infection, causes production of autoantibodies against the beta cells of the pancreas. The resultant destruction of the beta cells leads to a decline in and ultimate lack of insulin secretion. Insulin deficiency leads to hyperglycemia, enhanced lipolysis (decomposition of fat), and protein catabolism. These characteristics occur when more than 90% of the beta cells have been destroyed.

Type 2 diabetes mellitus is a chronic disease caused by one or more of the following factors: impaired insulin secretion, inappropriate hepatic glucose production, or peripheral insulin receptor insensitivity. Genetic factors are significant for both pancreatic beta-cell failure and insulin resistance, and onset is accelerated by obesity and a sedentary lifestyle. Again, added stress can be a pivotal factor. (See *Understanding type 2 diabetes,* page 478, and *How diabetes mellitus affects the body,* page 479.)

Gestational diabetes mellitus occurs when a woman not previously diagnosed with diabetes shows glucose intolerance during pregnancy. This may occur if placental hormones counteract insulin, causing insulin resistance. Gestational diabetes mellitus is a significant risk factor for the future occurrence of type 2 diabetes mellitus.

Signs and symptoms

⚠ **CLINICAL ALERT** *Type 1 diabetes usually presents rapidly, typically with polydipsia, polyuria, polyphagia, weakness, weight loss, dry skin, and ketoacidosis. Type 2 diabetes is typically slow and insidious in onset and usually unaccompanied by symptoms.*

◆ Polyuria and polydipsia due to high serum osmolality caused by a high blood glucose level

◆ Anorexia (common) resulting from an elevated blood glucose level or polyphagia (occasional)

(Text continues on page 479)

DISEASE BLOCK

Treatment of type 1 diabetes mellitus

The flowchart below shows the pathophysiologic process of diabetes and points for treatment intervention.

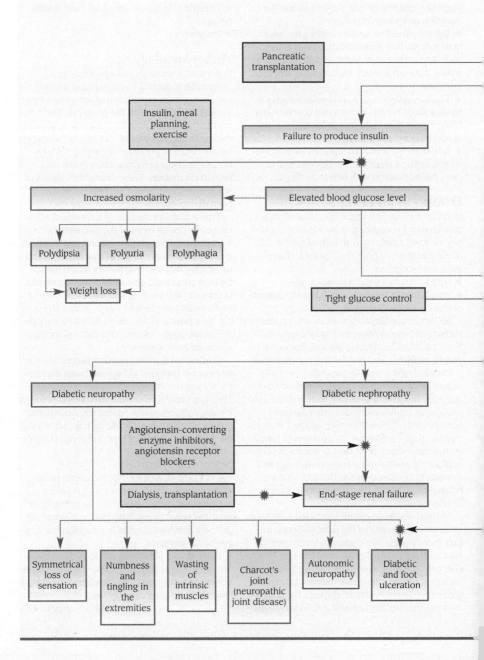

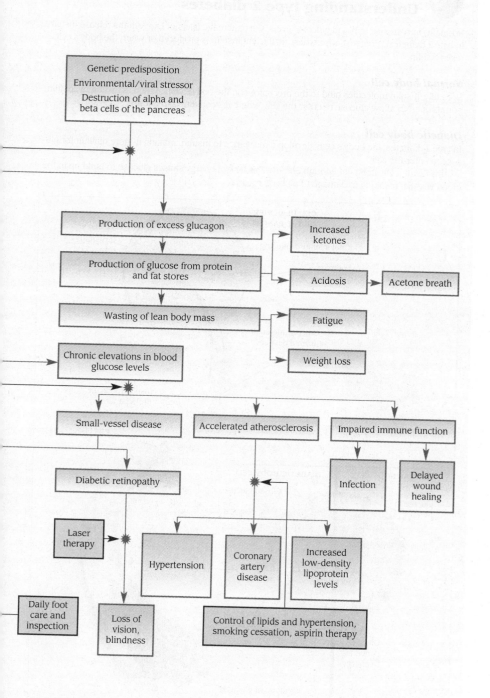

Genetic predisposition
Environmental/viral stressor
Destruction of alpha and beta cells of the pancreas

Production of excess glucagon

Increased ketones

Production of glucose from protein and fat stores

Acidosis → Acetone breath

Wasting of lean body mass

Fatigue

Chronic elevations in blood glucose levels

Weight loss

Small-vessel disease

Accelerated atherosclerosis

Impaired immune function

Diabetic retinopathy

Infection

Delayed wound healing

Laser therapy

Hypertension

Coronary artery disease

Increased low-density lipoprotein levels

Daily foot care and inspection

Loss of vision, blindness

Control of lipids and hypertension, smoking cessation, aspirin therapy

Key: ✳ = treatment

CLOSER LOOK
Understanding type 2 diabetes

Normally, in response to blood glucose levels, the pancreatic islets of Langerhans release insulin. In type 2 diabetes, problems arise when insufficient insulin is produced or when the body's cells resist insulin.

Normal body cell
Normally, insulin molecules bind to the preceptors on the body's cells. When activated by insulin, portals open to allow glucose to enter the cell, where it's converted to energy.

Diabetic body cell
In type 2 diabetes, the body's cells develop a resistance to insulin, making it more difficult for glucose to enter the cell.

As a result, cells don't get enough energy. This lack of energy causes glucose to build up in the blood vessels, resulting in damage to all body organs.

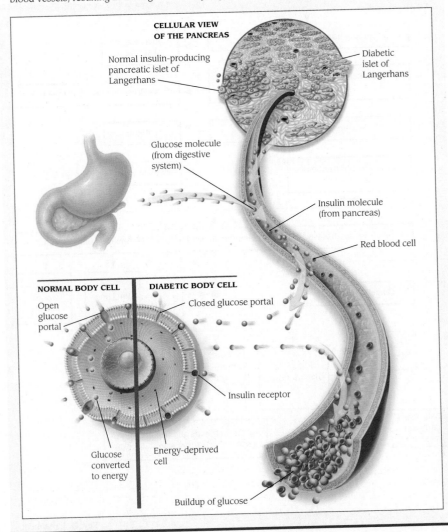

CELLULAR VIEW
OF THE PANCREAS

Normal insulin-producing
pancreatic islet of
Langerhans

Diabetic
islet of
Langerhans

Glucose molecule
(from digestive
system)

Insulin molecule
(from pancreas)

Red blood cell

NORMAL BODY CELL

DIABETIC BODY CELL

Open
glucose
portal

Closed glucose portal

Insulin receptor

Glucose
converted
to energy

Energy-deprived
cell

Buildup of glucose

MULTISYSTEM DISORDER
How diabetes mellitus affects the body

Diabetes mellitus can affect most major body systems. For this reason, a team approach to management and care is needed.

Cardiovascular system
♦ Arterial thrombosis may develop due to persistent activated thrombogenic pathways and impaired fibrinolysis.

GI system
♦ Autonomic neuropathy leads to abdominal discomfort and pain, causing gastroparesis and constipation.
♦ Nausea, diarrhea, or constipation may develop due to dehydration, electrolyte imbalances, or autonomic neuropathy.

Metabolic system
♦ Impaired or absent insulin function prevents normal metabolism of carbohydrates, fats, and proteins, leading to weight loss.
♦ Muscle cramps, irritability, and emotional lability result from electrolyte imbalances.

Neurologic system
♦ A low intracellular glucose level may result in headaches, fatigue, lethargy, reduced energy levels, and impaired school and work performance.

♦ Vision changes, such as blurring, occur due to glucose-induced swelling.
♦ Numbness and tingling occur due to neural tissue damage.

Renal system
♦ Polyuria and polydipsia occur because of high serum osmolality caused by a high serum glucose level.

Collaborative management
The patient may be managed by an endocrinologist to help control the blood glucose level, rehydrate him, and restore electrolyte and acid-base balance. Depending on the severity of the symptoms, the patient may require a pulmonologist to assist with ventilatory support. Nutritional therapy is indicated to assist with dietary needs. A diabetes educator can be valuable in helping the patient learn about his disease and how to manage it. Social services may assist with identifying financial and community resources and with arranging follow-up care.

---

most likely caused by cellular starvation and cellular depletion of nutrient stores
♦ Weight loss (usually 10% to 30%; persons with type 1 diabetes typically have almost no body fat at time of diagnosis) due to prevention of normal metabolism of carbohydrates, fats, and proteins caused by impaired or absent insulin function
♦ Headaches, fatigue, lethargy, reduced energy levels, and impaired school and work performance due to low intracellular glucose levels
♦ Muscle cramps, irritability, and emotional lability due to electrolyte imbalance
♦ Vision changes, such as blurring, due to glucose-induced swelling
♦ Numbness and tingling due to neural tissue damage
♦ Abdominal discomfort and pain due to autonomic neuropathy, causing gastroparesis and constipation
♦ Nausea, diarrhea, or constipation due to dehydration and electrolyte imbalances or autonomic neuropathy

♦ Slow-healing skin infections or wounds and itching of skin due to impaired peripheral circulation
♦ Recurrent candidal infections of the vagina or anus due to hyperglycemia

Complications
♦ Microvascular disease, including retinopathy, nephropathy, and neuropathy
♦ Dyslipidemia
♦ Macrovascular disease, including coronary, peripheral, and cerebral artery disease
♦ Diabetic ketoacidosis
♦ Hyperosmolar hyperglycemic nonketotic syndrome
♦ Excessive weight gain
♦ Skin ulcerations
♦ Chronic renal failure

Diagnosis
In adult men and nonpregnant women, diabetes mellitus is diagnosed by one of the following criteria (in the absence of unequivocal

hyperglycemia, these criteria should be repeated on a different day to confirm the diagnosis):
♦ a fasting plasma glucose level of 126 mg/dl or more
♦ typical symptoms of uncontrolled diabetes and a random blood glucose level of 200 mg/dl or more
♦ a blood glucose level of 200 mg/dl or more 2 hours after ingesting 75 g of oral dextrose.

Patients may also be referred to as having "prediabetes," or a relatively high risk of developing diabetes, if blood tests reveal:
♦ a fasting plasma glucose level of 100 to 125 mg/dl
♦ 2-hour postload glucose level of 140 to 199 mg/dl.

Diagnosis may also be based on:
♦ diabetic retinopathy on ophthalmologic examination
♦ other diagnostic and monitoring tests, including urinalysis for acetone and glycosylated hemoglobin (reflects glycemic control over the past 2 to 3 months).

Treatment

Effective treatment of all types of diabetes optimizes blood glucose control and decreases complications.

Type 1 diabetes mellitus

♦ Insulin replacement, meal planning, and exercise (current forms of insulin replacement include single-dose, mixed-dose, split mixed-dose, and multiple daily injection regimens and continuous subcutaneous insulin infusions)
♦ Pancreas transplantation (requires long-term immunosuppression)

Type 2 diabetes mellitus

♦ An oral antidiabetic to stimulate endogenous insulin production, increase insulin sensitivity at the cellular level, suppress hepatic gluconeogenesis, and delay GI absorption of carbohydrates (drug combinations may be used)
♦ Insulin therapy as appropriate to help manage glucose levels
♦ Beta-adrenergic blockers and angiotensin-converting enzyme inhibitors to control blood pressure
♦ Statins, fibrates, and niacin to treat dyslipidemia (particularly high levels of triglycerides and low levels of high-density lipoprotein cholesterol)

Both types

♦ Careful monitoring of the blood glucose level
♦ Individualized meal plan designed to meet nutritional needs, control blood glucose and lipid levels, and reach and maintain appropriate body weight (plan to be followed consistently with meals eaten at regular times)
♦ Weight reduction (obese patient with type 2 diabetes mellitus) or high calorie allotment, depending on growth stage and activity level (type 1 diabetes mellitus)
♦ Regular physical activity program (adapted for those with complications as needed)
♦ Psychological assessment to determine the impact of the disorder on the patient and family (If needed, psychological treatment should be incorporated into the patient's routine medical care.)
♦ Annual influenza vaccine (for all diabetic patients ages 6 months and older and at least one lifetime pneumococcal vaccine for adult patients with diabetes)

Gestational diabetes

♦ Medical nutrition therapy
♦ Injectable insulin if blood glucose control isn't achieved with diet alone (because oral antidiabetics are teratogenic and, therefore, are contraindicated during pregnancy)
♦ Postpartum counseling to address the high risk of gestational diabetes in subsequent pregnancies and type 2 diabetes later in life
♦ Regular exercise and prevention of weight gain to help prevent type 2 diabetes

Special considerations

Stress the importance of complying with the prescribed treatment program. Tailor your teaching to the patient's needs, abilities, and developmental stage. Include diet; purpose, administration, and possible adverse effects of medications; exercise; monitoring; hygiene; and the prevention, recognition, and treatment of hypoglycemia and hyperglycemia. Stress the effect of blood glucose control on long-term health.

⚠ **CLINICAL ALERT** *Watch for acute complications of diabetic therapy, especially hypoglycemia (vagueness, slow cerebration, dizziness, weakness, pallor, tachycardia, diaphoresis, seizures, and coma); immediately give carbohydrates, ideally in the form of fruit juice, hard candy, honey or, if the patient is unconscious, glucagon or dextrose I.V. Also, be alert for signs and symptoms of ketoacidosis (acetone breath, dehydration, weak and rapid pulse, Kussmaul's respirations) and hyperosmolar coma (polyuria, thirst, neurologic abnormalities, stupor). These hyperglycemic crises require I.V. fluids and regular insulin.*
♦ Monitor diabetes control by obtaining blood glucose, glycosylated hemoglobin, and lipid levels, and blood pressure measurements regularly.

🚫 PREVENTION
Preventing diabetes complications

Although diabetes mellitus itself cannot be prevented, several things can be done to prevent serious complications, such as blindness, kidney damage, and limb amputations.

Managing glucose
♦ Managing glucose levels is important for preventing complications because wildly fluctuating blood glucose levels place the patient at much higher risk. High levels of glucose can cause arteriosclerosis, which can lead to heart attack and stroke. By exercising and maintaining blood sugar at or near normal levels, the risk can be reduced.
♦ High glucose levels can cause blockage of the small blood vessels that supply the limbs with blood. This can cause nerve damage with a loss of sensation. In addition, the patient with diabetes has slow tissue repair, which makes him more prone to infections and amputation of the limbs. The patient with diabetes should never walk around barefoot. Even the smallest cut can cause problems.
♦ Following the prescribed diet (with weight loss if needed), medication regimen (if prescribed), and the recommended exercise program are the keys to controlling glucose levels.

Managing blood pressure
♦ Because an elevated glucose level causes elevated blood pressure, the patient with

diabetes who also has hypertension is at greater risk for developing kidney disease. The continuing high blood pressure can damage the kidney's filtration mechanism and cause kidney failure.
♦ Blood pressure control can reduce heart disease and stroke by about one-third to one-half and can reduce eye, kidney, and nerve disease by about a third.

Preventive care
♦ The patient with diabetes should check his feet every day for swelling, redness, and warmth. These are signs that he should notify his practitioner about immediately. In addition, the patient should have his feet checked at least once a year by his practitioner.
♦ Diabetes can damage the retina of the eye, called retinal neuropathy, which can lead to blindness. Eye examinations should be done once a year and any blurred vision should be reported to the practitioner immediately.

♦ Watch for diabetic effects on the cardiovascular system, such as cerebrovascular, coronary artery, and peripheral vascular impairment, and the peripheral and autonomic nervous systems. Treat all injuries, cuts, and blisters (particularly on the legs or feet) meticulously. Monitor the patient for signs and symptoms of cellulitis. Be alert for signs of urinary tract infection and renal disease. Tell the patient he will need a yearly microalbumin test.
♦ Urge the patient to have regular ophthalmologic examinations to detect diabetic retinopathy.
♦ Assess for signs and symptoms of diabetic neuropathy (numbness or pain in hands and feet, footdrop, neurogenic bladder). Stress the need for personal safety precautions because decreased sensation can mask injuries. Minimize complications by maintaining strict blood glucose control.
♦ Teach the patient to care for his feet by washing them daily, drying carefully between toes, and inspecting for corns, calluses, redness, swelling, bruises, and breaks in the skin. Urge him to report

any changes to the physician. Advise him to wear nonconstricting shoes and to avoid walking barefoot. Instruct him to use over-the-counter athlete's foot remedies and seek professional care should athlete's foot not improve. Encourage periodic visits to a podiatrist.
♦ Teach the patient how to manage his diabetes when he has a minor illness, such as a cold, flu, or upset stomach. (See *Preventing diabetes complications.*)
♦ To delay the clinical onset of diabetes, teach people at high risk to avoid risk factors. Advise genetic counseling for young adults with diabetes who are planning families.
♦ Further information may be obtained from the Juvenile Diabetes Research Foundation, the American Diabetes Association, and the American Association of Diabetes Educators.

GONADOTROPIN DEFICIENCY
Gonadotropin deficiency is a lack of hormones (follicle-stimulating hormone [FSH] and luteinizing hormone [LH]) that stimulate the sex glands,

primarily the testes and ovaries. Chronic gonadotropin deficiency, if not treated, can cause infertility and osteopenia (decreased bone mass). A decrease in testosterone results in decreased bone cell formation.

Causes

♦ Autoimmune pituitary destruction
♦ Genetics
♦ Hypothalamic suppression of gonadotropin-releasing hormone (Gn-RH) during periods of physical or emotional stress, obesity, starvation, or opioid use
♦ Oversecretion of target gland hormone, such as estrogen, progesterone, or testosterone
♦ Pituitary tumor or hemorrhage
♦ Prolactin-secreting tumor

Pathophysiology

Gn-RH is secreted by the hypothalamus and causes the anterior pituitary to secrete the gonadotropins FSH and LH. Estrogen, progesterone, and testosterone, produced by the gonads, function in a negative-feedback loop that regulates Gn-RH secretion.

Testosterone, which is responsible for masculine sex characteristics and sperm production, also functions in bone, muscle, and red blood cell (RBC) formation as well as having a role in neural signaling. Estrogen serves many functions, among them cognitive, bone, and vaginal maintenance. FSH and LH function to maintain the corpus luteum and pregnancy.

Several mechanisms can cause Gn-RH deficiency, including:
♦ pituitary tumor producing another hormone that impinges on the gonadotropin-producing cells and physically impairs Gn-RH biosynthesis
♦ medical treatments, such as radiation (impairs Gn-RH–producing cells) or chronic opioid treatment
♦ oversecretion of estrogen, progesterone, or testosterone by dysfunctional target glands, causing Gn-RH inhibition through the negative-feedback loop
♦ prolactin (inhibits pituitary secretion of Gn-RH; prolactin-secreting tumors can cause Gn-RH deficiency)
♦ reduced Gn-RH secretion due to response of hypothalamus to physical stress, obesity, or starvation (for example, females in competitive athletics may not enter menarche or may cease menstruation for extended periods of time).

Signs and symptoms

Many symptoms are directly related to a reduction in the differentiating sexual characteristics that are caused and maintained by the gonadotropins

(FSH and LH) and the hormones they stimulate, androgens and estrogen. These signs and symptoms vary with the degree and length of Gn-RH deficiency, and may include:
♦ decreased libido, strength, and body hair, and fine wrinkles around the eyes and lips (adults)
♦ amenorrhea; vaginal, uterine, and breast atrophy; clitoral enlargement; voice deepening; and beard growth (women)
♦ testicular atrophy, reduction in beard growth, and erectile dysfunction (men)
♦ decreased RBC count and loss of bone and muscle mass due to a low testosterone level
♦ mood and behavior changes due to changes in the testosterone level
♦ anosmia, which is the absence of a sense of smell (genetic cases).

The age of onset of Gn-RH deficiency affects the presentation in children:
♦ inadequate sexual differentiation shown by ambiguity, pseudohermaphroditism (individual showing one or more contraindications of the morphologic sex criteria), or normal-appearing female genitalia with male genetic coding (first trimester)
♦ microphallus and partial or complete lack of testicular descent (second and third trimesters)
♦ poor secondary sex characteristics and muscle development, lack of deepening voice in males, sparse body hair, gynecomastia (enlarged breast tissue), delayed fusion of epiphyseal plates, and continued long-bone growth (childhood through puberty).

Complications

♦ Infertility

Diagnosis

♦ Serum prolactin, estrogen, testosterone, and Gn-RH levels to differentiate between dysfunction of the hypothalamus or of the ovaries or testicles
♦ Low testosterone and high Gn-RH levels (primary testicular failure)
♦ Low estrogen and high Gn-RH levels (primary ovarian failure)
♦ Low Gn-RH and testosterone or estrogen levels (hypothalamic or pituitary dysfunction)
♦ Human chorionic gonadotropin (hCG) stimulation test (hCG, 500 IU/1.7 m^2 or 100 IU/kg in children, given after measuring baseline testosterone; after 3 to 4 days, the testosterone level should increase by 50% to 200% because hCG and LH stimulate Leydig's cells to stimulate testicular function)
♦ Clomiphene citrate test (normal response, 30% to 200% increase in FSH and 0% to 65% increase in testosterone) with impaired or

absent increase in hypothalamic and pituitary disorders
♦ Gn-RH stimulation test (rapid I.V. injection of Gn-RH stimulates the pituitary to secrete LH and FSH), with insufficient elevation of LH or FSH level, indicating pituitary or hypothalamic dysfunction

Treatment
♦ Surgery to remove tumors
♦ Gonadotropin, estrogen, or testosterone replacement
♦ Stress reduction and weight gain or loss

Special considerations
♦ Monitor the results of laboratory tests for hormonal deficiencies.
♦ Stress the need to take replacement medicines as directed and obtain ongoing follow-up care.

GROWTH HORMONE DEFICIENCY
Growth hormone (GH) deficiency results from hypofunction of the anterior pituitary gland with a resulting decreased secretion of GH. GH deficiency includes a group of childhood disorders characterized by subnormal growth velocity, delayed bone age, and a subnormal response to at least two stimuli for release of the hormone. GH deficiency in adults is characterized by general weakness and increased mortality.

Causes
♦ Autosomal recessive, autosomal dominant, or X-linked trait
♦ Biologically inactive GH
♦ GH receptor insensitivity
♦ Hematologic disorders
♦ Hypothalamic failure
♦ Idiopathic causes
♦ Pituitary hypoxic necrosis
♦ Pituitary inflammation
♦ Pituitary irradiation
♦ Pituitary or central nervous system tumor
♦ Trauma

Pathophysiology
The absence or deficiency of GH synthesis causes growth failure in children. In adults, metabolic derangements decrease GH response to stimulation.

Signs and symptoms
Signs and symptoms of GH deficiency are related to the lack of hormone production and include:
♦ short stature (two standard deviations less than the predicted mean for age and sex)

♦ reduced muscle mass and increased subcutaneous fat due to decreased protein synthesis and insufficient muscle anabolism
♦ hypoglycemia (usually in neonates)
♦ delayed or lack of sexual development.

Complications
♦ Short stature and, possibly, related psychosocial difficulties (if untreated)
♦ Fatal seizures, especially during periods of stress, due to fasting hypoglycemia
♦ Gonadotropin deficiency
♦ Multiple pituitary hormone deficiencies
♦ Increased mortality from cardiovascular disease (adults)

Diagnosis
Diagnosis of GH deficiency is based on decreased serum GH and somatomedin C levels. Low values of insulin-like growth factor (IGF)-1 and IGF binding protein-3 also suggest GH deficiency.

Treatment
Treatment of GH deficiency includes exogenous GH given subcutaneously up to several times weekly during puberty.

Special considerations
♦ After pubertal changes have occurred, the effects of GH therapy are limited. Thus, GH deficiency must be diagnosed and treated early in life so the child can achieve optimal height before epiphyseal closure occurs.
♦ Stress the need to take replacement GH as directed and to obtain ongoing follow-up care.

GROWTH HORMONE EXCESS
Growth hormone (GH) excess that begins in adulthood (after epiphyseal closure) is called *acromegaly.* GH excess that's present before closure of the epiphyseal growth plates of the long bones causes pituitary gigantism. In both cases, the result is increased growth of bone, cartilage, and other tissues as well as increased catabolism of carbohydrates and protein synthesis. Acromegaly is rare, with a prevalence of about 70 people per million in the United States. Although typically diagnosed between ages 40 and 50, acromegaly is usually present for years before diagnosis. GH excess is a slow but progressive disease that decreases longevity if untreated. Morbidity and mortality tend to be related to coronary artery disease and hypertension.

The earliest clinical sign of acromegaly is soft-tissue swelling of the extremities, which causes coarsening and hypertrophy of the facial features.

In gigantism, a proportional overgrowth of all body tissues starts before epiphyseal closure. This causes remarkable height increases—as much as 6″ (15.2 cm) per year. Gigantism affects infants and children, causing them to reach as much as three times the normal height for their age. As adults, they may reach a height of more than 7½′ (228.6 cm).

Causes

♦ Eosinophilic or mixed-cell adenomas of the anterior pituitary gland

Pathophysiology

A GH-secreting tumor creates an unpredictable GH secretion pattern, which replaces the usual peaks that occur 1 to 4 hours after the onset of sleep. Elevated GH and somatomedin levels stimulate tissue growth. In pituitary gigantism, because the epiphyseal plates aren't closed, the excess GH stimulates linear growth. It also increases the bulk of bones and joints and causes enlargement of internal organs and metabolic abnormalities. In acromegaly, the excess GH increases bone density and width, and the proliferation of connective and soft tissues.

Signs and symptoms

Acromegaly develops slowly, and gigantism is characterized by rapid growth.

Acromegaly

♦ Diaphoresis, oily skin, hypermetabolism, hypertrichosis (excessive hair growth), weakness, arthralgias, malocclusion of the teeth, and new skin tags (typical) due to excess growth hormone
♦ Severe headache, central nervous system impairment, bitemporal hemianopia (defective vision), loss of visual acuity, and blindness (if the intrasellar tumor compresses the optic chiasm or nerves)
♦ Cartilaginous and connective tissue overgrowth, causing the characteristic hulking appearance, with an enlarged supraorbital ridge and thickened ears and nose
♦ Marked prognathism (projection of the jaw) that may interfere with chewing
♦ Laryngeal hypertrophy, paranasal sinus enlargement, and thickening of the tongue causing the voice to sound deep and hollow
♦ Arrowhead appearance of distal phalanges on X-rays, thickened fingers
♦ Irritability, hostility, and various psychological disturbances
♦ Bowlegs, barrel chest, arthritis, osteoporosis, kyphosis, hypertension, and arteriosclerosis (prolonged effects of excessive GH secretion)

♦ Glucose intolerance and clinical diabetes mellitus due to action of GH as an insulin antagonist

Gigantism

♦ Backache, arthralgia, and arthritis due to rapid bone growth
♦ Excessive height due to rapid growth before epiphyseal plate closure
♦ Headache, vomiting, seizure activity, visual disturbances, and papilledema (edema where the optic nerve enters the eye chamber) due to tumor compressing nerves and tissue in surrounding structures
♦ Deficiencies of other hormone systems (if GH-producing tumor destroys other hormone-secreting cells)
♦ Glucose intolerance and diabetes mellitus due to insulin-antagonistic actions of GH

Complications

♦ Cardiomegaly
♦ Hypertension
♦ Diabetes mellitus

Diagnosis

♦ An elevated plasma GH level after oral administration of 100 g of glucose, measured by radioimmunoassay (results of random sampling may be misleading because of pulsatile GH secretion)
♦ Somatomedin C, which reflects the integrated production of GH (a better diagnostic alternative)
♦ IGF-1 values to guage integrated GH production and screen for acromegaly
♦ Glucose suppression test (glucose normally suppresses GH secretion; if glucose infusion doesn't suppress GH to less than 2 ng/ml and the patient has characteristic clinical features, hyperpituitarism is likely)
♦ Computed tomography scan or magnetic resonance imaging to show the presence and extent of pituitary lesion
♦ Bone X-rays showing a thickening of the cranium (especially frontal, occipital, and parietal bones) and long bones, and osteoarthritis in the spine (support the diagnosis)
♦ An elevated blood glucose level

Treatment

♦ Tumor removal by cranial or transsphenoidal hypophysectomy or pituitary radiation therapy
♦ Mandatory surgery for a tumor causing blindness or other severe neurologic disturbances (acromegaly)
♦ Replacement of thyroid, cortisone, and gonadal hormones (postoperative therapy)

◆ Somatostatin analogs (octreotide) and dopamine agonists to inhibit GH synthesis
◆ Radiotherapy (adjunctive treatment) for large invasive tumors or when surgery is contraindicated

Special considerations

◆ The striking body changes characteristic of GH excess can cause severe psychological stress. Provide emotional support to help the patient cope with an altered body image.
◆ Perform or assist with range-of-motion exercises to promote maximal joint mobility and prevent injury. Evaluate muscle weakness, especially in the patient with late-stage acromegaly.
◆ Keep the skin dry. Avoid using an oily lotion because the skin is already oily.
◆ A pituitary tumor may cause vision problems. If the patient has a hemianopsia, stand where he can see you. Remember that hyperpituitarism can cause inexplicable mood changes. Reassure the family that these mood changes result from the disease and can be modified with treatment.
◆ If the patient is a child, explain to the parents beforehand that surgery prevents permanent soft-tissue deformities but doesn't correct bone changes that have occurred. Arrange for counseling, if necessary, to help the child and parents cope with these permanent alterations. Diligently monitor vital signs and neurologic status after surgery.
◆ Before discharge, emphasize the importance of continuing hormone replacement therapy. Advise the patient to wear a medical identification bracelet at all times and to bring his hormone replacement schedule with him whenever he returns for follow-up care. Instruct him to have follow-up examinations at least once per year for the rest of his life because a slight risk exists that the tumor that caused his hyperpituitarism may recur.

HYPERALDOSTERONISM

In hyperaldosteronism, hypersecretion of the mineralocorticoid aldosterone by the adrenal cortex causes excessive reabsorption of sodium and water, and excessive renal excretion of potassium.

Incidence of hyperaldosteronism is three times higher in women than in men and is highest between ages 30 and 50.

Causes

◆ Benign aldosterone producing adrenal adenoma, in 70% of patients
◆ Bilateral adrenocortical hyperplasia (in children) or carcinoma (rarely)
◆ Unknown in 15% to 30% of patients

Pathophysiology

Hyperaldosteronism may be primary (uncommon) or secondary. In primary hyperaldosteronism (Conn's syndrome), chronic excessive secretion of aldosterone is independent of the renin-angiotensin system and, in fact, suppresses plasma renin activity. This aldosterone excess enhances sodium and water reabsorption and potassium loss by the kidneys, which leads to mild hypernatremia and, simultaneously, hypokalemia and increased extracellular fluid volume. Expansion of intravascular fluid volume also occurs and results in volume-dependent hypertension and increased cardiac output. Excessive ingestion of natural licorice can produce a syndrome similar to primary hyperaldosteronism. Natural licorice contains glycyrrhizic acid, which acts as a mineralocorticoid. There's currently little or no natural licorice in licorice-flavored foods sold in the United States.

Secondary hyperaldosteronism results from an extra-adrenal abnormality that stimulates the adrenal gland to increase aldosterone production. For example, conditions that reduce renal blood flow (renal artery stenosis) and extracellular fluid volume or produce a sodium deficit activate the renin-angiotensin system and, subsequently, increase aldosterone secretion. Thus, secondary hyperaldosteronism may result from conditions that induce hypertension through increased renin production (such as Wilms' tumor), ingestion of hormonal contraceptives, and pregnancy.

However, secondary hyperaldosteronism may also result from disorders unrelated to edema, such as Bartter's syndrome and salt-losing nephritis; or those that induce edema, such as nephrotic syndrome, hepatic cirrhosis with ascites, and heart failure.

Signs and symptoms

Hyperaldosteronism results in both hypokalemia and hypertension. The hypokalemia increases neuromuscular irritability and can result in muscle weakness and fatigue, headaches, abdominal distention and ileus, paresthesias, and tetany. Hypertension can produce signs of heart failure, stroke, carotid or abdominal bruits, renal insufficiency, hypertensive encephalopathy, and retinal changes.

Other characteristic findings of hyperaldosteronism include:
◆ loss of renal concentrating ability, resulting in nocturnal polyuria and polydipsia
◆ azotemia, indicating chronic potassium depletion nephropathy.

Complications

♦ Neuromuscular irritability, tetany, paresthesia
♦ Seizures
♦ Left ventricular hypertrophy, heart failure, death
♦ Metabolic alkalosis, nephropathy, azotemia

Diagnosis

In a nonedematous patient who isn't taking a diuretic, doesn't have obvious GI losses (from vomiting or diarrhea), and has a normal sodium intake, a persistently low serum potassium level suggests hyperaldosteronism. If hypokalemia develops in a hypertensive patient shortly after starting treatment with a potassium-wasting diuretic (such as a thiazide), and if it persists after the diuretic has been discontinued and potassium replacement therapy has been instituted, evaluation for hyperaldosteronism is necessary.

♦ A low plasma renin level that fails to increase appropriately during volume depletion (upright posture, sodium depletion) and a high plasma aldosterone level during volume expansion by salt loading confirm primary hyperaldosteronism in a hypertensive patient without edema.

♦ The serum bicarbonate level is usually elevated, with ensuing alkalosis due to hydrogen and potassium ion loss in the distal renal tubules.

♦ Other tests show a markedly increased urine aldosterone level, an increased plasma aldosterone level and, in secondary hyperaldosteronism, an increased plasma renin level.

♦ A suppression test is useful to differentiate between primary and secondary hyperaldosteronism. During this test, the patient receives oral desoxycorticosterone for 3 days while the plasma aldosterone level and the urinary metabolites level are continuously measured. These levels decrease in secondary hyperaldosteronism but remain the same in primary hyperaldosteronism. Simultaneously, the renin level are low in primary hyperaldosteronism and high in secondary hyperaldosteronism.

♦ Other helpful diagnostic evidence includes an increase in plasma volume of 30% to 50% above normal, electrocardiogram signs of hypokalemia (ST-segment depression and U waves), chest X-ray showing left ventricular hypertrophy from chronic hypertension, and localization of the tumor by adrenal angiography or computed tomography scan.

Treatment

Although treatment of primary hyperaldosteronism may include unilateral adrenalectomy, administration of a potassium-sparing diuretic — spironolactone — and sodium restriction may control hyperaldosteronism without surgery. For bilateral adrenal hyperplasia, spironolactone is the drug of choice. Treatment of secondary hyperaldosteronism must include correction of the underlying cause.

Special considerations

Patient care includes careful monitoring and recording of urine output, blood pressure, weight, and the serum potassium level.

♦ Watch for signs of tetany (muscle twitching, Chvostek's sign, Trousseau's sign) and for hypokalemia-induced cardiac arrhythmias, paresthesia, or weakness. Give potassium replacement, as ordered, and keep I.V. calcium gluconate available.

♦ Ask the dietitian to provide a low-sodium, high-potassium diet.

♦ After adrenalectomy, watch for weakness, hyponatremia, a rising serum potassium level, and signs of adrenal hypofunction, especially hypotension.

♦ If the patient is taking spironolactone, advise him to watch for signs of hyperkalemia. Tell him that impotence and gynecomastia may follow long-term use.

♦ Tell the patient who must take steroid hormone replacement to wear a medical identification bracelet.

HYPERPARATHYROIDISM

Hyperparathyroidism results from excessive secretion of parathyroid hormone (PTH) from one or more of the four parathyroid glands. PTH promotes bone resorption, and hypersecretion leads to hypercalcemia and hypophosphatemia. Renal and GI absorption of calcium increase.

Primary hyperparathyroidism is commonly diagnosed based on an elevated calcium level found on laboratory test results in asymptomatic patients. It's two to three times more common in women than in men.

Causes

Hyperparathyroidism may be primary or secondary. In primary hyperparathyroidism:

♦ one or more parathyroid glands enlarge and increase PTH secretion and the serum calcium level, most commonly caused by a single adenoma, but this may be a component of multiple endocrine neoplasia (all four glands usually involved).

In secondary hyperparathyroidism, a hypocalcemia-producing abnormality outside the parathyroid glands causes excessive compensatory production of PTH. Causes include:

♦ chronic renal failure
♦ osteomalacia due to phenytoin (Dilantin)
♦ rickets
♦ vitamin D deficiency.

Pathophysiology

Overproduction of PTH by a tumor or hyperplastic tissue increases intestinal calcium absorption, reduces renal calcium clearance, and increases bone calcium release. Response to this excess varies for each patient for an unknown reason.

Hypophosphatemia results when excessive PTH inhibits renal tubular phosphate reabsorption. The hypophosphatemia aggravates hypercalcemia by increasing the sensitivity of the bone to PTH.

Signs and symptoms

Signs and symptoms of primary hyperparathyroidism result from hypercalcemia and are typically present in several body systems. Signs and symptoms may include:

◆ polyuria, nephrocalcinosis, nocturia, polydipsia, dehydration, uremia symptoms, renal colic pain, nephrolithiasis, and renal insufficiency
◆ vague aches and pains, arthralgias, localized swellings
◆ chronic low back pain and easy fracturing due to bone degeneration; bone tenderness; chondrocalcinosis (streaking of soft tissues with calcium); osteopenia and osteoporosis, especially on the vertebrae; erosions of the juxta-articular (adjoining joint) surface; subchondral fractures; traumatic synovitis; and pseudogout (skeletal and articular systems)
◆ pancreatitis causing constant, severe epigastric pain that radiates to the back; peptic ulcers, causing abdominal pain, anorexia, nausea, and vomiting (GI system)
◆ muscle weakness and atrophy, particularly in the legs (neuromuscular system)
◆ psychomotor and personality disturbances, emotional lability, depression, slow mentation, poor memory, drowsiness, ataxia, overt psychosis, stupor and, possibly, coma
◆ pruritus caused by ectopic calcifications in the skin
◆ skin necrosis, cataracts, calcium microthrombi to lungs and pancreas, anemia, and subcutaneous calcification (other systems).

Secondary hyperparathyroidism may produce the same features of calcium imbalance with skeletal deformities of the long bones (such as rickets) as well as symptoms of the underlying disease.

Complications

◆ Pathologic fractures
◆ Renal damage
◆ Urinary tract infections
◆ Hypertension
◆ Cardiac arrhythmias

◆ Insulin hypersecretion, decreased insulin sensitivity
◆ Pseudogout

Diagnosis

Findings differ in primary and secondary disease.

In primary disease

◆ Hypercalcemia and high levels of serum PTH on radioimmunoassay (confirms the diagnosis)
◆ X-rays showing diffuse demineralization of bones, bone cysts, outer cortical bone absorption, and subperiosteal erosion of the phalanges and distal clavicles
◆ Microscopic bone examination by X-ray spectrophotometry typically showing increased bone turnover
◆ Elevated urine and serum calcium, chloride, and alkaline phosphatase levels; a decreased serum phosphorus level
◆ Elevated uric acid and creatinine levels, which may also increase basal gastric acid secretion and serum immunoreactive gastrin
◆ An increased serum amylase level (may indicate acute pancreatitis)

In secondary disease

◆ A normal or slightly decreased serum calcium level, and a variable serum phosphorus level, especially when the cause is rickets, osteomalacia, or kidney disease
◆ Vitamin D deficiency (a 25-hydroxyvitamin D level of less than 20 ng/ml or less than 50 nmol/L)
◆ Patient history possibly showing familial kidney disease, a seizure disorder, or drug ingestion

Treatment

Effective treatment varies, depending on the cause of the disease. In primary hyperparathyroidism, surgery is the only definitive therapy. The only effective long-term medical therapy is maintaining hydration in mild hyperparathyroidism.

For primary disease

◆ Surgery to remove the adenoma or, depending on the extent of hyperplasia, all but one-half of one gland, to provide a normal PTH level (may relieve bone pain within 3 days, but renal damage may be irreversible)
◆ Treatments to decrease the calcium level, such as forcing fluids, limiting dietary intake of calcium, and promoting sodium and calcium excretion through forced diuresis (using as much as 6 L of urine output in life-threatening circumstances), and use of furosemide (Lasix)

or ethacrynic acid (Edecrin) (preoperatively or if surgery isn't feasible or necessary)

♦ Oral sodium or potassium phosphate; subcutaneous calcitonin (Calcimar); I.V. plicamycin

♦ I.V. magnesium and phosphate or sodium phosphate solution by mouth or retention enema (for potential postoperative magnesium and phosphate deficiencies), possibly supplemental calcium, vitamin D, or calcitriol (Calcijex) (serum calcium level decreases to low-normal range during the first 4 to 5 days after surgery)

♦ Bisphosphonates (alendronate) given I.V. before surgical treatment to improve bone mineral density

For secondary disease

♦ Vitamin D to correct the underlying cause of parathyroid hyperplasia; aluminum hydroxide preparation to correct hyperphosphatemia in the patient with kidney disease

♦ Dialysis in the patient with renal failure to decrease the phosphorus level (may be lifelong)

♦ Enlarged glands may not revert to normal size and function even after the calcium level has been controlled in the patient with chronic secondary hyperparathyroidism

♦ For severe hypercalcemia (a serum calcium level greater than 14 mg/dl) or for the patient with severe symptoms, administration of calcitonin, a rapid-acting agent, along with hydration; possible initiation of pamidronate, a slower-acting agent, to provide a longer-lasting effect

Special considerations

Care emphasizes prevention of complications from the underlying disease and its treatment.

♦ Obtain pretreatment baseline serum potassium, calcium, phosphate, and magnesium levels because these values may change abruptly during treatment.

♦ During hydration to reduce the serum calcium level, record intake and output accurately. Strain urine to check for calculi. Provide at least 3 qt (3 L) of fluid per day, including cranberry or prune juice to increase urine acidity and help prevent calculus formation. As ordered, obtain blood samples and urine specimens to measure sodium, potassium, and magnesium levels, especially for the patient taking furosemide.

♦ Auscultate for breath sounds often. Listen for signs of pulmonary edema in the patient receiving large amounts of saline solution I.V., especially if he has pulmonary or cardiac disease. Carefully monitor the patient taking a cardiac glycoside because an elevated calcium level can rapidly produce toxic effects.

♦ Because the patient is predisposed to pathologic fractures, take safety precautions to minimize the risk of injury. Assist him with walking, keep the bed at its lowest position, and raise the side rails. Lift the immobilized patient carefully to minimize bone stress. Schedule care to allow the patient with muscle weakness as much rest as possible.

After parathyroidectomy

♦ Check frequently for respiratory distress, and keep a tracheotomy tray at the bedside. Watch for postoperative complications, such as laryngeal nerve damage or, rarely, hemorrhage. Carefully monitor intake and output.

♦ Check for swelling at the surgical site. Place the patient in semi-Fowler's position, and support his head and neck with sandbags to decrease edema, which may cause pressure on the trachea.

♦ Watch for signs of mild tetany, such as complaints of tingling in the hands and around the mouth. These symptoms should subside quickly but may be prodromal signs of tetany, so keep calcium gluconate or calcium chloride I.V. available for emergency administration. Watch for increased neuromuscular irritability and other signs of severe tetany, and report them immediately.

♦ Help the patient ambulate as soon as possible postoperatively, even though he may find this uncomfortable, because pressure on bones speeds up bone recalcification.

♦ Check laboratory results for low serum calcium and magnesium levels.

♦ Monitor mental status and watch for listlessness. In the patient with persistent hypercalcemia, check for muscle weakness and psychiatric symptoms.

♦ Before discharge, advise the patient of the possible adverse effects of drug therapy. Emphasize the need for periodic follow-up through laboratory blood tests. If hyperparathyroidism wasn't corrected surgically, warn the patient to avoid antacids and thiazide diuretics because they cause calcium retention.

HYPERTHYROIDISM

Hyperthyroidism, or *thyrotoxicosis*, is a metabolic imbalance that results from the overproduction of thyroid hormone. The most common form is Graves' disease, which increases thyroxine (T_4) production, enlarges the thyroid gland (goiter), and causes multiple system changes. (See *Other forms of hyperthyroidism.*)

AGE ALERT *The incidence of Graves' disease is greatest between ages 30 and 40, especially in those with a family history of thyroid abnormalities; only 5% of the patients are younger than age 15.*

With treatment, most patients can lead normal lives. However, thyroid storm — an acute, severe exacerbation of thyrotoxicosis — is a medical emergency that may have life-threatening cardiac, hepatic, or renal consequences.

Causes

Thyrotoxicosis may result from both genetic and immunologic factors, including:
◆ clinical thyrotoxicosis precipitated by excessive dietary intake of iodine or possibly stress (patients with latent disease)
◆ defect in suppressor-cell function, permitting production of autoantibodies (thyroid-stimulating immunoglobulin and thyroid-stimulating hormone [TSH]–binding inhibitory immunoglobulin)
◆ increased incidence in monozygotic twins, pointing to an inherited factor, probably autosomal recessive gene
◆ medications, such as lithium and amiodarone
◆ occasional coexistence with other endocrine abnormalities, such as type 1 diabetes mellitus, thyroiditis, and hyperparathyroidism
◆ stress, such as surgery, infection, toxemia of pregnancy, or diabetic ketoacidosis, can precipitate thyroid storm (inadequately treated thyrotoxicosis)
◆ toxic nodules or tumors.

Pathophysiology

The thyroid gland secretes the thyroid precursor, T_4, thyroid hormone or triiodothyronine (T_3), and calcitonin. T_4 and T_3 stimulate protein, lipid, and carbohydrate metabolism primarily through catabolic pathways. Calcitonin removes calcium from the blood and incorporates it into bone.

Biosynthesis, storage, and release of thyroid hormones are controlled by the hypothalamic-pituitary axis through a negative-feedback loop. Thyrotropin-releasing hormone (TRH) from the hypothalamus stimulates the release of TSH by the pituitary. Circulating T_3 provides negative feedback through the hypothalamus to decrease the TRH level and through the pituitary to decrease the TSH level.

Although the exact mechanism isn't understood, hyperthyroidism has a hereditary component, and about 50% of cases are associated with other autoimmune endocrinopathies.

Graves' disease is an autoimmune disorder characterized by the production of autoantibodies that attach to and then stimulate TSH receptors on the thyroid gland. A goiter is an enlarged thyroid gland, either the result of increased stimulation or a response to increased metabolic demand. The latter occurs in iodine-deficient areas of the world, where the incidence of goiter increases during puberty (a time of increased

Other forms of hyperthyroidism

◆ *Toxic adenoma,* a small, benign nodule in the thyroid gland that secretes thyroid hormone, is the second most common cause of hyperthyroidism. The cause of toxic adenoma is unknown; incidence is highest in elderly people. Clinical effects are essentially similar to those of Graves' disease, except that toxic adenoma doesn't induce ophthalmopathy, pretibial myxedema, or acropachy. Presence of adenoma is confirmed by radioactive iodine (^{131}I) uptake and thyroid scan, which show a single hyperfunctioning nodule suppressing the rest of the gland. Treatment includes either ^{131}I therapy or surgery to remove adenoma after antithyroid drug therapy achieves a euthyroid state.
◆ *Thyrotoxicosis factitia* results from chronic ingestion of thyroid hormone for thyrotropin suppression in patients with thyroid carcinoma or from thyroid hormone abuse by people who are trying to lose weight.
◆ *Functioning metastatic thyroid carcinoma* is a rare disease that causes excess production of thyroid hormone.
◆ *Thyroid-stimulating hormone-secreting pituitary tumor* causes overproduction of thyroid hormone.
◆ *Subacute thyroiditis* is a virus-induced granulomatous inflammation of the thyroid, producing transient hyperthyroidism associated with fever, pain, pharyngitis, and tenderness in the thyroid gland.
◆ *Silent thyroiditis* is a self-limiting, transient form of hyperthyroidism, with histologic thyroiditis but no inflammatory symptoms.

metabolic demand). These goiters commonly regress to normal size after puberty in males, but not in females. Sporadic goiter in non–iodine-deficient areas is of unknown origin. Endemic and sporadic goiters are nontoxic and may be diffuse or nodular. Toxic goiters may be uninodular or multinodular and may secrete excess thyroid hormone.

Pituitary tumors with TSH-producing cells are rare, as is hypothalamic disease causing TRH excess.

Signs and symptoms

Signs and symptoms of hyperthyroidism include:
◆ enlarged thyroid (goiter) resulting from increased stimulation of the thyroid gland or a

Recognizing hyperthyroidism

Below illustrates the common signs of an overactive thyroid.

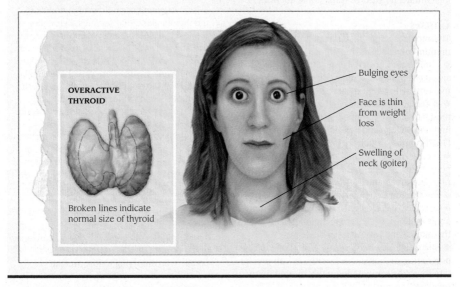

OVERACTIVE THYROID

Broken lines indicate normal size of thyroid

Bulging eyes

Face is thin from weight loss

Swelling of neck (goiter)

response to increased metabolic demand (See *Recognizing hyperthyroidism.*)

♦ nervousness caused by hypermetabolic state

♦ heat intolerance and sweating caused by hypermetabolic state and subsequent increase in vasodilation

♦ weight loss despite increased appetite resulting from hypermetabolic state

♦ frequent bowel movements resulting from sympathetic nervous stimulation and stimulation of GI motility

♦ tremor and palpitations caused by increased sympathetic nervous system activity and possible increased sensitivity of neural synapses

♦ exophthalmos (characteristic, but absent in many patients with thyrotoxicosis).

Other signs and symptoms, common because thyrotoxicosis profoundly affects virtually every body system, include:

♦ difficulty concentrating due to accelerated cerebral function; excitability or nervousness caused by increased basal metabolic rate from T_4; fine tremor, shaky handwriting, and clumsiness from increased activity in the spinal cord area that controls muscle tone; emotional instability and mood swings ranging from occasional outbursts to overt psychosis (central nervous system)

♦ moist, smooth, warm, flushed skin (patient sleeps with minimal covers and little clothing); fine, soft hair; premature patchy graying and

increased hair loss in both sexes; friable nails and onycholysis (distal nail separated from the bed); pretibial myxedema (nonpitting edema of the anterior surface of the legs, dermopathy), producing thickened skin; accentuated hair follicles; sometimes itchy or painful raised red patches of skin with occasional nodule formation; microscopic examination showing increased mucin deposits (integumentary system)

♦ systolic hypertension, tachycardia, full bounding pulse, wide pulse pressure, cardiomegaly, increased cardiac output and blood volume, visible point of maximal impulse, paroxysmal supraventricular tachycardia and atrial fibrillation (especially in elderly people), and occasional systolic murmur at the left sternal border (cardiovascular system)

♦ increased respiratory rate, dyspnea on exertion and at rest, possibly due to cardiac decompensation and increased cellular oxygen use (respiratory system)

♦ excessive oral intake with weight loss; nausea and vomiting due to increased GI motility and peristalsis; increased defecation; soft stools or, in severe disease, diarrhea; liver enlargement (GI system)

♦ weakness, fatigue, and muscle atrophy; rare coexistence with myasthenia gravis; possibly generalized or localized paralysis associated with hypokalemia; and, rarely, acropachy (soft-tissue swelling accompanied by underlying bone changes where new bone formation occurs) (musculoskeletal system)

♦ oligomenorrhea or amenorrhea, decreased fertility, increased incidence of spontaneous abortion (women), gynecomastia due to an increased estrogen level (men), diminished libido (both sexes) (reproductive system)

♦ exophthalmos due to combined effects of accumulated mucopolysaccharides and fluids in the retro-orbital tissues, forcing the eyeball outward and lid retraction, thereby producing characteristic staring gaze; occasional inflammation of conjunctivae, corneas, or eye muscles; diplopia; and increased tearing (eyes).

When thyrotoxicosis escalates to thyroid storm, these signs and symptoms may initially occur:

♦ extreme irritability
♦ hypertension
♦ marked tachycardia
♦ vomiting
♦ stupor.

If left untreated, the patient may experience:
♦ high fever (up to 106° F)
♦ vascular collapse, hypotension, angina, pulmonary edema
♦ tremors, emotional lability, extreme irritability, confusion, delirium, psychosis, apathy, stupor, coma, death
♦ diarrhea, abdominal pain, nausea and vomiting, jaundice, hyperglycemia.

AGE ALERT *Consider apathetic thyrotoxicosis, a morbid condition resulting from overactive thyroid, in elderly patients with atrial fibrillation or depression.*

Complications

♦ Muscle wasting, atrophy, and paralysis
♦ Visual loss or diplopia
♦ Heart failure, arrhythmias
♦ Excess bone calcium loss
♦ Hypoparathyroidism after surgical removal of thyroid
♦ Hypothyroidism after radioiodine treatment

Diagnosis

The diagnosis of thyrotoxicosis is usually straightforward. It depends on a careful clinical history and physical examination, a high index of suspicion, and routine hormone determinations. The following test results confirm the disorder:

♦ radioimmunoassay showing increased serum T_4 and T_3 levels
♦ a low TSH level
♦ thyroid scan showing increased uptake of radioactive iodine (^{131}I) in Graves' disease and, usually, in toxic multinodular goiter and toxic adenoma; low radioactive uptake in thyroiditis

and thyrotoxic factitia (test contraindicated in pregnancy)

♦ ultrasonography confirming subclinical ophthalmopathy.

Treatment

The primary forms of therapy include:
♦ an antithyroid drug
♦ single oral dose of [131]I
♦ surgery.

Appropriate treatment depends on:
♦ severity of thyrotoxicosis
♦ causes
♦ patient age and parity
♦ how long surgery will be delayed (if patient is appropriate candidate for surgery).

Antithyroid therapy includes an antithyroid drug for children, young adults, pregnant patients, and patients who refuse surgery or ^{131}I treatment. Antithyroid drugs are preferred in patients with new-onset Graves' disease because of spontaneous remission in many of these patients; they're also used to correct the thyrotoxic state in preparation for ^{131}I treatment or surgery. Treatment options include:

♦ a thyroid hormone antagonist, such as propylthiouracil (PTU) or methimazole (Tapazole), to block thyroid hormone synthesis (hypermetabolic symptoms subside within 4 to 8 weeks after therapy begins, but remission of Graves' disease requires continued therapy for 6 months to 2 years)

♦ propranolol (Inderal) until the antithyroid drug reaches its full effect, to manage tachycardia and other peripheral effects of excessive hypersympathetic activity resulting from blocking the conversion of T_4 to the active T_3 hormone

♦ minimum dosage needed to keep maternal thyroid function within the high-normal range until delivery, and to minimize the risk of fetal hypothyroidism; PTU is the preferred agent (during pregnancy)

♦ possibly an antithyroid drug and propranolol for neonates for 2 to 3 months because most infants of hyperthyroid mothers are born with mild and transient thyrotoxicosis caused by placental transfer of thyroid-stimulating immunoglobulins (neonatal thyrotoxicosis)

♦ continuous control of maternal thyroid function because thyrotoxicosis is sometimes exacerbated in the puerperal period; the antithyroid drug gradually tapered and thyroid function reassessed after 3 to 6 months postpartum

♦ periodic checks of infant's thyroid function with a breast-feeding mother on low-dose antithyroid treatment due to possible presence of small amounts of the drug in breast milk, which can rapidly lead to goiter in the neonate

single oral dose of ^{131}I (treatment of choice for patients not planning to have children; patients of reproductive age must give informed consent for this treatment, because ^{131}I concentrates in the gonads).

During treatment with ^{131}I, the thyroid gland picks up the radioactive element as it would regular iodine. The radioactivity destroys some of the cells that normally concentrate iodine and produce T_4, thus decreasing thyroid hormone production and normalizing thyroid size and function.

In most patients, hypermetabolic symptoms diminish 6 to 8 weeks after such treatment. However, some patients may require a second dose. Almost all patients treated with ^{131}I eventually develop hypothyroidism.

Treatment with surgery includes:
◆ subtotal thyroidectomy to decrease the thyroid gland's capacity for hormone production (patients who refuse or aren't candidates for ^{131}I treatment)
◆ an iodide (Lugol's solution or saturated solution of potassium iodide), an antithyroid drug, and propranolol to relieve hyperthyroidism preoperatively (if patient doesn't become euthyroid, surgery should be delayed and the antithyroid drug and propranolol given to decrease the systemic effects [cardiac arrhythmias] of thyrotoxicosis)
◆ lifelong regular medical supervision because most patients develop hypothyroidism, sometimes as long as several years after surgery.

Treatment of ophthalmopathy includes:
◆ local application of a topical medication, such as prednisone acetate suspension, but may require high doses of a corticosteroid
◆ a calcium channel blocker, such as diltiazem or verapamil, to block the peripheral effects of thyroid hormones
◆ external-beam radiation therapy or surgical decompression (severe exophthalmos causing pressure on optic nerve and orbital contents).

Emergency treatment of thyroid storm includes:
◆ an antithyroid drug to stop conversion of T_4 to T_3 and to block sympathetic effect; a corticosteroid to inhibit the conversion of T_4 to T_3; and iodide to block the release of thyroid hormone
◆ supportive measures, including the administration of nutrients, vitamins, fluids, oxygen, hypothermia blankets, and a sedative.

Special considerations

Patients with hyperthyroidism require vigilant care to prevent acute exacerbations and complications.
◆ Record vital signs and weight.

◆ Monitor serum electrolyte levels, and check periodically for hyperglycemia and glycosuria.
◆ Carefully monitor cardiac function if the patient is elderly or has coronary artery disease. If the heart rate is more than 100 beats/minute, check blood pressure and pulse rate often. Monitor the patient's ECG for arrhythmias and changes in the ST segment.
◆ Check level of consciousness and urine output.
◆ If the patient is pregnant, tell her to watch closely during the first trimester for signs of spontaneous abortion and to report such signs immediately.
◆ Encourage bed rest, and keep the patient's room cool, quiet, and dark. The patient with dyspnea will be most comfortable sitting upright or in high Fowler's position.
◆ Remember, extreme nervousness may produce bizarre behavior. Reassure the patient and his family that such behavior will probably subside with treatment. Provide a sedative as necessary.
◆ To promote weight gain, provide a balanced diet with six meals per day. If the patient has edema, suggest a low-sodium diet.
◆ If iodide is part of the treatment, mix it with milk, juice, or water to prevent GI distress, and administer it through a straw to prevent tooth discoloration.
◆ Watch for signs of thyroid storm (tachycardia, hyperkinesis, fever, vomiting, hypertension).
◆ Check intake and output carefully to ensure adequate hydration and fluid balance.
◆ Closely monitor blood pressure, heart rate and rhythm, and temperature. If the patient has a high fever, reduce it with appropriate hypothermic measures. Maintain an I.V. line and give drugs as ordered.
◆ If the patient has exophthalmos or other ophthalmopathy, suggest sunglasses or eye patches to protect his eyes from light. Moisten the conjunctivae often with isotonic eyedrops. Warn the patient with severe lid retraction to avoid sudden physical movements that might cause the lid to slip behind the eyeball.
◆ Avoid excessive palpation of the thyroid to avoid precipitating thyroid storm.

Thyroidectomy necessitates meticulous postoperative care to prevent complications:
◆ Check often for respiratory distress, and keep a tracheotomy tray at the bedside.
◆ Watch for evidence of hemorrhage into the neck, such as a tight dressing with no blood on it. Change dressings and perform wound care as ordered; check the back of the dressing for drainage. Keep the patient in semi-Fowler's position, and support his head and neck with sandbags to ease tension on the incision.

◆ Check for dysphagia or hoarseness from possible laryngeal nerve injury.

◆ Watch for signs of hypocalcemia (tetany, numbness), a complication that results from accidental removal of the parathyroid glands during surgery.

◆ Stress the importance of regular medical follow-up after discharge because hypothyroidism may develop 2 to 4 weeks postoperatively.

Drug therapy and ^{131}I therapy require careful monitoring and comprehensive patient teaching:

◆ After ^{131}I therapy, tell the patient not to expectorate or cough freely because his saliva will be radioactive for 24 hours. Stress the need for repeated measurement of the serum T_4 level. The patient shouldn't resume antithyroid therapy.

◆ If the patient is taking PTU and methimazole, monitor complete blood count periodically to detect leukopenia, thrombocytopenia, and agranulocytosis. Instruct him to take these medications with meals to minimize GI distress and to avoid over-the-counter cough preparations because many contain iodine.

◆ Tell the patient to report fever, enlarged cervical lymph nodes, sore throat, mouth sores, and other signs of blood dyscrasias and any rash or skin eruptions — signs of hypersensitivity.

◆ Watch the patient taking propranolol for signs and symptoms of hypotension (dizziness, decreased urine output). Tell him to rise slowly after sitting or lying down to prevent orthostatic syncope.

◆ Instruct the patient receiving an antithyroid drug or ^{131}I therapy to report any symptoms of hypothyroidism.

HYPOPARATHYROIDISM

Hypoparathyroidism is caused by disease, injury, or congenital malfunction of the parathyroid glands. Because the parathyroid glands primarily regulate calcium balance, hypoparathyroidism causes hypocalcemia and consequent neuromuscular symptoms ranging from paresthesia to tetany.

The clinical effects of hypoparathyroidism are usually correctable with replacement therapy. Some complications of long-term hypocalcemia, such as cataracts and basal ganglion calcifications, are irreversible.

Causes

Hypoparathyroidism may be acute or chronic and is classified as idiopathic or acquired. Possible causes include:

◆ accidental removal of or injury to the parathyroid glands during thyroidectomy or other neck surgery or, rarely, from massive thyroid irradiation (acquired)

◆ acute pancreatitis or malabsorption

◆ autoimmune genetic disorder or congenital absence of the parathyroid glands (idiopathic)

◆ impairment of hormone synthesis and release due to hypomagnesemia, suppression of normal gland function due to hypercalcemia, and delayed maturation of parathyroid function (acquired, reversible)

◆ ischemic infarction of the parathyroid glands during surgery, amyloidosis, neoplasms, or trauma (acquired)

◆ osteomalacia

◆ renal failure.

Parathyroid hormone (PTH) is regulated directly by the serum calcium level, not by the pituitary or hypothalamus. It normally maintains normocalcemia by regulating bone resorption and GI absorption of calcium. It also maintains an inverse relationship between serum calcium and phosphate levels by inhibiting phosphate reabsorption in the renal tubules.

AGE ALERT *The incidence of the idiopathic and reversible forms of hypoparathyroidism is greatest in children; the incidence of the irreversible acquired form is greatest in adults who have undergone surgery for hyperthyroidism or other head and neck conditions.*

Pathophysiology

Underproduction of PTH causes hypocalcemia and hyperphosphatemia. Surgical manipulation of the neck may damage the parathyroid glands, possibly by causing ischemia. The degree of hypoparathyroidism can vary from decreased reserve to frank tetany. Hypomagnesemia can prevent PTH secretion in patients with chronic GI magnesium losses, nutritional deficiencies, and renal magnesium wasting.

Signs and symptoms

Signs and symptoms vary depending on the onset and severity of disease.

Mild hypoparathyroidism

◆ May be asymptomatic but usually causes hypocalcemia and a high serum phosphate level affecting the central nervous system (CNS) and other systems

Chronic hypoparathyroidism

◆ Neuromuscular irritability, increased deep tendon reflexes, Chvostek's sign (spasm of the hyperirritable facial nerve when it's tapped), dysphagia, organic brain syndrome, psychosis, mental deficiency in children, and tetany caused by hypocalcemia and hyperphosphatemia

◆ Difficulty walking and a tendency to fall (chronic tetany)

Acute hypoparathyroidism

◆ Tingling in the fingertips, around the mouth, and occasionally in the feet (first symptom); spreading and becoming more severe, producing muscle tension and spasms and consequent adduction of the thumbs, wrists, and elbows; pain varying with the degree of muscle tension but seldom affecting the face, legs, and feet (acute overt tetany)

◆ Laryngospasm, stridor, cyanosis, and seizures (CNS abnormalities); worst during hyperventilation, pregnancy, infection, withdrawal of thyroid hormone, or administration of a diuretic and before menstruation (acute tetany)

◆ Abdominal pain; intestinal malabsorption with steatorrhea; dry, lusterless hair; spontaneous hair loss; brittle fingernails developing ridges or falling out; dry, scaly skin; exfoliative dermatitis; candidal infections; cataracts; and weakened tooth enamel, causing teeth to stain, crack, and decay easily (effects of hypocalcemia)

Complications

◆ Cardiac arrhythmias, heart failure
◆ Cataracts
◆ Basal ganglia calcifications
◆ Stunted growth, teeth malformation, and mental retardation
◆ Parkinson's symptoms
◆ Hypothyroidism

Diagnosis

◆ Radioimmunoassay for PTH showing a decreased serum PTH level
◆ Decreased serum (total and ionized) and urine calcium levels
◆ An increased serum phosphorus level
◆ A decreased magnesium level
◆ Electrocardiography (ECG) showing prolonged QT interval and ST segment due to hypocalcemia
◆ Inflating a blood pressure cuff on the upper arm to between diastolic and systolic blood pressure and maintaining this inflation for 3 minutes, eliciting Trousseau's sign (carpal spasm), to show clinical evidence of hypoparathyroidism

Treatment

◆ Immediate I.V. calcium salts, such as 10% calcium gluconate, to increase the ionized serum calcium level (acute, life-threatening tetany)
◆ Breathing into a paper bag and inhaling one's own carbon dioxide causes a mild respiratory acidosis that increases the serum calcium level (awake patient can cooperate)
◆ A sedative and an anticonvulsant to control spasms until the calcium level increases
◆ Increased dietary intake of calcium

◆ Maintenance therapy with oral calcium and vitamin D supplements (chronic tetany)
◆ Vitamin D and a calcium supplement because of calcium absorption from the small intestine requiring the presence of vitamin D (treatment of reversible disease, usually lifelong)
◆ Calcitriol (Calcijex) if hepatic or renal problems make the patient unable to tolerate vitamin D

Special considerations

While awaiting diagnosis of hypoparathyroidism in a patient with a history of tetany, maintain a patent I.V. line and keep I.V. calcium available. Because the patient is vulnerable to seizures, maintain seizure precautions. Also, keep a tracheotomy tray and endotracheal tube at the bedside because laryngospasm may result from hypocalcemia.

◆ Instruct the patient to follow a high-calcium, low-phosphorus diet.

◆ When caring for the patient with chronic disease, particularly a child, stay alert for minor muscle twitching and for signs of laryngospasm because these effects may signal the onset of tetany.

◆ For the patient on drug therapy, emphasize the importance of checking the serum calcium level at least three times per year. Instruct the patient to watch for signs of hypercalcemia and to keep medications away from light and heat.

◆ Dental changes, cataracts, and brain calcifications are permanent. These can be prevented with early detection and periodic calcium determinations.

◆ Because the patient with chronic disease has a prolonged QT interval on ECG, watch for heart block and signs of decreasing cardiac output. Because calcium potentiates the effect of cardiac glycosides, closely monitor the patient receiving both a cardiac glycoside and calcium. Stay alert for signs and symptoms of digoxin toxicity (arrhythmias, nausea, fatigue, visual changes).

◆ Instruct the patient with scaly skin to use creams to soften his skin. Also, tell him to keep his nails trimmed to prevent them from splitting.

◆ Hyperventilation or recent blood transfusions may worsen tetany. (Anticoagulant in stored blood binds calcium.)

◆ For the patient with tetany, administer 10% calcium gluconate by slow I.V. infusion (1 ml/ minute), and maintain a patent airway. The patient may also require intubation and sedation with I.V. diazepam. Monitor vital signs often after administration of diazepam to make certain that blood pressure and heart rate return to normal.

HYPOPITUITARISM

Hypopituitarism, also known as *panhypopituitarism*, is a complex syndrome marked by metabolic dysfunction, sexual immaturity, and growth retardation (when it occurs in childhood). The cause is a deficiency of the hormones secreted by the anterior pituitary gland. Panhypopituitarism is a partial or total failure of all six of this gland's vital hormones—corticotropin, thyroid-stimulating hormone (TSH), luteinizing hormone (LH), follicle-stimulating hormone (FSH), human growth hormone, and prolactin. Partial and complete forms of hypopituitarism affect adults and children; in children, these diseases may cause dwarfism and delayed puberty. The prognosis may be good with adequate replacement therapy and correction of the underlying cause.

Primary hypopituitarism usually develops in a predictable pattern. It generally starts with decreased gonadotropin (FSH and LH) levels and consequent hypogonadism, reflected by cessation of menses in women and impotence in men. Growth hormone deficiency follows, causing short stature, delayed growth, and delayed puberty in children. Subsequently, a decreased TSH level causes hypothyroidism and, finally, a decreased corticotropin level results in adrenal insufficiency. When hypopituitarism follows surgical ablation or trauma, the pattern of hormonal events may not necessarily follow that sequence. Damage to the hypothalamus or neurohypophysis may cause diabetes insipidus.

Causes

Hypopituitarism may be primary or secondary. Primary hypopituitarism may be caused by:
◆ congenital defects (hypoplasia or aplasia of the pituitary gland)
◆ granulomatous disease, such as tuberculosis (rare)
◆ idiopathic or autoimmune origin (occasionally)
◆ partial or total hypophysectomy by surgery, irradiation, or chemical agents
◆ pituitary infarction (most commonly from postpartum hemorrhage)
◆ tumor of the pituitary gland.

Secondary hypopituitarism is caused by:
◆ deficiency of releasing hormones produced by the hypothalamus, either idiopathic or resulting from infection, trauma, or a tumor.

Pathophysiology

Hypopituitarism is the low secretion of an anterior pituitary hormone, and panhypopituitarism is the low secretion of *all* anterior pituitary hormones. Both can result from malfunction of the pituitary gland or the hypothalamus. The result is a lack of stimulation of target endocrine organs and some degree of deficiency of the target organ hormone, which may not be discovered until the body is stressed and the expected increases in secretions from the target organs don't occur.

Signs and symptoms

◆ Corticotropin deficiency, causing weakness, fatigue, weight loss, fasting hypoglycemia, altered mental function, and depigmentation of skin due to hypocortisolism; loss of axillary and pubic hair due to androgen deficiency in women; orthostatic hypotension and hyponatremia due to aldosterone deficiency
◆ TSH deficiency, causing weight gain, constipation, cold intolerance, fatigue, coarse hair, slow thought process, and growth retardation in children
◆ Gonadotropin (FSH and LH) deficiency, causing amenorrhea, sexual dysfunction, and infertility
◆ Antidiuretic hormone deficiency, causing diabetes insipidus
◆ Prolactin deficiency, causing lactation dysfunction or gynecomastia

Complications

◆ Blindness
◆ Adrenal crisis

Diagnosis

◆ Hormonal deficiency of the tropic and target organ hormones affected, chosen after evaluation of clinical picture (testing includes adrenocorticotropic hormone and cosyntropin stimulation; TSH and thyroxine; FSH, LH, estradiol, or testosterone; prolactin; and growth hormone)
◆ Hypoglycemia (caused by insulin administration), stimulating secretion of corticotropin (consistently low levels of corticotropin indicate pituitary and hypothalamic failure)
◆ Computed tomography or magnetic resonance imaging of pituitary and target glands, showing destruction of the anterior pituitary or atrophy of target glands (adrenal cortex, thyroid, or gonads)

Treatment

◆ Replacement of hormones secreted by the target glands (cortisol, thyroxine, and androgen or cyclic estrogen); prolactin not replaced
◆ Clomiphene or cyclic gonadotropin-releasing hormone to induce ovulation in the patient of reproductive age

Special considerations

Caring for patients with hypopituitarism requires an understanding of hormonal effects and skilled physical and psychological support.
◆ Monitor the results of all laboratory tests for hormonal deficiencies, and know what they mean. Until hormone replacement therapy is

complete, check for signs and symptoms of thyroid deficiency (increasing lethargy), adrenal deficiency (weakness, ortho-static hypotension, hypoglycemia, fatigue, and weight loss), and gonadotropin deficiency (decreased libido, lethargy, and apathy).

♦ Watch for anorexia in the patient with panhypopituitarism. Help plan a menu containing favorite foods—ideally, high-calorie foods. Monitor for weight loss or gain.

♦ If the patient has trouble sleeping, encourage him to exercise during the day.

♦ Record temperature, blood pressure, and heart rate every 4 to 8 hours. Check eyelids, nail beds, and skin for pallor, which indicates anemia.

♦ Prevent infection by giving meticulous skin care. Because the patient's skin is probably dry, use oil or lotion instead of soap. If body temperature is low, provide additional clothing and covers, as needed, to keep the patient warm.

♦ Darken the room if the patient has a tumor that's causing headaches and vision disturbances. Help with any activity that requires good vision, such as reading the menu. The patient with bilateral hemianopsia has impaired peripheral vision, so be sure to stand where he can see you, and advise the family to do the same.

♦ During insulin testing, monitor closely for signs of hypoglycemia (initially, slow cerebration, tachycardia, diaphoresis, and nervousness, progressing to seizures). Keep dextrose 50% in water available for I.V. administration to correct hypoglycemia rapidly.

♦ Instruct the patient to wear a medical identification bracelet. Teach him and family members how to administer steroids parenterally in case of an emergency.

♦ Refer the family of a child with dwarfism to appropriate community resources for psychological counseling because the emotional stress caused by this disorder increases as the child becomes more aware of his condition.

HYPOTHYROIDISM IN ADULTS

Hypothyroidism results from hypothalamic, pituitary, or thyroid insufficiency or resistance to thyroid hormone. The disorder can progress to life-threatening myxedema coma. Hypothyroidism is more prevalent in women than men; in the United States, the incidence is increasing significantly in people ages 40 to 50.

⚠ **CLINICAL ALERT** *Hypothyroidism occurs primarily after age 40. After age 65, the prevalence increases to as much as 10% in women and 3% in men.*

Causes

♦ Inadequate production of thyroid hormone, usually after thyroidectomy or radiation therapy (particularly with iodine 131), or due to inflammation, chronic autoimmune thyroiditis (Hashimoto's disease), or such conditions as amyloidosis and sarcoidosis (rare)

♦ Pituitary failure to produce thyroid-stimulating hormone (TSH), hypothalamic failure to produce thyrotropin-releasing hormone (TRH), inborn errors of thyroid hormone synthesis, iodine deficiency (usually dietary), or use of such antithyroid medications as propylthiouracil

Pathophysiology

Hypothyroidism may reflect a malfunction of the hypothalamus, pituitary, or thyroid gland, all of which are part of the same negative-feedback mechanism. However, disorders of the hypothalamus and pituitary rarely cause hypothyroidism; when they do, the condition is known as *secondary hypothyroidism*. Primary hypothyroidism, a disorder of the gland itself, is most common. (See *How hypothyroidism affects the body*.)

Chronic autoimmune thyroiditis, also called chronic lymphocytic thyroiditis, occurs when autoantibodies destroy thyroid gland tissue. Chronic autoimmune thyroiditis associated with goiter is called Hashimoto's disease. The cause of this autoimmune process is unknown, although heredity has a role, and specific human leukocyte antigen subtypes are associated with greater risk.

Outside the thyroid, antibodies can reduce the effect of thyroid hormone in two ways. First, antibodies can block the TSH receptor and prevent the production of TSH. Second, cytotoxic antithyroid antibodies may attack thyroid cells.

Subacute thyroiditis, painless thyroiditis, and postpartum thyroiditis are self-limited conditions that usually follow an episode of hyperthyroidism. Untreated subclinical hypothyroidism in adults is likely to become overt at a rate of 5% to 20% per year.

Signs and symptoms

Signs and symptoms of hypothyroidism result from insufficiency or resistance to thyroid hormone, and may include:

♦ weakness, fatigue, forgetfulness, sensitivity to cold, unexplained weight gain, and constipation (typical, vague, early clinical features)

♦ characteristic myxedematous signs and symptoms of decreasing mental stability; coarse, dry, flaky, inelastic skin; puffy face, hands, and feet; hoarseness; periorbital edema; upper eyelid droop; dry, sparse hair; and thick, brittle nails (as the disorder progresses)

♦ cardiovascular involvement, including decreased cardiac output, slow pulse rate, signs of poor peripheral circulation and, occasionally, an enlarged heart.

How hypothyroidism affects the body

Because thyroid hormones are necessary for normal growth and development and act on many tissues to increase metabolic activity and protein synthesis, the effects of hypothyroidism are widespread. For this reason, a multidisciplinary approach to care is needed.

Cardiovascular system
◆ Cardiovascular involvement includes decreased cardiac output resulting in slow pulse rate, signs of poor peripheral circulation and, occasionally, an enlarged heart, eventually leading to heart failure.
◆ Fluid retention may lead to periorbital edema.

GI system
◆ Unexplained weight gain may be attributed to fluid retention in the myxedematous tissues.
◆ Constipation, anorexia, and abdominal distention occur; these conditions may eventually lead to megacolon.

Genitourinary system
◆ Menorrhagia and decreased libido occur because of an altered prolactin level; these conditions may lead to infertility.

Integumentary system
◆ Decreased sweating occurs.
◆ The epidermis thins and hyperkeratosis occurs.
◆ Increased dermal glycoaminoglycan content traps water and gives rise to skin thickening without pitting (myxedema).
◆ Dry, flaky, inelastic skin develops.
◆ Hair patterns and eyebrows change.
◆ Nails become dry and brittle.

Musculoskeletal system
◆ Ataxia, nystagmus, and reflexes with delayed relaxation time (especially in the Achilles tendon) occur because of endocrine effects.

Neurologic system
◆ Metabolic effects disrupt the central nervous system (CNS), leading to weakness, fatigue, forgetfulness, sensitivity to the cold, and decreased mental stability.
◆ CNS effects can progress to myxedema coma. Progression is usually gradual but may develop abruptly. Such stresses as hypoventilation, hypoglycemia, hyponatremia, hypotension, and hypothermia in those with severe or prolonged hypothyroidism increase the risk.

Collaborative management
An endocrinologist may be needed to help the patient obtain and maintain normal thyroid levels. A cardiologist may be necessary to help the patient improve cardiac output. A GI specialist may be consulted if the patient experiences chronic bowel problems. Counselors may be needed to assist the patient and his family with psychosocial needs.

Other common effects include:
◆ anorexia, abdominal distention, menorrhagia, decreased libido, infertility, paresthesia, joint stiffness, muscle cramping, ataxia, and nystagmus; reflexes with delayed relaxation time (especially in the Achilles tendon)
◆ progression to myxedema coma, usually gradual but may develop abruptly, with stress aggravating severe or prolonged hypothyroidism, including progressive stupor, hypoventilation, hypoglycemia, hyponatremia, hypotension, and hypothermia.

Complications
◆ Heart failure
◆ Myxedema coma
◆ Infection
◆ Megacolon
◆ Organic psychosis
◆ Infertility

Diagnosis
◆ Radioimmunoassay showing low triiodothyronine and thyroxine levels
◆ An increased TSH level with primary hypothyroidism; a decreased level with secondary hypothyroidism
◆ Thyroid panel differentiating primary hypothyroidism (thyroid gland hypofunction), secondary hypothyroidism (pituitary hyposecretion of TSH), tertiary hypothyroidism (hypothalamic hyposecretion of TSH), and euthyroid sick syndrome (impaired peripheral conversion of thyroid hormone due to a suprathyroidal illness such as severe infection) (See *Thyroid test results in hypothyroidism,* page 498.)
◆ Elevated serum cholesterol, alkaline phosphatase, and triglyceride levels
◆ Normocytic, normochromic anemia

Thyroid test results in hypothyroidism

Dysfunction involves	Thyrotropin-releasing hormone	Thyroid-stimulating hormone	Thyroid hormones (triiodothyronine [T_3] and thyroxine [T_4])
Hypothalamus	Low	Low	Low
Pituitary gland	High	Low	Low
Thyroid gland	High	High	Low
Peripheral conversion of thyroid hormones	High	Low or normal	T_3 and T_4 low, but reverse T_3 elevated

◆ A low serum sodium level, decreased pH, and increased partial pressure of carbon dioxide, indicating respiratory acidosis (myxedema coma)

Treatment
◆ Gradual thyroid hormone replacement with the synthetic hormone levothyroxine

■ **AGE ALERT** *Elderly patients should be started on a low dose of levothyroxine to avoid cardiac problems; the TSH level guides gradual increases in the dose.*
◆ Surgical excision, chemotherapy, or radiation for tumors

Special considerations
To manage the patient with hypothyroidism:
◆ Provide a high-bulk, low-calorie diet, and encourage activity to combat constipation and promote weight loss. Administer a cathartic and a stool softener as needed.
◆ After thyroid replacement begins, watch for signs and symptoms of hyperthyroidism, such as restlessness, sweating, and excessive weight loss.
◆ Tell the patient to report any signs and symptoms of aggravated cardiovascular disease, such as chest pain and tachycardia.
◆ To prevent myxedema coma, tell the patient to continue his course of thyroid medication even if his symptoms subside.
◆ Warn the patient to report infection immediately and to make sure any physician who prescribes a drug for him knows about the underlying hypothyroidism.
    Treatment of myxedema coma requires supportive care:
◆ Check frequently for signs of decreasing cardiac output (such as decreased urine output).
◆ Monitor temperature until stable. Provide extra blankets and clothing and a warm room to compensate for hypothermia. Rapid rewarming may cause vasodilation and vascular collapse.

◆ Record intake and output and daily weight. As treatment begins, urine output should increase and body weight decrease; if not, report this immediately.
◆ Avoid sedation when possible or reduce the dose because hypothyroidism delays metabolism of many drugs.
◆ Monitor vital signs carefully when administering levothyroxine because rapid correction of hypothyroidism can cause adverse cardiac reactions. Report chest pain or tachycardia immediately. If the patient is elderly, watch for hypertension and heart failure.
◆ Check arterial blood gas values for hypercapnia, metabolic acidosis, and hypoxia to determine whether the patient who's severely myxedematous requires ventilatory assistance.
◆ Administer a corticosteroid as ordered.
◆ Because myxedema coma may have been precipitated by an infection, check possible sources of the infection, such as blood and urine, and obtain sputum cultures.

HYPOTHYROIDISM IN CHILDREN
A deficiency of thyroid hormone secretion during fetal development and early infancy results in congenital hypothyroidism. Hypothyroidism in infants is seen as respiratory difficulties, cyanosis, persistent jaundice, lethargy, somnolence, large tongue, abdominal distention, poor feeding, and hoarse crying. Prompt identification and treatment of hypothyroidism in infants prevents physical and mental retardation. Older children who develop hypothyroidism have symptoms similar to those of adults, plus poor skeletal growth and late epiphyseal maturation and dental development. Sexual maturation may be accelerated in younger children and delayed in older children.

Hypothyroidism is three times more common in girls than boys. Early diagnosis and treatment allow the best prognosis; infants treated before age 3 months usually grow and develop normally. Athyroid children who remain untreated beyond age 3 months and children with acquired hypothyroidism who remain untreated beyond age 2 have irreversible mental retardation; their skeletal abnormalities are reversible with treatment.

Causes

◆ An antithyroid drug taken during pregnancy (less common)
◆ Chronic autoimmune thyroiditis (hypothyroidism after age 2)
◆ Defective embryonic development (most common cause), causing congenital absence or underdevelopment of the thyroid gland
◆ Inherited autosomal recessive defect in the synthesis of thyroxine (next most common cause)
◆ Iodine deficiency during pregnancy

Pathophysiology

Hypothyroidism in infants and children is related to decreased thyroid hormone production or secretion. Loss of functional thyroid tissue can be caused by an autoimmune process. Defective thyroid synthesis may be related to congenital defects, with thyroid dysgenesis (defective development) the most common. Iodine deficiency or an antithyroid drug used by the mother during pregnancy can also contribute. Hypothyroidism may also be related to decreased thyroid-stimulating hormone (TSH) secretion or resistance to TSH.

Signs and symptoms

Signs and symptoms result from insufficient thyroid hormone. The infant will have normal weight and length at birth, with characteristic signs developing within 3 to 6 months if no treatment is initiated; delayed onset of most symptoms until weaning from breast-feeding due to small amounts of thyroid hormone in breast milk. Signs and symptoms may include:
◆ typically, an infant with hypothyroidism sleeps excessively, seldom cries (except for occasional hoarse crying), and is inactive; parents may describe the infant as a "good baby — no trouble at all" (behavior actually due to reduced metabolism and progressive mental impairment)
◆ abnormal deep tendon reflexes, hypotonic abdominal muscles, protruding abdomen, and slow, awkward movements
◆ feeding difficulties, constipation, and jaundice because the immature liver can't conjugate bilirubin

◆ a large, protruding tongue obstructing respiration; loud, noisy mouth breathing; dyspnea on exertion; anemia; and abnormal facial features (such as a short forehead; puffy, wide-set eyes [periorbital edema]; wrinkled eyelids; a broad, short, upturned nose; and a dull expression, reflecting mental retardation)
◆ cold, mottled skin due to poor circulation; and dry, brittle, and dull hair
◆ teeth erupting late and decaying early, below-normal body temperature, and slow pulse rate
◆ growth retardation shown as short stature, due to delayed epiphyseal maturation, particularly in the legs; obesity; and head appearing abnormally large due to stunted arms and legs; delayed or accelerated sexual development; mental retardation can be prevented by appropriate treatment if child acquires hypothyroidism after age 2.

Complications

◆ Skeletal malformations and irreversible mental retardation (for hypothyroid infant not treated by age 3 months; early treatment prevents retardation)
◆ Learning disabilities
◆ Accelerated or delayed sexual maturation

Diagnosis

◆ An elevated TSH level associated with low triiodothyronine and thyroxine (T_4) levels pointing to cretinism (because early detection and treatment can minimize the effects of congenital hypothyroidism, all states require measurement of infant thyroid hormone levels at birth through neonatal screening tests)
◆ Thyroid scan and radioactive iodine uptake tests showing decreased uptake and confirming the absence of thyroid tissue in athyroid children
◆ Increased gonadotropin levels compatible with sexual precocity in older children may co-exist with hypothyroidism
◆ Electrocardiogram showing bradycardia and flat or inverted T waves in untreated infants
◆ Hip, knee, and thigh X-rays showing absence of the femoral or tibial epiphyseal line and markedly delayed skeletal development relative to chronological age
◆ Low T_4 and normal TSH levels suggesting hypothyroidism secondary to hypothalamic or pituitary disease (rare)

Treatment

Early detection is mandatory to prevent irreversible mental retardation and permit normal physical development. Treatment includes:
◆ oral levothyroxine (Synthroid), beginning with moderate doses and gradually increasing

to levels sufficient for lifelong maintenance (rapid increase in dose may precipitate thyrotoxicity); children require proportionately higher doses than adults because children metabolize thyroid hormone more quickly (infants younger than age 1).

Special considerations

Prevention, early detection, comprehensive parent teaching, and psychological support are essential. Know the early signs. Be especially wary if parents emphasize how good and how quiet their neonate is.

♦ During early management of infantile hypothyroidism, monitor blood pressure and pulse rate; report hypertension and tachycardia immediately. Remember, however, that a normal infant heart rate is about 120 beats/minute. If the infant's tongue is unusually large, position him on his side and observe him frequently to prevent airway obstruction. Check rectal temperature every 2 to 4 hours. Keep the infant warm and his skin moist.

♦ Inform parents that the child will require lifelong treatment with thyroid supplements. Teach them to recognize signs and symptoms of overdose, such as rapid pulse rate, irritability, insomnia, fever, sweating, and weight loss. Stress the need to comply with the treatment regimen to prevent further mental impairment.

♦ Provide support to help parents deal with a child who may be mentally retarded. Help them adopt a positive but realistic attitude and focus on their child's strengths rather than his weaknesses. Encourage them to provide stimulating activities to help the child reach his maximal potential. Refer them to appropriate community resources for support.

♦ To prevent congenital hypothyroidism, emphasize the importance of adequate nutrition during pregnancy, including iodine-rich foods and the use of iodized salt or, in case of sodium restriction, an iodine supplement.

METABOLIC SYNDROME

Metabolic syndrome — also called *syndrome X, insulin resistance syndrome, dysmetabolic syndrome,* and *multiple metabolic syndrome* — is a cluster of conditions characterized by abdominal obesity, a high blood glucose level (type 2 diabetes mellitus), insulin resistance, high blood cholesterol and triglyceride levels, and high blood pressure. More than 22% of people in the United States meet three or more of these criteria, raising their risk of heart disease and stroke and placing them at high risk for dying of a myocardial infarction.

Causes

♦ Abdominal obesity (A strong predictor because intra-abdominal fat tends to be more resistant to insulin than fat in other areas. This increases the release of free fatty acid into the portal system, leading to increased apolipoprotein B, low-density-lipoprotein [LDL], and triglyceride levels and a decreased high-density-lipoprotein [HDL] level. As a result, the risk of cardiovascular disease is increased.)

♦ Genetic predisposition (possible)

♦ High blood pressure (The combination of insulin resistance, hyperinsulinemia, and abdominal obesity leads to hypertension and its harmful cardiovascular effects. Moreover, insulin resistance promotes salt sensitivity in people with high blood pressure.)

♦ Insulin resistance and dyslipidemia (Insulin resistance leads to hyperinsulinemia, hyperglycemia, abnormal glucose and lipid metabolism, damaged endothelium, and cardiovascular disease. Insulin is also responsible for reducing the amount of free fatty acids in the liver. However, people with insulin resistance have an increased amount of free fatty acids reaching the liver, resulting in high triglyceride and LDL levels and producing an abnormal endothelium and atherosclerosis.)

♦ Type 2 diabetes mellitus (This is a hallmark of metabolic syndrome indicated by a fasting glucose level greater than 110 mg/dl. People with diabetes develop atherosclerotic heart disease at a younger age than other people and are also at increased risk for macrovascular disease, including ischemic heart disease, stroke, and peripheral vascular disease. Diabetes is a coronary heart disease risk equivalent.)

Pathophysiology

In the normal digestion process, the intestines break down food into its basic components, one of which is glucose. Glucose provides energy for cellular activity, and excess glucose is stored in cells for future use. Insulin, a hormone secreted in the pancreas, guides glucose into storage cells. However, in people with metabolic syndrome, glucose is insulin resistant and doesn't respond to insulin's attempt to guide it into storage cells. Excess insulin is then required to overcome this resistance. This excess in quantity and force of insulin causes damage to the lining of the arteries, promotes fat storage deposits, and prevents fat breakdown. This series of events can lead to diabetes, blood clots, and coronary events.

Signs and symptoms
◆ Abdominal obesity (evidenced by a waist of more than 40″ [101.6 cm] in men and 35″ [88.9 cm in women) caused by poor diet and sedentary lifestyle
◆ Blood pressure 130/85 mm Hg or higher due to a history of hypertension
◆ A fasting blood glucose level that's 100 mg/dl or higher due to diabetes or prediabetes

Complications
If metabolic syndrome is left untreated, complications may include:
◆ coronary artery disease
◆ diabetes
◆ hyperlipidemia
◆ stroke
◆ premature death.

Diagnosis
◆ Blood studies typically indicate an elevated blood glucose level, hyperinsulinemia, and an elevated serum uric acid level.
◆ Use of lipid profile studies reveal an elevated LDL level, a low HDL level, and an elevated triglyceride level.
◆ Further diagnostic procedures are nonspecific, but may be performed to detect hypertension, diabetes, hyperlipidemia, and hyperinsulinemia.

Treatment
◆ Lifestyle modification, focusing on weight reduction and exercise (Modest weight reduction through diet and exercise considerably improves the hemoglobin A_{1c} level, reduces insulin resistance, improves blood lipid levels, and decreases blood pressure. Recent studies have shown that in patients with impaired glucose tolerance, losing an average of 7% of body weight reduced the risk of developing type 2 diabetes by 58%.)
◆ A diet rich in vegetables, fruits, whole grains, fish, and low-fat dairy products combined with regular exercise (Moreover, nutrient-dense, low-energy foods should replace low-nutrient, high-calorie foods. Meal replacements and shakes may also reduce risk factors for metabolic syndrome and improve weight loss.)
◆ A regular exercise program of moderate physical activity — in addition to dietary modifications — to promote weight loss, improve insulin sensitivity, and reduce the blood glucose level (According to the Surgeon General's Report on Physical Activity and Health, a person should exercise moderately for a minimum of 30 minutes on most, if not all, days of the week. The selected exercise program should improve cardiovascular conditioning, increase strength

through resistance training, and improve flexibility.)
◆ Drug therapy for patients who have a body mass index (BMI) of 27 kg/m² or greater in the presence of other risk factors (such as diabetes, hypertension, and hyperlipidemia) or for patients with a BMI of 30 kg/m² or greater without other risk factors; may also be added to lifestyle changes if the patient hasn't achieved significant weight loss after 12 weeks
◆ Drug therapy including phentermine for short-term treatment of obesity in conjunction with diet and exercise
◆ Orlistat (Approved for long-term weight loss, it works by decreasing the absorption of dietary fat by inhibiting pancreatic lipase, which is needed for fat breakdown and absorption. However, because absorption of fat-soluble vitamins is reduced, the patient may require a vitamin supplement. Studies show that when obese patients take orlistat in conjunction with dieting, they achieve greater weight loss and serum glucose control than by dieting alone.)
◆ Sibutramine (Approved for long-term weight loss, it promotes weight loss by inhibiting the reuptake of serotonin, norepinephrine, and dopamine and increases the satiety-producing effects of serotonin. Further, it reduces the drop in metabolic rate that commonly occurs with weight loss.)
◆ Surgical treatment of obesity, such as through gastric bypass procedures, to produce a greater degree and duration of weight loss than other therapies and improve or resolve most of the factors of metabolic syndrome (Candidates include patients with a BMI greater than 40 kg/m² or those with a BMI greater than 35 kg/m² with obesity-related medical conditions. Gastric bypass procedures produce permanent weight loss in the majority of patients.)

Special considerations
◆ Monitor the patient's blood pressure, blood glucose, blood cholesterol, and insulin levels.
◆ To improve compliance, schedule frequent follow-up appointments with the patient. At that time, review his food diary and exercise log. Be positive and promote his active participation and partnership in his treatment plan.
◆ Because research indicates that longer lifestyle modification programs are associated with improved weight loss maintenance, encourage patients with metabolic syndrome to begin an exercise and weight loss program with a friend or family member. Help him explore options, and support his efforts.

Massive goiter

Massive multinodular goiter causes gross distention and swelling of the neck.

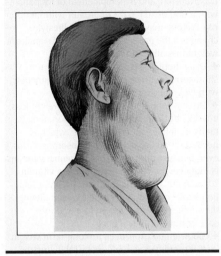

SIMPLE GOITER

Simple (or *nontoxic*) goiter is a thyroid gland enlargement that isn't caused by inflammation or a neoplasm, and is commonly classified as endemic or sporadic. Inherited defects may be responsible for insufficient thyroxine (T_4) synthesis or impaired iodine metabolism. Because families tend to congregate in a single geographic area, this familial factor may contribute to the incidence of endemic and sporadic goiters.

Simple goiter affects more females than males, especially during adolescence, pregnancy, and menopause, when the body's demand for thyroid hormone increases. Sporadic goiter affects no particular population segment. With appropriate treatment, the prognosis is good for either type of goiter.

Causes

Causes of endemic goiter include inadequate dietary intake of iodine. Causes of sporadic goiter include:
◆ ingestion by a pregnant woman of certain drugs, such as propylthiouracil, iodides, phenylbutazone, para-aminosalicylic acid, cobalt, and lithium, which may cross the placental barrier and affect the fetus
◆ ingestion of large amounts of foods containing agents that inhibit T_4 production, such as rutabagas, cabbage, soybeans, peanuts, peaches, peas, strawberries, spinach, and radishes.

Pathophysiology

Goiters can occur in the presence of hypothyroidism, hyperthyroidism, or normal levels of thyroid hormone. In the presence of a severe underlying disorder, compensatory responses may cause both thyroid enlargement (goiter) and hypothyroidism. Simple goiter occurs when the thyroid gland can't secrete enough thyroid hormone to meet metabolic requirements. As a result, the thyroid gland enlarges to compensate for inadequate hormone synthesis, a compensation that usually overcomes mild to moderate hormonal impairment.

Endemic goiter usually results from inadequate secretion of thyroid hormone caused by inadequate dietary intake of iodine associated with such factors as iodine-depleted soil or malnutrition. Since the introduction of iodized salt in the United States, cases of endemic goiter have virtually disappeared.

Sporadic goiter is triggered by certain drugs or foods that inhibit or block production of thyroid hormones.

Signs and symptoms

Thyroid enlargement may range from a mildly enlarged gland to a massive, multinodular goiter. (See *Massive goiter*.)

Complications

Because simple goiter doesn't alter the patient's metabolic state, complications arise solely from enlargement of the thyroid gland compressing adjacent tissues, including:
◆ stridor and respiratory distress
◆ dysphagia
◆ venous engorgement; development of collateral venous circulation in the chest
◆ congestion of the face, some cyanosis and, lastly, distress (Pemberton's sign) when the patient raises her arms until they touch the side of her head.

Diagnosis

Diagnosis of simple goiter requires a thorough patient history and physical examination to rule out disorders with similar clinical effects, such as Graves' disease, Hashimoto's disease, and thyroid carcinoma. A detailed patient history may also reveal goitrogenic medications or foods or endemic influence. The results of diagnostic laboratory tests include:
◆ a normal serum thyroid level
◆ a high or normal TSH level
◆ a low-normal or normal serum T_4 level

◆ normal or increased radioactive iodine uptake (50% of the dose at 24 hours).

Treatment
The goal of treatment is to reduce thyroid hyperplasia.
◆ Exogenous thyroid hormone replacement with levothyroxine (treatment of choice) inhibits thyroid-stimulating hormone secretion and allows the gland to rest.
◆ Small doses of iodide (Lugol's iodine or potassium iodide solution) commonly relieves goiter due to iodine deficiency.
◆ Avoidance of known goitrogenic drugs and foods.
◆ For large goiter that's unresponsive to treatment, subtotal thyroidectomy may be necessary.

Special considerations
◆ Measure the patient's neck circumference daily to check for progressive thyroid gland enlargement, and check for the development of hard nodules in the gland, which may indicate carcinoma.
◆ To maintain constant hormone levels, instruct the patient to take prescribed thyroid hormone preparations at the same time each day. Advise her to avoid taking the medicine at the same time as an iron-containing supplement (including a prenatal vitamin), calcium supplements, psyllium hydrophilic mucilloid (Metamucil), or grapefruit juice. Teach the patient and her family to identify and immediately report signs and symptoms of thyrotoxicosis, including increased pulse rate, palpitations, diarrhea, sweating, tremors, agitation, and shortness of breath.
◆ Instruct the patient with endemic goiter to use iodized salt to supply the daily 150 to 300 mcg of iodine necessary to prevent goiter.
◆ Monitor the patient taking goitrogenic drugs for signs of sporadic goiter.

SYNDROME OF INAPPROPRIATE ANTIDIURETIC HORMONE
Syndrome of inappropriate antidiuretic hormone (SIADH) results when excessive antidiuretic hormone (ADH) secretion is triggered by stimuli other than increased extracellular fluid osmolarity and decreased extracellular fluid volume, reflected by hypotension. SIADH is a relatively common complication of surgery or critical illness. The prognosis varies with the degree of disease and the speed at which it develops. SIADH usually resolves within 3 days of effective treatment.

Causes
The most common cause of SIADH is oat cell carcinoma of the lung, which secretes excessive levels of ADH or vasopressin-like substances. Other neoplastic diseases—such as pancreatic and prostate cancer, Hodgkin's disease, thymoma (tumor on the thymus), and renal carcinoma—may also trigger SIADH.

Less common causes include:
◆ central nervous system disorders, including brain tumor or abscess, stroke, head injury, and Guillain-Barré syndrome
◆ drugs that either increase ADH production or potentiate ADH action, such as antidepressants, nonsteroidal anti-inflammatory drugs, chlorpropamide (Diabinese), vincristine (Oncovin), cyclophosphamide (Cytoxan), carbamazepine (Tegretol), clofibrate (Atromid-S), metoclopramide (Reglan), and morphine
◆ miscellaneous conditions, including psychosis, myxedema, acquired immunodeficiency syndrome, physiologic stress, and pain
◆ pulmonary disorders, including pneumonia, tuberculosis, lung abscess, aspergillosis, bronchiectasis, and positive-pressure ventilation.

Pathophysiology
In the presence of excessive ADH, excessive water reabsorption from the distal convoluted tubule and collecting ducts causes hyponatremia and normal to slightly increased extracellular fluid volume.

Signs and symptoms
◆ Thirst, anorexia, fatigue, and lethargy (the first signs and symptoms), followed by vomiting and intestinal cramping due to hyponatremia and electrolyte imbalance
◆ Weight gain, edema, water retention and decreased urine output due to hyponatremia
◆ Additional neurologic signs and symptoms, such as restlessness, confusion, anorexia, headache, irritability, decreasing reflexes, seizures, and coma, due to electrolyte imbalances, and worsening with the degree of water intoxication
◆ Decreased deep tendon reflexes

Complications
◆ Cerebral edema
◆ Coma
◆ Severe hyponatremia
◆ Water intoxification

Diagnosis
SIADH is diagnosed by the following laboratory results:
◆ serum osmolality less than 280 mOsm/kg of water

◆ hyponatremia (a serum sodium level less than 135 mEq/L); lower values indicating worse condition
◆ an elevated urinary sodium level (more than 20 mEq/L) and increased osmolality (greater than 150 mOsm/kg)
◆ an elevated serum ADH level
◆ a normal blood urea nitrogen level.

Treatment
◆ Restricted water intake (16 to 32 oz [500 to 1,000 ml]/day) (symptomatic treatment)
◆ Administration of 200 to 300 ml of 3% saline solution to slowly and steadily increase the serum sodium level (severe water intoxication); if too rapid a rise, cerebral edema may result
◆ Correction of underlying cause of SIADH when possible
◆ Surgical resection, irradiation, or chemotherapy to alleviate water retention for SIADH resulting from cancer
◆ Demeclocycline or lithium to block the renal response to ADH (if fluid restriction is ineffective)

Special considerations
◆ Closely monitor and record intake and output, vital signs, and daily weight. Watch for hyponatremia.
◆ Observe for restlessness, irritability, seizures, heart failure, and unresponsiveness due to hyponatremia and water intoxication.
◆ To prevent water intoxication, explain to the patient and his family why he must restrict his intake.

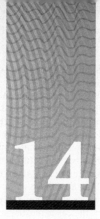

Renal System

The components of the renal system are the kidneys, ureters, bladder, and urethra. The kidneys, located retroperitoneally in the lumbar area, produce and excrete urine to maintain homeostasis. They regulate the volume, electrolyte concentration, and acid-base balance of body fluids; detoxify the blood and eliminate wastes; regulate blood pressure; and support red blood cell (RBC) production (*erythropoiesis*). The ureters are tubes that extend from the kidneys to the bladder; their only function is to transport urine to the bladder. The bladder is a muscular bag that serves as reservoir for urine until it leaves the body through the urethra.

Pathophysiologic changes

Wastes are eliminated from the body by urine formation. The process of urine formation occurs in the nephron, the functional unit of the kidney. Glomerular filtration, tubular reabsorption, and tubular secretion and excretion are all necessary for urine formation. Glomerular filtration is the process of filtering the blood as it flows through the kidneys. The glomerulus, a capillary network, filters plasma; the filtrate is either reabsorbed in the renal tubules or excreted as urine. Glomerular function depends on the permeability of the capillary walls, vascular pressure, and hydrostatic pressure. The normal glomerular filtration rate (GFR) is about 120 ml/minute. To prevent too much fluid from leaving the vascular system, tubular reabsorption opposes capillary filtration. Reabsorption takes place as capillary filtration progresses.

When fluid filters through the capillaries, albumin, which doesn't pass through capillary walls, remains behind. As the albumin concentration inside the capillaries increases, the capillaries begin to draw water back in by osmosis. This osmotic force controls the quantities of water and diffusible solutes that enter and leave the capillaries.

Factors that affect filtration or reabsorption affect total filtration effort. Capillary pressure and interstitial fluid colloid osmotic pressure affect filtration. Interstitial fluid pressure and plasma colloid osmotic pressure affect reabsorption.

Various factors can slow the GFR—altered renal perfusion; renal disease affecting the vessels, glomeruli, or tubules; or obstruction to urine flow. The results are retention of nitrogenous wastes (*azotemia*), such as blood urea nitrogen and creatinine, which can lead to acute renal failure.

CAPILLARY PRESSURE

The renal arteries branch into five segmental arteries, which supply different areas of the kidneys. The segmental arteries then branch into several divisions from which the afferent arterioles and vasa recta arise. Renal veins follow a similar branching pattern—characterized by stellate vessels and segmental branches—and empty into the inferior vena cava. The tubular system receives its blood supply from a peritubular capillary network. The ureteral veins follow the arteries and drain into the renal vein. The bladder receives blood through vesical arteries. Vesical veins unite to form the pudendal plexus, which empties into the iliac veins. A rich lymphatic system drains the renal cortex, kidneys, ureters, and bladder.

Capillary pressure reflects mean arterial pressure (MAP). Increased MAP increases capillary pressure, which in turn increases the GFR. When MAP decreases, so do capillary pressure and GFR. Autoregulation of afferent and efferent arterioles minimizes and controls changes in capillary pressure, unless MAP exceeds 180 mm Hg or is less than 80 mm Hg.

The kidneys are innervated by sympathetic branches from the celiac plexus, upper lumbar splanchnic and thoracic nerves, and the intermesenteric and superior hypogastric plexuses, which surround the kidneys. Similar numbers of sympathetic and parasympathetic nerves from the renal plexus, superior hypogastric plexus, and intermesenteric plexus innervate the ureters. Nerves that arise from the inferior hypogastric plexus innervate the bladder. The parasympathetic nerve supply to the bladder controls urination.

Increased sympathetic activity and angiotensin II constrict afferent and efferent arterioles, decreasing the capillary pressure. Because these changes affect both the afferent and efferent arterioles, they have no net effect on GFR.

Inadequate renal perfusion accounts for 40% to 80% of cases of acute renal failure. Volume loss (as with GI hemorrhage, burns, diarrhea, and diuretic use), volume sequestration (as in pancreatitis, peritonitis, and rhabdomyolysis), or decreased effective circulating volume (as in cardiogenic shock and sepsis) may reduce circulating blood volume. Decreased cardiac output due to peripheral vasodilation (by sepsis or drugs) or profound renal vasoconstriction (as in severe heart failure, hepatorenal syndrome, or with such drugs as nonsteroidal anti-inflammatory drugs [NSAIDs]) also diminish renal perfusion.

Hypovolemia causes a decrease in MAP that triggers a series of neural and humoral responses: activation of the sympathetic nervous system and renin-angiotensin-aldosterone system, and release of arginine vasopressin. Prostaglandin-mediated relaxation of afferent arterioles and angiotensin II–mediated constriction of efferent arterioles maintain GFR. GFR decreases steeply if MAP decreases to less than 80 mm Hg. Drugs that block prostaglandin production (such as NSAIDs) can cause severe vasoconstriction and acute renal failure during hypotension.

Prolonged renal hypoperfusion causes acute tubular necrosis. Processes involving large renal vessels, microvasculature, glomeruli, or tubular interstitium cause intrinsic renal disease. Emboli or thrombi, aortic dissection, or vasculitis can occlude renal arteries. Cholesterol-rich atheroemboli can occur spontaneously or follow aortic instrumentation. If they lodge in medium and small renal arteries, they trigger an eosinophil-rich inflammatory reaction.

AGE ALERT *After age 40, a person's renal function begins to diminish. If he lives to age 90, it may have decreased by as much as 50%. This change is reflected in a decreased GFR and is caused by age-related changes in the renal vasculature that disturb glomerular hemodynamics as well as by reduced cardiac output and atherosclerotic changes that reduce renal blood flow by more than 50%.*

INTERSTITIAL FLUID COLLOID OSMOTIC PRESSURE

Few plasma proteins and RBCs are filtered out of the glomeruli, so interstitial fluid colloid osmotic pressure (the force of albumin in the interstitial fluid) remains low. Large quantities of plasma protein flow through glomerular capillaries. Size and surface charge keep albumin, globulin, and other large proteins from crossing the glomerular wall. Smaller proteins leave the glomerulus but are absorbed by the proximal tubule.

Injury to the glomeruli or peritubular capillaries can increase interstitial fluid colloid osmotic pressure, drawing fluid out of the glomerulus and the peritubular capillaries. Swelling and edema occur in Bowman's space and the interstitial space surrounding the tubule. Increased interstitial fluid pressure opposes glomerular filtration, causes collapse of the surrounding nephrons and peritubular capillaries, and leads to hypoxia and renal cell injury or death. When cells die, intracellular enzymes that stimulate immune and inflammatory reactions are released. This further contributes to swelling and edema.

The resulting increase in interstitial fluid pressure can interfere with glomerular filtration and tubular reabsorption. Loss of glomerular filtration renders the kidney incapable of regulating blood volume and electrolyte composition. Diseases that damage the tubules alter their permeability, causing tubular proteinuria because small proteins can move from capillaries into tubules.

Normal glomerular cells, which are endothelial in nature, form a barrier that prevents cells and other particles from crossing the membrane. The basement membrane typically traps larger proteins. The channels of the basement membrane are coated with glycoproteins that are rich in glutamate, aspartate, and sialic acid.

CLOSER LOOK
The glomerulus

The normal internal structures separating the capillary lumen and the urinary space in the glomerulus are shown below.

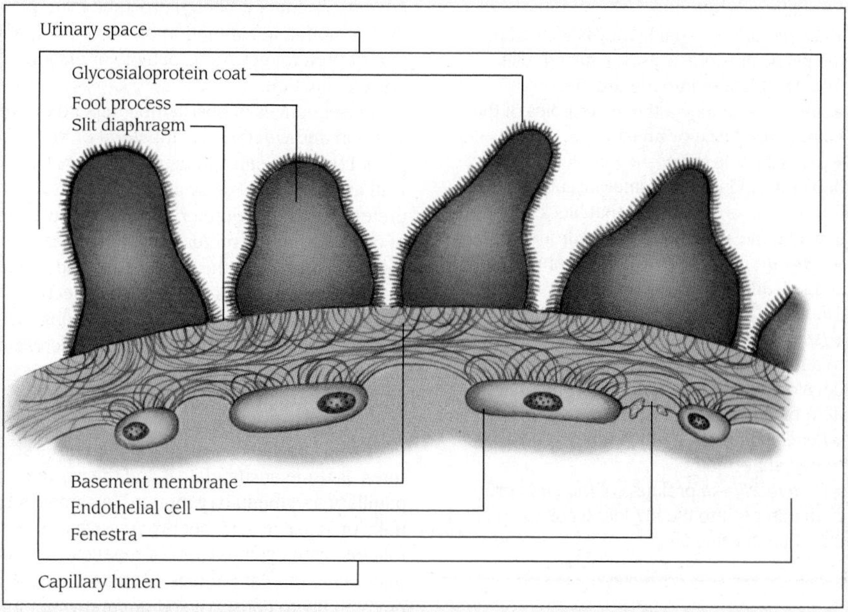

This produces a negative charge barrier that impedes the passage of such anionic molecules as albumin. (See *The glomerulus.*)

Glomerular disease disrupts the basement membrane, allowing large proteins to leak out. Damage to epithelial cells permits albumin leakage. Hypoalbuminemia, as in nephrotic syndrome, is the result of excessive loss of albumin in the urine, increased renal catabolism, and inadequate hepatic synthesis of albumin. Plasma oncotic pressure decreases and edema results as fluid moves from capillaries into the interstitium. Consequent activation of the renin-angiotensin system, arginine-vasopressin release, and sympathetic nervous system stimulation increases renal salt and water reabsorption, which further contributes to edema. The severity of edema is directly related to the degree of hypoalbuminemia, and is exacerbated by heart disease or peripheral vascular disease.

PLASMA COLLOID PRESSURE
Protein concentration of the plasma determines the plasma colloid pressure (the pulling force of albumin in the intravascular fluid), the major

force influencing reabsorption of fluid into the capillaries. The plasma protein level can decrease as a result of liver disease, protein loss in the urine, and protein malnutrition.

As oncotic pressure decreases, less fluid moves back into the capillaries and fluid begins to accumulate in the tubular and peritubular areas. Swelling around the tubule causes collapse of the tubule and peritubular capillaries, hypoxia, and death of the nephrons.

Diminished plasma oncotic pressure and urine protein loss stimulate hepatic lipoprotein synthesis, and the resulting hyperlipidemia manifests as lipid bodies (fatty casts, oval fat bodies) in the urine. Metabolic disturbances result as other proteins are lost in the urine, including thyroxine-binding globulin, cholecalciferol-binding protein, transferrin, and metal-binding proteins. Urine losses of antithrombin III, decreased serum levels of proteins S and C, hyperfibrinogenemia, and enhanced platelet aggregation lead to a hypercoagulable state, as in nephrotic syndrome. Some patients also develop severe immunoglobulin G deficiency, which increases susceptibility to infection.

Congenital nephropathies and uropathies

The following congenital conditions can affect kidney function:

♦ *Ectopic kidney* — the kidney is located in the pelvic or thoracic area, causing reflux from the bladder into the ureters.

♦ *Horseshoe kidney* — the lower poles of the kidneys are fused by an isthmus.

♦ *Obstructive uropathy* — a pathologic condition of the kidney (abnormal vasculature, adhesions, kinks, or masses) that blocks the flow of urine, usually causing hydronephrosis.

♦ *Renal dysplasia* — the kidney is abnormally shaped, and the involved areas are nonfunctional.

♦ *Renal hypoplasia* — the kidney is small due to a reduction in the number of normally developed nephrons, and it may be unilateral or bilateral.

♦ *Renal malrotation* — the kidney is positioned abnormally.

♦ *Ureterocele* — a prolapse of the end portion of the ureter into the bladder leads to an obstruction in urine flow.

STRUCTURAL VARIATIONS

Variations in normal anatomic structure of the urinary tract occur in 10% to 15% of the total population and range from minor and easily correctable to lethal. Ectopic kidneys, which result if the embryonic kidneys don't ascend from the pelvis to the abdomen, function normally. If the embryonic kidneys fuse as they ascend, a single u-shaped kidney results, causing no symptoms in about one-third of affected people. The most common problems associated with horseshoe kidneys include hydronephrosis, infection, and calculus formation.

■ **AGE ALERT** *Structural abnormalities of the renal system account for about 45% of renal failure in children.*

Urinary tract malformations are commonly associated with certain nonrenal anomalies. These characteristics include low-set and malformed ears, chromosomal disorders (especially trisomies 13 and 18), absent abdominal muscles, spinal cord and lower-extremity anomalies, imperforate anus or genital deviation, Wilms' tumor, congenital ascites, cystic disease of the liver, and positive family history of renal disease (hereditary nephritis or cystic disease). (See *Congenital nephropathies and uropathies.*)

OBSTRUCTION

Obstruction along the urinary tract causes urine to accumulate behind the source of obstruction, leading to infection or damage. Obstructions may be congenital or acquired. Causes include tumors, calculi (stones), trauma, strictures (secondary to surgical intervention and scarring), edema, pregnancy, benign prostatic hyperplasia or carcinoma, inflammation of the GI tract, and loss of ureteral peristaltic activity or bladder muscle function.

Consequences of obstruction depend on the location and whether it's unilateral or bilateral, partial or complete, and acute or chronic, as well as the cause. For example, obstruction of a ureter causes hydroureter, or an accumulation of urine within the ureter, which increases retrograde pressure to the renal pelvis and calyces. As urine accumulates in the renal collection system, hydronephrosis results. If the obstruction is complete and acute in nature, increasing pressure transmitted to the proximal tubule inhibits glomerular filtration. If the GFR declines to zero, the result is renal failure.

Chronic partial obstruction compresses structures as urine accumulates, and the result is papillary and medullary infarct. The kidneys initially increase in size, but progressive atrophy follows, with eventual loss of renal mass. The underlying tubular damage decreases the kidney's ability to conserve sodium and water and excrete hydrogen ions and potassium; sodium and bicarbonate are wasted. Urine volume is excessive, even though the GFR has declined. The result is an increased risk of dehydration and metabolic acidosis.

Tubular obstruction, caused by renal calculi or scarring from repeated infection, can increase interstitial fluid pressure. As fluid accumulates in the nephron, it backs up into Bowman's capsule and space. If the obstruction isn't relieved, nephrons and capillaries collapse, and renal damage is irreversible. The papillae, which are the final site of urine concentration, are particularly affected.

Relief of the obstruction is usually followed by copious diuresis of sodium and water retained during the period of obstruction, and a return to a normal GFR. Excessive loss of sodium and water (more than 10 L/ day) is uncommon. If a GFR doesn't recover quickly, diuresis may not be significant after the obstruction is relieved.

Unresolved obstruction can result in infection or even renal failure. Obstructions below the bladder cause urine to accumulate, forming a medium for bacterial growth.

AGE ALERT *Urinary tract infections are most common in girls ages 7 to 11. This is a result of bacteria ascending the urethra.*

Cystitis is an infection of the bladder that results in mucosal inflammation and congestion. The detrusor muscle becomes hyperactive, decreasing bladder capacity and leading to reflux into the ureters. This transient reflux can cause acute or chronic pyelonephritis if bacteria ascend to the kidney.

Bilateral obstruction of the ureters not relieved within 1 week of onset causes acute or chronic renal failure. Chronic renal failure progresses over weeks to months without symptoms until 90% of renal function is lost.

Disorders

Renal disorders include acute pyelonephritis, acute and chronic renal failure, acute tubular necrosis, congenital anomalies, glomerulonephritis, nephrotic syndrome, neurogenic bladder, polycystic kidney, renal calculi, renovascular hypotension, and vesicoureteral reflux.

ACUTE PYELONEPHRITIS

Acute pyelonephritis, also known as *acute infective tubulointerstitial nephritis,* is a sudden inflammation caused by bacteria that primarily affects the interstitial area and the renal pelvis or, less commonly, the renal tubules. It's one of the most common renal diseases and may affect one or both kidneys. With treatment and continued follow-up care, the prognosis is good, and extensive permanent damage is rare.

Pyelonephritis is more common in females, probably because of a shorter urethra and the proximity of the urinary meatus to the vagina and the rectum — both conditions allow bacteria to reach the bladder more easily — and a lack of the antibacterial prostatic secretions produced in the male. Incidence increases with age and is higher in the following groups:

♦ sexually active women — intercourse increases the risk of bacterial contamination
♦ pregnant women — about 5% develop asymptomatic bacteriuria; if untreated, about 40% develop pyelonephritis
♦ people with diabetes — neurogenic bladder causes incomplete emptying and urinary stasis; glycosuria may support bacterial growth in the urine
♦ people with other renal diseases — compromised renal function aggravates susceptibility.

Causes

Acute pyelonephritis results from bacterial infection of the kidneys. Infecting bacteria usually are normal intestinal and fecal flora that grow readily in urine. The most common causative organism is *Escherichia coli,* but *Klebsiella, Proteus, Pseudomonas, Staphylococcus aureus,* and *Enterococcus faecalis* (formerly *Streptococcus faecalis*) may also cause this infection.

Pathophysiology

Typically, the infection spreads from the bladder to the ureters, then to the kidneys, as in vesicoureteral reflux. Vesicoureteral reflux may result from congenital weakness at the junction of the ureter and the bladder. Bacteria refluxed to intrarenal tissues may create colonies of infection within 24 to 48 hours. Infection may also result from instrumentation (such as catheterization, cystoscopy, or urologic surgery), from a hematogenic infection (as in septicemia or endocarditis), or possibly from lymphatic infection.

Pyelonephritis may also result from an inability to empty the bladder (for example, in patients with neurogenic bladder), urinary stasis, or urinary obstruction due to tumors, strictures, or benign prostatic hyperplasia.

Signs and symptoms

Typical clinical features include:
♦ urinary urgency and frequency, burning during urination, dysuria, nocturia, and hematuria (usually microscopic but may be gross) caused by urinary tract irritation
♦ cloudy urine that has an ammonia-like or fishy odor resulting from bacteria in the urine and subsequent leukocyte response
♦ a temperature of 102° F (38.9° C) or higher, shaking chills, nausea and vomiting, flank pain, anorexia, and general fatigue caused by the infection.

These signs and symptoms characteristically develop rapidly over a few hours or a few days. Although they may disappear within days, even without treatment, residual bacterial infection is likely and may cause the signs and symptoms to recur later.

AGE ALERT *Elderly patients may exhibit GI or pulmonary symptoms rather than the usual febrile responses to pyelonephritis. In children younger than age 2, fever, vomiting, nonspecific abdominal complaints, or failure to thrive may be the only signs of acute pyelonephritis.*

Complications

♦ Septic shock
♦ Chronic pyelonephritis
♦ Chronic renal insufficiency

Chronic pyelonephritis

Chronic pyelonephritis is a persistent kidney inflammation that can scar the kidneys and may lead to chronic renal failure. Its cause may be bacterial, metastatic, or urogenous. This disease is most common in patients who are predisposed to recurrent acute pyelonephritis, such as those with urinary obstructions or vesicoureteral reflux.

Patients with chronic pyelonephritis may have a childhood history of unexplained fevers or bed-wetting. Clinical effects may include flank pain, anemia, low urine specific gravity, proteinuria, leukocytes in urine and, especially in late stages, hypertension. Uremia rarely develops from chronic pyelonephritis unless structural abnormalities exist in the excretory system. Bacteriuria may be intermittent. When no bacteria are found in the urine, diagnosis depends on excretory urography (renal pelvis may appear small and flattened) and renal biopsy.

Effective treatment of chronic pyelonephritis requires control of hypertension, elimination of the existing obstruction (when possible), and long-term antimicrobial therapy.

Diagnosis

Diagnosis requires urinalysis and culture. Typical findings include:
◆ pyuria (pus in urine) — Urine sediment reveals the presence of leukocytes singly, in clumps, and in casts and, possibly, a few red blood cells.
◆ significant bacteriuria — Urine culture reveals more than 100,000 organisms per microliter of urine.
◆ low specific gravity and osmolality — These findings result from a temporarily decreased ability to concentrate urine.
◆ slightly alkaline urine pH — These findings result from a temporarily decreased ability to concentrate urine.
◆ proteinuria, glycosuria, and ketonuria — These conditions are less common.

Computed tomography (CT) scan also helps in the evaluation of acute pyelonephritis. CT scan of the kidneys, ureters, and bladder may reveal calculi, tumors, or cysts in the kidneys and the urinary tract. Excretory urography may show asymmetrical kidneys.

Treatment

Treatment centers on antibiotic therapy appropriate to the specific infecting organism after identification by urine culture and sensitivity studies.

When the infecting organism can't be identified, therapy usually consists of a broad-spectrum antibiotic, such as ampicillin or cephalexin. If the patient is pregnant or elderly, antibiotics must be prescribed cautiously. A urinary analgesic, such as phenazopyridine, is also appropriate.

Symptoms may disappear after several days of antibiotic therapy. Although urine usually becomes sterile within 48 to 72 hours, the course of such therapy is 10 to 14 days. Follow-up treatment includes reculturing urine 1 week after drug therapy stops, then periodically for the next year to detect residual or recurring infection. Most patients with uncomplicated infections respond well to therapy and don't suffer reinfection.

If infection is caused by an obstruction or a vesicoureteral reflux, an antibiotic may be less effective; surgery may then be necessary to relieve the obstruction or correct the anomaly. Patients at high risk for recurring urinary tract and kidney infections, such as those with prolonged use of an indwelling catheter or maintenance antibiotic therapy, require long-term follow-up. Recurrent episodes of acute pyelonephritis can eventually result in chronic pyelonephritis. (See *Chronic pyelonephritis.*)

Special considerations

Patient care is supportive during antibiotic treatment of underlying infection.
◆ Administer an antipyretic for fever.
◆ Force fluids to achieve urine output of more than 2,000 ml/day. This helps to empty the bladder of contaminated urine and prevents calculi formation. Don't encourage intake of more than 3 qt (3 L) because this may decrease the effectiveness of the antibiotic.
◆ Provide a diet to prevent calculus formation (low sodium, low meat [all types], and increased potassium).
◆ Teach proper technique for collecting a clean-catch urine specimen. Be sure to refrigerate or culture a urine specimen within 30 minutes of collection to prevent overgrowth of bacteria.
◆ Stress the need to complete prescribed antibiotic therapy even after symptoms subside. Encourage long-term follow-up care for high-risk patients. (See *Preventing acute pyelonephritis.*)

||| LIFE-THREATENING DISORDER

ACUTE RENAL FAILURE

Acute renal failure, the sudden interruption of renal function, can be caused by obstruction, poor circulation, or underlying kidney disease. Whether prerenal, intrarenal, or postrenal, it usually passes through three distinct phases: oliguric, diuretic, and recovery. About 2% to 5% of hospitalized patients develop acute renal failure. The condition is usually reversible with treatment, but if not treated, it may progress to end-stage renal disease, prerenal azotemia, and death.

Causes
Acute renal failure may be prerenal, intrarenal, or postrenal.

Prerenal failure
♦ Antihypertensive medications (angiotensin-converting enzyme inhibitors and angiotensin receptor blockers)
♦ Arrhythmias that cause reduced cardiac output
♦ Arterial embolism
♦ Arterial or venous thrombosis
♦ Ascites
♦ Burns
♦ Cardiac tamponade
♦ Cardiogenic shock
♦ Dehydration
♦ Disseminated intravascular coagulation
♦ Diuretic overuse
♦ Eclampsia
♦ Heart failure
♦ Hemorrhage
♦ Hypercalcemia
♦ Hypoalbuminemia
♦ Hypotension
♦ Hypovolemic shock
♦ Malignant hypertension
♦ Myocardial infarction
♦ Nephrotoxic antibiotics (amphotericin)
♦ Nonsteroidal anti-inflammatory agents
♦ Pulmonary embolism
♦ Radiocontrast agents
♦ Sepsis
♦ Trauma
♦ Tumor
♦ Vasculitis
♦ Vasopressor agents (epinephrine)

Intrarenal failure
♦ Acute glomerulonephritis
♦ Acute interstitial nephritis
♦ Acute pyelonephritis
♦ Acute tubular necrosis
♦ Bilateral renal vein thrombosis
♦ Crush injuries
♦ Disseminated intravascular coagulation
♦ Malignant nephrosclerosis
♦ Myopathy
♦ Nephrotoxins

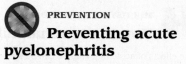

♦ Obstetric complications
♦ Papillary necrosis
♦ Polyarteritis nodosa
♦ Poorly treated prerenal failure
♦ Rapidly progressive glomerulonephritis
♦ Renal myeloma
♦ Scleroderma
♦ Sickle cell disease
♦ Systemic lupus erythematosus
♦ Transfusion reaction
♦ Vasculitis

Postrenal failure
♦ Benign prostatic hyperplasia
♦ Bladder obstruction
♦ Ureteral obstruction
♦ Urethral obstruction

Pathophysiology
The pathophysiology of prerenal, intrarenal, and postrenal failure differs.

Prerenal failure
Prerenal failure ensues when a condition that diminishes blood flow to the kidneys leads to hypoperfusion. Examples include hypovolemia, hypotension, vasoconstriction, or inadequate cardiac output. Azotemia (excess nitrogenous waste products in the blood) develops in 40% to 80% of acute renal failure cases.

When renal blood flow is interrupted, so is oxygen delivery. The ensuing hypoxemia and ischemia can rapidly and irreversibly damage the kidney. The tubules are most susceptible to hypoxemia's effects.

MULTISYSTEM DISORDER
How acute renal failure affects the body

The effects of acute renal failure can be seen across most body systems. For this reason, a multidisciplinary approach to care is needed.

Renal system
♦ Oliguria occurs as a result of a decreased glomerular filtration rate (GFR).
♦ Hyperkalemia occurs as a result of a decreased GFR and metabolic acidosis.
♦ Hyperphosphatemia and hypocalcemia occur because the kidney can't excrete phosphorus.
♦ Hypotension and dehydration may occur during the diuretic phase and lead to further ischemia of the kidneys. .

Cardiovascular system
♦ Hypertension and edema occur with fluid accumulation and hypervolemia.
♦ Fluid overload may cause pulmonary and peripheral edema, possibly leading to heart failure because of how these conditions increase the heart's workload.,
♦ Acute pulmonary edema and hypertensive crisis may result from nephron loss and decreased kidney size, causing decreased blood flow to the kidneys.
♦ Arrhythmias and cardiac arrest may result from hyperkalemia.

Endocrine and metabolic systems
♦ A hypermetabolic state caused by energy demands causes tissue catabolism and alterations in the blood glucose level.
♦ Metabolic acidosis occurs because the kidney can't excrete hydrogen ions and reabsorb sodium and bicarbonate.

GI system
♦ Nausea, vomiting, and anorexia occur with uremia.
♦ GI bleeding may occur with coagulation abnormalities and uremic gastric irritation.

Immune and hematologic systems
♦ Anemia occurs because of decreased erythropoiesis, glomerular filtration of erythrocytes, or bleeding associated with platelet dysfunction.
♦ Infection and sepsis may occur because of decreased white blood cell–mediated immunity.
♦ A hypercoagulable state results from anticoagulant abnormalities, which leads to bleeding and clotting difficulties.

Integumentary system
♦ Accumulation of uremic toxins leads to dryness, pruritus, pallor, purpura, and (rarely) the deposition of the uremic toxins on the skin (uremic frost).

Musculoskeletal system
♦ Muscle weakness may result from hyperkalemia.
♦ Pathologic bone fractures may be caused by prolonged hypocalcemia.

Neurologic system
♦ Altered mental status and peripheral neuropathies are related to the effects of uremic toxins on the highly sensitive nerve cells.

Azotemia is a consequence of renal hypoperfusion. The impaired blood flow results in a decreased glomerular filtration rate (GFR) and increased tubular reabsorption of sodium and water. A decrease in the GFR causes electrolyte imbalance and metabolic acidosis. Usually, restoring renal blood flow and glomerular filtration reverses azotemia.

Intrarenal failure
Intrarenal failure, also called intrinsic or parenchymal renal failure, results from damage to the filtering structures of the kidneys. Causes of intrarenal failure are classified as nephrotoxic, inflammatory, or ischemic. When the damage is caused by nephrotoxicity or inflammation, the

delicate layer under the epithelium (the basement membrane) becomes irreparably damaged, typically leading to chronic renal failure. Severe or prolonged lack of blood flow caused by ischemia may lead to renal damage (ischemic parenchymal injury) and excess nitrogen in the blood (intrinsic renal azotemia).

Acute tubular necrosis, the precursor to intrarenal failure, can result from ischemic damage to renal parenchyma during unrecognized or poorly treated prerenal failure; or from obstetric complications, such as eclampsia, postpartum renal failure, septic abortion, or uterine hemorrhage.

The fluid loss causes hypotension, which leads to ischemia. The ischemic tissue

♦ Headache, drowsiness, irritability, and seizures result from central nervous system involvement and, without treatment, may progress to coma.

Respiratory system
♦ Tachypnea and labored breathing result from anemia, causing tissue hypoxia. Respiratory rate and effort also increase to compensate for metabolic acidosis.

Collaborative management
A renal specialist or nephrologist can help evaluate, treat, and manage the patient's kidney function. Respiratory and cardiology specialists may be consulted depending on the patient's history and complications he may develop. Nutritional therapy may be involved to help institute necessary restrictions or supplementations. Physical and occupational therapy may be necessary to help with energy conservation and rehabilitation, depending on the patient's condition and length of stay. If a prolonged hospital stay is expected and the patient requires long-term or home care, social services may be consulted early on in the patient's care. The patient may also benefit from psychological or spiritual counseling if he's acutely ill or if he'll require continued care on discharge.

generates toxic oxygen-free radicals, which cause swelling, injury, and necrosis.

Another cause of acute failure is the use of nephrotoxins, including analgesics, anesthetics, heavy metals, radiographic contrast media, organic solvents, and antimicrobials, particularly aminoglycoside antibiotics. These drugs accumulate in the renal cortex, causing renal failure that manifests well after treatment or other toxin exposure. The necrosis caused by nephrotoxins tends to be uniform and limited to the proximal tubules, whereas ischemia necrosis tends to be patchy and distributed along various parts of the nephron.

Postrenal failure
Bilateral obstruction of urine outflow leads to postrenal failure. The cause may be in the bladder, ureters, or urethra.

Bladder obstruction can result from:
♦ anticholinergic use
♦ autonomic nerve dysfunction
♦ infection
♦ tumors.

Ureteral obstructions, which restrict urine flow from kidneys to bladder, can result from:
♦ blood clots
♦ calculi
♦ edema or inflammation
♦ necrotic renal papillae
♦ retroperitoneal fibrosis or hemorrhage
♦ surgery (accidental ligation and strictures)
♦ tumor or uric acid crystals.

Urethral obstruction can result from prostatic hyperplasia, tumor, or strictures.

The three types of acute renal failure (prerenal, intrarenal, or postrenal) usually pass through three distinct phases: oliguric, diuretic, and recovery. (See *How acute renal failure affects the body.*)

Oliguric phase
Oliguria may result from one or several factors. Necrosis of the tubules can cause sloughing of cells, cast formations, and ischemic edema. The resulting tubular obstruction causes a retrograde increase in pressure and a decrease in GFR. Renal failure can occur within 24 hours from this effect. Glomerular filtration may remain normal in some cases of renal failure, but tubular reabsorption of filtrate may be accelerated. In this instance, ischemia may increase tubular permeability and cause backleak. Another concept is that intrarenal release of angiotensin II or redistribution of blood flow from the cortex to the medulla may constrict the afferent arterioles, increasing glomerular permeability and decreasing the GFR.

Urine output may remain at less than 30 ml/hour or 400 ml/day for a few days to weeks. Before damage occurs, the kidneys respond to decreased blood flow by conserving sodium and water.

Damage impairs the kidney's ability to conserve sodium. Fluid (water) volume excess, azotemia (elevated serum levels of urea, creatinine, and uric acid), and electrolyte imbalance occur. Ischemic or toxic injury leads to the release of mediators and intrarenal vasoconstriction. Medullary hypoxia results in the swelling of tubular and endothelial cells, adherence of neutrophils to capillaries and venules, and inappropriate platelet activation. Increasing ischemia and vasoconstriction further limit perfusion.

Injured cells lose polarity, and the ensuing disruption of tight junctions between the cells promotes backleak of filtrate. Ischemia impairs the function of energy-dependent membrane pumps, and calcium accumulates in the cells. This excess calcium further stimulates vasoconstriction and activates proteases and other enzymes. Untreated prerenal oliguria may lead to acute tubular necrosis.

Diuretic phase

As the kidneys become unable to conserve sodium and water, the diuretic phase, marked by increased urine secretion of more than 400 ml/24 hours, ensues. The GFR may be normal or increased, but tubular support mechanisms are abnormal. Excretion of dilute urine causes dehydration and electrolyte imbalances. A high blood urea nitrogen (BUN) level produces osmotic diuresis and consequent deficits of potassium, sodium, and water. The diuretic phase may last days or weeks.

Recovery phase

If the cause of the diuresis is corrected, azotemia gradually disappears and recovery occurs. The recovery phase is a gradual return to normal or near-normal renal function over 3 to 12 months.

AGE ALERT *Even with treatment, the elderly patient is particularly susceptible to volume overload, precipitating acute pulmonary edema, hypertensive crisis, hyperkalemia, and infection.*

Signs and symptoms

Acute renal failure is a critical illness. Its early signs and symptoms are oliguria, azotemia and, rarely, anuria. Electrolyte imbalance, metabolic acidosis, and other severe effects follow, as the patient becomes increasingly uremic and renal dysfunction disrupts other body systems.

◆ GI — anorexia, nausea, vomiting, diarrhea or constipation, stomatitis, bleeding, hematemesis, dry mucous membranes, uremic breath
◆ Central nervous system — headache, drowsiness, irritability, confusion, peripheral neuropathy, seizures, coma
◆ Integumentary — dryness, pruritus, pallor, purpura and, rarely, uremic frost
◆ Cardiovascular — early in the disease, hypotension; later, hypertension, arrhythmias, fluid overload, heart failure, systemic edema
◆ Respiratory — pulmonary edema, Kussmaul's respirations
◆ Hematologic — anemia, altered clotting mechanisms.

Complications

Renal failure affects many body processes. Complications may include:
◆ fever and chills (common), which indicate infection
◆ metabolic acidosis, due to decreased excretion of hydrogen ions
◆ anemia due to erythropoietinemia, glomerular filtration of erythrocytes, or bleeding associated with platelet dysfunction; tissue hypoxia, stimulating increased ventilation and work of breathing
◆ sepsis because of decreased white blood cell–mediated immunity
◆ heart failure due to fluid overload and anemia, which cause additional workload to the heart
◆ hypercoagulable state due to abnormalities in quantities or function of anticoagulant proteins, coagulation factor, platelet, or endothelial mediators, resulting in bleeding or clotting difficulties
◆ altered mental status and peripheral sensation due to effects on the highly sensitive cells of nerves secondary to retained toxins, hypoxia, electrolyte imbalance, and acidosis.

Diagnosis

◆ Blood studies showing elevated BUN, serum creatinine, and potassium levels; decreased hematocrit and bicarbonate and hemoglobin levels; and low blood pH
◆ Urine studies showing casts, cellular debris, and decreased specific gravity; in glomerular diseases, proteinuria and urine osmolality close to serum osmolality; a urine sodium level less than 20 mEq/L if oliguria results from decreased perfusion, and more than 40 mEq/L if the cause is intrarenal
◆ Creatinine clearance test measuring the GFR and reflecting the number of remaining functioning nephrons
◆ Electrocardiogram (ECG) showing tall, peaked T waves; widening QRS complex; and disappearing P waves if hyperkalemia is present
◆ Ultrasonography, plain films of the abdomen, kidney-ureter-bladder radiography, excretory urography, renal scan, retrograde pyelography, computed tomographic scans, and nephrotomography

Treatment

◆ High-calorie diet low in sodium and potassium and with restricted protein to meet metabolic needs (protein intake must be adequate enough to prevent malnourishment)
◆ Careful monitoring of electrolyte levels; I.V. therapy to maintain and correct fluid and electrolyte balance

◆ Fluid restriction to minimize edema (although fluid restoration and maintenance may be needed during the diuretic phase)
◆ Renal-dose dopamine (1 to 5 mcg/kg/ minute) given I.V. to enhance renal perfusion
◆ Diuretic therapy to treat oliguric phase
◆ Sodium polystyrene sulfonate (Kayexalate) by mouth or enema to reverse hyperkalemia with mild hyperkalemic symptoms (malaise, loss of appetite, muscle weakness)
◆ Hypertonic glucose with insulin I.V., for more severe hyperkalemic symptoms (numbness and tingling and ECG changes)
◆ Sodium bicarbonate I.V. to treat metabolic acidosis
◆ Hemodialysis, continuous renal replacement therapy, or peritoneal dialysis to correct electrolyte and fluid imbalances
◆ Discontinuation of nephrotoxic agents (antibiotics, radioactive agents, and other such drugs)
◆ Discontinuation or adjustment of all medications cleared by renal excretion

Special considerations

Patient care includes careful monitoring and dietary education.
◆ Measure and record intake and output, including body fluids, such as wound drainage, nasogastric output, and diarrhea. Weigh the patient daily.
◆ Assess the hemoglobin level and hematocrit, and administer packed red blood cells, as ordered.
◆ Monitor vital signs. Watch for and report signs and symptoms of pericarditis (pleuritic chest pain, tachycardia, pericardial friction rub), inadequate renal perfusion (hypotension), and acidosis.
◆ Maintain proper electrolyte balance. Strictly monitor the potassium level.

⚠ **CLINICAL ALERT** *Watch the patient for symptoms of hyperkalemia (malaise, anorexia, paresthesia, or muscle weakness) and ECG changes (tall, peaked T waves; widening QRS complex; and disappearing P waves), and report them immediately. Avoid administering medications that contain potassium.*

◆ Assess the patient frequently, especially during emergency treatment to lower the potassium level. If the patient receives hypertonic glucose and insulin infusions, monitor potassium and glucose levels. If you give sodium polystyrene sulfonate rectally, make sure the patient doesn't retain it and become constipated, to prevent bowel perforation.
◆ Maintain nutritional status. Provide a high-calorie, restricted-protein, low-sodium, and low-potassium diet, with vitamin supplements. Give the anorexic patient small, frequent meals.
◆ Use sterile technique because the patient with acute renal failure is highly susceptible to infection. Don't allow personnel with upper respiratory tract infections to care for the patient.
◆ Prevent complications of immobility by encouraging frequent coughing and deep breathing and by performing passive range-of-motion exercises. Help the patient walk as soon as possible. Add lubricating lotion to the patient's bath water to combat skin dryness.
◆ Provide good mouth care frequently because mucous membranes are dry. If stomatitis occurs, an antibiotic solution may be ordered. Have the patient swish the solution around in his mouth before swallowing.
◆ Monitor for GI bleeding by guaiac-testing stools for blood. Administer medications carefully, especially antacids and stool softeners. Use aluminum hydroxide–based antacids; magnesium-based antacids can cause the serum magnesium level to rise to a critical level.
◆ Use appropriate safety measures, such as side rails and restraints (only when absolutely necessary), because the patient with central nervous system involvement may be dizzy or confused.
◆ Provide emotional support to the patient and his family. Reassure them by clearly explaining procedures.
◆ During peritoneal dialysis, position the patient carefully. Elevate the head of the bed to reduce pressure on the diaphragm and aid respiration. Be alert for signs of infection (cloudy drainage, elevated temperature) and, rarely, bleeding. If pain occurs, reduce the amount of dialysate. If the patient has diabetes, monitor his blood glucose level periodically and administer insulin, as ordered. Watch for complications, such as peritonitis, atelectasis, hypokalemia, pneumonia, and shock.
◆ If the patient requires hemodialysis, or continuous renal replacement therapy (CRRT), check the blood access site (arteriovenous fistula, subclavian or femoral catheter) every 2 hours for patency and signs of clotting (palpate for a thrill; auscultate for a bruit). Don't use the arm with the shunt or fistula for taking blood pressures or drawing blood. Weigh the patient before beginning dialysis. During dialysis and CRRT, monitor vital signs, clotting times, blood flow, the function of the vascular access site, and arterial and venous pressures. Watch for complications, such as septicemia, embolism, hepatitis, and rapid fluid and electrolyte loss. After dialysis, monitor vital signs and the vascular access site; weigh the patient;

watch for signs of fluid and electrolyte imbalances.
♦ Use standard precautions when handling blood and body fluids.

ACUTE TUBULAR NECROSIS

Acute tubular necrosis (ATN), also known as *acute tubulointerstitial nephritis,* is the most common cause of acute renal failure in critically ill patients. ATN injures the nephron's tubular segment, causing renal failure and uremic syndrome. Mortality ranges from 40% to 70%, depending on complications from underlying diseases. Nonoliguric forms of ATN have a better prognosis.

Causes

♦ Diseased tubular epithelium that allows leakage of glomerular filtrate across the membranes and reabsorption of filtrate into the blood
♦ Obstruction of urine flow by the collection of damaged cells, casts, red blood cells (RBCs), and other cellular debris within the tubular walls
♦ Ischemic injury to glomerular epithelial cells, resulting in cellular collapse and decreased glomerular capillary permeability
♦ Ischemic injury to vascular endothelium, eventually resulting in cellular swelling and tubular obstruction

Pathophysiology

ATN results from ischemic or nephrotoxic injury, most commonly in debilitated patients, such as the critically ill or those who have undergone extensive surgery. In ischemic injury, disruption of blood flow to the kidneys may result from circulatory collapse, severe hypotension, trauma, hemorrhage, dehydration, cardiogenic or septic shock, surgery, anesthetics, or reactions to transfusions. Nephrotoxic injury may follow ingestion of certain chemical agents, such as contrasts administered during radiologic procedures or administration of antibiotics (aminoglycosides), or result from a hypersensitive reaction of the kidneys. Because nephrotoxic ATN doesn't damage the basement membrane of the nephron, it's potentially reversible. However, ischemic ATN can damage the epithelial and basement membranes and can cause lesions in the renal interstitium. (See *Understanding acute tubular necrosis.*)

Signs and symptoms

ATN is usually difficult to recognize in its early stages because effects of the critically ill patient's primary disease may mask the symptoms of ATN. However, signs and symptoms may include:

♦ decreased urine output, generally the first recognizable effect because of reduced renal blood flow and glomerular filtration
♦ hyperkalemia because of disturbed renal tubular absorption
♦ uremic syndrome with oliguria (or, rarely, anuria) and confusion, which may progress to uremic coma caused by renal failure
♦ dry mucous membranes and skin due to the accumulation of uremic toxins
♦ central nervous system signs and symptoms, such as lethargy, twitching, or seizures resulting from effects of uremic toxins on highly sensitive nerve cells
♦ bibasilar crackles, tachycardia, and other signs of fluid overload.

Complications

♦ Heart failure
♦ Uremic pericarditis
♦ Pulmonary edema
♦ Uremic lung
♦ Metabolic acidosis
♦ Anemia
♦ Anorexia, intractable vomiting
♦ Poor wound healing due to debilitation

⚠ **CLINICAL ALERT** *Fever and chills may signal the onset of an infection, which is the leading cause of death in ATN.*

Diagnosis

Diagnosis is usually delayed until the condition has progressed to an advanced stage.
♦ The most significant laboratory clues are urinary sediment containing RBCs and casts, and dilute urine of a low specific gravity (1.010), low osmolality (less than 400 mOsm/kg), and high sodium level (40 to 60 mEq/L).
♦ Blood studies reveal elevated blood urea nitrogen and serum creatinine levels, anemia, defects in platelet adherence, metabolic acidosis, and hyperkalemia.
♦ An electrocardiogram may show arrhythmias (due to electrolyte imbalances) and, with hyperkalemia, widening QRS complex, disappearing P waves, and tall, peaked T waves.

Treatment

In the acute phase of ATN:
♦ identifying and treating underlying cause of ATN
♦ vigorous supportive measures until normal kidney function resumes
♦ initially, possible administration of a diuretic and infusion of a large volume of fluids to flush tubules of cellular casts and debris and to replace fluid loss (risk of fluid overload with this treatment).

Understanding acute tubular necrosis

Necrosis and sloughing of epithelial cells result in the formation of casts, which causes obstruction and an increase in the intraluminal pressure, reducing the glomerular filtration rate. Vasoconstriction of the afferent arteriole, caused by tubuloglomerular feedback, results in decreased glomerular capillary filtration pressure. Injury to the tubule results and the increased intraluminal pressure causes fluid to leak back from the lumen into the interstitium.

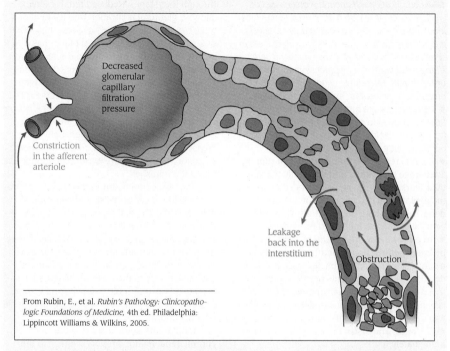

Decreased glomerular capillary filtration pressure

Constriction in the afferent arteriole

Leakage back into the interstitium

Obstruction

From Rubin, E., et al. *Rubin's Pathology: Clinicopathologic Foundations of Medicine*, 4th ed. Philadelphia: Lippincott Williams & Wilkins, 2005.

Long-term fluid management includes daily replacement of projected and calculated losses (including insensible loss).

Other appropriate measures to control complications include:
◆ transfusion of packed RBCs for anemia; epoetin alfa to stimulate RBC production as an alternative to blood transfusion
◆ administration of an antibiotic for infection
◆ emergency I.V. administration of 50% glucose, regular insulin, and sodium bicarbonate for hyperkalemia
◆ sodium polystyrene sulfonate with sorbitol by mouth or by enema to reduce the extracellular potassium level
◆ peritoneal dialysis or hemodialysis if the patient is catabolic or if hyperkalemia and fluid volume overload aren't controlled by other measures.

Special considerations

Patient care is largely supportive.
◆ Maintain fluid balance. Watch for fluid overload, a common complication of therapy. Accurately record intake and output, including wound drainage, nasogastric output, and hemodialysis and peritoneal dialysis balances. Weigh the patient daily.
◆ Monitor the hemoglobin level and hematocrit, and administer blood products as needed. Use fresh packed cells instead of whole blood to prevent fluid overload and heart failure.
◆ Maintain electrolyte balance. Monitor laboratory results, and report imbalances. Enforce dietary restriction of foods containing sodium and potassium, such as bananas, orange juice, and baked potatoes. Check for potassium content in prescribed medications (for example, potassium penicillin). Provide adequate calories and essential amino acids, while restricting protein intake to maintain an anabolic state. Total parenteral

nutrition may be indicated in the severely debilitated or catabolic patient.

◆ Use sterile technique, particularly when handling catheters because the debilitated patient is vulnerable to infection. Immediately report fever, chills, delayed wound healing, or flank pain if the patient has an indwelling catheter.

⚠ **CLINICAL ALERT** *Watch the patient for complications. If anemia worsens (pallor, weakness, lethargy with a decreased hemoglobin level), administer RBCs as ordered. For acidosis, give sodium bicarbonate or assist with dialysis in severe cases, as ordered. Watch for signs of diminishing renal perfusion (hypotension and decreased urine output). Encourage coughing and deep breathing to prevent pulmonary complications.*

◆ Perform passive range-of-motion exercises. Provide good skin care; apply lotion or bath oil for dry skin. Help the patient walk as soon as possible, but guard against exhaustion.

◆ Provide reassurance and emotional support. Encourage the patient and his family to express their fears. Fully explain each procedure; repeat the explanation each time the procedure is done. Help the patient and family set realistic goals according to individual prognosis.

◆ To prevent ATN, make sure patients are well hydrated before surgery or after X-rays that use a contrast medium. Administer mannitol, as ordered, to high-risk patients before and during these procedures. Carefully monitor patients receiving blood transfusions to detect early signs and symptoms of transfusion reaction (fever, rash, chills), and discontinue such transfusions immediately.

CHRONIC RENAL FAILURE

Chronic renal failure represents a destruction of renal tissue with irreversible sclerosis and loss of nephron function. It can result from chronic illness or from a rapidly progressing disease.

Few symptoms develop until less than 25% of glomerular filtration remains. The normal parenchyma deteriorates and symptoms worsen as renal function decreases. This condition is fatal without treatment, but maintenance on dialysis or a kidney transplant can sustain life.

Causes

◆ Chronic glomerular disease (glomerulonephritis)
◆ Chronic infection (such as chronic pyelonephritis and tuberculosis)
◆ Collagen disease (lupus erythematosus)
◆ Congenital anomalies (polycystic kidney disease)
◆ Endocrine disease (diabetic neuropathy)
◆ Nephrotoxic agents (long-term aminoglycoside therapy)
◆ Obstruction (renal calculi)
◆ Vascular disease (hypertension, nephrosclerosis)

Pathophysiology

Chronic renal failure typically progresses through four stages. Reduced renal reserve shows a glomerular filtration rate (GFR) of 35% to 50% of normal; renal insufficiency has a GFR of 20% to 35% of normal; renal failure has a GFR of 20% to 25% of normal; and end-stage renal disease has a GFR of less than 20% of normal.

Nephron damage is progressive; damaged nephrons can't function and don't recover. The kidneys can maintain relatively normal function until about 75% of the nephrons are nonfunctional. Surviving nephrons hypertrophy and increase their rate of filtration, reabsorption, and secretion. Compensatory excretion continues as the GFR diminishes.

Urine may contain abnormal amounts of protein, red blood cells (RBCs), and white blood cells or casts. The major end products of excretion remain essentially normal, and nephron loss becomes significant. As the GFR decreases, the plasma creatinine level increases proportionately, without regulatory adjustment. As sodium delivery to the nephron increases, less is reabsorbed, and sodium deficits and volume depletion follow. The kidney becomes incapable of concentrating and diluting urine.

If tubular interstitial disease is the cause of chronic renal failure, primary damage to the tubules—the medullary portion of the nephron—precedes failure, as do such problems as renal tubular acidosis, salt wasting, and difficulty diluting and concentrating urine. If vascular or glomerular damage is the primary cause, proteinuria, hematuria, and nephrotic syndrome are more prominent.

Changes in acid-base balance affect phosphorus and calcium balance. Renal phosphate excretion and $1,25(OH)_2$ vitamin D_3 synthesis are diminished. Hypocalcemia results in secondary hypoparathyroidism, diminished GFR, and progressive hyperphosphatemia, hypocalcemia, and dissolution of bone. In early renal insufficiency, acid excretion and phosphate reabsorption increase to maintain normal pH. When GFR decreases by 30% to 40%, progressive metabolic acidosis ensues and tubular secretion of potassium increases. The total-body potassium level may increase to a life-threatening level, requiring dialysis.

In glomerulosclerosis, distortion of filtration slits and erosion of the glomerular epithelial cells lead to increased fluid transport across the glomerular wall. Large proteins traverse the slits but become trapped in glomerular basement membranes, obstructing the glomerular capillaries. Epithelial and endothelial injury cause proteinuria. Mesangial-cell proliferation, increased production of extracellular matrix, and intraglomerular coagulation cause the sclerosis.

Tubulointerstitial injury occurs from toxic or ischemic tubular damage, as with acute tubular necrosis. Debris and calcium deposits obstruct the tubules. The resulting defective tubular transport is associated with interstitial edema, leukocyte infiltration, and tubular necrosis. Vascular injury causes diffuse or focal ischemia of renal parenchyma, associated with thickening, fibrosis, or focal lesions of renal blood vessels. Decreased blood flow then leads to tubular atrophy, interstitial fibrosis, and functional disruption of glomerular filtration, medullary gradients, and concentration.

The structural changes trigger an inflammatory response. Fibrin deposits begin to form around the interstitium. Microaneurysms result from vascular wall damage and increased pressure secondary to obstruction or hypertension. Eventual loss of the nephron triggers compensatory hyperfunction of uninjured nephrons, which initiates a positive-feedback loop of increasing vulnerability.

Eventually, the healthy glomeruli are so overburdened that they become sclerotic, stiff, and necrotic. Toxins accumulate and potentially fatal changes ensue in all major organ systems.

Extrarenal consequences

Physiologic changes affect more than one system, and the presence and severity of manifestations depend on the duration of renal failure and its response to treatment. In some fluid and electrolyte imbalances, the kidneys can't retain salt, and hyponatremia results. Dry mouth, fatigue, nausea, hypotension, loss of skin turgor, and listlessness can progress to somnolence and confusion. Later, as the number of functioning nephrons decreases, so does the capacity to excrete sodium and potassium. Sodium retention leads to fluid overload and edema; the potassium overload leads to muscle irritability and weakness, and life-threatening cardiac arrhythmias.

As the cardiovascular system becomes involved, hypertension occurs, and irregular distant heart sounds may be auscultated if pericardial effusion occurs. Bibasilar crackles in the lungs and peripheral edema reflect heart failure.

Pulmonary changes include reduced macrophage activity and increasing susceptibility to infection. Decreased breath sounds in areas of consolidation reflect the presence of pneumonia. As the pleurae become more involved, the patient may experience pleuritic pain and friction rubs.

Kussmaul's respirations may be noted as a result of metabolic acidosis. The GI mucosa becomes inflamed and ulcerated, and gums may also be ulcerated and bleeding. Stomatitis, uremic fetor (an ammonia smell to the breath), hiccups, peptic ulcer, and pancreatitis in end-stage renal failure are believed to be caused by the retention of metabolic acids and other metabolic waste products. Malnutrition may be secondary to anorexia, malaise, and reduced dietary intake of protein. The reduced protein intake also affects capillary fragility and results in decreased immune functioning and poor wound healing.

Normochromic normocytic anemia and platelet disorders with prolonged bleeding time ensue. Diminished erythropoietin secretion leads to reduced RBC production in the bone marrow. Uremic toxins associated with chronic renal failure shorten RBC survival time. The patient experiences lethargy and dizziness.

Demineralization of the bone (renal osteodystrophy) manifested by bone pain and pathologic fractures is due to several factors:
◆ decreased renal activation of vitamin D, decreasing absorption of dietary calcium
◆ retention of phosphate resulting in a decrease in serum calcium
◆ increased circulation of parathyroid hormone due to decreased urinary excretion.

The skin acquires a grayish yellow tint as urine pigments (urochromes) accumulate. Inflammatory mediators released by retained toxins in the skin cause pruritus. Uric acid and other substances in the sweat crystallize and accumulate on the skin as uremic frost. A high plasma calcium level is also associated with pruritus.

Restless leg syndrome (abnormal sensation and spontaneous movement of the feet and lower legs), muscle weakness, and decreased deep tendon reflexes are believed to result from the effect of toxins on the nervous system.

⚠ **CLINICAL ALERT** *Restless leg syndrome is one of the first signs of peripheral neuropathy. This condition will eventually progress to paresthesia and motor nerve dysfunction (bilateral footdrop) unless dialysis is initiated.*

Chronic renal failure increases the risk of death from infection. This is related to suppression of cell-mediated immunity and a reduction in the number and function of lymphocytes and phagocytes.

All hormone levels are impaired in excretion and activation. Women may be anovulatory, amenorrheic, or unable to carry pregnancy to full term. Men tend to have a decreased sperm count and impotence.

Signs and symptoms

♦ Hypervolemia due to sodium retention
♦ Hyperphosphatemia and hyperkalemia due to inability to balance electrolytes
♦ Hypocalcemia due to decreased intestinal calcium absorption and hyperphosphatemia
♦ Azotemia due to retention of nitrogenous wastes
♦ Metabolic acidosis due to loss of bicarbonate
♦ Bone and muscle pain and fractures caused by calcium-phosphorus imbalance and consequent parathyroid hormone imbalances
♦ Peripheral neuropathy due to accumulation of toxins
♦ Dry mouth, fatigue, and nausea due to hyponatremia
♦ Hypotension due to sodium loss
♦ Altered mental state due to hyponatremia and toxin accumulation
♦ Irregular heart rate due to hyperkalemia
♦ Hypertension due to fluid overload
♦ Gum sores and bleeding due to coagulopathies
♦ Yellow-bronze skin due to altered metabolic processes
♦ Dry, scaly skin and severe itching due to uremic frost
♦ Muscle cramps and twitching, including cardiac irritability, due to hyperkalemia
♦ Malnutrition, failure to thrive, fatigue, and somnolence due to uremia
♦ Kussmaul's respirations due to metabolic acidosis

■ **AGE ALERT** *Growth retardation in children occurs from endocrine abnormalities induced by renal failure. Impaired bone growth and bowlegs in children are also due to rickets.*

♦ Infertility, decreased libido, amenorrhea, and impotence due to endocrine disturbances
♦ GI bleeding, hemorrhage, and bruising due to thrombocytopenia and platelet defects
♦ Pain, burning, and itching in legs and feet associated with peripheral neuropathy
♦ Infection related to decreased macrophage activity

Complications

♦ Anemia
♦ Peripheral neuropathy
♦ Cardiopulmonary complications
♦ GI complications
♦ Hepatitis C (dialysis patients)
♦ Sexual dysfunction

♦ Skeletal defects
♦ Paresthesia
♦ Motor nerve dysfunction, such as footdrop and flaccid paralysis
♦ Pathologic fractures

Diagnosis

Blood study results that help diagnose chronic renal failure include:

♦ decreased arterial pH and bicarbonate, a low hemoglobin level and hematocrit
♦ decreased RBC survival time, mild thrombocytopenia, platelet defects
♦ elevated blood urea nitrogen, serum creatinine, sodium, and potassium levels
♦ increased aldosterone secretion related to increased renin production
♦ hyperglycemia (a sign of impaired carbohydrate metabolism)
♦ hypertriglyceridemia and a low level of high-density lipoproteins.

Urinalysis results aiding in diagnosis include:
♦ specific gravity fixed at 1.010
♦ proteinuria, glycosuria, RBC and leukocyte counts, casts, or crystals, depending on the cause.

Other study results used to diagnose chronic renal failure include:
♦ reduced kidney size on kidney-ureter-bladder radiography, excretory urography, nephrotomography, renal scan, or renal arteriography
♦ renal biopsy to identify underlying disease
♦ EEG to identify metabolic encephalopathy.

Treatment

♦ Restricted-protein diet, to limit accumulation of end products of protein metabolism that the kidneys can't excrete
♦ High-protein diet for patients on continuous peritoneal dialysis
♦ High-calorie diet, to prevent ketoacidosis and tissue atrophy
♦ Sodium, phosphorus, and potassium restrictions, to prevent elevated levels
♦ Fluid restrictions, to maintain fluid balance
♦ A loop diuretic, such as furosemide (Lasix), to maintain fluid balance
♦ A cardiac glycoside, such as digoxin, to strengthen myocardial contraction
♦ Calcium carbonate (Caltrate) or calcium acetate (PhosLo), to treat renal osteodystrophy by binding to and excreting phosphate and supplementing calcium
♦ An antihypertensive, to control blood pressure and edema
♦ Insulin, oral antidiabetic agents, or both to aggressively control hyperglycemia

◆ Avoidance of nephrotoxins (aminoglycosides, nonsteroidal anti-inflammatory agents, I.V. radiocontrast agents)
◆ An antiemetic, to relieve nausea and vomiting
◆ Famotidine (Pepcid) or ranitidine (Zantac), to decrease gastric irritation
◆ Methylcellulose or docusate, to prevent constipation
◆ Iron and folate supplements or RBC transfusion for anemia
◆ Synthetic erythropoietin, to stimulate the bone marrow to produce RBCs; supplemental iron, conjugated estrogens, and desmopressin, to combat hematologic effects
◆ An antipruritic, such as trimeprazine (Temaril) or diphenhydramine (Benadryl), to relieve itching
◆ Aluminum hydroxide gel, to reduce the serum phosphate level
◆ Supplementary vitamins, particularly B and D, and essential amino acids
◆ Dialysis for hyperkalemia and fluid imbalances
◆ Oral or rectal administration of cation exchange resins, such as sodium polystyrene sulfonate (Kayexalate), and I.V. administration of 50% dextrose and regular insulin, to reverse hyperkalemia
◆ Calcium gluconate to protect the heart from hyperkalemia
◆ Sodium bicarbonate to treat metabolic acidosis
◆ Emergency pericardiocentesis or surgery for cardiac tamponade
◆ Peritoneal or hemodialysis, to help control end-stage renal disease
◆ Renal transplantation (usually the treatment of choice if a donor is available)

Special considerations

Because chronic renal failure has such widespread clinical effects, it requires meticulous and carefully coordinated supportive care.
◆ Good skin care is important. Bathe the patient daily using superfatted soaps, oatmeal baths, and skin lotion without alcohol to ease pruritus. Don't use glycerin-containing soaps because they cause skin drying. Give good perineal care using mild soap and water. Pad the side rails to guard against ecchymoses. Turn the patient often, and use a convoluted foam mattress to prevent skin breakdown.
◆ Provide good oral hygiene. Brush the patient's teeth often with a soft brush or sponge tip to reduce breath odor. Sugarless hard candy and mouthwash minimize metallic taste in the mouth and alleviate thirst.

◆ Offer small, palatable meals that are also nutritious; try to provide favorite foods within dietary restrictions. Encourage intake of high-calorie foods. Instruct the outpatient to avoid high-sodium foods and high-potassium foods. Encourage adherence to fluid and protein restrictions. To prevent constipation, stress the need for exercise and sufficient dietary bulk.
◆ Encourage the patient who smokes to stop smoking.
◆ Watch for hyperkalemia. Observe for cramping of the legs and abdomen, and diarrhea. As the potassium level rises, watch for muscle irritability and a weak pulse rate. Monitor the electrocardiogram for tall, peaked T waves; a widening QRS complex; a prolonged PR interval; and disappearance of P waves, indicating hyperkalemia.
◆ Assess hydration status carefully. Check for jugular vein distention, and auscultate the lungs for crackles. Measure daily intake and output carefully, including drainage, vomitus, diarrhea, and blood loss. Record daily weight, presence or absence of thirst, axillary sweat, dryness of tongue, hypertension, and peripheral edema.
◆ Monitor for bone or joint complications. Prevent pathologic fractures by turning the patient carefully and ensuring his safety. Provide passive range-of-motion exercises for the bedridden patient.
◆ Encourage deep breathing and coughing to prevent pulmonary congestion. Listen often for crackles, rhonchi, and decreased breath sounds. Be alert for clinical effects of pulmonary edema (dyspnea, restlessness, crackles). Administer a diuretic and other medications as ordered.
◆ Maintain strict sterile technique. Use a micropore filter during I.V. therapy. Watch for signs of infection (listlessness, high fever, leukocytosis). Urge the outpatient to avoid contact with infected people during the cold and flu season.
◆ Carefully observe and document seizure activity. Infuse sodium bicarbonate for acidosis, and a sedative or an anticonvulsant for seizures, as ordered. Pad the side rails and keep an oral airway and suction setup at the bedside. Assess neurologic status periodically, and check for Chvostek's and Trousseau's signs, indicators of a low serum calcium level.
◆ Observe for signs of bleeding. Watch for prolonged bleeding at puncture sites and at the vascular access site used for hemodialysis. Monitor the hemoglobin level and hematocrit, and check stool, urine, and vomitus for blood.
◆ Report signs of pericarditis, such as a pericardial friction rub and chest pain.

⚠ **CLINICAL ALERT** *Also, watch the patient for the disappearance of friction rub, with a drop of 15 to 20 mm Hg in blood pressure during inspiration (paradoxical pulse)—an early sign of pericardial tamponade.*

♦ Schedule medications carefully. Give iron before meals, aluminum hydroxide gels after meals, and an antiemetic, as necessary, a half hour before meals. Administer an antihypertensive at appropriate intervals. If the patient requires a rectal infusion of sodium polystyrene sulfonate for a dangerously high potassium level, apply an emollient to soothe the perianal area. Make sure the sodium polystyrene sulfonate enema is expelled; otherwise, it will cause constipation and won't lower the potassium level. Recommend antacid cookies as an alternative to aluminum hydroxide gels needed to bind GI phosphate.

For dialysis

♦ Prepare the patient by fully explaining the procedure. Make sure that he understands how to protect and care for the arteriovenous shunt, fistula, or other vascular access. Check the vascular access site every 2 hours for patency and the extremity for adequate blood supply and intact nervous function (temperature, pulse rate, capillary refill time, and sensation). If a fistula is present, feel for a thrill and listen for a bruit. Use a gentle touch to avoid occluding the fistula. Report signs of possible clotting. Don't use the arm with the vascular access site to take blood pressure readings, draw blood, or give injections because these procedures may rupture the fistula or occlude blood flow.

♦ Withhold the morning dose of antihypertensive on the morning of dialysis, and instruct the outpatient to do the same.

♦ Use standard precautions when handling body fluids and needles.

♦ Monitor the hemoglobin level and hematocrit. Assess the patient's tolerance of his levels. Some individuals are more sensitive to lower levels than others. Instruct the anemic patient to conserve energy and to rest frequently.

♦ After dialysis, check for disequilibrium syndrome, a result of sudden correction of blood chemistry abnormalities. Symptoms range from a headache to seizures. Also, check for excessive bleeding from the dialysis site. Apply pressure dressing or absorbable gelatin sponge, as indicated. Monitor blood pressure carefully after dialysis.

♦ A patient undergoing dialysis is under a great deal of stress, as is his family. Refer him to appropriate counseling agencies for assistance in coping with chronic renal failure.

CONGENITAL ANOMALIES OF THE URETER, BLADDER, AND URETHRA

Congenital anomalies of the ureter, bladder, and urethra are among the most common birth defects, occurring in about 5% of births. Some of these abnormalities are obvious at birth; others aren't apparent and are recognized only after they produce symptoms.

Causes

Causes of these congenital anomalies are unknown.

Pathophysiology

The most common malformations include duplicated ureter, retrocaval ureter, ectopic orifice of the ureter, stricture or stenosis of the ureter, ureterocele, exstrophy of the bladder, congenital bladder diverticulum, hypospadias, and epispadias. Their pathophysiology, signs and symptoms, diagnosis, and treatment vary. (See *Congenital urologic anomalies.*)

Special considerations

⚠ **CLINICAL ALERT** *Because these anomalies aren't always obvious at birth, carefully evaluate the neonate's urogenital function. Document the amount and color of urine, voiding pattern, strength of stream, and any indications of infection, such as fever and urine odor. Tell parents to watch for these signs at home. In all children, watch for signs of obstruction, such as dribbling, oliguria or anuria, abdominal mass, hypertension, fever, bacteriuria, or pyuria.*

♦ Monitor renal function daily; record intake and output accurately. Weigh diapers, if necessary.

♦ Follow strict sterile technique in handling cystostomy tubes or indwelling urinary catheters.

♦ Make sure that ureteral, suprapubic, or urethral catheters remain in place and don't become contaminated. Document type, color, and amount of drainage.

♦ Apply sterile saline pads to protect the exposed mucosa of the neonate with bladder exstrophy. Don't use heavy clamps on the umbilical cord, and avoid dressing or diapering the infant. Place the infant in an isolette, and direct a stream of saline mist onto the bladder to keep it moist. Use warm water and mild soap to keep the surrounding skin clean. Rinse well, and keep the area as dry as possible to prevent excoriation.

♦ Provide reassurance and emotional support to the parents. When possible, allow them to participate in their child's care to promote normal

Congenital urologic anomalies

Anomoly	Pathophysiology	Clinical features	Diagnosis and treatment
Duplicated ureter	◆ Most common ureteral anomaly ◆ Complete, a double collecting system with two separate pelves, each with its own ureter and orifice ◆ Incomplete, two separate ureters join before entering bladder	◆ Persistent or recurrent infection ◆ Frequency, urgency, or burning on urination ◆ Diminished urine output ◆ Flank pain, fever, and chills	◆ Excretory urography ◆ Voiding cystoscopy ◆ Cystoureterography ◆ Retrograde pyelography ◆ Surgery for obstruction, reflux, or severe renal damage
Retrocaval ureter (preureteral vena cava)	◆ Right ureter passes behind the inferior vena cava before entering the bladder (Compression of the ureter between the vena cava and the spine causes dilation and elongation of the pelvis; hydroureter, hydronephrosis; fibrosis and stenosis of ureter in the compressed area.) ◆ Relatively uncommon; higher incidence in males	◆ Right flank pain ◆ Recurrent urinary tract infection ◆ Renal calculi ◆ Hematuria	◆ Excretory urography demonstrating superior ureteral enlargement with spiral appearance ◆ Surgical resection and anastomosis of ureter with renal pelvis, or reimplantation into bladder
Ectopic orifice of ureter	◆ Ureters single or duplicated in females, ureteral orifice usually inserts in urethra or vaginal vestibule, beyond external urethral sphincter; in males, in prostatic urethra, or in seminal vesicles or vas deferens	◆ Symptoms rare when ureteral orifice opens between the trigone and the bladder neck ◆ Obstruction, reflux, and incontinence (dribbling) in 50% of females ◆ In males, flank pain, frequency, urgency	◆ Excretory urography ◆ Urethroscopy, vaginoscopy ◆ Voiding cystourethrography ◆ Resection and ureteral reimplantation into bladder for incontinence
Strictures or stenosis of ureter	◆ Most common site, the distal ureter above ureterovesical junction; less common, ureteropelvic junction; rare, the midureter	◆ Megaloureter or hydroureter (enlarged ureter), with hydronephrosis when stenosis occurs in distal ureter	◆ Ultrasound ◆ Excretory urography ◆ Voiding cystography

(continued)

Congenital urologic anomalies (continued)

Anomoly	Pathophysiology	Clinical features	Diagnosis and treatment
	◆ Discovered during infancy in 25% of patients; before puberty in most ◆ More common in males	◆ Hydronephrosis alone when stenosis occurs at ureteropelvic junction	◆ Surgical repair of stricture; nephrectomy for severe renal damage
Ureterocele	◆ Bulging of submucosal ureter into bladder can be 1 to 2 cm, or can almost fill bladder ◆ Unilateral, bilateral, ectopic with resulting hydroureter and hydronephrosis	◆ Obstruction ◆ Persistent or recurrent infection	◆ Voiding cystourethrography ◆ Excretory urography and cystoscopy showing a thin, translucent mass ◆ Surgical excision or resection of ureterocele, with reimplantation of ureter
Exstrophy of bladder	◆ Absence of anterior abdominal and bladder wall allowing the bladder to protrude onto abdomen ◆ In males, associated undescended testes and epispadias; in females, cleft clitoris, separated labia, or absent vagina ◆ Skeletal or intestinal anomalies possible	◆ Obvious at birth, with urine seeping onto abdominal wall from abnormal ureteral orifices ◆ Surrounding skin excoriated; exposed bladder mucosa ulcerated; infection; related abnormalities	◆ Excretory urography ◆ Surgical closure of defect, and bladder and urethra reconstruction during infancy to allow pubic bone fusion; alternative treatment: protective dressing and diapering; urinary diversion eventually necessary for most patients
Congenital bladder diverticulum	◆ Circumscribed pouch or sac (diverticulum) of bladder wall ◆ Can occur anywhere in the bladder, usually lateral to a ureteral orifice (Large diverticulum at orifice can cause reflux.)	◆ Fever, frequency, and painful urination ◆ Urinary tract infection ◆ Cystitis, particularly in males	◆ Excretory urography showing diverticulum ◆ Retrograde cystography showing vesicoureteral reflux in ureter ◆ Surgical correction for reflux
Hypospadias	◆ Urethral opening is on ventral surface of penis or, in females (rare), within the vagina ◆ Occurs in 1 in 300 live male births (Genetic factor suspected in less severe cases.)	◆ Usually associated with chordee, making normal urination with penis elevated impossible ◆ Absence of ventral prepuce ◆ Vaginal discharge in females	◆ Mild disorder — no treatment ◆ Surgical repair of severe anomaly usually necessary before child reaches school age

Congenital urologic anomalies *(continued)*

Anomoly	Pathophysiology	Clinical features	Diagnosis and treatment
Epispadias	◆ Urethral opening on dorsal surface of penis; in females, a fissure of the upper wall of the urethra ◆ A rare anomaly; usually developing in males; commonly accompanies bladder exstrophy	◆ In mild cases, orifice appears along dorsum of glans; in severe cases, along dorsum of penis ◆ In females, bifid clitoris and short, wide urethra	◆ Surgical repair, in several stages, almost always necessary

bonding. As appropriate, suggest or arrange for genetic counseling.

GLOMERULONEPHRITIS

Glomerulonephritis is a bilateral inflammation of the glomeruli, typically following a streptococcal infection. Acute glomerulonephritis is also called *acute poststreptococcal glomerulonephritis.*

Acute glomerulonephritis is most common in boys ages 3 to 7, but it can occur at any age. Up to 95% of children and 70% of adults recover fully; the rest, especially elderly patients, may progress to chronic renal failure within months.

Rapidly progressive glomerulonephritis (RPGN) — also called *subacute, crescentic,* or *extracapillary glomerulonephritis* — most commonly occurs between ages 50 and 60. It may be idiopathic or associated with a proliferative glomerular disease, such as poststreptococcal glomerulonephritis.

AGE ALERT *Goodpasture's syndrome, a type of rapidly progressive glomerulonephritis, is rare, but is most common in men between ages 20 and 30.*

Chronic glomerulonephritis is a slowly progressive disease characterized by inflammation, sclerosis, scarring and, eventually, renal failure. It usually remains undetected until the progressive phase, which is usually irreversible.

Causes

Causes of acute and RPGN include:
◆ immunoglobulin (Ig) A nephropathy (Berger's disease)
◆ impetigo
◆ lipoid nephrosis
◆ streptococcal infection of the respiratory tract.

Chronic glomerulonephritis is caused by:
◆ focal glomerulosclerosis
◆ Goodpasture's syndrome
◆ hemolytic uremic syndrome
◆ membranoproliferative glomerulonephritis
◆ membranous glomerulopathy
◆ poststreptococcal glomerulonephritis
◆ RPGN
◆ systemic lupus erythematosus.

Pathophysiology

In nearly all types of glomerulonephritis, the epithelial or podocyte layer of the glomerular membrane is disturbed. This results in a loss of negative charge. (See *Characteristics of glomerular lesions,* page 526.)

Acute poststreptococcal glomerulonephritis results from the entrapment and collection of antigen-antibody complexes in the glomerular capillary membranes, after infection with a group A beta-hemolytic streptococcus. The antigens, which are endogenous or exogenous, stimulate the formation of antibodies. Circulating antigen-antibody complexes become lodged in the glomerular capillaries. Glomerular injury occurs when the complexes initiate complement activation and the release of immunologic substances that lyse cells and increase membrane permeability. Antibody damage to basement membranes causes crescent formation. The severity of glomerular damage and renal insufficiency is related to the size, number, location (focal or diffuse), duration of exposure, and type of antigen-antibody complexes. (See *Immune complex deposits on the glomerulus,* page 527.)

Characteristics of glomerular lesions

The types of glomerular lesions and their characteristics include:
◆ *crescent lesions* — accumulation of proliferating cells in Bowman's space
◆ *diffuse lesions* — relatively uniform, involve most of all glomeruli (for example, glomerulonephritis)
◆ *focal lesions* — involve only some glomeruli; others normal
◆ *membranous lesions* — thickening of glomerular capillary wall
◆ *mesangial lesions* — deposits of immunoglobulins in mesangial matrix
◆ *proliferative lesions* — increased number of glomerular cells
◆ *sclerotic lesions* — glomerular scarring from previous glomerular injury
◆ *segmental-local lesions* — involve only one part of the glomerulus.

Antibody or antigen-antibody complexes in the glomerular capillary wall activate biochemical mediators of inflammation — complement, leukocytes, and fibrin. Activated complement attracts neutrophils and monocytes, which release lysosomal enzymes that damage the glomerular cell walls and cause a proliferation of the extracellular matrix, affecting glomerular blood flow. Those events increase membrane permeability, which causes a loss of negative charge across the glomerular membrane as well as enhanced protein filtration.

Membrane damage leads to platelet aggregation, and platelet degranulation releases substances that increase glomerular permeability. Protein molecules and red blood cells (RBCs) can now pass into the urine, resulting in proteinuria or hematuria. Activation of the coagulation system leads to fibrin deposits in Bowman's space. The result is crescent formation and diminished renal blood flow and glomerular filtration rate (GFR). Glomerular bleeding causes acidic urine, which transforms hemoglobin to methemoglobin and results in brown urine without clots.

The inflammatory response decreases the GFR, which causes fluid retention, decreased urine output, extracellular fluid volume expansion, and hypertension. Gross proteinuria is associated with nephrotic syndrome. After 10 to 20 years, renal insufficiency develops, followed by nephrotic syndrome and end-stage renal failure.

Goodpasture's syndrome is an RPGN in which antibodies are produced against the pulmonary capillaries and glomerular basement membrane. Diffuse intracellular antibody proliferation in Bowman's space leads to a crescent-shaped structure that obliterates the space. The crescent is composed of fibrin and endothelial, mesangial, and phagocytic cells, which compress the glomerular capillaries, diminish blood flow, and cause extensive scarring of the glomeruli. The GFR is reduced, and renal failure occurs within weeks or months.

IgA nephropathy, or Berger's disease, is usually idiopathic. Plasma IgA level is elevated, and IgA and inflammatory cells are deposited into Bowman's space. The result is sclerosis and fibrosis of the glomerulus and a reduced GFR.

Lipid nephrosis causes disruption of the capillary filtration membrane and loss of its negative charge. This increased permeability with resultant loss of protein leads to nephrotic syndrome.

Systemic diseases, such as hepatitis B virus, systemic lupus erythematosus, and solid malignant tumors, cause a membranous nephropathy. An inflammatory process causes thickening of the glomerular capillary wall. Increased permeability and proteinuria lead to nephrotic syndrome.

Sometimes the immune complement further damages the glomerular membrane. The damaged and inflamed glomeruli lose the ability to be selectively permeable so that RBCs and proteins filter through as the GFR decreases. Uremic poisoning may result. Renal function may deteriorate, especially in adults with sporadic acute poststreptococcal glomerulonephritis, commonly in the form of glomerulosclerosis accompanied by hypertension. The more severe the disorder, the more likely the occurrence of complications. Hypervolemia leads to hypertension, resulting from either sodium and water retention (caused by the decreased GFR) or inappropriate renin release. The patient develops pulmonary edema and heart failure. (See *Averting renal failure in glomerulonephritis,* page 528.)

Signs and symptoms
◆ Decreased urination or oliguria due to a decreased GFR
◆ Smoky or coffee-colored urine due to hematuria
◆ Dyspnea and orthopnea due to pulmonary edema secondary to hypervolemia
◆ Periorbital edema due to hypervolemia
◆ Mild to severe hypertension due to decreased GFR, sodium or water retention, and inappropriate release of renin

CLOSER LOOK
Immune complex deposits on the glomerulus

The illustrations below show where the immune complex deposits appear in the glomerulus in glomerulonephritis.

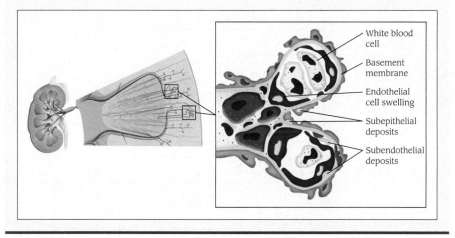

White blood cell

Basement membrane

Endothelial cell swelling

Subepithelial deposits

Subendothelial deposits

◆ Headache and confusion secondary to hypertension
◆ Bibasilar crackles due to heart failure

🟦 **AGE ALERT** *In children, the presenting features of glomerulonephritis may be encephalopathy with seizures and local neurologic deficits. An elderly patient with glomerulonephritis may report vague, nonspecific symptoms, such as nausea, malaise, and arthralgia.*

Complications
◆ Pulmonary edema
◆ Heart failure
◆ Sepsis
◆ Renal failure
◆ Severe hypertension
◆ Cardiac hypertrophy

Diagnosis
Blood study results that aid in diagnosis include:
◆ elevated electrolyte, blood urea nitrogen, and creatinine levels
◆ a decreased serum protein level
◆ a decreased hemoglobin level in chronic glomerulonephritis
◆ elevated antistreptolysin-O titers in 80% of patients, elevated streptozyme (a hemagglutination test that detects antibodies to several streptococcal antigens) and anti-DNase B (a test to determine a previous infection of group A beta-hemolytic streptococcus) titers, low serum complement levels indicating recent streptococcal infection.

Urinalysis results that help diagnose glomerulonephritis include:
◆ RBCs, white blood cells, mixed cell casts, and protein indicating renal failure
◆ fibrin-degradation products and C3 protein.

🟦 **AGE ALERT** *Significant proteinuria isn't a common finding in an elderly patient.*

Other results that help diagnose glomerulonephritis are:
◆ throat culture showing group A beta-hemolytic streptococcus
◆ bilateral kidney enlargement on kidney-ureter-bladder X-ray (acute glomerulonephritis)
◆ symmetric contraction with normal pelves and calyces (chronic glomerulonephritis) as seen on X-ray
◆ renal biopsy confirming the diagnosis or assessing renal tissue status.
◆ chest X-ray and echocardiogram ruling out cardiopulmonary involvement

Treatment
◆ Treating the primary disease to alter immunologic cascade
◆ An antibiotic for 7 to 10 days to treat infections contributing to ongoing antigen-antibody response
◆ An anticoagulant to control fibrin crescent formation in RPGN

DISEASE BLOCK

Averting renal failure in glomerulonephritis

The flowchart below shows the pathophysiologic process and the treatments that can alter the course of glomerulonephritis.

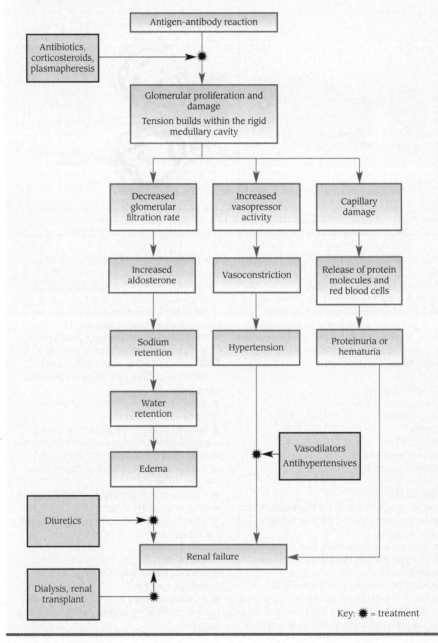

Antigen-antibody reaction

Antibiotics, corticosteroids, plasmapheresis

Glomerular proliferation and damage

Tension builds within the rigid medullary cavity

Decreased glomerular filtration rate

Increased vasopressor activity

Capillary damage

Increased aldosterone

Vasoconstriction

Release of protein molecules and red blood cells

Sodium retention

Hypertension

Proteinuria or hematuria

Water retention

Vasodilators Antihypertensives

Edema

Diuretics

Renal failure

Dialysis, renal transplant

Key: ✳ = treatment

◆ Avoiding strenuous activity; light activity as tolerated
◆ Fluid restriction to decrease edema
◆ Dietary sodium restriction to prevent fluid retention
◆ Correction of electrolyte imbalances
◆ A loop diuretic, such as metolazone (Zaroxolyn) or furosemide (Lasix), to reduce extracellular fluid overload
◆ A vasodilator such as hydralazine or an antihypertensive such as a beta-adrenergic blocker with a cardioselective alpha$_1$ blocker (labetalol) to decrease hypertension
◆ Dialysis or kidney transplantation for chronic glomerulonephritis progressing to chronic renal failure
◆ A corticosteroid to decrease antibody synthesis and suppress inflammatory response
◆ Plasmapheresis in RPGN to suppress rebound antibody production, possibly combined with a corticosteroid and cyclophosphamide (Cytoxan)

Special considerations

For patients with acute or chronic glomerulonephritis, care is primarily supportive.
◆ Check vital signs and electrolyte values. Monitor intake and output and daily weight. Assess renal function daily through serum creatinine, blood urea nitrogen, and urine creatinine clearance levels. Watch for and immediately report signs of acute renal failure (oliguria, azotemia, and acidosis). Monitor for ascites and edema.
◆ Consult the dietitian to provide a diet high in calories and low in protein, sodium, potassium, and fluids.
◆ Administer medications as ordered, and provide good skin care (because of pruritus and edema) and oral hygiene. Instruct the patient to continue taking the prescribed antihypertensive as scheduled, even if he's feeling better, and to report any adverse reactions. Advise him to take the diuretic in the morning so he won't have to disrupt his sleep to void. Teach him how to assess ankle edema.
◆ Protect the debilitated patient against secondary infection by providing good nutrition, using good hygienic technique, and preventing contact with infected people.
◆ Encourage bed rest with minimal activity during the acute phase. Allow the patient to gradually resume normal activities as symptoms subside.
◆ Advise the patient with a history of chronic upper respiratory tract infections to immediately report signs and symptoms of infection (fever, sore throat).

◆ Tell the patient that follow-up examinations are necessary to detect chronic renal failure. Stress the need for regular blood pressure, urinary protein, and renal function assessments during the convalescent months to detect recurrence. After acute glomerulonephritis, gross hematuria may recur during nonspecific viral infections; abnormal urinary findings may persist for years.
◆ Encourage pregnant women with a history of glomerulonephritis to have frequent medical evaluations because pregnancy further stresses the kidneys and increases the risk of chronic renal failure.
◆ Help the patient adjust to this illness by encouraging him to express his feelings. Explain all necessary procedures beforehand, and answer the patient's questions about them.

NEPHROTIC SYNDROME

Marked proteinuria, hypoalbuminemia, hyperlipidemia, and edema characterize nephrotic syndrome. It results from a defect in the permeability of glomerular vessels. About 75% of the cases result from primary (idiopathic) glomerulonephritis. The prognosis varies, depending on the underlying cause.

AGE ALERT *Age has no part in the progression or prognosis of nephrotic syndrome. Primary nephrotic syndrome is found predominantly in preschool children. Incidence peaks between ages 2 and 3 and is rare after age 8.*

Primary nephrotic syndrome is more common in boys than in girls; incidence ranges from 2 to 5 per 100,000 children under 16 years of age per year. Some forms of nephrotic syndrome may eventually progress to end-stage renal failure.

Causes

◆ Allergic reactions
◆ Circulatory diseases, such as heart failure, sickle cell anemia, and renal vein thrombosis
◆ Collagen-vascular disorders, such as systemic lupus erythematosus and periarteritis nodosa
◆ Focal glomerulosclerosis
◆ Hereditary nephritis
◆ Infections, such as tuberculosis and enteritis
◆ Lipid nephrosis (nil lesions)

AGE ALERT *Lipid nephrosis is the main cause of nephrotic syndrome in children younger than age 8.*
◆ Membranoproliferative glomerulonephritis
◆ Membranous glomerulonephritis

AGE ALERT *Membranous glomerulonephritis is the most common lesion in adult idiopathic nephrotic syndrome.*

◆ Metabolic diseases such as diabetes mellitus
◆ Neoplastic diseases such as multiple myeloma
◆ Nephrotoxins such as mercury, gold, and bismuth
◆ Pregnancy

Pathophysiology

In lipid nephrosis, the glomeruli appear normal by light microscopy, and some tubules may contain increased lipid deposits. Membranous glomerulonephritis is characterized by the appearance of immune complexes, seen as dense deposits in the glomerular basement membrane, and by the uniform thickening of the basement membrane. It eventually progresses to renal failure.

Focal glomerulosclerosis can develop spontaneously at any age, can occur after kidney transplantation, or may result from heroin injection. Some 10% of children and up to 20% of adults with nephrotic syndrome develop this condition. Lesions initially affect some of the deeper glomeruli, causing hyaline sclerosis. Involvement of the superficial glomeruli occurs later. These lesions usually cause slowly progressive deterioration in renal function, although remission may occur in children.

Membranoproliferative glomerulonephritis causes slowly progressive lesions in the subendothelial region of the basement membrane. This disorder may follow infection, particularly streptococcal infection, and occurs primarily in children and young adults.

Regardless of the cause, the injured glomerular filtration membrane allows the loss of plasma proteins, especially albumin and immunoglobulin. In addition, metabolic, biochemical, or physiochemical disturbances in the glomerular basement membrane result in the loss of negative charge as well as increased permeability to protein. Hypoalbuminemia results not only from urinary loss but also from decreased hepatic synthesis of replacement albumin. Increased plasma concentration and low molecular weight accentuate albumin loss. Hypoalbuminemia stimulates the liver to synthesize lipoprotein, with consequent hyperlipidemia, and clotting factors. Decreased dietary intake, as with anorexia, malnutrition, or concomitant disease, further contributes to a decreased plasma albumin level. Loss of immunoglobulin also increases susceptibility to infections.

Extensive proteinuria (more than 3.5 g/day) and a low serum albumin level, secondary to renal loss, lead to low serum colloid osmotic pressure and edema. The low serum albumin level also leads to hypovolemia and compensatory salt and water retention. Consequent hypertension may precipitate heart failure in compromised patients.

Signs and symptoms

◆ Periorbital edema, due to fluid overload (generally occurs in the morning)
◆ Mild to severe dependent edema of the ankles or sacrum resulting from fluid overload
◆ Orthostatic hypotension due to fluid imbalance
◆ Hypertension related to fluid overload (in 30% of patients)
◆ Ascites due to fluid imbalance
◆ Swollen external genitalia due to edema in dependent areas
◆ Respiratory difficulty due to pleural effusion
◆ Anorexia due to edema of intestinal mucosa
◆ Pallor and shiny skin with prominent veins due to edema
◆ Diarrhea due to edema of intestinal mucosa
◆ Frothy urine in children due to proteinuria
◆ Change in quality of hair related to protein deficiency
◆ Pneumonia due to susceptibility to infections

Complications

◆ Malnutrition
◆ Infection
◆ Coagulation disorders
◆ Thromboembolic vascular occlusion (especially in the lungs and legs)
◆ Accelerated atherosclerosis
◆ Hypochromic anemia, due to excessive urinary excretion of transferrin
◆ Acute renal failure

Diagnosis

◆ Consistent heavy proteinuria (24-hour protein more than 3.5 mg/dl)
◆ Urinalysis showing hyaline, granular and waxy fatty casts, and oval fat bodies
◆ Increased serum cholesterol, phospholipid (especially low-density and very-low-density lipoproteins), and triglyceride levels, and a decreased albumin level
◆ Renal biopsy for histologic identification of the lesion

Treatment

◆ Correction of underlying cause, if possible
◆ Nutritious diet, including 0.6 g of protein per kilogram of body weight
◆ Restricted sodium intake, to reduce edema
◆ A diuretic, to diminish edema
◆ An antibiotic, to treat infection

- An 8-week course of a corticosteroid, such as prednisone (Deltasone), followed by maintenance therapy or a combination of prednisone and azathioprine (Imuran) or cyclophosphamide (Cytoxan)
- Treatment of hyperlipidemia (usually unsuccessful)
- Paracentesis for ascites
- Thorocentesis for pleural effusion

Special considerations

Patient care includes identification and treatment of underlying cause accompanied by supportive care during treatment.
- Frequently check urine protein. (Urine containing protein appears frothy.)
- Measure blood pressure while the patient is in a supine position and while he's standing; immediately report a drop in blood pressure that exceeds 20 mm Hg.
- Monitor and document location and degree of edema.
- After kidney biopsy, watch for bleeding and shock.
- Monitor intake and output and check weight at the same time each morning—after the patient voids and before he eats—and while he's wearing the same kind of clothing. Ask the dietitian to plan a moderate-protein, low-sodium diet.
- Provide good skin care because the patient with nephrotic syndrome usually has edema.
- To avoid thrombophlebitis, encourage activity and exercise, and provide antiembolism stockings as ordered.
- Encourage normal activity, but limit exposure to those with respiratory infections to reduce the risk of exacerbations.

⚠ **CLINICAL ALERT** *Watch for and teach the patient and family how to recognize adverse drug reactions, such as bone marrow toxicity from cytotoxic immunosuppressants and cushingoid signs and symptoms (muscle weakness, mental changes, acne, moon face, hirsutism, girdle obesity, purple striae, amenorrhea) from long-term steroid therapy. Other steroid complications include masked infections, increased susceptibility to infections, ulcers, GI bleeding, and steroid-induced diabetes; a steroid crisis may occur if the drug is discontinued abruptly. To prevent GI complications, administer the steroid with an antacid or with cimetidine or ranitidine. Explain that steroid adverse effects will subside when therapy stops.*
- Offer the patient and his family reassurance and support, especially during the acute phase, when edema is severe and the patient's body image changes.

NEUROGENIC BLADDER

All types of bladder dysfunction caused by an interruption of normal bladder innervation by the nervous system are referred to as neurogenic bladder. Other names for this disorder include *neuromuscular dysfunction of the lower urinary tract, neurologic bladder dysfunction,* and *neuropathic bladder.* Neurogenic bladder can be hyperreflexic (hypertonic, spastic, or automatic) or flaccid (hypotonic, atonic, or autonomous).

Causes

Many factors can interrupt bladder innervation. Cerebral disorders causing neurogenic bladder include:
- brain tumor (meningioma and glioma)
- dementia
- diabetes mellitus
- incontinence associated with aging
- multiple sclerosis
- Parkinson's disease
- stroke.
  Spinal cord disease or trauma can also cause neurogenic bladder, including:
- arachnoiditis (inflammation of the membrane between the dura mater and the pia mater) causing adhesions between membranes covering the cord
- cervical spondylosis
- disorders of peripheral innervation, including autonomic neuropathies, due to endocrine disturbances, such as diabetes mellitus (most common)
- myelopathies from hereditary or nutritional deficiencies
- poliomyelitis
- spina bifida
- spinal stenosis causing cord compression
- tabes dorsalis (degeneration of the dorsal columns of the spinal cord).
  Other causes include:
- acute infectious diseases, such as Guillain-Barré syndrome or transverse myelitis (pathologic changes extending across the spinal cord)
- chronic alcoholism
- collagen diseases such as systemic lupus erythematosus
- distant effects of certain cancers such as primary oat cell carcinoma of the lung
- heavy metal toxicity
- herpes zoster
- metabolic disturbances, such as hypothyroidism or uremia
- sacral agenesis (absence of a completely formed sacrum)
- vascular diseases such as atherosclerosis.

Types of neurogenic bladder

Neural lesion	Type	Cause
Upper motor	Uninhibited	◆ Lack of voluntary control in infancy ◆ Multiple sclerosis
	Reflex or automatic	◆ Spinal cord transection ◆ Cord tumors ◆ Multiple sclerosis
Lower motor	Autonomous	◆ Sacral cord trauma ◆ Tumors ◆ Herniated disk ◆ Abdominal surgery with transection of pelvic parasympathetic nerves
	Motor paralysis	◆ Lesions at levels S2, S3, S4 ◆ Poliomyelitis ◆ Trauma ◆ Tumors
	Sensory paralysis	◆ Posterior lumbar nerve roots ◆ Diabetes mellitus ◆ Tabes dorsalis

Pathophysiology

An upper motor neuron lesion (at or above T12) causes spastic neurogenic bladder, with spontaneous contractions of detrusor muscles, increased intravesical voiding pressure, bladder wall hypertrophy with trabeculation, and urinary sphincter spasms. The patient may experience small urine volume, incomplete emptying, and loss of voluntary control of voiding. Urine retention also sets the stage for infection.

A lower motor neuron lesion (at or below S2 to S4) affects the spinal reflex that controls micturition. The result is a flaccid neurogenic bladder with decreased intravesical pressure, and increased bladder capacity, residual urine retention, and poor detrusor contraction. The bladder may not empty spontaneously. The patient experiences loss of voluntary and involuntary control of urination. Lower motor neuron lesions lead to overflow incontinence. When sensory neurons are interrupted, the patient can't perceive the need to void.

Interruption of the efferent nerves at the cortical, or upper motor neuron, level results in loss of voluntary control. Higher centers also control micturition, and voiding may be incomplete. Sensory neuron interruption leads to dribbling and overflow incontinence. (See *Types of neurogenic bladder*.) Altered bladder sensation often makes symptoms difficult to discern.

Urine retention contributes to renal calculi as well as infection. Neurogenic bladder can lead to deterioration of renal function if not promptly diagnosed and treated.

Signs and symptoms

◆ Some degree of incontinence, changes in initiation or interruption of micturition, inability to completely empty the bladder caused by interrupted nerve impulse transmission
◆ Frequent urinary tract infections (UTIs) due to urine retention
◆ Hyperactive autonomic reflexes (autonomic dysreflexia) when the bladder is distended and the lesion is at upper thoracic or cervical level
◆ Severe hypertension, bradycardia, and vasodilation (blotchy skin) above the level of the lesion
◆ Piloerection and profuse sweating above the level of the lesion
◆ Involuntary or frequent, scant urination without a feeling of bladder fullness due to hyperreflexic neurogenic bladder
◆ Spontaneous spasms (caused by voiding) of the arms and legs due to hyperreflexic neurogenic bladder
◆ Increased anal sphincter tone due to hyperreflexic neurogenic bladder
◆ Voiding and spontaneous contractions of the arms and legs due to tactile stimulation of the abdomen, thighs, or genitalia

◆ Overflow incontinence and diminished anal sphincter tone due to flaccid neurogenic bladder
◆ Greatly distended bladder without feeling of bladder fullness due to sensory impairment

Complications
◆ Incontinence
◆ Residual urine retention
◆ UTI
◆ Calculi formation
◆ Renal failure

Diagnosis
◆ Voiding cystourethrography, to evaluate bladder neck function, vesicoureteral reflux, and continence
◆ Urodynamic studies, to evaluate how urine is stored in the bladder, how well the bladder empties urine, and how quickly urine flows from the bladder during voiding
◆ Urine flow study (uroflow), to show diminished or impaired urine flow
◆ Cystometry, to evaluate bladder nerve supply, detrusor muscle tone, and intravesical pressures during bladder filling and contraction
◆ Urethral pressure profile, to determine urethral function with respect to the urethra's length and outlet pressure resistance
◆ Sphincter electromyelography, to correlate neuromuscular function of the external sphincter with bladder muscle function during bladder filling and contraction, and to evaluate how well the bladder and urinary sphincter muscles work together
◆ Videourodynamic studies, to correlate visual documentation of bladder function with pressure studies
◆ Retrograde urethrography, to show strictures and diverticula

Treatment
◆ Intermittent self-catheterization, to empty the bladder
◆ An alpha-anticholinergic and an adrenergic stimulator for the patient with hyperreflexic neurogenic bladder, until intermittent self-catheterization is performed
◆ Terazosin (Hytrin) and doxazosin (Cardura), to facilitate bladder emptying in neurogenic bladder
◆ Propantheline (Pro-Banthine), methantheline, flavoxate (Urispas), dicyclomine (Bentyl), imipramine (Tofranil), amitriptyline (Elavil), and pseudoephedrine (Sudafed), to facilitate urine storage
◆ Darifenacin (Enablex) and solifenacin succinate (VESIcare) to reduce bladder smooth-muscle contractions

◆ Oxybutynin chloride (Ditropan) and tolterodine L-tartrate (Detrol) to reduce symptoms of overactive or irritable bladder
◆ Surgery, to correct structural impairment through transurethral resection of the bladder neck, urethral dilation, external sphincterotomy, or urinary diversion procedures
◆ Implantation of an artificial urinary sphincter may be necessary if permanent incontinence follows surgery

Special considerations
Care for patients with neurogenic bladder varies according to the underlying cause and the treatment method.
◆ Explain diagnostic tests clearly so the patient understands the procedure, the time involved, and the possible results. Assure the patient that the lengthy diagnostic process is necessary to identify the most effective treatment plan. After the treatment plan is chosen, explain it to the patient in detail.
◆ Use strict sterile technique during insertion of an indwelling catheter (a temporary measure to drain the incontinent patient's bladder). Don't interrupt the closed drainage system for any reason. Obtain urine specimens with a syringe and small-bore needle inserted through the aspirating port of the catheter itself (below the junction of the balloon instillation site). Irrigate in the same manner if ordered.
◆ Clean the catheter insertion site with soap and water at least twice per day. Don't allow the catheter to become encrusted. Use a sterile applicator to apply antibiotic ointment around the meatus after catheter care. Keep the drainage bag below the tubing, and don't raise the bag above the level of the bladder. Clamp the tubing or empty the bag before transferring the patient to a wheelchair or stretcher to prevent accidental urine reflux. If urine output is considerable, empty the bag more frequently than once every 8 hours because bacteria can multiply in standing urine and migrate up the catheter and into the bladder.
◆ Watch for signs of infection (fever, cloudy or foul-smelling urine). Encourage the patient to drink plenty of fluids to prevent calculi formation and infection from urinary stasis. Try to keep the patient as mobile as possible. Perform passive range-of-motion exercises if necessary.
◆ If a urinary diversion procedure is to be performed, arrange for consultation with an enterostomal therapist, and coordinate the care plans.
◆ Tell the patient to avoid spicy foods, citrus fruits and juices, chocolate, and caffeine because they tend to exacerbate symptoms.

◆ Before discharge, teach the patient and his family evacuation techniques, as necessary (Credé's method, intermittent catheterization). Counsel him about sexual activities. Remember, the incontinent patient feels embarrassed and distressed. Provide emotional support.

POLYCYSTIC KIDNEY DISEASE

Polycystic kidney disease is an inherited disorder characterized by multiple, bilateral, grape-like clusters of fluid-filled cysts that enlarge the kidneys, compressing and eventually replacing functioning renal tissue. (See *Polycystic kidney*.) The disease affects males and females equally and appears in two distinct forms. Autosomal dominant polycystic kidney disease (ADPKD) occurs in 1 in 1,000 to 1 in 3,000 people and accounts for about 10% of end-stage renal disease in the United States. The rare infantile form causes stillbirth or early neonatal death. The adult form has an insidious onset but usually becomes obvious between ages 30 and 50; rarely, it remains asymptomatic until the patient is in his 70s.

AGE ALERT *Renal deterioration is more gradual in adults than infants, but in both age-groups the disease progresses relentlessly to fatal uremia.*

The prognosis in adults varies widely. Progression may be slow, even after symptoms of renal insufficiency appear. After uremia symptoms develop, polycystic disease usually is fatal within 4 years, unless the patient receives dialysis. Three genetic variants of the autosomal dominant form have been identified.

Causes

Polycystic kidney disease is inherited as an:
◆ autosomal dominant trait (adult type)
◆ autosomal recessive trait (infantile type).

Pathophysiology

Autosomal recessive polycystic kidney disease occurs in 1 in 1,000 Americans and has been localized to chromosome 6.

Grossly enlarged kidneys are caused by multiple spherical cysts, a few millimeters to centimeters in diameter, that contain straw-colored or hemorrhagic fluid. The cysts are distributed evenly throughout the cortex and medulla. Hyperplastic polyps and renal adenomas are common. Renal parenchyma may have varying degrees of tubular atrophy, interstitial fibrosis, and nephrosclerosis. The cysts cause elongation of the pelvis, flattening of the calyces, and indentations in the kidney.

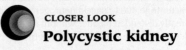

CLOSER LOOK
Polycystic kidney

This cross-sectional drawing shows multiple areas of cystic damage. Each indentation depicts a cyst.

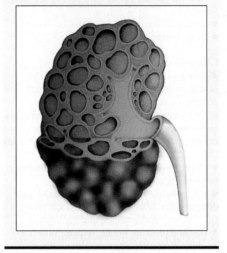

Characteristically, an affected infant shows signs of respiratory distress, heart failure and, eventually, uremia and renal failure. Accompanying hepatic fibrosis and intrahepatic bile duct abnormalities may cause portal hypertension and bleeding varices.

In most cases, about 10 years after symptoms appear, progressive compression of kidney structures by the enlarging mass causes renal failure.

Cysts also form elsewhere—such as on the liver, spleen, pancreas, and ovaries. Intracranial aneurysms, colonic diverticula, and mitral valve prolapse also occur.

In the autosomal recessive form, death in the neonatal period is most commonly due to pulmonary hypoplasia.

Signs and symptoms
In neonates
◆ Pronounced epicanthic folds (vertical fold of skin on either side of the nose); a pointed nose; small chin; and floppy, low-set ears (Potter facies), due to genetic abnormalities
◆ Huge, bilateral, symmetrical masses on the flanks that are tense and can't be transilluminated, due to kidney enlargement
◆ Respiratory distress related to impaired renal function and fluid imbalance
◆ Uremia, due to renal failure

In adults
◆ Hypertension, due to activation of the renin-angiotensin system
◆ Lumbar pain, due to enlarging kidney mass
◆ Widening abdominal girth, due to enlarged kidneys
◆ Swollen or tender abdomen caused by the enlarging kidney mass, worsened by exertion and relieved by lying down
◆ Grossly enlarged kidneys on palpation

Complications
AGE ALERT *A few infants with polycystic kidney disease survive for 2 years, and then die of hepatic complications or renal, heart, or respiratory failure.*
◆ Pyelonephritis
◆ Recurrent hematuria
◆ Life-threatening retroperitoneal bleeding from cyst rupture
◆ Proteinuria
◆ Colicky abdominal pain from ureteral passage of clots or calculi
◆ Renal failure

Diagnosis
◆ Excretory or retrograde urography showing enlarged kidneys, with elongation of the pelvis, flattening of the calyces, and indentations in the kidney caused by cysts
◆ Excretory urography of the neonate showing poor excretion of contrast medium
◆ Ultrasonography, tomography, and radioisotope scans showing kidney enlargement and cysts; tomography, computed tomography, and magnetic resonance imaging showing multiple areas of cystic damage
◆ Urinalysis and creatinine clearance tests showing nonspecific results indicating abnormalities

Treatment
◆ An antibiotic for infections
◆ Angiotensin-converting enzyme inhibitors or angiotensin II receptor antagonists for hypertension (calcium channel blockers aren't recommended)
◆ Lanthanum carbonate (Fosrenol) and sevelamer hydrochloride (Renagel) to reduce high phosphorus levels
◆ Adequate hydration to maintain fluid balance
◆ Surgical drainage of cystic abscess or retroperitoneal bleeding
◆ Surgery for intractable pain (uncommon symptom) or an analgesic for abdominal pain
◆ Dialysis or kidney transplantation for progressive renal failure
◆ Nephrectomy not recommended (polycystic kidney disease occurs bilaterally, and the infection could recur in the remaining kidney)

Special considerations
Because polycystic kidney disease is usually relentlessly progressive, comprehensive patient teaching and emotional support are essential.
◆ Refer the young adult patient or the parents of infants with polycystic kidney disease for genetic counseling. Parents will probably have many questions about the risk to other offspring.
◆ Provide supportive care to minimize any associated symptoms. Carefully assess the patient's lifestyle and his physical and mental status; determine how rapidly the disease is progressing. Use this information to plan individualized patient care.
◆ Acquaint yourself with all aspects of end-stage renal disease, including dialysis and transplantation, so you can provide appropriate care and patient teaching as the disease progresses.
◆ Explain all diagnostic procedures to the patient or to his family if the patient is an infant. Before beginning excretory urography or other procedures that use an iodine-based contrast medium, determine whether the patient has ever had an allergic reaction to iodine or shellfish. Even if the patient has no history of allergy, watch him for an allergic reaction during and after undergoing the procedures.
◆ Administer an antibiotic, as ordered, for urinary tract infection. Stress to the patient the need to take the medication exactly as prescribed, even if symptoms are minimal or absent.

RENAL CALCULI
Renal calculi, or stones (nephrolithiasis), can form anywhere in the urinary tract, although they most commonly develop on the renal pelves or calyces. They may vary in size and may be solitary or multiple. (See *Understanding renal calculi,* page 536.)

Renal calculi are more common in men than in women and rarely occur in children. Calcium calculi generally occur in middle-aged men with a family history of calculi formation.

Renal calculi rarely occur in blacks. They're prevalent in certain geographic areas, such as the southeastern United States (called the Stone Belt), possibly because a hot climate promotes dehydration and concentrates calculi-forming substances, or because of regional dietary habits.

Understanding renal calculi

Renal calculi vary in size and type. Small calculi may remain in the renal pelvis or pass down the ureter. A staghorn calculus (a cast of the calyceal and pelvic collecting system) may develop from a calculus that stays in the kidney.

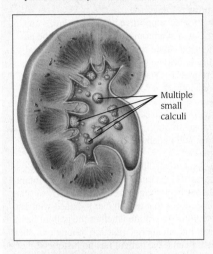

Multiple small calculi

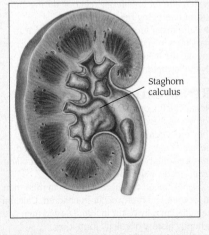

Staghorn calculus

Causes

Although the exact cause is unknown, predisposing factors of renal calculi include:
♦ changes in urine pH (calcium carbonate calculi, high pH; uric acid calculi, lower pH)
♦ dehydration
♦ dietary factors

♦ gout (a disease of increased uric acid production or decreased excretion)
♦ immobilization causing calcium to be released into the blood, which is filtered by the kidneys
♦ infection
♦ metabolic factors
♦ obstruction to urine flow leading to stasis in the urinary tract
♦ renal disease.

Pathophysiology

The major types of renal calculi are calcium oxalate and calcium phosphate, accounting for 75% to 80% of calculi; struvite (magnesium, ammonium, and phosphate), 15%; and uric acid, 7%. Cystine calculi are relatively rare, making up 1% of all renal calculi.

Calculi form when substances that are normally dissolved in the urine, such as calcium oxalate and calcium phosphate, precipitate. Dehydration may lead to renal calculi as calculi-forming substances concentrate in urine.

Calculi form around a nucleus or nidus in the appropriate environment. A crystal evolves in the presence of calculus-forming substances (calcium oxalate, calcium carbonate, magnesium, ammonium, phosphate, or uric acid) and becomes trapped in the urinary tract, where it attracts other crystals to form a calculus. A high urine saturation of these substances encourages crystal formation and results in calculus growth.

Calculi may be composed of different substances, and the pH of the urine affects the solubility of many calculi-forming substances. Formation of calcium oxalate and cystine calculi is independent of urine pH.

Calculi may occur on the papillae, renal tubules, calyces, renal pelves, ureter, or bladder. Many calculi are less than 5 mm in diameter and are usually passed in the urine. Staghorn calculi can continue to grow in the pelvis, extending to the calyces, forming a branching calculus, and ultimately resulting in renal failure if not surgically removed.

Calcium calculi are the smallest. Most are calcium oxalate or a combination of oxalate and phosphate. Although 80% are idiopathic, they commonly occur with hyperuricosuria (a high level of uric acid in the urine). Prolonged immobilization can lead to bone demineralization, hypercalciuria, and calculi formation. In addition, hyperparathyroidism, renal tubular acidosis, and excessive intake of vitamin D or dietary calcium may predispose to renal calculi.

Struvite calculi are typically precipitated by an infection, particularly with *Pseudomonas* or *Proteus* species. These urea-splitting organisms are more common in women. Struvite calculi can destroy renal parenchyma.

Gout results in a high uric acid production, hyperuricosuria, and uric acid calculi. Diets high in purine (such as meat, fish, and poultry) elevate the level of uric acid in the body. Regional enteritis and ulcerative colitis can precipitate the formation of uric acid calculi. These diseases commonly result in fluid loss and loss of bicarbonate, leading to metabolic acidosis. Acidic urine enhances the formation of uric acid calculi.

Cystinuria is a rare hereditary disorder in which a metabolic error causes decreased tubular reabsorption of cystine. This causes an increased amount of cystine in the urine. Because cystine is a relatively insoluble substance, its presence contributes to calculi formation.

Infected, scarred tissue may be an ideal site for calculi development. In addition, infected calculi (usually magnesium ammonium phosphate or staghorn calculi) may develop if bacteria serve as the nucleus in calculi formation.

Urinary stasis allows calculi constituents to collect and adhere and encourages infection, which compounds the obstruction.

Calculi may either enter the ureter or remain in the renal pelvis, where they damage or destroy renal parenchyma and may cause pressure necrosis.

In ureters, calculi cause obstruction with resulting hydronephrosis and tend to recur. Intractable pain and serious bleeding also can result from calculi and the damage they cause. Large, rough calculi occlude the opening to the ureteropelvic junction and increase the frequency and force of peristaltic contractions, causing hematuria from trauma. The patient usually reports pain traveling from the costovertebral angle to the flank and then to the suprapubic region and external genitalia (classic renal colic pain). Pain intensity fluctuates and may be excruciating at its peak. The patient with calculi in the renal pelvis and calyces may report a constant dull pain. He may also report back pain if calculi are causing obstruction within a kidney and severe abdominal pain from calculi traveling down a ureter. Infection can develop in static urine or after trauma as the calculus abrades surfaces. If the calculi lodge and block urine, hydronephrosis can occur.

Signs and symptoms
◆ Pain resulting from obstruction (may be mild to severe, deep flank pain or tenderness; or abrupt, severe colicky flank pain)
◆ Nausea and vomiting
◆ Fever and chills from infection
◆ Hematuria when calculi abrade a ureter
◆ Urinary hesitancy and dysuria due to obstruction
◆ Abdominal distention
◆ Anuria from bilateral obstruction, or obstruction of a patient's only kidney

Complications
◆ Damage or destruction of renal parenchyma
◆ Pressure necrosis
◆ Obstruction by the calculus
◆ Hydronephrosis
◆ Bleeding
◆ Pain
◆ Infection

Diagnosis
◆ Kidney-ureter-bladder (KUB) radiography or computed tomography scan of the kidneys to show most renal calculi
◆ For pregnant women, magnetic resonance imaging to diagnose calculi because it doesn't use radiation
◆ Excretory urography, to help confirm the diagnosis and determine the size and location of calculi
◆ Kidney ultrasonography, to detect obstructive changes, such as unilateral or bilateral hydronephrosis and radiolucent calculi not seen on KUB radiography
◆ Urinalysis showing pyuria, a sign of urinary tract infection; and to determine urine pH
◆ Urine culture to detect causative organism, if indicated
◆ 24-hour urine collection, for calcium oxalate, phosphorus, and uric acid excretion levels
◆ Calculi analysis, for mineral content
◆ Serial blood calcium and phosphorus levels, to diagnose hyperparathyroidism and increased calcium, relative to normal serum protein
◆ Blood protein levels, to determine the level of free calcium unbound to protein

Treatment
◆ Increasing fluid intake to more than 3 qt (3 L)/day to promote hydration
◆ An antimicrobial to treat infection, varying with the cultured organism
◆ An analgesic, such as morphine or ketorolac (Toradol), for pain

◆ Oral alpha blockers and calcium channel blockers in combination with oral steroids to increase the rate and decrease the time for spontaneous stone passage
◆ An antiemetic for nausea and vomiting
◆ An antibiotic to treat infection (if present)
◆ A diuretic to prevent urinary stasis and further calculi formation; a thiazide to decrease calcium excretion into the urine
◆ Methenamine to suppress calculi formation when infection is present
◆ Low-calcium diet to prevent recurrence
◆ Oxalate-binding cholestyramine for absorptive hypercalciuria
◆ Parathyroidectomy for hyperparathyroidism
◆ Allopurinol (Zyloprim) for uric acid calculi
◆ Daily small doses of ascorbic acid to acidify urine
◆ Cystoscope with manipulation of the calculi to remove any that are too large for natural passage
◆ Percutaneous ultrasonic lithotripsy and extracorporeal shock wave lithotripsy or laser therapy to shatter calculi into fragments for removal by suction or natural passage
◆ Surgical removal of cystine calculi or large calculi or placement of urinary diversion around the calculus to relieve obstruction

Special considerations

Patient care includes confirming the diagnosis, facilitating passage of calculi, and helping to prevent future occurrences. (See *Preventing renal calculi.*)

◆ To aid diagnosis, maintain a 24- to 48-hour record of urine pH, with nitrazine pH paper; strain all urine through gauze or a tea strainer, and save all solid material recovered for analysis.
◆ To facilitate spontaneous passage of calculi, encourage the patient to walk, if possible. Also, promote sufficient intake of fluids to maintain a urine output of 2 to 4 L/day (urine should be very dilute and colorless). To help acidify urine, offer fruit juices, particularly cranberry juice. If the patient can't drink the required amount of fluid, supplemental I.V. fluids may be given. Record intake and output and daily weight to assess fluid status and renal function.
◆ Stress the importance of proper diet and compliance with drug therapy. For example, if the patient's calculi are caused by a hyperuricemic condition, advise the patient or whoever prepares his meals which foods are high in purine.

◆ If surgery is necessary, give reassurance by supplementing and reinforcing what the surgeon has told the patient about the procedure. The patient is apt to be fearful, especially if surgery includes removal of a kidney, so emphasize the fact that the body can adapt well to one kidney. If he needs to have an abdominal or flank incision, teach deep-breathing and coughing exercises.
◆ After surgery, the patient will probably have an indwelling catheter or a nephrostomy tube. Unless one of his kidneys was removed, expect bloody drainage from the catheter. Never irrigate the catheter without a physician's order. Check dressings regularly for bloody drainage, and know how much drainage to expect. Immediately report suspected hemorrhage (excessive drainage, rising pulse rate). Use sterile technique when changing dressings or providing catheter care.
◆ Watch for signs and symptoms of infection (rising fever, chills), and give an antibiotic as ordered. To prevent pneumonia, encourage frequent position changes, and ambulate the patient as soon as possible. Have him hold a small pillow over the incision site to splint it and thereby facilitate deep-breathing and coughing exercises.
◆ Before discharge, teach the patient and his family the importance of following the prescribed dietary and medication regimens to prevent recurrence of calculi. Encourage increased fluid intake. If appropriate, show the patient how to check his urine pH, and instruct him to keep a daily record. Tell him to immediately report symptoms of acute obstruction (pain, inability to void).

RENOVASCULAR HYPERTENSION

Renovascular hypertension occurs when systemic blood pressure increases because of stenosis of the major renal arteries or their branches, or because of intrarenal atherosclerosis. This narrowing (*sclerosis*) may be partial or complete, and the resulting blood pressure elevation may be benign or malignant. Renovascular hypertension is the most common type of secondary hypertension.

Causes

In about 95% of patients, renovascular hypertension results from either atherosclerosis (especially in older men) or fibromuscular diseases of the renal artery wall layers (for example, medial fibroplasia and, less commonly, intimal and

PREVENTION

Preventing renal calculi

The formation of kidney stones may be prevented by making certain lifestyle changes. If these lifestyles changes don't help in the prevention of kidney stone formation, drugs are needed. Advise your patient to make these changes.

Maintain hydration
The most important lifestyle change is drinking plenty of fluids, especially water. An adult needs to drink at least 3½ quarts per day. Drinking plenty of fluids helps to flush out the kidneys.

Adjust diet
For a patient who tends to form calcium and oxalate stones, suggest an oxalate-restricted diet. Foods that are high in oxalate should be avoided. These foods include rhubarb, star fruit, beets, beet greens, collards, okra, refried beans, spinach, swiss chard, sweet potatoes, sesame seeds, almonds, and soy products. Restricting calcium in the diet doesn't seem to reduce the risk of kidney stones. Diets high in calcium actually help reduce the risk of oxalate stone formation. Calcium binds with oxalate so it can't be absorbed in the gastrointestinal tract and excreted by the kidneys.

All patients who form kidney stones should be on low-sodium diets. Sodium intake should be restricted to 3 to 4 grams of sodium per day. Also, diets very low in animal proteins may help reduce the risk of stones.

Take prescribed drugs
Drugs can be helpful in preventing stone formation. The drugs prescribed depend on the type of stone. Some stones, such as calcium stones, develop more easily in more alkaline environments, and some stones, such as uric acid stones, develop in an acid environment. Patients with struvite stones are treated with antibiotics to prevent infection. Cystine stones are the hardest to treat, and they're treated with a urine alkalinizer and chelator (D-Penicillamine and Thiola).

---

subadventitial fibroplasia). Other causes may include:
- anomalies of the renal arteries
- arteritis
- dissecting aneurysm
- embolism
- trauma
- tumor.

Pathophysiology
Stenosis or a renal artery occlusion stimulates the affected kidney to release renin, an enzyme that converts angiotensinogen (a plasma protein) to angiotensin I. As angiotensin I circulates through the lungs and liver, it converts to angiotensin II, which causes peripheral vasoconstriction, increased arterial pressure and aldosterone secretion and, eventually, hypertension. (See *What happens in renovascular hypertension,* page 540.)

Signs and symptoms
- Onset of hypertension in patients under age 30 without risk factors
- Abrupt onset of severe hypertension (greater than 160/100 mm Hg) patients over age 55
- Flank pain, systolic bruit over the epigastric vein in the upper abdomen, and reduced urine output due to reduced blood flow to the kidneys
- Headache, nausea, anorexia, anxiety, and hypertension due to the vasoconstricting effects of angiotensin II
- Alterations in the patient's level of consciousness and pitting edema if renal failure occurs

Complications
- Heart failure
- Myocardial infarction
- Stroke
- Renal failure

Diagnosis
- Isotopic renal blood flow scan and rapid-sequence excretory urography to identify renal blood flow abnormalities and discrepancies of kidney size and shape
- Renal arteriography to reveal the actual arterial stenosis or obstruction
- Magnetic resonance angiography to detect main renal artery stenosis of greater than 50%
- Plasma renin activity level to identify increased plasma renin levels
- Captopril test to differentiate renovascular hypertension from essential hypertension

CLOSER LOOK

What happens in renovascular hypertension

The kidneys normally play a key role in maintaining blood pressure and volume by vasoconstriction and regulation of sodium and fluid levels. In renovascular hypertension, these regulatory mechanisms fail.

Certain conditions, such as renal artery stenosis and tumors, reduce blood flow to the kidneys. This causes juxtaglomerular cells to continuously secrete renin.

In this stage, be alert for flank pain, systolic bruit in the epigastric vein over the upper abdomen, reduced urine output, and an elevated renin level.

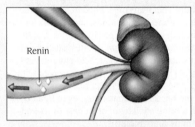

In the liver, renin and angiotensinogen combine to form angiotensin I, which converts to angiotensin II in the lungs. This potent vasoconstrictor heightens peripheral resistance and blood pressure.

Check for headache, nausea, anorexia, an elevated renin level, and hypertension.

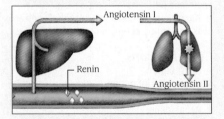

Angiotensin II acts directly on the kidneys, causing them to reabsorb sodium and water.

Assess for hypertension, diminished urine output, albuminuria, hypokalemia, and hypernatremia.

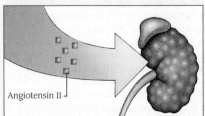

Angiotensin II stimulates the adrenal cortex to secrete aldosterone. This also causes the kidneys to retain sodium and water, elevating blood volume and pressure.

Expect worsening symptoms.

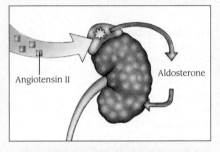

Intermittent pressure diuresis causes excretion of sodium and water, reduced blood volume, and decreasing cardiac output.

Check for blood pressure that increases slowly, drops (but not as low as before), and then increases again. Headache, high urine specific gravity, hyponatremia, fatigue, and heart failure also occur.

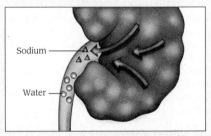

A high aldosterone level causes further sodium retention, but it can't curtail renin secretion. Excessive aldosterone and angiotensin II can damage renal tissue, leading to renal failure. Expect to find hypertension, pitting edema, anemia, decreased level of consciousness, and elevated blood urea nitrogen and serum creatinine levels.

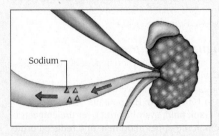

◆ Renal vein renin measurements to compare renin release from each kidney and to predict the potential success of surgical revascularization

Treatment
◆ Medications to control blood pressure, the most effective of which are angiotensin-converting enzyme inhibitors, which minimize the ischemia-induced increase in angiotensin production; other medications include beta-adrenergic blockers, calcium channel blockers, angiotensin receptor blockers, alpha blockers, and direct rennin inhibitors.
◆ Percutaneous transluminal renal angioplasty to open stenotic renal arteries; intravascular stents may be placed during angioplasty to prevent restenosis
◆ Surgical revascularization procedures to restore adequate renal circulation, control severe hypertension, and improve severely impaired renal function

Special considerations
◆ Prepare the patient for diagnostic tests. For example, adequately hydrate him before tests that use a contrast medium, and make sure he isn't allergic to the medium used. Watch for complications after excretory urography or arteriography.
◆ Accurately monitor and record intake and output and daily weight. Weigh the patient at the same time each day (before a meal) and when he's wearing the same amount of clothing.
◆ Frequently assess urine specific gravity, blood urea nitrogen, serum creatinine, and protein levels.
◆ Check blood pressure in both arms regularly, with the patient lying down and standing. A drop of 20 mm Hg or more in either systolic or diastolic pressure on arising may necessitate that the dosage of his antihypertensive be adjusted.
◆ Administer drugs as ordered. Adequately medicate the patient for pain to decrease anxiety and increase comfort.
◆ Maintain fluid and sodium restrictions.
◆ If the patient is anorexic, offer appetizing, high-calorie meals to ensure adequate nutrition.
◆ Encourage cardiovascular fitness, and work with the physician and patient to develop a beneficial program.
◆ Encourage the patient to perform stress-relieving exercises.

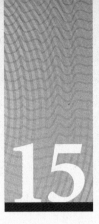

SENSORY SYSTEM

Through the sensory system, a person receives stimuli that facilitate interaction with the surrounding world. Afferent pathways connect specialized sensory receptors in the eyes, ears, nose, and mouth to the brain — the final station for continuous processing of sensory stimuli. Alterations in sensory function may lead to dysfunctions of sight and hearing as well as smell, taste, balance, and coordination.

Pathophysiologic changes

Alterations can occur in sight, hearing, smell, taste, balance, and coordination.

VISION

Disorders of vision include alterations in ocular movement, visual acuity, accommodation, refraction, and color vision.

Ocular movement

The eyes constantly move to keep objects being viewed on the fovea, which is a small area of the retina that contains only cones and is responsible for the best peripheral visual acuity. The six extraocular muscles that move each eye are innervated by the oculomotor (III), trochlear (IV), and abducens (VI) cranial nerves. Alterations in ocular movement include strabismus, diplopia, and nystagmus.

Strabismus

Strabismus occurs when one eye deviates from its normal position due to the absence of normal, parallel, or coordinated movement. The eyes may have an uncoordinated appearance, and the person may experience diplopia.

In children, types of strabismus are:
◆ *concomitant* (or *nonparalytic*), in which the degree of deviation doesn't vary with the direction of gaze
◆ *nonconcomitant* (or *paralytic*), in which the degree of deviation varies with the direction of gaze
◆ *congenital* (present at birth or during the first 6 months)
◆ *acquired* (present during the first 2½ years)
◆ *latent* (phoria; apparent only when the child is tired or sick)
◆ *constant.*

Tropia, or constant strabismus, is divided into four categories: esotropia (inward deviation), exotropia (outward deviation), hypertropia (upward deviation), and hypotropia (downward deviation).

Strabismic amblyopia, lazy eye, is characterized by the loss of central vision in one eye; it typically results in esotropia (due to fixation in the dominant eye and suppression of images in the deviating eye). Strabismic amblyopia may result from hyperopia (farsightedness) or anisometropia (unequal refractive power).

Esotropia may result from muscle imbalance and may be congenital or acquired. In accommodative esotropia, the child's attempt to compensate for the farsightedness affects the convergent reflex, and the eyes cross.

Strabismus is usually inherited, but its cause is unknown. In adults, strabismus may result from trauma. The incidence of strabismus is higher in patients with central nervous system disorders, such as cerebral palsy, mental retardation, and Down syndrome.

Muscle imbalances may be corrected by glasses, patching, or surgery, depending on the cause. However, residual defects in vision and extraocular muscle alignment may persist even after treatment.

AGE ALERT *Without early intervention, children with strabismus may develop amblyopia as a result of cerebral suppression of visual stimuli. Deviation of an eye is the second most common symptom in a child with retinoblastoma. Therefore, acquired strabismus should always be checked.*

Diplopia

Diplopia, or double vision, results when the extraocular muscles fail to work together and images fall on noncorresponding parts of the retinas. Diplopia usually begins intermittently or affects near or far vision exclusively. It can be classified as monocular (persisting when one eye is covered) or, more commonly, binocular (clearing when one eye is covered). Monocular diplopia may result from an early cataract, retinal edema or scarring, subluxated lens (partial dislocation of the lens of the eye), poorly fitting contact lens, or uncorrected refractive error. Binocular diplopia may result from ocular deviation or displacement, extraocular muscle palsies, or psychoneurosis, or after retinal surgery. Other causes of binocular diplopia include infection, neoplastic disease, metabolic disorders, degenerative disease, inflammatory disorders, and vascular disease.

Nystagmus

Nystagmus refers to involuntary oscillations or alternating movements of one or both eyes. These oscillations are usually rhythmic and may be horizontal, vertical, rotary, or mixed. They may be transient or sustained and may occur spontaneously or on deviation or fixation. Nystagmus may be classified as pendular (oscillations are equal in rate in both directions) or jerk (faster movements in one direction than in the opposite direction). Nystagmoid movements usually have a fast and a slow component. The direction of the nystagmus is given by the fast component. (See *Classifying nystagmus,* page 544.)

Nystagmus is a supranuclear ocular palsy resulting from pathology in the visual perceptual area, vestibular system, or cerebellum. Causes of nystagmus include brain stem or cerebellar lesions, labyrinthine disease, stroke, encephalitis, Ménière's disease, multiple sclerosis, trauma, and alcohol and drug toxicity, including

barbiturate, phenytoin (Dilantin), or carbamazepine (Tegretol) toxicity.

AGE ALERT *In children, pendular nystagmus may be idiopathic or may result from early impairment of vision associated with such disorders as optic atrophy, albinism, congenital cataracts, and severe astigmatism.*

Visual acuity

Visual acuity refers to the ability to see clearly. A lack of visual acuity is commonly associated with refractive errors. In nearsightedness, or myopia, the eye focuses the visual image in front of the retina, causing objects in close view to be seen clearly and those at a distance to be blurry. In farsightedness, or hyperopia, the eye focuses the visual image behind the retina, causing objects in close view to be blurry and those at a distance to be clear. Both these problems are caused by an alteration in the shape of the eyeball. Other causes of reduced visual acuity include aging, amblyopia, cataracts, glaucoma, papilledema, dark adaptation, and scotoma (an area of diminished visual acuity surrounded by an area of normal vision within the visual field).

Amblyopia is severely decreased visual acuity or virtual blindness in a structurally intact eye. It occurs when there is interference in the stimulation of the vision-receptive cells in the brain. When normally stimulated, these cells allow for sensory development of visual acuity. Amblyopia is a form of treatable vision loss if recognized early. Causes may include strabismus, congenital cataract, abnormal refractive error, tumor, trauma, or infection.

AGE ALERT *If amblyopia is detected and treated before age 5, cure is almost assured. Treatment begun after age 10 is rarely successful.*

AGE ALERT *With age, the pupil becomes smaller, which decreases the amount of light that reaches the retina. Older adults need about three times as much light as a younger person to see objects clearly.*

Accommodation

Accommodation occurs as the thickness of the eye's lens changes to maintain visual acuity. For near vision, the ciliary body contracts and relaxes the zonules, the lens becomes spherical, the pupil constricts, and the eyes converge. For far vision, the ciliary body relaxes, the zonules tighten, the lens becomes flatter, the eyes straighten, and the pupils dilate. The oculomotor nerve and coordinated brain stem pathways account for accommodation. Alterations in accommodation may be caused by pressure, inflammation, aging, or disorders affecting the

CLOSER LOOK
Classifying nystagmus

Nystagmus is classified as pendular or jerk. Each type has further classifications.

Pendular nystagmus
Oscillating: slow, steady oscillations of equal velocity around a center point; caused by congenital loss of visual acuity or multiple sclerosis.

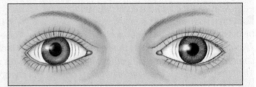

Vertical or seesaw: rapid, seesaw movement in which one eye appears to rise while the other appears to fall; suggests an optic chiasm lesion.

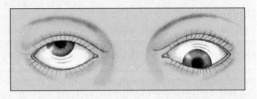

Jerk nystagmus
Convergence-retraction: irregular jerking of the eyes back into the orbit during upward gaze; can reflect midbrain tegmental (roof of the midbrain) damage.

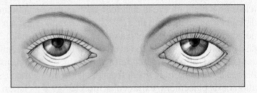

Downbeat: irregular downward jerking of the eyes during downward gaze; can signal lower medullary damage.

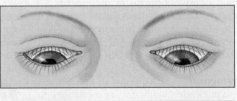

Vestibular: horizontal or rotary movements of the eyes; suggests vestibular disease or cochlear dysfunction.

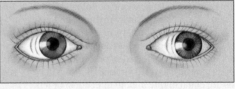

oculomotor nerve. The result of impaired accommodation may be diplopia, blurred vision, or headache.

Refraction

Refraction is the process of bending light rays so that they fall on the retina. As rays of light reach the surface of the cornea from all directions, the cornea directs them toward the lens. The lens further bends the light and directs the light rays to one spot on the retina. The greater the refractive power, the more the light rays are bent. Emmetropia is a condition in which light rays fall exactly on the retina. Alterations in refraction occur when light isn't properly focused. Causes include abnormalities in curvature of the cornea, focusing of the lens, and eye length. Results include myopia, hyperopia, and astigmatism. (See *Refractive errors.*)

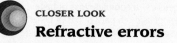

CLOSER LOOK
Refractive errors

Normal refraction
In the normal eye, light rays focus exactly on the retina.

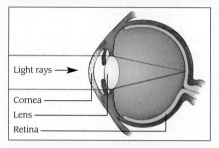

Hyperopia
In hyperopia, light rays focus behind the retina.

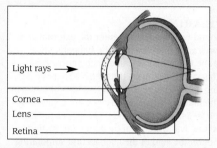

Myopia
In myopia, light rays focus in front of the retina.

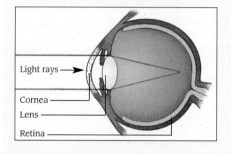

Astigmatism
In astigmatism, light rays don't come to a single focus on the retina.

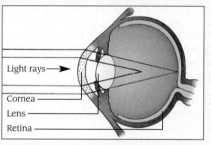

Myopia
Myopia, or nearsightedness, occurs when light rays focus in front of the retina. Near objects can be seen clearly, and distant objects appear blurry. This condition may occur if the eye is too long or the refractive power of the cornea or lens is too great.

Myopia may also occur if hyperglycemia in uncontrolled diabetes causes lens swelling. A concave lens that bends light rays outward is used to correct myopia.

Hyperopia
Hyperopia, or farsightedness, occurs when light rays focus behind the retina. Distant objects appear clear, and nearby objects are blurred. This condition occurs when the eye is too short or the refractive power of the cornea or lens is too low. It may be corrected with a convex lens that bends light rays inward.

 AGE ALERT *Presbyopia is a form of hyperopia that begins in middle age as the lens*

becomes firm and loses its elasticity. As a result, the refractive power of the lens is reduced, the eye loses its ability to accommodate, and near objects appear blurred. This condition is treated with a convex lens that bends light rays in different directions so they focus in a single point.

Astigmatism
Astigmatism occurs when unequal curvature of the cornea or eyeball causes light rays to focus on different points on the retina, resulting in distorted images. Astigmatism may occur in conjunction with other refractive disorders.

Color vision
The retina's cones are responsible for color vision. Each cone contains one of three different pigments (red, green, or blue) that absorb light waves of different wavelengths.

Color blindness is inherited on the X chromosome and therefore usually affects males. Acquired color blindness may also be due to diabetes, bilateral strokes affecting the ventral portion of the occipital lobe, or disease of the macula or optic nerve.

AGE ALERT *Older adults typically experience impaired color vision, especially in the blue and green ranges, because cones in the retina deteriorate. Yellowing of the aging lens also impairs color vision.*

HEARING

Sound waves normally enter the external auditory canal, then travel to the tympanic membrane in the middle ear, causing it to vibrate. This vibration causes the malleus to move, setting in motion the incus and, in turn, the stapes. The malleus, incus, and stapes are collectively referred to as the ossicles. The stapes presses on the oval window of the inner ear, setting in motion the fluid of the cochlea and stimulating hair cells. The hair cells carry impulses through the cochlear division of the auditory cranial nerve (VIII) to the brain. This type of sound transmission to the inner ear, called air conduction, is usually better than transmission through bone (bone conduction).

Alterations in hearing are classified as conductive or sensorineural. Mixed hearing loss combines aspects of conductive and sensorineural hearing loss.

TASTE AND SMELL

The senses of taste and smell are also subject to alterations.

Taste

The sensory receptors for taste are the taste buds, concentrated over the surface of the tongue and scattered over the palate, pharynx, and larynx. These buds can differentiate among sweet, salty, sour, and bitter stimuli. Taste and olfactory receptors together perceive more complex flavors. Much of what's considered taste is actually smell; food odors typically stimulate the olfactory system more strongly than related food tastes stimulate the taste buds.

A factor interrupting the transmission of taste stimuli to the brain may cause taste abnormalities. Taste abnormalities may result from trauma, infection, vitamin or mineral deficiencies, neurologic or oral disorders, and the effects of drugs. Moreover, because tastes are most accurately perceived in a fluid medium, dryness of the mouth may interfere with taste. Two major pathologic causes of impaired taste are aging, which normally reduces the number of taste buds, and heavy smoking (especially pipe smoking), which dries the tongue.

Alterations in taste may include:
- ◆ *ageusia* — a complete loss of taste
- ◆ *hypogeusia* — a partial loss of taste
- ◆ *dysgeusia* — a distorted sense of taste
- ◆ *cacogeusia* — an unpleasant or revolting taste of food.

AGE ALERT *Young children typically can't differentiate between an abnormal taste sensation and a simple taste dislike.*

Smell

As air travels between the septum and the turbinates of the nose, it touches sensory hairs (cilia) and olfactory nerve endings in the mucosal surface. The resultant stimulation of cranial nerve I sends impulses to the olfactory-receiving area, primarily in the frontal cortex. Temporary impairment in the sense of smell can result from a condition that irritates and causes swelling of the nasal mucosa and obstructs the olfactory area in the nose, such as heavy smoking, rhinitis, or sinusitis. Permanent alterations in the sense of smell usually result when the olfactory neuroepithelium or a part of the olfactory nerve is destroyed. Permanent or temporary loss can also result from inhaling irritants, such as cocaine or acid fumes, that paralyze nasal cilia. Conditions such as aging, Parkinson's disease, Alzheimer's disease, or Kallmann's syndrome (a congenital disorder) also may alter the sense of smell. Because combined stimulation of taste buds and olfactory cells produces the sense of taste, the loss of the sense of smell is usually accompanied by the loss of the sense of taste.

Alterations in smell include:
- ◆ *anosmia* — a total loss of the sense of smell
- ◆ *hyposmia* — an impaired sense of smell
- ◆ *parosmia* — an abnormal sense of smell.

Disordes

The most common disorders of vision are age-related macular degeneration, cataract, and glaucoma. Other common sensory disorders include hearing loss, Ménière's disease, and otosclerosis.

AGE-RELATED MACULAR DEGENERATION

Macular degeneration — *atrophy or degeneration of the macular disk* — is the most common cause of legal blindness in adults age 50 and older. It's also one of the causes of severe irreversible and unpreventable loss of central vision in elderly people.

Two types of age-related macular degeneration occur. The dry, or atrophic, form is characterized by atrophic pigment epithelial changes and typically causes mild, gradual visual loss. The wet, exudative form rapidly causes severe vision loss. It's characterized by the subretinal formation of new blood vessels (*neovascularization*) that cause leakage, hemorrhage, and fibrovascular scar formation.

Causes
The causes of macular degeneration are unknown but may include:
◆ aging
◆ infection
◆ inflammation
◆ injury
◆ nutrition.

Pathophysiology
Age-related macular degeneration results from hardening and obstruction of retinal arteries, which probably reflect normal degenerative changes. The formation of new blood vessels in the macular area obscures central vision. Underlying pathologic changes occur primarily in the retinal pigment epithelium, Bruch's membrane, and choriocapillaries in the macular region.

The dry form develops as yellow extracellular deposits, or drusen, accumulate beneath the pigment epithelium of the retina; they may be prominent in the macula. Drusen are common in elderly people. Over time, drusen grow and become more numerous. Vision loss occurs as the retinal pigment epithelium detaches and becomes atrophic.

Exudative macular degeneration develops as new blood vessels in the choroid project through abnormalities in Bruch's membrane and invade the potential space underneath the retinal pigment epithelium. As these vessels leak, fluid in the retinal pigment epithelium is increased, resulting in blurry vision.

Signs and symptoms
◆ Changes in central vision due to neovascularization such as a blank spot (scotoma) in the center of a page when reading
◆ Distorted appearance of straight lines caused by relocation of retinal receptors
◆ Worsening intermittent blurred vision due to vessel leakage in the retinal pigment epithelium

Complications
◆ Vision impairment progressing to blindness
◆ Nystagmus (if the macular degeneration is bilateral)

Diagnosis
◆ Indirect ophthalmoscopy, to show gross macular changes, opacities, hemorrhage, neovascularization, retinal pallor, or retinal detachment
◆ I.V. fluorescein angiography sequential photographs, to show leaking vessels as fluorescein dye flows into the tissues from the subretinal neovascular net
◆ Amsler's grid test, to show central visual field loss

Treatment
◆ Laser photocoagulation, to reduce the incidence of severe visual loss in patients with subretinal neovascularization (exudative form)
◆ Photodynamic therapy for wet macular degeneration, in which verteporfin is injected I.V., followed by a laser focused into the eyes to destroy abnormal vessels.

Special considerations
◆ Inform patients with bilateral central vision loss of the visual rehabilitation services available to them.
◆ Special devices, such as low-vision optical aids, are available to improve the quality of life in patients with good peripheral vision.
◆ Assist the patient to identify ways to modify his home to maintain safety.
◆ Encourage early detection through regular eye exams.

CATARACT
A cataract is a gradually developing opacity of the lens or lens capsule of the eye. Light shining through the cornea is blocked by this opacity, and a blurred image is cast onto the retina. As a result, the brain interprets a hazy image. Cataracts commonly occur bilaterally, and each progresses independently. Exceptions are traumatic cataracts, which are usually unilateral, and congenital cataracts, which may remain stationary. Cataracts are most prevalent in people older than age 70, as part of the aging process. The prognosis is generally good; surgery improves vision in 95% of affected people.

Causes
◆ Aging (senile cataracts)
◆ Atopic dermatitis
◆ Complicated cataracts
◆ Congenital disorders
◆ Diabetes mellitus
◆ Drugs that are toxic to the lens
– dinitrophenol
– ergot alkaloids
– exposure to ultraviolet rays

Congenital cataracts

Congenital cataracts may be caused by:
♦ chromosomal abnormalities
♦ infection during pregnancy (such as rubella)
♦ intrauterine nutritional deficiencies
♦ metabolic disease (such as galactosemia).
 Congenital cataracts may not be apparent at birth unless the eye is examined by funduscope.
 If the cataract is removed within a few months of birth, the infant will be able to develop proper retinal fixation and cortical visual responses. After surgery, the child is likely to favor the normal eye; the brain suppresses the poor image from the affected eye, leading to underdeveloped vision (amblyopia) in that eye. Postoperatively, in the child with bilateral cataracts, vision develops equally in both eyes.

– naphthalene
– phenothiazines
– pilocarpine
– prednisone (Deltasone)
♦ Exposure to ionizing radiation or infrared rays
♦ Foreign body injury
♦ Genetic abnormalities
♦ Glaucoma
♦ Hypoparathyroidism
♦ Maternal rubella during the first trimester of pregnancy
♦ Myotonic dystrophy
♦ Retinal detachment
♦ Retinitis pigmentosa
♦ Traumatic cataracts
♦ Uveitis

Pathophysiology

Pathophysiology may vary with each form of cataract. Congenital cataracts are particularly challenging. (See *Congenital cataracts*.) Senile cataracts show evidence of protein aggregation, oxidative injury, and increased pigmentation in the center of the lens. In traumatic cataracts, phagocytosis of the lens or inflammation may occur when a lens ruptures. The mechanism of a complicated cataract varies with the disease process — for example, in diabetes, increased glucose in the lens causes it to absorb water.
 Typically, cataract development progresses through four stages:
♦ *immature* — the lens isn't totally opaque
♦ *mature* — the lens is completely opaque and vision loss is significant

♦ *tumescent* — the lens is filled with water; may lead to glaucoma
♦ *hypermature* — the lens proteins deteriorate, causing peptides to leak through the lens capsule; glaucoma may develop if intraocular fluid outflow is obstructed.

Signs and symptoms

♦ Gradual painless blurring and loss of vision due to lens opacity
♦ Milky white pupil due to lens opacity
♦ Blinding glare from headlights at night due to the inefficient reflection of light rays by the opacities
♦ Poor reading vision caused by reduced clarity of images
♦ Better vision in dim light than in bright light in patients with central opacity; as pupils dilate, patients can see around the opacity

AGE ALERT *Elderly patients with reduced vision may become depressed and withdraw from social activities rather than complain about reduced vision.*

Complications

♦ Blindness
♦ Glaucoma

Surgical

♦ Loss of vitreous humor
♦ Wound dehiscence from loosening of sutures and flat anterior chamber or iris prolapse into the wound
♦ Hyphema, which is a hemorrhage into the eye's anterior chamber
♦ Vitreous-block glaucoma
♦ Retinal detachment
♦ Infection

Diagnosis

♦ Physical examination (shining a penlight on the pupil to show the white area behind the pupil, which remains unnoticeable until the cataract is advanced)
♦ Indirect ophthalmoscopy and slit-lamp examination to show a dark area in the normally homogeneous red reflex
♦ Visual acuity test to confirm vision loss

Treatment

♦ Extracapsular cataract extraction to remove the anterior lens capsule, and cortex and intraocular lens (IOL) implant in the posterior chamber, typically performed by using phacoemulsification to fragment the lens with ultrasonic vibrations, then aspirating the pieces (See *Comparing methods of cataract removal.*)

Comparing methods of cataract removal

Cataracts can be removed by extracapsular or intracapsular techniques.

Extracapsular cataract extraction

The surgeon may use irrigation and aspiration or phacoemulsification.

To irrigate and aspirate, he makes an incision at the limbus, opens the anterior lens capsule with a cystotome, and exerts pressure from below to express the lens. He then irrigates and suctions the remaining lens cortex.

In phacoemulsification, he uses an ultrasonic probe to break the lens into minute particles and aspirates the particles.

IRRIGATION AND ASPIRATION

Cystotome

Lens

Cortical and nuclear cataract material aspirated through needle

PHACOEMULSIFICATION

Ultrasonic probe

Lens

Nucleus and cortex fragmented and aspirated by probe

Intracapsular cataract extraction

The surgeon makes a partial incision at the superior limbus arc. He then removes the lens using specially designed forceps or a cryoprobe, which adheres to the frozen lens to facilitate its removal.

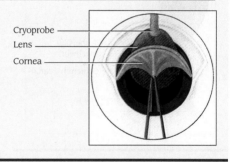

Cryoprobe

Lens

Cornea

◆ Intracapsular cataract extraction to remove the entire lens within the intact capsule by cryoextraction (The moist lens sticks to an extremely cold metal probe for easy and safe extraction; rarely performed today. An IOL may be placed in the anterior or posterior chamber after lens removal; or, a contact lens or aphakic glasses may be used to enhance vision.)
◆ Laser surgery after an extracapsular cataract extraction to restore visual acuity when a secondary membrane forms in the posterior lens capsule that has been left intact
◆ Discission (an incision) and aspiration may still be used in children with soft cataracts
◆ Contact lenses or lens implantation after surgery to improve visual acuity, binocular vision, and depth perception

Special considerations

After surgery

◆ Because the patient will be discharged after he recovers from anesthesia, remind him to return for a checkup the next day, and warn him to avoid activities that increase intraocular pressure such as straining.
◆ Urge the patient to protect the eye from accidental injury at night by wearing a plastic or metal shield with perforations; a shield or glasses should be worn for protection during the day.
◆ Before discharge, teach the patient to administer antibiotic ointment or drops to prevent infection and a steroid to reduce inflammation; combination steroid-antibiotic eyedrops can also be used.
◆ Advise the patient to watch for complications, such as a sharp pain in the eye uncontrolled by an analgesic as a result of hyphema,

CLOSER LOOK

Normal flow of aqueous humor

Aqueous humor, a transparent fluid produced by the ciliary epithelium of the ciliary body, flows from the posterior chamber through the pupil to the anterior chamber. It then flows peripherally and filters through the trabecular meshwork to Schlemm's canal, through which the fluid ultimately enters venous circulation.

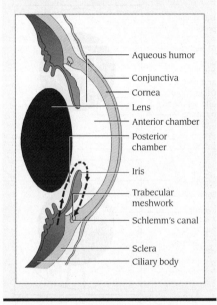

- Aqueous humor
- Conjunctiva
- Cornea
- Lens
- Anterior chamber
- Posterior chamber
- Iris
- Trabecular meshwork
- Schlemm's canal
- Sclera
- Ciliary body

or clouding in the anterior chamber (which may herald an infection), and to report them immediately.

♦ Caution the patient about activity restrictions, and advise him that he'll receive his corrective reading glasses or lenses in several weeks.

♦ Encourage the patient to wear sunglasses, and refer him to a smoking cessation program as appropriate.

GLAUCOMA

Glaucoma is a group of disorders characterized by an abnormally high intraocular pressure (IOP) that damages the optic nerve and other intraocular structures. Untreated, it leads to a gradual loss of vision and, ultimately, blindness. Glaucoma occurs in several forms: chronic open-angle (primary), acute angle-closure, congenital (inherited as an autosomal recessive trait), and secondary to other causes. Chronic

open-angle glaucoma is usually bilateral, with insidious onset and a slowly progressive course. Acute angle-closure glaucoma typically has a rapid onset, constituting an ophthalmic emergency. Unless treated promptly, this acute form of glaucoma causes blindness in 3 to 5 days.

Blacks are four times more likely to have the disorder as Whites, and people with a family history of open-angle glaucoma are twice as likely to develop it as those without a family history of the disorder.

Causes
Chronic open-angle glaucoma
♦ Aging
♦ Black ethnicity
♦ Diabetes mellitus
♦ Genetics
♦ Hypertension
♦ Severe myopia

Acute angle-closure glaucoma
♦ Drug-induced mydriasis (extreme dilation of the pupil)
♦ Emotional excitement, which can lead to hypertension

Secondary glaucoma
♦ Diabetes
♦ Infections
♦ Steroids
♦ Surgery
♦ Trauma
♦ Uveitis

Pathophysiology
Chronic open-angle glaucoma results from overproduction or obstruction of the outflow of aqueous humor through the trabecular meshwork or Schlemm's canal, causing increased IOP and damage to the optic nerve. (See *Normal flow of aqueous humor*.) In secondary glaucoma, conditions such as trauma and surgery increase the risk of obstruction of intraocular fluid outflow caused by edema or other abnormal processes.

Acute angle-closure glaucoma results from obstruction to the outflow of aqueous humor. Obstruction may be caused by anatomically narrow angles between the anterior iris and the posterior corneal surface, shallow anterior chambers, a thickened iris that causes angle closure on pupil dilation, or a bulging iris that presses on the trabeculae, closing the angle (peripheral anterior synechiae). Any of these may cause IOP to increase suddenly. (See *Congenital glaucoma*.)

■ **AGE ALERT** *In older patients, partial clo-sure of the angle may also occur, so two forms of glaucoma may coexist.*

Signs and symptoms

Clinical manifestations of chronic open-angle glaucoma typically are bilateral and include:
♦ mild aching in the eyes caused by increased IOP
♦ loss of peripheral vision due to compression of retinal rods and nerve fibers
♦ halos around lights as a result of corneal edema
♦ reduced visual acuity, especially at night, not correctable with glasses.

Clinical manifestations of acute angle-closure glaucoma have a rapid onset, are usually unilateral, and include:
♦ inflammation and red, painful eye caused by an abrupt elevation of IOP
♦ sensation of pressure over the eye due to increased IOP
♦ moderate pupillary dilation nonreactive to light due to a thickened or bulging iris
♦ cloudy cornea due to compression of intraocular components
♦ blurring and decreased visual acuity due to aberrant neural conduction
♦ photophobia due to abnormal intraocular pressures
♦ halos around lights due to corneal edema
♦ nausea and vomiting caused by increased IOP.

Complications

Glaucoma may be complicated by blindness.

Diagnosis

♦ Pressure measurement tonometry using an applanation or air puff tonometer (normal IOP is 8 to 21 mm Hg); fingertip tension to estimate IOP (on gentle palpation of closed eyelids, one eye feels harder than the other in acute angle-closure glaucoma)
♦ Slit-lamp examination of the eye's anterior structures, including the cornea, iris, and lens
♦ Gonioscopy, to determine the angle of the eye's anterior chamber, enabling differentiation between chronic open-angle glaucoma and acute angle-closure glaucoma (normal angle in chronic open-angle glaucoma and abnormal angle in acute angle-closure glaucoma) (See *Optic disk changes in chronic glaucoma,* page 552.)
♦ Ophthalmoscopy, to show cupping of the optic disk in chronic open-angle glaucoma; pale disk suggesting acute angle-closure glaucoma
♦ Perimetry or visual field tests, to detect loss of peripheral vision due to chronic open-angle glaucoma

Congenital glaucoma

Congenital glaucoma, a rare disease, occurs when a congenital defect in the angle of the anterior chamber obstructs the outflow of aqueous humor. Congenital glaucoma is usually bilateral, with an enlarged cornea that may be cloudy and bulging. Signs and symptoms in a neonate, though difficult to assess, may include tearing, pain, and photophobia.

Untreated, congenital glaucoma causes damage to the optic nerve and blindness. Surgical intervention (such as goniotomy, goniopuncture, trabeculotomy, or trabeculectomy) is necessary to reduce intraocular pressure and prevent vision loss.

♦ Fundus photography, to monitor the disk for changes

Treatment

Treatment of chronic open-angle glaucoma may include:
♦ a beta-adrenergic blocker, such as timolol or betaxolol (a beta₁-receptor antagonist), to decrease aqueous humor production
♦ an alpha agonist, such as brimonidine or apraclonidine, to reduce intraocular pressure
♦ a carbonic anhydrase inhibitor, such as dorzolamide or acetazolamide, to decrease the formation and secretion of aqueous humor
♦ epinephrine, to reduce IOP by improving aqueous outflow
♦ a prostaglandin, such as latanoprost, to reduce IOP
♦ miotic eyedrops, such as pilocarpine, to reduce IOP by facilitating the outflow of aqueous humor.

When medical therapy fails to reduce IOP, the following surgical procedures may be performed:
♦ argon laser trabeculoplasty of the trabecular meshwork of an open angle, to produce a thermal burn that changes the surface of the meshwork and increases the outflow of aqueous humor
♦ trabeculectomy, to remove scleral tissue, followed by a peripheral iridectomy, to produce an opening for aqueous outflow under the conjunctiva, creating a filtering bleb.

Acute angle-closure glaucoma is an ocular emergency requiring immediate intervention to reduce high IOP, including:
♦ I.V. mannitol (20%) or oral glycerin (50%), to reduce IOP by creating an osmotic pressure gradient between the blood and intraocular fluid

Optic disk changes in chronic glaucoma

Ophthalmoscopy and slit-lamp examination show cupping of the optic disk, which is characteristic of chronic glaucoma.

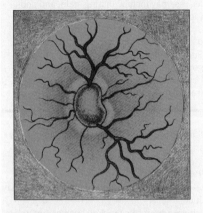

◆ steroid drops, to reduce inflammation
◆ acetazolamide, a carbonic anhydrase inhibitor, to reduce IOP by decreasing the formation and secretion of aqueous humor
◆ pilocarpine, to constrict the pupil, forcing the iris away from the trabeculae and allowing fluid to escape
◆ timolol, a beta-adrenergic blocker, to decrease IOP
◆ an opioid analgesic, to reduce pain if necessary
◆ laser iridotomy or surgical peripheral iridectomy, if drug therapy doesn't reduce IOP, to relieve pressure and preserve vision by promoting outflow of aqueous humor
◆ cycloplegic drops, such as apraclonidine, in the affected eye (only after laser peripheral iridectomy), to relax the ciliary muscle and reduce inflammation to prevent adhesions.

Special considerations
◆ Stress the importance of meticulous compliance with prescribed drug therapy to prevent an increase in IOP, resulting in disk changes and loss of vision.
◆ For the patient with acute angle-closure glaucoma, give medications as ordered, and prepare him physically and psychologically for laser iridotomy or surgery.

◆ Postoperative care after peripheral iridectomy includes cycloplegic eyedrops to relax the ciliary muscle and to decrease inflammation, thus preventing adhesions. *Note:* Cycloplegics must be used only in the affected eye. The use of these drops in the normal eye may precipitate an attack of acute angle-closure glaucoma in this eye, threatening the patient's residual vision.
◆ Encourage ambulation immediately after surgery.
◆ After surgical filtering, postoperative care includes dilation and a topical steroid to rest the pupil.
◆ Stress the importance of glaucoma screening for early detection and prevention. All people older than age 35, especially those with family histories of glaucoma, should have an annual tonometric examination.

HEARING LOSS
Hearing loss, or deafness, results from a mechanical or nervous impediment to the transmission of sound waves and is the most common pathologic process associated with hearing alteration. Hearing loss is further defined as an inability to perceive the range of sounds audible to an individual with normal hearing. Types of hearing loss include congenital hearing loss, sudden deafness, noise-induced hearing loss, and presbycusis.

Causes
Congenital hearing loss may be transmitted as a dominant, autosomal dominant, autosomal recessive, or sex-linked recessive trait. Hearing loss in neonates may also result from trauma, toxicity, or infection during pregnancy or delivery.
  Predisposing factors include:
◆ congenital abnormalities of the ears, nose, or throat
◆ maternal exposure to rubella or syphilis during pregnancy
◆ prematurity or low birth weight
◆ serum bilirubin level above 20 mg/dl
◆ trauma or prolonged fetal anoxia during delivery
◆ use of ototoxic drugs during pregnancy.
  Sudden deafness refers to sudden hearing loss in a person with no prior hearing impairment. This condition is considered a medical emergency because prompt treatment may restore full hearing. Its causes and predisposing factors may include:
◆ acute infections, especially mumps (most common cause of unilateral sensorineural hearing loss in children); other bacterial and viral infections, such as rubella, rubeola, influenza,

herpes zoster, and infectious mononucleosis; and *Mycoplasma* infections
◆ blood dyscrasias (leukemia, hypercoagulation)
◆ head trauma or brain tumors
◆ metabolic disorders (diabetes mellitus, hypothyroidism, hyperlipoproteinemia)
◆ neurologic disorders (multiple sclerosis, neurosyphilis)
◆ ototoxic drugs (tobramycin, streptomycin, quinine, gentamicin, furosemide, ethacrynic acid)
◆ vascular disorders (hypertension, arteriosclerosis).

Noise-induced hearing loss, which may be transient or permanent, may follow:
◆ brief exposure to extremely loud noise (greater than 90 dB)
◆ prolonged exposure to loud noise (85 to 90 dB).

Such hearing loss is common in workers subjected to constant industrial noise and in military personnel, hunters, and rock musicians.

AGE ALERT *Presbycusis, an otologic effect of aging, results from a loss of hair cells in the organ of Corti. This disorder causes progressive, symmetrical, bilateral sensorineural hearing loss, usually of high-frequency tones.*

Pathophysiology

The major forms of hearing loss are classified as:
◆ *conductive loss*—interrupted passage of sound from the external ear to the junction of the stapes and oval window due to wax, or otitis media or externa
◆ *sensorineural loss*—impaired cochlea or acoustic (eighth cranial) nerve dysfunction causing failure of transmission of sound impulses within the inner ear or brain
◆ *mixed loss*—combined dysfunction of conduction and sensorineural transmission.

Hearing loss may be partial or total and is calculated using this American Medical Association formula: Hearing is 1.5% impaired for every decibel that the pure tone average exceeds 25 dB.

Signs and symptoms

Although congenital hearing loss may produce no obvious signs of hearing impairment at birth, a deficient response to auditory stimuli generally becomes apparent within 2 to 3 days.

Other clinical features of hearing loss include:
◆ impaired speech development caused by inability to discriminate sounds

◆ loss of perception of certain frequencies (around 4,000 Hz), depending on severity of hearing loss
◆ tinnitus due to damaged hair cells
◆ inability to understand the spoken word.

AGE ALERT *A deaf infant's behavior can appear normal and mislead the parents as well as the professional, especially if the infant has autosomal recessive deafness and is the first child of carrier parents.*

Complications
◆ Increased hearing loss
◆ Total deafness
◆ Chronic ear problems
◆ Chronic tinnitus

Diagnosis
◆ Patient, family, and occupational histories and a complete audiologic examination usually provide ample evidence of hearing loss and suggest possible causes or predisposing factors.
◆ Weber, Rinne, and specialized audiologic tests differentiate between conductive and sensorineural hearing loss.

Treatment

After the underlying cause is identified, therapy for congenital hearing loss not treatable with surgery consists of:
◆ developing the patient's ability to communicate through sign language, speech reading, or other effective means
◆ phototherapy and exchange transfusions for hyperbilirubinemia
◆ aggressively immunizing children against rubella to reduce the risk of maternal exposure during pregnancy; educating pregnant women about the dangers of exposure to drugs, chemicals, or infection; and careful monitoring during labor and delivery to prevent fetal anoxia.

Treatment of sudden deafness requires prompt identification of the underlying cause. Prevention necessitates educating patients and health care professionals about the many causes of sudden deafness and the ways to recognize and treat them.

For patients with noise-induced hearing loss:
◆ Overnight rest usually restores normal hearing in those who have been exposed to noise levels greater than 90 dB for several hours.
◆ Reduction of exposure to loud noises generally prevents high-frequency hearing loss.
◆ Repeated exposure to such noise may require speech and hearing rehabilitation; hearing aids are seldom helpful.

Normal vestibular function

The semicircular canals and vestibule of the inner ear are responsible for equilibrium and balance. Each of the three semicircular canals lies at a 90-degree angle to the others. When the head moves, endolymph inside each semicircular canal moves in an opposite direction. The movement stimulates hair cells, which send electrical impulses to the brain through the vestibular portion of cranial nerve VIII. Head motion also causes movement of the vestibular otoliths (crystals of calcium salts) in their gel medium, which tugs on hair cells, initiating the transmission of electrical impulses to the brain through the vestibular nerve. Together, these two organs help detect the body's present position as well as a change in direction or motion.

For patients with presbycusis:
◆ Amplifying sound, as with a hearing aid, helps some patients.
◆ Many patients are intolerant of loud noise and aren't helped by a hearing aid.

Special considerations
◆ When speaking to a patient with hearing loss who can read lips, stand directly in front of him, with the light on your face, and speak slowly and distinctly. If possible, speak to him at eye level. Approach the patient within his visual range, and elicit his attention by raising your arm or waving; touching him may be unnecessarily startling.
◆ Make other staff members and hospital personnel aware of the patient's disability and his established method of communication. Carefully explain all diagnostic tests and hospital procedures in a way the patient understands.
◆ Make sure the patient with a hearing loss is in an area where he can observe unit activities and people approaching because such a patient depends on visual clues.
◆ When addressing an older patient, speak slowly and distinctly in a low tone; avoid shouting.
◆ Provide emotional support and encouragement to the patient learning to use a hearing aid. Teach him how the aid works and how to maintain it.
◆ Refer children with suspected hearing loss to an audiologist or otolaryngologist for further

evaluation. Any child who fails a language screening examination should be referred to a speech pathologist for language evaluation. The child with a mild language delay may be involved with a home language enrichment program.
◆ To help prevent hearing loss, watch for signs of hearing impairment in patients receiving ototoxic drugs. Emphasize the danger of excessive exposure to noise; stress the danger to pregnant women of exposure to drugs, chemicals, and infection (especially rubella); and encourage the use of protective devices in a noisy environment.

MÉNIÈRE'S DISEASE
Ménière's disease, an inner ear disease that results from a labyrinthine dysfunction (also known as *endolymphatic hydrops*), causes severe vertigo, sensorineural hearing loss, and tinnitus.

AGE ALERT *It usually affects adults between ages 30 and 60, is slightly more common in men than in women, and rarely occurs in children. Usually, only one ear is involved. After multiple attacks over several years, residual tinnitus and hearing loss can be incapacitating.*

Causes
The cause of Ménière's disease is unknown. It may be associated with:
◆ autonomic nervous system dysfunction
◆ family history
◆ head trauma
◆ immune disorder
◆ middle ear infection
◆ migraine headaches
◆ premenstrual edema.

Pathophysiology
Ménière's disease may result from overproduction or decreased absorption of endolymph—the fluid contained in the labyrinth of the ear. Accumulated endolymph dilates the semicircular canals, utricle, and saccule and causes degeneration of the vestibular and cochlear hair cells. Overstimulation of the vestibular branch of cranial nerve VIII impairs postural reflexes and stimulates the vomiting reflex. (See *Normal vestibular function*.) Perception of sound is impaired as a result of this excessive cranial nerve stimulation, and injury to sensory receptors for hearing may affect auditory acuity.

This condition may also stem from autonomic nervous system dysfunction that produces a temporary constriction of blood vessels supplying the inner ear.

CLINICAL ALERT *In some women, premenstrual edema may precipitate outbreaks of Ménière's disease.*

Signs and symptoms

◆ Sudden severe spinning, whirling vertigo, lasting from 10 minutes to several hours, due to increased endolymph (attacks may occur several times per year, or remissions may last as long as several years)

◆ Tinnitus caused by altered firing of sensory auditory neurons (may have residual tinnitus between attacks)

◆ Hearing impairment due to sensorineural loss (hearing may be normal between attacks, but repeated attacks may progressively cause permanent hearing loss)

◆ Feeling of fullness or blockage in the affected ear preceding an attack, a result of changing sensitivity of pressure receptors

◆ Severe nausea, vomiting, sweating, and pallor during an acute attack due to autonomic dysfunction

◆ Nystagmus due to asymmetry and intensity of impulses reaching the brain stem

◆ Loss of balance and falling to the affected side due to vertigo

Complications

◆ Continued tinnitus
◆ Hearing loss

Diagnosis

◆ Patient history of signs and symptoms
◆ Audiometric testing showing a sensorineural hearing loss and loss of discrimination and recruitment

◆ Electronystagmography showing normal or reduced vestibular response on the affected side

◆ Cold caloric testing showing impairment of oculovestibular reflex

◆ Electrocochleography showing increased ratio of summating potential to action potential

◆ Brain stem evoked response audiometry test, to rule out acoustic neuroma, brain tumor, and vascular lesions in the brain stem

◆ Computed tomography scan and magnetic resonance imaging, to rule out acoustic neuroma as a cause of symptoms

Treatment

During an acute attack, treatment may include:
◆ lying down to minimize head movement, and avoiding sudden movements and glaring lights to reduce dizziness

◆ promethazine (Phenergan) or prochlorperazine (Compazine) to relieve nausea and vomiting

◆ atropine to control an attack by reducing autonomic nervous system function

◆ dimenhydrinate (Dramamine), to control vertigo and nausea

◆ a central nervous system depressant, such as lorazepam (Ativan) or diazepam (Valium), during an acute attack to reduce excitability of vestibular nuclei

◆ an antihistamine, such as meclizine (Antivert) or diphenhydramine (Benadryl), to reduce dizziness and vomiting.

Long-term management may include:
◆ a diuretic, such as triamterene (Dyrenium) or acetazolamide (Diamox), to reduce endolymph pressure

◆ betahistine dihydrochloride to alleviate vertigo, hearing loss, and tinnitus

◆ a vasodilator to dilate blood vessels supplying the inner ear

◆ sodium restriction to reduce endolymphatic hydrops

◆ an antihistamine or a mild sedative to prevent attacks

◆ gentamicin, an ototoxic antibiotic, administered directly into the middle ear to control vertigo.

In Ménière's disease that persists despite medical treatment or produces incapacitating vertigo, the following surgical procedures may be performed:

◆ endolymphatic drainage and shunt procedures, to reduce pressure on the hair cells of the cochlea and prevent further sensorineural hearing loss

◆ vestibular nerve resection in patients with intact hearing, to reduce vertigo and prevent further hearing loss

◆ labyrinthectomy for relief of vertigo in patients with incapacitating symptoms and poor or no hearing, because destruction of the cochlea results in a total loss of hearing in the affected ear

◆ cochlear implantation, to improve hearing in patients with profound deafness due to Ménière's disease.

Special considerations

If the patient is in the hospital during an attack of Ménière's disease:

◆ Advise him against reading and exposure to glaring lights, to reduce dizziness.

◆ Keep the side rails of the patient's bed up to prevent falls. Tell him not to get out of bed or walk without assistance.

◆ Instruct the patient to avoid sudden position changes and any tasks that vertigo makes hazardous because an attack can begin quite suddenly.

◆ Before surgery, if the patient is vomiting, record fluid intake and output and characteristics of vomitus. Administer an antiemetic, as ordered, and give small amounts of fluid frequently.

◆ After surgery, record intake and output carefully. Tell the patient to expect dizziness and nausea for 1 to 2 days after surgery. Give a prophylactic antibiotic and an antiemetic as ordered.

OTOSCLEROSIS

The most common cause of chronic, progressive, conductive hearing loss, otosclerosis is the slow formation of spongy bone in the otic capsule, particularly at the oval window. It occurs in at least 10% of people of European descent and is three times as prevalent in women as in men; onset is usually between ages 15 and 30. Occurring unilaterally at first, the disorder may progress to bilateral conductive hearing loss. With surgery, the prognosis is good.

Causes
◆ Autosomal dominant trait
◆ Pregnancy

AGE ALERT *Children with osteogenesis imperfecta, an inherited condition characterized by brittle bones, may also have otosclerosis.*

Pathophysiology

In otosclerosis, the normal bone of the otic capsule is gradually replaced with a highly vascular spongy bone. This spongy bone immobilizes the footplate of the normally mobile stapes, disrupting the conduction of vibrations from the tympanic membrane to the cochlea. Because the sound pressure vibrations aren't transmitted to the fluid of the inner ear, the result is conductive hearing loss. If the inner ear becomes involved, sensorineural hearing loss may develop.

Signs and symptoms

◆ Progressive hearing loss, which starts unilaterally and may become bilateral without evidence of a middle ear infection caused by interference with vibration transmission
◆ Bilateral conductive hearing loss due to the disruption of the conduction of vibrations from the tympanic membrane to the cochlea
◆ Tinnitus due to overstimulation of cranial nerve VIII afferents
◆ Ability to hear a conversation better in a noisy environment than in a quiet one (paracusis of Willis) as a result of masking effects

Complications

A complication of otosclerosis is deafness.

Diagnosis

◆ Otoscopic examination showing a normal-appearing tympanic membrane; occasionally, the tympanic membrane may appear pinkish-orange (Schwartze's sign) as a result of vascular and bony changes in the middle ear
◆ Rinne test showing bone conduction lasting longer than air conduction (normally, the reverse is true); as otosclerosis progresses, bone conduction also deteriorates
◆ Audiometric testing showing hearing loss ranging from 60 dB in early stages to total loss
◆ Weber's test to detect sounds lateralizing to the more affected ear

AGE ALERT *Audiometric testing should be performed in late adolescence when otosclerosis and noise-induced hearing may start to occur.*

Treatment

◆ Prevention of infection with a prophylactic antibiotic
◆ Stapedectomy (removal of the stapes) and insertion of a prosthesis to restore partial or total hearing
◆ Stapedotomy (creation of a small hole in the footplate of the stapes) and insertion of a wire and piston as a prosthesis to help restore hearing
◆ Hearing aid (air conduction aid with molded ear insertion receiver) if surgery isn't possible to permit hearing of conversation in normal surroundings

Special considerations

◆ During the first 24 hours after surgery, keep the patient lying flat, with the affected ear facing upward (to maintain the position of the graft). Enforce bed rest with bathroom privileges for 48 hours. Because the patient may be dizzy, keep the side rails up and assist him with ambulation. Assess for pain and vertigo, which may be relieved with repositioning or prescribed medication.
◆ Tell the patient that his hearing won't return until edema subsides and packing is removed.
◆ Before discharge, instruct the patient to avoid loud noises and sudden pressure changes (such as those that occur while diving or flying) until healing is complete (usually 6 months). Advise the patient not to blow his nose for at least 1 week to prevent contaminated air and bacteria from entering the eustachian tube.
◆ Stress the importance of protecting the ears against cold; avoiding activities that provoke dizziness, such as straining, bending, or heavy lifting; and, if possible, avoiding contact with anyone who has an upper respiratory tract infection. Teach the patient and his family how to change the external ear dressing (eye or gauze pad) and care for the incision. Emphasize the need to complete the prescribed antibiotic regimen and return for scheduled follow-up care.

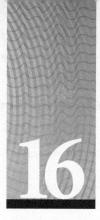

INTEGUMENTARY SYSTEM

The integumentary system, the largest and heaviest body system, includes the skin—the *integument,* or *external covering of the body*—and the epidermal appendages, including the hair, nails, and sebaceous, eccrine, and apocrine glands. It protects the body against injury and invasion of microorganisms, harmful substances, and radiation; regulates body temperature; serves as a reservoir for food and water; and synthesizes vitamin D. Emotional well-being, including one's responses to the daily stresses of life, is reflected in the skin.

Skin

The skin is composed of three layers: the epidermis, dermis, and subcutaneous tissues. The epidermis—the outermost layer—is thin and contains sensory receptors for pain, temperature, touch, vibration, pressure detection, and itching sensation. The epidermal layer has no blood vessels and relies on the dermal layer for nutrition. The dermis contains connective tissue, the sebaceous glands, and some hair follicles. The subcutaneous tissue lies beneath the dermis; it contains fat and sweat glands and the rest of the hair follicles. The subcutaneous layer can store calories for future use in the body. (See *Close-up view of the skin,* page 558.)

Hair and nails

The hair and nails are considered appendages of the skin. Both have protective functions in addition to their cosmetic appeal. The cuticle of the nail, for example, functions as a seal, protecting the area between two portions of the nail from external hazards. (See *Nail structure,* page 558.)

Glands

The sebaceous glands, found on all areas of the skin except the palms and soles, produce sebum, a semifluid material composed of fat and epithelial cells. Sebum is secreted into the hair follicle and exits to the skin surface. It helps waterproof the hair and skin and promotes the absorption of fat-soluble substances into the dermis.

The eccrine glands produce sweat, an odorless, watery fluid. Glands in the palms and soles secrete sweat primarily in response to emotional stress. The other remaining eccrine glands respond mainly to thermal stress, effectively regulating body temperature.

Located mainly in the axillary and anogenital areas, apocrine glands have a coiled secretory portion that lies deeper in the dermis than the eccrine glands. These glands begin to function at puberty and have no known biological function. Bacterial decomposition of the apocrine fluid produced by these glands causes body odor.

Skin color depends on four pigments: melanin, carotene, oxyhemoglobin, and deoxyhemoglobin. Each pigment is unique in its function and effect on the skin. For example, melanin, the brownish pigment of the skin, is

557

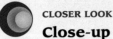

CLOSER LOOK
Close-up view of the skin

The skin is composed of two major layers—the epidermis and dermis. The epidermis consists of four strata, shown below. Subcutaneous tissue lying beneath the dermis consists of loose connective tissue that attaches the skin to underlying structures.

SKIN CROSS SECTION

Epidermis
- Stratum corneum
- Stratum granulosum
- Stratum spinosum
- Stratum basale

Dermis
- Papillary dermis
- Reticular dermis
- Arrector pili muscle
- Eccrine sweat gland

Subcutaneous layer
- Hair follicle

CLOSER LOOK
Nail structure

This illustration shows the anatomic components of a fingernail.

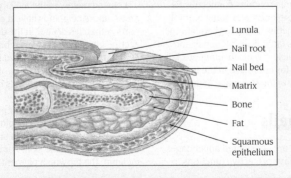

- Lunula
- Nail root
- Nail bed
- Matrix
- Bone
- Fat
- Squamous epithelium

genetically determined, although it can be altered by exposure to sunlight. Excessive dietary carotene (from carrots, sweet potatoes, and green, leafy vegetables) causes a yellowing of the skin. Excessive oxyhemoglobin in the blood causes a reddening of the skin, and excessive deoxyhemoglobin (not bound to oxygen) causes a bluish discoloration.

Pathophysiologic changes

Clinical manifestations of skin dysfunction include the inflammatory reaction of the skin and the formation of lesions.

INFLAMMATORY REACTION
An inflammatory reaction occurs with injury to the skin. The reaction can occur only in living organisms. Although a beneficial response, it's usually accompanied by some degree of discomfort at the site. Irritation changes the epidermal structure and consequent increase of immunoglobulin E activity. Other classic signs of inflammatory skin responses are erythema, edema, and warmth, due to bioamines released from the granules of tissue mast cells and basophils.

FORMATION OF LESIONS
Primary skin lesions appear on previously healthy skin in response to disease or external irritation. They're classified by their appearance as macules, papules, plaques, patches, nodules, tumors, wheals, comedos, cysts, vesicles, pustules, or bullae.

Modified lesions are described as secondary skin lesions. These lesions occur as a result of rupture, mechanical irritation, extension, invasion, or normal or abnormal healing of primary lesions. These include atrophy, erosions, ulcers, scales, crusts, excoriation, fissures, lichenification, and scars.

Disorders

Trauma, abnormal cellular function, infection, and systemic disease may cause disruptions in skin integrity. Integumentary disorders include acne; burns; cellulitis; dermatitis; folliculitis, furuncles, and carbuncles; fungal infections; pressure ulcers; psoriasis; scleroderma; toxic epidermal necrolysis; and warts.

ACNE
Acne is a chronic inflammatory disease of the sebaceous glands. It's usually associated with a high rate of sebum secretion and occurs on areas of the body that have sebaceous glands,

such as the face, neck, chest, back, and shoulders.

AGE ALERT *Acne occurs in both males and females. Acne vulgaris develops in 80% to 90% of adolescents or young adults, primarily between ages 15 and 18. Although the lesions can appear as early as age 8, acne primarily affects adolescents.*

Although the severity and overall incidence of acne is usually greater in males, it tends to start at an earlier age and lasts longer in females.

The prognosis varies and depends on the severity and underlying causes; with treatment, the prognosis is usually good.

Causes
The cause of acne is multifactorial. Diet isn't believed to be a precipitating factor. Possible causes of acne include increased activity of sebaceous glands and blockage of the *pilosebaceous ducts* (hair follicles).

Factors that may predispose a patient to acne include:
◆ cobalt irradiation
◆ cosmetics
◆ drugs, including androgens, bromides, corticosteroids, corticotropin (ACTH), halothane, iodides, isoniazid (Laniazid), lithium (Eskalith), phenytoin (Dilantin), striadril (Stri-Vectin SD), and trimethadione
◆ emotional stress
◆ exposure to greases, heavy oils, or tars
◆ heredity
◆ hormonal contraceptive use (Many women experience acne flare-up during their first few menses after starting or discontinuing hormonal contraceptives.)
◆ hormones (A decreased estrogen level or an increased testosterone level can exacerbate acne outbreaks.)
◆ hyperalimentation
◆ trauma or rubbing from tight clothing
◆ tropical climate.

Pathophysiology
There are two types of acne: *inflammatory,* in which the hair follicle is blocked by sebum, causing bacteria to grow and eventually rupture the follicle; and *noninflammatory,* in which the follicle doesn't rupture but remains dilated. (See *Understanding acne,* page 560.)

Signs and symptoms
The acne plug may appear as:
◆ a closed comedo, or whitehead (may be protruding from the follicle and covered by the epidermis)

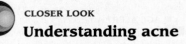

CLOSER LOOK

Understanding acne

The illustrations below show how acne lesions develop.

1. Excessive sebum production
Androgens stimulate sebaceous gland growth and the production of sebum, which is secreted into dilated hair follicles that contain bacteria.

2. Increased shedding of epithelial cells
The bacteria, usually *Propionibacterium acne* and *Staphylococcus epidermidis*, are normal skin flora that secrete the enzyme lipase. This enzyme interacts with sebum to produce free fatty acids, which provoke inflammation.

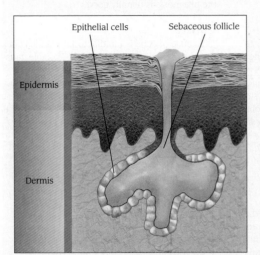

Epithelial cells   Sebaceous follicle

Epidermis

Dermis

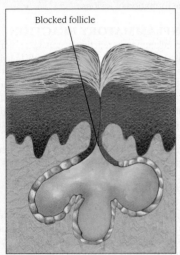

Blocked follicle

3. Inflammatory response in follicle
Hair follicles also produce more keratin, which joins with the sebum to form a plug in the dilated follicle.

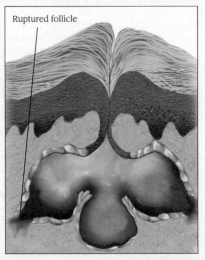

Ruptured follicle

◆ an open comedo, or blackhead (protruding from the follicle and not covered by the epidermis; melanin or pigment of the follicle causes the black color).

Rupture or leakage of an enlarged plug into the epidermis produces inflammation, characteristic acne pustules, papules or, in severe forms, acne cysts or abscesses (chronic, recurring lesions producing acne scars).

In women, signs and symptoms may include increased severity just before or during menstruation when the estrogen level is at its lowest. Additionally, an increased testosterone level, which occurs in both males and females during puberty, may also trigger an acne outbreak.

Complications
◆ Acne conglobata
◆ Scarring (when acne is severe)
◆ Impaired self-esteem
◆ Abscesses or secondary bacterial infections

Diagnosis
Diagnosis of acne vulgaris is confirmed by characteristic acne lesions, especially in adolescents.

Treatment
Topical treatment for noninflammatory acne includes the application of retinoic acid (tretinoin) on open and closed comedones. For inflammatory acne, an antibacterial such as benzoyl peroxide is effective. Topical and systemic antibiotics and systemic retinoids help reduce the effects of acne.

Systemic therapy consists primarily of:
◆ an antibiotic, usually tetracycline, to decrease bacterial growth (Dosage is reduced for long-term maintenance when the acne in remission.)
◆ oral isotretinoin (Accutane) to inhibit sebaceous gland function and keratinization (A 16- to 20-week course of isotretinoin is limited to patients with severe papulopustular or cystic acne not responding to conventional therapy because of its severe adverse effects. Also, because this drug is known to cause birth defects, the manufacturer, with U.S. Food and Drug Administration approval, recommends the following precautions: pregnancy testing before dispensing; dispensing only a 30-day supply, repeat pregnancy testing throughout the treatment period, effective contraception during treatment, and informed consent. Finally, because of the drug's effects on the liver, a serum triglyceride level should be drawn before and periodically during treatment.)

◆ for females, estrogens to inhibit androgen activity
◆ other treatments, including intralesional and oral corticosteroids, vitamin A and zinc supplements, exposure to ultraviolet light (although not when the patient is using a photosensitizing agent such as tretinoin), cryotherapy, and surgery.

Special considerations
The main focus of your care is teaching about the disorder, its treatment, and its prevention.
◆ Check the patient's drug history because certain medications, such as hormonal contraceptives, may cause an acne flare-up.
◆ Try to identify predisposing factors that may be eliminated or modified.
◆ Try to identify eruption patterns (seasonal or monthly).
◆ Explain the causes of acne to the patient and his family. Make sure they understand that the prescribed treatment is more likely to improve acne than a strict diet and fanatical scrubbing with soap and water. Provide written instructions regarding treatment.
◆ Describe the importance of not picking lesions and practicing good personal hygiene to prevent secondary infections.
◆ Instruct the patient receiving tretinoin to apply it at least 30 minutes after washing his face and at least 1 hour before bedtime. Warn against using it around the eyes or lips. After treatments, the skin should look pink and dry. If it appears red or starts to peel, the preparation may have to be weakened or applied less often. Advise the patient to avoid exposure to sunlight or to use a sunscreen. If the prescribed regimen includes tretinoin and benzoyl peroxide, avoid skin irritation by using one preparation in the morning and the other at night.
◆ Instruct the patient to take tetracycline on an empty stomach and not to take it with an antacid or milk because both have metallic ions, and tetracycline interacts with these ions and is then poorly absorbed.
◆ Tell the patient who is taking isotretinoin to avoid vitamin A supplements, which can worsen any adverse reactions. Also, teach the patient how to deal with the dry skin and mucous membranes that usually occur during treatment. Tell the female patient about the severe risk of teratogenicity. Monitor liver enzyme and lipid levels.
◆ Inform the patient that acne takes a long time to clear—even years for complete resolution. Encourage continued local skin care even after

acne clears. Explain the adverse effects of all drugs.
♦ Pay special attention to the patient's perception of his physical appearance, and offer emotional support.

BURNS

Burns are classified as first-degree, second-degree superficial, second-degree deep partial thickness, third-degree full thickness, and fourth degree. A first-degree burn is limited to the epidermis. The most common example of a first-degree burn is sunburn, which results from overexposure to the sun. In a second-degree burn, the epidermis and part of the dermis are damaged. A third-degree burn damages the epidermis and dermis, and vessels and tissue are visible. In a fourth-degree burn, the damage extends through deeply charred subcutaneous tissue to muscle and bone. Severe burns require immediate pain management and commonly result in permanent disability, requiring lengthy periods of rehabilitation.

Each year in the United States, about 2.4 million persons receive burn injuries. Most significant burns occur in the home; home fires account for the highest burn fatality rate.

In victims younger than age 4 and older than age 60, there's a higher incidence of complications and thus a higher mortality rate. Immediate, aggressive burn treatment increases the patient's chance for survival. Supportive measures and strict sterile technique can minimize infection. Survival and recovery from a major burn are more likely once the burn wound is reduced to less than 20% of the total body surface area (BSA).

Causes

More than 75% of all burn injuries and those that result in death are preventable.

Thermal burns, the most common type, typically result from:
♦ automobile accidents
♦ clothes that have caught on fire
♦ improper handling of firecrackers and gasoline
♦ kitchen and scalding accidents (such as a child climbing on top of a stove or grabbing a hot iron)
♦ parental abuse (of children or elderly people)
♦ playing with matches
♦ residential fires.

Chemical burns result from contact, ingestion, inhalation, or injection of acids, alkalis, or vesicants.

Electrical burns usually result from contact with faulty electrical wiring or high-voltage power lines. Sometimes young children chew electrical cords.

Friction or abrasion burns occur when the skin rubs harshly against a coarse surface.

Sunburn results from excessive exposure to sunlight. Sunlamp use may also result in burns.

Pathophysiology

The injuring agent denatures cellular proteins. Some cells die because of traumatic or ischemic necrosis. Loss of collagen cross-linking also occurs with denaturation, creating abnormal osmotic and hydrostatic pressure gradients, which cause the movement of intravascular fluid into interstitial spaces. Cellular injury triggers the release of mediators of inflammation, contributing to local and, in the case of major burns, systemic increases in capillary permeability. Specific pathophysiologic events depend on the cause and classification of the burn. (See *Classifications of burns.*)

First-degree burns

A first-degree burn causes localized injury or destruction to the skin (epidermis only) by direct (such as chemical spill) or indirect (such as sunlight) contact. The barrier function of the skin remains intact, and these burns aren't life-threatening.

Second-degree superficial partial-thickness burns

Second-degree superficial partial-thickness burns involve destruction of the epidermis and some of dermis. Thin-walled, fluid-filled blisters develop within a few minutes of the injury. As these blisters break, the nerve endings become exposed to the air. Because pain and tactile responses remain intact, subsequent treatments are very painful. The barrier function of the skin is lost.

Second-degree deep partial-thickness burns

Second-degree deep partial-thickness burns involve destruction of the epidermis and dermis, producing blisters and mild to moderate edema and pain. The hair follicles are still intact, so hair will grow again. Compared with second-degree superficial partial-thickness burns, there's less pain sensation with this burn because the sensory neurons have undergone extensive destruction. The areas around the burn injury remain very sensitive to pain. The barrier function of the skin is lost.

Classifications of burns

The depth of skin and tissue damage determines burn classification. This illustration shows the four degrees of burn classifications

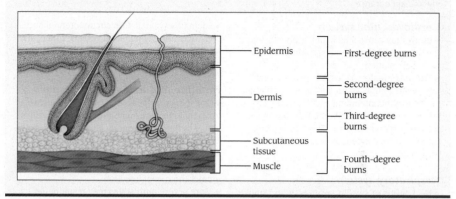

Third- and fourth-degree full-thickness burns

A major burn affects every body system and organ. A third-degree burn extends through the epidermis and dermis and into the subcutaneous tissue layer. A fourth-degree burn involves muscle, bone, and interstitial tissues. Within only hours, fluids and protein shift from capillary to interstitial spaces, causing edema. There's an immediate immunologic response to a burn injury, making burn wound sepsis a potential threat. Finally, an increase in calorie demand after a burn injury increases the metabolic rate. (See *How burns affect the body,* page 564.)

Signs and symptoms

Signs and symptoms depend on the type of burn and may include:

◆ localized pain and erythema, usually without blisters in the first 24 hours, caused by injury from direct or indirect contact with a burn source (first-degree burn)

◆ chills, headache, localized edema, and nausea and vomiting (more severe first-degree burn)

◆ thin-walled, fluid-filled blisters appearing within minutes of the injury, with mild to moderate edema and pain (second-degree superficial partial-thickness burn)

◆ white, waxy appearance to damaged area (second-degree deep partial-thickness burn)

◆ white, brown, or black leathery tissue and visible thrombosed vessels due to destruction of skin elasticity (dorsum of hand most common

site of thrombosed veins), without blisters (third-degree burn)

◆ silver-colored, raised area, usually at the site of electrical contact (electrical burn)

◆ singed nasal hairs, mucosal burns, voice changes, coughing, wheezing, soot in mouth or nose, and darkened sputum (with smoke inhalation and pulmonary damage).

Complications

◆ Infection (signs and symptoms including fever, increased pain, redness, swelling, drainage, pus, lymphadenopathy, and red streaks from the burn site)

◆ Dehydration (signs and symptoms including thirst, dry skin, dizziness, headache, lightheadedness, and decreased urine output)

◆ Loss of function (burns to face, hands, feet, and genitalia)

◆ Total occlusion of circulation in extremity (due to edema from circumferential burns)

◆ Airway obstruction (neck burns) or restricted respiratory expansion (chest burns)

◆ Pulmonary injury (from smoke inhalation or pulmonary embolism)

◆ Acute respiratory distress syndrome (due to left-sided heart failure or a myocardial infarction)

◆ Greater damage than indicated by the surface burn (electrical and chemical burns) or internal tissue damage along the conduction pathway (electrical burns)

◆ Cardiac arrhythmias (due to electrical shock and fluid shifts)

MULTISYSTEM DISORDER

How burns affect the body

Many changes occur as a result of a burn injury, affecting almost every body system. Multidisciplinary care can improve healing and maximize the patient's return to normal functioning and appearance.

Cardiovascular system

♦ Burns may cause fluid shifts or directly injure the heart and blood vessels, leading to impaired circulation.

♦ The inflammatory response increases capillary permeability. As a result, intravascular fluid shifts to the interstitial spaces, leading to edema, decreased circulating fluid volume, and increased blood viscosity. This hemoconcentration places the patient at risk for thrombus formation.

Respiratory system

♦ Neck burns or swelling from heat and smoke exposure or chemical injury to the mucosa of the respiratory tract can lead to respiratory distress.

♦ Restricted respiratory expansion from chest burns or eschar formation can lead to respiratory distress.

♦ Smoke inhalation or inhalation of other caustic substances results in pulmonary injury, such as bronchitis or respiratory distress.

♦ Hypoxia may result from a decreased amount of oxygen circulating through the blood, which may be caused by inhalation of carbon monoxide, a by-product of combustion that displaces oxygen from hemoglobin molecules.

GI system

♦ As blood is shunted away from the abdominal area and GI tract, peristalsis is slowed or absent altogether.

♦ Gastric dilation and vomiting may occur, possibly increasing the risk of aspiration.

♦ Curling's ulcers may result (stomach and intestinal ulcerations and hemorrhage).

Integumentary system

♦ Impaired skin integrity increases the risk of infection and causes hypothermia and rapid fluid losses.

♦ Contractures and impaired range-of-motion in extremities may result from hypertrophic scar formation.

♦ Edema associated with circumferential burns constricts underlying blood vessels, tissue, and muscle, impairing circulation to the affected area or extremity.

Immune and hematologic systems

♦ One theory suggests that burn cells release a toxin that interferes with the immune system's ability to function properly. Subsequently, major burns may result in immunosuppression.

♦ Generalized sepsis is a common and serious complication—the larger the wound, the greater the risk of infection.

♦ More severe burn states may result in the development of disseminated intravascular coagulation.

Renal system

♦ Hemoconcentration and decreased intravascular volumes cause decreased renal perfusion and decreased urine output.

♦ Prolonged decreased renal perfusion leads to acute tubular necrosis and renal failure.

Collaborative management

If the burn involves a large surface area or critical body parts, it usually requires treatment at a specialized burn center. Surgeons may be needed to perform escharotomy and fasciotomy to remove burn tissue. Wound care specialists may be needed to prevent wound infections and complications and promote wound healing. Respiratory therapy is needed to maximize respiratory function in cases of inhalation injury.

As the patient improves, physical therapy is necessary to maintain or improve range-of-motion and prevent contractures. Nutritional therapists can prescribe an optimal diet to promote wound healing. Referral to a therapist and a support group may help the patient deal with psychological effects of the traumatic injury. Similar referrals are needed if severe scarring or disfigurement is anticipated.

◆ Hypotension, secondary to shock or hypovolemia
◆ Stroke, heart attack, or pulmonary embolism (due to formation of blood clots resulting from slower blood flow)
◆ Burn shock (due to fluid shifts out of the vascular compartments, possibly leading to kidney damage and renal failure)
◆ Peptic ulcer disease or ileus (due to decreased blood supply in the abdominal area)
◆ Disseminated intravascular coagulation (more severe burn states)
◆ Added pain, depression, and financial burden (due to psychological component of disfigurement)

Diagnosis

Diagnosis involves determining the size and classifying the wound. The following methods are used to determine size:
◆ percentage of BSA covered by the burn using the rule of nines chart
◆ Lund-Browder chart (more accurate because it allows BSA changes with age); correlation of the burn's depth and size to estimate its severity. (See *Using the Rule of Nines and the Lund-Browder chart,* pages 566 and 567.)
  Major burns are classified as:
◆ third-degree burns over more than 10% of BSA
◆ second-degree burns over more than 25% of adult BSA (over 20% in children)
◆ burns of hands, face, feet, or genitalia
◆ burns complicated by fractures or respiratory damage
◆ electrical burns
◆ all burns in poor-risk patients.
  Moderate burns are classified as:
◆ third-degree burns over 2% to 10% of BSA
◆ second-degree burns over 15% to 25% of adult BSA (10% to 20% in children).
  Minor burns are classified as:
◆ third-degree burns over less than 2% of BSA
◆ second-degree burns over less than 15% of adult BSA (10% in children).

Treatment

Initial burn treatments are based on the type of burn and may include:
◆ immersing the burned area in cool water (55° F [12.8° C]) or applying cool compresses (minor burns)
◆ administering pain medication, as needed, or an anti-inflammatory
◆ covering the area with an antimicrobial and a nonstick bulky dressing (after debridement); prophylactic tetanus injection as needed

◆ not disturbing blisters or dead skin (increases risk of infection)
◆ preventing hypoxia by maintaining an open airway; assessing airway, breathing, and circulation; checking for smoke inhalation immediately when the patient presents; assisting with endotracheal intubation; and giving 100% oxygen (first immediate treatment for moderate and major burns)
◆ controlling active bleeding
◆ covering partial-thickness burns over 30% of BSA or full-thickness burns over 5% of BSA with a clean, dry, sterile bedsheet (because of drastic reduction in body temperature, *don't* cover large burns with saline-soaked dressings)
◆ removing smoldering clothing (first soaking the clothing in saline solution if it's stuck to the patient's skin), rings, and other constricting items
◆ immediate I.V. therapy to prevent hypovolemic shock and maintain cardiac output (lactated Ringer's solution or a fluid replacement formula; additional I.V. lines may be needed)
◆ antimicrobial therapy (all patients with major burns)
◆ correction of electrolyte imbalances, transfusion and replacement blood products as indicated by laboratory results, and dialysis for renal failure or myoglobinuria
◆ closely monitoring intake and output, frequently checking vital signs (every 15 minutes), possibly inserting an indwelling urinary catheter
◆ nasogastric tube to decompress the stomach and avoid aspiration of stomach contents
◆ irrigating the wound with copious amounts of normal saline solution (chemical burns)
◆ surgical intervention, including skin grafts and more thorough surgical cleaning (major burns).

Special considerations

◆ Don't treat the burn wound for a patient being transferred to a specialty facility within 4 hours. Maintain airway, breathing, and circulation. Wrap the patient in a sterile sheet and blanket for warmth, elevate the burned extremity, and prepare the patient for transport.
  Upon discharge or during prolonged care:
◆ Ensure increased caloric intake due to increased metabolic rate to promote healing and recovery.
◆ Give the patient complete discharge instructions, teaching him what he needs to know about home care; stress the importance of keeping the dressing clean and dry, elevating the burned extremity for the first 24 hours, and having the wound rechecked in 1 to 2 days. Also

Using the Rule of Nines and the Lund-Browder chart

You can quickly estimate the extent of an adult patient's burn by using the Rule of Nines. This method divides an adult's body surface area (BSA) into percentages. To use this method, mentally transfer your patient's burns to the body chart shown below, then add up the corresponding percentages for each burned body section. The total, an estimate of the extent of your patient's burns, enters into the formula to determine his initial fluid replacement needs.

You can't use the Rule of Nines for infants and children because their body section percentages differ from those of adults. For example, an infant's head accounts for about 17% at the total BSA compared with 7% for an adult. Instead, use the Lund-Browder chart.

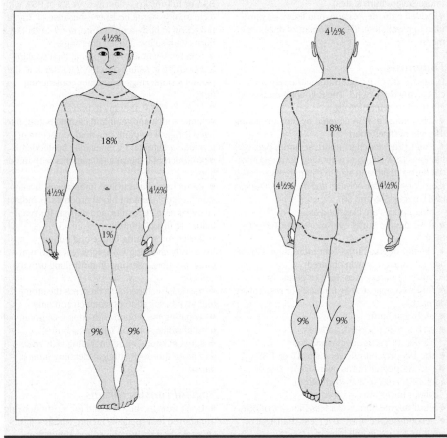

stress the importance of taking pain medication as needed, especially before dressing changes.

CELLULITIS

Cellulitis is an infection of the dermis or subcutaneous layer of the skin. It may follow damage to the skin, such as a bite or wound. As the cellulitis spreads, fever, erythema, and lymphangitis may occur.

If treated in a timely manner, the prognosis is usually good. Persons with other contributing health factors, such as diabetes, immuno-deficiency, impaired circulation, or neuropathy, have an increased risk of developing or spreading cellulitis.

Causes

Possible causes of cellulitis are bacterial and fungal infections, commonly group A streptococcus and *Staphylococcus aureus*.

Pathophysiology

As the offending organism invades the compromised area, it overwhelms the defensive cells

Lund-Browder chart

To determine the extent of an infant's or a child's burns, use the Lund-Browder chart shown here.

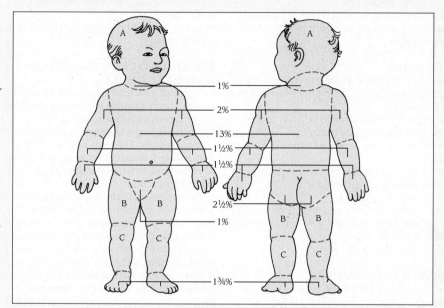

Relative percentages of areas affected by growth

	At birth	0 to 1 yr	1 to 4 yr	5 to 9 yr	10 to 15 yr	Adult
A: Half of head						
	9½%	8½%	6½%	5½%	4½%	3½%
B: Half of thigh						
	2¾%	3¼%	4%	4¼%	4½%	4¾%
C: Half of leg						
	2½%	2½%	2¾%	3%	3¼%	3½%

(neutrophils, eosinophils, basophils, and mast cells) that break down the cellular components, which normally contain and localize the inflammation. As cellulitis progresses, the organism invades tissue around the initial wound site.

Signs and symptoms

♦ Erythema and edema due to inflammatory responses to the injury (classic signs)
♦ Pain at the site and possibly surrounding area due to edema and subsequent increased pressure

♦ Fever and warmth due to temperature increase caused by infection

Complications

♦ Sepsis (untreated cellulitis)
♦ Progression of cellulitis to involve more tissue area
♦ Local abscesses
♦ Thrombophlebitis
♦ Lymphangitis in recurrent cellulitis

Diagnosis

◆ Visual examination and inspection of the affected area reveal the disorder.
◆ White blood cell count shows mild leukocytosis with a left shift.
◆ Blood studies show mildly elevated erythrocyte sedimentation rate.
◆ Culture and gram stain results of fluid from abscesses and bulla are positive for the offending organism.

Treatment

◆ Oral or I.V. penicillin (drug of choice for initial treatment) unless the patient has a known penicillin allergy
◆ Warm soaks to the site to help relieve pain and decrease edema by increasing vasodilation
◆ Pain medication as needed to promote comfort
◆ Elevation of infected extremity to promote comfort and decrease edema
◆ Modified bed rest
◆ Protective footwear for ambulation

AGE ALERT *Cellulitis of the lower extremity is more likely to develop into thrombophlebitis in an elderly patient.*

Special considerations

◆ Assess the patient for an increase in size of the affected area or a worsening of pain. Administer an antibiotic, an analgesic, and warm soak as ordered.
◆ Emphasize the importance of complying with treatment to prevent relapse.
◆ Instruct the patient to use the shower instead of the bathtub until the skin problem has healed to prevent spreading the infection.
◆ To prevent recurrent cellulitis, teach the patient to maintain good general hygiene and to carefully clean abrasions and cuts. Urge early treatment to prevent the spread of infection.
◆ Describe the importance of range-of-motion exercises to prevent deep vein thrombosis.
◆ Encourage patients with diabetes and neuropathy to see a podiatrist on a regular basis.

DERMATITIS

Dermatitis is an inflammation of the skin that occurs in several forms: atopic (see "Atopic dermatitis" in chapter 12), seborrheic, nummular eczematous, contact, chronic, localized neurodermatitis (lichen simplex chronicus), exfoliative, and stasis. (See *Types of dermatitis,* pages 570 to 573.)

Special considerations

◆ Warn the patient that drowsiness is possible with the use of antihistamines to relieve day-

time itching. If nocturnal itching interferes with sleep, suggest methods for inducing natural sleep, such as drinking a glass of warm milk, to prevent overuse of sedatives.
◆ Assist the patient in scheduling daily skin care. Keep his fingernails short to limit excoriation and secondary infections caused by scratching.
◆ Apply cool, moist compresses to relieve itching and burning.

FOLLICULITIS, FURUNCLES, AND CARBUNCLES

Folliculitis is a bacterial infection of a hair follicle that causes a pustule to form. The infection can be superficial (*follicular impetigo* or *Bockhart's impetigo*) or deep (*sycosis barbae*).

Furuncles, also known as boils, are another form of deep folliculitis. Carbuncles are a group of interconnected furuncles. (See *Follicular skin infection,* page 573.)

The incidence of folliculitis in the general population is difficult to determine because many of those affected never seek treatment.

With appropriate treatment, the prognosis for patients with folliculitis is good. The disorder usually resolves within 2 to 3 weeks. The prognosis for patients with carbuncles depends on the severity of the infection and the patient's physical condition and ability to resist infection.

Causes

The most common cause of folliculitis, furuncles, and carbuncles is coagulase-positive *Staphylococcus aureus.*

Other causes may include:
◆ *Enterobacter, Klebsiella,* or *Proteus* organisms (These organisms cause gram-negative folliculitis in patients on long-term antibiotic therapy, such as for acne.)
◆ *Methicillin-resistant staphylococcus aureus* (MRSA) (MRSA should be suspected in chronic skin lesions not responsive to antibiotics.)
◆ *Pseudomonas aeruginosa.* (This organism thrives in a warm environment with a high pH and low chlorine content — "hot tub folliculitis.")

Predisposing risk factors include:
◆ debilitation
◆ diabetes
◆ exposure to certain solvents
◆ friction
◆ immunosuppressant therapy
◆ infected wound
◆ poor hygiene
◆ tight clothes.

Pathophysiology

The affecting organism enters the body, usually at a break in the skin barrier (such as a wound site). The organism then causes an inflammatory reaction within the hair follicle.

Signs and symptoms

Folliculitis, furuncles, and carbuncles have different signs and symptoms depending on the degree of the inflammatory reaction involving the hair follicle.

◆ Folliculitis shows as pustules on the scalp, arms, and legs in children and the trunk, buttocks, and legs in adults.

◆ Furuncles show as hard, painful nodules, commonly on the neck, face, axillae, and buttocks. The nodules enlarge for several days, then rupture, discharging pus and necrotic material; after the nodules rupture, pain subsides but erythema and edema persist for days or weeks.

◆ Carbuncles show as extremely painful, deep abscesses draining through multiple openings onto the skin surface, usually around several hair follicles, with accompanying fever and malaise. Carbuncles are now rare.

Complications

◆ Scarring
◆ Bacteremia or cellulitis
◆ Metastatic seeding of a cardiac valve defect or arthritic joint

Diagnosis

◆ Patient history shows preexistent furuncles (carbuncles).
◆ Physical examination reveals the presence of the skin lesion (folliculitis or carbuncle).
◆ Wound cultures of the infected site usually show *S. aureus.*
◆ Blood studies may reveal elevated white blood cell count (leukocytosis).

Treatment

Appropriate treatments include:
◆ cleaning the infected area thoroughly with antibacterial soap and water
◆ applying warm, wet compresses to promote vasodilation and drainage from the lesions
◆ applying a topical antibiotic, such as mupirocin ointment or clindamycin or erythromycin solution.

Specific treatments include:
◆ folliculitis (extensive infection) — giving a systemic antibiotic, such as a cephalosporin (Ancef) or dicloxacillin (Dycill)
◆ furuncles — incision and drainage of ripe lesions after applying warm, wet compresses,

then giving a systemic antibiotic based on results of culture and sensitivity testing
◆ carbuncles — systemic antibiotic therapy and incision and drainage based on results of culture and sensitivity testing.

Special considerations

Care for patients with folliculitis, furunculosis, and carbunculosis is basically supportive and emphasizes teaching the patient scrupulous personal and family hygiene measures. Taking the necessary precautions to prevent the spread of infection is also an important part of care. (See *Preventing the spread of follicular skin lesions,* page 574.)

◆ Caution the patient never to squeeze a boil because this may cause it to rupture into the surrounding area and cause scarring.

◆ Advise the patient with recurrent furunculosis to have a physical examination because an underlying disease, such as diabetes, may be present or the patient may have an impaired immune system.

◆ Trauma resulting from hairstyles, such as cornrowing (gathering the hair into tight braids or tufts), can cause folliculitis.

FUNGAL INFECTIONS

Fungal infections of the skin are commonly regarded as superficial infections affecting the hair, nails, and *dermatophytes* (the dead top layer of the skin). They are unique in that they infect and survive on the keratin within these structures. The most common fungal infections are tinea and candidiasis.

Tinea infections are classified by the body location in which they occur. Tinea commonly infects children and adolescents. Obese patients are also at greater risk for these infections, especially in skin folds that are constantly moist. Some forms, such as *tinea cruris* (a fungal infection of the groin), infect one sex more than the other. Tinea cruris is more common in men.

Candidiasis can infect the skin or mucous membranes. These infections are also classified according to the infected site or area. *Candida* organisms are the normal flora found in some people (on the skin, in the mouth, GI tract, and genitalia).

Candidiasis usually occurs in children and immunosuppressed individuals. There are also higher rates of candidiasis in pregnant women and in patients with diabetes mellitus, as well as those with indwelling catheters and I.V. lines.

The prognosis for tinea and candidiasis is good. Both usually respond well to appropriate drug therapy and resolve completely. It's also

(Text continues on page 572.)

Types of dermatitis

Type	Cause
Contact dermatitis Often sharply demarcated inflammation of the skin resulting from contact with an irritating chemical or atopic allergen (a substance producing an allergic reaction in the skin) and irritation of the skin resulting from contact with concentrated substances to which the skin is sensitive, such as perfumes, soaps, chemicals, or metals and alloys (such as nickel used in jewelry)	◆ Mild irritants: chronic exposure to detergents or solvents ◆ Strong irritants: damage on contact with acids or alkalis ◆ Allergens: sensitization after repeated exposure
Exfoliative dermatitis Severe skin inflammation characterized by redness and widespread erythema and scaling, covering virtually the entire skin surface	◆ Preexisting skin lesions progressing to exfoliative stage, such as in contact dermatitis, drug reaction, lymphoma, leukemia, or atopic dermatitis ◆ May be idiopathic
Hand or foot dermatitis A skin disease characterized by inflammatory eruptions of the hands or feet	◆ In many cases unknown, but may result from irritant or allergic contact ◆ Excessively dry skin can be a contributing factor ◆ 50% of patients are atopic
Localized neurodermatitis (lichen simplex chronicus, essential pruritus) Superficial inflammation of the skin characterized by itching and papular eruptions that appear on thickened, hyperpigmented skin	◆ Chronic scratching or rubbing of a primary lesion or insect bite or other skin irritation ◆ May be psychogenic
Nummular eczematous dermatitis A chronic form of dermatitis characterized by inflammation in coin-shaped, scaling, or vesicular patches, usually pruritic	◆ Possibly precipitated by stress, dry skin, irritants, or scratching
Seborrheic dermatitis A subacute skin disease affecting the scalp, face, and occasionally other areas that's characterized by lesions covered with yellow or brownish gray scales	◆ Unknown; stress, immunodeficiency, and neurologic conditions may be predisposing factors; related to the yeast *Pityrosporum ovale* (normal flora)

Signs and symptoms	Treatment and intervention
◆ Mild irritants and allergens: erythema and small vesicles that ooze, scale, and itch ◆ Strong irritants: blisters and ulcerations ◆ Classic allergic response: clearly defined lesions, with straight lines following points of contact ◆ Severe allergic reaction: marked erythema, blistering, and edema of affected areas	◆ Eliminating known allergens and decreasing exposure to irritants; wearing protective clothing, such as gloves; and washing immediately after contact with irritants or allergens ◆ A topical anti-inflammatory (including a corticosteroid), a systemic corticosteroid for edema and bullae, an antihistamine, and local applications of Burow's solution (for blisters)
◆ Generalized dermatitis, with acute loss of stratum corneum, erythema, and scaling ◆ Sensation of tight skin ◆ Hair loss ◆ Possible fever, sensitivity to cold, shivering, gynecomastia, and lymphadenopathy	◆ Hospitalization, with protective isolation and hygienic measures to prevent secondary bacterial infection ◆ Open wet dressings, with colloidal baths ◆ Bland lotions over a topical corticosteroid ◆ Maintenance of constant environmental temperature to prevent chilling or overheating ◆ Careful monitoring of renal and cardiac status ◆ A systemic antibiotic and a steroid
◆ Redness and scaling of the palms or soles ◆ May produce painful fissures ◆ Some cases present with blisters (dyshidrotic eczema)	◆ Same as for nummular eczematous dermatitis ◆ Severe cases may require a systemic steroid
◆ Intense, sometimes continual scratching ◆ Thick, sharp-bordered, possibly dry, scaly lesions with raised papules and accentuated skin lines (lichenification) ◆ Usually affects easy-to-reach areas, such as ankles, lower legs, anogenital area, back of neck, and ears ◆ One or several lesions may be present; asymmetric distribution	◆ Scratching must stop; then lesions disappear in about 2 weeks ◆ Fixed dressings or Unna's boot to cover affected areas ◆ A topical corticosteroid under occlusion or by intralesional injection ◆ An antihistamine and open wet dressings ◆ Emollients ◆ Patient informed about underlying cause
◆ Round, nummular (coin-shaped), red lesions, usually on arms and legs, with distinct borders of crusts and scales ◆ Possible oozing and severe itching ◆ Summertime remissions common, with wintertime recurrence	◆ Elimination of known irritants ◆ Measures to relieve dry skin: increased humidification, limited frequency of baths, use of bland soap and bath oils, and application of emollients ◆ Application of wet dressings in acute phase ◆ A topical corticosteroid (occlusive dressings or intralesional injections) for persistent lesions ◆ A tar preparation and an antihistamine to control itching ◆ An antibiotic for secondary infection
◆ Eruptions in areas with many sebaceous glands (usually scalp, face, chest, axillae, and groin) and in skin folds ◆ Itching, redness, and inflammation of affected areas; lesions may appear greasy; fissures may occur ◆ Indistinct, occasionally yellowish scaly patches from excess stratum corneum (dandruff may be a mild seborrheic dermatitis)	◆ Removal of scales with frequent washing and shampooing with selenium sulfide suspension (most effective), zinc pyrithione, ketoconazole 2%, or tar and salicylic acid shampoo ◆ Application of a topical corticosteroid and an antifungal to the involved area

(continued)

Types of dermatitis *(continued)*

Type	Cause
Stasis dermatitis A condition usually caused by impaired circulation and characterized by eczema of the legs with edema, hyperpigmentation, and persistent inflammation	◆ Secondary to peripheral vascular diseases affecting the legs, such as recurrent thrombophlebitis and resultant chronic venous insufficiency

---

important to reduce risk factors to obtain a good outcome from the infection. Antifungal therapy usually resolves candidiasis, but if risk factors aren't avoided, a chronic condition can develop.

Causes
Causes of candidiasis include:
◆ bone marrow suppression and neutropenia in immunocompromised patients (at greater risk for the disseminating form)
◆ *Candida* overgrowth in the mouth (thrush)
◆ *Candida albicans,* normal GI flora (causes candidiasis in susceptible patients)
◆ overgrowth of *Candida* organisms and infection due to depletion of the normal flora (such as with antibiotic therapy).
   Tinea infections are caused by:
◆ contact with contaminated objects or surfaces
◆ *Epidermophyton, Microsporum,* or *Trichophyton* organisms.
   Risk factors for tinea include:
◆ antibiotic therapy with suppression of normal flora
◆ exposure to the causative organisms
◆ obesity
◆ softened skin from prolonged water contact, such as with water sports or diaphoresis.

Pathophysiology
In tinea infections, fungi attack the outer, dead skin layers. Fungi prefer a dark, warm, moist environment. Tinea infections can be spread from human to human, animal to human, or soil to human. Tinea corpis, for example, can be contracted from animals infected with *Microsporum canis* or *Trichophyton mentagrophytes,* and also from humans infected with *Trichophyton rubrum.*
   In candidiasis, the *Candida* organism penetrates the epidermis after it binds to integrin re-

ceptors and adhesion molecules. The secretion of proteolytic enzymes facilitates tissue invasion. An inflammatory response results from the attraction of neutrophils to the area and from activation of the complement cascade.

Signs and symptoms
Tinea
◆ Erythema and pustules in a ringlike formation
◆ Itching, commonly severe

Candidiasis
◆ Superficial papules and pustules caused by proteolytic enzyme destruction of keratin
◆ Erythematous and edematous areas of the infected epidermis or mucous membrane (with progression of inflammation, a white-yellow, curdlike crust covering the infected area) caused by the release of possible toxins by the fungus
◆ Severe pruritus and pain at the lesion sites (common) caused by inflammation
◆ White coating of the tongue and possibly lesions in the mouth (thrush)

Complications
◆ Secondary bacterial infections of wounds opened by scratching
◆ Ulcers with chronic forms (candidiasis lesions)
◆ Candidal meningitis, endocarditis, or septicemia due to systemic disseminating candidiasis

Diagnosis
◆ Culture determines the causative organism and suggests the mode of infection transmission (tinea infection).
◆ Microscopic examination of a potassium hydroxide–treated skin scraping and culture reveals tinea and candidal infections.

Signs and symptoms

◆ Varicosities and edema common, but obvious vascular insufficiency not always present
◆ Usually affects the lower leg just above internal malleolus or sites of trauma or irritation
◆ Early signs: dusky-red deposits of hemosiderin in skin, with itching and dimpling of subcutaneous tissue
◆ Later signs: edema, redness, and scaling of large areas of legs
◆ Possible fissures, crusts, and ulcers

Treatment and intervention

◆ Measures to prevent venous stasis: avoidance of prolonged sitting or standing, use of support stockings, weight reduction in obesity, and leg elevation
◆ Corrective surgery for underlying cause
◆ After ulcer develops, encourage rest periods with legs elevated, open wet dressings, Unna's boot (zinc gelatin dressing provides continuous pressure to affected areas), and an antibiotic for secondary infection after wound culture

CLOSER LOOK

Follicular skin infection

The degree of hair follicle involvement in bacterial skin infection ranges from superficial erythema and pustule of a single follicle to deep abscesses (carbuncles) involving several follicles.

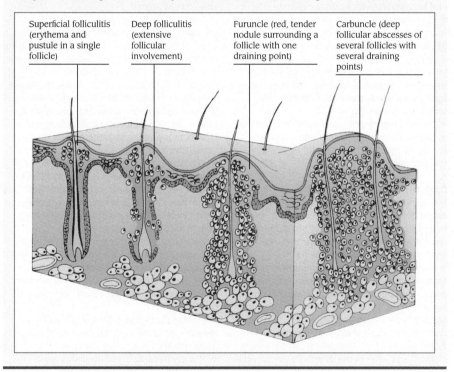

Superficial folliculitis (erythema and pustule in a single follicle)

Deep folliculitis (extensive follicular involvement)

Furuncle (red, tender nodule surrounding a follicle with one draining point)

Carbuncle (deep follicular abscesses of several follicles with several draining points)

PREVENTION

Preventing the spread of follicular skin lesions

To help prevent bacteria from spreading to family members, explain that the patient shouldn't share towels or washcloths and should change clothes and bedding daily. Recommend washing all the patient's towels, washcloths, bedding, and clothes in hot water and cleaning the bathtub he uses with bleach or a strong disinfectant. Encourage the patient to change dressings frequently and to discard them promplty in a paper bag.

Treatment

◆ For tinea, topical seleniumsulfide lotion 2.5%, topical sodium thiosulfate 25%, zinc pyrithione shampoo 1%, or imidazole antifungal agents

◆ A topical antifungal, such as ketoconazole or oral ketoconazole for extensive disease

◆ Oral therapy with griseofulvin if no response to topical treatment to arrest fungal cell activity by disrupting its miotic spindle structure (tinea)

◆ Oral ketoconazole for infections resistant to griseofulvin therapy to make the fungus more susceptible to osmotic pressure; other oral medications include fluconazole (Diflucan) and terbinafine (Lamisil)

◆ Eliminating risk factors (tinea and candidiasis)

◆ Oral nystatin (Mycostatin) and a topical antifungal, such as miconazole (Monistat) (candidiasis)

Special considerations

Management of tinea infections requires application of a topical agent, observation for sensitivity reactions, observation for secondary bacterial infections, and patient teaching. Specific care varies by site of infection:

◆ For tinea capitis — Perform treatments or take medications as directed. Discontinue medications if the condition worsens, and notify the physician. Use good hand-washing technique, and teach the patient to do the same. Spores of tinea capitis are shed in the air around an infected patient or may spread on contaminated clothing and other personal articles. To prevent spread of infection to others, advise the patient to wash his towels, bedding, and combs frequently in hot water and to avoid sharing them. Suggest that family members be checked for tinea capitis.

◆ For tinea corporis — Use abdominal pads between skin folds for the patient with excessive abdominal girth; change pads frequently. Check the patient daily for excoriated, newly denuded areas of skin. Apply wet Burrow's compresses two or three times daily to decrease inflammation and help remove scales.

◆ For tinea unguium — Keep nails short and straight. Gently remove debris under the nails with an orangewood stick. Prepare the patient for prolonged therapy and possible adverse effects of griseofulvin, such as headache, nausea, vomiting, and photosensitivity. If using ketoconazole or terbinafine, monitor liver function test results.

◆ For tinea pedis — Encourage the patient to expose his feet to air whenever possible, and to wear sandals or leather shoes and clean cotton socks. Instruct the patient to wash his feet twice daily and, after drying them thoroughly, to apply antifungal cream followed by antifungal powder to absorb perspiration and prevent excoriation. Socks should be washed in hot water. Sandals or beach slippers should be worn in public places, such as showers and locker rooms, and shouldn't be shared.

◆ For tinea cruris — Instruct the patient to dry the affected area thoroughly after bathing and to evenly apply antifungal powder after applying the topical antifungal agent. Advise him to wear loose-fitting clothing, which should be changed frequently and washed in hot water. Encourage the patient to take sitz baths to reduce itching.

◆ Use of griseofulvin doesn't require routine monitoring of liver function test results unless treatment is prolonged or the dosage is exceptionally high.

For the patient with candidiasis:

◆ Instruct a patient using nystatin solution to swish it around in his mouth for several minutes before he swallows it. Instruct the patient not to drink or eat for at least 30 minutes after drug administration.

◆ Swab nystatin on the oral mucosa of an infant with thrush. Treat the infant after a feeding because feedings will wash the medication away. The infant's mother should also be treated to prevent the infection from being passed back and forth.

◆ Provide the patient with a nonirritating mouthwash to loosen tenacious secretions and a soft toothbrush to avoid irritation.

◆ Use dry padding in intertriginous areas of obese patients to prevent irritation.

◆ Note dates of insertion of I.V. catheters, and replace them according to facility policy to prevent phlebitis. Do the same with indwelling urinary catheters.

◆ Assess the patient with candidiasis for underlying causes, such as diabetes mellitus. If the patient is receiving amphotericin B for systemic candidiasis, he may have severe chills, fever, anorexia, nausea, and vomiting. Premedicate with acetaminophen, an antihistamine, or an antiemetic, as ordered, to help minimize adverse reactions.

◆ Frequently check vital signs of patients with systemic infections. Provide appropriate supportive care. In patients with renal involvement, carefully monitor intake and output and urine blood and protein levels.

◆ Check high-risk patients daily, especially those receiving an antibiotic, for patchy areas, irritation, sore throat, bleeding of mouth or gums, or other signs of superinfection. Check for vaginal discharge; record color and amount.

◆ Encourage women in their third trimester of pregnancy to be examined for vaginal candidiasis to protect their infants from infection at birth.

PRESSURE ULCERS

Pressure ulcers, commonly called *pressure sores* or *bedsores,* are localized areas of cellular necrosis that are most common in the skin and subcutaneous tissue over bony prominences. These ulcers may be superficial, caused by local skin irritation with subsequent surface maceration, or deep, originating in underlying tissue. Deep lesions commonly go undetected until they penetrate the skin, but by then they have usually caused subcutaneous damage. (See *Staging pressure ulcers,* pages 576 and 577.)

Most pressure ulcers develop over five body locations: sacral area, greater trochanter, ischial tuberosity, heel, and lateral malleolus. Collectively, these areas account for 95% of all pressure ulcer sites. Patients who have contractures are at an increased risk for developing pressure ulcers because of the added pressure on the tissue and the alignment of the bones.

AGE ALERT *Age also has a role in the incidence of pressure ulcers. Muscle is lost with aging, and skin elasticity decreases. Both of these factors increase the risk of developing pressure ulcers.*

Partial-thickness ulcers usually involve the dermis and epidermis; with treatment, these wounds heal within a few weeks. Full-thickness ulcers also involve the dermis and epidermis, but in these wounds the damage is more severe and complete. There may also be damage to the deeper tissue layers. Ulcers of the subcutaneous tissue and muscle may require several months to heal. If the damage has affected the bone in addition to the skin layers, osteomyelitis may occur, which will prolong healing time.

Causes

◆ Constant moisture on the skin causing tissue maceration

◆ Friction or shearing forces causing damage to the epidermal and upper dermal skin layers

◆ Immobility and decreased level of activity

◆ Impaired hygiene status, such as with urinary or fecal incontinence, leading to skin breakdown

◆ Malnutrition (associated with pressure ulcer development)

◆ Medical conditions, such as diabetes and orthopedic injuries (These conditions may predispose the patient to pressure ulcer development.)

◆ Psychological factors, such as depression and chronic emotional stresses (Certain psychological factors may have a role in pressure ulcer development.)

Pathophysiology

A pressure ulcer is caused by an injury to the skin and its underlying tissues. The pressure exerted on the area causes ischemia and hypoxemia to the affected tissues because of decreased blood flow to the site. As the capillaries collapse, thrombosis occurs, which subsequently leads to tissue edema and progression to tissue necrosis. Ischemia also adds to an accumulation of waste products at the site, which in turn leads to the production of toxins. The toxins further break down the tissue and eventually lead to cell death.

Signs and symptoms

◆ Blanching erythema, varying from pink to bright red depending on the patient's skin color; in dark-skinned people, purple discoloration or a darkening of normal skin color (first clinical sign); when the examiner presses a finger on the reddened area, the "pressed on" area whitens and color returns within 1 to 3 seconds if capillary refill is good

◆ Pain at the site and surrounding area caused by increased pressure from edema

◆ Localized edema due to the inflammatory response

◆ Increased body temperature due to initial inflammatory response (in more severe cases, cool skin due to more severe damage or necrosis)

◆ Nonblanching erythema (more severe cases) ranging from dark red to purple or cyanotic; indicates deeper dermal involvement

◆ Blisters, crusts, or scaling as the skin deteriorates and the ulcer progresses

Staging pressure ulcers

The National Pressure Ulcer Advisory Panel has updated the staging of pressure ulcers to include the original four stages but also has added two other stages called *suspected deep tissue injury* and *unstageable.*

Suspected deep tissue injury

Suspected deep tissue injury involves maroon or purple intact skin or a blood-filled blister due to damage from shearing or pressure on the underlying soft tissue. Before the discoloration occurs, the area may be painful; mushy, firm, or boggy; and warmer or cooler as compared to other tissue.

Stage I

A stage I pressure ulcer is an area of intact skin that does not blanch and is usually over a bony prominence. Skin that is darkly pigmented may not show blanching but its color may differ from surrounding area. The area may be painful, firm or soft, or warmer or cooler when compared to the surrounding tissue.

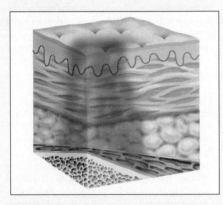

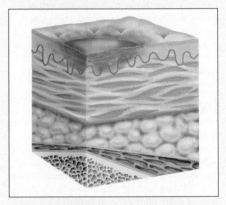

Stage III

A stage III pressure ulcer is a full-thickness wound with tissue loss. The subcutaneous tissue may be visible but muscle, tendon, or bone is not exposed. Slough may be present but it does not hide the depth of the tissue loss. Undermining and tunneling may be present.

Stage IV

A stage IV pressure ulcer involves full-thickness skin loss with exposed muscle, bone, and tendon. Eschar and sloughing may be present as well as undermining and tunneling.

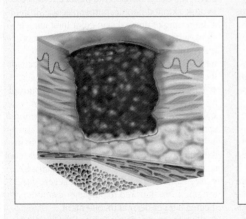

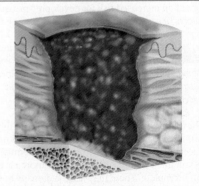

Stage II

A stage II pressure ulcer is a superficial partial-thickness wound that presents clinically as a shallow, open ulcer without slough and with a red and pink wound bed. This term shouldn't be used to describe perineal dermatitis, maceration, tape burns, skin tears or excoriation. It should only be used to describe an abrasion, a blister, or a shallow crater that involves the epidermis and dermis.

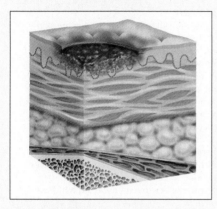

Unstageable

An unstageable pressure ulcer involves full-thickness tissue loss. The base of the ulcer is covered by yellow, tan, gray, green, or brown slough or tan, brown, or black eschar. Some may have both slough and eschar. The pressure ulcer cannot be staged until enough eschar or slough is removed to expose the base of the wound.

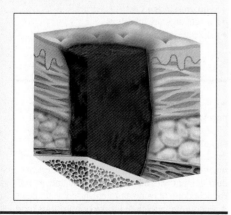

◆ Usually, dusky red appearance, doesn't bleed easily, warm to the touch, and possibly mottled (deep ulcer originating at the bony prominence below the skin surface)
◆ Possibly, foul-smelling and purulent drainage from the ulcerated lesion
◆ Eschar tissue on and around the lesion due to the necrotic tissue that prevents healthy tissue growth

Complications

◆ Progression of the pressure ulcer to a more severe state (greatest risk)
◆ Secondary infections, such as sepsis
◆ Loss of limb from bone involvement, or osteomyelitis

Diagnosis

Diagnosis is based on:
◆ physical examination showing presence of ulcer
◆ wound culture with exudate or evidence of infection
◆ elevated white blood cell count with infection
◆ possibly elevated erythrocyte sedimentation rate
◆ total serum protein and serum albumin levels showing severe hypoproteinemia
◆ elevated temperature with infection.

Treatment

◆ Successful treatment relieves pressure on the affected area, keeps the area clean and dry, and promotes healing. (See *Preventing pressure ulcers*, page 578.)

Special considerations

◆ During each shift, check the skin of bedridden or high-risk patients for possible changes in color, turgor, temperature, and sensation. Assess the patient for pain. Examine an existing ulcer for any change in size or degree of damage. When using pressure relief aids or topical agents, explain their function to the patient.
◆ Prevent pressure ulcers by repositioning the bedridden patient at least every 2 hours around the clock. To minimize the effects of a shearing force, use a footboard and raise the head of the bed to an angle not exceeding 60 degrees. Also, use a draw or pull sheet to turn the patient or to pull him up. Keep the patient's knees slightly flexed for short periods. Perform passive ROM exercises, or encourage the patient to do active exercises, if possible.
◆ To prevent pressure ulcers in immobilized patients, use pressure relief aids on their beds.
◆ Provide meticulous skin care. Keep the skin clean and dry without the use of harsh soaps.

Preventing pressure ulcers

Prevent pressure ulcers by repositioning the bedridden patient at least every 2 hours around the clock. To minimize the effects of a shearing force, use a footboard and raise the head of the bed to an angle not exceeding 60 degrees. Also, use a draw or pull sheet to turn the patient or to pull him up. Keep the patient's knees slightly flexed for short periods. Perform passive range-of-motion exercises, or encourage the patient to do active exercises if possible.

Pressure relief aids

To prevent pressure ulcers in immobilized patients, use pressure relief aids on their beds.

♦ *Gel flotation pads* disperse pressure over a greater skin surface area; they're convenient and adaptable for home and wheelchair use.

♦ *Alternating pressure mattress* contains tube-like sections, running lengthwise, that deflate and reinflate, changing areas of pressure. Use the mattress with a single, untucked sheet because layers of linen decrease its effectiveness.

♦ *Convoluted foam mattress* minimizes area of skin pressure with its alternating areas of depression and elevation: soft, elevated foam areas cushion skin; depressed areas relieve pressure. This mattress should be used with a single, loosely tucked sheet and is adaptable for home and wheelchair use. If the patient is incontinent, cover the mattress with a plastic sleeve.

♦ *Spanco mattress* has polyester fibers with silicon tubes to decrease pressure without limiting the patient's position. It has no weight limitations.

♦ *Sheepskin* is soft, dry, absorbent, and easy to clean. It should be in direct contact with the patient's skin. It's available in sizes to fit elbows and heels and is adaptable for home use.

♦ *Air-fluidized bed* supports the patient at a subcapillary pressure point and provides a warm, relaxing, therapeutic airflow. It eliminates friction and maceration.

♦ *Low air-loss beds*, such as Flexicare and Accucare, slow the drying of any saline soaks, and elderly patients often experience less disorientation than with high air-loss beds. The head of the bed can be elevated so there's less chance of aspiration, especially in patients who require tube feeding. Patients can get out of bed more easily on low air-loss surfaces.

Skin care

Provide meticulous skin care. Keep the skin clean and dry without the use of harsh soaps. Gently massaging the skin around the affected area—not on it—promotes healing. Thoroughly rub moisturizing lotions into the skin to prevent maceration of the skin surface. Change bed linens frequently for patients who are diaphoretic or incontinent. Use a fecal incontinence bag for incontinent patients.

Skin-damaging agents to avoid include:

♦ harsh alkaline soaps
♦ alcohol-based products (can cause vasoconstriction)
♦ tincture of benzoin (may cause painful erosions)
♦ hexachlorophene (may irritate the central nervous system)
♦ petroleum gauze.

Topical dressings

Types of topical dressings that aid in prevention and treatment of pressure ulcers include:

♦ transparent films
♦ hydrocolloid dressings
♦ hydrogel dressings
♦ foam dressings
♦ calcium alginate dressings
♦ gauze dressings.

Gently massaging the skin around the affected area—not on it—promotes healing. Thoroughly rub moisturizing lotions into the skin to prevent maceration of the skin surface. Change bedding frequently for patients who are diaphoretic or incontinent or who have large amounts of drainage from wounds, suture lines, or drain sites. Use a fecal incontinence bag for incontinent patients.

♦ Clean open lesions with a normal saline solution. Dressings, if needed, should be porous and lightly taped to healthy skin. Debridement of necrotic tissue may be necessary to allow healing. One method is to apply open wet dressings and allow them to dry on the ulcer. Removal of the dressings mechanically debrides exudate and necrotic tissue. Other methods include surgical debridement with a fine scalpel blade and chemical debridement using a proteolytic enzyme agent.

♦ Encourage adequate intake of nutritious food and fluids to maintain body weight and promote healing. Consult with the dietitian to provide a diet that promotes granulation of new tissue. Encourage the debilitated patient to eat frequent, small meals that provide protein and are calorie rich. Assist weakened patients with their meals.

PSORIASIS

Psoriasis is a chronic, recurrent disease marked by epidermal proliferation and characterized by recurring partial remissions and exacerbations. Flare-ups are commonly related to specific systemic and environmental factors, but may be unpredictable. Widespread involvement is called exfoliative, or erythrodermic, psoriasis.

Psoriasis affects about 2% of the population in the United States. Although this disorder usually affects young adults, it may strike at any age, including infancy. Genetic factors predetermine the incidence of psoriasis; researchers have discovered a significantly greater incidence of certain human leukocyte antigens (HLAs) in families with psoriasis.

Flare-ups can usually be controlled with therapy. Appropriate treatment depends on the type of psoriasis, extent of the disease, the patient's response, and the effect of the disease on the patient's lifestyle. No permanent cure exists, and all methods of treatment are palliative.

Causes

Causes of psoriasis include:
◆ environmental factors
◆ flare-up of guttate (drop-shaped) lesions due to infections, especially beta-hemolytic streptococci
◆ genetically determined tendency to develop the disorder
◆ immune disorder, as shown in the HLA type in families
◆ isomorphic effect or Koebner's phenomenon, in which lesions develop at sites of injury due to trauma.

Other contributing factors include:
◆ climate (cold weather tends to exacerbate psoriasis)
◆ emotional stress
◆ endocrine changes
◆ pregnancy
◆ smoking.

Pathophysiology

A skin cell normally takes 14 days to move from the basal layer to the stratum corneum, where it's sloughed off after 14 days of normal wear and tear. Thus, the life cycle of a normal skin cell is 28 days compared with only 4 days for a psoriatic skin cell. This markedly shortened cycle doesn't allow time for the cell to mature.

Consequently, the stratum corneum becomes thick and flaky, producing the cardinal manifestations of psoriasis. Recent research suggests that psoriasis may be a T-cell mediated autoimmune response to an unidentified antigen.

Signs and symptoms

◆ Itching and occasional pain from dry, cracked, encrusted lesions (most common)
◆ Erythematous and usually well-defined plaques, sometimes covering large areas of the body (psoriatic lesions)
◆ Lesions most commonly on the scalp, chest, elbows, knees, back, and buttocks
◆ Plaques with characteristic silver scales that either flake off easily or thicken, covering the lesion; scale removal can produce fine bleeding
◆ Occasional small guttate lesions (usually thin and erythematous, with few scales), either alone or with plaques

Complications

◆ Spread to fingernails, producing small indentations or pits and yellow or brown discoloration (about 60% of patients)
◆ Accumulation of thick, crumbly debris under the nail, causing it to separate from the nail bed (onycholysis)
◆ Infection from excoriations, secondary to itching

Rarely, psoriasis becomes pustular, taking one of two forms:
◆ localized pustular psoriasis, with pustules on the palms and soles that remain sterile until opened
◆ generalized pustular (von Zumbusch) psoriasis, typically occurring with fever, leukocytosis, and malaise, with groups of pustules coalescing to form lakes of pus on red skin (also remain sterile until opened), commonly involving the tongue and oral mucosa
◆ erythrodermic psoriasis (least common form), which is an inflammatory form of the disorder characterized by periodic fiery erythema and exfoliation of the skin with severe itching and pain
◆ arthritic symptoms, usually in one or more joints of the fingers or toes, the larger joints, or sometimes the sacroiliac joints, which may progress to spondylitis, and morning stiffness (occurring in 7% to 42% of patients with the disorder).

Diagnosis

◆ Patient history, appearance of the lesions and, if needed, the results of skin biopsy reveal the disorder.

♦ Serum uric acid level is usually elevated in severe cases due to accelerated nucleic acid degradation, but without indications of gout.
♦ HLA-Cw6, -B13, and -Bw57 may be present in early-onset familial psoriasis.

Treatment

♦ Topical agents, including corticosteroids, coal tar, anthralin, calcipotriene, and tazarotene, to resolve psoriasis in 6 to 8 weeks; agents may be rotated, with effects evident in 2 to 3 weeks; keratolytics may be added
♦ Ultraviolet B (UVB) phototherapy, excimer lasers (new high-intensity UVB devices) or natural sunlight exposure to retard rapid cell production to the point of minimal erythema
♦ Psoralen plus ultraviolet A (PUVA) photochemotherapy using the photosensitizing drug methoxsalen in combination with UVA to treat more extensive disease
♦ Excimer laser UVB for high-dose light to limited plaques
♦ Systemic treatment with agents such as methotrexate or cyclosporine if topical and phototherapy prove unsuccessful
♦ Moisturizers to keep the skin moist and well lubricated
♦ Intralesional steroid injection for small, stubborn plaques
♦ Cytotoxin, usually methotrexate (Mexate) (last-resort treatment for refractory psoriasis)
♦ A retinoid, such as tazarotene or acitretin, to inhibit malignant transformation of the skin
♦ Cyclosporine (Neoral), an immunosuppressant (in resistive cases)
♦ A low-dose antihistamine, oatmeal baths, emollients, and open wet dressings to help relieve pruritus
♦ Aspirin and local heat to help alleviate the pain of psoriatic arthritis; a nonsteroidal anti-inflammatory in severe cases
♦ A biologic agent, such as etanercept or alefacept, that uses immunology to inhibit cytokine release and target T cells in severe, recalcitrant cases

Special considerations

Design your patient's care plan to include patient teaching and careful monitoring for adverse reactions to therapy.
♦ Make sure the patient understands his prescribed therapy; provide written instructions to avoid confusion. Teach correct application of prescribed ointments, creams, and lotions. A steroid cream, for example, should be applied in a thin film and rubbed gently into the skin until the cream disappears. All topical medications, especially those containing anthralin and tar,

should be applied with a downward motion to avoid rubbing them into the follicles. Gloves must be worn because anthralin stains and injures the skin. After application, the patient may dust himself with powder to prevent anthralin from rubbing off on his clothes. Warn the patient never to put an occlusive dressing over anthralin. Suggest use of mineral oil, then soap and water, to remove anthralin. Caution the patient to avoid scrubbing his skin vigorously to prevent Koebner's phenomenon. If a medication has been applied to the scales to soften them, suggest the patient use a soft brush to remove them.
♦ Watch for adverse reactions, especially allergic reactions to anthralin, atrophy and acne from a steroid, and burning, itching, nausea, and squamous cell epitheliomas from PUVA.
♦ Initially evaluate the patient on methotrexate weekly, then monthly for red blood cell, white blood cell, and platelet counts because cytotoxins may cause hepatic or bone marrow toxicity. Liver biopsy may be done to assess the effects of methotrexate. Patients taking methotrexate shouldn't drink alcohol because of the increased risk of hepatotoxicity.
♦ Caution the patient receiving PUVA therapy to stay out of the sun on the day of treatment, and to protect his eyes with sunglasses that block out UVA rays for 24 hours after treatment. Tell him to wear goggles during exposure to this light.
♦ Be aware that psoriasis can cause psychological problems. Assure the patient that psoriasis isn't contagious and, although exacerbations and remissions occur, they're controllable with treatment. However, be sure he understands that there's no cure. Also, because stressful situations tend to exacerbate psoriasis, help the patient learn effective stress management techniques and coping mechanisms. Explain the relationship between psoriasis and arthritis, but point out that psoriasis causes no other systemic disturbances. Refer all patients to the National Psoriasis Foundation, which provides information and directs patients to local chapters.

SCLERODERMA

Scleroderma (also known as *systemic sclerosis*) is an uncommon disease of diffuse connective tissue disease characterized by inflammatory and then degenerative and fibrotic changes in the skin, blood vessels, synovial membranes, skeletal muscles, and internal organs (especially the esophagus, intestinal tract, thyroid, heart, lungs, and kidneys). There are several forms of scleroderma, including systemic sclerosis (diffuse and limited forms), localized, linear, chemically induced localized, eosinophilia myalgia syndrome, toxic oil syndrome, and graft-versus-host disease.

Scleroderma affects 300,000 people in the United States. More women than men develop the disorder, especially those between ages 30 and 50.

Scleroderma usually progresses slowly. When the condition is limited to the skin, the prognosis is usually favorable. However, about 30% of patients with scleroderma die within 5 years of onset. Death is usually caused by infection or renal or heart failure.

Causes
The cause of scleroderma is unknown, but some possible causes include:
◆ anticancer drugs, such as bleomycin (Blenoxane), or nonopioid analgesics such as pentazocine (Talwin)
◆ environmental exposure to glues, organic solvents, coating materials, or viruses
◆ fibrosis due to an abnormal immune system response
◆ systemic exposure to silica dust or polyvinyl chloride
◆ underlying vascular cause with tissue changes initiated by a persistent perfusion.

Pathophysiology
Scleroderma usually begins in the fingers and extends proximally to the upper arms, shoulders, neck, and face. The skin atrophies, edema and infiltrates containing CD4+ T cells surround the blood vessels, and inflamed collagen fibers become edematous, losing strength and elasticity, and degenerative. The dermis becomes tightly bound to the underlying structures, resulting in atrophy of the affected dermal appendages and destruction of the distal phalanges by osteoporosis. As the disease progresses, this atrophy can affect other areas. For example, in some patients, muscles and joints become fibrotic.

Signs and symptoms
◆ Skin thickening, commonly limited to the distal extremities and face, but which can also involve internal organs (limited systemic sclerosis)
◆ CREST syndrome (a benign subtype of limited systemic sclerosis), which is characterized by calcinosis, Raynaud's phenomenon, esophageal dysfunction, sclerodactyly, and telangiectasia
◆ Generalized skin thickening and involvement of internal organs (diffuse systemic sclerosis)
◆ Patchy skin changes with a teardrop-like appearance known as morphea (localized scleroderma)

◆ Band of thickened skin on the face or extremities that severely damages underlying tissues, causing atrophy and deformity (linear scleroderma)

AGE ALERT *Atrophy and deformity with scleroderma are most common in childhood.*

◆ Raynaud's phenomenon (blanching, cyanosis, and erythema of the fingers and toes when exposed to cold or stress); progressive phalangeal resorption may shorten the fingers (early symptoms)
◆ Pain, stiffness, and swelling of fingers and joints (later symptoms)
◆ Taut, shiny skin over the entire hand and forearm due to skin thickening
◆ Tight and inelastic facial skin, causing a masklike appearance and "pinching" of the mouth; contractures with progressive tightening
◆ Thickened skin over proximal limbs and trunk (diffuse systemic sclerosis)
◆ Frequent reflux, heartburn, dysphagia, and bloating after meals due to GI dysfunction
◆ Abdominal distention, diarrhea, constipation, and malodorous floating stool

Complications
◆ Compromised circulation due to abnormal thickening of the arterial intima, possibly causing slowly healing ulcerations on fingertips or toes leading to gangrene
◆ Decreased food intake and weight loss due to GI symptoms
◆ Arrhythmias and dyspnea due to cardiac and pulmonary fibrosis; malignant hypertension due to renal involvement, called renal crisis (may be fatal if untreated; advanced disease)

Diagnosis
◆ Typical cutaneous changes are the first clue to diagnosis.
◆ Blood studies reveal slightly elevated erythrocyte sedimentation rate, positive rheumatoid factor in 25% to 35% of patients, and positive antinuclear antibody test results.
◆ Urinalysis shows proteinuria, microscopic hematuria, and casts (with renal involvement).
◆ Hand X-rays show terminal phalangeal tuft resorption, subcutaneous calcification, and joint space narrowing and erosion.
◆ Chest X-rays show bilateral basilar pulmonary fibrosis.
◆ GI X-rays reveal distal esophageal hypomotility and stricture, duodenal loop dilation, small-bowel malabsorption pattern, and large diverticula.
◆ Pulmonary function studies show decreased diffusion and vital capacity.

♦ Electrocardiogram reveals nonspecific abnormalities related to myocardial fibrosis.
♦ Skin biopsy shows changes consistent with disease progression, such as marked thickening of the dermis and occlusive vessel changes.

Treatment

There's no cure for scleroderma. Treatment aims to preserve normal body functions and minimize complications and may include:
♦ an immunosuppressant, such as cyclosporine (Neoral) or chlorambucil (Leukeran) (common palliative medications)
♦ a vasodilator and an antihypertensive, such as nifedipine (Adalat), prazosin (Minipress), or topical nitroglycerin (Nitrol); digital sympathectomy; or, rarely, cervical sympathetic blockade to treat Raynaud's phenomenon
♦ digital plaster cast to immobilize the area, minimize trauma, and maintain cleanliness; possible surgical debridement for chronic digital ulceration
♦ an antacid to reduce total acid level in GI tract; proton pump inhibitor, such as omeprazole (prilosec), to block the formation of gastric acid); periodic dilation, and a soft, bland diet for esophagitis with stricture
♦ a broad-spectrum antibiotic to treat small-bowel involvement with erythromycin or tetracycline (preferred drugs) to counteract the bacterial overgrowth in the duodenum and jejunum related to hypomotility
♦ short-term benefit from a vasodilator, such as nifedipine (Adalat) or hydralazine (Apresoline), to decrease contractility and oxygen demand and cause vasodilation (for pulmonary hypertension)
♦ an angiotensin-converting enzyme inhibitor to preserve renal function (early intervention in renal crisis)
♦ physical therapy to maintain function and promote muscle strength, heat therapy to relieve joint stiffness, and patient teaching to make performance of daily activities easier (for hand debilitation).

Special considerations

♦ Assess motion restrictions, pain, vital signs, intake and output, respiratory function, and daily weight.
♦ Because of compromised circulation, warn against finger-stick blood tests.
♦ Remember that air conditioning may aggravate Raynaud's phenomenon.
♦ Help the patient and family adjust to the patient's new body image and to the limitations and dependence that these changes cause.
♦ Teach the patient to avoid fatigue by pacing activities and organizing schedules to include necessary rest.

♦ The patient and family need to accept the fact that this condition is incurable. Encourage them to express their feelings, and help them cope with their fears and frustrations by offering information about the disease, its treatment, and relevant diagnostic tests.
♦ Whenever possible, let the patient participate in treatment by measuring his own intake and output, planning his own diet, giving himself heat therapy, and doing prescribed exercises.
♦ Direct the patient to seek out support groups, which can be found in every state. Instruct the patient to contact the Scleroderma Foundation at 1-800-722-HOPE or to go to *www. scleroderma.org* to find the closest local chapter.

WARTS

Warts, also known as verrucae, are common, benign, viral infections of the skin and adjacent mucous membranes. Although their incidence is greatest in children and young adults, warts can occur at any age. The prognosis varies; many types of warts resolve spontaneously, whereas others need more vigorous and prolonged treatment. Most people eventually develop an immune response to the papillomavirus that causes the warts to disappear spontaneously. An immune response to certain types of warts may develop, but this immune response can be delayed for many years.

Causes

♦ Human papillomavirus (HPV)
♦ Spread on the affected person by auto-inoculation
♦ Transmission by touch and skin-to-skin contact

Pathophysiology

HPV replicates in the epidermal cells, causing irregular thickening of the stratum corneum in the infected areas. People who lack the virus-specific immunity are susceptible to the virus.

Signs and symptoms

Signs and symptoms depend on the type of wart and its location and may include:
♦ rough, elevated, rounded surface, usually occurring on extremities, particularly hands and fingers; most prevalent in children and young adults (common warts [verruca vulgaris])
♦ single, thin, threadlike projection; commonly occurring around the face and neck (filiform)
♦ rough, irregularly shaped, elevated surface, occurring around edges of fingernails and toenails (when severe, extending under the nail and lifting it off the nail bed, causing pain [periungual])

◆ multiple groupings of up to several hundred slightly raised lesions with smooth, flat, or slightly rounded tops, common on the face, neck, chest, knees, dorsa of hands, wrists, and flexor surfaces of the forearms (usually occur in children but can affect adults); often linear distribution due to spread by scratching or shaving (flat or juvenile)
◆ slightly elevated or flat; occurring singly or in large clusters (mosaic warts), primarily at pressure points of the feet (plantar)
◆ fingerlike, horny projection arising from a pea-shaped base, occurring on scalp or near hairline (digitate)
◆ usually small, pink to red, moist, and soft, occurring singly or in large cauliflower-like clusters on the penis, scrotum, vulva, and anus; although transmitted through sexual contact, it isn't always venereal in origin (condyloma acuminatum [moist wart]).

Complications
◆ Autoinoculation
◆ Scar formation
◆ Chronic pain after plantar wart removal and scar formation
◆ Nail deformity after injury to nail matrix
◆ Cervical cancer, with increased risk if a woman smokes (certain strains of HPV)
◆ Esophageal warts (in neonates exposed to genital warts)

AGE ALERT *The presence of perianal warts in children may be a sign of sexual abuse.*

Diagnosis
◆ Physical examination of the patient reveals warts.
◆ Sigmoidoscopy with recurrent anal warts rules out internal involvement necessitating surgery.

Treatment
If immunity develops, warts resolve by themselves. Treatments may include:
◆ a skin irritant, such as salicylic acid or formaldehyde, applied to the wart to try to stimulate an immune response
◆ curettage or cryosurgery (cryosurgical kits are available over-the-counter)
◆ 25% podophyllin in compound with tincture of benzoin for venereal warts
◆ carbon dioxide laser treatment for recalcitrant warts of on the feet, groin, or nail bed
◆ abstinence or condom use until warts are eradicated; partners should also be examined and treated as needed (genital warts).

Special considerations
◆ The use of an antiviral is under investigation; suggestion and hypnosis are occasionally successful, especially with children.
◆ Conscientious adherence to prescribed therapy is essential. The patient's sex partner may also require treatment.

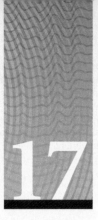

REPRODUCTIVE
SYSTEM

The reproductive system must function properly to ensure survival of the species. The male reproductive system produces sperm and delivers them to the female reproductive tract. The female reproductive system produces the ovum. If a sperm fertilizes an ovum, this system also nurtures and protects the embryo and developing fetus and delivers it at birth. The functioning of the reproductive system is determined not only by anatomic structure but also by complex hormonal, neurologic, vascular, and psychogenic factors.

Anatomically, the main distinction between the male and female is the presence of conspicuous external genitalia in the male. In contrast, the major reproductive organs of the female lie within the pelvic cavity.

Male reproductive system

The male reproductive system consists of the organs that produce and maintain sperm, transfer mature sperm from the testes, and introduce them into the female reproductive tract, where fertilization occurs.

Besides supplying male sex cells (in a process called *spermatogenesis*), the male reproductive system plays a part in the secretion of male sex hormones. The penis also functions in urine elimination.

In males, the reproductive and urinary systems are structurally integrated; most disorders, therefore, affect both systems. Congenital abnormalities or prostate enlargement may impair both sexual and urinary function. Abnormal findings

in the pelvic area may result from pathologic changes in other organ systems, such as the upper urinary and GI tracts, endocrine glands, and neuromusculoskeletal system.

REPRODUCTIVE ORGANS

The male reproductive organs include the penis, scrotum, testes, duct system, and accessory reproductive glands.

Penis

The penis consists of three cylinders of erectile tissue: two corpora cavernosa, and the corpus spongiosum, which contains the urethra. The glans, or tip, of the penis contains the urethral meatus, through which urine and semen pass to the exterior, and many nerve endings for sexual sensation. In uncircumcised males, the glans is covered by a loose, hoodlike fold of skin called the *prepuce* or *foreskin*. Smegma, a secretion of the glans, may collect in this area.

Scrotum

The scrotum, which contains the testes, epididymis, and lower spermatic cords, maintains the proper testicular temperature for spermatogenesis through relaxation and contraction. This is important because excessive heat reduces the sperm count.

Testes

The testes (also called *gonads,* which is a term for any reproductive organ, or testicles) produce sperm in the seminiferous tubules. Complete spermatogenesis develops in most males by age 15 or 16.

The testes form in the abdominal cavity of the fetus and complete final descent into the scrotum during the 7th month of gestation.

The testes produce and secrete hormones, especially testosterone, in their interstitial cells (Leydig's cells). Testosterone affects the development and maintenance of secondary sex characteristics and sex drive. It also regulates metabolism, stimulates protein anabolism (encouraging skeletal growth and muscular development), inhibits pituitary secretion of the gonadotropins (follicle-stimulating hormone and interstitial cell-stimulating hormone), promotes potassium excretion, and mildly influences renal sodium reabsorption.

Duct system

The vas deferens connects the epididymis, in which sperm mature and ripen for up to 6 weeks, and the ejaculatory ducts. The seminal vesicles—two convoluted membranous pouches—secrete a viscous liquid of fructose-rich semen, which provides energy for sperm; and prostaglandins, which probably facilitate fertilization.

Accessory reproductive glands

The prostate gland secretes the thin alkaline substance that comprises most of the seminal fluid; this fluid also protects sperm from acidity in the male urethra and in the vagina, thus increasing sperm motility.

The bulbourethral (*Cowper's*) glands secrete an alkaline ejaculatory fluid, probably similar in function to that produced by the prostate gland. The spermatic cords are cylindrical fibrous coverings in the inguinal canal containing the vas deferens, blood vessels, and nerves.

Female reproductive system

Female reproductive structures include the mammary glands, external genitalia, and internal genitalia. Hormonal influences determine the development and function of these structures and affect fertility, childbearing, and the ability to experience sexual pleasure.

In no other part of the body do so many interrelated physiologic functions occur in such proximity as in the area of the female reproductive tract. Besides the internal genitalia, the female pelvis contains the organs of the urinary and GI systems (bladder, ureters, urethra, sigmoid colon, and rectum). The reproductive tract and its surrounding area are thus the site of urination, defecation, menstruation, ovulation, copulation, impregnation, and parturition.

MAMMARY GLANDS

Located in the breasts, the mammary glands are specialized accessory glands that secrete milk. Although present in both sexes, they normally function only in females.

EXTERNAL STRUCTURES

Female genitalia include the following external structures, collectively known as the vulva: mons pubis (or *mons veneris*), labia majora, labia minora, clitoris, and the vestibule. The perineum is the external region between the vulva and the anus. The size, shape, and color of these structures—as well as pubic hair distribution and skin texture and pigmentation—vary greatly among individuals. Furthermore, these external structures undergo distinct changes during the life cycle.

Mons pubis

The mons pubis is the pad of fat over the symphysis pubis (pubic bone), which is usually covered by the base of the inverted triangular patch of pubic hair that grows over the vulva after puberty.

Labia majora

The labia majora are the two thick, longitudinal folds of fatty tissue that extend from the mons pubis to the posterior aspect of the perineum. The labia majora protect the perineum and contain large sebaceous glands that help maintain lubrication. Virtually absent in the young child, their development is a characteristic sign of onset of puberty. The skin of the more prominent parts of the labia majora is pigmented and darkens after puberty.

Labia minora

The labia minora are the two thin, longitudinal folds of skin that border the vestibule. Firmer than the labia majora, they extend from the clitoris to the posterior fourchette.

Clitoris

The clitoris is the small, protuberant organ located just beneath the arch of the mons pubis. The clitoris contains erectile tissue, venous cavernous spaces, and specialized sensory corpuscles that are stimulated during coitus. It's homologous to the male penis.

Vestibule

The vestibule is the oval space bordered by the clitoris, labia minora, and fourchette. The urethral meatus is located in the anterior portion of the vestibule, and the vaginal meatus is in the posterior portion. The hymen is the elastic membrane that partially obstructs the vaginal meatus in virgins. Its absence doesn't necessarily imply a history of coitus, nor does its presence obstruct menstrual blood flow.

Several glands lubricate the vestibule. Skene's glands (also known as the *paraurethral glands*) open on both sides of the urethral meatus; Bartholin's glands, on both sides of the vaginal meatus.

The fourchette is the posterior junction of the labia majora and labia minora. The perineum, which includes the underlying muscles and fascia, is the external surface of the floor of the pelvis, extending from the fourchette to the anus.

INTERNAL STRUCTURES

The internal structures of the female genitalia include the vagina, cervix, uterus, fallopian tubes (or *oviducts*), and ovaries.

Vagina

The vagina occupies the space between the bladder and the rectum. A muscular, membranous tube 2″ to 3″ (5 to 7.5 cm) in length, the vagina connects the uterus with the vestibule of the external genitalia. It serves as a passageway for sperm to the fallopian tubes, a conduit for the discharge of menstrual fluid, and the birth canal during parturition.

Cervix

The cervix, the narrow neck of the uterus, is the most inferior part of the vagina, protruding into the vaginal canal. The cervix provides a passageway between the vagina and the uterine cavity.

Uterus

The uterus is the hollow, pear-shaped organ in which the fetus grows during pregnancy. The thick uterine wall consists of mucosal, muscular, and serous layers. The inner mucosal lining (the *endometrium*) undergoes cyclic changes (based on hormonal activity) to facilitate and maintain pregnancy.

The smooth-muscle middle layer (the *myometrium*) interlaces the uterine and ovarian arteries and veins that circulate blood through the uterus. During pregnancy, this vascular system expands dramatically. After abortion or childbirth, the myometrium contracts to constrict the vasculature and control loss of blood.

The outer serous layer (the *parietal peritoneum*) covers all of the fundus, part of the corpus, but none of the cervix. This incompleteness allows surgical entry into the uterus without incision of the peritoneum, thus reducing the risk of peritonitis in the days before effective antibiotic therapy.

Fallopian tubes

The two fallopian tubes extend from the sides of the fundus and terminate near the ovaries. Each tube has a fimbriated (fringelike) end adjacent to the ovary that serves to capture an oocyte after ovulation. Through ciliary and muscular action, these small tubes carry ova from the ovaries to the uterus and facilitate the movement of sperm from the uterus toward the ovaries. The same ciliary and muscular action helps move a zygote (fertilized ovum) down to the uterus, where it may implant in the blood-rich inner uterine lining, the endometrium.

Ovaries

The ovaries are two almond-shaped organs, one on either side of the pelvis, situated behind and below the fallopian tubes. The ovaries produce ova and two primary hormones — estrogen and progesterone — in addition to small amounts of androgen. These hormones in turn produce and maintain secondary sex characteristics, prepare the uterus for pregnancy, and stimulate mammary gland development. The ovaries are connected to the uterus by the utero-ovarian ligament.

In the 30th week of gestation, the fetus has about 7 million follicles, which degenerate, leaving about 2 million present at birth. By puberty, only 400,000 remain, and these ova precursors become graafian follicles in response to the effects of pituitary gonadotropic hormones (follicle-stimulating hormone [FSH] and luteinizing hormone [LH]). Fewer than 500 of each woman's ova mature and become potentially fertile.

THE MENSTRUAL CYCLE

Maturation of the hypothalamus and the resultant increase in hormone levels initiate puberty. In the young girl, the appearance of pubic and axillary hair (pubarche) and the characteristic adolescent growth spurt follow breast development (thelarche) — the first sign of puberty. The reproductive system begins to undergo a series of hormone-induced changes that result in menarche, or the onset of menstruation (or *menses*).

The menstrual cycle consists of three different phases: menstrual, proliferative (estrogen dominated), and secretory (progesterone dominated). (See *Understanding the menstrual cycle*.)

At the end of the secretory phase, the uterine lining is ready to receive and nourish a zygote. If fertilization doesn't occur, increasing estrogen and progesterone levels decrease LH and FSH production. Because LH is needed to maintain

CLOSER LOOK
Understanding the menstrual cycle

The menstrual cycle is divided into three distinct phases.

◆ During the *menstrual phase,* which starts on the first day of menstruation, the top layer of the endometrium breaks down and flows out of the body. This flow, the menses, consists of blood, mucus, and unneeded tissue.

◆ During the *proliferative (follicular) phase,* the endometrium begins to thicken, and the level of estrogen in the blood increases, surging at midcycle. Then estrogen production decreases, the follicle matures, and ovulation occurs.

◆ During the *secretory (luteal) phase,* the endometrium begins to thicken to nourish an embryo should fertilization occur. Without fertilization, the top layer of the endometrium breaks down and the menstrual phase of the cycle begins again.

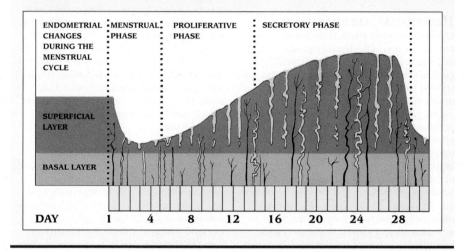

the corpus luteum, a decrease in LH production causes the corpus luteum to atrophy and halt the secretion of estrogen and progesterone. The thickened uterine lining then begins to slough off, and menstruation begins.

In the nonpregnant female, LH controls the secretions of the corpus luteum, thereby increasing the amount of progesterone in the bloodstream. In the pregnant woman, human chorionic gonadotropin (hCG), produced by the nascent placenta, controls these secretions.

If fertilization and pregnancy occur, the endometrium grows even thicker and vascular ingrowth occurs. After implantation of the zygote (5 to 6 days after fertilization), the endometrium becomes the decidua. Trophoblastic cells produce hCG soon after implantation, stimulating the corpus luteum to continue secreting estrogen and progesterone, which prevents further ovulation and menstruation.

hCG continues to stimulate the corpus luteum until the placenta (the vascular organ

that develops to transport materials to and from the fetus) forms and starts producing its own estrogen and progesterone. After the placenta takes over hormone production, secretions of the corpus luteum are no longer needed to maintain the pregnancy, and the corpus luteum gradually decreases its function and begins to degenerate. This is termed *luteoplacental shift* and commonly occurs by the end of the first trimester.

Pathophysiologic changes

Alterations may occur in the structure, process, or function of both the male and female reproductive systems.

SEXUAL MATURATION ALTERATIONS

Sexual maturation, or puberty, can be affected by various congenital and endocrine disorders. The timing of puberty may be too early (precocious puberty) or too late (delayed puberty). Precocious puberty is the onset of sexual maturation before age 9 in boys and before age 6 in girls. It's more common in girls than in boys. The cause is usually idiopathic but can result from central nervous system or congenital abnormalities.

In delayed puberty, there's no evidence of the development of secondary sex characteristics in boys by age 14 or girls by age 13. There's usually no evidence of hormonal abnormalities. The hypothalamic-pituitary-ovarian axis, a system that stimulates and regulates the production of hormones necessary for normal sexual development and function, is intact, but maturation is slow. The cause is unknown.

HORMONAL ALTERATIONS

Complex hormonal interactions determine the normal function of the female reproductive tract and require an intact hypothalamic-pituitary-ovarian axis. A defect or malfunction of this system can cause infertility due to insufficient gonadotropin secretions (both LH and FSH). The ovary controls—and is controlled by—the hypothalamus through a system of negative and positive feedback mediated by estrogen production. Insufficient gonadotropin levels may result from infections, tumors, or neurologic disease of the hypothalamus or pituitary gland. A mild hormonal imbalance in gonadotropin production and regulation, possibly caused by polycystic disease of the ovary or abnormalities in the adrenal or thyroid gland that adversely affect hypothalamic-pituitary functioning, may sporadically inhibit ovulation. Because gonadotropins are released in a pulsatile fashion, a significant disturbance in this pulsatility will adversely affect ovulatory function. Marijuana use can delay the onset of puberty because it blocks the release of gonadotropin-releasing hormone from the hypothalamus, which ultimately delays gonadal function.

Male hypogonadism, or an abnormal decrease in gonad size and function, results from decreased androgen production in males, which may impair spermatogenesis (causing infertility) and inhibit the development of normal secondary sex characteristics. The clinical effects of androgen deficiency depend on age at onset. Primary hypogonadism results directly from interstitial (Leydig's cell) cellular or seminiferous tubular damage of the testes due to faulty development or mechanical damage. Androgen deficiency causes increased secretion of gonadotropins by the pituitary in an attempt to increase the testicular functional state and is therefore termed *hypergonadotropic hypogonadism*. This form of hypogonadism includes Klinefelter's syndrome (47 XXY), Reifenstein's syndrome, male Turner's syndrome, Sertoli-cell-only syndrome, anorchism, orchitis, and aftereffects of irradiation.

Secondary hypogonadism is due to faulty interaction within the hypothalamic-pituitary axis, resulting in failure to secrete a normal level of gonadotropins, and is therefore termed *hypogonadotropic hypogonadism*. This form of hypogonadism includes hypopituitarism, isolated FSH deficiency, isolated LH deficiency, Kallmann's syndrome, and Prader-Willi syndrome. Depending on the patient's age at onset, hypogonadism may cause eunuchism (complete gonadal failure) or eunuchoidism (partial failure).

Signs and symptoms vary depending on the specific cause of hypogonadism. Some characteristic findings may include delayed bone maturation; delayed puberty; infantile penis and small, soft testes; less than average muscle development and strength; fine, sparse facial hair; scant or absent axillary, pubic, and body hair; and a high-pitched, effeminate voice. In an adult, hypogonadism diminishes sex drive and potency and causes regression of secondary sex characteristics.

MENSTRUAL ALTERATIONS

Alterations in menstruation include the absence of menses, abnormal bleeding patterns, or painful menstruation. Menopause is the cessation of menstruation. It results from a complex continuum of physiologic changes—the climacteric—caused by declining ovarian function. The climacteric produces various changes in the body, the most dramatic being the cessation of menses.

AGE ALERT *The climacteric, a normal gradual reduction in ovarian function due to aging, begins in most women between ages 45 and 50. Perimenopause begins 5 to 10 years (sometimes more) before menopause and commences with vasomotor symptoms and irregular menses. Menopause begins 12 months after final menses and is characterized by the continuation of vasomotor symptoms as well as urogenital symptoms (vaginal dryness and dyspareunia).*

Premature ovarian failure, or premature menopause, the gradual or abrupt cessation of menstruation before age 40, occurs without apparent cause in about 1% of women in the United States. Factors that may precipitate premature ovarian failure include malnutrition, debilitation, extreme emotional stress, pelvic irradiation, viral agents, and surgical procedures that impair ovarian blood supply. Artificial menopause may follow radiation therapy or surgical procedures, such as removal of both ovaries (bilateral oophorectomy). Other causes of premature ovarian failure include a decreased number of germ cells, chromosomal abnormalities, gonadotropin secretion defects, and autoimmune disorders. Hysterectomy decreases the interval before menopause, even when the ovaries aren't removed. It's speculated that hysterectomy may decrease ovarian blood flow in some fashion.

Ovarian failure, in which no ova are produced, may result from a functional ovarian disorder from premature ovarian failure. Amenorrhea is a natural consequence of ovarian failure.

Pain is commonly associated with the menstrual cycle; in many common diseases of the female reproductive tract, such pain may follow a cyclic pattern. A patient with endometriosis, for example, may report increasing premenstrual pain that decreases at the end of menstruation. For a description of the types of abnormal menstrual bleeding, (see *Abnormal premenopausal bleeding*.)

SEXUAL DYSFUNCTION

Sexual dysfunction includes arousal problems, orgasmic problems, and sexual pain (dyspareunia, vaginismus). Dysfunction may be caused by a general medical condition, psychological condition, substance use or abuse, or a combination of these factors.

Arousal disorder is an inability to experience sexual pleasure. According to the *Diagnostic and Statistical Manual of Mental Disorders*, 4th edition, Text Revision (*DSM-IV-TR*), the essential feature is a persistent or recurrent inability to attain or to maintain an adequate lubrication-swelling response of sexual excitement until completion of the sexual act. Orgasmic disorder, according to the *DSM-IV-TR*, is a persistent or recurrent delay in or absence of orgasm after a normal sexual excitement phase.

Both arousal and orgasmic disorders are considered primary if they exist in a female who has never experienced sexual arousal or orgasm; they're secondary when a physical, mental, or situational condition has inhibited or obliterated a previously normal sexual function. The prognosis is good for temporary or mild disorders resulting from misinformation or situational stress but is guarded for disorders that result from intense anxiety, chronically discordant relationships, psychological disturbances, or drug or alcohol abuse in either partner.

The following factors, alone or in combination, may cause an arousal or orgasmic disorder:
◆ certain drugs, including central nervous system depressants, alcohol, street drugs and, rarely, hormonal contraceptives

Abnormal premenopausal bleeding

Causes of abnormal premenopausal bleeding vary with the type of bleeding:
◆ *Cryptomenorrhea* (no external bleeding, although menstrual symptoms are experienced) may result from an imperforate hymen or cervical stenosis.
◆ *Hypermenorrhea* (excessive bleeding occurring at regular intervals) usually results from local lesions, such as uterine leiomyomas, endometrial polyps, and endometrial hyperplasia. It may also result from endometritis, salpingitis, or anovulation.
◆ *Hypomenorrhea* (decreased amount of menstrual fluid) results from local, endocrine, or systemic disorders or blockage caused by partial obstruction by the hymen or cervical obstruction.
◆ *Metrorrhagia* (bleeding occurring at irregular intervals) usually results from slight physiologic bleeding from the endometrium during ovulation but may also result from local disorders, such as uterine malignancy, cervical erosions, polyps (which tend to bleed after intercourse), or inappropriate estrogen therapy.
◆ *Oligomenorrhea* (infrequent menses) and polymenorrhea (menses occurring too frequently) usually result from anovulation due to an endocrine or systemic disorder.

Complications of pregnancy can also cause premenopausal bleeding, which may be as mild as spotting or as severe as hypermenorrhea.

◆ general systemic illnesses, diseases of the endocrine or nervous system, or diseases that impair muscle tone or contractility
◆ gynecologic factors, such as chronic vaginal or pelvic infection or pain, congenital anomalies, and genital cancer
◆ inadequate or ineffective stimulation
◆ psychological factors, such as performance anxiety, early traumatic sexual experiences, guilt, depression, or unconscious conflicts about sexuality
◆ relationship problems, such as poor communication, hostility, interpersonal disharmony, or ambivalence toward the partner, fear of abandonment or independence, or boredom with sex
◆ stress and fatigue.

All of these factors may contribute to involuntary inhibition of the orgasmic reflex. Another crucial factor is the fear of losing control of feelings or behavior. Whether these factors produce sexual dysfunction — as well as the type of dysfunction they produce — depends on how well the woman copes with the resulting pressures. Physical factors may also cause arousal or orgasmic disorder.

Female sexual function and responses decline, along with estrogen levels, in the perimenopausal period. The decrease in estradiol levels during menopause affects nerve transmission and response in the peripheral vascular system. As a result, the timing and degree of vasoconstriction during the sexual response is affected, vasocongestion decreases, muscle tension decreases, lubrication decreases, and contractions are fewer and less intense during orgasm.

A female with arousal disorder has limited or absent sexual desire and experiences little or no pleasure from sexual stimulation. Physical signs of this disorder include lack of vaginal lubrication or absence of signs of genital vasocongestion.

Dyspareunia is genital pain associated with intercourse. Insufficient lubrication is the most common cause. Other physical causes of dyspareunia include:
◆ disorders of the surrounding viscera (including residual effects of pelvic inflammatory disease or disease of the adnexal and broad ligaments)
◆ endometriosis
◆ genital, rectal, or pelvic scar tissue
◆ infections of the genitourinary tract (acute or chronic).

Other possible physical causes include:
◆ allergic reactions to diaphragms, condoms, or other contraceptives
◆ benign and malignant growths and tumors
◆ deformities or lesions of the introitus or vagina
◆ intact hymen
◆ radiation to the pelvis.

Psychological causes include:
◆ anxiety caused by a new sexual partner or technique
◆ fear of pain or injury during intercourse
◆ fear of pregnancy or injury to the fetus during pregnancy
◆ guilty feelings about sex
◆ mental or physical fatigue
◆ previous painful experience, including sexual abuse.

Vaginismus is an involuntary spastic constriction of the lower vaginal muscles, usually from fear of vaginal penetration. This disorder may coexist with dyspareunia and, if severe, may prevent intercourse (a common cause of

unconsummated marriages). Vaginismus may be physical or psychological in origin. It may occur spontaneously as a protective reflex to pain or result from organic causes, such as hymenal abnormalities, genital herpes, obstetric trauma, and atrophic vaginitis.

Psychological causes may include:
◆ childhood and adolescent exposure to rigid, punitive, and guilt-ridden attitudes toward sex
◆ early traumatic experience with pelvic examinations
◆ fear of pregnancy, sexually transmitted disease, or cancer
◆ fear resulting from painful or traumatic sexual experiences, such as incest or rape.

In males, the normal sexual response involves erection, emission, and ejaculation. Sexual dysfunction is the impairment of one or all of these processes.

Erectile disorder, or impotence, refers to inability to attain or maintain penile erection sufficient to complete intercourse. Transient periods of impotence aren't considered dysfunction and probably occur in half the adult males. Erectile disorder affects all age-groups but increases in frequency with age.

AGE ALERT *With aging, males experience a gradual decline in their serum total and free testosterone levels. This decline may affect both the male libido and sexual function.*

Psychogenic factors (guilt, fear, depression) are responsible for 50% to 60% of the cases of erectile dysfunction; organic factors, for the rest. In some patients, psychogenic and organic factors (chronic disease, paralysis, consequence of a surgical procedure) coexist, making isolation of the primary cause difficult.

Most problems with emission and ejaculation usually have structural causes.

MALE STRUCTURAL ALTERATIONS
Structural defects of the male reproductive system may be congenital or acquired. Testicular disorders, such as cryptorchidism or torsion, may result in infertility.

In cryptorchidism, a congenital disorder, one or both testes fail to descend into the scrotum, remaining in the abdomen or inguinal canal or at the external ring. If bilateral cryptorchidism persists untreated into adolescence, it may result in sterility, make the testes more vulnerable to trauma, and significantly increase the risk for testicular cancer, particularly germ cell tumors. It should be corrected between the ages of 12 and 24 months to reduce the risk of male infertility. In about 75% of affected infants, the testes descend spontaneously during the first year; in the rest, the testes may descend through puberty.

■ **AGE ALERT** *The testes of an older male may be slightly smaller than those of a younger male, but they should be equal in size, smooth, freely moveable, and soft, without nodules. The left testis is commonly lower than the right.*

Benign prostatic hyperplasia is a disorder of prostate enlargement due to androgen-induced growth of prostate cells. It's more prevalent with aging and may result in urinary obstructive symptoms.

Hypospadias is the most common penile structural abnormality. The midline fusion of the urethral folds is incomplete, so the urethral meatus opens on the ventral (anterior, or "belly") surface of the penis. In epispadias, the urethral meatus is located on the dorsal (posterior, or "back") surface of the penis.

Priapism is prolonged, painful erection in the absence of sexual stimulation. It results from arteriovenous shunting within the corpus cavernosum that leads to obstructed venous outflow from the penis. The most common cause is drug therapy for erectile dysfunction. It's also associated with the use of antihypertensives, anticoagulants, cocaine, corticosteroids, and amphetamines. In children it may be associated with sickle cell disease, leukemia, blood clots, or pelvic tumors. Without prompt treatment it can lead to ischemic fibrosis and infertility.

A urethral stricture is a narrowing of the urethra caused by scarring. It may result from trauma, surgery (adhesions), or infection. Common complications include prostatitis and secondary infection.

During the first 3 years of life, congenital adhesions between the foreskin and the glans penis separate naturally with penile erections. Phimosis is a condition in which the foreskin can't be retracted over the glans penis; it can be congenital or acquired (from forceful retraction) or can result from poor hygiene or chronic infection. Paraphimosis is a condition in which the foreskin is retracted behind the coronal sulcus; the penis becomes constricted, causing edema of the glans. Severe paraphimosis is a surgical emergency.

To prevent threatened spontaneous abortion, millions of women took diethylstilbestrol (DES) between 1946 and 1971. Men whose mothers took DES during their 8th to 16th weeks of pregnancy experienced structural abnormalities, such as urethral meatal stenosis, hypospadias, epididymal cysts, varicoceles, cryptorchidism, and decreased fertility.

Disorders

Disorders of the reproductive system may affect sexual, reproductive, or urinary function. Reproductive system disorders include abnormal uterine bleeding, amenorrhea, benign prostatic hyperplasia, cryptorchidism, dysmenorrhea, endometriosis, erectile dysfunction, gynecomastia, hydrocele, ovarian cysts, polycystic ovarian syndrome, premenstrual syndrome, precocious puberty, prostatitis, testicular torsion, uterine fibroids, and varicocele.

ABNORMAL UTERINE BLEEDING

Abnormal uterine bleeding refers to abnormal endometrial bleeding without recognizable organic lesions. Abnormal uterine bleeding is the indication for almost 25% of gynecologic surgical procedures. The prognosis varies with the cause. Correction of hormonal imbalance or structural abnormality yields a good prognosis.

Causes

Abnormal uterine bleeding usually results from an imbalance in the hormonal-endometrial relationship in which persistent and unopposed stimulation of the endometrium by estrogen occurs. Before menarche, it may also result from malignancy, trauma, or sexual abuse.

Disorders that cause sustained a high estrogen level include:
◆ anovulation (women in their late 30s to early 40s)
◆ immaturity of the hypothalamic-pituitary-ovarian mechanism (postpubertal teenagers)
◆ obesity (because enzymes present in peripheral adipose tissue convert the androgen androstenedione to estrogen precursors)
◆ polycystic ovary syndrome.

Other causes of abnormal uterine bleeding include:
◆ coagulopathy, such as thrombocytopenia or leukemia (rare)
◆ drug-induced coagulopathy, adrenal hyperplasia, or Cushing's disease
◆ endometriosis
◆ genital tract infections, neoplasms, or other pathology
◆ liver, renal, or thyroid disease
◆ medications and iatrogenic causes
◆ trauma (foreign object insertion or direct trauma)
◆ von Willebrand's disease.

Pathophysiology

Irregular bleeding is associated with hormonal imbalance and anovulation (failure of ovulation to occur). When progesterone secretion is absent but estrogen secretion continues, the endometrium proliferates and becomes hypervascular. When ovulation doesn't occur, the endometrium is randomly broken down, and exposed vascular channels cause prolonged, excessive bleeding. In most cases of abnormal uterine bleeding, the endometrium shows no pathologic changes. However, in chronic unopposed estrogen stimulation (as from a hormone-producing ovarian tumor), the endometrium may show hyperplastic or malignant changes.

Signs and symptoms

◆ Metrorrhagia (episodes of vaginal bleeding between menses)
◆ Hypermenorrhea (heavy or prolonged menses, longer than 8 days)
◆ Chronic polymenorrhea (menstrual cycle less than 18 days) or oligomenorrhea (infrequent menses)
◆ Fatigue due to anemia
◆ Oligomenorrhea and infertility due to anovulation
◆ Postcoital bleeding
◆ Pelvic pain
◆ Weight changes

Complications

◆ Iron-deficiency anemia (blood loss of more than 1.6 L over a short time) and hemorrhagic shock or right-sided heart failure (rare)
◆ Endometrial adenocarcinoma due to chronic estrogen stimulation

⚠ **CLINICAL ALERT** *There's an association between abnormal uterine bleeding and obesity. These patients are at risk for concomitant diabetes, heart disease, and endometrial hyperplasia or carcinoma.*

Diagnosis

Abnormal uterine bleeding may be caused by anovulation. Diagnosis of anovulation is based on:
◆ history of abnormal bleeding, bleeding in response to a brief course of progesterone, absence of ovulatory cycle body temperature changes, and a low serum progesterone level (A "bleeding calendar" may be helpful to define the pattern of bleeding and to record the number of pads and tampons used.)
◆ diagnostic studies ruling out other causes of excessive vaginal bleeding, such as organic, systemic, psychogenic, and endocrine causes, including certain cancers, polyps, pregnancy, and infection
◆ dilatation and curettage (D&C) or endometrial biopsy to rule out endometrial hyperplasia and cancer in women older than age 35

◆ imaging studies, such as transvaginal ultrasonography to determine endometrial thickness and sonohysterography to evaluate the endometrial cavity and identify structural problems
◆ hemoglobin level and hematocrit to determine the need for blood transfusion or iron supplementation.

Treatment

◆ High-dose estrogen-progestogen combination therapy (a hormonal contraceptive) to control endometrial growth and reestablish a normal cyclic pattern of menstruation; maintenance therapy with lower-dose combination hormonal contraceptives
◆ Endometrial biopsy to rule out endometrial adenocarcinoma (patients age 35 and older)
◆ Progestogen therapy (alternative in many women, such as those susceptible to such adverse effects of estrogen as thrombophlebitis)
◆ I.V. estrogen followed by progesterone or combination hormonal contraceptives if the patient is young (more likely to be anovulatory) and severely anemic (if oral drug therapy is ineffective)
◆ D&C (short-lived treatment and not clinically useful, but an important diagnostic tool) with hysteroscopy as a useful adjunct
◆ Iron supplementation or transfusions of packed cells or whole blood, as indicated, due to anemia caused by recurrent or excessive bleeding
◆ Explaining the importance of following the prescribed hormonal therapy; explaining D&C or endometrial biopsy procedure and purpose (if ordered)
◆ Stressing the need for regular checkups to assess the effectiveness of treatment

Special considerations

◆ If a patient complains of abnormal bleeding, tell her to record the dates of the bleeding and the number of sanitary pads she saturates per day. This helps in assessing the pattern and the amount of bleeding. Instruct the patient not to use tampons.
◆ Instruct the patient to immediately report abnormal bleeding to help rule out major hemorrhagic disorders, such as those that occur in abnormal pregnancy.
◆ To prevent abnormal bleeding due to organic causes and to ensure early detection of malignancy, encourage the patient to have a Papanicolaou test and a pelvic examination annually.
◆ Offer reassurance and support. The patient may be particularly anxious about excessive or frequent blood loss and passage of clots.

Suggest that she minimize blood flow by avoiding strenuous activity and by lying down with her feet elevated.

AMENORRHEA

Amenorrhea is the abnormal absence or suppression of menstruation. Absence of menstruation is normal before puberty, after menopause, or during pregnancy and lactation; it's abnormal — and therefore pathologic — at any other time. Primary amenorrhea is the absence of menarche in an adolescent (age 16 and older). Secondary amenorrhea is the failure of menstruation for at least 3 cycle intervals or 6 months after the normal onset of menarche. Primary amenorrhea occurs in 0.3% of women; secondary amenorrhea is seen in 1% to 3% of women. Prognosis varies, depending on the specific cause. Surgical correction of outflow tract obstruction is usually curative.

Causes

Amenorrhea usually results from:
♦ anovulation due to hormonal abnormalities, such as decreased secretion of estrogen, follicle-stimulating hormone (FSH), gonadotropins, and luteinizing hormone
♦ constant presence of progesterone or other endocrine abnormalities
♦ lack of ovarian response to gonadotropins.
   Amenorrhea may also result from:
♦ absence of a uterus, cervix, or vagina, or of more than one of these structures
♦ adrenal, ovarian, or pituitary tumors
♦ emotional disorders (common in patients with severe disorders, such as depression and anorexia nervosa); mild emotional disturbances tending to distort the ovulatory cycle; severe psychic trauma abruptly changing the bleeding pattern or completely suppressing one or more full ovulatory cycles
♦ endometrial damage
♦ malnutrition and intense exercise, causing an inadequate hypothalamic response
♦ systemic disorders, such as hypothyroidism or pituitary disease
♦ a transverse vaginal septum or imperforate hymen.

Pathophysiology

The mechanism varies depending on the cause and whether the defect is structural, hormonal, or both. Women who have an adequate estrogen level but a progesterone deficiency don't ovulate and are thus infertile. In primary amenorrhea, the hypothalamic-pituitary-ovarian axis is dysfunctional. Because of anatomic defects of the central nervous system, the ovary doesn't receive the hormonal signals that normally initiate the development of secondary sex characteristics and the beginning of menstruation.

Secondary amenorrhea can result from several central factors (hypogonadotropic hypoestrogenic anovulation), uterine factors (as with Asherman syndrome, in which the endometrium is sufficiently scarred that no functional endometrium exists), cervical stenosis, premature ovarian failure, and others.

Signs and symptoms

Amenorrhea may result from many disorders. Signs and symptoms depend on the specific cause, and include:
♦ absence of menstruation
♦ vasomotor flushes, vaginal atrophy, hirsutism (abnormal hairiness), and acne (secondary amenorrhea).

Complications

♦ Infertility
♦ Osteoporosis (associated with long-term amenorrhea)
♦ Endometrial adenocarcinoma (amenorrhea associated with anovulation that gives rise to unopposed estrogen stimulation of the endometrium)

Diagnosis

♦ History of failure to menstruate in females age 16 and older, if consistent with bone age confirms primary amenorrhea.
♦ Absence of menstruation for 3 cycle intervals or 6 months in a previously established menstrual pattern confirms secondary amenorrhea.
♦ Breast development absence or presence is a marker of estrogen action and function of the ovary.
♦ Physical and pelvic examination and sensitive pregnancy test rule out pregnancy, as well as anatomic abnormalities (such as cervical stenosis) that may cause false amenorrhea (cryptomenorrhea), in which menstruation occurs without external bleeding.
♦ Onset of menstruation (spotting) within 1 week after giving pure progestational agents, such as medroxyprogesterone (Provera), indicates that there's enough estrogen to stimulate the lining of the uterus. If menstruation doesn't occur, special diagnostic studies, such as gonadotropin levels, are indicated.
♦ Blood and urine studies show hormonal imbalances, such as lack of ovarian response to gonadotropins (an elevated pituitary gonadotropin level), failure of gonadotropin secretion (a low pituitary gonadotropin level), and abnormal thyroid levels. Without suspicion of premature

ovarian failure or central hypogonadotropism, gonadotropin levels aren't clinically meaningful because they're released in a pulsatile fashion; at a given time of day, levels may be elevated, low, or average.

♦ Complete medical workup, including pelvic ultrasound, appropriate X-rays, laparoscopy, and a biopsy, identify ovarian, adrenal, and pituitary tumors.

Tests to identify dominant or missing hormones include:

♦ "ferning" of cervical mucus on microscopic examination (an estrogen effect)
♦ vaginal cytologic examination
♦ endometrial biopsy
♦ low serum progesterone level
♦ high serum androgen level
♦ an elevated urinary 17-ketosteroid level with excessive androgen secretions
♦ a plasma FSH level more than 50 IU/L, depending on the laboratory (suggests primary ovarian failure); or normal or low FSH level (possible hypothalamic or pituitary abnormality, depending on the clinical situation).

Treatment

♦ Appropriate hormone replacement to reestablish menstruation
♦ Treatment of the cause of amenorrhea not related to hormone deficiency (for example, surgery for amenorrhea due to a tumor or obstruction)
♦ Inducing ovulation; with intact pituitary gland, clomiphene citrate (Clomid) may induce ovulation in women with secondary amenorrhea due to gonadotropin deficiency, polycystic ovarian disease, or excessive weight loss or gain if it's reversed
♦ FSH and human menopausal gonadotropins (Pergonal) for women with pituitary disease
♦ Improving nutritional status
♦ Modification of exercise routine

Special considerations

♦ Explain all diagnostic procedures to the patient.
♦ Provide reassurance and emotional support. Psychiatric counseling may be necessary if amenorrhea results from emotional disturbances.
♦ After treatment, teach the patient how to keep an accurate record of her menstrual cycles to aid early detection of recurrent amenorrhea.

BENIGN PROSTATIC HYPERPLASIA

Although most men age 50 and older have some prostatic enlargement, in benign prostatic hyperplasia (BPH) — also known as *benign prostatic hypertrophy* or *nodular hyperplasia* — the prostate gland enlarges enough to compress the urethra and cause overt urinary obstruction. (See *Prostatic enlargement.*) Depending on the size of the enlarged prostate, the age and health of the patient, and the extent of obstruction, BPH is treated symptomatically or surgically. BPH is common, affecting 40% to 50% of men ages 50 to 60, and more than 80% of men age 80 and older. It also affects about 8% of men ages 31 to 40.

Causes

The main cause of BPH may be age-associated changes in hormone activity. Androgenic hormone production decreases with age, causing imbalance in androgen and estrogen levels and a high level of dihydrotestosterone, the main prostatic intracellular androgen. A genetic predisposition (most likely an autosomal dominant trait) may be responsible for 10% of cases.

Pathophysiology

Regardless of the cause, BPH begins with non-malignant changes in periurethral glandular tissue. The growth of the fibroadenomatous nodules (masses of fibrous glandular tissue) progresses to compress the remaining normal gland (nodular hyperplasia). The hyperplastic tissue is mostly glandular, with some fibrous stroma and smooth muscle. As the prostate enlarges, it may extend into the bladder and obstruct urinary outflow by compressing or distorting the prostatic urethra. There are periodic increases in sympathetic stimulation of the smooth muscle of the prostatic urethra and bladder neck. Progressive bladder distention may also cause a pouch to form in the bladder that retains urine when the rest of the bladder empties. This retained urine may lead to calculus formation or cystitis.

Signs and symptoms

Clinical features of BPH depend on the extent of prostatic enlargement and the lobes affected. Characteristically, the condition starts with a group of symptoms known as prostatism, which are caused by enlargement, and include:
♦ reduced urine stream caliber and force
♦ urinary hesitancy
♦ difficulty starting micturition (resulting in straining, feeling of incomplete voiding, and an interrupted stream).

As the obstruction increases, it causes:
♦ frequent urination with nocturia
♦ sense of urgency
♦ dribbling
♦ urine retention
♦ incontinence
♦ possible hematuria.

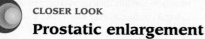

CLOSER LOOK
Prostatic enlargement

As the prostate gland enlarges, the urethra becomes compressed, causing overt urinary obstruction.

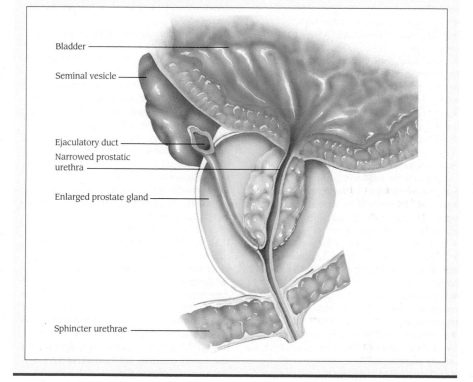

Complications

As BPH worsens, a common complication is complete urinary obstruction after infection or while using decongestants, tranquilizers, alcohol, antidepressants, or anticholinergics.

Other complications include:
◆ infection
◆ hydronephrosis, renal insufficiency and, if untreated, renal failure
◆ urinary calculi
◆ hemorrhage
◆ shock.

Diagnosis

Diagnosis includes physical examination showing:
◆ visible or palpable midline mass above the symphysis pubis (This is a sign of an incompletely emptied bladder.)
◆ enlarged prostate with rectal palpation.

Clinical features and a rectal examination are usually sufficient for diagnosis. Other findings that help confirm BPH may include:

◆ excretory urography to rule out urinary tract obstruction, hydronephrosis (distention of the renal pelvis and calices due to obstruction of the ureter and consequent retention of urine), calculi or tumors, and filling and emptying defects in the bladder
◆ alternatively, if the patient isn't cooperative, cystoscopy to rule out other causes of urinary tract obstruction (neoplasm, calculi)
◆ elevated blood urea nitrogen and serum creatinine levels (suggest renal dysfunction)
◆ an elevated prostate-specific antigen (PSA) level (Prostatic carcinoma must be ruled out.)
◆ urinalysis and urine cultures showing hematuria, pyuria and, with bacterial count more than 100,000/µl, urinary tract infection (UTI)
◆ cystourethroscopy for severe symptoms (definitive diagnosis) showing prostate enlargement, bladder wall changes, and a raised bladder. (Cystourethroscopy is only done immediately before surgery to help determine the best procedure.)

Treatment

Conservative therapy includes:
◆ prostate massages
◆ sitz baths
◆ avoiding fluids before bedtime and completely emptying the bladder to prevent bladder distention
◆ an antimicrobial to treat infection
◆ regular ejaculation to help relieve prostatic congestion
◆ alpha-adrenergic blockers to improve urine flow rates to relieve bladder outlet obstruction by preventing contractions of the prostatic capsule and bladder neck
◆ 6-alpha reductase inhibitors to possibly reduce the size of the prostate in some patients
◆ continuous drainage with an indwelling urinary catheter to alleviate urine retention (high-risk patients).

Surgery is the only effective therapy to relieve acute urine retention, hydronephrosis, severe hematuria, recurrent UTIs, and other intolerable signs and symptoms. The following procedures involve open surgical removal:
◆ transurethral resection (if the prostate weighs less than 2 oz [56.7 g]); tissue removed with a wire loop and electric current using a resectoscope
◆ suprapubic (transvesical) resection (Most common and useful for prostatic enlargement remaining within the bladder.)
◆ retropubic (extravesical) resection allowing direct visualization (Potency and continence are usually maintained.)
◆ balloon dilation of the urethra and prostatic stents to maintain urethral patency (occasionally)
◆ laser excision to relieve prostatic enlargement
◆ nerve-sparing surgical techniques to reduce common complications, such as erectile dysfunction.

Minimally invasive outpatient procedures may be appropriate to help moderate symptoms without hospitalization and include:
◆ transurethral microwave thermotherapy for heating and coagulation of prostatic tissue
◆ transurethral needle ablation, which uses radiofrequency needles that are placed within the prostate for heating and coagulation of prostatic tissue.

Special considerations

◆ Monitor and record the patient's vital signs, intake and output, and daily weight, watching closely for signs of postobstructive diuresis (such as increased urine output and hypotension) that may lead to serious dehydration, reduced blood volume, shock, electrolyte loss, and anuria.

◆ Insert an indwelling urinary catheter for urine retention (usually difficult in a patient with BPH). Using a coude catheter may make insertion easier.
◆ If the catheter can't be passed transurethrally, assist with suprapubic cystostomy under local anesthetic (watching for rapid bladder decompression).

After prostatic surgery, interventions may include:
◆ Maintain patient comfort; watch for and prevent postoperative complications; observe for immediate dangers of prostatic bleeding (shock, hemorrhage); check the catheter often (every 15 minutes for the first 2 to 3 hours) for patency and urine color; check dressings for bleeding.
◆ Postoperatively, many urologists insert a three-way catheter and establish continuous bladder irrigation. Keep the catheter open at a rate sufficient to maintain clear, light-pink returns; watch for fluid overload from absorption of the irrigating fluid into systemic circulation; observe an indwelling regular catheter closely (if used); irrigate a catheter with stopped drainage due to clots with 80 to 100 ml of normal saline solution, as ordered, maintaining strict sterile technique.
◆ Watch for septic shock (most serious complication of prostatic surgery); immediately report severe chills, sudden fever, tachycardia, hypotension, or other signs and symptoms of shock; start rapid infusion of an I.V. antibiotic, as ordered; watch for signs and symptoms of a pulmonary embolus, heart failure, and renal failure; monitor vital signs, central venous pressure, and arterial pressure continuously. (Supportive care in the intensive care unit may be needed.)
◆ Administer belladonna and opium suppositories or another anticholinergic as ordered to relieve painful bladder spasms that often occur after transurethral resection.
◆ After an open procedure, take patient comfort measures, such as providing suppositories (except after perineal prostatectomy), analgesic medication to control incision pain, and frequent dressing changes. Suppositories and rectal temperatures are sometimes contraindicated following open prostatic procedures — confirm orders with the physician.
◆ Continue infusing I.V. fluids until the patient can drink a sufficient amount of fluids (2 to 3 qt [2 to 3 L]/day) to maintain adequate hydration.
◆ Administer a stool softener and a laxative, as ordered, to prevent straining. (Don't check for fecal impaction because a rectal examination may precipitate bleeding.)

◆ Reassure the patient that temporary frequency, dribbling, and occasional hematuria will likely occur after the catheter is removed.

◆ Reinforce prescribed limits on activity, such as lifting, strenuous exercise, and long automobile rides that increase bleeding tendency; caution the patient to restrict sexual activity for several weeks after discharge.

◆ Instruct the patient about the prescribed oral antibiotic regimen and indications for using a gentle laxative.

◆ Tell the patient to avoid diuretics, such as caffeine and alcohol, to reduce the frequency of urination.

◆ Urge the patient to seek medical care immediately if he can't void, passes bloody urine, or develops a fever.

◆ Encourage annual digital rectal examinations and screening for PSA to identify a possible malignancy.

CRYPTORCHIDISM

Cryptorchidism is a congenital disorder in which one or both testes fail to descend into the scrotum, remaining in the abdomen or inguinal canal or at the external ring. Although this condition may be bilateral, it more commonly affects the left testis. True undescended testes remain along the path of normal descent, while ectopic testis deviate to an aberrant position.

Cryptorchidism occurs in 30% of premature male neonates, but in only about 3% of those born at term. In about 80% of affected infants, the testes descend spontaneously during the 1st year; in the rest, the testes may descend later. If indicated, surgical therapy is successful in up to 95% of the cases if the infant is treated early enough.

Causes

The mechanism by which the testes descend into the scrotum is still unexplained, but cryptorchidism occurs more commonly among those with congenital disorders. Possible causes of cryptorchidism include:

◆ genetic predisposition in a small number of cases (greater incidence of cryptorchidism in infants with neural tube defects)

◆ hormonal factors, most likely androgenic hormones from the placenta, maternal or fetal adrenals, or the immature fetal testis and possibly maternal progesterone or gonadotropic hormones from the maternal pituitary

◆ premature neonates most commonly affected due to normal descent of testes into the scrotum during the 7th month of gestation

◆ structural factors impeding gonadal descent, such as ectopic location of the testis or short spermatic cord

◆ testosterone deficiency resulting in a defect in the hypothalamic-pituitary-gonadal axis, causing failure of gonadal differentiation and gonadal descent.

Pathophysiology

A prevalent but still unsubstantiated theory links undescended testes to the development of the gubernaculum, a fibromuscular band that connects the testes to the scrotal floor. Normally, in the male fetus, testosterone stimulates the formation of the gubernaculum. This band probably helps pull the testes into the scrotum by shortening as the fetus grows. Thus, cryptorchidism may result from inadequate testosterone levels or a defect in the testes or the gubernaculum. Because the testis is maintained at a higher temperature, spermatogenesis is impaired, leading to reduced fertility.

Signs and symptoms

◆ Testis on the affected side not palpable in the scrotum; underdeveloped scrotum (unilateral cryptorchidism)

◆ Scrotum enlarged on the unaffected side due to compensatory hypertrophy (occasionally)

◆ Infertility after puberty due to prevention of spermatogenesis (uncorrected bilateral cryptorchidism) despite a normal testosterone level

Complications

Bilateral cryptorchidism that's untreated into adolescence may result in:

◆ sterility because of testicular temperature higher than optimal for spermatogenesis

◆ significantly increased risk of testicular cancer because the higher temperatures can cause abnormal division of germ cells

◆ increased vulnerability of the testes to trauma.

Diagnosis

Physical examination confirms cryptorchidism after sex is determined by the following laboratory tests:

◆ buccal smear (cells from oral mucosa) to determine genetic sex (a male sex chromatin pattern)

◆ serum gonadotropin to confirm the presence of testes by showing presence of circulating hormone; luteinizing hormone, follicle-stimulating hormone, and testosterone levels as well as other laboratory studies to confirm the diagnosis

◆ imaging studies (ultrasound, computed tomography scanning, magnetic resonance imagining) may be used to assess for nonpalpable testes;

however, the sensitivity of these studies for this purpose isn't that reliable.

Treatment

If the testes don't descend spontaneously by age 1, surgical correction is generally indicated. Surgery should be performed by age 2 because by this time about 40% of undescended testes can no longer produce viable sperm. Treatment includes:

◆ orchiopexy to secure the testes in the scrotum and to prevent sterility, excessive trauma from abnormal positioning, and harmful psychological effects (usually before age 4; optimum age, 1 to 2 years)

◆ human chorionic gonadotropin I.M. to stimulate descent.

Special considerations

◆ Encourage parents of the child with undescended testes to express their concern about his condition.

◆ Provide information on causes, available treatments, and effect on reproduction. Emphasize that testes may descend spontaneously (especially in premature infants).

◆ If orchiopexy is necessary, explain the surgery to the child, using terms he understands. Tell him that a rubber band may be taped to his thigh for about 1 week after surgery to keep the testis in place. Explain that his scrotum may swell but shouldn't be painful.

After orchiopexy:

◆ Monitor vital signs, intake, and output. Check dressings. Encourage coughing and deep breathing. Watch for urine retention.

◆ Keep the operative site clean, telling the child to wipe from front to back after defecating.

◆ Maintain tension on the rubber band that was applied to keep the testis in place. Make sure that it isn't too tight.

◆ Encourage parents to participate in postoperative care, such as bathing and feeding the child. Urge the child to do as much for himself as possible.

DYSMENORRHEA

Dysmenorrhea is painful menstruation associated with ovulation that isn't related to pelvic disease. It's the most common gynecologic complaint and a leading cause of absenteeism from school (affecting 10% of high school girls each month) and work (estimated 140 million work hours lost annually). The incidence peaks in women in their early 20s and then slowly decreases.

Dysmenorrhea can occur as a primary disorder or secondary to an underlying disease. Because primary dysmenorrhea is self-limiting,

the prognosis is generally good. The prognosis for secondary dysmenorrhea depends on the underlying disorder.

Causes

Although primary dysmenorrhea is unrelated to an identifiable cause, possible contributing factors include:

◆ hormonal imbalance

◆ psychogenic factors.

Dysmenorrhea may also be secondary to such gynecologic disorders as:

◆ cervical stenosis

◆ endometriosis

◆ pelvic inflammatory disease

◆ pelvic tumors

◆ uterine fibroids (benign fibroid tumors).

Pathophysiology

The pain of dysmenorrhea probably results from increased prostaglandin secretion in menstrual blood, which intensifies normal uterine contractions. Prostaglandins intensify myometrial smooth-muscle contraction and uterine blood vessel constriction, thereby worsening the uterine hypoxia normally associated with menstruation. This combination of intense muscle contractions and hypoxia causes the intense pain of dysmenorrhea. Prostaglandins and their metabolites can also cause GI disturbances, headache, and syncope.

Because dysmenorrhea almost always follows an ovulatory cycle, both the primary and secondary forms are rare during the anovulatory cycle of menses. Primary dysmenorrhea typically begins 1 to 2 years after the onset of menses. After age 20, dysmenorrhea is generally secondary.

Signs and symptoms

Possible signs and symptoms of dysmenorrhea include sharp, intermittent cramping and lower abdominal or pelvic pain, usually radiating to the back, thighs, groin, and vulva, and typically start with or immediately before menstrual flow and peaking within 24 hours.

Dysmenorrhea may also be associated with signs and symptoms suggestive of premenstrual syndrome, including:

◆ urinary frequency

◆ nausea

◆ vomiting

◆ diarrhea

◆ headache

◆ backache

◆ chills

◆ abdominal bloating

◆ painful breasts

◆ depression
◆ irritability.

Complications

A possible but rare complication is dehydration due to nausea, vomiting, and diarrhea.

Diagnosis

◆ Pelvic examination and a detailed patient history help suggest the cause.
◆ Rule out secondary causes for menses causing pain since menarche (primary dysmenorrhea).
◆ Tests, such as laparoscopy, hysteroscopy, and pelvic ultrasound, can aid diagnosis of underlying disorders in secondary dysmenorrhea.

Treatment

Initial treatment aims to relieve pain and may include:
◆ an analgesic, such as a nonsteroidal anti-inflammatory drug (NSAID), for mild to moderate pain, especially effective due to inhibition of prostaglandin synthesis through inhibition of the enzyme cyclooxygenase

⚠ CLINICAL ALERT *If the patient's pain is uncontrollable with an NSAID or another over-the-counter product, an evaluation for a secondary cause of the pain should be investigated. Opioids should be avoided.*

◆ a prostaglandin inhibitor (such as mefenamic acid or ibuprofen) to relieve pain by decreasing the severity of uterine contractions
◆ heat applied locally to the lower abdomen (may relieve discomfort in mature women), used cautiously in young adolescents because appendicitis may mimic dysmenorrhea
◆ alternative therapies, including vitamins, dietary changes, herbal supplements, biofeedback, and relaxation techniques to help alleviate discomfort.

For primary dysmenorrhea:
◆ a sex steroid (effective alternative to treatment with an antiprostaglandin or an analgesic), such as a hormonal contraceptive to relieve pain by suppressing ovulation and inhibiting endometrial prostaglandin synthesis (patients attempting pregnancy should rely on antiprostaglandin therapy)
◆ psychological evaluation and appropriate counseling due to possible psychogenic cause of persistently severe dysmenorrhea.

Treatment of secondary dysmenorrhea is designed to identify and correct the underlying cause and may include surgical treatment of underlying disorders, such as endometriosis or uterine fibroids (after conservative therapy fails).

Special considerations

Effective management of the patient with dysmenorrhea focuses on relief of symptoms, emotional support, and appropriate patient teaching, especially for the adolescent.

◆ Obtain a complete history focusing on the patient's gynecologic complaints, including detailed information on symptoms of pelvic disease, such as excessive bleeding, changes in bleeding pattern, vaginal discharge, and dyspareunia (painful intercourse).
◆ Provide thorough patient teaching, including explanation of normal female anatomy and physiology as well as the nature of dysmenorrhea (depending on circumstances, providing the adolescent patient with information on pregnancy and contraception).
◆ Encourage the patient to keep a detailed record of her menstrual cycle and symptoms and to seek medical care if symptoms persist.

ENDOMETRIOSIS

Endometriosis is the presence of endometrial tissue outside the lining of the uterine cavity. Ectopic tissue is generally confined to the pelvic area, usually around the ovaries, uterovesical peritoneum, uterosacral ligaments, and cul de sac, but it can appear anywhere in the body. (See *Common sites of endometriosis,* page 600.)

Active endometriosis may occur at any age, including adolescence. About 30% to 40% of infertile women may have endometriosis, although the true incidence in both fertile and infertile women remains unknown.

Severe symptoms of endometriosis may have an abrupt onset or may develop over many years. Infertility occurs in 30% to 40% of women with endometriosis. Endometriosis usually manifests during the menstrual years; after menopause, it tends to subside. Hormonal treatment of endometriosis (continuous use of a hormonal contraceptive, danazol [Danocrine], and a gonadotropin-releasing hormone [GnRH] antagonist) is potentially effective in relieving discomfort, although treatment of advanced stages of endometriosis usually isn't as successful because of impaired follicular development. However, nonsurgical treatment of endometriosis generally remains inadequate. Surgery appears to be the more effective way to enhance fertility, although definitive class I evidence doesn't currently exist. Pharmacologic and surgical treatment of endometriosis may be beneficial for managing chronic pelvic pain.

Causes

The cause of endometriosis remains unknown. The main theories to explain this disorder (one

CLOSER LOOK

Common sites of endometriosis

Ectopic endometrial tissue can implant almost anywhere in the pelvic peritoneum. It can even invade distant sites such as the lungs.

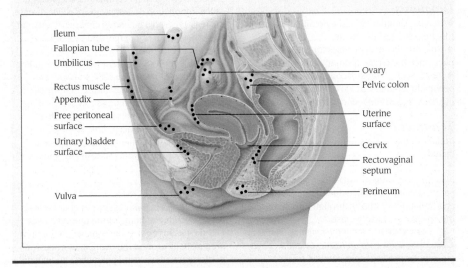

Labels: Ileum, Fallopian tube, Umbilicus, Rectus muscle, Appendix, Free peritoneal surface, Urinary bladder surface, Vulva, Ovary, Pelvic colon, Uterine surface, Cervix, Rectovaginal septum, Perineum

or more are perhaps true for certain populations of women) include:

◆ coelomic metaplasia (repeated inflammation inducing metaplasia of mesothelial cells to the endometrial epithelium)
◆ genetic predisposition and depressed immune system (may predispose certain females to endometriosis)
◆ lymphatic or hematogenous spread (extraperitoneal disease)
◆ retrograde menstruation with implantation at ectopic sites (retrograde menstruation alone may not be sufficient for endometriosis to occur because it occurs in women with no clinical evidence of endometriosis).

Pathophysiology

The ectopic endometrial tissue responds to normal stimulation in the same way as the endometrium, but more unpredictably. The endometrial cells respond to estrogen and progesterone with proliferation and secretion. During menstruation, the ectopic tissue bleeds, which causes inflammation of the surrounding tissues. This inflammation causes fibrosis, leading to adhesions that produce pain and infertility.

Signs and symptoms

Signs and symptoms of endometriosis include:

◆ dysmenorrhea, abnormal uterine bleeding, and infertility (classic symptoms) caused by inflammation from bleeding ectopic tissue
◆ pain that begins 2 to 7 days before menses peaks and lasts for 2 to 3 days (varies among patients); severity of pain not indicative of extent of disease.

Other signs and symptoms depend on the location of the ectopic tissue and may include:
◆ infertility and profuse menses (ovaries and oviducts)
◆ deep-thrust dyspareunia (ovaries or cul de sac)
◆ suprapubic pain, dysuria, and hematuria (bladder)
◆ abdominal cramps, pain on defecation, constipation; bloody stools due to bleeding of ectopic endometrium in the rectosigmoid musculature (large bowel and appendix)
◆ bleeding from endometrial deposits in these areas during menses; pain during intercourse (cervix, vagina, and perineum)
◆ rectal pain.

Complications

◆ Infertility due to fibrosis, scarring, and adhesions (major complication)
◆ Chronic pelvic pain
◆ Ovarian carcinoma (rare)

Diagnosis

The only definitive way to diagnose endometriosis is through laparoscopy or laparotomy. Pelvic examination may suggest endometriosis or be unremarkable. Findings suggestive of endometriosis include:

◆ multiple tender nodules on uterosacral ligaments or in the rectovaginal septum (in one-third of the patients)

◆ ovarian enlargement in the presence of endometrial cysts on the ovaries.

Although laparoscopy is recommended to diagnose and determine the extent of disease, some clinicians recommend:

◆ empiric trial of GnRH agonist therapy to confirm or refute the impression of endometriosis before resorting to laparoscopy (controversial, but may be cost-effective)

◆ biopsy at the time of laparoscopy (helpful to confirm the diagnosis), although in some instances, diagnosis is confirmed by visual inspection.

Treatment

Treatment of endometriosis varies according to the stage of the disease and the patient's age and desire to have children. Conservative therapy for young women who want to have children includes:

◆ an androgen, such as danazol (Danocrine)

◆ a progestin and continuous, combined hormonal contraceptives (pseudopregnancy regimen) to relieve symptoms by causing a regression of endometrial tissue

◆ a GnRH agonist to induce pseudomenopause (medical oophorectomy), causing remission of the disease (commonly used).

When ovarian masses are present, surgery must rule out cancer. Conservative surgery includes:

◆ laparoscopic removal of endometrial implants with conventional or laser techniques (no benefit shown for laser laparoscopy over electrocautery or suture methods)

◆ presacral neurectomy for central pelvic pain; effective in about 50% or less of appropriate candidates

◆ laparoscopic uterosacral nerve ablation (LUNA) also for central pelvic pain, although definitive studies supporting the efficacy of LUNA are lacking

◆ total abdominal hysterectomy with or without bilateral salpingo-oophorectomy; although success rates vary, it's unclear whether ovarian conservation is appropriate (treatment of last resort for women who don't want to have children or for extensive disease).

Special considerations

◆ Minor gynecologic procedures are contraindicated immediately before and during menstruation.

◆ Advise adolescents to use sanitary pads instead of tampons; this can help prevent retrograde flow in girls with a narrow vagina or small introitus.

◆ Because infertility is a possible complication, advise the patient who wants children not to postpone childbearing.

◆ Recommend an annual pelvic examination and Papanicolaou test to all patients.

ERECTILE DYSFUNCTION

Erectile dysfunction refers to a male's inability to attain or maintain penile erection sufficient to complete intercourse. The patient with primary impotence has never achieved a sufficient erection. Secondary impotence is more common but no less disturbing than the primary form, and implies that the patient has succeeded in completing intercourse in the past.

Transient periods of impotence aren't considered dysfunction and probably occur in half of adult males. Erectile disorder affects all age-groups but increases in frequency with age. The prognosis for erectile dysfunction patients depends on the severity and duration of their impotence and the underlying causes.

Causes

Causes of erectile dysfunction include psychogenic factors (50% to 60% of cases), organic causes, or both psychogenic and organic factors in some patients. This complexity makes the isolation of the primary cause difficult.

Psychogenic causes of erectile dysfunction include:

◆ intrapersonal psychogenic causes reflecting personal sexual anxieties and generally involving guilt, fear, depression, or feelings of inadequacy resulting from previous traumatic sexual experience, rejection by parents or peers, exaggerated religious orthodoxy, abnormal mother-son intimacy, or homosexual experiences

◆ psychogenic factors reflecting a disturbed sexual relationship, possibly stemming from differences in sexual preferences between partners, lack of communication, insufficient knowledge of sexual function, or nonsexual personal conflicts

◆ situational impotence, a temporary condition in response to stress.

Organic causes include:

◆ chronic diseases that cause neurologic and vascular impairment, such as cardiopulmonary disease, neurogenic diseases, chronic obstructive

pulmonary disease, sleep apnea, endocrine conditions (diabetes mellitus, hyperthyroidism, hypothyroidism, hypogonadism), malnutrition, or renal failure
◆ complications of surgery, particularly radical prostatectomy
◆ drug- or alcohol-induced dysfunction
◆ genital anomalies or central nervous system defects
◆ some medications (antidepressants, antipsychotics, antihypertensives, antiulcer medications, 5-alpha reductase inhibitors, and cholesterol-lowering agents).

Pathophysiology

Dysfunction results in lack of the autonomic signal and—in combination with organic, physiologic, endocrine, or psychogenic factors—interferes with the ability to obtain or sustain an erection. The blood is shunted around the sacs of the corpus cavernosum into medium-sized veins, which prevents the sacs from filling completely. Also, perfusion of the corpus cavernosum is initially compromised because of partial obstruction of small arteries, leading to loss of erection before ejaculation.

Psychogenic causes may exacerbate emotional problems in a circular pattern; anxiety causes fear of erectile dysfunction, which causes further emotional problems.

Signs and symptoms

Secondary erectile disorder is classified as:
◆ *partial*—inability to achieve or sustain a full erection
◆ *intermittent*—sometimes potent with the same partner
◆ *selective*—potent only with certain partners.

Some men lose erectile function suddenly, whereas others lose it gradually. If the cause isn't organic, erection may still be achieved through masturbation.

Immediately before a sexual encounter, patients with psychogenic impotence may:
◆ feel anxious
◆ perspire
◆ have palpitations
◆ lose interest in sexual activity.

Complications

A complication of erectile dysfunction is severe depression (patients with psychogenic or organic drug-induced erectile dysfunction), causing the impotence or resulting from it. It may also place a strain on sexual relationships.

Diagnosis

A detailed history, including a sexual and interpersonal relationship history, helps differentiate between organic and psychogenic factors and primary and secondary impotence.

Diagnosis also includes:
◆ ruling out chronic diseases and congenital or traumatic causes
◆ performing hormonal testing it symptoms include a diminished or absent libido
◆ carrying out imaging studies if pelvic trauma or surgery occurred
◆ evaluating vascular function within the penis with duplex ultrasound
◆ evaluating penile function by direct injection of prostaglandin E1 into the corpora to judge the quality of erection
◆ testing nerve function in the penis.

Treatment

Treatment of psychogenic impotence includes:
◆ sex therapy including both partners (course and content of therapy depend on the specific cause of dysfunction and nature of the partner relationship)
◆ teaching or helping the patient to improve verbal communication skills, eliminate unreasonable guilt, or reevaluate attitudes toward sex and sexual roles.

Treatment of organic impotence includes:
◆ reversing the cause, if possible
◆ arterial reconstruction (for patients with disorders of the arterial system)
◆ psychological counseling to help the couple deal realistically with their situation and explore alternatives for sexual expression if reversing the cause isn't possible
◆ phosphodiesterase inhibitors such as sildenafil (Viagra), vardenafil (Levitra), or tadalafil (Cialis) to cause vasodilation within the penis (This may effectively manage erectile dysfunction in appropriate patients.)
◆ an adrenergic antagonist or yohimbine to enhance parasympathetic neurotransmission
◆ testosterone supplementation for hypogonadal men (This isn't given to men with prostate cancer.)
◆ prostaglandin E injected directly into the corpus cavernosum (This may induce an erection for 30 to 60 minutes in some men.)
◆ vacuum constriction device (allows for an erect penis via induction of a vacuum within the cylinder)
◆ surgically inserted inflatable or noninflatable penile implants. (Used in some patients with organic impotence.)

Special considerations

◆ When you identify a patient with impotence, help him feel comfortable about discussing his sexuality. Assess his sexual health during your initial nursing history. When appropriate, refer him for further evaluation or treatment.

◆ After penile implant surgery, instruct the patient to avoid intercourse until the incision heals, usually in 6 weeks.

To help prevent impotence:

◆ Promote establishment of responsible health and sex education programs at primary, secondary, and college levels.

◆ Provide information about resuming sexual activity as part of discharge instructions for any patient with a condition that requires modification of daily activities. Such patients include those with cardiac disease, diabetes, hypertension, and chronic obstructive pulmonary disease and all postoperative patients.

GYNECOMASTIA

Gynecomastia is the enlargement of breast tissue in males. Gynecomastia can occur unilaterally or bilaterally. Infants can have a nascent gynecomastia that regresses in 2 to 3 weeks. Pubertal gynecomastia typically occurs between ages 10 and 12 and peaks between ages 13 and 14. The disorder generally regresses within 18 months and is uncommon after age 17. The cause is typically physiologic.

Causes

Excessive estrogen production from conditions including:

◆ some hypogonadism syndromes
◆ obesity
◆ pituitary tumors
◆ testicular tumors.

Systemic disorders associated with gynecomastia that may alter the estrogen-testosterone ratio include:

◆ chronic obstructive lung disease
◆ chronic renal failure
◆ liver disease causing inability to break down normal male estrogen secretions.

Pharmacologic agents that may cause gynecomastia include marijuana and exogenous estrogen, as given for prostatic malignancy. Medications that inhibit androgen synthesis (ketoconazole) or action (spironolactone) may also lead to gynecomastia.

Pathophysiology

Gynecomastia results from altered estrogen and androgen balances, or from increased sensitivity to normal estrogen levels. An imbalance between the stimulating effects of estrogen and the inhibitory effects of androgen results in a stimulation of the ductile system and fibroblasts of the breast tissue and an increase in vascularity.

Signs and symptoms

◆ Enlarged breast tissue (at least ¾" [2 cm] in diameter), either unilateral or bilateral, beneath the areola
◆ Bilateral enlargement (hormone-induced gynecomastia)

Complications

A possible complication of gynecomastia is malignant changes in the breast tissue.

Diagnosis

◆ Biopsy rules out malignancy.
◆ An excessively high estrogen level and a normal testosterone level reveal drug- and tumor-induced hyperestrogenism.
◆ A very low testosterone level and a normal estrogen level reveal hypergonadism.

Treatment

Gynecomastia usually resolves spontaneously without treatment. If indicated, treatments include:

◆ treatment of the cause to reduce excess breast tissue
◆ tamoxifen for patients with painful gynecomastia
◆ an aromatase inhibitor (such as letrozole, anastrozole, and exemestane) to reduce the estrogen level
◆ resection of extra breast tissue for cosmetic reasons.

Special considerations

◆ To make the patient as comfortable as possible, apply cold compresses to his breasts and administer an analgesic. Prepare him for diagnostic tests, including chest and skull X-rays and blood hormone levels.
◆ Because gynecomastia may alter the patient's body image, provide emotional support. Reassure the patient that treatment can reduce gynecomastia.

HYDROCELE

A hydrocele is a collection of fluid between the visceral and parietal layers of the tunica vaginalis of the testicle or along the spermatic cord. It's the most common cause of scrotal swelling.

Causes

◆ Congenital malformation (infants)
◆ Infection of the testes or epididymis
◆ Testicular tumor
◆ Trauma to the testes or epididymis

Pathophysiology

Congenital hydrocele occurs because of a patency between the scrotal sac and the peritoneal cavity, allowing peritoneal fluids to collect in the scrotum. The exact mechanism of congenital hydrocele is unknown, although it's thought by some to be a protective mechanism.

In adults, the fluid accumulation may be caused by infection, trauma, tumor, an imbalance between the secreting and absorptive capacities of scrotal tissue, or an obstruction of lymphatic or venous drainage in the spermatic cord. This leads to a displacement of fluid in the scrotum, outside the testes. Subsequent swelling results, leading to reduced blood flow to the testes.

Signs and symptoms

◆ Scrotal swelling and feeling of heaviness caused by fluid accumulation
◆ Inguinal hernia (typically present in congenital hydrocele)
◆ Size from slightly larger than the testes to the size of a grapefruit or larger
◆ Fluid collection with either flaccid or tense mass
◆ Pain with acute epididymal infection or testicular torsion
◆ Scrotal tenderness due to severe swelling

Complications

◆ Epididymitis
◆ Testicular atrophy

Diagnosis

◆ Transillumination distinguishes fluid-filled from solid mass (a tumor doesn't transilluminate).
◆ Ultrasound visualizes the testes and determines the presence of a tumor.
◆ Fluid biopsy determines the cause and differentiates between normal cells and malignant ones.

Treatment

Usually, no treatment of congenital hydrocele is indicated, because this condition typically resolves spontaneously by age 1. Otherwise, possible treatments for hydrocele include:
◆ surgical repair to avoid strangulation of the bowel (inguinal hernia with bowel present in the sac)
◆ aspiration of fluid and injection of sclerosing drug into the scrotal sac for a tense hydrocele that impedes blood circulation or causes pain
◆ excision of the tunica vaginalis for recurrent hydroceles
◆ suprainguinal excision for testicular tumor detected by ultrasound.

Special considerations

◆ Place a rolled towel between the patient's legs and elevate the scrotum to help reduce severe swelling. Or, if the patient has mild or moderate swelling, advise him to wear a loose-fitting athletic supporter lined with soft cotton dressings.
◆ Encourage sitz baths, and apply heat or ice packs to decrease inflammation.

OVARIAN CYSTS

Ovarian cysts are usually nonneoplastic sacs on an ovary that contain fluid or semisolid material. Although these cysts are usually small and produce no symptoms, they may require thorough investigation as possible sites of malignant change. Cysts may be single or multiple (polycystic ovarian disease). Common physiologic ovarian cysts include follicular cysts, theca-lutein cysts, and corpus luteum cysts. Ovarian cysts can develop any time between puberty and menopause, including during pregnancy. The prognosis for nonneoplastic ovarian cysts is excellent. The risk of ovarian malignancy isn't increased with a functional (physiologic) ovarian cyst.

Causes

◆ Granulosa-lutein cysts, which occur within the corpus luteum, are functional (arising during some variation of the ovulatory process), nonneoplastic enlargements of the ovaries caused by excessive accumulation of blood during the hemorrhagic phase of the menstrual cycle
◆ Theca-lutein cysts, which are commonly bilateral and filled with clear, straw-colored liquid; they're usually associated with hydatidiform mole, choriocarcinoma, or hormone therapy (with human chorionic gonadotropin [hCG] or clomiphene citrate)

Pathophysiology

Follicular cysts are generally very small and arise from follicles that overdistend, either because they haven't ruptured or have ruptured and resealed before their fluid was reabsorbed. (See *Follicular cyst.*) Luteal cysts develop if a mature corpus luteum persists abnormally and continues to secrete progesterone. They consist of blood or fluid that accumulates in the cavity of the corpus luteum and are typically more symptomatic than follicular cysts. When such cysts persist into menopause, they secrete excessive amounts of estrogen in response to the hypersecretion of follicle-stimulating hormone and luteinizing hormone that normally occurs during menopause.

Signs and symptoms

♦ No symptoms (small ovarian cysts such as follicular cysts)
♦ Mild pelvic discomfort, lower back pain, dyspareunia, or abnormal uterine bleeding, secondary to a disturbed ovulatory pattern (large or multiple cysts)
♦ Acute abdominal pain similar to that of appendicitis (ovarian cysts with torsion)
♦ Unilateral pelvic discomfort (from granulosalutein cysts appearing early in pregnancy and growing as large as 2″ to 2¼″ [5 to 6 cm] in diameter), delayed menses, followed by prolonged or irregular bleeding (granulosalutein cysts in nonpregnant women)
♦ Urinary frequency and constipation if the cyst is large

Complications

♦ Torsion or rupture causing signs of an acute abdomen (abdominal tenderness, distention, and rigidity) due to massive intraperitoneal hemorrhage or peritonitis
♦ Infertility and amenorrhea

Diagnosis

Generally, characteristic clinical features suggest ovarian cysts. They're confirmed by visualization of the ovary through ultrasound, laparoscopy, or surgery (usually for another condition).

Treatment

Treatment depends on the type of cyst and symptoms and may include:
♦ no treatment due to tendency of cyst to disappear spontaneously within one to two menstrual cycles; persisting cyst indicates excision to rule out malignancy (follicular cysts)
♦ hormonal treatment (commonly used, but has minimal benefit in ovarian cyst management)
♦ an analgesic to relieve symptoms (functional cysts that occur during pregnancy); cysts usually diminish during the third trimester (rarely needing surgery)
♦ elimination of the hydatidiform mole, destruction of choriocarcinoma, or discontinuation of hCG or clomiphene citrate (Clomid) therapy (theca-lutein cysts)
♦ laparoscopy or exploratory laparotomy with possible ovarian cystectomy or oophorectomy for persistent or suspicious ovarian cyst (These may be performed during pregnancy, if necessary. Optimal timing for surgery is the second trimester; laparoscopic management during pregnancy is promising.)
♦ surgery for ongoing hemorrhage from ruptured corpus luteum cyst. (Otherwise, ruptured ovarian cysts may be treated by

CLOSER LOOK

Follicular cyst

A common type of ovarian cyst, a follicular cyst is usually semitransparent and overdistended, with watery fluid visible through its thin walls.

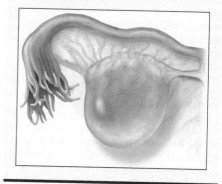

draining intraperitoneal fluid through culdocentesis in the emergency department or office setting.)

Special considerations

Counseling and support required by surgical cyst patients may include:
♦ explaining the nature of the cyst; describing of postprocedural discomfort, if any; and informing the patient how long condition may last
♦ preoperatively, watching for signs and symptoms of cyst rupture, such as increasing abdominal pain, distention, and rigidity; monitoring vital signs for fever, tachypnea, or hypotension (possibly indicating peritonitis or intraperitoneal hemorrhage)
♦ postoperatively, encouraging frequent movement in bed and early ambulation, as ordered, to prevent pulmonary embolism
♦ providing emotional support; offering appropriate reassurance if the patient fears cancer or infertility
♦ advising the patient to gradually increase her activities at home over 4 to 6 weeks after surgery.

POLYCYSTIC OVARIAN SYNDROME

Polycystic ovarian syndrome is a metabolic disorder characterized by multiple ovarian cysts. About 22% of the women in the United States have the disorder, and obesity is present in 50% to 80% of these women. Among those who seek treatment for infertility, more than 75% have some degree of polycystic ovarian syndrome, usually manifested by anovulation alone. Prognosis is good for ovulation and fertility with appropriate treatment.

Causes

The precise cause of polycystic ovarian syndrome is unknown. Theories include:
◆ abnormal enzyme activity triggering excess androgen secretion from the ovaries and adrenal glands
◆ endocrine abnormalities causing all of the signs and symptoms of polycystic ovarian disease; amenorrhea, polycystic ovaries on ultrasound, hyperandrogenism (part of the Stein-Leventhal syndrome).

Pathophysiology

A general feature of all anovulation syndromes is a lack of pulsatile release of gonadotropin-releasing hormone. Initial ovarian follicle development is normal. Many small follicles begin to accumulate because there's no selection of a dominant follicle. These follicles may respond abnormally to the hormonal stimulation, causing an abnormal pattern of estrogen secretion during the menstrual cycle. Endocrine abnormalities may be the cause of polycystic ovarian syndrome or cystic abnormalities; muscle and adipose tissue are resistant to the effects of insulin, and lipid metabolism is abnormal.

Signs and symptoms

Signs and symptoms of classic polycystic ovarian syndrome (Stein-Leventhal syndrome) are related to abnormal hormonal secretions that occur during the menstrual cycle and include:
◆ mild pelvic discomfort
◆ lower back pain
◆ dyspareunia
◆ abnormal uterine bleeding secondary to disturbed ovulatory pattern
◆ hirsutism
◆ acne
◆ male-pattern hair loss
◆ obesity.

Complications

Possible complications of polycystic ovarian syndrome include:
◆ malignancy due to sustained estrogenic stimulation of the endometrium
◆ increased risk for cardiovascular disease and type 2 diabetes mellitus due to insulin resistance.
Polycystic ovarian disease may produce:
◆ secondary amenorrhea
◆ oligomenorrhea
◆ infertility
◆ metabolic syndrome.

Diagnosis

◆ History and physical examination show bilaterally enlarged polycystic ovaries and menstrual disturbance, usually dating back to menarche.
◆ Visualization of the ovary through ultrasound, laparoscopy, or surgery may confirm ovarian cysts.
◆ A slightly elevated urinary 17-ketosteroid level and anovulation are shown by basal body temperature graphs and endometrial biopsy.
◆ An elevated ratio of luteinizing hormone to follicle-stimulating hormone (usually 3:1 or greater) and elevated levels of testosterone and androstenedione reveal the disorder.
◆ Unopposed estrogen action during the menstrual cycle due to anovulation reveals the disorder.
◆ Direct visualization by laparoscopy rules out paraovarian cysts of the broad ligament, salpingitis, endometriosis, and neoplastic cysts.

Treatment

Treatment of polycystic ovarian syndrome includes monitoring patient's weight to maintain a normal body mass index in order to reduce risks associated with insulin resistance, which may cause spontaneous ovulation in some women.

Treatment of polycystic ovarian syndrome may include such drugs as:
◆ clomiphene (Clomid) to induce ovulation
◆ medroxyprogesterone (Provera) for 10 days each month for a patient wanting to become pregnant
◆ a low-dose hormonal contraceptive to treat abnormal bleeding for the patient needing reliable contraception.

Special considerations

◆ Preoperatively, watch for signs and symptoms of cyst rupture, such as increasing abdominal pain, distention, and rigidity; monitor vital signs for fever, tachypnea, or hypotension (possibly indicating peritonitis or intraperitoneal hemorrhage).
◆ Postoperatively, encourage frequent movement in bed and early ambulation as ordered to prevent pulmonary embolism.
◆ Provide emotional support, offering appropriate reassurance if the patient fears cancer or infertility.

PRECOCIOUS PUBERTY

Precocious puberty may occur in males or females. Males begin to mature sexually before age 9. This disorder occurs most commonly as true precocious puberty—early maturation of the hypothalamic-pituitary-gonadal axis, development of secondary sex characteristics, gonadal development, and spermatogenesis—or as pseudoprecocious puberty, marked by development of secondary sex characteristics without gonadal development. Males with true precocious puberty have fathered children as early as age 7.

In most males with precocious puberty, sexual characteristics develop in essentially normal sequence; these children function normally when they reach adulthood.

In females, precocious puberty is the early onset of pubertal changes, such as breast development, pubic and axillary hair development, and menarche, before age 8. The occurrence is five times more common in females than males. Normally, the mean age for menarche is 13, although the exact age may vary based on race, ethnicity, and weight. In true precocious puberty, the ovaries mature and pubertal changes progress in an orderly manner.

In pseudoprecocious puberty, pubertal changes occur without corresponding ovarian maturation. (See *Precocious puberty,* pages 608 to 610.) In many cases, precocious puberty can be reversed.

PREMENSTRUAL SYNDROME

Characterized by varying symptoms, premenstrual syndrome (PMS) appears 7 to 14 days before menses and usually subsides with its onset. The effects of PMS range from minimal discomfort to severe, disruptive signs and symptoms and can include nervousness, irritability, depression, and multiple somatic complaints.

Researchers believe that 70% to 90% of women experience PMS at some time during their childbearing years, usually between ages 25 and 45.

Causes

The causes of PMS aren't yet clear. Although stress may exacerbate PMS, it doesn't cause it.

Pathophysiology

The biological theories offered to explain the cause of PMS include such conditions as a progesterone deficiency in the luteal phase of the menstrual cycle and vitamin deficiencies. Many theories have been discredited.

Failure to identify a specific disorder with a specific mechanism suggests that the signs and symptoms of PMS are triggered by normal physiologic hormonal changes.

Signs and symptoms

Clinical features vary widely among patients and may include any combination of the following:

◆ behavioral—mild to severe personality changes, nervousness, hostility, irritability, agitation, sleep disturbances, fatigue, lethargy, depression and increased appetite

◆ somatic—breast tenderness or swelling, abdominal tenderness or bloating, joint pain, headache, edema, diarrhea or constipation, and exacerbations of skin problems (such as acne or rashes), respiratory problems (such as asthma), or neurologic problems (such as seizures)

◆ other symptoms—headache, heart palpitations, and dizziness.

Complications

Women affected by PMS may experience psychosocial complications, such as:

◆ reduced self-esteem
◆ depression
◆ the inability to function in home, work, or school settings.

Diagnosis

The patient's history shows typical symptoms related to the menstrual cycle.

◆ To help ensure an accurate history, the patient may be asked to record menstrual symptoms and body temperature on a calendar for 2 to 3 months before diagnosis.

◆ Estrogen and progesterone blood levels aren't clinically useful.

◆ A psychological evaluation is recommended to rule out or detect an underlying psychiatric disorder.

Treatment

Education and reassurance that PMS is a real physiologic syndrome are important parts of treatment. Because treatment is predominantly symptomatic, each patient must learn to cope with her specific symptoms. Treatment may include:

◆ an antidepressant (particularly a selective serotonin reuptake inhibitor)
◆ a prostaglandin inhibitor
◆ a nonsteroidal anti-inflammatory.

For effective treatment, the patient may have to maintain a diet that's low in simple sugars, caffeine, alcohol, and salt.

Special considerations

◆ Inform the patient that self-help groups exist for women with PMS; if appropriate, help her contact such a group.

(Text continues on page 610.)

Precocious puberty

Although precocious puberty occurs in both female and male children, the origins of the disorder are different, so treatment varies.

	Female	Male
Causes	About 85% of the cases of true precocious puberty in girls are idiopathic. Other causes of true precocious puberty are pathologic, including central nervous system (CNS) disorders resulting from tumors, trauma, infection, other lesions, primary hypothyroidism, and irradiation therapy. Pseudoprecocious puberty may result from: ♦ increased levels of sex hormones due to ovarian and adrenocortical tumors ♦ adrenal cortical virilizing hyperplasia ♦ estrogen or androgen ingestion ♦ increased end-organ sensitivity to low levels of circulating sex hormones (estrogens promoting premature breast development, androgens promoting premature pubic and axillary hair growth).	True precocious puberty may be: ♦ idiopathic and genetically transmitted as a dominant trait ♦ cerebral (neurogenic). Pseudoprecocious puberty may result from: ♦ testicular tumors (hyperplasia, adenoma, or carcinoma) that produce excessive testosterone levels ♦ congenital adrenogenital syndrome, producing high levels of adrenocortical steroids.
Patho-physiology	Idiopathic precocious puberty results from early development and activation of the endocrine glands without corresponding abnormality.	Idiopathic precocious puberty results from pituitary or hypothalamic intracranial lesions that cause excessive secretion of gonadotropin.
Signs and symptoms	Changes that may occur independently or simultaneously before age 8 include: ♦ rapid growth spurt ♦ thelarche (breast development) ♦ pubarche (pubic hair development) ♦ menarche.	All boys with precocious puberty experience: ♦ early bone development, causing an initial growth spurt ♦ early muscle development ♦ premature closure of the epiphyses, thus stunted adult stature ♦ adult hair pattern, penile growth, bilateral enlarged testes. Signs and symptoms of precocity due to cerebral lesions include: ♦ nausea, vomiting ♦ headache, vision disturbances ♦ internal hydrocephalus. Signs and symptoms of pseudoprecocity due to testicular tumors include: ♦ adult hair patterns, acne ♦ discrepancy in testis size (enlarged testis feels hard or contains a palpable, isolated nodule). Adrenogenital syndrome produces: ♦ adult skin tone, excessive hair and beard, deepened voice ♦ stocky, muscular appearance ♦ penile, scrotal sac, and prostate enlargement (but not the testes).

Precocious puberty *(continued)*

	Female	Male
Complications	Development of ovarian or adrenal malignancy.	Testicular tumors or, in precocious puberty caused by a brain tumor, possibly death.
Diagnosis	Diagnosis requires: ♦ complete patient history ♦ thorough physical examination ♦ special tests to differentiate between true and pseudoprecocious puberty and to indicate the necessary treatment ♦ X-rays of the hands, wrists, knees, and hips to determine bone age and possible premature epiphyseal closure ♦ ultrasound, laparoscopy, or exploratory laparotomy to verify a suspected abdominal lesion ♦ EEG, ventriculography, pneumoencephalography, computed axial tomography scan, or angiography to detect CNS disorders. 　Other tests detect abnormally high hormonal levels for the patient's age and may include: ♦ vaginal smear for estrogen secretion ♦ urinary tests for gonadotropic activity and excretion of 17-keto-steroids ♦ radioimmunoassay for both luteinizing and follicle-stimulating hormones. ♦ complete physical examination	Diagnosis requires: ♦ detailed patient history to evaluate the patient's recent growth pattern, behavior changes, family history of precocious puberty, or ingestion of hormones. In true precocity, laboratory results include: ♦ elevated serum levels of luteinizing and follicle-stimulating hormones and corticotropin ♦ an elevated plasma testosterone level (equal to an adult male's) ♦ ejaculate showing the presence of live spermatozoa ♦ possible CNS tumors on brain scan, skull X-rays, and EEG ♦ skull and hand X-rays showing advanced bone age. 　In pseudoprecocity, diagnosis includes: ♦ chromosomal karyotype analysis showing abnormal pattern of autosomes and sex chromosomes ♦ elevated levels of 24-hour urinary 17-ketosteroids and other steroids.
Treatment	Treatment of constitutional true precocious puberty may include medroxyprogesterone (Provera) to reduce gonadotropin secretion and prevent menstruation and gonadotropin-releasing hormone (GnRH) analogue therapy to slow accelerated puberty. Other therapy depends on the cause of precocious puberty and its stage of development and includes: ♦ cortical or adrenocortical steroid replacement for adrenogenital syndrome ♦ surgery to remove ovarian and adrenal tumors, resulting in regression of secondary sex characteristics, especially in young children ♦ surgery and chemotherapy for choriocarcinomas ♦ thyroid extract or levothyroxine to decrease gonadotropic secretions in hypothyroidism ♦ discontinuation of medication for drug ingestion ♦ no treatment in precocious thelarche and pubarche.	Boys with idiopathic precocious puberty generally require no medical treatment and have no physical complications in adulthood. Supportive psychological counseling is the most important therapy. GnRH analogue therapy can slow accelerated puberty. 　Interventions for specific conditions include: ♦ regular reassessment for possible tumors in a child with an initial diagnosis of idiopathic precocious puberty ♦ neurosurgery for brain tumors (they commonly resist treatment) ♦ removal of the affected testis (orchiectomy) for testicular tumors; chemotherapy and lymphatic radiation therapy for malignant tumors (poor prognosis) ♦ lifelong therapy with maintenance doses of a glucocorticoid (cortisol) to inhibit corticotropin production in adrenogenital syndrome causing precocious puberty.

(continued)

Precocious puberty *(continued)*

	Female	Male
Special considerations	Interventions to help the child undergoing these changes and his family include: ◆ encouraging the patient and family to express their feelings about these changes ◆ explaining all diagnostic procedures and telling patient and family that surgery may be necessary ◆ explaining the condition to the child in terms she can understand to prevent feelings of shame and loss of self-esteem ◆ providing appropriate sex education, including information on menstruation and related hygiene ◆ emphasizing to parents that the child's social and emotional development should remain consistent with her chronological age, not with physical development; advising parents not to place unrealistic demands on the child ◆ suggesting that parents continue to dress their daughter in clothes appropriate for her age that don't call attention to her physical development ◆ reassuring parents that precocious puberty doesn't usually precipitate precocious sexual behavior.	Interventions to help the child undergoing these changes and his family include: ◆ emphasizing to parents that the child's social and emotional development should remain consistent with his chronological age, not with his physical development; advising parents not to place unrealistic demands on the child ◆ reassuring the child that although his body is changing more rapidly than those of other boys, they'll eventually experience the same changes ◆ helping him feel less self-conscious about his changing body; suggesting clothing that de-emphasizes sexual development ◆ providing sex education for the child with true precocity ◆ explaining adverse effects of medication (cushingoid symptoms) to family if a child must take a glucocorticoid for the rest of his life.

◆ Obtain a complete patient history to help identify any emotional problems that may contribute to PMS. If necessary, refer the patient for psychological counseling.

⚠ **CLINICAL ALERT** *Suggest that the patient seek further medical consultation if symptoms are severe and interfere with her normal lifestyle. (See* Premenstrual dysphoric disorder.*)*
◆ If possible, discuss ways in which the patient can modify her lifestyle, such as making changes in her diet and avoiding stimulants and alcohol. Tell her to keep a diary of her symptoms and menstrual cycle.
◆ Encourage the patient to get regular exercise and adequate rest.

PROSTATITIS

Prostatitis, or inflammation of the prostate gland, may be acute or chronic. Acute prostatitis most commonly results from gram-negative bacteria and is easy to recognize and treat. However, chronic prostatitis, the most common cause of recurrent urinary tract infections (UTIs) in men,

is less easy to recognize. As many as 35% of men age 50 and older have chronic prostatitis. Granulomatous prostatitis (tuberculous prostatitis), nonbacterial prostatitis, and prostatodynia (painful prostate) are other classifications of the disease.

Causes

Bacterial prostatitis is caused by:
◆ *Enterobacter, Klebsiella, Proteus, Pseudomonas, Staphylococcus,* or *Streptococcus* organisms (about 20% of cases)
◆ *Escherichia coli* (65% to 80% of cases).
These organisms probably spread to the prostate by:
◆ an ascending urethral infection or through the bloodstream
◆ bacterial invasion from the urethra (chronic prostatitis)
◆ infrequent or excessive sexual intercourse
◆ invasion of rectal bacteria through lymphatics
◆ procedures, such as cystoscopy or catheterization (less commonly)

Premenstrual dysphoric disorder

Premenstrual dysphoric disorder (PMDD) is a severe form of premenstrual syndrome (PMS) that has a cyclical occurrence of psychiatric symptoms (such as anger, irritability, and internal tension) that starts after ovulation (usually the week before the onset of menstruation) and ends within the first day or two of menses. Its underlying cause and pathophysiology remain unclear. However, researchers theorize that normal cyclic changes in the body cause abnormal responses to neurotransmitters, such as serotonin, resulting in physical and behavioral signs and symptoms.

PMDD affects as many as 1 in 20 American women who have regular menstrual periods. It's unclear why some women are affected and others aren't.

How PMDD and PMS differ

PMDD is characterized by severe monthly mood swings and physical signs and symptoms that interfere with everyday life. Compared with PMS, its signs and symptoms are abnormal and unmanageable. Although depression, anxiety, and sadness are common with PMS, in patients with PMDD, these symptoms are extreme. Some women may feel the urge to hurt or kill themselves or others.

The Diagnostic and Statistical Manual of Mental Disorders, 4th edition, Text Revision, sets these criteria for diagnosing PMDD:

♦ functional impairment
♦ predominant mood symptoms, with one being affective
♦ symptoms beginning 1 week before the onset of menstruation
♦ symptoms that don't result from any underlying primary mood disorder.

In addition, at least five of the following symptoms must be present during the week before menses and resolving within a few days after menses starts:

♦ appetite changes
♦ decreased interests
♦ difficulty concentrating
♦ fatigue
♦ feelings of being overwhelmed, sad, and self-deprecating
♦ insomnia or hypersomnia
♦ irritability
♦ "low mood"
♦ mood swings and frequent tearfulness
♦ physical symptoms
♦ tension, anger, and interpersonal conflicts.

♦ reflux of infected bladder urine into prostate ducts.

Granulomatous prostatitis is caused by *Mycobacterium tuberculosis.* The cause of nonbacterial prostatitis is unknown but possible causes include infection by a protozoa or virus. The cause of prostatodynia is also unknown.

■ **AGE ALERT** *In older men, acute prostatitis is associated with benign prostatic hyperplasia.*

Pathophysiology

Spasms in the genitourinary tract or tension in the pelvic floor muscles may cause inflammation and nonbacterial prostatitis.

Bacterial prostatic infections can be the result of a previous or concurrent infection. The bacteria ascend from the infected urethra, bladder, lymphatics, or blood through the prostatic ducts and into the prostate. Infection stimulates an inflammatory response in which the prostate becomes larger, tender, and firm. Inflammation is usually limited to a few of the gland's excretory ducts.

Signs and symptoms

Acute prostatitis begins with:
♦ chills
♦ lower back pain, especially when standing, due to compression of the prostate gland
♦ perineal fullness and suprapubic tenderness caused by inflammation and prostatic enlargement
♦ frequent and urgent urination caused by pressure from enlarged prostate
♦ dysuria, nocturia, and urinary obstruction due to blocked urethra by enlarged prostate
♦ cloudy urine due to infection.

Signs of systemic infection include:
♦ fever
♦ myalgia
♦ fatigue
♦ arthralgia.

Patients with chronic prostatitis may be asymptomatic between acute episodes, but may exhibit symptoms of chronic pelvic pain syndrome (suprapubic and perineal pain and pain that may occur in the penis, groin, testes, or lower back). Other signs and symptoms of chronic bacterial prostatitis may include:

♦ the same urinary symptoms as the acute form but to a lesser degree
♦ recurrent symptomatic cystitis.
Other possible signs and symptoms include:
♦ evidence of UTI, such as urinary frequency, burning, cloudy urine
♦ painful ejaculation
♦ bloody semen
♦ persistent urethral discharge
♦ sexual dysfunction.

Complications
♦ UTI (common)
♦ Bacterial prostatis, bacterial epididymitis, or prostatic abscess
♦ Infected and abscessed testis (removed surgically)

Diagnosis
♦ Rectal examination finds evidence of acute prostatitis, such as a very tender, warm, and enlarged prostate (characteristic).
♦ Rectal examination finds a firm, irregularly shaped, and slightly enlarged prostate due to fibrosis (chronic bacterial prostatitis).
♦ Palpation shows a normal prostate by exclusion (nonbacterial prostatitis).
♦ Pelvic X-ray shows prostatic calculi.
♦ Transrectal ultrasonography evaluates prostate disease and provides ultrasound guidance of biopsy needles.
♦ Urine culture and gram stain identify the causative infectious organism.
♦ Urine culture identifies no UTI or causative organism (nonbacterial prostatitis).
♦ Increased serum prostate-specific antigen may indicate acute prostatitis.
Firm diagnosis depends on a comparison of urine cultures of specimens obtained by the Meares-Stamey four-glass test. A significant increase in colony count in the prostatic specimens confirms prostatitis. This test requires four specimens:
♦ first specimen when the patient starts voiding (voided bladder one [VB1])
♦ second specimen midstream (VB2)
♦ third specimen after the patient stops voiding and the physician massages the prostate to produce secretions (expressed prostate secretions [EPS])
♦ final voided specimen (VB3).
However, the two-glass test (including premassage and postmassage specimens) is gaining popularity as a more simple and cost-effective diagnostic tool.

Treatment
Systemic antibiotic therapy is the treatment of choice for acute prostatitis is based on the

results of culture and sensitivity testing. Therapy may include fluoroquinolones, trimethoprim-sulfamethoxazole, and ampicillin with gentamicin.
Supportive therapy includes:
♦ bed rest
♦ adequate hydration
♦ an analgesic
♦ an antipyretic
♦ sitz baths
♦ a stool softener as necessary.
In symptomatic chronic prostatitis, treatment may include:
♦ instructing patient to drink at least eight glasses of water daily
♦ regular careful massage of the prostate to relieve discomfort (vigorous massage may cause secondary epididymitis or septicemia)
♦ regular ejaculation to help promote drainage of prostatic secretions
♦ a fluoroquinolone (for chronic prostatitis caused by *E. coli* and other Enterobacteriaceae, but not when caused by *P. aeruginosa* or enterocci)
♦ an anticholinergic and an analgesic to help relieve nonbacterial prostatitis symptoms
♦ an alpha-adrenergic blocker and a muscle relaxant to relieve pain
♦ continuous low-dose anabolic steroid therapy (effective in some men).
If drug therapy is unsuccessful, surgical treatment may include:
♦ transurethral resection of the prostate removing all infected tissue (not usually performed on young adults; may cause retrograde ejaculation and sterility)
♦ total prostatectomy (curative but may cause impotence and incontinence).

Special considerations
Patient care is primarily supportive.
♦ Ensure bed rest and adequate hydration. Provide a stool softener and administer sitz baths, as ordered.
♦ As necessary, prepare to assist with suprapubic needle aspiration of the bladder or a suprapubic cystostomy.
♦ Emphasize the need for strict adherence to the prescribed drug regimen. Instruct the patient to drink at least eight glasses of water per day. Have him report adverse drug reactions (rash, nausea, vomiting, fever, chills, and GI irritation).

TESTICULAR TORSION
Testicular torsion is an abnormal twisting of the spermatic cord due to rotation of a testis or the mesorchium (a fold in the area between

the testis and epididymis), which causes strangulation and, if left untreated, eventual infarction of the testis. Onset may be spontaneous or may follow physical exertion or trauma. This condition is almost always (90%) unilateral. The greatest risk occurs during the neonatal period and again between ages 12 and 18 (puberty), but it may occur at any age. Infants with torsion of one testis have a greater incidence of torsion of the other testis later in life than do males in the general population. The prognosis is good with early detection and prompt treatment.

Causes
In intravaginal torsion (the most common type of testicular torsion in adolescents), testicular twisting may result from:
◆ abnormality of the coverings of the testis and abnormally positioned testis
◆ incomplete attachment of the testis and spermatic fascia to the scrotal wall, leaving the testis free to rotate around its vascular pedicle.
   In extravaginal torsion (most common in neonates):
◆ loose attachment of the tunica vaginalis to the scrotal lining causing spermatic cord rotation above the testis
◆ sudden forceful contraction of the cremaster muscle (may precipitate this condition).

Pathophysiology
Normally, the tunica vaginalis envelops the testis and attaches to the epididymis and spermatic cord. Normal contraction of the cremaster muscle causes the left testis to rotate counterclockwise and the right testis to rotate clockwise. In testicular torsion, the testis rotates on its vascular pedicle and twists the arteries and vein in the spermatic cord, causing an interruption of circulation to the testis. Vascular engorgement and ischemia develop, causing scrotal swelling unrelieved by rest or elevation of the scrotum. If manual reduction is unsuccessful, it must be surgically corrected within 6 hours after the onset of symptoms to preserve testicular function (70% salvage rate). After 12 hours, the testis becomes dysfunctional and necrotic. (See *Extravaginal torsion.*)

Signs and symptoms
Signs and symptoms of testicular torsion include:
◆ excruciating pain in the affected testis or iliac fossa of the pelvis due to tissue ischemia (although painless testicular swelling may occur in 10% of cases)

CLOSER LOOK
Extravaginal torsion

In extravaginal torsion, rotation of the spermatic cord above the testis causes strangulation and, eventually, infarction of the testis.

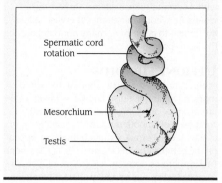

Spermatic cord rotation

Mesorchium

Testis

◆ edematous, elevated, and ecchymotic scrotum with loss of the cremasteric reflex (stimulation of the skin on the inner thigh retracts the testis on the same side) on the affected side.
   Associated signs and symptoms include:
◆ abdominal pain
◆ nausea and vomiting.

Complications
◆ Testicular infarction and necrosis
◆ Infertility

Diagnosis
◆ Physical examination while the patient is standing shows tense, tender swelling in the scrotum or inguinal canal; persistent reddening of the overlying skin; possibly palpable twisting of the spermatic cord (when examined before severe edema develops).
◆ Doppler ultrasonography helps distinguish testicular torsion from strangulated hernia, undescended testes, or epididymitis (absent blood flow and avascular testis in torsion).

Treatment
Treatment consists of immediate surgical repair by:
◆ orchiopexy (fixation of a viable testis to the scrotum and prophylactic fixation of the contralateral testis)
◆ orchiectomy (excision of a nonviable testis) to decrease the risk for autoimmune response to necrotic testis and its contents, damage to unaffected testis, and subsequent infertility

♦ manual manipulation of the testis counterclockwise to improve blood flow before surgery (not always possible).

Special considerations

♦ Promote the patient's comfort before and after surgery.

♦ After surgery, administer pain medication as ordered. Monitor voiding, and apply an ice bag with a cover to reduce edema. Protect the wound from contamination. Otherwise, allow the patient to perform as many normal daily activities as possible.

UTERINE FIBROIDS

Uterine fibroids, the most common benign tumors in women, are also known as myomas, fibromyomas, or leiomyomas. They're tumors composed of smooth muscle that usually occur in the uterine corpus, although they may appear on the cervix or on the round or broad ligament. Uterine fibroids occur in 20% to 25% of women of reproductive age and may affect three times as many Blacks as Whites, although the true incidence in either population is unknown.

The tumors become malignant (leiomyosarcoma) in less than 0.1% of patients, which should serve to comfort women concerned with the possibility of a uterine malignancy in association with a fibroid.

Causes

The cause of uterine fibroids is unknown, but some factors implicated as regulators of fibroid growth include:

♦ several growth factors, including epidermal growth factor

♦ steroid hormones, including estrogen and progesterone (fibroids typically arise after menarche and regress after menopause, implicating estrogen as a promoter of fibroid growth).

Pathophysiology

Fibroids are classified according to location. They may be located within the uterine wall (intramural) or protrude into the endometrial cavity (submucous) or from the serosal surface of the uterus (subserous). Their size varies greatly. They're usually firm and surrounded by a pseudocapsule composed of compressed but otherwise normal uterine myometrium. The uterine cavity may become larger, increasing the endometrial surface area. This can cause increased uterine bleeding.

Signs and symptoms

Most fibroids are asymptomatic. Signs and symptoms of fibroids include:

♦ abnormal bleeding, typically menorrhagia with disrupted submucosal vessels (most common sign)

♦ pain only associated with torsion of a pedunculated (stemmed) subserous tumor or fibroid undergoing degeneration (The fibroid outgrows its blood supply and shrinks down in size. This can be artificially induced through myolysis, a laparoscopic procedure to shrink fibroids, or uterine artery embolization.)

♦ pelvic pressure and impingement on adjacent viscera (indications for treatment, depending on severity) resulting in mild hydronephrosis. (This isn't believed to be an indication for treatment because renal failure rarely, if ever, results.)

Complications

Various disorders have been attributed to uterine fibroids, including:

♦ recurrent spontaneous abortion
♦ preterm labor
♦ malposition of the fetus
♦ anemia secondary to excessive bleeding
♦ bladder compression
♦ infection (if tumor protrudes out of the vaginal opening)
♦ secondary infertility (rare)
♦ bowel obstruction.

Diagnosis

♦ Clinical findings (enlarged uterus) and patient history suggest uterine fibroids.

♦ Blood studies show anemia from abnormal bleeding and may support the diagnosis.

♦ Bimanual examination shows enlarged, firm, nontender, and irregularly contoured uterus (also seen with adenomyosis and other pelvic abnormalities).

♦ Ultrasound accurately assesses the dimension, number, and location of the tumors.

♦ Magnetic resonance imaging (especially sensitive with regard to fibroid imaging) reveals fibroids.

Other diagnostic procedures include:

♦ hysterosalpingography
♦ hysteroscopy
♦ endometrial biopsy (to rule out endometrial cancer in patients older than age 35 with abnormal uterine bleeding)
♦ laparoscopy.

Treatment

Treatment depends on the severity of symptoms, size and location of the tumors, and the patient's age, parity, pregnancy status, desire to have children, and general health.

Treatment options include nonsurgical as well as surgical procedures. Pharmacologic treatment generally isn't effective in the long term for fibroids. Although usually prescribed by gynecologists, progestational agents are ineffective as primary treatment for fibroids.

Besides observation, nonsurgical methods include:
◆ a gonadotropin-releasing hormone agonist to decrease uterine volume (it also decreases blood loss when used before surgery.)
◆ mifepristone, an antihormonal agent, to slow or stop the growth of fibroids
◆ a nonsteroidal anti-inflammatory for dysmenorrhea or pelvic discomfort.

Surgical procedures include:
◆ abdominal, laparoscopic, or hysteroscopic myomectomy (removal of tumors in the uterine muscle) for patients of any age who want to preserve their uterus
◆ myolysis (a laparoscopic procedure to treat fibroids without hysterectomy or major surgery, performed on an outpatient basis) to coagulate the fibroids and preserve the uterus and childbearing potential
◆ uterine artery embolization (radiologic procedure) to block uterine arteries using small pieces of polyvinyl chloride (This is a promising alternative to surgery in many women, but no existing long-term studies confirm long-term success or any potential adverse effects of the procedure. There are also no long-term studies to determine if this procedure is appropriate in women who anticipate becoming pregnant in the near future. Recent anecdotal data suggest decreased time to menopause after embolization.)
◆ hysterectomy (Although this is the definitive treatment for symptomatic women who have completed childbearing, it's critical to inform women of all their choices because hysterectomy usually isn't the only available option.)
◆ blood transfusions (with severe anemia due to excessive bleeding).

Before undergoing surgery, patients should be helped to understand the effects of hysterectomy or oophorectomy, if indicated, on menstruation, menopause, sexual activity, and hormonal balance. Patients should also understand that pregnancy is still possible if multiple myomectomy is necessary, although cesarean delivery may be necessary. Extensive scar tissue may rupture during the contractions of vaginal delivery. (Violation of the endometrial cavity is the classic indication for cesarean delivery in such patients, but it's unclear why a cell layer one to two cells thick would protect against uterine dehiscence in subsequent pregnancy.)

Special considerations
◆ Tell the patient to report abnormal bleeding or pelvic pain immediately.
◆ Reassure the patient that she won't experience premature menopause if her ovaries are left intact.
◆ In a patient with severe anemia due to excessive bleeding, administer an iron supplement and blood transfusions, as ordered.
◆ Encourage the patient to verbalize her feelings and concerns related to the disease process and its effects on her lifestyle.

VARICOCELE
A mass of dilated and tortuous varicose veins in the spermatic cord is called a varicocele. It's classically described as a "bag of worms." Between 20% and 40% of all men diagnosed with infertility have a varicocele. Varicocele occurs in the left spermatic cord 95% of the time. It occurs in 10% to 15% of all males, usually between ages 13 and 18.

Causes
Causes of varicocele include:
◆ incompetent or congenitally absent valves in the spermatic veins
◆ tumor or thrombus obstructing the inferior vena cava (unilateral left-sided varicocele).

Pathophysiology
Because of a valvular disorder in the spermatic vein, blood pools in the pampiniform plexus of veins that drain each testis rather than flowing into the venous system. One function of the pampiniform plexus is to keep the testes slightly cooler than body temperature, which is the optimal temperature for sperm production. Incomplete blood flow through the testis thus interferes with spermatogenesis. Testicular atrophy also may occur because of the reduced blood flow.

Signs and symptoms
Usually, no symptoms are associated with the presence of a varicocele. Occasionally, symptoms may include:
◆ feeling of heaviness on the affected side due to blood pooling
◆ testicular pain and tenderness on palpation.

Complications
◆ Infertility due to the elevated temperature caused by increased blood flow to the testes
◆ Metastasis from a renal tumor leading to sudden development of a varicocele in an older man (late sign)

Diagnosis
Physical examination shows:
◆ palpation of "bag of worms" when the patient is upright
◆ drained varicocele can't be felt when the patient is recumbent.

Treatment
◆ Conservative treatment with a scrotal support to relieve discomfort (mild varicocele and fertility not an issue)
◆ Surgical repair or removal involving ligation of the spermatic cord at the internal inguinal ring (if infertility is an issue)

Special considerations
◆ Promote the patient's comfort before and after surgery.
◆ After surgery, administer pain medication, as ordered. Monitor voiding, and apply an ice bag with a cover to reduce edema. Protect the wound from contamination. Otherwise, allow the patient to perform as many normal daily activities as possible.

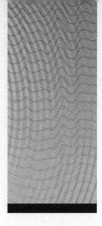

LESS COMMON DISORDERS

SELECTED REFERENCES

INDEX

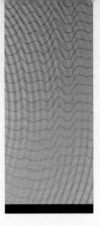

LESS COMMON DISORDERS

Disease and causes	Pathophysiology	Signs and symptom
Adenoid hyperplasia ♦ Cause unknown; may be hereditary or due to chronic infections or irritations	Increased mitosis leads to an increase in cell numbers in adenoid tissue resulting in chronic enlargement of the adenoid glands.	♦ Respiratory obstruction, especially mouth breathing, snoring at night, and frequent, prolonged nasal congestion ♦ Persistent mouth breathing during the formative years ♦ Sinusitis, frequent otitis media
Albinism ♦ Autosomal recessive inheritance	Absence of the enzyme tyrosine results in a defect in melanin formation. There can be a partial or total lack of melanin pigment.	♦ Extremely fair skin color ♦ Fine, white hair ♦ Gray or blue irises of the eye ♦ Strabismus, nystagmus, photophobia ♦ Persistent loss of visual acuity
Amblyopia ♦ Strabismus in children ♦ Excessive alcohol or tobacco use in adults	Acuity is reduced due to a toxic reaction in the orbital portion of the optic nerve or by cerebral blockage of the visual stimuli.	♦ Visual dimness, photophobia, and ocular discomfort ♦ Small central or pericentral scotoma enlarges slowly ♦ Temporal disk pallor ♦ Possible blindness
Amyloidosis ♦ Pressure due to accumulation and infiltration of amyloid causes atrophy of nearby cells (Abnormal immunoglobulin synthesis and reticuloendothelial cell dysfunction may occur.) ♦ Familial inheritance in persons with Portuguese ancestry	A rare, chronic disease of abnormal fibrillar scleroprotein (a waxy, starchlike glycoprotein) accumulation that infiltrates body organs and soft tissues. Perireticular type affects the inner coats of blood vessels, whereas pericollagen type affects the outer coats. Amyloidosis can result in permanent, even life-threatening, organ damage.	♦ Proteinuria, leading to nephrotic syndrome, eventually to renal failure ♦ Heart failure due to cardiomegaly, arrhythmias, and amyloid deposits in subendocardium, endocardium, and myocardium ♦ Stiffness and enlargement of tongue, decreased intestinal motility, malabsorption, bleeding, abdominal pain, constipation, and diarrhea ♦ Appearance of peripheral neuropathy ♦ Liver enlargement, commonly with azotemia, anemia, albuminuria and, rarely, jaundice

Disease and causes	Pathophysiology	Signs and symptoms
Amyloidosis *(continued)* ♦ May occur with tuberculosis, chronic infection, rheumatoid arthritis, multiple myeloma, Hodgkin's disease, paraplegia, brucellosis, and Alzheimer's disease		
Ankylosing spondylitis ♦ Cause unknown; strongly associated with presence of human leukocyte antigen (HLA)-B27 ♦ Familial inheritance	Fibrous tissue of the joint capsule is infiltrated by inflammatory cells that erode the bone and fibrocartilage. Repair of the cartilaginous structures begins with the proliferation of fibroblasts, which synthesize and secrete collagen. The collagen forms fibrous scar tissue that eventually undergoes calcification and ossification, causing the joint to fuse or lose flexibility.	♦ Intermittent low back pain that's most severe following inactivity or in the morning ♦ Stiffness, limited lumbar spine motion ♦ Pain and limited expansion of chest ♦ Peripheral arthritis in shoulders, hips, and knees ♦ Kyphosis in advanced stages ♦ Hip deformity and limited range of motion ♦ Mild fatigue, fever, and anorexia or weight loss ♦ Dyspnea if the costovertebral joints are involved
Aspergillosis ♦ Fungal infection due to *Aspergillus* species; transmitted by inhalation of fungal spores or invasion of spores through wounds or injured tissue ♦ Usually occurs in immunocompromised individuals	*Aspergillus* species produce extracellular enzymes, such as proteases and peptidases that contribute to tissue invasion, leading to hemorrhage and necrosis.	♦ Incubation period is a few days to weeks; may be asymptomatic or mimic tuberculosis, causing a productive cough and purulent or blood-tinged sputum, dyspnea, empyema, and lung abscesses ♦ Allergic aspergillosis causes wheezing, dyspnea, pleural pain, and fever ♦ Aspergillosis endophthalmitis appears 2 to 3 weeks after eye surgery ♦ Cloudy vision, eye pain, reddened conjunctiva, and purulent exudate
Behçet's syndrome ♦ Cause unknown; environmental factor or unknown virus can initiate process if genetic predisposition exists (presence of HLA-B51 is a risk factor) ♦ Family members may exhibit similar symptoms	Overactive immune system produces sudden inflammation of small blood vessels; symptoms based on location of inflammation. Behçet's syndrome is more apparent in persons with Mediterranean, Middle East, or Far East ancestry. Onset usually occurs in the late 20s to early 30s; five times more common in males.	♦ Recurrent genital ulcerations ♦ Recurrent oral ulcerations ♦ Eye inflammation and skin lesions ♦ Subcutaneous thrombophlebitis ♦ Epididymitis and deep vein thrombosis ♦ Arterial occlusion and aneurysm ♦ Severe headache and fatigue ♦ Bloating, diarrhea, cramping, and bloody stools ♦ Movement and speech difficulties
Blastomycosis ♦ Fungal infection due to *Blastomyces dermatitidis;* usually infects the lungs and produces bronchopneumonia ♦ May disseminate through blood causing osteomyelitis and central nervous system (CNS), skin, and genital disorders	Inhalation of the conidia leads to clearing of the organism by alveolar macrophages that kill conidia. Conidia that aren't killed convert to yeast forms that trigger an inflammatory response resulting in the formation of noncaseating granulomas.	♦ Dry, hacking, or productive cough ♦ Pleuritic chest pain, dyspnea ♦ Fever, shaking, chills, night sweats, malaise, and anorexia ♦ Small, painless, nonpruritic, and nondistinctive macules or papules on exposed body parts ♦ Painful swelling of testes, epididymis, or prostate; deep perineal pain, pyuria, and hematuria

Disease and causes	Pathophysiology	Signs and symptoms
Bronchiectasis ♦ Conditions associated with continued damage to bronchial walls and abnormal mucociliary clearance cause tissue breakdown to adjacent airways; such conditions include cystic fibrosis, immunologic disorders, and recurrent bacterial respiratory tract infections	Inflammation and destruction of the structural components of the bronchial wall lead to chronic abnormal dilation.	*In early stages:* ♦ Asymptomatic with complaints of frequent pneumonia or hemoptysis ♦ Chronic cough producing copious, foul-smelling, mucopurulent secretions, hemoptysis ♦ Coarse crackles during inspiration ♦ Wheezing, dyspnea, sinusitis, fever, and chills *In advanced stage:* ♦ Chronic malnutrition and right-sided heart failure due to hypoxic pulmonary vasoconstriction
Bronchiolitis ♦ Acute viral infection of the lower respiratory tract; most common cause is infection with respiratory syncytial virus or parainfluenza virus; may be associated with specific diseases or conditions, such as bone marrow, heart, or lung transplants; rheumatoid arthritis; lupus erythematosus; and Crohn's disease	Infection or other unknown factors cause necrosis of the bronchial epithelium and destruction of ciliated epithelial cells. As the submucosa becomes edematous, cellular debris and fibrin form plugs in the bronchioles.	*Subacute symptoms:* ♦ Fever, persistent nonproductive cough, dyspnea, malaise, and anorexia ♦ Physical assessment reveals dry crackles *Less common:* ♦ Tachypnea, tachycardia, intercostal and subcostal retractions ♦ Productive cough, hemoptysis, chest pain, general aches, and night sweats ♦ Wheezing and respiratory distress in late stages
Brucellosis ♦ Caused by gram-negative, aerobic *Brucella bacterium* that's transmitted by consumption of unpasteurized dairy products and meat or contact with infected animals or their secretions or excretions	Nonmotile, nonspore-forming, gram-negative coccobacilli of *Brucella* species cause an acute febrile illness.	Usually insidious *In acute phase:* ♦ Fever, chills, profuse sweating, fatigue, headache, backache, enlarged lymph nodes ♦ Anorexia, joint pain, and enlarged spleen *In chronic phase:* ♦ Endocarditis and cerebral abscesses ♦ Depression, sleep disturbances, and sexual impotence
Celiac disease ♦ Results from a complex interaction involving dietary, genetic, and immunologic factors	The body can't hydrolyze peptides contained in gluten. Ingestion of gluten causes injury to the villi in the upper small intestine, leading to a decreased surface area and malabsorption of most nutrients. Inflammatory enteritis also results, leading to osmotic diarrhea and secretory diarrhea.	♦ Recurrent diarrhea, abdominal distention, stomach cramps, weakness, muscle wasting, or increased appetite without weight gain ♦ Normochromic, hypochromic, or macrocytic anemia ♦ Osteomalacia, osteoporosis, tetany, and bone pain in lower back, rib cage, and pelvis ♦ Peripheral neuropathy, paresthesia, or seizures ♦ Dry skin, eczema, psoriasis, dermatitis herpetiformis, and acne rosacea ♦ Amenorrhea, hypometabolism, and adrenocortical insufficiency ♦ Extreme lethargy, mood changes and irritability

Disease and causes	Pathophysiology	Signs and symptoms
Cholera ♦ Acute enterotoxin-mediated GI infection due to gram-negative bacillus (*Vibrio cholerae*), which is transmitted through water and food contamination with fecal material from carriers or people with active infections incubation period several hours to 5 days	After ingestion of a significant inoculum, colonization of the small intestine occurs. The secretion of a potent enterotoxin results in a massive outpouring of isotonic fluid from the mucosal surface of the small intestine. Profuse diarrhea, vomiting, and fluid and electrolyte loss occurs and may lead to hypovolemic shock, metabolic acidosis, or death.	♦ Incubation period is several hours to 5 days ♦ Acute, painless, profuse watery diarrhea, and vomiting ♦ Intense thirst, weakness, loss of skin tone; dehydration; electrolyte imbalances; oliguria ♦ Muscle cramps ♦ Cyanosis ♦ Tachycardia ♦ Falling blood pressure, fever, and hypoactive bowel sounds
Chronic fatigue and immune dysfunction syndrome ♦ Cause unknown; may be found in HHV-6 or other herpesviruses, enteroviruses, or retroviruses	Infectious agents or environmental factors trigger an abnormal immune response and hormonal alterations.	♦ Constellation of symptoms including myalgia, arthralgia with arthritis, low grade fever, pain, cervical adenopathy, sore throat, headache, memory deficits, and sleep disturbances ♦ Prolonged, overwhelming fatigue
Coccidioidomycosis ♦ Fungal infection due to possible inhalation of *Coccidioides iimmitis* spores from the soil or in plaster casts or dressing of infected people	*C. immitis* induces a granulomatous reaction that results in caseous necrosis.	♦ Dry cough, pleuritic chest pain, dyspnea, pleural effusion ♦ Fever, sore throat, chills, malaise, headache, and itchy macular rash ♦ Tender red nodules on legs with joint pain in knees and ankles in white women ♦ Chronic pulmonary cavitation ♦ Anorexia and weight loss
Colorado tick fever ♦ Virus transmitted to human by a hard-shelled wood tick, *Dermacentor andersoni* (Tick acquires the virus when it bites an infected rodent and remains a permanently infected vector.)	Virus circulates inside of erythropoietic cells, producing typical febrile symptoms.	♦ Incubation period is 3 to 6 days; symptoms begin abruptly ♦ Chills, high temperature, severe back, arm and leg aches, and lethargy ♦ Headache with ocular movement ♦ Photophobia, abdominal pain, nausea, and vomiting
Complement deficiencies ♦ Primary complement deficiencies inherited as autosomal recessive traits; however, C1 esterase inhibitor is autosomal dominant ♦ Secondary deficiencies may follow complement-fixing reactions ♦ May be associated with such illnesses as acute poststreptococcal glomerolonephritis or acute systemic lupus erythematosus	Series of circulating enzymatic serum proteins with nine functional components labeled C1 through C9. Deficiencies may increase susceptibility to infections and certain autoimmune disorders.	♦ Clinical effects vary with deficiency *C5 deficiency (familial defect in infants):* ♦ Diarrhea and seborrheic dermatitis *C1 esterase inhibitor deficiency:* ♦ Swelling in face, hands, abdomen, or throat; possible fatal laryngeal edema *C2 and C3 deficiencies and C5 familial dysfunction:* ♦ Increased susceptibility to bacterial infection *C2 and C4 deficiencies:* ♦ Collagen vascular disease (lupus and chronic renal failure)

Disease and causes	Pathophysiology	Signs and symptoms
Congenital adrenal hyperplasia ♦ Autosomal recessive disorder that causes a 21-hydroxylase deficiency or 11-ß hydroxylase deficiency ♦ Tumor of the adrenal glands	Lack of an enzyme needed to synthesize cortisol causes an excessive corticotropin response through the negative feedback loop to the pituitary. The continual corticotropin message to the adrenal glands results in hyperplasia of adrenal tissue. Excessive androgen production is stimulated because the adrenal pathway to androgen production isn't blocked. Hypersecretion of androgens results in somatic masculinization.	♦ Enlarged external genitalia in neonate due to excessive androgen production; female neonates may have slightly enlarged clitoris or clitoris with a penile shape and labia fused to appear as a scrotum, whereas males have enlarged genitals ♦ Severe electrolyte imbalance, dehydration, vomiting, wasting, and shock due to adrenal crisis at 5 to 10 days
Costochondritis ♦ Cause unknown; may be trauma related	An inflammatory process of the costochondral or costosternal joints is initiated, causing localized pain and tenderness.	♦ Sharp pain in chest wall ♦ Area is sensitive to touch ♦ Pain may radiate into arm ♦ Pain worsens with movement ♦ Reproducible pain
Cryptococcosis ♦ Fungal infection due to *Cryptococcus neoformans,* which is transmitted in particles of dust contamination by pigeon feces ♦ Transmission by inhalation of cryptococci ♦ Most commonly occurs in patients with acquired immunodeficiency syndrome (AIDS)	An asymptomatic pulmonary infection disseminates to extrapulmonary sites, usually the CNS, but also skin, bones, prostate gland, liver, or kidneys. If untreated, infection progresses from coma to death due to cerebral edema or hydrocephalus.	♦ Fever, cough with pleuritic pain, and weight loss ♦ Severe frontal and temporal headache, diplopia, blurred vision, dizziness, aphasia, and vomiting ♦ Skin abscesses and painful lesions of the long bones, skull, spine, and joints
DiGeorge syndrome ♦ Caused by microdeletion of chromosome 22 ♦ Partial or total absence of cell-mediated immunity that results from a deficiency of T-lymphocytes	Abnormal fetal development of the third and fourth pharyngeal pouches interferes with thymus formation. The thymus is absent or partially present in an abnormal site, causing deficient cell-mediated immunity. Without a fetal thymus transplant, patients die by age 2.	At birth: ♦ Low-set ears, notches in ear pinna, fish-shaped mouth, bifid uvula, high-arched palate, an undersized jaw and abnormally wide-set eyes ♦ Great vessel anomalies and tetralogy of Fallot ♦ Hypocalcemia ♦ CNS and early heart failure
Encephalitis ♦ Severe inflammation of the brain, usually caused by a mosquito- or tick-borne virus; also by ingestion of infected goat's milk and accidental injection or inhalation of the virus	Intense lymphocytic infiltration of brain tissues and the leptomeninges causes cerebral edema, degeneration of the brain's ganglion cells, and diffuse nerve cell destruction.	♦ Acute illness begins with sudden onset of fever, headache, and vomiting ♦ Progresses to signs and symptoms of meningeal irritation (stiff neck and back) and neuronal damage (drowsiness, coma, paralysis, seizures, ataxia, tremors, nausea, vomiting, and organic psychoses) ♦ After acute illness, coma may persist for days or weeks

Disease and causes	Pathophysiology	Signs and symptoms
Encephalitis *(continued)* ♦ Results from infection with arboviruses, enteroviruses, herpesvirus, mumps virus, human immunodeficiency virus (HIV), adenoviruses, and demyelinating diseases after measles, varicella, rubella, or vaccination		
Epicondylitis ♦ Inflammation of the extensor tendons of the forearm or inflammation at the origin of the flexor muscles of the wrist ♦ Common among tennis players or persons whose activities require a forceful grasp, wrist extension against resistance, or frequent forearm rotation	This disorder probably begins as a partial tear of the tendon or muscle. Untreated epicondylitis may become disabling as adherent fibers form between the tendons and the elbow capsule.	♦ Elbow pain that gradually worsens and usually radiates to the forearm and back of the hand whenever grasping an object or twisting the elbow ♦ Tenderness over the involved lateral or medial epicondyle or over the head of the radius and a weak grasp
Epidermolysis bullosa ♦ Cause unknown ♦ Nonscarring forms result from an autosomal dominant inheritance, except for junctional epidermolysis bullosa (recessively inherited) and dystrophic epidermolysis bullosa (results from X-linked recessive inheritance)	Vesicles and bullae occur from frictional trauma or heat; prognosis depends on severity. Fatal in infants and children, but becomes less severe with maturity.	♦ Vesicles and bullae appear on hands, feet, knees, or elbows, and occur in the GI, respiratory, or genitourinary tracts ♦ Eyelid blisters, conjunctivitis, adhesions, and corneal opacities ♦ Sloughing of large areas of newborn skin ♦ Scars and contractures may result upon healing
Epiglottiditis ♦ Acute inflammation of the epiglottis that tends to cause airway obstruction; typically strikes children between ages 2 and 8 ♦ Usually results from infection with *Haemophilus influenzae* type B and, occasionally, pneumococci and group A streptococci	Sometimes preceded by an upper respiratory tract infection, epiglottiditis may rapidly progress to complete upper airway obstruction within 2 to 5 hours. Laryngeal obstruction results from inflammation and edema of the epiglottis.	♦ High fever, stridor, sore throat, dysphagia, irritability, restlessness, and drooling ♦ To relieve severe respiratory distress, child may hyperextend his neck, sit up, and lean forward with his mouth open, tongue protruding, and nostrils flaring ♦ Inspiratory retractions and rhonchi
Esophageal varices ♦ Portal hypertension	Shunting of blood to the venae cavae due to portal hypertension leads to a complex of enlarged, swollen, and tortuous veins at the lower end of the esophagus.	♦ Hemorrhage and subsequent hypotension ♦ Compromised oxygen supply ♦ Altered level of consciousness ♦ Hematemesis

Disease and causes	Pathophysiology	Signs and symptoms
Fanconi's syndrome ♦ Inherited renal tubular transport disorder ♦ May also result from exposure to certain environmental toxins such as heavy metals	Changes in the proximal renal tubules due to atrophy of epithelial cells and loss of proximal tube volume results in a shortened connection to glomeruli by an unusually narrow segment. Malfunction of the proximal renal tubules leads to hyperkalemia, hypernatremia, glycosuria, phosphaturia, aminoaciduria, uricosuria, acidosis, retarded growth, and rickets.	♦ Mostly normal appearance at birth with slightly lower birth weight ♦ After 6 months: weakness, failure to thrive, dehydration, cystine crystals in the corners of the eye, and retinal pigment degeneration ♦ Yellow skin with little pigmentation ♦ Slow linear growth
Galactosemia ♦ Inherited autosomal recessive defects ♦ Inability to metabolize galactose (a sugar formed mainly by digestion of the disaccharaide lactose that's present in milk)	Galactose-1-phosphate and galactose accumulate in the tissues, leading to decreased hepatic output of glucose and hypoglycemia.	♦ Poor growth in the first few weeks of life ♦ Nausea, vomiting, and diarrhea ♦ Renal failure ♦ Jaundice and hepatomegaly ♦ Mental retardation, malnourishment, progressive hepatic failure, and death
Gallbladder and bile duct carcinoma ♦ Rare cancer in patients with cholecystitis ♦ Rapidly progressive and fatal ♦ Cause of extrahepatic bile duct carcinoma unknown	Direct extension to liver, cystic and common bile ducts, stomach, and colon causes obstructions and consequent progressive, profound jaundice and epigastric and right upper quadrant pain.	♦ Presents with ulcerative colitis; difficult to distinguish from cholecystitis ♦ Pain in epigastrium or upper right quadrant ♦ Weight loss, anorexia, chills, and fever ♦ Nausea, vomiting, and jaundice ♦ Pruritus and skin excoriations
Gas gangrene ♦ Local infection in devitalized tissue due to *Clostridium perfringens*	Bacteria produce hydrolytic enzymes and toxins that destroy connective tissue and cellular membranes and cause gas bubbles to form in muscle cells. Enzymes also lyse red blood cell (RBC) membranes, destroying their oxygen-carrying capacity.	♦ Myositis and soft-tissue anaerobic cellulitis ♦ Crepitus ♦ Severe localized pain, swelling, and distortion ♦ Bullae and necrosis form after 36 hours ♦ Skin over wound may rupture, exposing dark red or black necrotic muscle and a foul-smelling watery or frothy discharge ♦ Intravascular hemolysis, thrombosis of blood vessels, toxemia, and hypovolemia ♦ Toxic delirium

Disease and causes	Pathophysiology	Signs and symptoms
Giant cell arteritis ♦ Immune-mediated process ♦ Possible infectious cause ♦ Genetic factors apparent with HLA-DR4 genotype; twice as common in women; incidence increases sharply with age	Lymphocytes, plasma cells, and multinucleated giant cells infiltrate affected vessels. Patchy or segmental changes overcome the medium and large arteries of the head and neck and may extend into the carotids and aorta. A cell-mediated immune response directed toward antigens in or near the elastic tissue component of the arterial wall may account for this disorder.	♦ Continuous, throbbing, intractable temporal headache ♦ Ischemia of masseter muscles, tongue, and pharynx ♦ Necrosis and ulceration of scalp ♦ Ocular or orbital pain ♦ Transient loss of vision, visual field defects, blurring, and hallucinations ♦ Tender, red, swollen, and nodular temporal arteries with diminished pulses ♦ Sudden blindness ♦ Pale, swollen optic disk surrounded by pericapillary hemorrhage ♦ Depression, difficulty in chewing, weight loss, and fever
Goodpasture's syndrome ♦ Cause unknown; may result from a genetic predisposition or environmental insult	Abnormal production of autoantibodies directed against alveolar and glomerular basement membranes leads to immune-mediated inflammation of lung and kidney tissues.	♦ Cough, bloody sputum, and dyspnea ♦ Anemia ♦ Peripheral edema ♦ Hematuria, elevated serum creatinine and protein levels, progressive renal failure
Hand, foot, and mouth disease ♦ Highly contagious, common disease in infants and children due to coxsackievirus A 16 or enterovirus 71	RNA virus produces fever and vesicles in the oropharynx and on the hands and feet.	♦ Fever, poor appetite, malaise, and sore throat ♦ Painful vesicular lesions on the mouth, tongue, hands, and feet
Hemothorax ♦ Blood in the chest that usually results from blunt or penetrating chest trauma	Blood from damaged intercostal, pleural, mediastinal, and (infrequently) lung parenchymal vessels enters the pleural cavity. Depending on the amount of bleeding and the underlying cause, hemothorax may be associated with varying degrees of lung collapse and mediastinal shift. Pneumothorax commonly accompanies hemothorax.	♦ Chest pain, tachypnea, and mild to severe dyspnea ♦ Marked blood loss producing hypotension and shock ♦ Affected side of the chest expands and stiffens, whereas the unaffected side rises and falls with the patient's breaths
Hiatal hernia ♦ Malformation or weakening of the diaphragm	Weakening of anchors from the gastroesophageal junction to the diaphragm or increased abdominal pressure allow herniation of part of the stomach through the esophageal hiatus in the diaphragm.	♦ Reflux of gastric contents with associated indigestion (heartburn) ♦ Dysphagia ♦ Chest pain

Disease and causes	Pathophysiology	Signs and symptoms
Hirsutism ♦ Androgen excess due to hereditary or endocrine (such as Cushing's or acromegaly) causes or pharmacologic adverse effects	Minoxidil, androgenic steroids, or testosterone ingestion can cause signs of masculinization, pituitary dysfunction (precocious puberty), or adrenal dysfunction (Cushing's syndrome).	♦ Excessive hair growth in women or children, typically in an adult male distribution pattern
Hydronephrosis ♦ An abnormal dilation of the renal pelvis and the calyces of one or both kidneys, caused by an obstruction of urine flow in the genitourinary tract (such as from benign prostatic hyperplasia, urethral strictures, or calculi)	Partial obstruction and hydronephrosis may not produce initial symptoms, but pressure built up behind the area of obstruction results in symptomatic renal dysfunction. Total obstruction of urine flow with dilation of the collecting system ultimately causes complete cortical atrophy and cessation of glomerular filtration.	*Clinical features include:* ♦ No symptoms or only mild pain and slightly decreased urine flow ♦ Severe, colicky renal pain or dull flank pain that may radiate to the groin and gross urinary abnormalities, such as hematuria, pyuria, dysuria, alternating oliguria and polyuria, or complete anuria *Other signs and symptoms include:* ♦ Nausea, vomiting, and abdominal fullness ♦ Pain on urination, dribbling, or hesitancy, and infection due to urinary stasis
Hyperbilirubinemia ♦ Rh or ABO mother/fetal incompatibility or intrauterine viral infection ♦ May also result from disease states that either increase the rate of bilirubin production or decrease the rate of bilirubin secretion into the bile ducts	Massive destruction of RBCs causes a high level of bilirubin in the blood.	♦ Elevated serum bilirubin level ♦ Jaundice
Hypersplenism ♦ Increased activity of the spleen, whereby all types of blood cells are removed from circulation due to chronic myelogenous leukemia, lymphomas, Gaucher's disease, hairy cell leukemia, or sarcoidosis ♦ May also be associated with portal hypertension, malaria, tuberculosis, and various connective tissue and inflammatory diseases	Spleen growth may be stimulated by an increase in its workload, such as the trapping and destroying of abnormal RBCs.	♦ Enlarged spleen ♦ Cytopenia ♦ Abdominal pain on left side ♦ Fullness after eating only a small amount of food
Idiopathic pulmonary fibrosis ♦ Chronic progressive lung disease associated with inflammation and fibrosis. ♦ Cause unknown, but may be associated with cigarette smoking, wood or metal dust exposure, or chronic gastroesophageal reflux disease	Interstitial inflammation consists of an alveolar septal infiltrate of lymphocytes, plasma cells, and histiocytes. Fibrotic areas are composed of dense acellular collagen. Areas of honeycombing that form are composed of cystic fibrotic air spaces, frequently lined with bronchiolar epithelium and filled with mucus. Smooth-muscle hyperplasia may occur in areas of fibrosis and honeycombing.	♦ Dyspnea ♦ Nonproductive cough ♦ Chest heaviness ♦ Wheezing ♦ Anorexia ♦ Weight loss

Disease and causes	Pathophysiology	Signs and symptoms
Intussusception ♦ A telescoping (invagination) of a portion of the bowel into an adjacent distal portion ♦ Cause of most cases unknown; may be linked to viral infection, alterations in intestinal motility, hemangioma, lymphosarcoma, lymphoid hyperplasia, or Meckel's diverticulum in children and benign or malignant tumors in adults	When a bowel segment invaginates, peristalsis propels it along the bowel, pulling more bowel along with it. This invagination produces edema, hemorrhage from venous engorgement, incarceration, and obstruction. If treatment is delayed for longer than 24 hours, strangulation of the intestine usually occurs, causing gangrene, shock, and perforation.	♦ Intermittent attacks of colicky pain ♦ Vomiting ♦ "Currant jelly" stools, containing a mixture of blood and mucus ♦ Tender, distended abdomen, with a palpable, sausage-shaped abdominal mass
Kaposi's sarcoma ♦ Malignant, AIDS-related cancer	Arising from vascular endothelial cells, Kaposi's sarcoma affects endothelial tissue, which compromises all blood vessels.	♦ Red-purple or brown circular lesions, slightly raised on the face, arms, neck, and legs ♦ Internal lesions, especially in GI tract, identified by biopsy
Keratitis ♦ Inflammation of cornea due to microorganisms, trauma, or an autoimmune disorder	Bacterial infection leads to ulceration of the cornea.	♦ Decreased visual acuity ♦ Pain ♦ Photophobia
Kidney cancer ♦ Renal cell carcinoma that results from structural alteration of the short arm of chromosome 3 (3p) ♦ Associated with obesity and cigarette smoking	Tumors of various cell types and patterns that are usually aggressive in growth and affect younger patients.	♦ Hematuria, flank pain, increased erythrocyte sedimentation rate ♦ Palpable mass ♦ Weight loss, anemia, fever, and hypertension
Lassa fever ♦ Highly contagious viral infection due to *Lassa* species	An epidemic hemorrhagic fever transmitted to humans by contact with infected rodent urine, feces, or saliva. Human-to-human transmission may occur through contact with the blood, tissue, or secretions of an infected person.	♦ Fever lasting 2 to 3 weeks ♦ Exudative pharyngitis, oral ulcers, dysphagia, and swelling of face and neck ♦ Lymphadenopathy ♦ Purpura, ecchymoses ♦ Conjunctivitis ♦ Bradycardia, shock, peripheral collapse ♦ Pleural effusion and renal involvement
Legionnaires' disease ♦ Infection caused by gram-negative bacillus *Legionella pneumophila*	Transmission occurs with inhalation of organism carried in aerosols produced by air-conditioning units, water faucets, shower heads, humidifiers, and contaminated respiratory equipment.	♦ Dry cough ♦ Myalgia ♦ GI distress, diarrhea ♦ Pneumonia ♦ Cardiovascular collapse
Leprosy ♦ Infection caused by *Mycobacterium leprae*	Chronic, systemic infection with progressive cutaneous lesions, attacking the peripheral nervous system.	♦ Skin lesions ♦ Anesthesia ♦ Muscle weakness ♦ Paralysis

Disease and causes	Pathophysiology	Signs and symptoms
Medullary sponge kidneys ♦ Genetic disorder	Collecting ducts in the renal pyramids dilate, forming cavities, clefts, and cysts that produce complications of calcium oxylate stones and infections.	♦ Renal calculi ♦ Hematuria ♦ Infection (fever, chills, and malaise)
Melasma ♦ Hypermelanotic skin disorder associated with increased hormonal levels with pregnancy, hormonal contraceptive use, or ovarian cancer	Thought to be due to the effects of estrogen and progesterone on melanin production.	♦ Patchy, nonraised, hypermelanotic rash
Myelitis and acute transverse myelitis ♦ Caused by acute infectious disease (measles or pneumonia) or primary lesions of the spinal cord (syphilis or acute disseminated encephalomyelitis); can accompany demyelinating diseases (acute multiple sclerosis) and inflammatory and necrotizing disorders of the spinal cord (hematoyelia) ♦ May result from certain toxic agents (such as carbon monoxide, lead, or arsenic); other infections, such as poliovirus, herpes zoster, or herpesvirus B; disorders that cause meningeal inflammation; smallpox or polio vaccination; or an autoimmune reaction	Myelitis is an inflammation of the spinal cord that can result from several diseases. Only the cord's gray matter may be affected, producing motor dysfunction, or the white matter may be affected, producing sensory dysfunction. These types of myelitis can attack any level of the spinal cord, causing partial destruction or scattered lesions. Acute transverse myelitis, which affects the entire thickness of the spinal cord, produces motor and sensory dysfunctions. It has a rapid onset and is the most devastating form of myelitis.	♦ Sensory or motor dysfunction, depending on the site of damage to the spinal cord *Acute transverse myelitis:* ♦ Rapid motor and sensory dysfunctions below the level of spinal cord damage appearing in 1 to 2 days ♦ Flaccid paralysis of the legs with loss of sensory and sphincter functions ♦ Reflexes disappear, but may reappear later ♦ Extent of damage depends on the level of the spinal cord affected ♦ If spinal cord damage is severe, shock may occur (hypotension and hypothermia)
Necrotizing enterocolitis ♦ Diffuse or patchy intestinal necrosis, accompanied by sepsis in about one-third of cases ♦ Exact cause unknown; suggested predisposing factors include birth asphyxia, postnatal hypotension, umbilical vessel catheterization, exchange transfusion, or patent ductus arteriosus; may also be a response to significant prenatal stress, such as premature rupture of membranes, placenta previa, preeclampsia, or maternal sepsis	According to current theory, necrotizing enterocolitis develops when the infant suffers perinatal hypoxemia due to shunting of blood from the gut to more vital organs. Subsequent mucosal ischemia provides an ideal medium for bacterial growth. As the bowel swells and breaks down, gas-forming bacteria invade damaged areas, producing free air in the intestinal wall. This may result in fatal perforation and peritonitis.	♦ Distended (especially tense or rigid) abdomen with gastric retention ♦ Increasing residual gastric contents, which may contain bile ♦ Bile-stained vomitus ♦ Occult blood in the stool ♦ Thermal instability, lethargy, metabolic acidosis, jaundice, and disseminated intravascular coagulation

Disease and causes	Pathophysiology	Signs and symptoms
Neurofibromatosis ♦ Inherited autosomal dominant disorder	Group of developmental disorders of the nervous system, muscles, bones, and skin that affects the cell growth of neural tissue.	♦ Café-au-lait spots ♦ Multiple, pediculated, soft tumors (neurofibromas) ♦ Hearing loss ♦ Bone changes and skeletal deformities
Orbital cellulitis ♦ Bacterial infection typically due to streptococcal, staphylococcal, and pneumococcal organisms	Inflammation and infection of the fatty orbital tissues and eyelids.	♦ Unilateral eyelid edema ♦ Hyperemia ♦ Redden eyelids and matted lashes
Osgood-Schlatter disease ♦ Probably results from trauma before the epiphysis has completely fused to the main bone (between ages 10 and 15); such trauma may be a single violent action or repeated knee flexion against a tight quadriceps muscle	This disorder is a painful, incomplete separation of the epiphysis of the tibial tubercle from the tibial shaft and is most common in active adolescent boys. Severe disease may cause permanent tubercle enlargement.	♦ Constant aching and pain and tenderness below the kneecap ♦ Obvious soft-tissue swelling and localized heat and tenderness
Pediculosis ♦ Infestation by the lice parasite	Louse attaches itself to the hair shaft with claws and feeds on blood several times daily; resides close to the scalp to maintain its body temperature. Itching may be due to an allergic reaction to louse saliva or irritability.	♦ Itching and inflammation ♦ Eczematous dermatitis ♦ Tiredness, irritability, and weakness ♦ Lice present in hair (head, axillae, and pubic area)
Penile cancer ♦ Preceded by chronic irritation, condylomata acuminata, or phimosis in uncircumcised men	Neoplasms may be benign or malignant; latter are usually squamous cell carcinomas.	♦ Painless ulcerations on the glans or foreskin; small, warty plaque ♦ Dysuria, purulent discharge, and obstruction
Phenylketonuria ♦ Inborn error in phenylalanine metabolism resulting in the accumulation of high serum phenylalanine levels ♦ Transmitted by an autosomal recessive gene	The patient with this disorder has insufficient hepatic phenylalanine hydroxylase, an enzyme that acts as a catalyst in the conversion of phenylalanine to tyrosine. As a result, phenylalanine and its metabolites accumulate in the blood, causing mental retardation if left untreated. The exact mechanism that causes this retardation is unclear.	♦ By age 4 months, infant shows signs of arrested brain development, including mental retardation and, later, personality disturbances (schizoid and antisocial personality patterns and uncontrollable temper) ♦ Lighter complexion and commonly has blue eyes ♦ Microcephaly; eczematous skin lesions or dry, rough skin; and a musty (mousy) odor ♦ Abnormal EEG patterns and, possibly, seizures
Pheochromocytoma ♦ Polyglandular multiple endocrine neoplasia ♦ Possible familial origin	Tumor of the chromaffin cells of the adrenal medulla that causes an increased production of catecholamines.	♦ Hypertension, high blood glucose and lipid levels ♦ Headache, palpitations, sweating, dizziness, syncope, anxiety, and constipation

Disease and causes	Pathophysiology	Signs and symptoms
Pilonidal disease ♦ May develop congenitally from a tendency to hirsutism, or it may be acquired from stretching or irritation of the sacrococcygeal area from prolonged rough exercise, heat, excessive perspiration, or constrictive clothing	A coccygeal cyst forms in the intergluteal cleft on the posterior surface of the lower sacrum. It usually contains hair and becomes infected, producing an abscess, a draining sinus, or a fistula.	♦ Generally, no signs or symptoms until the cyst becomes infected ♦ Local pain, tenderness, swelling, or heat ♦ Continuous or intermittent purulent drainage ♦ Abscess development, chills, fever, headache, and malaise
Pleurisy ♦ Several causes including lupus, rheumatoid arthritis, and tuberculosis	Inflammation of the visceral and parietal pleurae that line the inside of the thoracic cage and envelop the lungs.	♦ Sharp, stabbing chest pain ♦ Dyspnea ♦ Pleural friction rub ♦ Fever
Pneumoconioses ♦ Inhalation of dust particles, usually in an occupational setting	Chronic and permanent disposition of particles in the lungs causes a tissue reaction, which may be harmless or destructive.	♦ Shortness of breath and cough ♦ Fatigue and weakness ♦ Weight loss ♦ Emphysema
Polycythemia vera ♦ Cause unknown; possibly due to a multipotential stem cell defect	Increased production of RBCs, neutrophils, and platelets inhibits blood flow to microcirculation, resulting in intravascular thrombosis.	♦ Signs and symptoms usually absent in early stages; in later stages, related to expanded blood volume and system affected ♦ Weakness, headache, light-headedness, vision disturbances, and fatigue ♦ Hepatomegaly and splenomegaly ♦ Maroon or plum-color skin and mucous membranes ♦ Hypertension
Postherpetic neuralgia ♦ Complication of the chronic phase of herpes zoster	Varicella virus in ganglia of the posterior nerve roots reactivates, multiplies, and spreads down the sensory nerves to the skin.	♦ Intractable neurologic pain lasting for more than 6 weeks after disappearance of herpes zoster rash
Pseudogout ♦ Cause unknown; genetic predisposition for the disease exists ♦ Associated with conditions that cause degenerative or metabolic changes in cartilage	Calcium pyrophosphate crystals deposit in periarticular joint structures. It commonly invades knee joint.	♦ Sudden joint pain and swelling in larger peripheral joints; mimics other form of arthritis ♦ Presence of tophi
Pseudomembranous enterocolitis ♦ Acute inflammation and necrosis of the small and large intestines, usually affecting the mucosa but may extend into submucosa and, rarely, other layers ♦ Exact cause unknown; *Clostridium difficile* may produce a toxin that could play a role in development	Necrotic mucosa is replaced by a pseudomembrane filled with staphylococci, leukocytes, mucus, fibrin, and inflammatory cells.	♦ Copious watery or bloody diarrhea, abdominal pain, and fever ♦ Possible severe dehydration, electrolyte imbalance, hypotension, shock, and colonic perforation

Disease and causes	Pathophysiology	Signs and symptoms
Pyloric stenosis ♦ Congenital; cause unknown	Pyloric sphincter muscle fibers thicken and become inelastic, leading to a narrowed opening. The extra peristaltic effort needed leads to hypertrophied muscle layers of the stomach.	♦ Progressive nonbilious vomiting, leading to projectile vomiting at ages 2 to 4 weeks
Rectal prolapse ♦ Protrusion of one or more layers of mucous membrane through the anus due to conditions that affect the pelvic floor or rectum	Increased intra-abdominal pressure triggers the circumferential protrusion of one or more layers of the mucous membrane.	♦ Lower abdominal pain due to ulceration, bloody diarrhea, or tissue protruding from rectum during defecation or walking
Reiter's syndrome ♦ Cause unknown; typically follows a urogenital or enteric infection ♦ Genetic factor (HLA-B27) increases risk of acquiring disorder	An infection (caused by *Mycoplasma, Shigella, Salmonella, Yersinia,* or *Chlamydia* organisms) is thought to initiate an aberrant and hyperactive immune response that produces inflammation in involved target organs.	*General:* ♦ Low-grade fever and unexplained diarrhea ♦ Superficial lesions on palms or soles *Urogenital tract:* ♦ Burning sensation with urination, penile discharge, and prostatitis in men ♦ Cervicitis, urethritis, and vulvovaginitis in women *Joint symptoms or arthritis:* ♦ Affects knees, ankles, and feet ♦ Inflammation where tendon attaches to bone *Eye involvement:* ♦ Conjunctivitis and uveitis
Renal infarction ♦ Formation of a coagulated, necrotic area in one or both kidneys ♦ Caused by renal artery embolism in 75% of patients; less common causes include atherosclerosis, with or without thrombus formation; and thrombus from flank trauma, sickle cell anemia, scleroderma, polyarteritis nodosa, and arterionephrosclerosis	Results from renal blood vessel occlusion that reduces blood flow to renal tissue and leads to ischemia. The location and size of the infarction depend on the site of vascular occlusion; usually, infarction affects the renal cortex, but it can extend into the medulla. Residual renal function after infarction depends on the extent of the damage from the infarction.	♦ May be asymptomatic ♦ Typically, severe abdominal or gnawing flank pain and tenderness, costovertebral tenderness ♦ Fever, anorexia, nausea, and vomiting ♦ Possibly gross hematuria
Renal tubular acidosis ♦ *Distal (type I):* familial with another genetic disease or an isolated autosomal dominant disease ♦ *Proximal (type II):* accompanies several inherited diseases, multiple myeloma, vitamin D deficiency, and chronic hypocalcemia, and follows renal transplantation and treatment with certain drugs	In type I, the distal tubule is unable to secrete hydrogen ions across the tubular membrane, causing decreased excretion of titratable acids and ammonium and increased loss of potassium and bicarbonate. Prolonged acidosis leads to hypercalciuria and renal calculi. In type II, defective	*In infants:* ♦ Vomiting, fever, constipation, anorexia, weakness, polyuria, growth retardation, nephrocalcinosis, and rickets *In children and adults:* ♦ Growth problems, urinary tract infections, and rickets

Disease and causes	Pathophysiology	Signs and symptoms

Renal tubular acidosis *(continued)*

reabsorption of bicarbonate in proximal tubule causes bicarbonate to flood the distal tubule, leading to impaired formation of titratable acids and ammonium for excretion.

Renal vein thrombosis
♦ Clotting in the renal vein
♦ Caused by a tumor that obstructs the renal vein, thrombophlebitis of the inferior vena cava or blood vessels of the legs, heart failure, or periarteritis
♦ In infants, caused by diarrhea, leading to severe dehydration

Results in renal congestion, engorgement, possible infarction. Acute or chronic, may affect both kidneys. Chronic thrombosis usually impairs renal function, causing nephrotic syndrome. Abrupt onset with extensive damage may precipitate rapidly fatal renal infarction. Less severe thrombosis affecting only one kidney or gradual progression allowing circulation to develop may preserve partial renal function.

With rapid onset:
♦ Severe lumbar pain and tenderness in the epigastric region and at the costovertebral angle
♦ Fever, leukocytosis, pallor, hematuria, proteinuria, and peripheral edema
♦ Enlarged kidneys, easily palpable
With gradual onset:
♦ Symptoms of nephrotic syndrome
♦ Pain generally absent
♦ Proteinuria, hypoalbuminemia, and hyperlipidemia
In infants:
♦ Enlarged kidneys, and oliguria
♦ Renal insufficiency that may progress to acute or chronic renal failure

---

Retinal detachment
♦ Caused by trauma, cataract surgery, severe uveitis, and primary or metastatic choroidal tumors; may also occur as a result of internal changes in the vitreous chamber associated with aging

The neural retina separates from the underlying retinal pigment epithelium.

♦ Floaters, flashing lights, scotoma in peripheral visual field (painless) and, eventually, a curtain or veil occurs in the field of vision

---

Retinitis pigmentosa
♦ Autosomal recessive disorder in 80% of affected children
♦ Less commonly transmitted as an X-linked trait

Slow, degenerative changes in rods cause the retina and pigment epithelium to atrophy. Irregular black deposits of clumped pigment are in equatorial region of retina and eventually in the macular and peripheral areas.

♦ Progressive night blindness, visual field constriction with ring scotoma, and loss of acuity progressing to blindness

---

Rocky Mountain spotted fever
♦ Infection due to *Rickettsia rickettsii* carried by several tick species

R. rickettsii multiplies within endothelial cells and spreads via the bloodstream. Focal areas of infiltration lead to thrombosis and leakage of RBCs into surrounding tissue.

♦ Fever, headache, mental confusion, and myalgia
♦ Rash develops as small macules that progress to maculopapules and petechiae (Starts on wrists and ankles, spreads to trunk. Diagnostic rash on palms and soles.)
♦ Constipation and abdominal distention

Disease and causes	Pathophysiology	Signs and symptoms
Rosacea ♦ Cause unknown	Small facial blood vessels, usually in the nose and cheeks, become flushed and dilated.	♦ Pronounced flushing of nose, cheeks, and forehead ♦ Papules, pustules, and telangiectases can be superimposed
Sarcoidosis ♦ Cause unknown ♦ Evidence suggests that disease is result of exaggerated cellular immune response to limited class of antigens	Organ dysfunction results from an accumulation of T lymphocytes, mononuclear phagocytes, and nonsecreting epithelial granulomas, which distort normal tissue architecture.	♦ Mainly generalized, most commonly involving the lung with resulting respiratory symptoms such as shortness of breath ♦ Fever, fatigue, and malaise
Scabies ♦ Human itch mite (Sarcoptes scabiei var. hominis)	Mite burrows superficially beneath stratum corneum depositing eggs that hatch, mature, and reinvade the skin. Sensitization reaction against mite excreta results.	♦ Intense itching, worsens at night ♦ Threadlike lesions on wrists, between fingers, and on elbows, axillae, belt line, buttocks, and male genitalia ♦ Secondary bacterial infection may occur
Septic arthritis ♦ Infectious arthritis ♦ Common infecting organisms include gram-positive cocci and Staphylococcus aureus, Streptococcus pyogenes, and S. pneumoniae in children; Neisseria gonorrhoeae, S. aureus, and streptococci in adults ♦ Predisposing factors include concurrent bacterial infection or serious chronic illness, diseases that depress the immune system and immunosuppressant therapy, recent articular trauma, joint surgery, intra-articular injections, and local joint abnormalities	This disorder occurs when bacterial invasion of a joint causes inflammation of the synovial lining, effusion and pyogenesis, and destruction of bone and cartilage. Septic arthritis can lead to ankylosis and, without prompt treatment, even fatal septicemia.	♦ Intense pain, inflammation, and swelling of the affected joint ♦ Low-grade fever ♦ Migratory polyarthritis
Severe combined immmunodeficiency syndrome ♦ Both cell-mediated (T-cell) and humoral (B-cell) immunity are deficient or absent, resulting in susceptibility to infection from all classes of microorganisms during infancy ♦ Usually transmitted as an autosomal recessive trait, although it may be X-linked	In most cases, genetic defect seems associated with failure of the stem cell to differentiate into T and B lymphocytes. Many molecular defects, such as mutation of the kinase ZAP-70, can cause this disorder. X-linked severe combined immunodeficiency syndrome is due to a mutation of a subunit of the interleukin (IL)-2, IL-4, and IL-7 receptors. Less commonly, it results from an enzyme deficiency.	♦ Extreme susceptibility to infection ♦ Failure to thrive and chronic otitis, sepsis, watery diarrhea (associated with Salmonella or Escherichia coli), recurrent pulmonary infections, persistent oral candidiasis and, possibly, fatal viral infections (such as chickenpox) ♦ Pneumocystis carinii pneumonia

Disease and causes	Pathophysiology	Signs and symptoms
Silicosis ♦ Exposure to high concentrations of respirable silica dust	Alveolar macrophages engulf respirable particles of free silica, causing release of cytotoxic enzymes. This attracts other macrophages and produces fibrous tissue in the lung parenchyma. Note: Silicosis is associated with a high incidence of active tuberculosis.	*In simple nodular silicosis:* ♦ Cough and raise sputum, usually no symptoms *In conglomerate silicosis:* ♦ Severe shortness of breath, cough, and sputum; may lead to pulmonary hypertension and cor pulmonale
Sjögren's syndrome ♦ Autoimmune rheumatic disorder with unknown cause; genetic and environmental factors may be involved	Lymphocytic infiltration of exocrine glands causes tissue damage that results in xerostomia and dry eyes.	*In xerostomia:* ♦ Dry mouth; difficulty swallowing and speaking; ulcers of tongue, buccal mucosa and lips; severe dental caries *In ocular involvement:* ♦ Dry eyes; gritty, sandy feeling; decreased tearing; burning; itching; redness; and photosensitivity *Extraglandular:* ♦ Arthralgias, Raynaud's phenomenon, lymphadenopathy, and lung involvement
Sleep apnea ♦ Caused by occlusion of airway (obstructive), absence of respiratory effort (central), or both ♦ Associated with obesity	Airflow ceases due to upper-airway narrowing and glottal obstruction as a result of obesity or congenital abnormalities of the upper airway. When primary brain stem medullary failure occurs, sleeping patient may breathe insufficiently or not at all.	*In obstructive sleep apnea:* ♦ Snoring, excessive daytime sleepiness, intellectual impairment, memory loss, and cardiorespiratory symptoms *In central sleep apnea:* ♦ Sleeping poorly, morning headache, and daytime fatigue
Spinal cord ischemia or infarction ♦ Caused by direct vascular compression (tumors and acute disc compression) or by remote occlusion (aortic surgery and dissecting aneurysm)	Major arterial branches that supply the spinal cord become compressed or occluded, decreasing blood flow to the spinal cord, causing cord ischemia and motor and sensory deficiencies.	♦ If associated with spinal column injury, sudden back pain and pain in distribution of affected segment followed by bilateral flaccid weakness and dissociated sensory loss below level of infarct ♦ If associated with embolic infarct, no pain
Sporotrichosis ♦ Fungal infection caused by *Sporothrix schenckii*, which occurs in soil, wood, sphagnum moss, and decaying vegetation	Inflammatory response includes both the clustering of neutrophils and a marked granulomatous response, with epithelioid cells and giant cells producing nodular erythematous primary lesions and secondary lesions along lymphatic channels in cutaneous lymphatic type.	*In cutaneous or lymphatic sporotrichosis:* ♦ Subcutaneous, movable, painless nodule on hands or fingers that grows progressively larger, discolors, and eventually ulcerates; additional lesions form on the adjacent lymph node chain *In pulmonary sporotrichosis:* ♦ Productive cough, lung cavities and nodules, pleural effusion, fibrosis, and formation of fungus ball

Disease and causes	Pathophysiology	Signs and symptoms
Sporotrichosis *(continued)*	In pulmonary sporotrichosis, inflammatory response produces pulmonary lesions and nodules. In disseminated sporotrichosis, multifocal lesions spread from skin or lungs.	*In disseminated sporotrichosis:* ♦ Weight loss, anorexia, synovial or bony lesions and, possibly, arthritis or osteomyelitis
Stickler syndrome ♦ Autosomal dominant chondrodysplasia caused by structural defects in collagen, an essential component of connective tissue ♦ Characterized by ocular, skeletal, auditory, and craniofacial abnormalities	Collagen defect typically is caused by a mutation in the type II collagen gene (COL2A1) located on chromosome 12q13.11 to 12q13.2. Others show linkage to the COL11A2 gene located on chromosome 6p21.3 and others to COL11A1 gene located on chromosome 1p21. COL11A2 and COL11A1 are expressed in the hyaline cartilage, vitreous, intervertebral disc, and inner ear.	♦ Ocular signs and symptoms: myopia, vitreal abnormalities, and retinal detachment resulting in blindness ♦ Auditory signs and symptoms: conductive hearing loss or sensorineural hearing loss ♦ Craniofacial features: micrognathia and a flattened midface and nasal bridge ♦ Skeletal signs and symptoms: joint hypermobility, spondyloepiphyseal dysplasia, and degenerative arthropathy
Strabismus ♦ Eye malalignment that's commonly inherited; controversy exists whether amblyopia is caused by or results from strabismus	In paralytic (nonconcomitant) strabismus, paralysis of one or more ocular muscles may be due to oculomotor nerve lesion. In nonparalytic (concomitant) strabismus, unequal ocular muscle tone is due to supranuclear abnormality within the CNS.	♦ Noticeable eye malalignment by external eye examination, ophthalmoscopic observation of the corneal light reflex in center of pupils, diplopia, and other visual disturbances ♦ Visual acuity diminishes with decreased use of an eye
Tinea versicolor ♦ Caused by *Malassezia furfur,* which occurs normally in human skin ♦ Unclear whether disorder is due to infectious cause or a proliferation of normal skin fungi	Nondermatophyte dimorphic fungus converts to the hyphal form and causes characteristic lesions. Invasion of the stratum corneum by the yeast produces C9 and C11 dicarboxylic acids that inhibit tyrosinase in vitro.	♦ Asymptomatic, well-delineated, hyperpigmented or hypopigmented macules occur on upper trunk and arms
Tourette syndrome ♦ Autosomal dominant multipletic disorder	Obscure pathology; dopaminergic excess suggested because tics may respond to treatment with a dopamine blocker.	♦ Single or multiple motor tics that commonly affect the face, and phonic tics ♦ Involuntary arm and shoulder movements
Trachoma ♦ Infection caused by *Chlamydia trachomatis*	Chronic conjunctivitis due to *C. trachomatis* that leads to inflammatory leukocytic infiltration and superficial vascularization of the cornea,	♦ Mild infection resembling bacterial conjunctivitis; red and edematous eyelids, pain, photophobia, tearing, and exudation

Disease and causes	Pathophysiology	Signs and symptoms
Trachoma *(continued)*	conjunctival scarring, and eyelid distortion. This causes lashes to abrade the cornea, which progresses to corneal ulceration, scarring, and blindness.	
Trichomoniasis ♦ Infection of the genitourinary tract caused by *Trichomonas vaginalis*	*T. vaginalis* infects the vagina, urethra and, possibly, the endocervix, bladder, or Bartholin's or Skene's glands. In males, it infects the lower urethra and possibly the prostate gland, seminal vesicles, and epididymis.	*In females:* ♦ Malodorous, green-yellow vaginal discharge; irritation of vulva, perineum, and thighs; dyspareunia; and dysuria *In males:* ♦ Generally asymptomatic; some transient frothy or purulent urethral discharge with dysuria and frequency; and recurrent urethritis
Trigeminal neuralgia ♦ Cause unknown, possibly a compression neuropathy ♦ At surgery or autopsy, the intracranial arterial and venous loops are found to compress the trigeminal nerve root at the brain stem	Painful disorder along the distribution of one or more of the trigeminal nerve's sensory divisions, usually the maxillary.	♦ Searing or burning pain lasting seconds to 2 minutes at the trigeminal nerve distribution ♦ Touching a trigger point typically elicits pain
Uveitis ♦ Cause unknown but associated with many autoimmune diseases or from allergy, bacteria, viruses, fungi, chemicals, trauma, or surgery	An inflammation of any part of the uveal tract. Inflammatory cells floating in aqueous humor or deposited on corneal endothelium affect the uveal tract.	*Anterior:* ♦ Pain, redness, photophobia, and decreased vision *Intermediate:* ♦ Floaters and decreased vision *Posterior:* ♦ Diverse signs and symptoms, most commonly floaters and decreased vision
Vaginal cancer ♦ Cause unknown; tumor development has been linked to intrauterine exposure to diethylstilbestrol and to human papillomavirus	Presents mainly as squamous cell carcinoma (sometimes as melanoma, sarcoma, or adenocarcinoma), progresses from intraepithelial tumor to invasive cancer.	♦ Abnormal bleeding and discharge ♦ Firm, ulcerated lesion in the vagina
Vitiligo ♦ Cause unknown; usually acquired but may be familial (autosomal dominant) ♦ Possible immunologic and neurochemical basis	Destruction of melanocytes (humoral or cellular) and circulating antibodies against melanocytes results in hypopigmented areas.	♦ Progressive, symmetric areas of complete pigment loss with sharp borders, generally appearing in periorifical areas, flexor wrists, and extensor distal extremities

Disease and causes	Pathophysiology	Signs and symptoms
Volvulus ♦ May result from an anomaly of rotation, an ingested foreign body, or an adhesion, or cause may be unknown	Twisting of the intestinal tract at least 180 degrees on its mesentery causes blood vessel compression and ischemia. In adults, most common site is the sigmoid bowel; in children, the small bowel. Other common sites: stomach and cecum.	♦ Vomiting and rapid, marked abdominal distention ♦ Sudden onset of severe abdominal pain
Wiskott-Aldrich syndrome ♦ X-linked recessive immunodeficiency disorder resulting from genetic defect found on Xp11.22-23 ♦ Defective B-cell and T-cell functions	Deficiency in both B-cell and T-cell function allows for susceptibility to infection. Metabolic defect in platelet synthesis causes production of small, short-lived platelets, resulting in thrombocytopenia.	*In neonate:* ♦ Hemorrhagic symptoms such as bloody stools, bleeding from circumcision site, petechiae, and purpura *In older children:* ♦ Recurrent systemic infections and eczema ♦ Meningitis

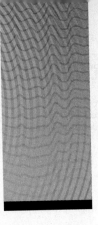

SELECTED REFERENCES

General

ACC Atlas of Pathophysiology, 3rd ed. Philadelphia: Lippincott Williams & Wilkins, 2009.

Fauci, A.S., et al., eds. Harrison's Principles of Internal Medicine, 17th ed. New York: McGraw-Hill Book Co., 2008.

Huether, S., and McCance, K. Understanding Pathophysiology, 4th ed. St. Louis: Mosby, 2008.

Nursing2009 Drug Handbook. Philadelphia: Lippincott Williams & Wilkins, 2009.

Porth, C.M. Essentials of Pathophysiology: Concepts of Altered Health States, 2nd ed. Philadelphia: Lippincott Williams & Wilkins, 2007.

Professional Guide to Diseases, 9th ed. Philadelphia: Lippincott Williams & Wilkins, 2009.

Seeley, R.R., et al. Anatomy and Physiology, 8th ed. New York: McGraw-Hill Book Co., 2007.

Smeltzer, S.C., et al. Brunner and Suddarth's Textbook of Medical-Surgical Nursing, 11th ed. Philadelphia: Lippincott Williams & Wilkins, 2006.

Cancer

Abraham, J., et al. Bethesda Handbook of Clinical Oncology, 2nd ed. Philadelphia: Lippincott Williams & Wilkins, 2005.

Chabner, B.A., and Longo, D.L. Cancer Chemotherapy and Biotherapy, 4th ed. Philadelphia: Lippincott Williams & Wilkins, 2005.

Kantarjian, H.M., et al. The MD Anderson Manual of Medical Oncology. New York: McGraw-Hill Book Co., 2006.

Kelsen, D.P., et al. Principles and Practice of Gastrointestinal Oncology, 2nd ed. Philadelphia: Lippincott Williams & Wilkins, 2007.

Pellegrino, A. "Looking at Liver Cancer," Nursing2006 36(10):52-55, October 2006.

Riehl, M. "Help Your Patient Cope with Pancreatic Cancer," Nursing2007 37(4):54-57, April 2007.

Schiech, L.S. "Looking at Laryngeal Cancer," Nursing2007 37(5):50-55, May 2007.

Wetherbee, S.L. "New Weapons to Snuff Out Kidney Cancer," Nursing2006 36(12):58-63, December 2006.

Infection

Delahanty, K.M., and Myers, F.E. "Nursing2007 Infection Control Survey Report," Nursing 37(6):28-37, June 2007.

Gantz, N.M., et al. Manual of Clinical Problems in Infectious Disease, 5th ed. Philadelphia: Lippincott Williams & Wilkins, 2005.

Goicoechea, M. "Human H5N1 Influenza," New England Journal of Medicine 356(13):1375, March 2007.

Goss, L.K. "Infection Control: It's in Your Hands," Nursing Management 38(6):56-57, June 2007.

Jarvis, W.R. Bennett and Brachman's Hospital Infections, 5th ed. Philadelphia: Lippincott Williams & Wilkins, 2007.

Knipe, D.M., et al. Fields Virology, 5th ed. Philadelphia: Lippincott Williams & Wilkins, 2006.

Krein, S.L., et al. "Use of Central Venous Catheter-Related Bloodstream Infection Prevention Practices by U.S. Hospitals," Mayo Clinic Proceedings 82(6):672-78, June 2007.

Menzies, D., et al. "Risk of Tuberculosis Infection and Disease Associated with Work in Health Care Settings," International Journal of Tuberculosis and Lung Disease 11(6):593-605, June 2007.

Miranda, J.A., et al. "Firm-Based Trial to Improve Central Venous Catheter Insertion Practices," Journal of Hospital Medicine 2(3):135-42, June 2007.

Spicuzza, L., et al. "New and Emerging Infectious Diseases," Allergy and Asthma Proceedings 28(1):28-34, January-February 2007.

Fluids and electrolytes

Coggon, J.M. "Arterial Blood Gas Analysis. 2: Compensatory Mechanisms," Nursing Times 104(19):24-25, May 2008.

Critical Care Nursing in a Flash. Philadelphia: Lippincott Williams & Wilkins, 2008.

Fluids and Electrolytes Made Incredibly Easy, 4th ed. Philadelphia: Lippincott Williams & Wilkins, 2007.

Gorski, L.A. "Infusion Nursing Standards of Practice," *Journal of Infusion Nursing* 30(3):151-52, May/June 2007.

Humphreys, M. "Potassium Disturbances and Associated Electrocardiogram Changes," *Emergency Nursing* 15(5):28-34, September 2007.

Owen, P., et al. "Implementing and Assessing an Evidence-Based Electrolyte Dosing Order Form in the Medical ICU," *Intensive and Critical Care Nursing* 24(1):8-19, February 2008.

Siow, E. "Enteral versus Parenteral Nutrition for Acute Pancreatitis," *Critical Care Nurse* 28(4):19-30, August 2008.

Vacca, V. "Hyperkalemia," *Nursing2008* 38(7):72, July 2008.

Wright, S.K., and Schroeter, S. "Hyponatremia as a Complication of Selective Serotonin Reuptake Inhibitors," *Journal of the American Academy of Nurse Practitioners* 20(1):47-51, January 2008.

Cardiovascular system

Dracup, K., et al. "Acute Coronary Syndrome: What Do Patients Know?" *Archives of Internal Medicine* 168(10):1049-54, May 2008.

Gendreau-Webb, R. "Is It a Kidney Stone or Abdominal Aortic Aneurysm?" *Nursing2006* 36(5 Suppl):22-24, Spring 2006.

Reckard, D., et al. "Mitral Valve Replacement: A Case Report," *AANA Journal* 76(2):125-29, April 2008.

Stephen, S.A., et al. "Symptoms of Acute Coronary Syndrome in Women with Diabetes: An Integrative Review of the Literature," *Heart & Lung* 37(3):179-89, May-June 2008.

Swart, S., and Tiffen, J. "Acute Pericarditis," *AAOHN Journal* 55(2):44-46, February 2007.

Washburn, S.C., and Hornberger, C.A. "Nurse Educator Guidelines for the Management of Heart Failure," *Journal of Continuing Education in Nursing* 39(6):263-67, June 2008.

Woods, S.L., et al. *Cardiac Nursing*, 5th ed. Philadelphia: Lippincott Williams & Wilkins, 2004.

Wung, S.F., and Kozik, T. "Electrocardiographic Evaluation of Cardiovascular Status," *Journal of Cardiovascular Nursing* 23(2):169-74, March-April 2008.

Yates, G., and Saunders, K. "Pulmonary Hypertension: A Review for Nurses," *Canadian Journal of Cardiovascular Nursing* 18(1):7-14, 2008.

Zeigler, V.L. "Congenital Heart Disease and Genetics," *Critical Care Nursing Clinics of North America* 20(2):159-69, June 2008.

Respiratory system

Alho, O., et al. "Tonsillectomy Versus Watchful Waiting in Recurrent Streptococcal Pharyngitis in Adults: Randomised Controlled Trial," *British Medical Journal* 334(7600):939, May 2007.

Alsaghir, A.H., and Martin, C.M. "Effect of Prone Positioning in Patients with Acute Respiratory Distress Syndrome: A Meta-Analysis," *Critical Care Medicine* 36(2):603-09, February 2008.

Baren, J.M., et al. "Randomized Controlled Trial of Emergency Department Interventions to Improve Primary Care Follow-up for Patients with Acute Asthma," *Chest* 129(2):257-65, February 2006.

Bjelakovic, G., et al. "Mortality in Randomized Trials of Antioxidant Supplements for Primary and Secondary Prevention: Systematic Review and Meta-Analysis," *JAMA* 297(8):842-57, February 2007.

Blasi, F., et al. "Prulifloxacin: A Brief Review of its Potential in the Treatment of Acute Exacerbation of Chronic Bronchitis," *International Journal of Chronic Obstructive Pulmonary Disease* 2(1):27-31, December 2007.

Bonay, M., et al. "Cytokines in Pulmonary Emphysema: Can Results in Mice Be Translated to Humans?" *American Journal of Respiratory and Critical Care Medicine* 177(2):238, January 2008.

Chawla, R., et al. "Guidelines for Noninvasive Ventilation in Acute Respiratory Failure," *Indian Journal of Critical Care Medicine* 10(2):117-47, April-June 2006.

Doz, E., et al. "Cigarette Smoke-Induced Pulmonary Inflammation Is TLR4/MyD88 and IL-1R1/MyD88 Signaling Dependent," *Journal of Immunology* 180(2):1169-78, January 2008.

Lee, K.S., et al. "Modulation of Airway Remodeling and Airway Inflammation by Peroxisome Proliferator-Activated Receptor Gamma in a Murine Model of Toluene Diisocyanate-Induced Asthma," *Journal of Immunology* 177(8):5248-57, October 2006.

Nervous system

Buhse, M. "Assessment of Caregiver Burden in Families of Persons with Multiple Sclerosis," *Journal of Neuroscience Nursing* 40(1): 25-31, February 2008.

Chen, H., and Boore, J. "Living with a Spinal Cord Injury: A Grounded Theory Approach," *Journal of Clinical Nursing* 17(5A):116-24, March 2008.

Gruber, R.A., et al. "Self-management Programs for People with Parkinson's Disease: A Program Evaluation Approach," *Topics in Geriatric Rehabilitation* 24(2):141-50, April/June 2008.

Keuscamp, J., et al, "High-dose Intraarterial Verapamil in the Treatment of Cerebral Vasospasm after Aneurysmal Subarachnoid Hemorrhage," *Journal of Neurosurgery* 108(3):458-63, March 2008.

Lee, E., and Armstrong, T. "Increased Intracranial Pressure," *Clinical Journal of Oncology Nursing* 12(1): 37-41; February 2008.

McElroy-Cox, C. "Caring for Patients with Epilepsy," *Nurse Practitioner* 32(10):34-40, October 2007.

Peters, M., et al. "Migraine and Chronic Daily Headache Management: Implications for Primary Care Practitioners," *Journal of Clinical Nursing* 16(7B):159-67, July 2007.

Rincon, F., and Sacco, R. "Secondary Stroke Prevention," *Journal of Cardiovascular Nursing* 23 (1): 34-41, January/February 2008.

RN Expert Guides: Neurologic Care. Philadelphia: Lippincott Williams & Wilkins, 2007.

Rowland, L. *Merritt's Neurology*, 11th ed. Philadelphia: Lippincott Williams & Wilkins, 2005.

Tilly, J., and Reed, P. "Falls, Wandering, and Physical Restraints: A Review of Interventions for Individuals with Dementia in Assisted Living and Nursing Homes," *Alzheimer's Care Today* 9(1):45-50, January/March 2008.

Valente, S., and Karp, J. "Life with Lou Gehrig's Disease: Managing ALS symptoms," *Nurse Practitioner* 32(12):26-33, December 2007.

Young, P., et al. *Basic Clinical Neuroscience*. Philadelphia: Lippincott Williams & Wilkins, 2007.

Gastrointestinal system

Baldi, F. "Key Points in the Management of Gastroesophageal Reflux Disease," *Current Gastroenterology Reports* 9(1):1-2, February 2007.

Buchman, A. *Clinical Nutrition in Gastrointestinal Disease*. Thorofare, N.J.: Slack Incorporated, 2006.

Irving, P., et al. *Clinical Dilemmas in Inflammatory Bowel Disease*. Hoboken, N.J.: Wiley-Blackwell, 2006.

McPhee, S.J., et al. *Current Medical Diagnosis and Treatment 2007*, 46th ed. New York: McGraw-Hill Book Co., 2006.

Sun, D.F., and Fang, J.Y. "Two Common Reasons of Malabsorption Syndromes: Celiac Disease and Whipple's Disease." *Digestion* 74(3-4): 174-83, March 2007.

Musculoskeletal system

Chung, E.K., et al. *Visual Diagnosis in Pediatrics*. Philadelphia: Lippincott Williams & Wilkins, 2006.

Manaster, B.J., et al. *Diagnostic and Surgical Imaging Anatomy: Musculoskeletal*. Philadelphia: Lippincott Williams & Wilkins, 2006.

Paget, S.A., et al. *Hospital for Special Surgery Manual of Rheumatology and Outpatient Disorders*, 5th ed. Philadelphia: Lippincott Williams & Wilkins, 2005.

Roposch, A., and Wright, J.G. "Increased Diagnostic Information and Understanding Disease: Uncertainty in the Diagnosis of Developmental Hip Dysplasia," *Radiology* 242(2): 355-59, February 2007.

Voight, M.L., et al. *Musculoskeletal Interventions: Techniques for Therapeutic Exercise*. New York: McGraw-Hill Book Co., 2006.

Hematologic system

Lichtman, M.A., et al. *Williams Hematology*, 7th ed. New York: McGraw-Hill Book Co., 2005.

McPhee, S.J., et al. *Current Medical Diagnosis and Treatment 2007*, 46th ed. New York: McGraw-Hill Book Co., 2007.

Rodgers, G.P., and Young, N.S. *Bethesda Handbook of Clinical Hematology*, 2nd ed. Philadelphia: Lippincott Williams & Wilkins, 2009.

Tkachuk, D., and Hirschmann, J. *Wintrobe's Atlas of Clinical Hematology*. Philadelphia: Lippincott Williams & Wilkins, 2006.

Immune system

Abbas, A.K., and Lichtman, A.H. *Basic Immunology: Functions and Disorders of the Immune System*, 3rd ed. Philadelphia: W.B. Saunders Co., 2008.

Cantani, A. *Pediatric Allergy, Asthma and Immunology*. New York: Springer Publishing Co., 2008.

Chapel, H., et al. *Essentials of Clinical Immunology*, 5th ed. Hoboken, N.J.: Wiley-Blackwell, 2006.

Coleman, C.L. "Revisiting HIV/AIDS," *Men in Nursing* 1(6):20-27. December 2006.

Mak, T. W., and Saunders, M. *The Immune Response: Basic and Clinical Principles*. St. Louis: Academic Press, 2005.

Endocrine system

Diabetes Mellitus: A Guide to Patient Care. Philadelphia: Lippincott Williams & Wilkins, 2006.

Gardner, D.G., and Shoback, D.M. *Greenspan's Basic & Clinical Endocrinology*, 8th edition. New York: McGraw-Hill Book Co., 2007.

Mugo, M., et al. "Association of Hepatitis C Virus Infection and Diabetes Mellitus," *Endocrinologist* 16(1):41-48, January/February 2006.

Wright, M.A., and Appel, S. "Inhaled Insulin: Breathing New Life into Diabetes Therapy," *Nursing2007* 37(1):46-48, January 2007.

Renal and Urinary system

Chisholm-Burns, M.A., et al. *Pharmacology Principles and Practice*. New York: McGraw-Hill Book Co., 2007.

Koeppen, B.M., and Stanton, B.A.. *Renal Physiology*, 4th ed. Philadelphia: Mosby, 2007.

Metcalfe, P.D., and Rink, R.C. "Bladder Augmentation: Complications in the Pediatric Population," *Current Urology Reports* 8(2): 152-56, March 2007.

Schrier, R.W. *Diseases of the Kidney and Urinary Tract*, 8th ed. Philadelphia: Lippincott Williams & Wilkins, 2006.

Sensory system

Bartlett, J.D., et al. *Ophthalmic Drug Facts 2009*, 20th ed. St. Louis: Facts and Comparisons, Inc., 2008.

Fickert, N.A. "Health Matters: Taking a Closer Look at Acute Otitis Media in Kids," *Nursing2006* 36(4):20-21, April 2006.

Kertes, P.J., and Johnson, T.M. *Evidence-Based Eye Care*. Philadelphia: Lippincott Williams & Wilkins, 2006.

Lalwani, A. *Current Diagnosis and Treatment in Otolaryngology—Head and Neck Surgery*, 2nd ed. New York: McGraw-Hill Book Co., 2007.

McPhee, S.J., et al. *Current Medical Diagnosis and Treatment 2007*, 46th ed. New York: McGraw-Hill Book Co., 2007.

Pavan-Langston, D. *Manual of Ocular Diagnosis and Therapy*, 6th ed. Philadelphia: Lippincott Williams & Wilkins, 2007.

Pullen, R.L. "Spin Control: Caring for a Patient with Inner Ear Disease," *Nursing2006* 36(5): 48-51, May 2006.

Shin, J., et al. *Evidenced-Based Otolaryngology*. New York: Springer Publishing Co., 2007.

Swartz, R., and Longwell, P. "Treatment of Vertigo," *American Family Physician* 71(6):1115-22, March 15, 2005.

Integumentary system

Ali, A. *Dermatology: A Pictorial Review*. New York: McGraw-Hill Book Co., 2006.

Hall, J.C. *Sauer's Manual of Skin Diseases*, 9th ed. Philadelphia: Lippincott Williams & Wilkins, 2006.

Roebuck, H.L. "Dermatology Discussion: Newer Treatment Options for Patients with Moderate-to-Severe Psoriatic Disease." *The Nurse Practitioner: The American Journal of Primary Health Care* 31(8):5-11, August 2006.

Weinberg, S., et al. *Color Atlas of Pediatric Dermatology*. New York: McGraw-Hill Book Co., 2007.

Reproductive system

Arafeh, J.M. "Preeclampsia: Pieces of the Puzzle Revealed," *Journal of Perinatal and Neonatal Nursing* 20(1):85-87, January/March 2006.

Berek, J.S. *Berek & Novak's Gynecology*, 14th ed. Philadelphia: Lippincott Williams & Wilkins, 2006.

DeCherney, A.H., et al. *Current Obstetrics and Gynecologic Diagnosis and Treatment*. New York: McGraw-Hill Book Co., 2006.

Evans, A.T. *Manual of Obstetrics*, 7th ed. Philadelphia: Lippincott Williams & Wilkins, 2007.

Ficorelli, C.T., and Weeks, B. "Health Matters: Untangling the Complexities of Male Infertility," *Nursing2007* 37(1):24-26, January, 2007.

Fortner, K.B., et al. *The Johns Hopkins Manual of Gynecology and Obstetrics*, 3rd ed. Philadelphia: Lippincott Williams & Wilkins, 2006.

Leveno, K.J., et al. *Williams Manual of Obstetrics*, 22nd ed. New York: McGraw-Hill Book Co., 2007.

Pillitteri, A. *Maternal and Child Health Nursing*, 6th ed. Philadelphia: Lippincott Williams & Wilkins, 2009.

Schwoebel, A., and Gennaro, S. "Neonatal Hyperbilirubinemia," *Journal of Perinatal and Neonatal Nursing* 20(1):103-07, January/March 2006.

Tanagho, E.A., and McAninch, J.W. *Smith's General Urology*. New York: McGraw-Hill Book Co., 2007.

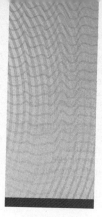

INDEX

i refers to an illustration; t refers to a table

i refers to an illustration; t refers to a table

i refers to an illustration; t refers to a table

i refers to an illustration; t refers to a table

i refers to an illustration; t refers to a table

i refers to an illustration; t refers to a table

i refers to an illustration; t refers to a table